NURSING PRACTICE
AND HEALTH CARE

NURSING PRACTICE AND HEALTH CARE

Second Edition

EDITED BY

Susan M. Hinchliff, BA, RGN, RNT,
Director of Studies, Distance Learning Centre,
South Bank University, London

Susan E. Norman, RGN, NDN. Cert, RNT, B.Ed (Hons),
Formerly Senior Nurse Teacher, The Nightingale School,
West Lambeth Health Authority

Jane E. Schober, MN, RGN, RCNT, Dip.N, Dip.N.Ed., RNT,
Principal Lecturer (Nursing), Department of Health and
Community Studies, De Montfort University

Edward Arnold
A division of Hodder & Stoughton
LONDON MELBOURNE AUCKLAND

© 1993 Edward Arnold

First published in Great Britain 1989
Second edition 1993

British Library Cataloguing in Publication Data

Nursing practice and health care.
  1. Medicine. Nursing – For student nurses
  Hinchliff, Susan M.
    Nursing Practice and Health Care. –
    2Rev.ed
    I. Title
    610.73

    ISBN 0-340-55788-5

Whilst the advice and information in this book is believed to be true and accurate at the date of going to press, neither the author nor the publisher can accept any legal responsibility or liability for any errors or omissions that may be made. In particular (but without limiting the generality of the preceding disclaimer) every effort has been made to check drug dosages; however, it is still possible that errors have been missed. Furthermore, dosage schedules are constantly being revised and new side effects recognised. For these reasons the reader is strongly urged to consult the drug companies' printed instructions before administering any of the drugs recommended in this book.

Typeset in 10/11pt Linotron Optima by
Rowland Phototypesetting Limited, Bury St Edmunds, Suffolk.
Printed and bound in Great Britain for Edward Arnold,
a division of Hodder and Stoughton Limited, Mill Road,
Dunton Green, Sevenoaks, Kent TN13 2YA by
Butler and Tanner Limited, Frome, Somerset.

PREFACE TO THE FIRST EDITION

The original idea for this book sprang from the implications for nurse education of the competencies set out in rule 18(1) of the Nurses, Midwives and Health Visitors Rules Approval Order 1983 (No. 873). The recommendations of the United Kingdom Central Council (Project 2000) and the Royal College of Nursing plus the English National Board's Guidelines for syllabus translation to curriculum augmented this idea.

The book is designed mainly as a course text for learners preparing for part 12 of the Register, but those preparing for other parts of the Register are by no means excluded. Its purpose is to enable them to promote health and to practise effective, individualised client/patient care from a sound knowledge base.

Most of the 27 chapter authors are themselves nurses; all of them are experienced in teaching nurses.

A multi-author text of this nature has the obvious advantage of bringing together a team of subject experts, but it does inevitably result in some differences between chapters in approach, style, level and presentation. This diversity in treatment of the various topics lends a freshness to the work, whose general cohesiveness has been secured by certain features common to most chapters.

(1) At the start of each chapter, the reader will find a clear statement of its aim.

(2) Following the aim, there is a brief review of the main topics covered in each chapter to help the reader find his/her way around the book more easily.

(3) Where appropriate, chapters end with a glossary defining terms not fully explained in their original context. Glossary terms are printed in **_bold italics_** where they first appear in the text, for ease of reference.

(4) The terminal references list, in each chapter, covers texts and journals which should be readily available in a College of Nursing and Higher Education establishment library. Every effort has been made not to include obscure references which might be difficult to find.

(5) Suggestions for further reading, to broaden the reader's understanding of issues considered in that chapter, are given.

(6) Where appropriate, chapters include a list of useful addresses relevant to the patient-groups or issues explored in that chapter. Readers may wish to seek further information from such sources, for themselves or for those needing care.

(7) Some chapters contain care plans which illustrate points relevant to the aspect of care under discussion. These care plans are not prescriptive; the reader should use them as a learning tool which attempts to illustrate aspects of care. Inevitably, the style of (and approach to) such plans will differ between chapter authors.

For convenience, the nurse is referred to throughout this book in the female gender. The patient is referred to in most chapters in the male gender, unless this is clearly inappropriate. Exceptions to the latter rule occur in Chapters 17 and 18:

Care of Women and Maternity Care (for obvious reasons): Chapter 19: The Care of Children; and, because of the proportions of the sexes in the elderly population, also in Chapter 26. The terms 'patient' 'person' and 'client' are used inter- changeably, as are the terms 'nurse learner' and 'student'.

Sue Hinchliff
Sue Norman
London, 1988
Jane Schober

PREFACE TO THE SECOND EDITION

The learning needs of students undertaking the new preparation for practice have become increasingly apparent since the first edition was published in 1989. All of the existing chapters have therefore undergone revision, with an increased focus on:

- presentation of material at Diploma level

- the perspective of health in the context of the 1990s

- the needs of the individual in the context of health care for the 1990s

- the promotion of critical awareness in the reader

- the inclusion of a range of research relevant to practice

- updated further reading.

In this second edition the number of chapters has been increased to 27 with the inclusion of new chapters on:

- The Social Context of Health

- Communicating for Health

- The Nature of Stress and Its Implications for Nursing Practice

Additionally, several of the chapters have had a new author as a result of changes in post of the original authors. This has, of necessity, resulted in a fresh approach to the subject matter and the presentation of different insights.

Throughout the preparation of this edition we have tried to respond to the evolving needs of a new generation of professional carers. We have enjoyed working to this end and hope that we have succeeded in making a worthwhile contribution to the education of nurses of the future.

Readers should note that the views expressed are those of the chapter authors and not necessarily those of the editors.

Sue Hinchliff
Sue Norman
London, 1992　　　　*Jane Schober*

CONTENTS

CONTRIBUTORS

Paul Barber, PhD, MSc, BA, RGN, RMN, RNMS, RNT, Director of The Human Potential Resource Group, Department of Educational Studies, University of Surrey

Anne Betts, BSc (Hons), MSc, RGN, RNT, Lecturer in Life Sciences, Institute of Advanced Nursing Education, Royal College of Nursing, London

Carol Blake, RGN, RCNT, Dip. Counselling, Nurse Teacher, Hertfordshire College of Health Care Studies

Elisabeth Clark, BA, PhD, Academic Coordinator for Health Services, Open Learning Foundation, and Principal Lecturer, School of Health Care Studies, Middlesex University

Janice Colson, MA, RSCN, RGN, RNT, Dip.N.Ed., Senior Education Manager – Child Care, Buckinghamshire College of Nursing and Midwifery, Stoke Mandeville Hospital, Aylesbury

Alan Cribb, PhD, Course Director, MSc Health Education and Visiting Fellow, Medical Ethics, King's College, London

John Foord, BA (Hons), MSc, Senior Lecturer in Biological Sciences for Nursing Studies, University of Brighton

Sally Glen, MA, Dip.Ed., RGN, RSCN, Dip.N., Dip.N.Ed., RNT, Head of Division, Nursing and Midwifery Education, School of Health and Education, South Bank University

Dinah Gould, BSc, M.Phil., RGN, Dip.N., Lecturer in Nursing Studies, King's College, London

Judith Hill, BSc, MSc, RGN, RNT, Regional Nursing Director, Wessex Regional Health Authority

Tom Keighley, BA (Hons), RGN, RMN, NDN. Cert., RCNT, Dip.N., Regional Director of Nursing and Quality, Yorkshire Health

Sally Kendall, BSc (Hons), PhD, RGN, RHV, Senior Lecturer in Nursing, Buckinghamshire College of Higher Education, Chalfont St Giles

Ann Mackenzie, MA, PhD, RGN, DN, RNT, Lecturer in Nursing Studies, Department of Nursing Studies, King's College, London

Kim Manley, MN, RGN, Dip.N., Dip.N.Ed., RNT, PGCEA, Lecturer in Nursing, Institute of Advanced Nursing Education, Royal College of Nursing, London and Clinical Nurse Specialist, Intensive Care Unit and Nursing Development Unit, Westminster Hospital, London

Meg Miller, MSc, RGN, RMN, Dip.N., Dip.N.Ed., Senior Lecturer (Nursing), South Bank University, London

Susan Montague, BSc (Hons), RGN, HV Dip., RNT, Senior Lecturer in Health Studies, University of Hertfordshire

Alan Myles, MA (Ed), RGN, Dip.Ed., RNT, Principal Lecturer in Education Studies, Institute of Advanced Nursing Education, Royal College of Nursing, London

Margaret Ostro, RGN, RM, Dip.N., Dip.N.Ed., RNT, Cert. Gerontology (London), Senior Tutor, The Nightingale and Guys College of Nursing and Midwifery, London

Elizabeth Raymond, B.Ed.(Hons), RGN, SCM, QN, HV.Tut.Cert., Cert.Ed., Senior Lecturer, Nursing and Community Health Studies, South Bank University, London

Marion Richardson, BA (Hons), RGN, RCNT, Dip.N., Nurse Teacher (Acute and Critical Care), Hertfordshire College of Health Care

Rosemary Rogers, BA, RGN, Editor, *Paediatric Nursing*

Jane Schober, MN, RGN, RCNT, Dip.N., Dip.N.Ed., RNT, Principal Lecturer (Nursing), Department of Health and Community Studies, De Montfort University

David Sines, BSc (Hons), PhD, FRCN, RMN, RNMH, Senior Lecturer (Mental Handicap), Department of Social and Health Sciences, University of Ulster, Northern Ireland

Beatrice Sofaer, BA, PhD, RN, Reader in Nursing, Director of Nursing Research Unit, University of Brighton

Sister Anne Thompson, B.Ed (Hons), RGN, RM, MTD, Senior Lecturer in Midwifery Studies, Royal College of Midwifery, London

Verena Tschudin, BSc (Hons), RGN, RM, Dip.Counselling Skills, Counsellor and Writer, London

Kate Ward, RGN, RSCN, FETC, Specialist Nurse Adviser, Infection Control, Department of Public Health and Medicine, Southern Derbyshire Health Authority

Paul Watt, BA (Hons), MSc, M.Phil, Cert.Ed., Senior Lecturer in Sociology, Buckinghamshire College of Higher Education, Chalfont St Giles

1

THE PHILOSOPHY OF HEALTH

Alan Cribb

The book begins with a chapter that aims to ask some fundamental questions about the meaning of health, and the ways in which our ideas about health affect health care.

The following issues are discussed:

- What are the meanings of 'health', 'healthy', 'holism', and 'well-being'?

- What are the advantages and disadvantages of using different ideas of health, e.g. 'broad' versus 'narrow', or 'positive' versus 'negative' ideas?

- What can we learn about health by starting from an individual's experience of health and illness?

- Is there a single, 'correct' definition or idea of health?

- How can we measure health or quality of life?

This chapter is about two things. It is about the idea of health and it is about the process of trying to understand this idea. Ideas are central to everything we do. Certain ideas will have had a profound effect on each of our lives: ideas about what it is to be a good person, to have an education, and to be a success in life. This certainly applies in the world of health care. Most people spend their lives working in settings in which ideas are built into the system. Their objectives, the shape of their day and all their tasks are defined by other people's ideas about what matters. All we can do to lessen this domination is to spend some time reflecting on these ideas, where they come from, and how far they make sense to us.

Vast quantities of time, energy and resources are spent in the name of ideas like 'health' and 'well-being'. Yet if we were to ask what these ideas mean most of us would probably look blank; fur-thermore we might be accused of fussing; 'Never mind what they *mean*, let's get on and do some work!'. I have a lot of sympathy with this attitude but I do not believe it can be left at that. We still have to decide what work health workers should do. How far, for example, should health workers spend time 'just talking' to people, or getting involved in community projects? Or are these things on the margins of health care? One way of approaching questions like this, and I stress only one way, is to ask about the meaning of health. What is it that health workers are trying to bring about; what is health?

The obvious problem is that different people have different ideas about what health is. Different groups of professionals, and different individuals inside and outside of health care, all tend to disagree. It has become customary in situations like this to ask for a definition. Unfortunately this is to misunderstand the situation in two important respects. First, definitions only work within a framework of agreement. If a number of people get together and agree to define the word 'paper' in a certain way this may prove to be useful, providing they do not expect others automatically to change the way they use the word. (As part of a scientific community this can work well, and these are called **stipulative definitions**.) Second, the whole business of definition does not work well with words that refer to abstract social concepts like 'equality', 'happiness' or 'health'. These concepts, which are closely tied in with people's emotions and values, have a number of conflicting meanings. They are inherently debatable or, to use the technical expression of philosophy, *essentially contestable* (Gallie, 1964). That is, we cannot reduce their meaning to a single definition without taking sides in an important debate. Any stipulative definition would not only be ignored by others, but would be attacked for missing 'the real meaning' of the concept.

Thus, in what follows, I will not be looking for the definition of health but rather exploring its meanings. In fact, I will only really consider three kinds of definition:

(1) health as disease-freedom;
(2) health as well-being;
(3) health as personal capacity or resources for living.

I will normally use the word **conception** rather than the word 'definition'. This is a word philosophers use to stand for the different meanings of a complex concept. It is a broader term than definition, and unlike the latter it makes no claim to be definitive in the sense of universal or final. It is possible for the same person to operate with several different conceptions of health, although they may have a preferred one. Indeed, I shall argue that this would be to their advantage.

But the chapter is not simply going to be a catalogue of the meanings of health. It is also about the process of clarifying these meanings and it raises a host of surrounding questions such as: 'How should we think about health, what attitudes, what types of knowledge are required?' and 'What are the implications of thinking about health for health care policy and practice?'. Let us begin with yet another question, which looks superficially the same as 'What is health?', but is in fact different: what do we mean by the word 'healthy'?

Three ways to be healthy

Many things are said to be 'healthy'. A run round the park, clean air, a glowing complexion, our pets or plants, and even some bank balances. Aristotle distinguished between the different senses of the word and also explained that all these senses are related: 'Everything which is healthy is related to health, one thing in the sense that it preserves health, another in the sense that it produces it, another in the sense that it is a symptom of health, another because it is capable of it' (1941, page 732). This does not account for metaphorical uses of 'healthy' such as the last example in the above list, but a bank balance can be seen as a potentially fruitful resource just as we tend to see health.

Some things preserve or produce health, and some things are symptoms of health. We could call the former determinants of health, and the latter aspects of quality of life. But this does not take us very far in understanding what health is. Aristotle's other category takes us a little further by indicating that some sorts of things are capable of having health. Thus pets, plants and people can literally be healthy whereas rocks, watches and tables cannot be. We can think of ways in which watches, for example, might, like bank balances, be described metaphorically as healthy, but we normally reserve the word 'health' for living things. Health and life are inextricably linked.

If we think of the biological characteristics of life – movement, reproduction, exchange with the environment, and growth – we see immediately that there are many things which can affect the quality of life. A rock does not share any of these characteristics, does not perform any complicated functions, does not have a biological identity, does not have any potential to realise and consequently cannot fail to realise potential.

Watches, and other designed objects, only have some of these characteristics. Objects can be good *for a purpose*: a rock may make a good doorstop, a table may be well or badly designed to do its job, but these things cannot simply *be* well. Living things may perform all sorts of tasks but in addition to this their life systems can work well (or badly), i.e. they are 'beings' which can *be* well or healthy. This gives us an idea of what it is to have health. But someone might object that this is too limited an idea. I am equating health with good biological functioning, but for humans growth and development are not merely biological but involve the growth of personality, of projects, of goals, and of autonomy.

If we are to seek to understand the 'good functioning' of a person, we need to consider more than biology; likewise, the causes and effects of 'good personal functioning' or 'well-being' will be much broader than the causes and effects of good biological functioning. The causes or determinants of good biological functioning are broad-ranging and include our genetic make-up, behaviours, relationships, and physical and social environment. But the range of causes relevant to our functioning successfully as a person is almost unlimited. Certainly factors like architecture, music and religion as well as politics and economics (and all of the others relating to biological health) seem potentially relevant. This is what lies behind the debate about narrow versus broad conceptions of health (which should not be confused with the debate about so-called 'negative' versus 'positive' conceptions of health).

Health can be used to refer to a relatively narrow range of characteristics – roughly all those characteristics which human beings share with plants and other animals. Alternatively it can be used to refer to a very wide range of characteristics such that we talk about things like a healthy personality or even a healthy attitude to life. Some people will only feel comfortable with the narrow usage and see the broader one as a kind of metaphorical extension of it. Others will take the broader usage to be equally valid.

The examples with which we began all relate to the narrow conception. A run round the park and clean air preserve or produce health. The person who runs can possess health, and a glowing complexion can be an effect, or sign, of health. We could call these three ways to be healthy:

(a) health causing;
(b) health possessing;
(c) health enjoying.

Many attempts to understand what it is to be healthy fail because they do not distinguish these aspects. It is worth noting that a person can be healthy in all three ways. If the parts of their life systems are working well, these are healthy ('health causing' to the person); the person can

function well as a whole (possess health), and thereby experience a high quality of life (be 'health enjoying').

Negative, positive, broad and narrow conceptions

A negative conception of something is a picture of what it is not. To paint a negative picture of poverty, we might talk about the characteristics of wealth. Wealth allows people choices, it enables them to live in comfort, it gives them some sense of security about the future. To be poor is not to have any wealth, it is not to be able to enjoy any of these benefits. There is a tradition of theologians that talks about God in negative terms: He is not made of matter, He is not petty or selfish. Similarly, political activists sometimes talk about an ideal future society in negative terms. There will be no oppression, no prejudice, and no discrimination. In some cases it is because of the lack of an appropriate language in which to couch a positive description that a negative one is used. Sometimes it is because a state of affairs is largely understood as the absence of something, as poverty is the absence of money, that a negative description seems appropriate. Some people define health this way; 'As a physician, I am content to define health as the absence of disease' (Scadding, 1988). This is a negative, and also a narrow, conception of health. It suggests that a living creature is healthy to the extent that it does not suffer from diseases or disability. It is a very clear and useful definition, and we should not be put off it completely just because it is fashionable (in some circles) to dismiss it.

It is possible to demonstrate its usefulness by making a simple analogy. Imagine someone employed to test and report the quality of jigsaw puzzles. She has to put each one together and jot down any comments. It is not difficult to imagine her ending up with two piles of boxes. In one pile every box would have 'Fine' or 'OK' marked on it, but the other pile would contain a range of labels – 'missing pieces', 'broken pieces', 'mis-shapen pieces', 'the wrong pieces', and so on. On the face of it there is not much to be said about the good quality puzzles but much more to be said about the puzzles that fall short in some way. There are countless ways that a person can fall short of being 'fine'. The whole of medicine depends upon the careful cataloguing and description of types of disease and disability. To define health as the absence of disease is to put the emphasis on the traditional role of medicine, i.e. the prevention, cure or alleviation of diseases. It also serves to rule out speculation about 'health' as some kind of mysterious substance or process. Just as darkness is not a special kind of stuff, but only the absence of light, health is just another word for being disease-free.

We can imagine negative but broader conceptions of health although they are not employed as commonly. There are many ways in which people can fall short of being 'fine' that do not amount to diseases. People can be ignorant, confused, frightened, alienated, exhausted and so on, and we might wish to conceive of health as the absence of these 'disabling states'. Are the narrow or the broader negative conceptions enough?

Let us take the narrow negative one first. Surely, health is not exactly like darkness in being only an absence of something? A brick wall is disease-free but it is not thereby healthy. Health thought of as good biological functioning can be catalogued and described in the same way as diseases. Indeed, the two processes of description are inseparable. Just as it would be impossible to recognise a poor jigsaw puzzle without having a picture of what a good jigsaw puzzle should be, it is impossible to understand disease without at the same time having an understanding of a healthy organism. They are two sides of the same coin. So when health is seen as the absence of disease, a normal background state of affairs is presupposed. This background norm can be summarised as 'biological fitness and efficient functioning'. It is a positive conception of health, a conception which aims to inform us about what health is, not simply what it is not.

It is, however, much more problematic to articulate a broad positive conception of health. Having noted that there are many ways in which a person can fall short of being 'fine', can we say what it is to be fine, to be functioning well, not just biologically but as a person? Does it not follow from the above arguments that here too we must have some picture of a normal or satisfactory state of affairs if we are prepared to identify certain states as falling short of it? This is what is often referred to as 'positive health' or 'personal and social health' and distinguished from a so-called medical model of

health which equates health with disease-freedom. Another way in which this point is made is to talk about the merits of a holistic approach, or a holistic conception of health. There is a danger here of confusing two distinct points. It is possible to advocate a holistic approach without necessarily wishing to *define* health in a very broad way. Let us look first at the approach, and then at a holistic definition.

Holism

Holism means paying regard to the whole. At one level this means we should not treat the different physical systems of the body as if they were really separate because in fact they make up an interconnected whole. It also means that we should not treat individuals as if they were separate from their immediate or total environment. For some practical purposes we can behave as if these separations were possible but unless we appreciate the artificiality of these distinctions we will never understand health.

At another level, to pay regard to the whole means recognising that people are part of a range of systems, not all of which are physical. It is now commonplace to hear about psychosocial factors in health and disease. These relate to the psychological and social components in the lives of people. Those who advocate holism are usually drawing our attention to the importance of these components. If we wish to look after people, it would be absurd not to have a concern for their states of mind, their relationships or their social circumstances. Yet a large part of what is intended in the critique of 'the medical model' is to say that this is precisely what can happen if we become narrowly focused on the need to diagnose and treat disease.

The narrow focus can come about in a number of different ways. It is sensible for health workers to focus on diseases; this is often the major preoccupation of all parties. The patient's life may be threatened, he may be in pain or substantially incapacitated. A high priority has to be attached to addressing these issues. It is not surprising that individual health workers get into the habit of giving these issues priority and sometimes do so when it is not appropriate. But it is too simple to see this only as a product of individual habit formation; it is normally a product of systems or policies of care. Take, for example, the case of screening for breast cancer. Here an elaborate system has been developed to enable the early detection and treatment of breast cancer. This is an expensive and an administratively and technically sophisticated task. It would be a waste of a good deal of human resources if it failed in its chief objective of early detection, and this must be the priority of the service. Yet by its very nature its clients are well women who have social and psychological needs other than those relating to breast cancer, and for whom an invitation to screening may be experienced as an additional burden and a source of disquiet or alarm. A holistic service would attempt to give a certain priority to meeting these concerns as well as the clinical ones, and fortunately there is some evidence of this happening in the UK (Gray and Austoker, 1989), but it is easy in this case to see that the service is essentially a disease-centred one. The same is true of most other systems and policies of the health service, leading to the much repeated complaint that it is really a 'disease service'.

So far we have added psychological and social components to biological ones. But this still treats people as complicated objects made up of interacting systems. Imagine someone who studied these systems coming up to you and saying, 'I understand what makes you tick'. What would she have to know about? She would presumably know something about biochemistry, anatomy and physiology. She would have to know something about psychology, sociology and other human sciences. Perhaps she has gone further and has interviewed your family, friends, teachers and so on. She now claims to be an expert on you. How would that claim make you feel? Despite the attention, it would make most people feel strangely disregarded, not only because someone had gone behind their back but also because they had been treated merely as an object of investigation, not as a full person. After all, you would expect to be consulted about who you are; you probably feel as if you are the expert about yourself.

Here we are touching on a very deep problem about the scientific study of human beings. To see someone as conforming to scientific generalisations is to some extent to 'reduce' their behaviour to these generalisations. ***Reductionism*** is the opposite of holism. There are times when it is useful and even necessary, but it can also lead to a dangerous partial-sightedness. The so-called medical model is criticised when it reduces people to bearers of

disease. But merely adding on psychological and social models does not get rid of reductionism. It is still possible to reduce a person to 'an introvert' or 'a single, white, middle-aged male', etc. Individuals are individuals, and we have our own sense of who and what we are; we are subjects as well as objects. Whatever we may say when we are being 'intellectual', we do not feel in our bones that our life and behaviour can be entirely explained by the generalisations of science; we feel that we are at least partly authors of our own life, and expect to be treated as such.

Thus a holistic stance entails bringing more and more into our gaze. Ultimately it means we have to encounter the person with whom we are dealing. As we enlarge our perspective, something new comes into focus. We move from a cold consideration of arrangements of matter to a meeting with a person, an equal who looks back at us with her own interests and concerns in mind.

Hence systems of care can fail to be holistic if they neglect properly to consider the psychological and social needs of people. But they can also fail to be holistic if they neglect to meet properly the individual concerns and needs as felt by, and voiced by, those who are receiving care. No system of care can claim to be holistic if it leaves the individual person (on his or her own terms) out of the picture.

It is because of the merits of a holistic approach that some people advocate the use of a holistic, or very broad, conception of health. The most famous of such conceptions is offered in the World Health Organisation Constitution; 'Health is a state of complete physical, mental and social well-being and not merely the absence of disease and infirmity' (WHO, 1947). If we put aside the word 'complete' – which would entail that nobody could ever qualify as healthy – this is another very useful, although rather imprecise definition. It offers a broad and positive conception of health. It equates health with well-being and it makes clear that this involves a good deal more than physical well-being or good biological functioning. But it does not make clear exactly what this 'more' is.

Hopefully, everyone is agreed that when we are dealing with people we should have regard to their whole well-being and not just their physical health. However it does not follow from this belief that we must operate with a holistic conception of health. Some people may prefer to restrict the use of the word 'health' to the narrower conceptions and use other words, like 'well-being' or 'welfare', to stand for the broader ones. There are advantages and disadvantages to both approaches. Using a broad conception of health makes it more difficult to fall into the trap of reducing people to mere bodies, but it can mean that health professionals lose sight of the limits to their responsibility and expertise in an effort to look after 'the whole person'. On the other hand, using a narrow conception keeps the focus on definite objectives, but this tends to encourage reductionism.

What is well-being?

What is well-being? This is a question that has been asked in many different forms through the centuries, and it is a question that each of us asks in our own way whenever we make major decisions in our life. What is a good life, a happy life, a full life? What is it to be fulfilled, to flourish, to make the most of things? I will not pretend to answer it here but rather to point to certain aspects of its scope and complexity. It is a very demanding question but at the same time it is a question which anyone who claims to care for people must confront.

A fashionable answer would be to say that a person's well-being is whatever he or she chooses it to be. You may value some things, I may value others. It is a matter of opinion, or subjective judgement. This is the kind of thing a child might say to her parents; 'You have your ideas about what's good for me, I have mine'. In many ways the view that it is all subjective seems plausible, yet it cannot be entirely right. The expression 'One man's meat is another man's poison' is used to sum up this stance, but we also know that in most cases this expression is not *literally* true. In broad terms it is possible to say what substances are poisonous to human beings, and these things are normally poisonous to all human beings. We would regard somebody who said that they could choose what was a poison as being stupid, as trying to ignore objective facts.

So it looks as if the answer to 'What is well-being?' is partly subjective and partly objective. This is one reason for using a fairly narrow and biological conception of health. Here it is possible to generalise about what is good and bad. Human beings have a definite physical constitution which has to be respected. At the other extreme there are many areas, such as our choice of wallpaper,

where it seems clear we are dealing with subjective judgements about what suits us. This suggests we can divide up the answer to the question about well-being into two parts: a part to do with facts and a part to do with values. It could be said that whether or not we identify our well-being with our family or money, etc. is a matter of values but that there are certain things like food and shelter which are simply good as a matter of fact. The further we move away from the biological facts of life the further we get into the realm of personal beliefs and values. Perhaps the best example of this is religious belief. Some Christians, for example, believe that no one can be fully well unless they have come to accept the 'Good News' of Christianity, and this remains so no matter how physically healthy they are, or how well they may feel. (Note that it may be essential to understand this if you knew you were caring for such a person.)

But this distinction between factual judgements and value judgements is too simple-minded, as a closer look at examples shows. The Christian and the atheist are not merely agreeing to differ over personal values, they are disagreeing about what the facts are. The former is claiming that it is objectively the case that human welfare will be improved by recognising the existence of God, the latter is claiming that there is no God. It is difficult to imagine a more important disagreement. For our purposes this disagreement also indicates something important. It indicates the sheer scope of the question about well-being, and that it is possible to subscribe to very broad conceptions of well-being as being of general, and not merely personal, applicability. There is a tradition, rooted in classical philosophy, of debating the nature of the good life. Plato debated the relative merits of a life based on the pursuit of pleasure, the pursuit of status or the pursuit of knowledge (Plato, 1982). And those who participate in such debates look to them for insights of general applicability.

It is worth stopping to take stock. We have identified two sorts of questions about well-being: some questions appear to be open to a generalisable answer, others appear to be a matter of personal judgement. Not only is there considerable disagreement about the answers to some of these questions, but there is also disagreement about which of the two categories they fall into. Whether or not we can live well without air clearly falls into the first category. Whether we enjoy drinking coffee or tea clearly falls into the second category.

Whether or not it is good to have many sexual partners, or take 'hard drugs', or have an abortion do not obviously fit into either category. People would not only disagree about the answers (even given a specific instance) but would disagree about whether or not these questions are entirely a matter for personal judgement. Many of the issues that health workers have to cope with fall into this in-between category where both factual evidence and value judgements are relevant. Hence it is necessary to look at what evidence there is about how, in general, these issues affect well-being, and it is necessary to be conscious about our own values and the values of those for whom we are caring.

Thus we return to the importance of recognising people as subjects and not merely as objects. Because there is so much scope for disagreement about well-being, we often place emphasis on the judgements people make about their own well-being. Some of the time this is because they are the best judge, the experts, about what seems to suit them. This is the case if we are getting them to choose the least bad side effects of different therapies. But some of the time it is because we are treating their views (with which we may disagree) about a debatable subject, like bringing up their children, with respect. It is not because any view, or any choice, about well-being is as good as any other.

So we can see that the idea of well-being is very unclear. Not only does it encompass all aspects of life, but its meaning is subject to the most profound disagreements about the nature of the world, of people and about what makes up a good or full life. However, perhaps it is possible to say something helpful about well-being. First, it does appear to have a subjective element – being well is surely connected in some way with believing or feeling that one is well. Second, we can say that at least some 'objective' social and environmental conditions, like the existence of food and shelter, are necessary for the existence of well-being. These are the subjects for the following two sections.

The subjective perspective

There is another starting point from which to begin thinking about health: our own subjective perspective. It follows from what has already been said about holism and well-being. Let us start from an experience which is fairly common: a time during which we feel we are becoming unwell. It would

be helpful to think about what goes through our minds at such a time. We might worry about our immediate commitments; perhaps there is something that has to be done for work, perhaps we are looking forward to going out. We might look around for explanations; perhaps we are overtired, perhaps we are imagining it, perhaps it is something we ate. We might start to look into the future; 'Should I buy in some provisions?', 'Will I miss next week's trip?'. Maybe we know exactly what it is; a condition we live with permanently which affects what we can and cannot do. Perhaps it is getting gradually worse and the whole future looks bleak and uncertain.

Thought experiments like this highlight a couple of key things about the nature of health and well-being. Firstly, there is a gap between how we feel and other people's assessment of how healthy we are. We may feel unwell and yet hesitate to talk to anyone else about it, least of all a health professional, for fear of not being taken seriously. Conversely, we may feel fine and happy but other people may see signs that make them concerned about our health. Secondly, feeling unhealthy, in however broad or narrow a sense, is never experienced as only physical symptoms. It is always experienced as a threat to, and a disturbance in, our life patterns, and sometimes as a threat to our life itself. Health is about changes in biography, not just biology.

For these reasons the distinction between broad and narrow conceptions of health seems less appropriate to the subjective perspective. Clearly there are very 'broad' phenomena like anxiety about the future of the world, and very 'narrow' phenomena like a headache. But on the whole feelings of 'dis-ease', broad or narrow, are actually experienced as affecting life as a whole. Disease and well-being cannot be easily separated out.

Also for these reasons, social scientists who are interested in studying experiences of health and illness have to use very different methods and conceptions from those working in the clinical and biological sciences. For a start they tend to talk about 'illness' rather than 'disease'. The latter refers to a clinically defined pathological abnormality, whereas the former refers to a person's subjective experience of ill health (Field, 1976). We are the authorities about whether or not we are ill in this sense, but we may not know whether we have a disease. It is possible to feel ill without having a disease, and to have a disease without feeling ill. It should be clear that if we see health as the 'absence of illness' we would have a much broader, but rather less definite conception of health than if we define it as 'the absence of disease'. Again it seems to me that what really matters here is not whether or not we operate with a broad or narrow definition of health but how we treat people. People who feel ill are manifestly in need of respect and care whether or not a pathological abnormality is detectable.

Another respect in which the sociological perspective differs from the perspective of clinical science is the context in which ill health is seen. Whilst studying disease you are interested in things like micro-organisms, the physical environment, and DNA. Whilst studying illness, which may be the consequence of disease, you must look at things like personal and working relationships, cultural beliefs, and social and economic structures. This is the shift from biology through biography to sociology. For the experience of illness is not only shaped by an individual's own decisions and beliefs; all experiences and beliefs are shaped by the social world in which we live. We have to live with the language, the values and the constraints which are more or less given to us and we experience ill health through this framework. This means that people of different cultures, or subcultures, might be expected to have rather different ways of making sense of experiences of health and illness. Norms and attitudes to the body, to personal space, to professional-client relationships, to gender expectations, to death, and to what is serious and so forth can vary between cultures. An awareness of this fact has to be balanced against the danger of 'labelling' people according to stereotypical beliefs about other cultures.

Hence it is crucial that those who participate in health care are aware of both the personal and social significance of ill health. Without this awareness they may totally miss the mark about what actually matters to people. This is why communication between health professionals and so-called 'lay people' or patients is so important. It is not about a mere 'transfer of information' so that the professional can check hypotheses about signs and symptoms. It is to find out how the patient feels, how they make sense of what is happening to them, what their hopes and fears are, and what they think should and should not be done. It is to try to see the world from their perspective. Even with the very best will in the world, such communication may be limited. It is important to understand that people tend to have a public version and a private version of their concerns (Cornwell, 1984). The latter may only be shared with trusted friends or family members or with others who 'speak the same language'. The formal situation of an encounter with health professionals normally entails the presentation of the public face. On occasions a 'transfer of information' approach will be enough, e.g. when prescribing reading glasses. On other occasions (e.g. counselling someone who is going blind), a patient-centred approach is essential. Most situations in health care involve a mixture of these demands, and a skilful communicator will know how to move between them and not get stuck in one mode.

Cross-cultural communication is particularly important. Here, where there is the greatest need for person-centred communication, there is the greatest danger of resorting to a 'transfer of information' stance in inappropriate circumstances. There may be barriers to both spoken and body language, and institutional or personal racism, as well as divergence of cultural beliefs and norms. There are no easy answers to these challenges, but there is always scope for positive action to increase access, uptake and satisfaction with services – but this will usually involve changing services.

This introduces another factor which underlines the value of the subjective perspective: the question of power. Enabling people to communicate, and treating what they say with respect, is enabling them to participate in care. Illness is often experienced as a loss of control over our affairs. It is possible to see health care as an attempt to restore control. Yet most health care settings are made up in such a way that they make non-professionals feel relatively powerless, thereby compounding the problem. Some of this is inevitable. An unfamiliar environment, bad memories or associations, and lack of technical expertise all lead to feelings of powerlessness. And patients normally lack real knowledge and power which others have, particularly knowledge and power connected to the management of disease. Yet there is a lot that can be done, through dialogue, to give patients greater control over their care. This power-sharing need not be confined to one-to-one interactions but can be built into the way institutions work, the ways in which the health care agenda is drawn up, and the way in which resources are allocated. As well as important differences, there are a lot of commonalities between the perspectives of individual patients. Taken together, and taken seriously, they would make for a different health service.

Social well-being

The famous WHO definition of health refers to 'social well-being' as part of health. Sometimes this is taken to refer to an aspect of personal well-being, i.e. that aspect of an individual's welfare that stems from the quantity and quality of social relationships and social support that they enjoy. But it is also possible to interpret it in a wider sense as the well-being of society. If so, is there more to a healthy society than the health of the individuals who make it up? Even if we operate with a narrow conception of health, these are important questions. Aristotle's distinctions are helpful here. Society itself cannot possess physical health, only individuals can do that, but it can be healthy in the sense of 'health causing'. This is the reason so much emphasis has come to be placed upon health promotion. As well as aiming to develop personal skills, health promotion seeks to 'build healthy public policy; create supportive environments; strengthen community action: and reorient health services' (WHO, 1986a). In other words, to help bring about a healthy social and physical environment. The following two chapters deal in depth with the social context of health and health promotion respectively, but it is worth introducing some issues about the relationship between individual and social well-being here.

One way into these issues is by looking at what has become the accepted technical usage of the terms 'impairment', 'disability' and 'handicap' (WHO, 1980). These terms are often fudged together in ordinary usage, but for the purposes of scientific classification and communication the WHO has produced three useful stipulative definitions. In brief, an *impairment* is a physical or psychological abnormality that may or may not lead to a disability. A *disability* is a loss of function experienced by the impaired person which in turn may or may not lead to a handicap. And a *handicap* is some social disadvantage suffered by a person because of their disability. Thus it is possible to have an impairment (such as slight damage to one ear) which does not cause any significant disability (such as loss of hearing) or handicap. It

is equally possible to have a disability (such as short-sightedness) which does not cause any significant handicap. Note that as we move from impairment to handicap we are moving from a medical through a functional to a social conception of health.

Leaving aside the exact technical specification of these three terms, the distinctions between them are most useful. It is plain that if we want to reduce handicap we must address social factors. Someone who cannot walk has, by definition, a substantial disability but they only have a substantial handicap if the world in which they live makes it impossible for them to enjoy equal opportunities. Just as we turn to physical remedies for disability, we need social action to address handicap. Often the cause of handicap is the attitudes of others, either individually or collectively embodied in institutions, policies or actions. These points do not only apply to those with recognised disabilities; they apply equally to anyone who is put at a social disadvantage. Some people are handicapped by physical disabilities, others by gender, race, social class or other factors.

The existence of discrimination and inequalities takes us on to social well-being in the broader sense, and to politics. It is well known that there are inequalities in patterns of disease and death, as well as in access to health care and health promotion. These inequalities are intimately tied in with more general inequalities such as those in material living and working conditions (Townsend *et al.*, 1988). It is very tempting for those interested in maximising health to assume that everything possible should be done to reduce all such inequalities. Unfortunately this is too simple-minded. If we take health to refer to something narrow, such as the absence of disease, then there are other social goods that we may also value (such as personal liberty and market competition) which might be undermined in the pursuit of equal health. However, if we see equality as part of what we mean by social well-being or 'a healthy society' then this is fine providing that we accept that it is a political judgement about the nature of a good society. There is always a danger of trying to smuggle in our moral or political values disguised as neutral-sounding references to health.

What is undoubtedly the case is that expectation and quality of life are related to divisions of wealth, status and power. For many, this is a forceful political argument. Even those who are quite happy to see inequalities in houses, cars and holidays often find it difficult to accept that one person should live for longer than another for reasons of wealth. This is because in most people's minds health is seen as a basic need, or even a basic entitlement. It is felt to be a minimum requirement of life, and it is uncomfortable to admit that our social or economic arrangements do not distribute this equitably. These feelings and judgements are not only important politically; they also indicate something about what health means to many people.

What is health?

Thus far we have explored some of the issues around narrow and broad conceptions of health. We have noted that it is possible to have negative and positive versions of these conceptions, and that it is possible to assess our state of health from an internal subjective perspective or from an external perspective. The only two definitions we have looked at, health as absence of disease and health as well-being, seem to be at two extreme poles. The former is a narrow negative conception and the latter a broad positive conception. The former would entail health assessment being made from an external perspective, the latter has a subjective as well as an objective dimension.

There are two main routes that can be taken from this point and they are both worthy of serious attention. On the one hand, it could be said that there is no need to look for a definitive conception of health. Individuals might have preferred definitions or conceptions; they may choose to use rather different conceptions in different circumstances. All that matters is that they are self-conscious about their use of the word 'health', and that they are willing and able to make clear how they are using it. On the other hand, it could be said that we do need to look for some more definitive conception. That there must be some compromise between, or common denominator lying beneath, the variety of conceptions. This way, by identifying the 'true' definition of health, we will not only clarify things further, but we will also provide a conception which everyone can come to share. It is worth spending some time pursuing this goal, even if some people see whatever

emerges as just one more conception.

The search for a compromise seems sensible, as disease-freedom seems too narrow and well-being too broad. Also, a compromise seems quite possible if we return to the idea with which we began, of health as 'good functioning' whether that be the good functioning of the body or of the person as a whole. The problem is that the general formula of 'good personal functioning' is useful at an abstract level but the minute we try to specify it further we get tangled in a web of value debates. There is a mass of moral, political and religious disagreements about what it is to function well as a person.

However, there is a way forward. Some authors have argued that there are certain basic elements in common between all conceptions of well-being. So although we may not be able to agree about the full meaning of well-being, we should be able to agree about a core meaning, that part which relates to essentials or basic needs (Plant et al., 1980). The argument is that whatever conception of the good life we have, there are certain requirements that need to be fulfilled in order for us to attain it. *Physical survival* is one of these requirements, and we saw in the section on well-being that conditions like food and shelter can be seen as 'objective' parts of well-being. But, it is argued, another such requirement is *autonomy* or self-determination (i.e. the capacity of an individual to make and carry out choices on his or her own behalf). For how could we say that someone was functioning well as a person, let alone that they were trying to meet their own conception of well-being, if they lacked any measure of autonomy? In turn we can see that there are conditions such as physical functioning, education, and some level of social and economic opportunity which are necessary conditions for autonomy.

These arguments, therefore, make space for a conception of health between the two extreme poles. Health could be seen as the state of having one's basic needs satisfied, or more positively as having the necessary resources to live one's life as one chooses. This is the kind of conception that the WHO has moved towards in recent years:

'Health is, therefore, seen as a resource for everyday life, not the objective of living; it is a positive concept emphasizing social and personal resources, as well as physical capacities'
(WHO, 1986b)

This is also the frame of reference that informs David Seedhouse's influential work on the meaning of health. His conception of health is a carefully articulated version of 'the resources for living' or what he calls 'the foundations for achievement' approach:

'A person's optimum state of health is equivalent to the state of the set of conditions which fulfil or enable a person to work to fulfil his or her realistic chosen and biological potentials'
(Seedhouse, 1986, page 61)

Although this is not offered as a final definition but as a way of delimiting the meaning of health, it is certainly very useful and thought-provoking. Anyone who is interested in this subject would do well to read the whole of the book from which this quotation is taken. But the essence of the conception is clear. Health is seen as the foundations or conditions necessary to live one's own life to the full. These conditions will include things like physical fitness, food and shelter but also things like education, self-confidence and access to opportunities. Although most of these necessary conditions will be the same for all people, some of them will vary according to the circumstances and the particular life goals individuals have. Finally, as with any sensible conception, there are degrees of health depending upon how many of the foundation conditions are realised. Remember the 'healthy bank balance' with which we began? It seems we have come full circle. This new conception of health sees health as 'personal and social wealth', where 'wealth' is understood in the broadest, and not merely monetary, sense.

This conception of health overlaps with a famous sociological definition of health as 'the state of optimum capacity of an individual for the effective role and tasks for which he has been socialised' (Parsons, 1981). It emphasises the idea of health as the capacity to function well. However, there is also a crucial difference. According to Seedhouse the yardstick for 'good functioning' depends partly upon the choice of the individual concerned, and not upon the norms or expectations prevailing in society at the time.

Perhaps we have arrived at the ultimate destination. It is up to you to decide. Here we have a relatively clear conception of health which is neither too narrow nor too broad. One clear advantage of this sort of conception over both the narrow and broad conceptions is the way they relate to mental health. According to the disease-freedom model, mental health only exists as the absence of pathological abnormality. This seems wrong for two reasons. First, there is the highly controversial reduction of mental ill health to physical pathology; mental illness seems better described in behavioural rather than physical language. Second, it seems that there is much more to the positive conception of mental health than the absence of mental illness, however the latter is understood. But the broad conception of complete mental well-being seems far too vague and all-encompassing. We would probably regard anyone who thought they had complete mental well-being as mad! Ideas like 'self-realisation' seem to demand too much. The conception of health as necessary resources for a full life suggests a compromise picture of mental health. To have mental health would require a certain level of autonomy, and in turn this would depend upon conditions like understanding one's environment, self-confidence, and a relatively supportive (as opposed to oppressive) social environment. All of these resources are necessary for adequate-to-good mental functioning. They are practical and positive considerations; more than just the absence of something, and less than perfection.

From this example we can see the practical implications of the 'resources conception'. It draws attention to those conditions which either enable or block the realisation of potentials. Thus health workers can put their own energies into providing those resources that are most needed. They need not be pre-occupied with diseases (although these can be important blocks to potential); neither need they be overwhelmed by the endless range of things that affect well-being.

It would be tidy to end this section here, but a concern for truth does not always coincide with tidiness. Indeed, when Seedhouse identifies work for health as the provision of 'foundations for achievement', he writes, 'The common factor is, on the face of it, blindingly simple, but on analysis the idea soon becomes plagued with difficulties' (1986, page 63). I will give a brief indication of two possible difficulties, the first arguably trivial but the second rather more important.

The first difficulty is this: how can food, shelter, clean air or employment be part of a person's health when they are 'outside' of the person? They are clearly 'health causing', and therefore have implications for health work, but it seems to be odd to see them as part of someone's health. I would prefer to see health as referring to an individual's physical and mental resources. That is, to personal resources, rather than to both personal and social resources (whilst noting that the former are dependent upon the latter). What do you think?

The second difficulty is more complicated and more challenging. Is the idea of basic resources or foundations really neutral between all the various conceptions of well-being? It can be argued that it is not; that this conception of health actually rests upon a particular conception of well-being, in which personal well-being is closely identified with the exercise of autonomy or choice. This is rather like the view that was questioned in the earlier section on well-being. According to this conception of health someone whose foundations are in place is in effect healthy and there is no reason, nor right, for health workers to interfere in their lives. This applies even if they use their autonomy to choose to smoke, or over-eat, or even to commit suicide. So long as they are autonomous they are healthy. Many people who have more definite views about health and well-being find this implication difficult to accept. Once again you must decide what you think.

Assessing ill health or quality of life

One of the main reasons for trying to clarify the meaning of health is so we can assess the health of individuals and populations. It should be clear by now that we cannot ask how healthy someone is without specifying a conception of health. So many apparent complications and paradoxes come about because this is ignored. Someone who is diseased may be healthy in the sense that they do not feel ill, and/or in the sense that they have the resources to function well, and/or in the sense that they are enjoying considerable personal well-being. It is possible to generate countless examples in which people can be judged to be unhealthy (according to some conceptions) *and* healthy (according to others). Even within a conception of health, individuals can be both healthy and unhealthy, just as a glass can be both half full and half empty, because health is always a matter of degree.

It seems, therefore, that it is important to understand the contestable meaning of health, and to be able to appreciate and move between the various conceptions discussed above. But from another point of view all of this seems most unhelpful. Suppose you were given a health care budget to manage. There would be two questions you would feel obliged to answer: 'On what, and on whom, should we spend this money?' and 'Having spent money, are we doing as much good as possible?'. These questions give rise to many complexities which it is not possible to explore here; however, we can see that these questions could be raised by asking about the health of populations before or after care. Imagine how you would feel faced with the reply, 'We cannot tell you what the health of this population is, there are a countless number of answers, it all depends what you mean'. This may well be true but it will not do as an answer. It is necessary to fasten upon some indicator, however crude, of whether or not health care or health care policies are improving health. Here we face a practical challenge which opens up all of the above theoretical discussions. Should our indicators be negative or positive, broad or narrow, subjective or objective? This question has to be tackled at policy level and at the level of practice.

We cannot avoid making some policy decision about the purposes and priorities of health care. These decisions are either 'made' implicitly by what happens to be provided, or they can be made explicitly. One way of doing so explicitly is by advocating a particular conception of health. Thus if we accept that health care is, in broad terms, the promotion of personal autonomy, we would look to increase some indicators of autonomy. Or we could say that health is, in broad terms, absence of medically defined pathology, and aim for lower indications of disease. However, although a decision about the purposes and priorities of health care is inevitable, it does not follow that this decision is the same as deciding upon a conception of health. It is worth making some effort trying to appreciate this. Take an individual who is a car mechanic. She may believe that it is part of her job to keep owners informed, reassured and satisfied. But no one would think that all this is part of the *meaning* of 'car maintenance'. Thus it is perfectly possible to subscribe to a narrow conception of health and to believe that health care should aim to meet other aspects of well-being. What matters, what is essential, is that the overall purposes or ends of health care are decided upon. Only then, when we have decided what we will count as a benefit, can we assess the costs and benefits of various patterns of provision. So although what we are assessing can be summarised in broad terms as 'ill health' or 'quality of life', in practice we will use a wide range of concepts like 'needs' or 'satisfaction' in the process of assessment.

These general questions of policy or philosophy are notoriously difficult, and in some ways things are easier at the level of practice. Any particular practitioner can focus in on his or her own medium and short term objectives and ask how far these are being met. Up to a point, appropriate indicators will be suggested by the objectives. If the objective of a particular intervention is pain relief then assessment will depend upon subjective reporting of pain; if it is to increase mobility, it will be possible to use more generalisable measures, and so on. This does not tell us how to combine such assessments into more holistic indicators. Nor can these limited indicators be used to justify forms of care, for it is always necessary to ask the general policy question, 'Why should we be doing this at all?'. But these sorts of narrow indicators do offer a start in the process of assessing ill health or quality of life. Also, it would be foolish in the extreme to rely on a very general conception of health to assess the outcome of specific interventions. Such a conception would form a valuable part of an overall evaluation, but we will also want to know whether the intervention meets its specific objectives.

There are two particularly influential approaches to the assessment of ill health which it is worth introducing, and which roughly correspond with the two questions raised above. In order to assess the health of populations so as to determine what kind of health care to offer, it is necessary to employ some form of **needs assessment**. In order to assess any improvement in the health of individuals or groups who have received care, it is possible to use a **quality of life measurement scale**.

As we have seen, the concept of need is intimately connected with the conception of health as personal resources. The negative version of this conception would be that health equals the absence of basic needs. Hence it is sensible to use the concept of need in order to identify what to provide, but many people would see it as too broad. They would want to distinguish between needs and health needs where the latter means the

ability to benefit from actual or potential health care (Stevens and Gabbay, 1991). Once again the scope of needs assessment depends upon whether we use broad or narrow, subjective or objective indicators. However interpreted, it depends upon systematic social and epidemiological research. In order to assess the needs of a local population, researchers will look at some combination of death and disease (mortality and morbidity) statistics, use of services, expressed needs or demands of patients, and subjective concerns of some sample of the population as a whole.

Most forms of needs assessment (like quality of life scales) involve *measurement*. This makes a special demand on those who practise it. Measures taken at different times and places have to be comparable. That is, they have to be **reliable**. They also have to be accurate, or **valid**, indicators of whatever they set out to measure. For these purposes a vague conception is not good enough; it is necessary to use a stipulative technical definition (sometimes called an **operational definition**). For example, and to oversimplify, we could choose to define someone's need for health care as 'the number of visits made to clinics or hospitals'. Even this would provide some kind of indication of need, and it would enable us to provide comparable and reliable measures. However, we can see that there would be a considerable gap between this measure and our conception of health need. The more sophisticated the measure the narrower this gap would become, but there would always be some gap. The challenge is to find practical and reliable measures which are as valid as possible. Above all, it is vital not to confuse a measure of needs or ill health with the full meaning of these concepts.

All of this applies equally to quality of life measures. Quality of life is a good shorthand phrase for the overall aim of health care; it is the effect of possessing health. Health care can only be properly evaluated if improvements in quality of life as well as quantity of life are taken into account. To this end a number of quality of life scales or measures have been developed and checked for their reliability and validity (Bowling, 1991). These are ways of estimating the overall quality of life of individuals according to combinations of narrow indicators. Some of these indicators, or criteria, are dependent upon professional observations, but most are decided by the subjective reporting of the patient. In this way, diverse criteria like mobility or depression or social support can be translated into an overall score or picture of quality of life. Many of these scales are very sophisticated and holistic in ambition. However, it should be clear how difficult it is fully to capture quality of life even with the most sophisticated measure. As with needs assessment, the only option is to choose an approach which best fits the purpose to which the measurement is going to be put.

Elsewhere I have argued that it is possible to see the elements of quality of life on a map which, roughly speaking, moves from the public to the personal (Cribb, 1985). At one extreme are the most public and generalisable determinants of quality of life, what might be called 'quality of lifestyle'. These relate to people's capacities and restrictions in their work, social and home life. These elements are the most easily quantified and compared, but they are too blunt to provide good assessment of quality of life as a whole. At the other extreme is what could be called 'sense of life'. This relates to the individual's subjective perspective on their life, its meaning and value. Experiences of health and illness are enmeshed in a web of fears, beliefs and commitments from the most mundane to the most profound. It would be impossible to understand, or assess, an individual's quality of life without taking this into account. But it does not lend itself to measurement. In between these extremes are less specific elements of outlook or subjective well-being, what might loosely be called 'mental health'. Here both measurement scales and more subjective forms of assessment are possible, and can be combined.

From this we can see that the process of measurement, which is essential if proper assessments and comparisons are to be done, pushes us towards a more generalisable, 'scientific' or reductionist stance. Thus there is a constant danger that we will forget the importance of the person-centred or subjective perspective.

Conclusions

Thinking about the meaning of health takes us in many different directions, and raises many questions and uncertainties. These complexities stem from the fact that thinking about health is thinking about the basic nature of life, of people, and of the world in which they live. We cannot neatly separate out health issues from non-health issues. Neither can we completely separate out factual questions about health from value questions.

For practical purposes we sometimes have to divide the world into supposed health domains (e.g. the local 'health' centre) and non-health domains (e.g. the local tax office). But it only takes a moment to see that this separation is false. There is no domain of activity which is not connected with health in the sense that it does not affect people's state of health, or their experience of health and illness. In order to avoid getting entangled in value debates about health we might decide to employ a narrow, 'scientific' conception or definition of health. We might choose to see health as the absence of disease, and thereby leave all the complications, abstractions and disagreements behind whilst we get on with clinical science and practice. I hope that what has been said above is enough to show why this 'trick' will not work.

There are many value questions which arise however we define health. Firstly, questions about the distribution of health, the targeting of health care, and the rectification of inequalities. The answers to these questions cannot be found in clinical science but only through moral and political reflection and analysis. Secondly, questions about *how* to behave towards people, and how to take their perspectives, their values and objectives into account. Once again there are no universal scientific solutions. Finally, there are questions about the general well-being of people, about what is in their overall interests. These arise whether or not individuals are well enough to express their own views or preferences. Focusing in on diseases does not make these larger concerns disappear.

There is yet another reason why the resort to scientific language does not avoid the need for value judgements. An important complication, which has not been discussed above, can be indicated briefly here in order to make clear that this chapter is the beginning rather than the end of the debate. That is, even apparently scientific classifications or descriptions of ill health are not entirely free from value judgement. The ideas of physical impairment or disease depend upon an idea of a range of normality, but the definition of this range of normality is arguably determined in part by cultural and value judgements (Kennedy, 1981; Scadding, 1988).

None of this is to say that the conception of health as the absence of disease is not useful. I have tried to show that there are advantages and disadvantages with this narrow conception, as with the broader conceptions of 'personal capacity or resources' and 'well-being'. It is merely to emphasise that we cannot solve the problem of health care by fastening upon a definition of health. Some of the time it is helpful to use a conception of health which concentrates on specific measurable objectives; some of the time it is helpful to be reminded of the infinite variety of elements that can contribute to life's quality; and it is always helpful to remember that health care involves enabling individuals to function well as people and not just as biological organisms.

Thinking about the meaning of health is necessary if we are to decide what kinds of knowledge, attitudes and values should be built into health care; but it is only a start.

Glossary

Conception: One of the various, debatable, meanings of a complex concept

Needs assessment: Researching, describing and measuring the health care needs of a population in order to plan the provision of care

Operational definition: A stipulative definition which is formulated in such a precise way that it enables the scientific community to 'isolate' and measure the defined phenomenon. Note, once again, that this will not coincide with common usage; an operational definition of 'class', for example, will not measure all the things we associate with class

Quality of life measurement scale: A research instrument which employs a set of criteria to assess people's quality of life. These can be used for needs assessment or to measure and compare the effectiveness of therapies

Reductionism: The process of 'reducing' a whole to some of its parts. In particular, it is the way in which human beings can be regarded as bodies or objects of study. In itself this is neither good nor bad, but it has the potential to cause problems

Reliability: A key dimension of the usefulness of a measurement scale. A reliable measure will consistently give the same measure to the same phenomenon, and will thereby enable comparisons across time and space

Stipulative definition: A definition of a word which is decided by agreement, and set out systematically and explicitly. For these reasons it may not coincide with the normal usage of the word, which is likely to vary and have less clear boundaries

Validity: The other key dimension of the usefulness of a measurement scale. A measure is valid if it gives a faithful and accurate picture of the phenomenon being measured

References

Aristotle. (1941). *The Basic Works of Aristotle*. Random House, New York.

Bowling, A. (1991). *Measuring Health*. Open University Press, Milton Keynes.

Cornwell, J. (1984). *Hard-Earned Lives*. Tavistock Publications, London.

Cribb, A. (1985). Quality of life. *Journal of Medical Ethics*, 11(3), 142–145.

Field, D. (1976). The social definition of illness. In *An Introduction to Medical Sociology*, Tuckett, D. (ed.). Tavistock Publications, London.

Gallie, W.B. (1964). *Philosophy and the Historical Understanding*. Chatto and Windus, London.

Gray, J.A.M. and Austoker, J. (1989). *Draft Guidelines on Improving Acceptability*. Screening Publications, Oxford.

Kennedy, I. (1981). *Unmasking Medicine*. Allen and Unwin, London.

Parsons, T. (1981). Definitions of health and illness in the light of American values and social structure. In *Concepts of Health and Disease*, Caplan, A.L., Engelhardt, H.T. and McCartney, J.J. (eds.). Addison-Wesley, New York.

Plant, R., Lesser, H. and Taylor-Gooby, P. (1980). *Political Philosophy and Social Welfare*. Routledge and Kegan Paul, London.

Plato. (1982). *Philebus*. Penguin Classics, Harmondsworth.

Scadding, J.G. (1988). Health and disease: what can medicine do for philosophy? *Journal of Medical Ethics*, 14(3), 118–124.

Seedhouse, D. (1986). *Health: The Foundations for*

Achievement. John Wiley and Sons, Chichester.

Stevens, A. and Gabbay, J. (1991). Needs assessment needs assessment. *Health Trends*, 23(1), 20–23.

Townsend, P., Davidson, N. and Whitehead, M. (1988). *Inequalities in Health*. Penguin, Harmondsworth.

World Health Organisation. (1947). *World Health Organisation: Constitution*. WHO, Geneva.

WHO. (1980). *International Classification of Impairments, Disabilities, and Handicaps*. WHO, Geneva

WHO. (1986a). *The Ottawa Charter of Health Promotion*. WHO, Geneva.

WHO. (1986b). A discussion document on the concept and principles of health promotion. *Health Promotion*, 1(1), 73–76.

Suggestions for further reading

Bowling, A. (1991). *Measuring Health*. Open University Press, Milton Keynes.

Morse, J.M. and Johnson, J.L. (eds.). (1991). *The Illness Experience*. Sage, London.

Plato. (1982). *Philebus*. Penguin Classics, Harmondsworth.

Seedhouse, D. (1986). *Health: The Foundations for Achievement*. John Wiley and Sons, Chichester.

2

THE SOCIAL CONTEXT OF HEALTH

Paul Watt

> The aim of this chapter is to examine the social context in which health and health care occur from a sociological perspective.
>
> The chapter includes the following topics:
>
> - Theoretical perspectives in sociology with reference to social stratification
>
> - Class and health
>
> - Gender and health
>
> - Ethnicity, racism and health
>
> - Poverty and health, including sections on elderly people, unemployment, lone parent families and homelessness

The previous chapter has explored the various ways in which health has been defined. In this chapter we will be considering how a person's health is affected by their social circumstances. The emphasis will be placed upon how health is linked to what sociologists call *social stratification*, more commonly referred to as social inequality.

Throughout this chapter, attention will be drawn to the manner in which individuals share common life experiences and problems with others and how these experiences follow certain social patterns. In so doing, we are developing what the American sociologist C. Wright Mills called 'the sociological imagination', in which we can see the connections between an individual's private troubles and what Mills (1970) refers to as, 'the public issues of social structure' (page 14). An individual's private troubles illuminate the social structure, but we cannot possibly hope either to understand or explain those private troubles without reference to that social structure of which the individual is a part. The rest of this chapter will deal with the manner in which various aspects of social inequality, namely *class*, gender, race and poverty, affect people's health.

This chapter is not intended to be a general introduction to sociology. There are several good books which provide such an introduction (see the suggestions for further reading at the end of the chapter). Nevertheless it is necessary to say something about the discipline of sociology itself. A prominent British sociologist defines sociology as follows:

'Sociology is the study of human social life, groups and societies'

(Giddens, 1989, page 7)

As such, sociology is concerned with the regularities and recurring patterns of social life, with describing and understanding these regularities and patterns, and crucially with *explaining* why these social patterns exist. One such regularity is that nurses as an occupational group are approximately 90% female. There is a range of socio-logical explanations which could be brought to bear on this 'social fact', as the French sociologist, Durkheim, called such patterns; for example, one could point to the way in which, in contemporary Western societies, girls are socialised in the family into the caring **role**. You might like to suggest your own explanations for this sociological phenomenon.

Sociological perspectives and social stratification

Within sociology there is a range of what are called *theoretical perspectives* which refer to the different ways in which sociologists look at social reality. In other words, sociologists differ in defining social reality and in how they understand and explain social phenomena. In broad terms, sociological perspectives can be divided into two: there are *macro-perspectives* which are concerned with understanding and explaining large-scale social processes usually in relation to an entire society, often defined as a nation state, but possibly in relation to the whole world. On the other hand, there are *micro-perspectives* which are concerned with small-scale social interaction involving a few people and these are the areas of sociology which are closest to psychology, especially social psychology. In this chapter, we will mainly be concerned with the macro-perspectives since it is these which have had most to say about social stratification.

Stratification, or the social structure of inequality, is generally regarded as playing a central role in the discipline of sociology:

> '. . . we can virtually define the core of sociology as an inquiry into the origins, characteristics and consequences of social inequality defined in terms of power, status and class'
>
> (Turner, 1986, page 30)

All known societies contain some form of stratification although the basis of the system of stratification varies from society to society. The various theoretical perspectives emphasise different aspects of stratification and we will briefly deal with some of these major approaches below, all of which, apart from **symbolic interactionism**, are macro-perspectives.

(1) Functionalism

Functionalism asks the question, 'What is the function of the component parts of the society in relation to the maintenance of order in the social system as a whole?' It uses an organic analogy: in a body, each particular organ plays a vital role in the maintenance of the whole body, and in a similar way each part of society fulfils a particular function for the whole society. An example is the system of stratification itself. Davis and Moore (1945) argued that not only is social stratification universal, in that it exists in all known societies, but that it plays a vital role in ensuring that the most talented people in a society are enticed into the most important positions; this is done since those positions receive more rewards, in terms of income and prestige, than less important positions. Therefore, social inequality is both universal and necessary in any society.

This functionalist theory assumes a *consensus* model of society in that society is said to be characterised by order and stability; this order is based upon agreement over the values held by the members of society. In contrast, the next three perspectives, Marxism, Weberian sociology and feminism, all assume a *conflict* model of society whereby society is said to be structured around the conflicts of interest arising out of the system of stratification itself. In this sense, social inequality is said to generate various forms of conflict and is not regarded in the same positive light as it is by functionalist sociologists.

(2) Marxism

Marxism derives from the work of Karl Marx, the 19th century German social theorist and revolutionary. Marx concentrated on the form of stratification which is called social class. For Marx, class refers, in a capitalist society, to the manner in which property, in the form of industry and commerce or, as Marx terms it, 'the means of production', is owned by a relatively small group of people called the *capitalist class*. According to Marx, this class only gains profits from its ownership of factories, offices and banks because it exploits a much larger class, the proletariat or *working class*, which, because it does not own the means of production, is compelled to sell its labour to the capitalist class in exchange for wages. The relationship between these two classes is an antagonistic one in Marxist theory and results in class conflict, and ultimately revolution.

Modern Marxism still uses this two-class model as the core of its analysis, but it does recognise that in 20th century Western capitalist societies, there has been a huge expansion in occupational groups which do not fit neatly into the simple two-class model; for example, professionals such as doctors.

(3) Weberian sociology

Unlike Marxism, **Weberian sociology** does not prioritise class over other forms of stratification, for example, inequality based upon racial or religious differences. Instead its founder, Weber, argued that stratification arises out of the distribution of power in a society and that there are three main forms of power: economic power which gives rise to classes, social power or status which gives rise to status groups, and political power which gives rise to political parties (Saunders, 1990). For the purposes of this analysis we will ignore the latter and concentrate on classes and status groups. Classes, for Weber, are phenomena which arise out of the distribution of property and occupational skills/qualifications in a market society, which means that using Weber's analysis one can identify several classes in modern society: an upper class of property owners, the middle classes consisting of small shopkeepers and entrepreneurs as well as professionals, and a lower or working class which possesses neither property nor qualifications (Saunders, 1990).

Status groups arise out of the possession of what Weber calls 'social honour' or prestige. Examples of such status groups can be seen in the **caste system** in India or the racial division between 'whites', 'blacks' and 'coloureds' in South Africa. Such status groups are not classes because their position does not depend upon economic factors, but instead on possession of some socially significant marker which distinguishes that group from others. Skin colour or other physical characteristics can form the basis for such status groups and we will explore this aspect of stratification further when we discuss racism and ethnicity later in the chapter. Social conflict, in Weberian theory, can

arise out of any of the different forms of stratification within a particular society and is not solely based on class conflict, as it tends to be in Marxist sociology.

(4) Feminism

Feminism, like Marxist and Weberian approaches, is also a conflict theory. Feminists have been responsible for highlighting two issues which have provoked important insights into the social context of health. The first is that a distinction is made between the categories of *sex* and *gender*. The former refers to the biological differences between males and females. The latter refers to the social construction of masculine and feminine behaviour; that is, the socially acceptable behaviour which is expected of the two sexes in different societies. Feminism has pointed out how males and females are socialised into their respective **gender roles** and how these roles are irreducible to biological differences between the sexes. The second issue feminism has raised is that gender is regarded as being about more than merely the playing of roles; instead it is argued that gender relations are based upon inequality of power between men and women and that this power takes the form of **patriarchy** or the oppression of women by men. Such oppression can take the form of domestic violence, for example, and we will discuss the relevance of patriarchy for health when we go on to look at gender in more detail later in the chapter.

The above provides a very brief outline of how the major perspectives theorise stratification. We will be referring to some of their ideas in the rest of the chapter, primarily from the three conflict approaches rather than functionalism, since most of the work on health and inequality utilises elements of Marxist, Weberian and feminist theory.

(5) Symbolic interactionism

A micro-level perspective which has been very influential in the sociology of health, particularly in relation to mental illness, is symbolic interactionism. According to this perspective, people interact with their fellows on the basis of symbols and language which are modified in the process of interaction itself. Using mental illness as an example, symbolic interactionists are not concerned with the social structural causes of mental illness, which Marxists might say are related to class inequality, but instead with the social processes by which certain people's behaviour comes to be interpreted as mental illness. Interactionists regard mental illness as a form of **deviance**; that is, behaviour which breaks the social rules. Interactionists are concerned to show how certain behaviour comes to be seen by others as deviant and, importantly, what is the role of those people, in this example psychiatrists, who 'label' others as deviant. The emphasis on the labelling of deviance by people in authority is termed **labelling theory** and has been usefully applied in relation to the mental health of women and ethnic minorities, as we will see in later sections. An excellent example of an interactionist account of life inside a mental hospital is *Asylums* by Goffman (1968).

Defining and measuring health

The previous chapter was concerned with identifying the various concepts of health which have been used in the past and currently. In the sociological literature on health, a variety of measures of health is used including **mortality rates** and **morbidity rates**. The latter cover both disease as assessed by medical practitioners and also people's own subjective assessment of their health, which can be measured both negatively in terms of how ill people feel, or positively in terms of how healthy they feel. One example of a morbidity rate is the number of people in a given population who have been diagnosed by their GP as having chickenpox. The General Household Survey, a national survey carried out annually by the Office of Population Censuses and Surveys (OPCS), includes another measure of morbidity based upon people's own assessment of whether they have a 'long-standing illness' (OPCS, 1990). Whichever measure of health is used, sociologists have drawn attention to the fact that such measures are social constructions themselves: in other words, they are the creations of researchers, employed in particular organisations, who have specific objectives in mind. We will be commenting on the limitations of various measures of health throughout this chapter.

Class and health

Class

We have already seen that class is a key element of stratification for both Marxist and Weberian sociologists. However, many empirical studies of the relationship between class and health use a model of class based upon the government's own classification of occupations: the Registrar General's (RG) social class schema (see Table 2.1). This schema has been in existence since 1911, and in 1980 occupations were allotted to a particular social class on the basis of sharing a similar level of occupational skill, with the higher classes said to possess more skills than those lower down the scale.

Table 2.1. *The Registrar General's social class schema (OPCS, 1980)*

Class I	Professional occupations (for example, doctor, lawyer)
Class II	Intermediate occupations (for example, nurse, manager)
Class IIIN	Skilled non-manual occupations (for example, secretary, clerical worker)
Class IIIM	Skilled manual occupations (for example, electrician, bus driver)
Class IV	Partly skilled occupations (for example, postman/woman, bus conductor)
Class V	Unskilled occupations (for example, labourer, cleaner)

From a sociological point of view, one problem with this class scale is that its theoretical basis is unclear; while it is obviously not based upon Marxism because it is not concerned with the ownership/non-ownership of property, neither is it firmly based upon Weberian theory, although it is closer to the latter since it differentiates classes as occupational groupings based upon their level of skill (Saunders, 1990). Feminists have also criticised this model of class since it allots married women a class position based upon their husband's occupation and not their own if they are in employment, as in fact the majority of married women are.

The social context of health 21

Notwithstanding the many criticisms of the RG schema, it has been widely used in research investigating the relationship between class and health and as a result we will refer to it here. Using the RG scale, the *middle class* are usually taken to be classes I, II and IIIN, whilst the *working class* are in classes IIIM, IV and V. It is worth noting that some sociologists would query such a simple middle class/working class distinction based on the non-manual/manual divide between occupations (see Saunders, 1990).

Evidence on class and health

The links between class and ill health were documented during the 19th century by a range of social reformers, as well as revolutionaries such as Marx. They all addressed the appalling living and working conditions of the working class during the early phase of industrial capitalism, which led either directly or indirectly to illness, disease and death. A series of state welfare reforms were introduced this century to combat the poverty and ill health of the working class, including the creation of the National Health Service in 1948 by the Labour government. Given that the NHS provided free health care at the point of delivery, it was commonly assumed that the links between ill health and class would be broken. In addition, the **full employment** which Britain had during the 1950s and 1960s and the gradual improvement in living standards should have also meant that the relationship between class and ill health would become a thing of the past.

The Black Report on health inequalities gathered data on class and health for the period of the early 1970s and was published in 1980. The Report showed that wide class variations in mortality rates existed for all age groups, so that as one moved down the RG class scale, from class I (professional) to V (unskilled manual), the mortality rate increased. Not only that, the Report also found that rather than such class inequalities diminishing in size, they had in fact increased for the period 1930–1972. So the Report confounded expectations that, after 20 years of the NHS, class inequalities would have diminished. The newly elected Conservative government in 1979, under Mrs Thatcher, responded very coolly to the Report's findings, especially the suggestion that the government should embark on a comprehensive anti-poverty campaign if the class differentials

were to be reduced (see the Introduction in Townsend, Davidson and Whitehead, 1988).

A second report on health inequalities was published in 1987 by Margaret Whitehead, called *The Health Divide*. This report looked at morbidity rates and mortality rates and found that significant class inequalities existed in both. All of the major diseases follow class gradients, with the lower social classes being far more likely to have such diseases at every stage of life, the exception being malignant melanoma: skin cancer usually caused by too many holidays in the sun! *The Health Divide* found that not only did significant class variations in mortality and morbidity exist, but that the mortality differentials had in fact widened since the Black Report (both reports can be found in *Inequalities in Health* by Townsend, Davidson and Whitehead, 1988).

A recent survey of the evidence (Smith, Bartley and Blane, 1990) suggests that further widening of class differentials in mortality can be expected. The tables below provide evidence on both mortality (Table 2.2) and chronic sickness (Table 2.3).

Explanations of health inequalities

The Black Report offered four possible explanations for the health inequalities which it found and *The Health Divide* replicated these explanations. We will briefly consider these four: the artefact explanation, theories of natural and social selection, cultural/behavioural, and materialist/structuralist explanations. We will then add a fifth which has recently received attention from sociologists, namely social support.

(1) The artefact explanation

This explanation suggests that the method of measuring social class using the RG schema artificially inflates the size and importance of mortality differentials. Jones and Cameron (1984) have pointed out the limitations of the RG scale by demonstrating that there are substantial differences in standardised mortality ratios (SMRs) *within* each social class, which means that the SMR for each class is only a crude average. They suggest that such problems render use of the scale illegitimate and stem from its inadequate theoretical base which, as we have mentioned above, is not firmly rooted in a sociological theory of class. Carr-Hill (1987) has suggested that there are problems with

Table 2.2 Social class mortality differentials for men aged 20–64, Great Britain, 1979–83 (OPCS, 1986, page 113).

Social class		*Standardised mortality ratios (all persons = 100)
I	Professional occupations	66
II	Intermediate occupations	76
IIIN	Skilled non-manual occupations	94
IIIM	Skilled manual occupations	106
IV	Partly skilled occupations	116
V	Unskilled occupations	165

* The average **standardised mortality ratio** for the population as a whole is 100. Ratios below 100 indicate lower than average chances of death and ratios above 100 indicate higher than average chances of death.

Table 2.3 Chronic sickness: percentage of all ages who reported long-standing illness by sex and socio-economic group, Great Britain, 1988 (OPCS, 1990, page 72)

Socio-economic group*	Males	Females
Professional	25	26
Employers and managers	32	29
Intermediate and junior non-manual	29	33
Skilled manual	33	33
Semi-skilled manual	38	40
Unskilled manual	40	47

* Socio-economic groups are groups of occupations with similar social and economic status (OPCS, 1980). They are not directly equivalent to the Registrar General's social classes.

utilising the RG class schema to measure changes in health inequalities over time, given that the size of the classes changed considerably between 1931 and 1981, notably that classes I and II have increased in size whilst classes IV and V have shrunk.

It would seem, then, that the RG schema is prob-

ably not the best measure of class for determining the nature of the relationship between class and health. However, this does not mean the relationship found in the Black Report is artificial. There is evidence that the use of the RG scale as a measure of socio-economic inequality actually underestimates the impact of such inequality on health. The Whitehall study of civil servants (Marmot, 1986) looked at the death rates of a cohort of male civil servants and found that the mortality gradient is actually much steeper than the Black Report found for the social classes, with the mortality rate of the lowest grade of civil servant being three times higher than that of the highest grade. Such results would suggest that the RG schema is simply not differentiated enough to pick up all of the impact of socio-economic inequality on health.

Recently the government has actually abandoned the RG classification in favour of a Standard Occupational Classification which operates on the basis of nine occupational groupings (Employment Department Group/OPCS, 1990). Whether this scheme will be as pertinent for analysing class inequalities in health as the RG scale, despite its faults, proved to be remains to be seen.

(2)   Theories of natural and social selection

This explanation accepts that social class inequalities in health exist, but argues that the inequalities are caused by a process of health selection. This means that people with poorer health are more likely to move down the class scale (they experience downward **social mobility**) and so concentrate in the lowest classes. This works in reverse for people in good health who would tend to travel up the class scale. The relationship between class and health occurs not because being a member of a lower social class causes ill health, but instead because having poor health causes individuals to move down the class scale; for example, illness in childhood can result in absence from school which in turn leads to educational failure and an unskilled job. The Health Divide did find some evidence to support the health selection explanation of health inequalities, but in itself this explanation has only a small effect on the overall class gradient in ill health.

(3) Cultural/behavioural explanations

According to these explanations, health in-equalities arise because the working class, particularly those in semi- and unskilled occupations, have adopted more health-damaging behaviour than the middle class and are also less likely to utilise preventive health services, including ante-natal care and vaccinations. We will examine use of such services later in this section on class. Attention here is focused on four aspects of behaviour which most epidemiologists agree have an inde-pendent impact on health: cigarette smoking, food and nutrition, exercise in leisure time, and alcohol consumption. All except the last, drinking alcohol, follow clear class gradients in that manual workers are more likely to smoke, eat more fatty foods and less fruit and fibre, and take less exercise. The pos-ition is somewhat reversed as regards alcohol, especially for women: professional women are more likely than women in semi/unskilled occupa-tions to drink more than the recommended sen-sible amount and are also less likely to be non-drinkers (OPCS, 1990). Apart from alcohol, working class people seem to lead less healthy lifestyles than the middle class and it is this which is said to cause their poorer health. Figure 2.1 illus-trates this in relation to smoking.

To say that the working class lead a less healthy lifestyle does not in itself explain why this might be the case. There are two very different theoretical interpretations of the evidence. The first is that the unhealthy lifestyles of manual workers stem from their actions as *individuals*; in other words, the lower classes have in some sense chosen to lead such unhealthy lifestyles by their choosing to smoke, eat fatty foods, etc. This view of human behaviour is individualistic since it locates the source of behaviour in the 'free' choice of indi-viduals. It is a view which historically is associated with conservatism, and more recently with monet-arist economics (Turner, 1986) and what has come to be known as the **New Right**. The argument is that manual workers are less healthy because they choose out of wilful ignorance to smoke cigarettes or eat white bread which they must know is un-healthy, so they only have themselves to blame. This individualistic approach to health forms the basis of much contemporary health education (Beattie, 1991) and it received some notoriety through the statements of Edwina Currie, a junior Health Minister in the 1980s, who described the links found in research between ill health and pov-erty in the following terms:

'I honestly don't think it has anything to do with

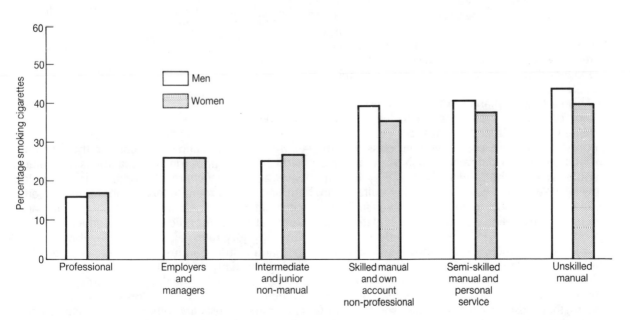

Fig. 2.1 *Cigarette smoking prevalence by sex and socio-economic group, Great Britain 1988 (OPCS, 1990; page 86)*

poverty. The problem very often for many people is just ignorance . . . and failing to realize they do have some control over their own lives'
(quoted in Townsend, Davidson and Whitehead, 1988, page 12)

As Smith and Nicolson (1991) demonstrate, this emphasis, by politicians and other people in authority, on the ignorance of the working class in relation to health goes back to the end of the 19th century. Such individualistic explanations for the unhealthy lifestyles of the working class do not generally find a great deal of support in sociology, largely because they tend to ignore the social nature of human behaviour; that is, what people share in common with others.

Because of this, most sociologists prefer a *cultural* explanation for the unhealthy lifestyles of the working class. This explanation emphasises how individuals share common beliefs and customs with each other; in other words, they share a common **culture**. According to this approach, behaviour such as smoking and drinking alcohol are not isolated aspects of working class life, but they derive their meanings from within working class culture as a whole. For example, smoking has a cultural acceptability amongst manual workers since it is seen as a form of leisure activity, as witnessed in pubs in working class areas and in factory canteens. During the last 20 years, smoking has become a form of despised activity amongst the middle class so that there is greater group pressure to give up the habit amongst professionals and managers compared with manual workers (Hart, 1985).

This cultural explanation for health inequalities is not one which has gone unchallenged. One problem with it is that it can abstract 'culture' from the rest of the lives of the working class, chiefly in relation to material factors such as the income people have or the kind of houses they live in. Several researchers have argued that culture can only be understood in relation to these material circumstances. For example in relation to smoking, Graham (1987a), in a study of young mothers on low incomes, has shown how smoking offers very positive benefits for such mothers in allowing them to cope in situations of little money but constant demands from children. Smoking means that these mothers can gain some form of psychological release from emotionally challenging situations which they cannot physically

escape from. Blaxter (1990) has pointed out that behavioural factors, such as smoking and drinking, actually have a greater influence on the health of the middle class compared with those in poor material circumstances. It would seem, then, that less healthy lifestyles cannot in themselves account for all of the health inequalities which the Black Report found and this is certainly the conclusion which both this report and *The Health Divide* came to.

Marxist sociologists would argue that the emphasis on culture only examines one dimension of class; that is, class in terms of consumption habits. As such it neglects the way in which consumption is related to what is produced and that such production is based upon what is profitable in capitalist society and not what is healthy. Marxists would point to the class-based nature of the production of cigarettes, alcohol, etc., and how powerful business interests are involved in ensuring the sale of such commodities (Doyal, 1979). As such, attention needs to be directed at the class structure as a whole, including the capitalist class, and not just the buying habits of the most disadvantaged section of the working class.

(4) Materialist/structuralist explanations

These types of explanations focus on the role of social structural factors in causing health inequalities; that is, the working and living conditions which arise out of people occupying a position in the class structure. The Black Report states that such materialist explanations are the most important and further evidence supports this claim (Blane, 1985).

(a) Work

Work itself, meaning here paid work, can be a cause of ill health and even death. In the 19th and early 20th centuries, deaths in factories and mines were a regular feature of working class life. Increased government intervention in health and safety at work, including the 1974 Health and Safety at Work Act, did lead to a reduction in industrial injury rates, although the level of injuries in manufacturing industry did rise considerably during the early 1980s (Tombs, 1990). Industrial accidents, including fatalities, are particularly high in the mining and construction industries. Chemicals, fumes, dusts and other toxic substances can cause industrial diseases, including direct poisoning, allergies, congenital abnormalities, or various forms of cancer (Doyal, 1979). Both industrial diseases and accidents are more likely to affect manual workers and this partially explains the class inequalities in health, particularly for men. Office workers also suffer from specific industrial hazards, such as **repetitive strain injury** which can occur in data processor operators and telephonists, amongst others (Ewan, Lowy and Reid, 1991). The level of control over their job experienced by workers could also be a factor in determining the higher mortality rates amongst junior as opposed to senior office workers (Marmot, 1986). Nurses themselves also suffer from various kinds of work-induced accidents and diseases and are even at risk from violent attack (McGrother, 1990).

(b) Income

The Black Report concluded that low income was one of the main reasons for the health inequalities which it found. Whilst by no means all manual workers are poor, those people with low incomes are most likely to be found employed in low skilled manual occupations (Townsend, 1979) and they are the people who are likely to be restricted in the kinds and even quantities of food which they can buy. Charles and Kerr (1988), in a study on food, commented that:

'Women who have to count every penny have less opportunity than women who are relatively comfortably off to concern themselves with issues of goodness; they are constrained to buy what they can afford to ensure that their families eat "properly"'

(page 169)

Given the links between diet and health, income would seem to play a major role in explaining the relationship between class and health.

(c) Housing

In the 1930s great attention was paid to the condition of slum housing in British cities and the effects of overcrowding and insanitary conditions on health. Considerable slum clearance took place in the 1930s and the large-scale building of council houses in the 1950s and 1960s was thought to have broken the links between working class health and housing.

However, the Black Report and *The Health Divide* both pointed to research which showed that such optimism was premature. Both reports made the general finding that mortality rates for all classes were highest in council and private rented dwellings compared with owner-occupied housing. Since the working class are more likely to live in council housing, this must explain some of the class differential in health. Byrne *et al.* (1986) found that there were significant differences in health within the council housing sector, with those people living in 'difficult to let' estates reporting the worst health.

Several studies (Martin *et al.*, 1987; Platt *et al.*, 1989) have noted the effects of damp and mould on health, particularly in relation to respiratory symptoms amongst children. Other health problems associated with poor quality housing include infestation, accidents, psychological distress and cold (Lowry, 1989, 1990b). One recent study carried out in West Belfast found that the health of children in particular was affected by living in a large, run-down, public sector block of flats and the report concluded that the 'Divis Flats is a contemporary public sector slum and supports the case for clearance and rehousing' (Blackman *et al.*, 1989, page 1). Unfortunately, these conditions are unlikely to be unique to West Belfast.

(d) Deprivation

The above three factors are likely to account for a large proportion of the class differences in mortality and morbidity rates. However, one problem with the use of the above factors to explain class differences in ill health is that while accidents at work, low income and poor housing are associated with class, so that manual workers are more likely to experience accidents at work, have low incomes and live in poor quality housing compared with the middle class, there is considerable variation in such material factors *within each class*. For example, there are very wide income differentials within each class as measured by the RG scale (Wilkinson, 1989). This means that a minority of people in the higher social classes will be more materially deprived than some of the better off people in the lowest social classes. In other words, class, as measured by the RG, is only an approximate measure of **material deprivation**.

Other research has tried to separate out measures of material deprivation from social class in order to see if it really is the material factors which play the largest part in explaining health inequalities. The study by Townsend, Phillimore and Beattie (1988) did exactly this by looking at the health of people living in 678 wards in the north of England. They constructed a health index and a deprivation index based on the following four factors: **unemployment** level, non-ownership of a car, non-ownership of a house, and over-crowding. They found that across the wards, variations in health tended to correspond closely with variations in material deprivation and certainly closer than with occupational class. It could be, then, that class inequalities in health are more specifically a result of material deprivation, which is linked to class but not adequately measured by class schemas such as that of the RG (Wilkinson, 1989).

(5) Social support

A fifth possible explanation for health inequalities is the amount and quality of social support people receive. The importance of social support in health and illness has been recognised ever since Durkheim's classic study *Suicide*, originally published in 1897, which linked suicide levels to the extent of social integration in a society. Durkheim (1952) argued that single, widowed and divorced people are more prone to suicide than married people because they have fewer social ties and are hence less integrated into the life of the community.

In a recent study of social support ties amongst a sample of 507 pregnant women in England, Oakley and Rajan (1991) found that:

'. . . our data conflict with the conventional picture of close-knit supportive social networks based on kin and neighbourhood among working class women'

(page 53)

They go on to say that they found that working class women were no more likely to be closely involved with their relatives than middle class women and that the latter had more support from both their friends and male partners than the former. Although this study is necessarily limited to a particular social group, it is suggestive in that the class differences in health may be due, in part, to differences in the levels of social support between the classes. The Whitehall civil servants study (Marmot, 1986) also found evidence of an association between social support and mortality rates and this is clearly an area for further research.

Class and the health service

The bulk of the evidence in the Black Report is concerned with those social conditions which could affect people's health and it has much less to say about the possible effects of the health service on inequalities in health. However, the Black Report does argue that the NHS can play a role in ameliorating the inequalities which it found, whilst it recognises that the root of the inequalities lies in social conditions which the NHS by itself cannot tackle. What do the Black Report and *The Health Divide* say about the manner in which the NHS is currently organised and used in relation to class inequalities?

As regards use of the health service, the evidence is not altogether consistent. On the one hand, the working class make more use of GP services than the middle class and they also seem to make more use of outpatient departments at hospitals. Against this must be balanced the evidence which suggests that, relative to their health needs, manual workers actually make less use of the health service than the middle class (Townsend, Davidson and Whitehead, 1988). It is difficult to be definitive about this because of the problems in measuring health need. The Black Report found that the use of preventive health services, such as family planning and maternity clinics, cancer screening facilities and dental services, did follow clear class gradients with the lower classes making less use of these services than the higher classes, although Blackburn (1991) argues that the evidence is ambiguous in relation to attendance at child health clinics.

Explanations for the differential patterns of use of the health service by the social classes tend to focus on either the users of the service or on the service itself. The former explanation argues that the working class makes less use of preventive health services than the middle class because the two classes hold different cultural beliefs about health with the former regarding health negatively, as the absence of disease, while the latter regard health as a sense of well-being. Blackburn (1991) has challenged this cultural explanation by arguing that mothers in deprived areas do not have negative attitudes towards preventive services, but that they may not attend child health clinics because of the difficulties of travelling to them or because of the manner in which the clinics are organised. This leads us on to consider the organisation of the health service.

Both the Black Report and *The Health Divide* suggest that the pattern of service use by the different social classes is linked to the accessibility of those services. This can be seen in two ways: firstly in terms of the physical location of the services and how easy it is for people to get to them, and secondly in terms of the times at which the services are available. So rather than saying that if women cannot get to a clinic then they are to blame themselves, the services should be designed in such a manner that working class people can gain access to them; this might mean, for example, having more clinics in a particular area, having 'outreach' services which take the service to the user, including mobile antenatal clinics, or that the services should be open at times when people can get to them, including evenings and weekends. Blackburn (1991) also notes the formality of child health clinics which may put some mothers off attending. The Black Report has a series of recommendations on how the health services could be planned so as to alleviate some of the health inequalities which the Report documented (Townsend, Davidson and Whitehead, 1988, Chapter 8). The later *Health Divide* does report that several health authorities and health workers themselves have set up initiatives to improve services, particularly for the most deprived sections of the population.

One of the most interesting developments in recent health care has been the links forged between health care workers and council house tenants over issues of health and housing conditions. In three recent cases, in the Easthall estate in Glasgow and the Divis and Moyard estates in West Belfast, partnerships have developed between the local residents and teams of health professionals, including district nurses, health visitors, doctors, social workers and health researchers (McShane, 1985; Lowry, 1990c; Seymour, 1991). The focus has been on how the residents perceive their own health in *public* not individual terms; in other words, their health is directly related to the social conditions in which they live instead of an individualistic approach which merely 'blames the victims' (see Chapter 3). This 'community development' approach to the health of the working class involves a change in the role of health professionals:

'The professional is required to become a partner with local people rather than the distant "expert" that he or she has been trained to become'
(McShane, 1985, page 81)

Health workers then respond to the health needs of local people who are active agents in the creation of their own health care, instead of being passive recipients of the knowledge of professional 'experts'. The other interesting aspect of this community development approach to health is the way in which health care is seen less as the preserve of a single professional group, either from the health or social services, but actually involves a multidisciplinary team sharing their particular knowledge and skills. In conclusion, such community development work provides one possible model for a more public health-oriented nursing practice.

Gender and health

Gender

As we saw earlier, gender refers to the socially constructed relations which appertain to the sexes. Feminists have drawn attention to the manner in which gender acts as a form of stratification which exists not only in the so-called private sphere of the family, but also in the public world of industry, commerce and politics. The nuclear family is structured along gender lines, with the vast bulk of domestic labour, in the form of housework and child care, being carried out by women (Leonard and Speakman, 1986). In the sphere of employment, it is clear that paid work is stratified by gender with women doing different kinds of jobs from men and frequently being employed in low paid and low status occupations (Beechey, 1986). Feminists have also looked at the way in which other areas of social life are structured by gender, for example, sexuality, violence and crime. This section will be concerned with the manner in which gender relations structure both health and health care.

Evidence on gender and health

The broad conclusion on gender differences in health is that, on average, women live longer than men, but that they suffer more ill health than men. In 1988 men in the United Kingdom could expect to live to 72.4 years of age compared with a life expectancy for women of 78.1 years (Central Statistical Office, 1991). Excess male mortality exists in every age group from birth upwards. Amongst young people, the main cause of the gap between the sexes is the greater incidence of accidents and violence. *The Health Divide* found evidence that the sex differences in mortality for certain causes of death may be narrowing in more recent years, for example in relation to deaths due to lung cancer in which the male/female ratio declined from 9:1 in 1960 to 4:1 in the late 1970s.

Does class make a difference to the mortality differences between men and women? As the Black Report showed, the death rates for men aged between 15 and 64 are nearly twice that of women in every occupational class, so the relationship between sex and mortality is not specific to any one class. However, there are class differences in the mortality rates of women as there are for men. Given the limitations of the RG class schema as applied to women, researchers have devised more complex measures of class for assessing inequality in women's mortality. One study utilised a composite measure of women's class position based upon their own employment, their **housing tenure** and whether they had use of a car, and this study found for women:

> 'High mortality is associated with working in manual occupations, living in rented housing, and with no car in the household. In contrast, low mortality is associated with non-manual occupations and living in owner-occupied housing with a car'
>
> (Pugh and Moser, 1990, page 110)

So far we have looked at mortality. What of the differences in morbidity rates? As we saw above, women on average have higher rates of both acute and chronic illness. However, *The Health Divide* found that age affects this relationship, with boys and young men more likely to have higher rates of serious illness than girls and young women, whilst women are more likely to record higher levels of illness than men from middle age. The differences in reported illness are particularly significant for mental illness, with men more likely to be admitted to mental hospital with a diagnosis of alcoholism or drug dependence, whilst women are more likely to be admitted with diagnoses of depression, senile dementia and neurotic disorders (Graham, 1984). We will explore mental illness and gender in greater detail in a later section. Arber (1990) found that morbidity is also affected by the social class

of the woman, with higher class women reporting less long-standing illness than lower class women. She found that marital status also seems to affect a woman's health, with married women having better health than single women, whilst divorced, separated and widowed women have the worst health of all.

Explanations of health inequalities

As with class inequalities, gender differences in mortality and morbidity have a variety of explanations offered for them. *The Health Divide* suggests that parallels can be drawn between the explanations for class inequalities and sex inequalities in health, with the four (artefact, natural selection, cultural/behavioural, materialist/structuralist) all being potential explanations for gender inequalities in health. We will examine each of these in turn and in addition we will consider a fifth possible explanation, that which focuses on patriarchy.

(1) The artefact explanation

The emphasis here is that the relationship between gender and health is actually an artificial one created by the measures of health used. Morbidity rates based upon use of the health services, for example number of visits to a GP, may not be an accurate indicator of women's own ill health, but may arise because women are more likely to visit the GP on behalf of others, notably children (Abbott and Wallace, 1990). *The Health Divide* suggests that it could be that women are more likely to report illness than men, either to the health service or to an interviewer asking questions about health. This could arise because women are more likely to adopt the **sick role** than men (Abbott and Wallace, 1990). This explanation suggests that the gender role into which women are socialised means that it is more acceptable for women to admit to illness and hence not to carry out their normal role obligations. Women's greater reporting of ill health may then reflect gender differences in the acceptability of going to seek medical assistance or in simply admitting to ill health, with men conforming to cultural **stereotypes** of masculinity and under-reporting ill health and women conforming to stereotypes of femininity and over-reporting ill health (for example, the stereotype of the 'neurotic female').

Other research has criticised this view and has suggested that consultation rates are deficient not because of conformity to cultural stereotypes, but rather the opposite; that, as summarised by Abbott and Wallace (1990), 'Women are more likely than men to suffer in silence' (page 100). This is because women have the major family responsibilities of domestic work, child care and care for other relatives, and therefore, 'tend to normalise and accommodate symptoms, stressing the importance of keeping going and coping with suffering' (Graham, 1987b, page 17). Here, then, we can see a more feminist interpretation of the gender differences in morbidity rates which suggests that such rates actually underestimate the extent of such differences. The oppressive nature of gender relations, in which women are expected to shoulder the burden of caring for other family members regardless of their own health, ensures that women's illnesses are less likely to reach the public attention of health service workers than are men's illnesses. Brown and Harris (1978) found a large **illness iceberg** of unreported depression amongst a sample of women in London which supports the view of women suffering in silence.

(2) Theories of natural selection

This explanation suggests that the differentials in health between the sexes are not a product of gender processes at all, but are simply the result of the biological differences between the sexes. There are clearly biological explanations for some of the differences in the *types* of illnesses experienced by men and women, most centring around the differences in the reproductive systems of the two sexes (see Chapter 17). The fact that only women can die in childbirth obviously accounts for differences in the cause of death. However, the incidence of illness and mortality associated with women's reproductive systems varies from society to society. The fact that, in all Western societies, women have a greater life expectancy than men should not blind us to the fact that in some Third World societies this position is reversed, largely due to the higher incidence of maternal mortality which is partly linked to levels of nutrition. Therefore, the so-called natural longevity of women is actually socially variable. In Britain, the fact that women live longer than men partly explains the higher rates of morbidity amongst women, since women are more likely than men to experience

those chronic illnesses which are associated with ageing (see Chapter 26).

Whilst it would be naive to discount the effect of biology on health differences between the sexes, it must also be remembered that feminists have argued that biological explanations for the health of women have frequently been used as a means of controlling women by the male-dominated medical profession. Many aspects of women's health, for example anorexia nervosa or premenstrual syndrome, are explained in biological terms, which may actually serve to ignore or play down the role of social factors in producing illness. On the other hand, feminists have also severely criticised the medical profession for what they regard as the **medicalisation** of women's lives, especially in relation to pregnancy and childbirth (Oakley, 1979, 1980). We will discuss medicalisation in greater detail when we go on to look at gender and mental illness. As this short discussion has suggested, it is not a simple matter to disentangle biological from social factors in relation to gender differences in health.

(3) Cultural/behavioural explanations

This approach, as we have seen in the section on class, focuses on those aspects of 'lifestyle' behaviour which are associated with health: cigarette smoking, excess alcohol consumption, poor diet and lack of exercise. Hart (1989) summarises the reason for the higher rates of male mortality, particularly after middle age:

> 'It is the greater male consumption of socially legitimate drugs, alcohol and cigarettes, which appears to underlie the vulnerability of men' [to an earlier death]
>
> (page 133)

As with men, the major causes of death amongst women are circulatory diseases (coronary heart disease and stroke) and cancers. The major 'risk factors' in relation to coronary heart disease are smoking, high blood cholesterol and high blood pressure (see Chapter 3). Cholesterol levels are linked to the amount of saturated fat in the diet, whilst blood pressure is influenced by several factors: 'Genetic factors, obesity, heavy drinking and a high dietary salt intake probably all play a part' (Smith and Jacobson, 1988, page 34). The two most important causes of cancer are smoking and diet, although breast cancer is linked to 'early men-arche (age at first period) and first pregnancy de-layed until after the age of 35' (Smith and Jacobson, 1988, page 52).

It would seem, then, that lifestyle factors such as smoking and diet play a significant role in re-lation to the major 'killer' diseases. The gender differences in mortality rates are probably simply a result of the fact that men tend to lead less healthy lifestyles than women.

Why might this be the case? From a feminist perspective, smoking cigarettes, drinking alcohol and taking exercise can only be understood in terms of the fact that leisure activities, along with most aspects of social relations, are structured along gender lines (Deem, 1990). Historically, most alcohol was drunk in public houses by working class men, or in gentlemen's clubs amongst the upper classes. Whilst in contemporary Britain women do go to the pub, they do so less than men and also, as Green et al. (1987) argue, they do so on male terms.

Smoking has also been historically linked to cul-tural notions of gender. During both world wars, cigarettes were a regular part of the ration of the soldier. Smoking was then symbolically associated with masculinity since it was the thing which 'brave' male soldiers did. Until the 1950s smoking amongst women was heavily stigmatised; it was seen as 'unfeminine'. The growth in female smoking in the 1950s and 1960s can be attributed to changes in gender relations, particularly to the increase in women in paid employment since the end of World War Two, giving women their own incomes and also changing women's sense of their own identities (Hart, 1989). The closing of the gap for male/female rates of death due to lung cancer mentioned earlier could be linked to the narrowing of the gap between male and female cigarette smoking as seen in Fig. 2.2.

Of course, this emphasis upon healthy lifestyles focuses solely on health as being a matter of con-sumption. From a Marxist or socialist feminist per-spective, issues of consumption cannot be divorced from issues of production. The increase in female smoking across the century can be linked to the enormous power of the tobacco industry in both advertising cigarettes and in attempting in various ways to blunt the effectiveness of anti-smoking campaigns (Jacobson, 1988). Similarly with food:

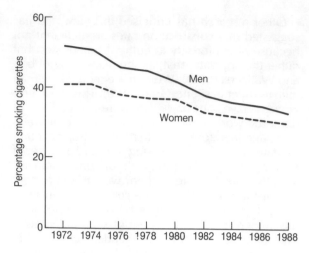

Fig. 2.2 *Cigarette smoking by sex, Great Britain 1972– 1988 (OPCS, 1990; page 84)*

'. . . when faced with the power of the food manufacturing industry and agribusiness to con-trol the food available in the shops, exhortations to individual women to make their families' diets more healthy without, at the same time, exhorting the food producers not to produce food which is dangerous to health, seem designed to divert attention from those who have the power to change things and increase women's burden of anxiety and guilt'

(Charles and Kerr, 1988, page 125)

So far we have concentrated on those aspects of health behaviour which are associated with some of the major degenerative and ultimately fatal dis-eases. However, to reduce health behaviour to smoking and drinking is in itself a very narrow and, one could even argue, a male-biased way of conceptualising the notion of a 'healthy lifestyle'. Graham (1985) has developed the idea that it is impossible to understand women's health ad-equately without also taking into account the fact that it is women who do most of the *health work* in society, both formally in terms of nursing care (the vast majority of nurses are women) and infor-mally in terms of the caring role which women adopt in the family by caring for children, hus-bands and other relatives. This health work reflects the sexual division of labour in the family with women carrying out most of the domestic tasks and men playing the 'breadwinner' role. The caring which women perform in the family can itself be detrimental to their health in terms of producing both physical and mental illness, largely due to stress, exhaustion and isolation (Lewis and Meredith, 1988). It is probably the demands of caring which partially account for the greater amount of morbidity amongst women.

Apart from the above, there is also mounting evidence that material factors should be taken into consideration when examining the relation between health and gender.

(4) Materialist/structuralist explanations

Here the emphasis is on material inequalities between men and women. Despite the 1970 Equal Pay Act, women who were full-time employees in 1990 on average earned only 77% of the hourly average earnings of male full-timers (Equal Opportunities Commission, 1991). Women are also far more likely than men to be in part-time employment, and in relation to poverty:

'One aspect of these inequalities [between women and men] is that women are at far greater risk of poverty than men; at any given stage in their lives, women are far more likely than men to be poor and their experience of poverty is also likely to be far more acute'

(Millar and Glendinning, 1989, page 363)

Women represent the vast majority of both the elderly and lone parents living on **income support**. However, it is not only that women are more represented amongst those groups who are prone to poverty. Glendinning and Millar (1991) point out how even within those households which are nominally above the poverty line, resources are not equitably distributed within the family. In low income households, men are likely to retain some money for their own personal use whereas the same is not true of women. Not only are women likely to have less command over household income than men, but they are likely to be responsible for the household expenses to a greater extent than men in terms of the day-to-day running of the household. In low income households it is women who are most likely to do without. Even in higher income households which possess large consumer durable items such as cars, these are more likely to be used by men than women (Beurat, 1991). There is not space here to go into the reasons for the gendering of poverty except to say that social policies in terms of benefits and child care pro-

vision, as well as the disadvantaged position of women in the labour market, are important factors (see Glendinning and Millar, 1987).

How does the material deprivation experienced by women affect their health? It affects it directly in terms of the fact that women on low incomes cut down on the amount and the quality of food (Charles and Kerr, 1988; Graham, 1990) which they consume and this has obvious health effects. It also means that women are less likely to make use of preventive health measures, such as screening services or antenatal classes, because they are difficult to get to without access to a car (Beurat, 1991). Graham's work (1990) on mothers caring for children on a low income demonstrates the manner in which women develop coping strategies which include such health-damaging behaviour as smoking themselves and giving sweets and crisps to their children. As Graham argues, it makes little sense to focus on women's health behaviour in purely individualistic terms since this fails to take into account the *health work* that women do for their families as a whole, often in situations of poverty. It is likely that the combined effects of caring for others on a low income accounts for a large proportion of the greater levels of morbidity experienced by women as opposed to men. Payne (1991) also points out that women tend to spend more time at home than men, both in terms of carrying out domestic labour and for leisure time, and so the ill health effects of poor quality housing are likely to affect women more than men.

(5) Patriarchy

Patriarchy is 'the generalized power of men over women' (Ramazanoglu, 1989, page 15). For radical feminists, the gender relations and the material inequalities discussed above are manifestations of patriarchal relations between women and men. However, whilst feminists recognise that women are subordinated to men in material ways, for example due to their occupying low paid and low status jobs, and also in ideological ways, for example the idea that 'a woman's place is in the home', they also argue that this is not all there is to patriarchy. This system of oppression is also based upon more overt forms of social control, chiefly those of violence against women by men. The definition of violence is not clear cut, but feminists have argued that it encompasses a broad range of behaviour including the following: rape, domestic battering, incest, sexual harassment and pornography (Edwards, 1987).

One important aspect of male violence is that the threat of violence can be as intimidating as the actual physical aggression itself. This threat can clearly have profound psychological and even physical effects on women's health. The peculiar feature of violence against women which feminists have pointed to is that, unlike the victims of other kinds of violence, female victims are somehow held to blame for the damage caused to themselves! As Orr (1988) says, nurses should not collude in this process of stigmatisation, but should instead attempt to give greater recognition to the problem of violence against women:

'Battering should be part of the differential diagnosis that nurses make, for the woman may be reluctant to state the problem overtly because of the stigma involved. Women who are victims of any form of male violence may be reluctant to be nursed by male nurses or to be in a mixed ward, but this is one area of patient choice which is not addressed'

(Orr, 1988, page 129)

Gender and mental health

Most of the above discussion on gender and health focuses on the structural determinants of ill health as they differentially affect women and men. Thus we saw how, for example, gender roles and material deprivation could be used to explain the differences in mortality and morbidity rates between the sexes. As regards mental health, several studies have suggested that women's higher susceptibility to neurotic mental illness, such as depression, occurs as a result of the more stressful lives which women lead. This stress can then be explained in terms of the burdens of caring for others, lack of support and material disadvantage. Brown and Harris's (1978) study of women in London (see Chapter 17) demonstrates that such a combination of factors explains the women's chances of becoming depressed. This approach argues that women's greater prevalence of depression is a social product. Whilst Brown and Harris do not adopt a feminist perspective and nor do they compare women and men, their study can be used by feminists as support for the argument that aspects of gender relations, along with class position,

oppress women and make them ill. Miles (1988) found that one important factor as to why women were more likely to develop neurosis than men was that married women receive far less emotional support from their husbands than the latter receive from their wives.

However, as Busfield (1989) argues, this is not the only way in which women's mental illness can be analysed. An alternative approach within feminism looks upon mental illness as a social construct; this approach turns its attention to the definitions of mental health and illness used by GPs and psychiatrists and at how the practice of psychiatry is carried out. In so doing, it draws upon ideas from labelling theory and symbolic interactionism. Labelling theory regards mental illness as a form of 'deviant' or rule-breaking behaviour. In this case, feminists argue that psychiatry itself operates with a sexist conception of mental health whereby women's behaviour is more likely to be considered deviant than that of men and is more likely to be defined as 'neurotic'.

Not only are women more likely to be labelled as 'mentally ill', but they are also more likely to be given psychotropic drugs in comparison with men. This is because psychiatrists are concerned to 'help' women play their domestic roles which are defined as 'normal' for women. Instead of regarding women's problems as arising out of the oppression which they experience in performing the domestic role, psychiatry acts so as to coerce women into accepting that role. As Penfold and Walker (1984) say, the paradox is that the psychiatry which women turn to for help acts in such a manner as to oppress them further. This feminist critique of psychiatry draws attention to the manner in which the medical profession can 'medicalise' women's problems with living and in so doing obscure the social origins of such problems by labelling the problems as 'illnesses' which must be treated with drugs. Pollock and West (1987) argue that a feminist approach to therapy dovetails with the emphasis upon **holistic care** in nursing, in that women are not just treated as bundles of symptoms but as people whose health needs can only be understood in a social context which includes the relation between the health worker and the client.

Gender and the health services

The above section on mental health is only part of

a substantial feminist critique of the structure and practices of the health care system as a whole in relation to women's health. This critique (adapted from Orr, 1988, and Foster, 1991) focuses on several areas:

(1) The medicalisation of women's health.
(2) The manner in which the medical profession exercises patriarchal control over its female patients and expects them to conform to its demands in a passive fashion.
(3) The lack of a holistic approach to health in which emotional and social aspects of women's lives are treated seriously.
(4) The manner in which the health care system itself reflects the sexual division of labour, with a largely female nursing workforce subordinate to a largely male medical profession.

Foster (1989) sets out several principles which should underpin a feminist model of health care delivery and Orr (1988) uses feminist ideas to suggest ways in which nurses can help to shape health care policies for women. She argues that nurses need to allow women to determine their own health needs in a manner which takes full account of their social circumstances. As Twomey (1987) suggests, this approach involves the sharing of knowledge with clients rather than an emphasis on the nurse being the health care 'expert'. In many ways, **well women clinics** are models of a feminist health care system. However, as Foster (1989, 1991) argues, the danger is that well women clinics are marginalised within the health care system as a whole and she suggests that feminist health care workers need to begin to tackle the much wider challenge posed by mainstream health services. Part of this challenge lies within nursing itself, given the fact that men form only 10% of the nursing workforce but they hold a much greater proportion of the senior posts. Changes in working practices, improved child care facilities and men taking on more child care responsibilities are necessary if equal opportunities for women in nursing are to become a reality (Hunt, 1991).

Ethnicity, racism and health

Ethnicity and racism

The idea that there are separate races based upon physical appearances is actually one which is highly dubious on both biological and sociological grounds. That is why sociologists tend to use the terms ethnicity and racism in preference to 'race'. *Ethnicity* refers to a group with a common cultural identity and sense of a shared heritage. An ethnic minority group refers to an ethnic group which constitutes a minority in a particular society: West Indians, Africans, Indians, Pakistanis, Bangladeshis, Chinese, Vietnamese, Arabs, Turkish Cypriots, Greek Cypriots, Irish, etc., all constitute minority groups within British society. Donovan (1984) explains the term *black people* thus:

> 'The term "black people" . . . is a political term, emphasizing unity and solidarity among minority groups. The term does not seek to exclude any minority ethnic groups, but in general it tends to refer to people of Asian or Afro-Caribbean descent who share the common experience of differentiation or **racial discrimination** in Britain because of the colour of their skin'
>
> (page 663)

In this section, we will be concentrating our attention on black people as defined by Donovan above, although we will be making occasional reference to other ethnic minority groups apart from Afro-Caribbeans and Asians.

As regards *racism*, it is usually divided into two types: *personal racism* refers to the way in which certain individuals are prejudiced against certain social groups on the basis of some physical characteristic, often, although not exclusively, skin colour; *institutional racism*, on the other hand, refers to the way in which one 'racial group' has a position of power over another. Hence in Britain today, institutional racism inheres in the fact that in all the major institutions of society, including government, the legal system, industry and commerce, education and the health service, white people are in dominant positions and black people are in subordinate positions. We will discuss the issue of racism in the health service later in this section. It is worth noting that this concept of institutional racism has been challenged by Marxist writers, such as Miles (1989), who argue that racism can only be adequately discussed in relation to the class structure. The relative importance of class and racism in understanding the social position of black people in Britain is a topic of much debate in sociology, with Marxists paying more attention to class relations and Weberians laying more emphasis on racism and ethnicity (Rex and Mason, 1986). However, most sociologists would agree that the place of the ethnic minority groups in Britain can only fully be understood historically in relation to the processes of slavery, *colonialism* and immigration (Fryer, 1984).

In modern British society, people from the Asian and Afro-Caribbean ethnic minorities are significantly socially disadvantaged in terms of employment and housing, and at least some of this is due to racial discrimination by the white majority (Brown, 1985).

Evidence on ethnicity, racism and health

Given the clear picture of social disadvantage faced by black people in Britain with evidence going back to the 1960s on employment and housing (Daniel, 1968; Rex and Moore, 1967), it is surprising that the study of ethnicity and health has had relatively little attention until recently: the Black Report devotes less than two pages to the topic! However, the 1980s witnessed a burgeoning of research in this field although, as Sheldon and Parker (1991) indicate, this work is of variable sociological quality.

Both the Black Report and *The Health Divide* concentrated their attention on studies which compared the health of immigrants with that of people born in England and Wales. A recent study by Balarajan (1991) found that deaths due to ischaemic heart disease were much higher in both men and women born in the Indian subcontinent compared with people born in England and Wales, whereas the rates for both men and women born in the Caribbean were much lower than those for the indigenous population. However, Caribbean-born men and women had the highest mortality from cerebrovascular disease. But there are problems in using such studies to assess the health of ethnic minorities, as we discuss below.

There is considerable evidence regarding the health of ethnic minorities in relation to specific health conditions. This evidence usually comes from the medical profession and does not necessarily reflect the complete health picture of the minority groups. As Donovan (1984) points out, there are five main areas of research:

(1) Rickets: Asians are more likely to develop rickets than the rest of the population.
(2) Tuberculosis: higher in all immigrant groups compared with the indigenous population.
(3) Inherited diseases: **sickle cell anaemia** is an inherited disease which affects Afro-Caribbeans, whilst **thalassaemia** affects a range of ethnic minority groups.
(4) Mental health: Asian people are less likely to suffer from any form of mental illness than white people, whilst Afro-Caribbeans experience less depression but have higher rates of schizophrenia compared with the rest of the population (we will return to the issue of mental illness in a later section).
(5) Family (usually children's) health: the **infant mortality rate** is higher amongst Asians and Asian babies have lower birth weights in comparison with white babies, whilst rates of childhood accidents are greater in Afro-Caribbean families.

These do not exhaust the health issues in relation to race and ethnicity, but they are topics which have generated a great deal of heated debate in the sociological and medical literature. Let us now look at the explanations which have been put forward for these health inequalities and differences.

Explanations of health inequalities

As with the previous two sections we will attempt to use the explanatory framework devised in the Black Report and we will also include a fifth possible explanation, that of racism.

(1) The artefact explanation

As Sheldon and Parker (1991) argue, there are considerable problems regarding the categories of ethnic group which researchers have used. Studies based upon comparing immigrants with people born in Britain are not really measuring the impact of ethnicity or racism on health at all, since they exclude those ethnic minority members born in this country and they include, in their immigrant category, white people emigrating from countries such as India. In Balarajan's (1991) paper quoted above, he groups immigrants born in India, Pakistan, Bangladesh and Sri Lanka together in an 'Indian subcontinent' category; given the distinctive cultural and other social differences between the migrants from these different countries, it would seem that this approach hides as much as it reveals. The question of ethnic categorisation is an extremely complex one and, moreover, it has considerable political implications. Some sociologists have expressed profound doubts about the validity of the term 'ethnicity' itself as granting a spurious homogeneity and fixity to cultural patterns which in reality are far more variable and fluid (Phoenix, 1988a; Westwood and Bhachu, 1988; Pearson, 1989; Sheldon and Parker, 1991). We will deal with this issue in more detail when we turn to look at the debate over the relative importance of culture and racism in relation to black people's use of the health services.

(2) Theories of natural selection

To say that there is a biological basis to ethnic groups falls back on the now discredited biological theories of race, as Sheldon and Parker (1991) argue. Nevertheless, there does seem to be a genetic basis to the two inherited diseases mentioned above; that is, sickle cell anaemia and thalassaemia. As Donovan (1984) says, the Sickle Cell Society has called for more training of health workers and for information on the subject to be more widely available.

(3) Cultural/behavioural explanations

Much of the work on the health of ethnic minorities has focused on the cultural differences between the minorities and the white majority. Probably the most famous example of this is the higher rates of rickets found amongst the Asian minorities and the consequent Stop Rickets Campaign launched in 1982. Most researchers agree that vitamin D deficiency is the major factor leading to rickets and the causes of this are said to be lack of sunshine and/or dietary deficiencies. As far as Asians in Britain are concerned, most attention was placed on dietary factors, notably the use of foods other than fortified margarine, as well as the eating of foods high in phytic acid including chappatis (Donovan, 1984; Pacy, 1989). Some researchers offered the following solution to what they saw as the problem:

'The long term answer to Asian rickets probably lies in health education and a change towards the Western diet and life-style'
(Goel et al., quoted in Donovan, 1984, page 664)

In effect, Asian culture itself is seen as a 'problem' which needs to be changed! Such an approach is clearly culturally elitist and it neglects the evidence that the Western diet is thought to be one factor behind circulatory diseases. There is a variety of other approaches to the phenomenon of rickets amongst Asians, including the provision of vitamin D supplements (Pacy, 1989; Ganatra, 1989) or more simply the fortification of chappati flour in the same way that margarine itself was fortified (Donovan, 1984).

Apart from rickets, one other health issue affecting the Asian minorities which has also led to a major health promotion campaign is that of a high **perinatal mortality rate** amongst Asian babies. The DHSS and the Save the Children Fund sponsored the Asian Mother and Baby Campaign which began in 1984 and was designed to reduce the perinatal mortality rate by helping pregnant Asian women to make more use of antenatal and maternity services. This campaign raises a number of important issues in relation to the provision of health services for ethnic minority groups and for an account of these, see Rocheron (1988). Certainly some commentators regard this campaign as being an improvement on the Stop Rickets Campaign since it is concerned with providing more responsive health services rather than simply with delivering health educational messages (Ahmad, 1989).

As with the debate over the relative importance of cultural and material factors in the explanation of class health inequalities, a parallel debate exists in relation to ethnicity and health. Several writers in this field (Donovan, 1984; Ahmad, 1989; Pearson, 1989; Sheldon and Parker, 1991) point out that cultural explanations of ethnic minority ill health are in effect 'victim-blaming' (see Chapter 3) in that they focus on the lifestyles of the minorities and neglect the material deprivation and racial discrimination suffered by Asians and Afro-Caribbeans in Britain. Let us turn first to the materialist explanations.

(4) Materialist/structuralist explanations

Despite the evidence of a growing black middle class, notably amongst the Indian and East African

Asian ethnic minorities (Robinson, 1988), it is still true to say that the ethnic minorities, on average, are significantly materially disadvantaged relative to the white population. They are more likely to live in the decaying inner city areas with their problems of multiple deprivation. Probably most notable has been the very high rates of unemployment amongst black people, with unemployment between 1987 and 1989 amongst the Pakistani and Bangladeshi ethnic groups, for example, being at over twice the rate for white people with equivalent educational qualifications (Central Statistical Office, 1991). It is likely that some of this difference is due to discriminatory practices by employers. Also noteworthy is the fact that many black people live in poor, often overcrowded housing (Brown, 1985). Given these factors, many researchers have argued that material deprivation is at the heart of the health issues faced by the ethnic minorities. Donovan (1984) suggests that of the five health issues focused upon by medical researchers, including TB, rickets, high infant mortality, mental illness and inherited diseases, only the last is unconnected to material deprivation. Other research in the deprived Tower Hamlets borough of east London confirms the effects of housing dampness on the general health of Bengalis living in the area (Hyndman, 1990).

(5) Racism

Nevertheless, many writers would add that whilst black people in inner city areas share the same material disadvantages as the poor white working class, they are subject to another form of social disadvantage, namely racism, which can have direct and indirect effects on health. The most obvious form of racism which can affect health is that of racial harassment which can include physical assaults, attacks on property, graffiti, arson, verbal abuse, racist phone calls, etc. It has been estimated that one in four Asians living in the east London borough of Newham has been the victim of a racial attack, whilst there were 960 racist attacks reported to the police across London as a whole in 1987 (Tompson, 1988). Such attacks, as Tompson illustrates, often leave tremendous physical and mental scarring. However, it is not just the actual physical attacks themselves but also the anxiety and fear generated by harassment. A study in Leeds by the Independent Commission of Enquiry into Racial Harassment (1987) found that

many of the Asians they spoke to were afraid to go out and that their children needed to be escorted because of fear of harassment, whilst 45% of the sample had changed the way they lived in some way because of potential harassment. Similarly, Fenton (1986) found that fear of racial attack was common amongst the Asians he studied in Bristol, as well as fear of repatriation. Given that nursing is moving towards a more positive holistic view of health in which the health service user is located within their social environment, it is important that nurses are aware of some of the uglier sides of British society: consider the effect on a person's sense of well-being of regularly having faeces pushed through his or her letterbox, as happens to some Asian people in certain inner city areas.

The above only provides a brief outline of the ways in which racial harassment can affect health. This is only the most graphic example of racism in society. As we mentioned at the start of this section on race and health, institutionalised racism permeates all the major institutions of society and included amongst these is the NHS. Pearson (1989) illustrates this in the following extract:

> 'While a walk around many hospitals would reveal a reasonable number of ethnic minority staff, a disproportionate number are in inferior positions. The majority are in low paid, ancillary and manual jobs, working night shifts and at weekends, in the less qualified echelons of nursing or in "twilight" areas such as geriatrics and psychiatry in the less prestigious non-teaching hospitals'
>
> (page 77)

Racism is documented in both nursing (Pearson, 1986a; Chudley and Smith, 1989; Carlisle, 1990; Trevelyan, 1990) and medicine (McKeigue et al., 1990). It could be argued, as Pearson (1986a) and Chevannes (1990) do, that tackling the issue of racial discrimination in the NHS and in nursing would seem to be an important part of making the health service more responsive to the health needs of Britain's black population.

Ethnicity, racism and mental health

One of the areas of health which has generated considerable research in relation to the ethnic minorities has been that of mental health. The available evidence suggests that, on the whole, Asian people have less reported mental illness than the rest of the population (Ineichen, 1990), whilst Afro-Caribbeans have less depression but more psychosis, especially schizophrenia, and the ethnic group with the highest rate of mental hospital admissions is the Irish (Littlewood and Lipsedge, 1989). In this section I will be concentrating on the question of Afro-Caribbeans and schizophrenia since it highlights a number of sociological issues in relation to mental health.

Whilst it is well established in the psychiatric literature that migrants have higher rates of mental illness than the indigenous populations, suggesting that the stress of migration is implicated, what has recently emerged is that second generation Afro-Caribbeans in Britain have higher rates of psychotic illness than their parents (Cope, 1989). Clearly this latter finding cannot be explained with reference to the strains of migration. It could be that socio-economic disadvantages, including racial discrimination, contribute towards the high rates of psychosis amongst second generation Afro-Caribbeans; this is an area which requires further research (Cope, 1989). Another possibility is in relation to labelling theory. This theory directs our attention to the fact that interpreting other people's behaviour is inherently a social process and that judgements about 'normal' and 'abnormal' behaviour imply socially created standards: what is considered 'normal' in one group or society may be considered 'bad' or even 'mad' in another. The problem is, how can mainly white male psychiatrists correctly understand the behaviour of someone from an ethnic minority group which has a different culture? Psychiatric diagnosis involves value judgements in relation to socially constructed standards of acceptable behaviour and there is evidence that white psychiatrists are more likely to apply the label 'schizophrenic' to Afro-Caribbeans (Knowles, 1991). Littlewood and Lipsedge (1989) give several illustrations of the way in which religious beliefs amongst Afro-Caribbeans in Britain can be misunderstood by psychiatrists if they operate within a strictly **medical model** of mental illness. The danger is that psychiatry feeds off and helps to maintain social stereotypes, particularly that of the 'alien' for Afro-Caribbeans:

> 'Whatever the empirical justification, the frequent diagnosis in black patients of schizophrenia (bizarre, irrational, outside) and the infrequent diagnosis of depression (acceptable, understandable, inside) validates the stereotypes'
>
> (Littlewood and Lipsedge, 1989, page 251)

However, other writers have challenged this emphasis on cultural differences and misunderstandings, arguing that it does not sufficiently recognise the importance of power between psychiatrist and patient and crucially the issue of racism (Black Health Workers and Patients Group, 1983; Knowles, 1991). The relative importance of culture and racism is discussed in the next section.

Ethnicity, racism and the health services

There are essentially two approaches to the issue of ethnicity, racism and the health services. The first is that of **multiculturalism** which argues that the main problem in relation to ethnic minorities and the health services is a lack of effective communication arising out of cultural differences between minority patients and the health service which reflects the majority 'white' culture. In particular, attention is drawn to language differences, dietary customs and religious practices. The multicultural approach suggests that health service workers need to familiarise themselves with the culture of the ethnic minorities in order that any communication barriers which prevent effective health care are removed. This involves health workers learning about the dietary customs and religious practices of the ethnic minorities, as well as instituting measures to overcome language barriers, such as the use of interpreters for non-English speaking patients and also link workers to improve take-up rates for preventive services. This multicultural approach focuses on the concept of *ethnicity* and in different ways is illustrated in the Stop Rickets Campaign and the Asian Mother and Baby Campaign mentioned above. There are parallels between this multicultural approach to health care and the concept of *transcultural nursing* developed by Leininger in the USA (for a summary and critique of transcultural nursing, see Stokes, 1991). In British nursing, multiculturalism has been prominent in the professional literature (Phillips, 1985; Dobson, 1988; Perry, 1988; Sen, 1989).

However, this multicultural approach has come in for a good deal of criticism from those sociologists and health workers who emphasise **anti-racism**. These writers do not argue that the multicultural approach is of no value whatsoever (although see Black Health Workers and Patients Group, 1983), but that it is limited. In particular, the multicultural approach assumes that there is an equality of power between the various ethnic groups, whereas antiracists argue that the white majority exercises power over the black minority through institutionalised racism and that it is the latter which needs tackling in terms of black people gaining more control and power within the NHS, both as the *users* of health services and as *employees* of the NHS. Thus Rocheron (1988) argues that the Asian Mother and Baby Campaign, by focusing on cultural factors, could have helped to alleviate personal racism, that is individuals' prejudices towards black people; however, it did not engage with institutionalised racism and issues of inequality and power (see McNaught, 1988, and Hugman, 1991, in relation to racism in the NHS).

One further potential problem with the multicultural approach to health care is that there is a danger that it provides a checklist of 'cultural differences' which are really no more than stereotypes. Examples of such stereotypes are that Asians in Britain all live in close-knit extended families, which Westwood and Bhachu (1988) show to be erroneous, or that Afro-Caribbean families are all headed by a single mother, again untrue (Phoenix, 1988b). Such stereotypes gloss over class, religious and regional variations within the black community in Britain. This is not to say that learning about cultural variation is not important for nurses, but that, as Henley (1986) points out:

'It is not a question of learning sets of inflexible facts or stereotypes about different groups, but rather of extending our sensitivity and awareness' (page 18)

Some researchers, for example Littlewood and Lipsedge (1989), argue that the 'either culture or racism' debate is a sterile one and that both ethnicity and racism need to be incorporated into an analysis of the health and health care of black people. This recognition of the importance of both cultural factors and the systematic disadvantages experienced by black people, as both users and employees of the NHS, is reflected in recent work in relation to nursing (Pearson, 1986a, 1986b, 1986c; Henley, 1986; Chevannes, 1990).

Poverty and health

Poverty

Having explored the relationship between health and class in an earlier section, one would have thought that it was unnecessary to include a separate section on poverty. However, class, as defined by the Registrar General and also by Weberian sociologists, is essentially assessed in terms of people's occupation and hence their participation in the labour market. This excludes those people without an occupation, including elderly people, the unemployed and many lone parent families and we will be investigating the health circumstances of these groups, along with the homeless, in this section.

There are usually two ways in which poverty is defined. The first is that of *absolute* poverty in which people are classified as poor if they have insufficient resources to acquire the basic essentials for a healthy life; that is, food, clothing and shelter. The poverty line, then, is the point at which people's resources fall below a level adequate to maintain their physical efficiency. The absolute definition of poverty is meant to be cross-cultural and trans-historical, but problems of making comparisons over time have led most poverty researchers to use a second definition of poverty, that is, a *relative* one. According to this definition, standards of poverty are relative to the general standards of living which exist in a society at a particular point in time. As those general living standards change historically, so should our conceptions of poverty. Relative poverty involves lacking the resources to participate fully in the life of the society. Peter Townsend has been a life-long champion of the relative approach to poverty and he defines it in the following terms:

'Individuals, families and groups in the population can be said to be in poverty when they lack the resources to obtain the type of diets, participate in the activities and have the living conditions and amenities which are customary, or at least widely encouraged or approved, in the societies to which they belong. Their resources are so seriously below those commanded by the average individual or family that they are, in effect, excluded from ordinary living patterns, customs and activities.'

(Townsend, 1979, page 31)

Having defined poverty, it is then necessary to say something about the extent of poverty in Britain. Clearly the extent of poverty which a researcher finds is linked to the definition used, with more absolute measures likely to find fewer poor people than more relative measures. In Britain there is not an 'official' poverty line, but one frequently used measure is the numbers of people receiving income support (supplementary benefit prior to April 1988). The latest available figures relate to the period when supplementary benefit was in use, and they show that 10.2 million people had incomes at or below this level in 1987, or 19% of the population of Britain; this is an increase from 6.07 million (12%) in 1979 (quoted in Blackburn, 1991). There is considerable dispute over the status of the income support/supplementary benefit level as to whether it is an accurate indicator of poverty, with right wing commentators arguing that people on this benefit are not poor, whereas most poverty researchers argue that the benefit income is considerably below the level at which deprivation occurs (Townsend, 1989; Blackburn, 1991). As a result, some poverty researchers use the figure of 140% of the income support/supplementary benefit level as being an indication of poverty.

The following groups of people are most likely to be in poverty today:

(1) Elderly people
(2) The unemployed
(3) Lone parent families
(4) Chronically sick and disabled people
(5) Workers in low paid occupations.

Of course, not everyone in these groups can be said to be in poverty. The Queen Mother in her nineties is clearly elderly, but by no stretch of the imagination could she be said to be poor! Poverty, like illness, does not strike randomly and it seems to be that the loss of an occupation through unemployment, retirement, disability or sickness is most likely to lead to poverty if the occupation lost was a manual one. In this sense class and poverty are linked (Townsend, 1979). As we have already seen, gender and poverty are also connected, whilst black people are more likely to be poor than white people due to racism in the labour market and in the operations of the welfare state (Cook and Watt, 1987).

Let us now turn to some of the groups most likely to experience poverty.

Elderly people and health

Readers also need to refer to Chapter 26 on care of the elderly person. Sociological work on old age suggests that several assumptions about elderly people need to be challenged. First of all is that they constitute a homogeneous group; in fact, there is considerable variation between elderly people in terms of class, income, gender, ethnicity, lifestyles, etc. Secondly, there is a common assumption that elderly people are a 'problem', usually because they are seen as being more likely to be disabled, sick or isolated. Sociologists point out that levels of chronic conditions are little greater between the ages of 65 and 74 compared with 55 to 64 and only rise rapidly after the age of 75 or even 80 (Fennell *et al.*, 1988); similarly, social isolation affects only a minority of elderly people, with just 2% in 1986 saying they never made or received visits from relatives or friends (OPCS, 1989). Freer (1988) challenges the negative stereotypes about old age:

'The majority of older people are well and live reasonably happy lives . . . and there is no evidence of a significant decline in happiness or life satisfaction with age'

(page 4)

Nevertheless, despite the fact that many old people in Britain today are far better off in material terms than their predecessors, it is still true to say that old age is often a time of poverty, especially for women and working class men, both of whom are less likely to have an occupational pension scheme. Walker (1990) argues that poverty in old age is linked to a person's economic status prior to retirement and also to the low level of state benefits. In 1985, nearly a third of elderly people were living on or below the poverty line, using the supplementary benefit level, compared with one-tenth of those under pension age (DHSS figures quoted by Walker, 1990). Not only are elderly people at greater risk of poverty, but their experience of poverty is likely to be an enduring one (Walker, 1990).

What of the health of elderly people? Recent research shows that there are significant class, gender and age differences in the mortality and morbidity rates for those aged over 65:

'Consistently, those elderly from the professional and managerial classes experience better health than their contemporaries from the manual occupational groups'

(Victor, 1991, page 33)

It could be that this finding reflects the fact that elderly working class people have experienced a lifetime of disadvantage, or that it is precisely these people who, in old age, are most likely to live in a state of poverty. Elderly people who are poor are likely to live in the worst housing and are least likely to have access to a car or household amenities such as a telephone. As Taylor (1988) demonstrates, they are also likely to have worse health than old people as a whole.

Unemployment and health

Mass unemployment returned to Britain during the 1980s, reaching a peak of 3.12 million officially unemployed in 1986 (Central Statistical Office, 1991), a condition which most people thought had disappeared for good since the Depression of the 1930s. Whilst unemployment declined during the late 1980s, it increased again to 2.47 million in October 1991 (Department of Employment, 1991) and is likely to go even higher as a result of the recession in the early 1990s. There is doubt from many commentators on the veracity of the official unemployment figures, with the Unemployment Unit (1989) suggesting that these figures actually underestimate the true amount by several hundred thousands.

What impact does unemployment have upon health? A recent article in the *British Medical Journal* presented a stark claim:

'The evidence that unemployment kills – particularly the middle aged – now verges on the irrefutable'

(Smith, 1991, page 606)

Surveys have shown that there is a higher incidence of mortality and morbidity amongst those who are unemployed compared with similar people who are in employment. However, this statistical relationship does not in itself prove that unemployment is the *cause* of ill health. It could be that the direction of causality is the other way around, so that it is not that unemployment causes ill health but that those who are sick are the ones who are most likely to become unemployed. Hence the poor health of unemployed people could be a cause not a consequence of unemployment (Hakim, 1982). Also, the health of some employees who work in particularly dangerous jobs could actually improve with a short spell of unemployment!

Some of the problems of the direction of causality can be ameliorated using what is called a longitudinal study in which a sample of those who are unemployed have their health re-assessed over a period of time. Using the OPCS Longitudinal Study, Moser et al. (1986) followed up men seeking work at the time of the 1971 census over a ten year period to 1981. They found a third higher mortality rate for these men compared with all men aged between 15 and 64. Part of this excess mortality is explained by the fact that people who are unemployed are more likely to be in classes IV and V, who as we have seen already have a higher mortality rate. Nevertheless, even when class is taken into account in the analysis, there is still an excess of between 20 and 30% deaths amongst these unemployed men. In a more recent study using the follow-up sample to the 1981 census, Moser et al. (1987) found a higher mortality rate in the period 1981–83 for men unemployed at the time of the 1981 census.

Whilst there is evidence of the effects of unemployment on mortality and morbidity, there is some debate as to the exact processes which have the most effect. Hakim (1982) suggests that two processes could be at work. One is the impact of economic instability and financial insecurity upon levels of stress, and the study by Mattiason et al. (1990) on the impact of the threat of unemployment on health would lend support to this argument. Also, Moser et al. (1986) found that deaths due to suicide and lung cancer were much higher amongst the unemployed and both of these are linked to stress and stress-related activity. The second process is the poverty associated with unemployment, particularly long-term unemployment. In 1988–1989 half the unemployed families had net incomes below £50 per week compared with 1 in 8 of the population as a whole (Atkinson, 1989). Such levels of income are likely to affect the quality of food consumed, as we have seen in previous sections.

What of the impact of unemployment on psychological well-being? Hakim (1982) argues that, 'The severity of the psychological consequences of job loss is determined by the degree of attachment to paid employment and/or occupation as a central focus of personal identity' (page 449). Thus the distress associated with unemployment is greatest amongst the middle-aged (45–54) and lowest amongst those under 25 and those over 55 who are approaching retirement. A minority of those who are unemployed may suffer from depression.

Unemployed people are more likely to make use of health services, including general practitioners (Yuen and Balarajan, 1989), and this is something which health workers need to take into account when planning services.

Lone parent families and health

One of the most striking demographic trends over the past 20 years in Britain and throughout the Western world has been the growth in the number of married couples who divorce. In England and Wales, the number of divorces per year stood at 25,000 in 1961, 74,000 in 1971 and reached 151,000 in 1989 (Central Statistical Office, 1991). Haskey (1989) estimated on the basis of the 1987 divorce rate that almost four out of ten couples would eventually divorce. One of the consequences of the increase in divorce has been the growth of lone parent families. They doubled in number from 570,000 in 1971 (Lewis, 1989) to nearly 1.1 million in 1988 (Haskey, 1991), a figure which represents 16% of the total families with dependent children (OPCS, 1990). Approximately nine out of ten lone parent families are headed by women.

Lone parent families are far more likely to be in poverty than two parent families. Using 140% of the supplementary benefit level as the measure of poverty, Millar and Glendinning (1987) found 61% of lone parent families headed by women to be in poverty in 1983, compared with 43% of lone fathers and 20% of couples with children. The greater extent of poverty amongst lone parent mothers compared with fathers is largely explicable in terms of the fact that lone fathers are more likely to be in full-time employment. The poverty of lone parents, and particularly mothers, cannot be separated from the employment position of women generally and aspects of social policy such as child care policy (Lewis, 1989).

Popay and Jones (1990), using the General Household Survey, found that lone parents were in poorer health on all measures than parents living in couples. However there are gender differences within lone parents, with mothers likely to have poorer health than fathers on all measures except that of long-standing illness. Lone fathers have less child care responsibility than lone mothers; this is because the children of fathers tend to be older on average and they are more likely to receive help from other people in the household. In contrast, many lone mothers have children under five and only half of these have any arrangement for child care, either formal or informal. Given the lower proportion of lone mothers with child care arrangements and their greater poverty, the parenting demands on lone mothers are likely to be greater than those on lone fathers. This is likely to result in greater rates of mortality and morbidity in later life. Apart from the impact of material circumstances upon health, Popay and Jones (1990) argue that social isolation is an important contributory factor in the poor health of both lone mothers and fathers.

The issue of social isolation was examined in more detail by Evason (1980) in an earlier study of lone parents in Northern Ireland. She looked at the proneness of lone parents to symptoms of depression, namely: sleep problems, feelings of lassitude, feelings of hopelessness and being overwhelmed, and loss of appetite. Out of the sample of 694 lone parents, more than three fifths experienced one or more symptoms of depression all or most of the time, whilst one parent in six experienced three or four symptoms all or most of the time. Evason's explanation of these findings is in terms of the following factors: social isolation, low income and non-employment. One third of the sample had no one to whom they felt they could talk about their problems.

It would seem, then, that the poorer health of both single parents and their children is largely explicable in terms of the material and social deprivation which lone parent families experience. A variety of policies has been suggested which could improve the material and social circumstances of lone parents, not least of which is to improve the access of lone mothers to paid employment in order to combat poverty and isolation. In turn, such policies would be likely over the long term to improve the health of single parents (see Popay and Jones, 1990, for a summary of these policies). It is important to note, as Popay and Jones do, that many lone parents provide positive and enjoyable lives for their children and themselves. The point of focusing on their health is not to increase the negative image which lone parent families can have, especially in the mass media, but to show how their efforts in providing a positive life can mean that they pay a high price in terms of their future health status.

Homelessness and health

If mass unemployment in the 1980s was in some ways an 'invisible' social problem with those who were unemployed suffering in isolated silence, homelessness was and is very much on public display in many of the major cities in Britain. The sight of young people huddled in shop doorways in London's West End has become an all too familiar sight in the capital. Those people sleeping rough, however, are only the most visible of those who are homeless. It is actually not a straightforward matter to define 'homelessness'. The narrowest definition is that of 'rooflessness' which means literally lacking a roof over one's head and this refers to those people who are sleeping rough on the streets. The 1991 census found 2703 people sleeping rough in England and Wales on census night, although CHAR (Campaign for the Homeless and Roofless) suggests that the total figure is actually higher than this (*The Guardian*, 23 July 1991). The statutory definition of homelessness is based on the 1985 Housing Act which local authorities use as a basis for deciding who they can house of the people who come to them and declare themselves as homeless. The number of families accepted as homeless by local authorities has gone up from 53,000 in 1978 to 126,680 in 1989 which Shelter estimates to be around 363,500 individuals (Miller, 1990). Because of the limitations of the statutory definition of homelessness, which tends to exclude certain categories of people, Shelter and other housing organisations argue the local authority figures are likely seriously to underestimate the total number of people who are homeless, particularly young single people. A study by the housing charity Centrepoint Soho estimates that there are 51,000 16–19 year olds living in temporary accommodation in London alone, including hostels and squats (Randall, 1988).

It is impossible here to give an account of the various explanations which have been put forward for homelessness. However, the shortage of affordable rented accommodation coupled with the recent changes in social security benefits, especially as affecting young people (Sanders, 1988; Randall,

1988, 1989), are both likely to be important factors.

How does homelessness affect health? For those sleeping rough, the effects on health are only too obvious:

> 'Once on the streets it is hard to keep healthy. The shelter, warmth, and privacy often taken for granted do not exist; good food may be hard to find or expensive; it is almost impossible to keep clean; "minor" illnesses are hard to cure'
> (Lowry, 1990a, page 32)

Evidence from young people living at the Centrepoint Night Shelter in London showed that 27% of a sample of 231 felt their health had deteriorated since they left their last settled home (Randall, 1988). A more detailed study of the health needs and problems of homeless people was carried out by Shelter (Miller, 1990) based on interviews with 105 homeless families living in temporary accommodation, for example, bed and breakfast hotels. In terms of health needs, 60% of respondents were seriously concerned about their children's health and development, with most accommodation lacking a place for children to play in. Many of the families were socially isolated, whilst the restrictions on visitors in hostels and hotels exacerbated this isolation. Cooking facilities were often negligible which meant families lived on expensive, poor quality take-away food. Living conditions were frequently unhygienic. Given this catalogue of material and social deprivation, it is unsurprising that nearly half of the respondents had health problems they believed were caused by their accommodation, including depression and physical illnesses such as asthma.

One of the main problems identified with health care of people who are homeless is that members of this group are less likely to be registered with a GP than those who are housed and they may well receive little actual health care despite their obvious needs. Lowry (1990a) suggests that existing services could be made more accessible and less intimidating, whilst Crane (1990), in discussing elderly homeless people, suggests that teams of workers from the psychiatric field and social services could take a more pro-active approach and seek out and liaise with elderly people in hostels and on the street about their health needs. It would seem that health and social services, including nursing, need to develop new ways of providing health care for homeless people (see Brown, 1987, for a summary of possible nursing strategies in relation to this group).

Conclusion

This chapter has outlined the social context of health in which nurses will be operating. There are many aspects of this social context which have either been neglected, such as the social position of disabled people or those with learning difficulties, or only briefly mentioned, such as old age and childhood. In addition, there is little reference to the social organisation of hospitals or the sociological nature of the nursing profession. For these topics, readers need to refer to the suggestions for further reading.

Because of the sociological approach adopted in this chapter, mainly a structural one in which the emphasis is on the way in which the stratification system affects people's health, readers may finish this chapter feeling rather impotent about the social context of health: 'The problems are so big; what can I as an individual nurse do about them?'. Sociology is not a discipline which suggests that analysing 'problems', such as inequalities in health, is a simple matter or which claims to provide easy solutions. Different sociological perspectives will provide different views on the possible directions social change should take if the health inequalities illustrated in this chapter are to be diminished, while some sociologists, notably Weberians, are sceptical about whether sociology even *should* make recommendations for social change at all.

One thing which this chapter has underemphasised but which follows out of the perspectives of feminism, Marxism and Weberianism is that, while people are located within a structure of stratification, they are also active agents who can, to some extent, modify and change that structure by their actions. Those groups we have singled out as being the most vulnerable to ill health, the working class, women, black people, poor and homeless people, are not just passive victims of their social position, but are actively engaged in shaping their lives and their health. We have indicated throughout this chapter that nurses need to work *with* their clients so as to allow these disadvantaged groups in particular to shape their own

health care agenda rather than having one imposed upon them by experts, no matter how well meaning. As Marx said, albeit in a different context, 'The educator must himself be educated' (Bottomore and Rubel, 1963, pages 82–3); in other words, those who are without power and social advantage can teach nurses about the circumstances of their lives and what they think their health needs are. Holistic care is not simply about seeing people in their social environment; it is also, ideally, about trying to shift the power balance towards those people who have least power in this society, so that they can truly fulfil their human potential and take genuine control of their lives; in other words, lead healthy lives.

There are various suggestions regarding possible directions for nursing practice scattered throughout the chapter, and for a forceful account of how nurses, both individually and collectively, can change the health care agenda, see Labelle (1986). A more focused approach to family health in relation to issues of social inequality can be found in Blackburn (1991).

This chapter has implicitly challenged the language of consumerism which frequently dominates discussions of the NHS, whereby health service users are described as 'consumers'. As this chapter has attempted to show, describing the population in such terms gives a spurious uniformity to what is in effect a deeply divided society. Henley sums up the dilemma facing the NHS and also of nurses within that system:

'We need to decide whether we are in the business of fitting people to the system (possibly high efficiency but low quality care) or of fitting the system to the people (possibly low efficiency but high quality care)'

(Henley, 1986, page 18)

Hopefully this chapter has contributed towards providing the sociological evidence which will stimulate debate amongst both trainee and qualified nurses.

Acknowledgements

The author would like to thank Dylan Tomlinson, Sally Kendall, Cathryn Britton and Shirley Koster for their comments on an earlier draft of this chapter.

Glossary

Antiracism: An approach to race relations which stresses the role of institutional racism in structuring the experiences of black people in Britain. Antiracists are politically committed to challenging racism in all the institutions of British society (see *multiculturalism*)

Caste system: A type of stratification based on the Hindu religion in India. A person is born into a caste and *social mobility* is impossible

Class: A grouping within a society which shares a common economic and social position. Classes are inherently unequal. The various sociological approaches emphasise different economic criteria in their identification of classes: Marxists stress property ownership; Weberians look at both property ownership and occupational skills; while the Registrar General in government surveys measures class on the basis of occupational skills. As well as being an objective social fact, class also has a subjective element to it in the sense that people can be aware of themselves as being members of a particular class

Colonialism: A historical process whereby European nations established their political rule over the rest of the world

Culture: A way of life, including customs, values and beliefs, as well as family and other social arrangements. Culture can refer to the way of life of an entire society or to a particular group within a society, for example a group based upon a shared ethnic identity

Deviance: Types of action which are said to go against the socially acceptable ways of behaving, that is, the 'norms' or informal rules of society. *Functionalism* and *symbolic interactionism* regard illness as a form of deviance

Feminism: A social theory which both attempts to explain why gender relations between women and men are unequal and to challenge this inequality politically. There are several variants of feminism: liberal, Marxist, socialist and radical (Abbott and Wallace, 1990). Liberal feminism argues for equal rights for women, whilst radical feminism emphasises *patriarchy* and hence male domination. Marxist and socialist feminism concentrate on the relations between patriarchy and other forms of *stratification*, notably *class* and racism

Full employment: An economic term usually taken to be an unemployment rate of 3%. The unemployment rate is the percentage of the labour force which is unemployed at a particular point in time. This rate reached a post-war peak of 13% in 1986 (see *unemployment*)

Functionalism: A theoretical perspective in sociology which is concerned with the question of how order and stability are maintained in a society. It concentrates upon the role of a shared value system in the maintenance of social consensus, and also on the manner in which the various parts of society contribute towards the efficient functioning of the society as a whole. The functionalist perspective was dominant in sociology in the post-war period up to the early 1960s, largely under the influence of the American sociologist Talcott Parsons (1902–79) who devised the concept of the *sick role*. Functionalism has declined in importance since the early 1960s under the critical onslaught of conflict perspectives and *symbolic interactionism*

Gender roles: The socially constructed set of expectations of male and female behaviour

Holistic care: An approach to health care which treats the individual as a whole person in relation to his or her environment

Housing tenure: The way in which properties are occupied, for example, rented or owned. There are three main housing tenures in Britain: owner-occupied, rented from local authorities, and rented from private landlords

Illness iceberg: That amount of illness which is socially 'invisible' because it is not reported to medical practitioners

Income support: A means-tested benefit for those aged over 18, who are either not in work or who work below a certain number of hours per week, and whose income falls below a minimum level set by Parliament. Income support replaced supplementary benefit in April 1988

Infant mortality rate: Number of deaths of children less than one year old per 1000 live births

Labelling theory: That part of *symbolic interactionism* which is concerned with *deviance*. Labelling theory argues that deviance is not a result of rule-breaking behaviour in itself, but is instead due to the social reaction of people in positions of authority who label certain behaviour as 'deviant'

Marxism: A social theory which attempts to explain social relations in capitalist society in terms of class exploitation and class conflict. It is also a political philosophy committed to changing society from one based upon capitalist property relations to one based upon the communal ownership of property. Marxism is based upon the works of Karl Marx (1818–1883)

Material deprivation: A state when people lack the material standards of living which are ordinarily available in their society, for example in relation to diet, clothing, housing and household amenities, working and living environments (Townsend, 1987)

Medical model: A model of health which suggests that health is the absence of disease in a person's body and that restoring a person to health is a matter of curing the disease. This model of health is associated with modern medicine and can be contrasted to the principles underlying *holistic care*

Medicalisation: The process whereby natural and social phenomena are turned into 'diseases' or are treated as diseases by the medical profession

Morbidity rates: Measures of the amount of illness or disease in a population

Mortality rates: Measures of the number of deaths in a population

Multiculturalism: An approach to race relations which stresses the role of ethnicity in relation to the position of black people in Britain. It is politically committed to the furtherance of both knowledge about and tolerance of the range of ethnic cultures in Britain (see *antiracism*)

New Right: A social theory which aims to explain social behaviour in terms of the actions of individuals. It is politically committed to the attempt to limit the role of the state in economic and social life in order for markets to operate in a manner free from state intervention

Patriarchy: The generalised power of men over women. The term is associated with *feminism* and is particularly prominent in radical feminism

Perinatal mortality rate: The number of deaths per 1000 live births that occur between the 28th week of pregnancy and the 4th week after the birth

Racial discrimination: The treatment of an individual or group of people less favourably than another on racial grounds, for example, skin colour

Repetitive strain injury: A term for a range of work-related disorders which affect the hand, arm and neck. They usually involve persistent pain and are often the result of rapid repetitive movements (e.g. typing)

Role: The social expectations which are attached to a person's occupancy of a particular social position. These expectations are not necessarily realised in practice

Sick role: A term devised by the functionalist sociologist Parsons to refer to the manner in which being ill is a *role* comprised of sets of expectations of acceptable behaviour, for example, the injunctions on someone who is sick to seek out and follow professional medical advice

Sickle cell anaemia: An inherited disease which affects the red blood cells and is found mainly amongst people of African or Caribbean descent

Social mobility: The movement of individuals either up or down the class structure

Social stratification: The social structure of inequality between groupings of people who are ranked along a hierarchy in relation to power, wealth and status. *Class*, gender and race are the main examples of social stratification

Standardised mortality ratios: A measure of death rates

Stereotype: A rigid and inflexible categorisation of people as members of a social group, usually with a negative connotation

Symbolic interactionism: A theoretical perspective in sociology which stresses the role of symbols and language in human interaction. It is derived from the ideas of the American sociologist George H. Mead (1861–1931)

Thalassaemia: An inherited disease which affects the red blood cells and is found mainly amongst Cypriot, Greek, Turkish and Indian people

Unemployment: A situation which exists when members of the labour force want to work but cannot get a job (see *full employment*)

Weberian sociology: The sociology which is derived from the work of the German sociologist Max Weber (1864–1920). He stressed the role played by social action in understanding society, and in relation to stratification he criticised Marxism for reducing all inequality to issues of class and neglecting the role of non-class factors, for example, race. Weber's ideas are particularly influential in contemporary studies of stratification

Well women clinics: Clinics run by and for

women with the aim of practising a holistic approach to women's health care needs. The emphasis is on allowing the female clients to determine their own health needs

References

Abbott, P. and Wallace, C. (1990). *An Introduction to Sociology: Feminist Perspectives*. Routledge, London.

Ahmad, W.I.U. (1989). Policies, pills and political wills: a critique of policies to improve the health status of ethnic minorities. *Lancet*, 1, 148–150.

Arber, S. (1990). Revealing women's health. In *Women's Health Counts*, Roberts, H. (ed.). Routledge, London.

Atkinson, A.B. (1989). *Poverty and Social Security*. Harvester Wheatsheaf, Hemel Hempstead.

Balarajan, R. (1991). Ethnic differences in mortality from ischaemic heart disease and cerebrovascular disease in England and Wales. *British Medical Journal*, 302, 560–564.

Beattie, A. (1991). Knowledge and control in health promotion: a test case for social policy and social theory. In *The Sociology of the Health Service*, Gabe, J., Calnan M. and Bury, M. (eds.). Routledge, London.

Beechey, V. (1986). Women's employment in contemporary Britain. In *Women in Britain Today*, Beechey, V. and Whitelegg, E. (eds.). Open University Press, Milton Keynes.

Beurat, K. (1991). Women and transport. In *Women's Issues in Social Policy*, Maclean, M. and Groves, D. (eds.). Routledge, London.

Black Health Workers and Patients Group. (1983). Psychiatry and the corporate state. *Race and Class*, XXV(2), 49–64.

Blackburn, C. (1991). *Poverty and Health*. Open University Press, Milton Keynes.

Blackman, T., Evason, E., Melaugh, M. and Woods, R. (1989). Housing and health: a case study of two areas in West Belfast. *Journal of Social Policy*, 18(1), 1–26.

Blane, D. (1985). An assessment of the Black Report's explanations of health inequalities. *Sociology of Health and Illness*, 7(3), 423–445.

Blaxter, M. (1990). *Health and Lifestyles*. Tavistock/Routledge, London and New York.

Bottomore, T.B. and Rubel, M. (1963). *Karl Marx: Selected Writings in Sociology and Social Philosophy*. Penguin Books, Harmondsworth.

Brown, C. (1985). *Black and White Britain: The 3rd PSI Survey*. Gower Publishing Co., Aldershot.

Brown, G.W. and Harris, T. (1978). *Social Origins of Depression*. Tavistock Publications, London.

Brown, P. (1987). A vulnerable minority: homeless families. *Senior Nurse*, 7(4), 33–35.

Busfield, J. (1989). Sexism and psychiatry. *Sociology*, 23(3), 343–364.

Byrne, D., Harrisson, S.P., Keithley, J. and McCarthy, P. (1986). *Housing and Health*. Gower Publishing Co., Aldershot.

Carlisle, D. (1990). Racism in nursing. *Nursing Times*, 86(14), 25–29.

Carr-Hill, R. (1987). The inequalities in health debate: a critical review of the issues. *Journal of Social Policy*, 16(4), 509–542.

Central Statistical Office. (1991). *Social Trends 21*, 1991 edition. HMSO, London.

Charles, N. and Kerr, M. (1988). *Women, Food and Families*. Manchester University Press, Manchester.

Chevannes, M. (1990). Stamping out inequality. *Nursing Times*, 86(42), 38–40.

Chudley, P. and Smith, S. (1989). Enrolled nurses: stuck on the career ladder. *Nursing Times*, 85(27), 36–38.

Cook, J. and Watt, S. (1987). Racism, women and poverty. In *Women and Poverty in Britain*, Glendinning, C. and Millar, J. (eds.). Wheatsheaf Books, Brighton.

Cope, R. (1989). The compulsory detention of Afro-Caribbeans under the Mental Health Act. *New Community*, 15(3), 343–356.

Crane, M. (1990). Old, homeless and unwanted. *Nursing Times*, 86(21), 44–46.

Daniel, W.W. (1968). *Racial Discrimination in England*. Penguin Books, Harmondsworth.

Davis, K. and Moore, W.F. (1945). Some principles of stratification. *American Sociological Review*, 10, 242–249.

Deem, R. (1990). Women and leisure – all work and no play? *Social Studies Review*, 5(4), 139–143.

Department of Employment. (1991). *Employment Gazette*, Labour Market Data, December 1991.

Dobson, S. (1988). Ethnic identity: a basis for care. *Midwife, Health Visitor and Community Nurse*, 24(5), 172, 176, 178.

Donovan, J. (1984). Ethnicity and health: a research review. *Social Science and Medicine*, 19(7), 663–670.

Doyal, L. (1979). *The Political Economy of Health*. Pluto Press, London.

Durkheim, E. (1952). *Suicide*. Routledge & Kegan Paul, London.

Edwards, A. (1987). Male violence in feminist theory: an analysis of the changing conceptions of sex/gender violence and male dominance. In *Women, Violence and Social Control*, Hanmer, J. and Maynard, M. (eds.). Macmillan Press, Basingstoke.

Employment Department Group/Office of Population Censuses and Surveys. (1990). *Standard Occupational Classification Vol. 1*. HMSO, London.

Equal Opportunities Commission. (1991). *Women and Men in Britain 1991*. HMSO, London.

Evason, E. (1980). *Just Me and the Kids: A Study of Single Parent Families in Northern Ireland*. (3rd ed.) Equal Opportunities Commission for Northern Ireland, Belfast.

Ewan, C., Lowy, E. and Reid, J. (1991). 'Falling out of culture': the effects of repetition strain injury on sufferers' roles and identity. *Sociology of Health and Illness*, 13(2), 168–192.

Fennell, G., Phillipson, C. and Evers, H. (1988). *The Sociology of Old Age*. Open University Press, Milton Keynes.

Fenton, S. (1986). *Race, Health and Welfare. Afro-Caribbean and South Asian People in Central Bristol: Health and Social Services*. Department of Sociology, University of Bristol, Bristol.

Foster, P. (1989). Improving the doctor-patient relationship: a feminist perspective. *Journal of Social Policy*, 18(3), 337–361.

Foster, P. (1991). Well women clinics. In *Women's Issues in Social Policy*, Maclean, M. and Groves, D. (eds.). Routledge, London.

Freer, C. (1988). Old myths: frequent misconceptions about the elderly. In *The Ageing Population: Burden or Challenge?*, Wells, N. and Freer, C. (eds.). Macmillan Press, Basingstoke.

Fryer, P. (1984). *Staying Power*. Pluto Press, London.

Ganatra, S. (1989). Features of Gujarati, Punjabi and Muslim diets in the UK. In *Ethnic Factors in Health and Disease*, Cruickshank, J.K. and Beevers, D.G. (eds.). Wright, London.

Giddens, A. (1989). *Sociology*. Polity Press, Cambridge.

Glendinning, C. and Millar, J. (1987). *Women and Poverty in Britain*. Wheatsheaf Books, Brighton.

Glendinning, C. and Millar, J. (1991). Poverty: the forgotten Englishwoman – reconstructing research and policy on poverty. In *Women's Issues in Social Policy*, Maclean, M. and Groves, D. (eds.). Routledge, London.

Goffman, E. (1968). *Asylums*. Penguin Books, Harmondsworth.

Graham, H. (1984). *Women, Health and the Family*. Wheatsheaf Books, Brighton.

Graham, H. (1985). Providers, negotiators and mediators: women as the hidden carers. In *Women, Health and Healing*, Lewin, E. and Olesen, V. (eds.). Tavistock Publications, London.

Graham, H. (1987a). Women's smoking and family health. *Social Science & Medicine*, 25(1), 47–56.

Graham, H. (1987b). Women, health and illness. *Social Studies Review*, 3(1), 15–20.

Graham, H. (1990). Behaving well: women's health behaviour in context. In *Women's Health Counts*, Roberts, H. (ed.). Routledge, London.

Green, E., Hebron, S. and Woodward, D. (1987). Women, leisure and social control. In *Women, Violence and Social Control*, Hanmer, J. and Maynard, M. (eds.). Macmillan Press, Basingstoke.

Hakim, C. (1982). The social consequences of high unemployment. *Journal of Social Policy*, 11(4), 433–467.

Hart, N. (1985). *The Sociology of Health and Medicine*. Causeway Books, Ormskirk.

Hart, N. (1989). Sex, gender and survival. In *Health Inequalities in European Countries*, Fox, J. (ed.). Gower Publishing Co., Aldershot.

Haskey, J. (1989). Current prospects for the proportion of marriages ending in divorce. *Population Trends*, 55, 34–37.

Haskey, J. (1991). Estimated numbers and demographic characteristics of one-parent families in Great Britain. *Population Trends*, 65, 35–43.

Henley, A. (1986). Nursing care in a multiracial society. *Senior Nurse*, 4(2), 18–20.

Hugman, R. (1991). *Power in Caring Professions*. Macmillan Press, Basingstoke.

Hunt, M. (1991). Men in nursing: who flies highest? *Nursing Times*, 87(7), 29–31.

Hyndman, S.J. (1990). Housing dampness and health amongst British Bengalis in East London. *Social Science and Medicine*, 30(1), 131–141.

Independent Commission of Enquiry into Racial Harassment (1987). *Racial Harassment in Leeds 1985–1986*. Leeds Community Relations Council, Leeds.

Ineichen, B. (1990). The mental health of Asians in Britain. *British Medical Journal*, 300, 1669–1670.

Jacobson, B. (1988). *Beating the Ladykillers: Women and Smoking*. Victor Gollancz Ltd, London.

Jones, I.G. and Cameron, D. (1984). Social class analysis: an embarrassment to epidemiology. *Community Medicine*, 6, 37–46.

Knowles, C. (1991). Afro-Caribbeans and schizophrenia: how does psychiatry deal with issues of race, culture and ethnicity? *Journal of Social Policy*, 20(2), 173–190.

Labelle, H. (1986). Nurses as a social force. *Journal of Advanced Nursing*, 11(3), 247–253.

Leonard, D. and Speakman, M.A. (1986). Women in the family: companions or caretakers? In *Women in Britain Today*, Beechey, V. and Whitelegg, E. (eds.). Open University Press, Milton Keynes.

Lewis, J. (1989). Lone parent families: politics and economics. *Journal of Social Policy*, 18(4), 595–600.

Lewis, J. and Meredith, B. (1988). *Daughters Who Care*. Routledge, London.

Littlewood R. and Lipsedge M. (1989). *Aliens and Alienists: Ethnic Minorities and Psychiatry*. (2nd ed.) Unwin Hyman, London.

Lowry, S. (1989). Housing and health: temperature and humidity. *British Medical Journal*, 299, 1326–1328.

Lowry, S. (1990a). Housing and health: health and homelessness. *British Medical Journal*, 300, 32–34.

Lowry, S. (1990b). Housing and health: families and flats. *British Medical Journal*, 300, 245–247.

Lowry, S. (1990c). Housing and health: getting things done. *British Medical Journal*, 300, 390–392.

Marmot, M.G. (1986). Social inequalities in mortality: the social environment. In *Class and Health*, Wilkinson, R.G. (ed.). Tavistock Publications, London.

Martin, C.J., Platt, S.D. and Hunt, S.M. (1987). Housing conditions and ill health. *British Medical Journal*, 294, 1125–1127.

Mattiason, I., Lindgarde, F., Nilsson, J.A. and Theorell, T. (1990). Threat of unemployment and cardiovascular risk factors: longitudinal study of quality of sleep and serum cholesterol concentrations in men threatened with redundancy. *British Medical Journal*, 301, 461–466.

McGrother, J. (1990). Does work make you sick? *Nursing Times*, 86(7), 38–39.

McKeigue, P.M., Richards, J.D.M. and Richards, P. (1990). Effects of discrimination by sex and race on the early careers of British medical graduates during 1981–7. *British Medical Journal*, 301, 961–964.

McNaught, A. (1988). *Race and Health Policy*. Croom Helm, London.

McShane, L. (1985). Health services in working class areas. *Critical Social Policy*, 5(2), 73–82.

Miles, A. (1988). *Women and Mental Illness*. Wheatsheaf Books, Brighton.

Miles, R. (1989). *Racism*. Routledge, London.

Millar, J. and Glendinning, C. (1987). Invisible women, invisible poverty. In *Women and Poverty in Britain*, Glendinning, C. and Millar, J. (eds.). Wheatsheaf Books, Brighton.

Millar, J. and Glendinning, C. (1989). Gender and poverty. *Journal of Social Policy*, 18(3), 363–381.

Miller, K. (1990). *Wasting Money, Wasting Lives: The Scandal of Temporary Homes*. Shelter, London.

Mills, C.W. (1970). *The Sociological Imagination*. Penguin Books, Harmondsworth.

Moser, K.A., Fox, A.J. and Jones D.R. (1986). Unemployment and mortality in the OPCS Longitudinal Study. In *Class and Health*, Wilkinson, R.G. (ed.). Tavistock Publications, London.

Moser, K.A., Goldblatt, P.O., Fox, A.J. and Jones, D.R. (1987). Unemployment and mortality: comparison of the 1971 and 1981 longitudinal study census samples. *British Medical Journal*, 294, 86–90.

Oakley, A. (1979). *Becoming a Mother*. Martin Robertson, Oxford.

Oakley, A. (1980). *Women Confined: Towards a Sociology of Childbirth*. Martin Robertson, Oxford.

Oakley, A. and Rajan, L. (1991). Social class and social support: the same or different? *Sociology*, 25(1), 31–59.

Office of Population Censuses and Surveys. (1980). *Classification of Occupations 1980*. HMSO, London.

Office of Population Censuses and Surveys. (1986). *Occupational Mortality: the Registrar General's Decennial Supplement for Great Britain, 1979–80, 1982–83*. Series DS6. HMSO, London.

Office of Population Censuses and Surveys. (1989). *General Household Survey 1986*. HMSO, London.

Office of Population Censuses and Surveys. (1990). *General Household Survey 1988*. HMSO, London.

Orr, J. (1988). Women's health: a nursing perspective. In *Political Issues in Nursing: Past, Present and Future, Volume 3*, White, R. (ed.). John Wiley and Sons, Chichester.

Pacy, P.C. (1989). Nutritional patterns and deficiencies. In *Ethnic Factors in Health and Disease*, Cruickshank, J. and Beevers, D. (eds.). Wright, London.

Payne, S. (1991). *Women, Health and Poverty*. Harvester Wheatsheaf, Hemel Hempstead.

Pearson, M. (1986a). Ten years on. *Senior Nurse*, 4(4), 18–19.

Pearson, M. (1986b). Less favourable treatment? *Senior Nurse*, 4(5), 15–17.

Pearson, M. (1986c). Fitting in. *Senior Nurse*, 4(6), 14–15.

Pearson, M. (1989). Sociology of race and health. In *Ethnic Factors in Health and Disease*, Cruickshank, J. and Beevers, D. (eds.). Wright, London.

Penfold, P.S. and Walker, G.A. (1984). *Women and the Psychiatric Paradox*. Open University Press, Milton Keynes.

Perry, F. (1988). Far from black and white. *Nursing Times*, 84(10), 40–41.

Phillips, K. (1985). Aspects of midwifery: Asians in Britain. *Midwife, Health Visitor and Community Nurse*, 21(4), 114–118.

Phoenix, A. (1988a). Narrow definitions of culture: the case of early motherhood. In *Enterprising Women: Ethnicity, Economy and Gender Relations*, Westwood, S. and Bhachu, P. (eds.). Routledge, London.

Phoenix, A. (1988b). The Afro-Caribbean myth. *New Society*, 83(1314), 10–13

Platt, S.D., Martin, C.J., Hunt, S.M. and Lewis, C.W. (1989). Damp housing, mould growth and symptomatic health state. *British Medical Journal*, 298, 1673–1678.

Pollock, L. and West, E. (1987). Women and psychiatry today. *Senior Nurse*, 6(6), 11–14.

Popay, J. and Jones, G. (1990). Patterns of health and illness amongst lone parents. *Journal of Social Policy*, 19(4), 499–534.

Pugh, H. and Moser, K. (1990). Measuring women's mortality differences. In *Women's Health Counts*, Roberts, H. (ed.). Routledge, London.

Ramazanoglu, C. (1989). *Feminism and the Contradictions of Oppression*. Routledge, London.

Randall, G. (1988). *No Way Home: Homeless Young People in Central London*. Centrepoint Soho, London.

Randall, G. (1989). *Homeless and Hungry: A Sign of the Times*. Centrepoint Soho, London.

Rex, J. and Mason, D. (1986). *Theories of Race and Ethnic Relations*. Cambridge University Press, Cambridge.

Rex, J. and Moore, R. (1967). *Race, Community and Conflict*. Oxford University Press, Oxford.

Robinson, V. (1988). The new Asian middle class in Britain. *Ethnic and Racial Studies*, 11(4), 456–473.

Rocheron, Y. (1988). The Asian Mother and Baby Campaign: the construction of ethnic minorities' health needs. *Critical Social Policy*, 8(1), 4–23.

Sanders, C. (1988). Thatcher's untouchables. *New Statesman and Society*, 1 (29–30), 13–15.

Saunders, P. (1990). *Social Class and Stratification*. Routledge, London.

Sen, D. (1989). Asian culture and communications in midwifery. *Midwife, Health Visitor and Community Nurse*, 25(1 & 2), 16–18.

Seymour, J. (1991). Whose health is it anyway? *Nursing Times*, 87(15), 16–18.

Sheldon, T.A. and Parker, H. (1991). *The Racialisation of Health Research*. Paper given at British Sociological Association Annual Conference, University of Manchester, March 25–28.

Smith, A. and Jacobson, B. (1988). *The Nation's Health*. King's Fund, London.

Smith, D. and Nicolson, M. (1991). *Health and Ignorance – Past and Present*. Paper given at British Sociological Association Annual Conference, University of Manchester, March 25–28.

Smith, G.D., Bartley, M. and Blane, D. (1990). The Black Report on socioeconomic inequalities in health 10 years on. *British Medical Journal*, 301, 373–377.

Smith, R. (1991). Unemployment: here we go again. *British Medical Journal*, 302, 606–607.

Stokes, G. (1991). A transcultural nurse is about. *Senior Nurse*, 11(1), 40–42.

Taylor, R. (1988). The elderly as members of society: an examination of social differences in an elderly population. In *The Ageing Population: Burden or Challenge?*, Wells, N. and Freer, C. (eds.). Macmillan Press, Basingstoke.

Tombs, S. (1990). Industrial injuries in British manufacturing industry. *Sociological Review*, 38(2), 324–343.

Tompson, K. (1988). *Under Siege: Racism and Violence in Britain Today*. Penguin Books, Harmondsworth.

Townsend, P. (1979). *Poverty in the United Kingdom*. Penguin Books, Harmondsworth.

Townsend, P. (1987). Deprivation. *Journal of Social Policy*, 16(2), 125–146.

Townsend, P. (1989). Slipping through the net. *The Guardian*, 29 November, 27.

Townsend, P., Davidson, N. and Whitehead, M. (1988). *Inequalities in Health: The Black Report* and *The Health Divide*. Penguin Books, Harmondsworth.

Townsend, P., Phillimore, P. and Beattie, A. (1988). *Health and Deprivation: Inequality and the North*. Routledge, London.

Trevelyan J. (1990). Racism in nursing: racism alert. *Nursing Times*, 86(24), 45–46.

Turner, B.S. (1986). *Equality*. Ellis Horwood and Tavistock Publications, Chichester and London.

Twomey, M. (1987). Working with women. *Senior Nurse*, 6(6), 15–16.

Unemployment Unit. (1989). *United Kingdom Unemployment Figures 1982–1988*. Unemployment Unit, London.

Victor, C.R. (1991). Continuity or change: inequalities in health in later life. *Ageing and Society*, 11(1), 23–39.

Walker, A. (1990). Poverty and inequality in old age. In *Ageing in Society*, Bond, J. and Coleman, P. (eds.). Sage Publications, London.

Westwood, S. and Bhachu, P. (1988). Images and realities. *New Society*, 84(1323), 20–22.

Wilkinson, R.G. (1989). Class mortality differentials, income distribution and trends in poverty 1921–81. *Journal of Social Policy*, 18(3), 307–335.

Yuen, P. and Balarajan, R. (1989). Unemployment and patterns of consultation with the general practitioner. *British Medical Journal*, 298, 1212–1214.

Suggestions for further reading

Abbott, P. and Wallace, C. (1990). *An Introduction to Sociology: Feminist Perspectives*. Routledge, London.

Abercrombie, N., Warde, A., Soothill, K., Urry, J. and Walby, S. (1988). *Contemporary British Society*. Polity Press, Cambridge.

Blackburn, C. (1991). *Poverty and Health*. Open University Press, Milton Keynes.

Bond, J. and Bond, S. (1986). *Sociology and Health Care*. Churchill Livingstone, Edinburgh.

Bond, J. and Coleman, P. (1990). *Ageing in Society: An Introduction to Social Gerontology*. Sage Publications, London.

Giddens, A. (1989). *Sociology*. Polity Press, Cambridge.

Henley, A. (1986). Nursing care in a multiracial society. *Senior Nurse*, 4(2), 18–20.

Karseras, P. and Hopkins, E. (1987). *British Asians – Health in the Community*. John Wiley and Sons, Chichester.

Labelle, H. (1986). Nurses as a social force. *Journal of Advanced Nursing*, 11(3), 247–253.

Mitchell, J. (1984). *What Is To Be Done About Illness and Health?* Penguin Books, Harmondsworth.

Orr, J. (1987). *Women's Health in the Community*. John Wiley and Sons, Chichester.

Salvage, J. (1985). *The Politics of Nursing*. Heinemann, London.

Saunders, P. (1990). *Social Class and Stratification*. Routledge, London.

Townsend, P., Davidson, N. and Whitehead, M. (1988). *Inequalities in Health: The Black Report and The Health Divide*. Penguin Books, Harmondsworth.

Webb, C. (1986). *Feminist Practice in Women's Health Care*. John Wiley and Sons, Chichester.

Wells, N. and Freer, C. (1988). *The Ageing Population*. Macmillan Press, Basingstoke.

3

PROMOTING HEALTH

Sally Kendall

The aim of this chapter is to examine ways of promoting and maintaining health which the nurse may apply in clinical practice.

The chapter will include consideration of the following topics:

- The relationship between nursing and the promotion of health

- The challenge of promoting health

- The use of a range of health promotion models including illness prevention, self-empowerment and radical models

- The importance of promoting human potential through the nurse working in partnership with the patient is a theme throughout this chapter

The previous chapter has explored in some depth the broad and varied concepts that people may hold about health and some of the possible influences on those conceptions. This chapter will be looking at how we, as nurses, can use our ideas about health and our skills (both in practical nursing and communication) to both promote and maintain health. Firstly, the relationship between nursing and health will be explored. This will be followed by a series of examples of how health can potentially be promoted.

The intention here is not to define health. You will by now be aware that health is an area of enormous subjectivity and as such is difficult to label or measure in such a way that it can be universally understood. However, it may be useful when thinking about health to refer to David Seedhouse's idea that:

'All theories of health and all approaches designed to increase health are intended to advise against, to prevent the creation of, or to remove, obstacles to the *achievement of human potential*. These obstacles may be biological, environmental, societal, familial or personal'

(Seedhouse, 1986, page 53, our emphasis)

Although we may each differ in our understanding of what constitutes human potential, it is at least a phrase unburdened by values related to sickness or wellness. Thus, it is possible to begin to understand how individuals may exist at any point along the wellness–sickness continuum and still be in a position to achieve potential. For example, a young woman disabled by multiple sclerosis may have come to terms with her illness and found a new and satisfying relationship with her family. Another woman of the same age might be physically fit, but finds it difficult to handle stress leading to difficulties in personal relationships and health behaviours such as smoking. Is it possible to say who is the healthier of these two women? Seen in terms of human potential we can see that they each have obstacles to overcome and each has managed to do so with different degrees of success.

The obstacles to achieving human potential, and the ways in which we as nurses may enable those in our care to overcome them, will form the main focus of this chapter.

Nursing and health promotion

Before addressing the nurse's role in health promotion, it is useful to consider what is meant by the term as there is some debate about the difference between health promotion and health education. In 1984 the World Health Organisation (WHO) produced some principles of health promotion which are summarised below:

(1)   Health promotion involves the population as a whole in the context of their everyday life, rather than focusing on people at risk for specific diseases
(2)   Health promotion is directed towards action on the determinants or causes of health
(3)   Health promotion combines diverse, but complementary methods or approaches
(4)   Health promotion aims particularly at effective and concrete public participation
(5)   While health promotion is not a medical service, health professionals – particularly in primary health care – have an important role in nurturing and enabling health promotion.

This involves action which:

(1)   Enhances equal access to health
(2)   Develops an environment conducive to health
(3)   Strengthens social networks and support
(4)   Promotes positive health behaviour and appropriate coping strategies
(5)   Increases knowledge and disseminates information.

These principles suggest that health promotion is an activity, which nurses, among others, may engage in. Some of these actions will be addressed later in the chapter. However, Baric (1985) has

argued that health promotion is not so much a specific activity as a 'movement towards the achievement of health as a basic right for all'. Whilst he acknowledges that the health care professions have an important part to play in this movement, he suggests that other professions such as economists and policy-makers should equally be part of promoting health for all. One could also argue that if public participation in health is to be realised, then lay people should form a part of that movement also. Baric's discussion concludes that, by defining health promotion as an activity rather than a movement, significant participants may be excluded or marginalised as professionals take on specific activities as part of their perceived role. On the other hand, Baric sees health education as a more active process which is concerned with raising individual competence and knowledge about health and illness, about the body and its functions, about prevention and coping and with raising awareness about social, political and environmental factors that influence health. Health *education* should ensure that people are competent and knowledgeable whilst health *promotion* should facilitate their active involvement in the decision-making process.

Not all authors agree on the difference between health promotion and health education. Tones (1986) has suggested that health promotion is often perceived to be about promoting positive health and well-being rather than just preventing disease. He warns that this could lead to people being promised an idealistic state of health which is unobtainable and also that it can lead to a form of 'healthism'. By this, he means that some elite individuals may manage to achieve a state of health which encompasses physical fitness, freedom from disease, coping skills, satisfactory social relationships, etc., leaving the majority who cannot achieve this feeling that they have failed in some way, whereas they may be constrained by their social and environmental context from achieving positive well-being. Williams (1984) has also cautioned against the over-enthusiastic use of the term 'health promotion' as this may be misinterpreted as a coercive 'sales' strategy to persuade people to 'buy' a health product which they may neither want nor need. Both Williams (1984) and Tones (1986) seem to agree that health education is an activity which promotes health-related learning. As Tones suggests, it may 'produce changes in belief or attitude and facilitate the acquisition of skills; or it may generate changes in behaviour or lifestyle.' Others see health education as a part of health promotion (French and Adams, 1986; Gott and O'Brien, 1990) and that the processes involved depend on the concept of health adopted and the approach to health promotion will evolve from this.

Clearly, there is no easy definition of health promotion, but for the purposes of this chapter health promotion is perceived to be the broader activities which enable people to achieve human potential, of which health education is a part.

Although there seems to be a general feeling in nursing that changes in approaches to practice, such as those promoted by Project 2000 (UKCC, 1986), are new and as such should be treated with caution, the principles underlying such innovations are scarcely original. Florence Nightingale not only introduced education and training for nurses but possessed an analytical and forward-thinking mind. Although nursing as we know it was only in its infancy under Miss Nightingale's influence, she was already planning for the future direction of nursing in relation to individual and societal change. In 1891 she wrote in one of her letters:

> 'I look forward to the day when there are no nurses of the sick, only nurses of the well'
>
> (Nightingale, 1891)

This may seem to us naive, but just over 50 years later Aneurin Bevan had a similar vision when he created the National Health Service. Florence Nightingale saw health in terms of prevention and eradication of disease because of the conditions she observed around her. She saw the main obstacles as bad hygiene, poor nutrition and poverty. It was her aim that nurses in both hospitals and the community should help people to overcome these obstacles. She gave papers at conferences in which she stressed the role of the nurse as a health educator, particularly in the home:

> 'Health nursing is to keep or put the constitution of the healthy child or human being in such a state as to have no disease'
>
> (Nightingale, 1893)

Are we any nearer nurses being truly active in health promotion and education than we were 100 years ago? Is it appropriate that nurses should take on this role? In answer to the first question, there

is evidence to show that nurses are not generally engaging in health promotion. There are, of course, particular areas of nursing such as health visiting, school nursing and practice nursing which do have health education within their brief. Often, however, it is viewed as an area of special interest which is introduced as an 'extra' if time allows, rather than as a continuous thread running throughout their work. Studies undertaken by the Health Education Council give some clues as to why this should be. In 1980 they found that less than one half of all schools of nursing in England and Wales had a working definition of health education. A later study in 1982 found that nurse tutors were themselves inadequately educated to prepare learner nurses for this role. Other studies have suggested possible inadequacies in nursing which may have contributed to nurses abdicating a health education role. Syred (1981) has argued that nurse education lacks a framework for health education. By this she means that nurses are not taught the necessary concepts or guidelines in order to function as health teachers. However, whilst Syred urges nurses to incorporate the Health Belief Model (Becker and Maiman, 1975) into their care planning, she does not present any empirical evidence on which to base her convictions.

Traditionally, nurses have been taught to nurse the sick within a medical framework, or model, which embodies the principles of diagnosis, treatment and cure. There is no analogous framework for health within nursing, probably because, until the advent of Project 2000, nursing has been unable to unleash itself from the medical model. Other studies (Faulkner and Ward, 1983; Macleod Clark *et al.*, 1990) have highlighted interpersonal skills as the factor most lacking in the nurses' ability to become health educators. The ability to ask questions sensitively and to listen and respond to the client's needs are undeniably important assets to the health educator. However, as Gott and O'Brien (1990) point out, it is not only communication skills which are relevant to health promotion activities. It is also the ability to understand health behaviour and the contextual nature of this as well as appreciating the meaning of health promotion. It could be, then, that nurses need both skills and a deeper knowledge of health and health beliefs in order to practise effectively.

In their own experience many nurses find aspects of the work stressful (Booth and Faulkner, 1986) and little value is placed upon their own health. For example, night duty, long shifts and coping with death all place stress on the nurse which if unacknowledged, as it frequently is, may leave the nurse feeling that her own health is undervalued and that she is powerless to remove the obstacles (Seedhouse, 1986). It is possible that, given the appropriate health-orientated environment within which to learn and practise, in conjunction with communication skills training, nurses could overcome some of the problems that currently militate against them becoming effective health promoters.

Turning to the second question, how appropriate is it for nursing to move in this direction? The World Health Organisation views health promotion as an important activity for all health professionals. At a world conference in 1977 a statement was made which has become known as the 'Declaration of Alma-Ata'. It reads:

> 'The main social target of governments and the World Health Organisation in the coming decades should be the attainment by all citizens of the world by the year 2000 of a level of health that will permit them to lead a socially and economically productive life. *Primary health care is the key to attaining this target'*
>
> (WHO, 1978, our emphasis)

Primary health care includes all health professionals working at the interface between the individual or community and the health care system in operation. Nurses are a very important part of primary health care, working in partnership with their medical and paramedical colleagues. The WHO has set targets (WHO, 1985) related to many aspects of health to be achieved on an international level by the year 2000. For example, one target is that all member nations will have a smoking population of not more than 20%. Other targets are related to environment, lifestyles and research, etc. Some of these targets have recently been adopted by the Department of Health in the UK (DoH, 1992). Nursing plays an increasingly important role in helping to achieve the WHO targets. There has been official acceptance by the DHSS since 1983 that nurses should be trained as health educators:

> 'Courses leading to a professional qualification should enable the nurse to acquire the competencies required to advise on the promotion of health and the prevention of illness'
>
> (DHSS, 1983)

Bureaucratic decrees are not in themselves reason enough for nurses to accept this challenging role. Indeed, Gott and O'Brien (1990) have suggested that health promotion policies frequently seem to misinterpret or ignore preceding documents, making it difficult for nurses to develop their own policy. An example of this is the Department of Health document *Promoting Better Health* (DoH, 1988) which claims that doctors are in the best position to promote health. It largely ignores the potential role of nurses except as handers-out of leaflets and adopts a 'victim-blaming' approach to health promotion which flies in the face of previous documents such as the Cumberlege Report (DHSS, 1986) on neighbourhood nursing and the Ottawa Charter for Health Promotion (1986) to which the UK was a signatory. Both of these documents acknowledge that nurses have an important role to play and that health promotion should be brought about through public participation and collaboration between different professions and institutions.

However, underlying both the WHO's (1978) and the DHSS's (1983) statements are the same principles that Florence Nightingale was applying back in the 1890s. The main principle is one of change – changes in economy, technology and lifestyle lead to changes in **demography** (the study of populations), environment and expectations. These factors are all closely related to the health of a community. For example, technological advances and economic growth since the Second World War have led to lifestyle changes. These include increased leisure time, dietary changes such as an overall increase in fat consumption, and environmental changes such as increases in lead levels. This means that the problems facing health workers are also changing and in today's society some of the main challenges are chronic illness, old age and care of the dying. The means of meeting these challenges lie in the promotion and maintenance of an acceptable level of health and the prevention of disease which can exacerbate the problems of an ageing population. Nursing cannot afford to turn its back on this challenge.

The challenge of promoting health

If we accept that it is desirable and appropriate for nurses to be engaged in health promotion, how then can we prepare to meet the challenge? The major part of this chapter will aim to demonstrate a variety of arenas within which nurses can practise health promotion. Each will be examined in terms of the potential of individuals or communities, the obstacles which work against them achieving these potentials, and the role of the nurse in enabling individuals or communities to overcome these obstacles.

In this context, it is useful to consider how the nurse might practise and not simply what she should do. It is useful at this stage to consider some possible approaches to health promotion. According to Tones (1986), there are three main approaches to health promotion. These can be seen as the traditional approach of health education to preventing illness, the self-empowering approach which enables people to make decisions, and the radical approach which works towards political and social change. Each of these approaches will be considered in more depth and their application to nursing explored.

The preventive approach

Prevention of ill health has traditionally been the aim of preventive medicine and health educationists. In the short term the aim of the preventive approach is to increase people's knowledge about a particular health issue such as smoking, thereby changing attitudes and behaviour. Ultimately, those using this approach to health promotion hope to achieve changes in **morbidity** and **mortality** statistics; in other words, to reduce the incidence and prevalence of certain diseases and subsequent deaths from them. This can be illustrated by much of the current publicity surrounding AIDS. Government literature and figures reproduced in newspapers and magazines constantly remind us of the number of people who are HIV-positive, the number of deaths from AIDS and the projected numbers for future years if people do not change their sexual and social behaviour. The aim of health educators using a preventive approach is to educate people about AIDS in the hope that this will deter them from having unsafe sex or using intravenous drugs, thereby curbing the increasing numbers of HIV-positive individuals. The educative processes involved may include individual counselling, mass media campaigns, group work, the availability of leaflets and posters, or a combination of these.

Caplan (1969) has identified three levels of prevention, the preventive approach being appropriate at any one of them. Caplan first suggested his conceptual framework in his discussion of promoting mental health in the community. However, it is fairly obvious how it can be applied to a wide range of physical and social conditions as well as mental health:

Primary prevention Reducing the risk of members of a community succumbing to a particular obstacle. For example, preventing disease by **immunisation**.

Secondary prevention Activities involved in reducing the duration of an established obstacle, thus reducing its **prevalence** in the community. For example, screening and early diagnosis of cervical cancer.

Tertiary prevention The prevention of further disability or suffering in those where an obstacle is already established. For example, preventing loss of dignity in the confused elderly patient.

Caplan's framework is not without its critics, primarily because it does appear to maintain the medical model of health care based on disease. However, Caplan's original work looked at mental health in the community and by this he was referring to:

'. . . the potential of a person to solve his problems in a reality based way'
(Caplan, 1969, page vii)

This seems to relate comfortably to Seedhouse's (1986) ideas about health and human potential as discussed earlier and thus, in its broadest sense, Caplan's framework can be seen as a useful tool for approaching health promotion.

The problem with the preventive approach to health promotion is that it takes a very narrow view of health, which is seen purely as the absence of disease. This ignores the more positive view of health proposed by the World Health Organisation (1946) and upheld in more recent documents such as the Ottawa Charter on Health Promotion (1986). It also ignores the views of health that lay people themselves may hold. In this sense it can be described as paternalistic in that the view is taken that health experts know what is best for the good of the people. It assumes, also, that if individuals do not take responsible action to prevent disease then they are themselves to blame for the consequences. This 'victim-blaming' approach has been criticised for its apparent ignorance of the social and environmental determinants of health and illness as described in the Black Report (Townsend and Davidson, 1982). In this respect it can be seen to be ethically questionable since the very things which the health educator seeks to prevent may in fact be caused by the political and economic fabric of society. For example, it could be argued that people turn to drugs in areas of high unemployment, thus increasing their risk of AIDS. But some of the underlying causes of unemployment may be outside the control of the individual. The preventive approach may also be seen as economically unsound since, to use Zola's metaphor (cited in McKinlay, 1979), it relies on intensive efforts at fishing people out of the river before they drown rather than concentrating on the factors upstream which are causing them to fall in. In other words, the problems of unemployment, poverty and racial discrimination should be addressed at a political level.

On the positive side, there may be occasions when individuals do want information in relation to their health and when learning something about their body or their environment may help them to change their behaviour and prevent ill health. This would be most likely in an acute situation where a life has been threatened, perhaps following a myocardial infarction or a road traffic accident.

Traditionally, where nurses have engaged in health-promoting activities it has been at the preventive level and to a large extent this is still the case. For example, the White Paper *Working for Patients* (DoH, 1989a) exhorts general practitioners to be more involved in screening and health assessment, which it suggests can be delegated to the practice nurse. The aim is to increase immunisation uptake and screening procedures for diseases such as cervical cancer and hypertension, thus preventing future disease. Whilst this appears to be an effective measure in which nurses can actively be involved, it appears to be limited by the problems mentioned above. It seems probable that nurses need to consider expanding their role in this area by developing the skills which will enable them to take a more self-empowering approach to health promotion. However, before dis-

cussing self-empowerment further, some in-depth examples of the preventive approach will be presented, which can be used to evaluate the method.

Promoting immunisation uptake – an example of primary prevention

Primary prevention involves activities which reduce the risk of members of a community succumbing to a particular obstacle. Some examples include the prevention of communicable disease by immunisation, the prevention of pregnancy by contraception and the prevention of serious injury and death on the roads by seatbelt legislation. You can probably think of other examples. It is the secondary obstacles that usually work against us achieving the potential we desire. For example, most of us in today's society would find the concept of planned parenthood desirable. However, our bodies are regulated by homeostatic mechanisms to produce fertile ova and sperm. We can overcome that primary obstacle to an unwanted pregnancy by using contraception, but experience tells us that the equation isn't that simple. A young woman, for example, may become pregnant in the belief that she was 'safe' the first time she had intercourse without using contraception. The obstacles facing her would be ignorance and possibly pressure from her partner. It is in helping people to overcome these secondary obstacles that the nurse can play a major role, using a nursing process approach to assess the individual's response to the obstacles facing them and planning care to meet these individual needs.

The discovery of immunological mechanisms and the development of *vaccines* means that, potentially, humankind can protect itself from any communicable disease of which it has knowledge. Thus, major diseases such as smallpox have been eradicated to an extent which makes immunisation unnecessary on a worldwide basis and other diseases such as tuberculosis are well controlled in the Western world. Immunisation policies are developed according to certain criteria such as severity and frequency of the disease and other important factors. So, for example, in the UK we do not immunise against yellow fever because although it can be severe, it is not very frequent. We do, however, have immunisation policies for infectious diseases such as measles, diphtheria and polio as they are all severe, particularly in childhood, and would be frequent if it were not for the high degree of immunity we now have in the community, known as *herd immunity*. To illustrate the issues which are raised when looking at immunisation as a means of primary prevention, whooping cough (*Bordatella pertussis*) immunisation will be used as an example.

Whooping cough is a highly communicable bacterial disease which primarily affects the trachea and bronchi. It is typified by paroxysmal coughing which may last for two to three months. The disease may be complicated by lung damage such as collapse or bronchopneumonia, and by cerebral anoxia which can cause brain damage. The majority of complications and deaths occur in infants under six months of age. As can be seen from Fig. 3.1, prevalence of the disease has fallen dramatically since 1957 when the vaccine was introduced.

It should be noted that notification of whooping cough (and other infectious diseases) is notoriously poor and it has been suggested that notifications represent the true number by only a third or a quarter (Bedford, 1991). In addition, dramatic declines in mortality from whooping cough (Fig. 3.2) have also been apparent. Note, however, that much of the decline in mortality was occurring before 1957, suggesting that improved nutritional standards and medical care after the Second World War may have also contributed to this.

The recommended schedule of vaccination is:

First dose – 2 months of age
Second dose – 3 months
Third dose – 4–6 months (DoH, 1990a)

In 1974 there was a fall-off in the uptake of immunisation which lead to major **epidemics** in 1977–1979 and 1981–1983 (DHSS, 1984). This **epidemiological** evidence suggests that immunisation against whooping cough contributes significantly to its prevention in the community.

So far, the straight facts about whooping cough have been presented. With this evidence it would be reasonable to assume that the vaccine is available, parents take it up for their children and whooping cough is well controlled. Unfortunately, it is not as simple as it at first appears. Despite the obvious beneficial effects of immunity against whooping cough, uptake in England has not approached 100%. The real problem with the uptake of whooping cough immunisation is that, although the overall figures have improved, there are still vast discrepancies between districts. Whilst some

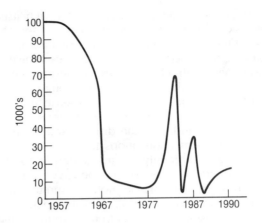

Fig. 3.1 *Notification of whooping cough 1957–1990 (DoH, 1990a)*

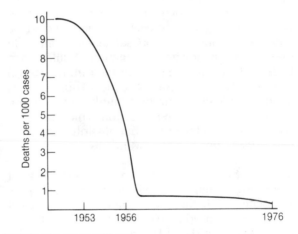

Fig. 3.2 *UK deaths per 1000 notified cases of whooping cough 1953–1976 (DHSS, 1984)*

may achieve immunisation levels of 80% or 90%, others are in the low 60s. Clearly, prevention of the disease is impossible whilst there are still large pockets of unprotected children.

As mentioned earlier, there was actually a fall in uptake in 1974 and this can largely be accounted for by the controversy surrounding the safety of the vaccine, when whooping cough vaccine was implicated as the cause of severe brain damage in some children. Some of the effects of this controversy continue today. The most recent assessment of risk from whooping cough vaccine (DoH, 1990a) suggests that neurological damage occurs so rarely that its frequency cannot be accurately measured. This has to be weighed up against the risks associated with whooping cough itself. The risk of dying from the disease is 1 in 5000 cases (DHSS, 1984). Whilst there is no information available on the long-term morbidity resulting from whooping cough, other factors to consider are the distress for a child with whooping cough and the long-term complications of the disease itself. In addition parents are put under considerable stress caring for a child with the disease and there are also longer term implications for the community as well as the family, such as caring for the handicapped child or for the bereaved parents. The implications for promoting immunisation are therefore very powerful. A further potentially forceful pressure on parents to take up immunisation may come as a result of recent health service legislation, the NHS and Community Care Act (DoH, 1990b). As part of the NHS reforms, contracts will be held by general practitioners which encourage targets in preventive medicine to be met. For example, it is proposed that immunisation rates for each practice population should reach 80%. GPs will not be paid for their immunisation services if the targets are not met. Thus, there is almost inevitably going to be further pressure on families to take up immunisation which may not come only from the doctor but possibly from practice nurses, health visitors and district nurses as well.

Given the evidence that immunisation against whooping cough is beneficial and that the risks associated with the vaccine are relatively small and are minimised by each individual child's history being considered before immunisation, why is it that the immunisation uptake is not nearer 100%? In other words, what are the secondary obstacles which prevent parents from having their children immunised and how can the nurse help them to overcome them?

Lack of knowledge of the disease and the vaccine

The potential to protect an individual from a communicable disease such as whooping cough may not be achieved through ignorance and fear. People do not always act on knowledge alone, but without accurate information they do not have the foundations on which to base a decision. Perkins (1982) found that parents often had incomplete or distorted knowledge of whooping cough and the effects of the vaccine. Nurses can help parents to reach their decision by assessing the parent's level of knowledge, discussing the arguments for and against immunisation and giving information where appropriate. As Perkins points out, helping the parents to sort out the information involves a partnership between nurse and client. This approach may also involve designing informative notice boards or posters in the clinical area, ensuring that the potential language barriers of those from ethnic minorities are addressed.

Restricted access to the vaccine

There could be several reasons for restricted access to the vaccine. There may be geographical difficulties, for example the clinic or surgery may be a long distance from home involving bus journeys, perhaps with awkward push chairs and toddlers. The cost of such a journey might be prohibitive. Nurses can help by being aware of local immunisation facilities and advising parents on the facilities nearest to them.

Lack of motivation

Some research studies have found (Townsend and Davidson, 1982; While, 1985) that there is a lower uptake of immunisation among the lower social classes. This is partly due to ignorance, but is more often due to a lack of motivation. This can be because of social and economic conditions such as poor housing and unemployment which may have a generally demoralising effect, leading to apathy and poor motivation. An awareness of these factors and an understanding of the interaction between social factors and health behaviour can enable the nurse to approach parents sensitively in the discussion of immunisation, responding to the individual needs as they arise. There does appear to be a need for more research into motivation and immunisation uptake so this is a further area in which nurses can be involved.

Promoting health screening – an example of secondary prevention

We now come on to the second part of Caplan's (1969) model of prevention. Secondary prevention can be seen as the activities involved in reducing the duration of an established obstacle. Some examples of secondary prevention are:

- The reduction of mortality from **invasive carcinoma** of the cervix by the early detection of **pre-invasive carcinoma**. This procedure is known as screening.
- The reduction of stroke incidence by screening for those with high blood pressure.
- Reduction of lung cancer mortality by stopping smoking.
- Reduction of antisocial behaviour, accidents and liver disease by stopping alcohol misuse.

Secondary prevention can be loosely broken down into screening procedures and reducing health-damaging behaviours. By routinely examining apparently healthy people, screening aims to detect either those who are likely to develop a particular disease or those in whom the disease is already present but not yet producing symptoms. There are many screening programmes advocated in the UK, among which are included screening for rubella immunity among pregnant women, for phenylketonuria in the newborn, for the developmental progress of children, and for hypertension. Cervical cancer screening will be used as an example of how screening can be effective, the obstacles that work against people being screened, and the nurse's role.

Cervical cancer continues to be a common cause of death among women. In 1987, 1763 women died from the disease (DoH, 1989b). Although some risk factors have been identified in its aetiology, for example herpes virus and several sexual partners (Hakama, 1983), there are no proven methods of primary prevention. The only practical way of controlling the disease is therefore early diagnosis by screening. Setting up any screening programme depends on several factors:

- The availability of a safe, repeatable and valid test.
- The effect of early treatment on the prognosis of the disease.
- The relative costs and benefits of the programme.
- The acceptability of the screening programme to the public (Open University, 1985).

In the case of cervical cancer screening, the smear test is available every five years to women between 20 and 65 years at family doctors, family planning clinics, well women clinics, and hospital inpatient and outpatient services. It is a safe test involving the removal of cells from the surface of the cervix. The cells are taken from the transformation zone where the columnar epithelium meets the squamous epithelium, with little or no risk to the individual. The test is repeatable and it is valid, i.e. it shows what it is supposed to show. The cost of surgery, radiotherapy and aftercare in the treatment of invasive carcinoma of the cervix is much higher than for the screening procedure and treatment of carcinoma in situ (the pre-invasive stage of the cancer). Of more importance, detection and early treatment of cervical cancer is of demonstrable benefit to the woman concerned. Carcinoma in situ can be treated by laser or surgically (by cone biopsy) which completely removes the altered cells. In almost all cases the woman will go on to lead a normal reproductive life, with no invasive stage of the carcinoma. The screening procedure for cervical cancer is therefore not misleading in its effects on outcomes, i.e. it does lead to early detection and effective treatment and not just an early diagnosis which could be used to exaggerate survival rates. In other words, women in whom carcinoma in situ has been identified and treated recover; they do not just live longer with the knowledge that they have cancer. Given this seemingly safe and effective screening programme, why is it that thousands of women continue to die of cervical cancer every year? The main reason is that many woman are not screened and there are a variety of possible reasons for this.

Fears and beliefs about cancer

One of the obstacles which prevents women taking up the screening service is their fears and beliefs about the nature of cancer. Accepting screening is an acknowledgement of cancer. Despite the fact that many forms of cancer are now curable, many people equate cancer with certain death and prefer to dissociate from it completely. Susan Sontag (1978) has described how it is the metaphoric invasion and destruction of the body by the advancing army of cancer which seems to differentiate it in people's minds from other diseases. Nurses also may find it difficult to discuss cancer, especially in cases where the client is unaware of her diagnosis. Even the discussion of screening can be hard if both nurse and client are trying to avoid the difficult issue of cancer. Being frank about the purpose of cervical screening brings cancer out into the open. It takes a great deal of skill on the part of the nurse if she is to help the client to overcome her fears. A study by King (1987) found that generally older women attributed cervical cancer to a 'germ' or 'smoking' and therefore resisted the test on the grounds that it did not apply to them. She also found that older women tended to resist screening as they felt that it reflected on their morality, as cervical cancer was thought to be a 'dirty' disease resulting from 'promiscuity'. Nurses can help to allay these worries by giving accurate and reassuring information.

Fear of the test

King's study also found that resistance to cervical screening among older women was often due to fear of the test itself. It was held to be a painful procedure and many were reluctant to be examined internally, particularly by a male doctor. King concludes that beliefs about the test are the strongest indicators of non-attendance. Nurses can use this research finding by helping women, especially in middle age, to understand the nature of the test and reinforcing its benefits to all age groups.

Organisation of the service

The organisation of cervical screening in the UK is such that if women are not screened at one of the existing centres or they do not attend their GP spontaneously for a smear test, they will not be automatically invited for screening. There is no centralisation of the programme so if a woman moves to another part of the country she is unlikely to be followed up for repeat screening. There have been cases reported in the media of women developing invasive carcinoma because they have never been informed that they had a positive smear. These are obviously obstacles outside the individual's control but women in general and nurses in particular should lobby for a more organised service. Potentially, the introduction of the GP contracts mentioned previously should have a positive effect on the organisation of screening tests. If doctors are aiming to meet targets for cervical screening then it is less likely that eligible women will be overlooked.

To summarise, immunisation and screening have been presented as examples of health promotion using the preventive approach. The aim is to pre-vent disease such as whooping cough and cervical cancer by informing individuals and communities about the possible health risks and the benefits to their health if they accept the services offered. However, as we have seen, information alone does not always motivate people to take health action. It may be that obstacles apparently or actually outside their control are operating and that a different approach to health promotion may be more appropriate. We will now turn to such an approach which encourages people to develop decision-making skills.

Self-empowerment

Tones (1986) argues that whilst understanding a health issue may be a precursor to action, it is not sufficient. Thus, health educationists have argued that provision of information should be accompanied by a process of belief and values clarification, which should be followed by development of decision-making skills. The overall aim of the self-empowerment approach is therefore to foster informed choice, which stems ideologically from the concept of autonomy (Harris, 1985). It is important to consider, however, that even in democratic communities people do not always have individual autonomy or a completely free choice about their health. An example in the UK would be the seatbelt legislation. Whilst the law relating to this was brought about within the democratic framework, some would argue that people should remain at liberty to choose whether they wear a seatbelt or not.

A second point in relation to choice is that self-empowerment is about enabling people to make their own decisions even if the decision finally arrived at is not that favoured by the health promoter. It is therefore important to remember that the perceived healthy option is not the only option and to ensure that education for health does not become indoctrination (Campbell, 1990) However, self-empowerment does not simply aim to make people more skilled in their decision-making, but to use those skills to empower themselves and others. In this way it is possible that social change can be brought about which would alter the environment in which people seek to become healthy.

Tones *et al.* (1990) suggest that such a process involves addressing issues such as self-esteem and self-efficacy as well as social skills. Self-esteem is important as individuals who do not perceive themselves favourably may find it more difficult to change or to take health action. Self-efficacy relates to a person's perceptions of his or her own capabilities, which according to Bandura (1977b) can be influenced by past experience and through self-mastery by accomplishment of specific actions.

Thus, the self-empowerment approach to health promotion involves much more than preventing disease through the provision of knowledge. The health promoter must be able to provide the information which people need to make an informed choice, but she also needs to be able to assess self-esteem and self-efficacy and to appreciate the health beliefs and values of others, as well as enabling people to develop skills in decision-making and assertiveness. This clearly requires a great deal of skill and initiative on the part of the health promoter and some nurses may not feel that they are prepared for such a role. For example, ideally, learning how to make decisions should be done in a safe environment (i.e. one where the wrong decision will not result in unfavourable outcomes) and should allow for practice through simulation and role play (Bond and Kendall, 1990). Preparation for general nursing remains limited in its scope for learner nurses to become skilled in group work and learning methods. However, this does not mean that a self-empowerment approach to health promotion should not be attempted, but it could be seen as an approach which may be employed by the more advanced practitioner.

The provision of health information could be seen as the first stage of the self-empowerment approach, and potentially all nurses could be involved at this stage.

Application of the self-empowerment approach to coronary heart disease (CHD)

Coronary heart disease (CHD) is a major health problem in the UK (British Cardiac Society, 1987). One way of reducing the prevalence of this condition and enhancing the quality of people's lives may be through the self-empowerment approach, thus enabling people to make informed decisions about their lifestyle. This may involve considerations of diet, exercise and smoking behaviour.

As Tones *et al.* (1990) suggest, the first stage of self-empowerment may be considered to be information giving in relation to people's beliefs and values. Some background information which may be useful to the nurse is summarised here, followed by discussion of how health may be promoted by enabling people to make informed choices. Smoking is considered as a separate health issue although it does have significant implications for coronary heart disease.

Background information to CHD

The term coronary heart disease (CHD) includes factors which predispose to acute manifestations such as **atherosclerosis** and those which precipitate the eventual myocardial infarction such as plaque rupture, thrombosis and coronary spasm. It is often thought of as a disease of affluence because of its prevalence in the Western world but this is deceptive because it is more likely to be people from the relatively poorer communities who die of it (Townsend and Davidson, 1982). However, it is likely to kill more people from any social group in the UK than any other single cause of death, including cancer. For example, in 1982, 31% of male deaths resulted from CHD compared to 24% from all cancers. For women, the figures were 23% for CHD and 21% for cancer (OPCS, 1982). Currently, England and Wales have the highest rate of death from CHD (about 600 per 100,000) after Finland and Scotland. The lowest rate is in Japan (about 100 per 100,000) (Marmot, 1985). The most recently available figures suggest that in 1987, 81,037 men and 63,824 women died from CHD (DoH, 1989b).

CHD is also responsible for substantial morbidity. Clearly, it is a cause of both individual suffering and community concern since treatment puts a strain on resources in terms of human resources in the health service, hours lost from work due to sickness, expensive surgical procedures, and drugs and rehabilitation. Prevention of CHD could reduce this considerably.

A report of a WHO meeting in 1984 (WHO, 1984b) stated that the debate is now about 'how, not whether CHD could be prevented'. The British Cardiac Society (1987) has recommended that prevention be implemented using both a population approach (i.e assuming that all members of a community are at risk) as well as a high risk approach (i.e. some members of a community are at higher risk than others and can be identified by screening procedures). The main risk factors which have been identified are raised serum **cholesterol** levels, smoking and high blood pressure. For the purposes of this part of the chapter we will concentrate on serum cholesterol and the role of diet in controlling it.

Serum cholesterol, dietary fat and CHD

Biochemically, cholesterol is an important steroid which forms the basis of many hormones such as the oestrogens and androgens. It is produced by the liver and its production appears to be related to dietary fat, particularly saturated fat. Atheromatous plaques in the blood vessels contain a high level of cholesterol (Datta and Ottaway, 1976). Geoffrey Rose, an epidemiologist, sees the role of serum cholesterol in CHD primarily as a population problem (Rose, 1987). In simple terms, he bases this proposal on the fact that among the Japanese (where CHD is not a problem) the mean serum cholesterol is less than 3 mmols per litre. In countries where the mean serum cholesterol level is above 5 mmols per litre, CHD is always a problem. In the UK, the average serum cholesterol level is 6 mmols per litre. Rose states that by old age, 90% of the UK population have developed a high degree of atherosclerosis and it is therefore everybody's problem. Even among individuals of relatively low risk the commonest cause of death is still CHD.

One way of lowering serum cholesterol levels in the population is through dietary change. Most experts (COMA, 1984; British Cardiac Society, 1987) agree that serum cholesterol levels can be controlled by changing the ratio of saturated fatty acids to polyunsaturated fatty acids in the diet. The terms *saturated* and *polyunsaturated* refer to the chemical bonding of the fatty acid and its reactivity with oxygen. Thus, polyunsaturates are oxidised much more readily than saturated fatty acids. Saturated fatty acids (SFA) are generally found in animal products such as meat and dairy produce whilst polyunsaturated fatty acids (PUFA) are found in vegetable and fish oils, although some are higher in PUFA than others. For example, among the vegetable oils safflower oil is higher in PUFA than olive oil. There are also exceptions — palm oil is composed mainly of SFA. This demonstrates the importance of accurate food labelling since foods containing vegetable oils may, on closer inspection, contain a high level of palmitic acid, the main component of palm oil.

The Committee on Medical Aspects of Food Policy (COMA, 1984) made recommendations to the government on how the national diet should change to make appreciable differences to the average serum cholesterol level. COMA recommended that 15% of food energy should be from SFA and 35% of food energy from total fat intake. The ratio of PUFA to SFA (the P/S ratio) should be increased to 0.45 (1:2.2) or more. The current average P/S ratio in the UK is 0.27 (1:3.7) compared with 0.5 (1:2) in the USA, where mortality from CHD has fallen dramatically over the past 20 years (Marmot, 1985). An analysis of food intake over a 20 year period in the USA appears to confirm the evidence that it is the protective effect of a high P/S ratio which is more important in the prevention of CHD than the harmful effect of saturated fatty acids.

Other recommendations put forward by COMA are an increase in fibre-rich **carbohydrates** (bread, cereals, fruit and vegetables) to compensate in energy for the reduced fat consumption, and that foods should be clearly labelled regarding their fat content. There are many areas of agreement between the NACNE report (1983) and the COMA report (1984).

Table 3.1. *Intake of foods and nutrients (g/day) 1965 and 1977 and % change in men aged 35–50, US Nationwide Food Consumption Survey (Stamler, 1981)*

Food or nutrient	1965	1977	% change
Milk and milk drinks	236	203	−14
Cheese	13	18	+38.4
Eggs	51	41	−19.6
Beef	102	79	−22.5
Pork	82	52	−30
Fish	13	17	+30.8
Fats and oils	39	19	−51.3
Total fat	132.4	109.3	−17.4

The role of exercise

Exercise can be considered alongside dietary factors since it is physical activity which determines how much of the energy provided by food is expended. It is the relationship between energy intake and energy expenditure which may determine the degree to which risk factors such as obesity and hypertension are present, although other factors such as basal metabolism and gender may also be important. Although the British Cardiac Society (1987) point out that there have been no controlled research studies of the role of exercise in primary prevention, there are some studies which appear to demonstrate the protective effect of exercise against CHD. A study by Morris et al. (1980) found that British civil servants were less likely to develop CHD if they undertook some vigorous exercise. A study on primates (Kramsch et al., 1981) found that the diameter of the coronary blood vessels was greater in monkeys who were more active and they developed less atherosclerosis than their inactive counterparts fed on the same diet. Although this type of evidence is not conclusive, it is widely accepted that exercise may have a protective effect, operating through various mechanisms. These include improved cardiopulmonary function and exercise tolerance and a possible decrease in blood pressure as well as weight being more easily controlled. The NACNE report (1983) recommends that physical activity should be promoted alongside dietary changes.

A joint document by the Health Education Authority and the Sports Council (1987) divides fitness into three major areas. *Suppleness* is the ability to bend, stretch and turn through a range of movements; *strength* is the ability to exert force for pushing, pulling and lifting; and *stamina* is the ability to keep going whilst running or walking without getting tired quickly. It is stamina that helps to protect against heart disease and aerobic exercise is recommended to improve stamina. This kind of exercise is usually fairly energetic, keeps the body moving for about 20 minutes at a time and makes the individual fairly breathless. It is known as aerobic exercise because enough oxygen is breathed in to supply working muscles so an oxygen debt is not incurred. Aerobic exercise includes brisk walking, jogging, swimming and cycling as well as the exercises included in 'aerobic classes'. To maintain weight and stamina, the Health Education Authority (1987) suggest that aerobic exercise should be taken for 20–30 minutes two or three times per week. As with everything else, people's individual needs and abilities will vary and it is important to take account of this when helping clients to plan their exercise.

Self-empowerment and risk factors associated with CHD

Although there have been many reports (COMA, 1984; DHSS, 1981; Royal College of Physicians/British Cardiac Society, 1976) on the dietary aspect of preventing CHD, very few of them address the problem of how the health promoters can encourage the population to change its diet. Even the National Advisory Committee on Nutrition Education (NACNE, 1983), which was led by a working party from the Health Education Council, fails to give any practical guidelines on how their suggested goals might be achieved. As you will by now be beginning to appreciate, health promotion is not simply a process of giving people information and people changing their behaviour on the basis of that information. Lack of information is only one of the obstacles in the prevention of CHD. We will now turn to those obstacles which influence whether people change their dietary and exercise behaviour or not and some possible ways in which the nurse can enable them to make the decision to change by using the self-empowerment approach.

Information giving

People need sufficient and accurate information on which to base a decision. The nurse can find out how much the client knows about his health by careful assessment and provide clear and accurate information as necessary. This depends on the nurse herself being aware of research findings and keeping up to date with new knowledge. There is a variety of approaches to providing information which range from the one-to-one interaction, to visual displays, the provision of books and leaflets and group work. The self-empowerment approach determines that where information is provided, it should not only be accurate but in accordance with the client's needs, values and beliefs. It is therefore imperative that these are established before any information is imparted. Nurses can equally be involved in groups such as preparation for retirement or women's groups where information can be exchanged. In relation to nutrition, women's groups are particularly significant as there is evidence that women are the main providers of food within British families (Charles and Kerr, 1986).

Beliefs and values

When trying to empower people to reach healthy decisions in relation to diet and exercise, it is crucial to understand and work with their beliefs and values in relation to food, exercise and the relationship between their bodies, mind and health. The Health Belief Model (Becker and Maiman, 1975) may be a useful tool in aiding the assessment and understanding of people's health behaviours in relation to their health beliefs. This model was originally constructed by Becker and Maiman to try to explain why people do not carry out preventive health action, and some elements of the model (see Fig. 3.3) have been shown to be of particular value in explaining health behaviour. For example, Champion (1987) and Stillman (1977) have both demonstrated the particular validity of the variable of perceived barriers to preventive action. These are considered below.

One obstacle which may prevent people from changing their behaviour is their financial situation. Many people believe that eating 'health foods' is more expensive than their usual diet and those in most need of change probably have the lowest income. The Black Report (Townsend and Davidson, 1982) and *The Health Divide* (Whitehead, 1988) both report inequalities in health leading to higher levels of ill health among the unemployed and low income groups. Re-

ducing SFA intake, increasing the P/S ratio and increasing the energy intake from carbohydrates need not be expensive if carefully planned. For example, oily fish such as mackerel is cheaper than many types of meat, polyunsaturated margarines are cheaper than butter. Wholemeal bread and fresh fruit and vegetables do tend to be slightly more expensive, but they are more satisfying and can be made to go further than the cheaper processed foods. For example, root vegetables are relatively cheap and can fill out a reduced-meat casserole. Simple changes in cooking methods can also reduce fat consumption without affecting the family budget; for example, changing from frying to grilling.

However, there is some evidence to show that people living in the most disadvantaged areas do have to pay more for items such as wholemeal bread. Graham's (1984) research found that large council estates were often built considerable distances from town centres so that shopping involved either expensive journeys by public transport into town or paying higher prices at a local store where healthy alternatives are frequently unavailable. Large supermarkets where foods tends be cheaper are frequently on the outskirts of towns and necessitate the use of a car which many poorer families do not possess. Graham found that women's knowledge in relation to healthy eating was not lacking — they felt pro-

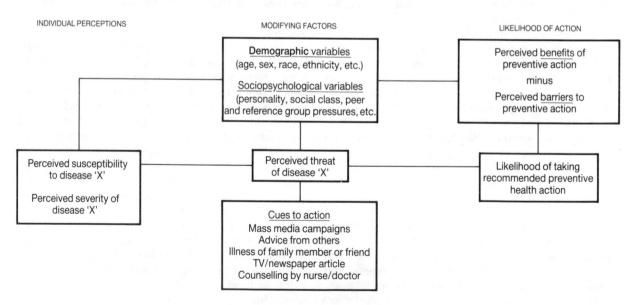

Fig. 3.3 *The health belief model (Becker and Maiman, 1975)*

hibited by the factors described and also that they were not doing their best for their families. Therefore, the belief that healthy eating is expensive is not entirely unfounded and it is important to consider these factors when planning for healthy eating with a client. Similarly, exercise can be perceived to be difficult because of expensive equipment, clothing or membership fees. Whilst it can be argued that exercise such as jogging or walking is free, women in particular may perceive themselves to have problems in carrying out these activities because of the need for child care.

Ultimately, the self-empowerment approach should enable people to assert their needs so that town planners and transport policy-makers, among others, take heed of the health of the community as well as the immediate goal of housing, transport and leisure provision, and child care facilities (Ottawa Charter, 1986).

The exploration of attitudes to food and exercise is an aspect of psychology which will not be considered here in detail. An *attitude* has been defined by Roediger *et al.* (1984, page 587) as 'a relatively stable tendency to respond consistently to particular people, objects or situations'. This suggests that attitudes can be held towards just about anything, including food, dietary behaviour and exercise, and that although they tend to be stable, they are not fixed. In other words, attitudes are amenable to change and are also open to conflict. Whilst a person may generally behave in accordance with the attitudes held, he may occasionally behave in a way which conflicts with his attitudes. For example, a person may hold favourable attitudes towards reducing saturated fats in his diet, but may also hold favourable attitudes towards cream cakes and chocolate. Therefore, making the decision to change the diet depends very much on how the individual thinks and behaves towards food and his attitude towards health. A fatalistic attitude, for example, would suggest a person who makes comments such as, 'We all have to die sometime so I may as well eat what I like now and enjoy it'. Part of the health promotion process is clarifying people's attitudes in order to enable change, if appropriate.

Attitudes can change but it tends to be a slow process. For example, the general attitude in the UK towards the consumption of polyunsaturated margarines is changing; butter is no longer seen as the only thing to spread on bread! How this change came about is probably due to a number of influences including information from a variety of sources (television, magazines, health personnel, etc.), changes in the availability of foodstuffs in the shops, advertising, and the social pressure to change. A study in Finland (Vartianinen *et al.*, 1987) has shown how a community approach to CHD has changed public attitudes to eating and lowered serum cholesterol levels, especially amongst adolescents. This has involved major changes in the Finnish way of life where dairy produce has traditionally been the staple diet of the population. Finnish nurses have been very active in this project, which has involved changes in school meals, reducing fat content of milk, encouraging retailers to stock less butter and more polyunsaturated margarines and providing farmers with incentives to produce fruit rather than dairy produce. Even if nurses are not taking part in formal research work, it is possible to help to change attitudes towards diet by finding out what the client's beliefs are about diet, exercise and health; using professional skills and knowledge to dispel any false ideas they may hold about dietary fat and its relationship to heart disease. It is not an uncommon belief, for example, that meat is an essential part of every main meal. You cannot force anybody to become vegetarian but healthy alternatives to red meat (such as fish and pulses) can be suggested. On a wider level, nurses can also be involved in hospital and school food policies and community group work, particularly with women as they do still tend to be the providers of food (Charles and Kerr, 1986).

Beliefs, attitudes and values may be cultural in origin. Culture can have a religious, ethnic or social origin. Cultural influences on diet are very strong and in a multicultural nation such as the UK, many of them are apparent. The influence of the Islamic culture, for example, is obvious in many communities where a halal butcher is present, reflecting the Muslim attitudes towards animal slaughter techniques. Within the indigenous British population, cultural attitudes to food are steeped in class tradition. The rather stereotyped view of the working man coming home to a 'good hot dinner' is based on cultural norms which responded to the needs of the manual labourer. As mines have closed down, farming becomes more technological and industry has moved from shipbuilding to light electronics, the need for heavy manual labour has decreased, but the cultural patterns take time to change. From the nursing point of view, it is important to take into account cultural attitudes to food before helping a client to plan his diet. This implies both finding out from the client what his cultural background is and being aware of the dietary preferences of that culture. In a multicultural society, no one could expect you to have a full knowledge of every cultural aspect of diet. Your most reliable source of such information is the client. However, people often need help in clarifying their own beliefs about aspects of their health and this is an important component of the self-empowerment approach, as self-awareness is necessary in facilitating the decision-making process.

Decision-making

Having provided and shared information about diet and exercise, explored and clarified beliefs and attitudes towards behavioural changes in these areas, the final stage of the self-empowerment approach is to facilitate decision-making. As a health promoter your aim is to enable decision-making, not to challenge the final decision reached. It is therefore important to be aware of your own attitudes towards diet and exercise and to separate those from the client's decision. In order to make effective decisions, people need to have the available options before them but they also need to have some idea about the potential outcomes of their decision and how this would relate to their own lifestyle and experience. As Tones *et al.* (1990) suggest, there is also an element of psychological control involved with decision-making which may include concepts such as self-esteem and self-efficacy. Whilst it is not possible to explore these concepts in detail here, it is important to recognise that an individual's health behaviour may be regulated by his or her feelings of personal mastery over a particular action, which Bandura (1977b) has suggested may be influenced by past experience, observation of others and persuasion. Thus, practice in decision-making should be a component of the self-empowerment process as it may develop or reinforce feelings of personal mastery. Simulation of real-life situations such as making a choice between walking or catching the bus, role-playing situations which might jeopardise a healthy decision such as being pressurised to eat high fat foods in a social situation, and rehearsing potential conflict within oneself, can all be useful techniques towards self-empowerment.

It is within such practice situations that self-esteem and self-efficacy can be enhanced, particularly where trust and confidence within a group have been established, as peer support can be very encouraging in making and sustaining a decision. It is not within the scope of this chapter to discuss skills in group work in any detail, but clearly in order to use the self-empowerment approach to health promotion it is a useful attribute to develop such skills, as well as skills in communication and understanding health behaviour. Tones *et al.* (1990) have argued that if the self-empowerment approach can lead to positive changes in self-esteem and self-efficacy then these are positive health-promoting achievements in themselves. In this sense, the self-empowerment approach can be seen not only as an approach to promoting changes in health behaviour, but as a way of directly and positively promoting health.

In summary, there is evidence to show that dietary fat and exercise play an important role in the development of CHD. CHD is thought to be a population problem, i.e. all members of our community are at risk. However, CHD is widely held to be a preventable condition and one of the factors in its aetiology, dietary fat, can be controlled, thus leading to a decrease in the incidence of the disease. Factors which work against people changing their diet in order to reduce serum cholesterol levels and increase the P/S ratio, and taking regular exercise, are lack of knowledge, existing beliefs and attitudes towards food and exercise, and a need to develop decision-making skills. The nurse has the potential to be influential in helping people to overcome or work around these obstacles by adopting a self-empowerment approach to health promotion.

Smoking and health

There are many behaviours in our society which could be seen as prejudicial to achieving human potential. Among them are misuse of drugs and alcohol, smoking and driving dangerously. Primary prevention of these behaviours begins before they have been started, as in the prevention of smoking among school children. Secondary prevention, however, involves helping people to give up the behaviour before any long-term damage is done. Usually, activities such as drinking and smoking are experienced as enjoyable by the participants and advice to give it up may be seen as an infringement on personal liberty. People are free to make their own choices, but nurses can help them to maintain personal autonomy whilst making the healthy choice and by supporting them in that decision.

As a further illustration of the self-empowerment approach, the use of tobacco will be used to illustrate the obstacles that prevent people from changing their behaviour and the nurse's role in helping them to overcome them.

Background information to smoking

Tobacco smoking is a widespread habit in the UK. The most recent figures suggest that 33% of men and 30% of women smoke (OPCS, 1990). It is responsible for a substantial degree of morbidity and mortality (Fig. 3.4). Research which was commenced in 1948 (Doll and Hill, 1952) demonstrated a relationship between smoking and lung cancer and it is now known to be associated with many other debilitating and life-threatening diseases such as chronic obstructive lung disease and coronary heart disease (Royal College of Physicians, 1983). Of a total of 600,000 deaths per year in the UK, 100,000 can be related to smoking. However, the onset of irreparable disease through smoking is relatively slow. Lung cancer may not be evident for 30 years or more after the commencement of smoking; giving up smoking even after 20 years is therefore going to be beneficial. This delay in the effects of smoking becoming evident accounts for the observable difference in lung cancer rates between men and women shown in Fig. 3.4. This is because women did not take up smoking seriously until after the Second World War – so its effects are only now becoming apparent – whereas men started smoking much earlier. The fact that lung cancer rates for men are declining as cigarette consumption falls is further evidence of the relationship between tobacco and lung cancer.

Apart from the long term consequences, there are immediate benefits of giving up smoking. Ex-smokers report feeling fitter, more energetic, having fewer coughs and colds and having more money available for other things. Given that smoking does have both these long-term and immediate effects on human potential, why don't people give up smoking more readily? There are a number of obstacles to this eventuality which

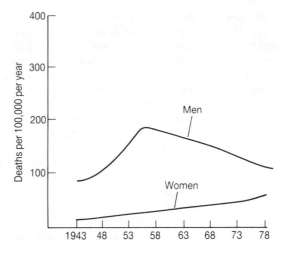

Fig. 3.4 *Death rates from lung cancer for men and women 1943–1978 (Royal College of Physicians, 1983)*

nurses should be aware of and which the self-empowerment approach may help to overcome.

Habituation/addition

Many smokers claim they cannot give up because they are '***addicted***'. There is still some debate as to whether nicotine is a physically addictive drug, but it is undoubtedly habit-forming and regular smoking maintains the blood level of nicotine. Smokers describe withdrawal effects such as irritability and depression when they stop smoking. Pharmacologically, nicotine has paradoxical effects on the body because of its action on both the central and autonomic nervous systems (Ashton and Stepney, 1982). The effects produced, for example, can be both relaxation and a greater ability to concentrate. Such effects appear to habituate the smoker into associating having a cigarette with other activities such as using the phone, sitting down after a meal or coping with stressful situations. Breaking these rituals can become extremely difficult.

Using the self-empowerment approach to enable a person to overcome this obstacle is appropriate since it involves not only the information necessary to make a decision, but also clarifying the individual's beliefs and attitudes to smoking and facilitating the decision-making process by enhancing self-esteem and self-efficacy. Again, the Health Belief Model (Becker and Maiman, 1975) may be helpful here in the assessment of people's beliefs and values about smoking. The nurse can start by helping a client to look more closely at the situations in which he is most likely to smoke and what alternative strategies can be utilised to overcome the need for a cigarette. This would also involve an analysis of the costs and benefits as perceived by the client of continuing to smoke and giving up, alongside the potential perceived costs and benefits of any alternative strategies. For example, the perceived stress related to giving up may be outweighed by the perceived benefits of saving money (Becker and Maiman, 1975).

It is important that the nurse uses her skill in assessment to ensure that decisions reached are, in fact, based on the client's perception of the situation rather than her own. For some individuals, support from a smoking cessation group or the use of nicotine chewing gum have been shown to be useful (Raw and Heller, 1984), but groups do not suit everybody and it appears that one-to-one support by a nurse can be very effective (Macleod Clark et al., 1990).

Motivation

People can only change their behaviour if they wish to do so. Research has shown that the intention of people to stop smoking is closely related to their desire to stop and this in turn is related to their attitude to smoking and health (Mattheson and Marsh, 1983). Attitudes to smoking vary between, 'This is the only thing I have which I enjoy' and 'It's too late to stop now'. Such attitudes may be changed by new knowledge or a new experience (such as the death of someone close from lung cancer) but information alone is unlikely to change attitudes. Attitudes can change under group pressure so that although smoking is often commenced and maintained under peer pressure, it can also be peers and social attitudes generally that make people want to stop. Public attitudes towards smoking have changed dramatically over the past 20 years – it is now unacceptable to smoke in many public places such as cinemas and on public transport and even some hospitals. The self-empowerment approach suggests that such attitudes and values should be clarified. As suggested earlier, attitudes are not fixed but people are unlikely to change if they have not thought about their attitude to their own smoking behaviour and that of others. For example, smokers commonly hold conflicting attitudes in that they feel positive

about their own smoking behaviour but negative towards being in a smoke-filled room. Such conflict in attitude can be explored, thus enabling the client to understand himself better and his motivations for continuing to smoke or wanting to give up.

Nurses can also help to raise public awareness and motivation to change smoking behaviour by being involved in smoking cessation initiatives in the community such as National No Smoking Day and hospital smoking policies.

Coping with emotions

Smokers frequently use their behaviour as a way of coping with emotions such as stress, anxiety and depression (Maclaine and Macleod Clark, 1991). Dealing with these emotions can be very difficult and may be related to feelings of low self-esteem and lack of personal mastery. Stress may be incurred by the fact that women may take on both domestic responsibilities as well as paid employment and this stress may be partially relieved by smoking. By exploring the underlying cause of the stress a nurse may be able to help an individual to identify the first step towards taking alternative stress management measures. One aspect of this may be to enable a person to feel that they can take some control over their lives by considering the alternatives. The nurse herself may be able to offer therapeutic interventions such as massage, relaxation or aromatherapy. There appears to be growing evidence that nursing itself is therapeutic (McMahon and Pearson, 1991). However, whilst a nurse may help a client to identify the cause of his stress or anxiety, it is important to be aware of the referral network, such as counselling, if the client needs more than relaxation exercises, for instance. It can be distressing for the client and arguably psychologically damaging if emotions are brought to the surface and then left unresolved.

Research has shown that nurses can be effective in helping people to give up smoking (Macleod Clark et al., 1990). This study suggests that the development of communication skills in nursing and health promotion is an important indicator of success. The research has shown that whilst the self-empowerment approach to enabling people to give up smoking does require some counselling skills, even with some fairly basic communication skills nurses can be effective. Exploring the client's perceptions by using open questions and listening skills, for example, were shown to be key indicators of success in enabling people to stop smoking.

In summary, the self-empowerment approach to health promotion has been illustrated by addressing two major health issues – CHD and smoking. The aim of the self-empowerment approach is to facilitate decision-making skills in the client which will potentially promote a healthy lifestyle. For the health promoter, this involves providing information which will enhance informed decision-making, clarifying attitudes and beliefs with the client, and facilitating the actual decision-making process. This may include analysing the client's perceptions of the costs and benefits of behaviour change, as well as considering such factors as self-esteem and self-efficacy.

The radical approach to health promotion

Tones *et al.* (1990) suggest that a third possible approach to health promotion is the radical option. This approach differs from both prevention and self-empowerment in that it attempts to tackle the determinants of health and illness at the social level rather than on an individual level. Whilst the preventive approach, and to a certain extent the self-empowerment approach, are derived ideologically from the concept of responsibility for self, the radical approach acknowledges that the social, environmental and political context have a major influence on the health of communities. This has been demonstrated by research into inequalities in health such as the Black Report (Townsend and Davidson, 1982) and upheld by more recent documents (Whitehead, 1988; Smith and Jacobson, 1988). For example, Whitehead highlights the problem of ill health related to poor nutrition among children and specifically targets the school meals service. Policy changes such as the abolition of price maintenance and national nutritional standards for children have resulted in a haphazard school meals service in which those children which are most needy often fare the worst. This is not an individual problem, but as Lang (1987, cited by Whitehead) puts it:

'Low income is the key link between food, poverty and health. Tackling low income goes entirely beyond the capacity of the local authority and into the realms of benefit policy. Above all, it needs national, not just local action'

But who is going to instigate such action and do nurses have any role to play here? Arguably, nurses are in a key position to take a radical approach to health promotion. They form a very large body of professionals who ought, through their professional organisations, trades unions and pressure groups, to be able to influence social and health policy. The potential for nurses taking the radical approach will be explored using two health issues as examples – these are alcohol abuse and mental health.

Background information to alcohol abuse

Over the past 20–30 years there has been a steady increase in the intake of alcohol in the British population (Smith, 1981). Well over 90% of the population drink alcohol to some extent (DHSS, 1985). It is therefore quite clearly a potential health issue which affects the vast majority. The increase in consumption is largely accounted for by the relative price of alcohol in an increasingly prosperous society. For example, in 1950 a bottle of whisky cost the equivalent of 659 minutes of manual work whilst in 1980 it cost only 153 minutes of manual work (NACNE, 1983). By comparison, the cost of a loaf of bread increased in these terms from the equivalent of nine minutes of work in 1950 to ten minutes in 1980. In other words, people are economically in a favourable position to purchase alcohol if they choose to do so.

Although the DHSS (1985) estimated that there are several hundred thousand alcoholics in the UK, which is undeniably both a health and social problem, the aim of the radical approach is to understand the causes of people drinking heavily and to take action to avert some of the determinants of alcoholism. Smith and Jacobson (1988) have differentiated between alcoholism and other types of problem drinking. They refer to 'heavy drinking' which may result in biochemical abnormalities such as toxic damage to the liver, 'problem drinking' which results in harm to self or others or arrest for drunkenness, and 'alcohol dependence' which results in a combination of the above effects.

Clearly, a great many people drink alcohol regularly although they may not be alcoholic in the sense that they are dependent on alcohol. They nevertheless expose themselves to health risks such as cirrhosis of the liver, gastrointestinal disturbances, degeneration of the central nervous system, metabolic disorders and an increased susceptibility to infection (Smith, 1981). In addition, there is the risk of accidental death or injury due to the effects of alcohol. The DHSS (1985) estimate that one third of all drivers and one quarter of all pedestrians killed on the roads had blood levels of alcohol exceeding the legal limit (80 mg per 100 ml). There are also the social consequences to consider – drunkenness contributes to aggressive and abusive behaviour which can be detrimental to the health of families and communities. Women are particularly at risk of violent attacks from alcoholic partners. The effect of alcohol on some physical disorders remains unclear. For example, it is uncertain how alcohol affects cardiovascular disease. Some epidemiological data suggests that those individuals who take some alcohol may be less susceptible to myocardial infarction than total abstainers (Marmot et al., 1981). However, overall the cost of misusing alcohol outweighs the possible benefits and the population as a whole would certainly benefit in health terms from a reduction in alcohol consumption.

Guidelines for alcohol consumption

Since drinking alcohol is a widespread social activity and since some studies seem to show that moderate consumption is not harmful, it would be difficult to set as a target a society where no alcohol is consumed. Smith and Jacobson (1988) suggest that we should set a target in the UK of reducing alcohol consumption by 20% by the year 2000. Guidelines for consumption have therefore been drawn up by the Health Education Authority based on the research mentioned and the legal requirements. All drinks are related by their alcohol content to a standard as follows:

1 standard drink
= Half a pint of ordinary beer or lager
= A single measure ($^1/_6$ of a gill) of spirits, e.g. whisky, gin, vodka
= 1 glass of wine
= 1 small glass of sherry
= 1 measure of vermouth or aperitif, e.g. Martini.

The HEA suggest that to drink safely the limits are:

Men: Four to six standard drinks two or three times per week, or 20 units a week

Women: Two or three standard drinks two or three times per week, or 14 units a week

The reason that the limits are different for men and women is because men have a higher water content in their bodies (55–65%) than women (45–55%) and absorbed alcohol is therefore more 'diluted'. Men also have larger livers than women and can metabolise alcohol more easily. Having given these guidelines the HEA recommend that anybody who is driving or operating machinery should avoid alcohol and it strongly advises against drinking during pregnancy. This is because alcohol is absorbed directly into the bloodstream and can cross the placenta into the fetal circulation, producing similar effects on the developing fetus as it does on the drinker. Babies born to alcoholic mothers may have developmental defects associated with fetal alcohol syndrome including growth retardation and microcephaly (Rubin et al., 1986). However, it has to be said that fetal alcohol syndrome is relatively rare in the UK.

There does appear to be evidence that income and social class are associated with alcohol consumption. In a recent lifestyles survey, Blaxter (1990) found that alcohol consumption was strongly correlated with other 'unhealthy' behaviours such as smoking and poor diet, particularly among younger men from the manual working groups. Low income was also a strong correlate of alcohol consumption. Power et al. (1991) have also found evidence to suggest that young men from the lower social classes are more likely to present with poor health outcomes as a result of alcohol consumption, among other health-related behaviours, than young men from the professional and managerial groups.

The reasons why people become problem drinkers are manifold and it is not appropriate in this chapter to enter a detailed discussion. Suffice it to say that the research is still unclear because alcohol-related problems such as violence, child abuse and divorce cannot be separated from the underlying cause or other contributing factors. For example, does drink cause divorce or does the trauma of divorce lead to problem drinking? What does appear to be evident is that the harmful effects of alcohol are most likely to occur among communities who are in most need in terms of income and employment and, by implication, housing, education and health facilities. This would suggest that at least some of the causes of problem drinking lie not within individual control, but rather at a political level. The radical approach to health promotion indicates that by taking political action to change inequalities in health, some of the problems associated with problem drinking could be averted.

Traditionally, nurses have not been very active politically. Butterworth (1988) has criticised nurses for their apparent lethargy towards social and national policy issues. The reasons for this seem unclear, but could be rooted in the historical development of nursing as a predominantly female profession with its associated powerlessness in relation to the male-dominated medical profession. This raises many issues about the way nurses perceive themselves and the way they are perceived by the public and professional colleagues. Despite history, some nurses have seen the value of taking collectivist, radical action to put pressure on policy-makers. Examples are the radical midwives group who have campaigned for women to have more choice in childbirth with some success and the radical health visitors who support issues such as the new public health movement which aims to reduce health problems through creating a safer and healthier social environment. It is difficult (though not impossible) for nurses to take a radical approach to health promotion single-handed. One person may be disregarded; a group of people have to be listened to at some level. For this reason, a collectivist approach to a health problem such as alcohol abuse may be most effectively tackled by campaigning and lobbying with other nurses. This could be in association with a professional organisation or trade union such as the Royal College of Nursing or the Health Visitors Association, or through a local pressure group. In relation to alcohol, the type of campaigns which could be organised include:

(1) Taxation on all alcoholic drinks to be maintained at the rate of inflation
(2) Advertising for alcohol to display clear information about alcoholic content and warnings about health risks of drinking
(3) An annual levy imposed on alcohol advertising which could be used to fund community education programmes

(4) Clarification and enforcement of the legislation relating to the sale of alcohol to under-18s and to roadside breathalysing
(5) Custodial sentences for offences such as dangerous and reckless driving under the influence of alcohol, particularly where the death of a third party is concerned.

The above campaigns could be seen as using the legislative framework to control drinking behaviour. Other, more general, political action which could potentially have a more far-reaching effect on all aspects of health would include lobbying for:

(1) The right to housing and tackling the problems of homelessness
(2) Increases in welfare benefits such as child benefit, and the state pension to be raised to a level commensurate with the cost of living
(3) Provision of state-funded child care for preschool children
(4) Reduction in unemployment
(5) Equal distribution of resources for services such as education and the health service
(6) Equal opportunities, regardless of gender, race, age or religion.

Nurses form a very large body of people. As individuals, they will have their own political views and will hold their own convictions about health and health promotion. As a profession, they are caring for people who may not have had the education, the wealth or the opportunity to take control of their health and it could be perceived as a professional duty to advocate publicly for the disadvantaged or powerless within our society.

Mental health

Mental health is notoriously difficult to define. It can be argued that it means more than just the absence of mental illness, that it refers to a state of well-being, an ability to make rational decisions, a feeling of self-worth. It is encompassed in Seedhouse's (1986) definition of health when he speaks of achieving human potential, but what is the full potential of the human psyche? In many ways, mental health is inseparable from physical health if we are referring to a holistic approach to health. Human potential has to be seen in terms of the whole being more than the sum of its parts; the mind and the body are inter-related and the determinants of physical health will to a great extent be the same as the determinants of mental health. For example, it has already been noted that poverty makes a significant contribution to ill health. Brown and Harris (1978) have argued that depression among women is much greater when certain vulnerability factors such as mother's unemployment are present, and more recently Blaxter (1990) has suggested that income is correlated with poor psychosocial health. These two studies will form the focus of this section as they both suggest ways in which mental health can be promoted through both radical and other measures.

Brown and Harris's (1978) study of depression among women in the community takes a sociological stance. In other words, it looks for causes of depression within the social context of women's lives rather than for a biochemical abnormality within individuals. Brown and Harris interviewed a random sample of women in the community who had not necessarily been clinically labelled as depressed and found that there was a high incidence of women who defined themselves as depressed. Brown and Harris acknowledge that this raises questions of diagnosis, but argue that just because people have not been labelled by the psychiatrist does not mean that they are not experiencing depression.

Having explored a large number of variables which could be related to depression, Brown and Harris put forward a model which proposed some social origins of depression. There is a greater likelihood of major life events such as a bereavement leading to depression in the presence of background social factors such as social class and what they term 'vulnerability factors'; these include unemployment of the woman, three or more children under 15 years, loss of her own mother before the age of 11 and lack of a close and trusting relationship with a partner. Low self-esteem will contribute to an outcome of depression in the presence of these factors. The absence of these vulnerability factors can also be seen as protective against depression, especially where the woman has high self-esteem. But where vulnerability factors lead to low self-esteem and where a life event or difficulty arises (such as death, divorce or separation from children) then depression is likely to occur as a result of a sense of hopelessness about the future and failure to work through grief. Women with high self-esteem are more able to find alternative sources of value and this enables them to resolve their sense of hopelessness.

Brown and Harris's findings appear to indicate that working class women are much more likely than middle class women to experience a severe psychiatric disorder in the presence of a life event, which they ascribe to the presence of the vulnerability factors and associated low self-esteem. In other words, working class women are more likely to be unemployed, without a supportive partner, to have three children under the age of 15 and to have lost their own mother before the age of 11 years. Whilst the authors acknowledge gaps in the research, such as the diagnostic label already mentioned and the difference between depression and the experience of grief, the findings seem to indicate clearly that depression has social origins which could potentially be prevented through political means, such as improving the employment status of women and providing a wider choice of child care facilities either free or at affordable cost. Brown and Harris do not mention housing as a vulnerability factor. Perhaps there was optimism about housing in the early 1970s when this research was conducted and a municipal housing programme was still in progress. It would be interesting in today's climate to test the model further to see whether housing would feature as a vulnerability factor.

Blaxter's more recent (1990) study was a comprehensive survey of health and lifestyles which was conducted by interviewing a random sample of 9003 people from England, Scotland and Wales. Whilst Blaxter was not attempting to provide a causative model of mental ill health, she was trying to establish some of the major correlates between many aspects of health and people's lifestyles. However, she found very similar relationships between what she terms psychosocial health and income. She found that women on low incomes with no social support were most likely to experience symptoms related to poor psychosocial health such as depression, worry or sleep disturbances. Overall, it was the young in the 18–39 age group, the unemployed, the divorced, separated and widowed and single parents of dependent children who were most likely to report high rates of psychosocial malaise.

These findings would appear to support Brown and Harris's thesis that mental ill health has social determinants. Blaxter is particularly concerned with the role that social support plays in the prevention of psychosocial symptoms and its relative protectiveness compared with 'healthy' lifestyles. Perhaps not surprisingly, she found that people with both low social support and 'unhealthy' lifestyles (smoking, drinking, poor diet and lack of fitness) were most likely to experience psychosocial symptoms but either social support or a healthy lifestyle was not protective on its own. A combination of social support and a healthy lifestyle was found to be protective although only a minority of the sample fulfilled all four lifestyle criteria. Smith and Jacobson (1988) have also explored the concept of social support as a determinant of mental health. Whilst there does appear to be evidence that intimate and trusting relationships can be protective against the negative effects of life events, these authors argue that more research is required into the qualitative nature of social support.

It appears from Blaxter's study that again it is those who are most disadvantaged who are most likely to experience psychosocial symptoms, and whilst the terms of reference and definitions differ from Brown and Harris's earlier study, there do appear to be some similarities. This would suggest that there are some aspects of mental health which can be approached using a radical approach to health promotion, with the emphasis on reducing poverty and unemployment. It seems that the causes of a lack of social support also need to be addressed – is there more divorce among poorer people and if so, is this precipitated by poverty and unemployment? Are the mortality rates higher among the poor and is this related to social isolation? We already know that social deprivation is strongly related to ill health (Townsend and Davidson, 1982; Whitehead, 1988); perhaps it is time for nurses to be more pro-active in their response to the research.

In summary, the radical approach to health promotion has been addressed by exploring two health issues – alcohol abuse and mental health. This approach sees the determinants of health and illness as being within the social and political arena, rather than within the direct control of the individual. It attempts, in this respect, to avoid 'victim-blaming' and to find ways through the democratic processes of lobbying, campaigning, protesting and voting to resolve some of today's major health issues. Nurses have not been very prominent in this arena and this may be related to their own position within the health service.

However, they do form a very large majority within the health service and there is potential for nurses to influence social policy.

The exemplary role of the nurse

If we accept that nurses should be active in health promotion, should we expect nurses also to set an example with their own lifestyle and behaviours? For example, does a nurse lose credibility if, when talking to a patient about the effects of smoking, he notices her fingers are stained with nicotine? It is probably true to say that patients and clients are less likely to be motivated to change their behaviour if the health educator is not able to demonstrate her personal commitment to health. Certainly, social learning theory (Bandura, 1977a) would suggest that role models form an important component of learned behaviour. However, there are other facets to this discussion. Reference was made at the beginning of the chapter to the possibility that nurses are not encouraged to value their own health. For example, there is evidence to suggest that nurses have to endure work conditions which give rise to stress and burn-out and for which little or no support is offered (Parkes, 1985; Dewe, 1988; Coffey *et al.*, 1988). Nurses face many obstacles of their own, both as individuals and within their working environment. For example, the pressure of work may make it difficult to eat at reasonable intervals, so that food which quickly fills a gap is more likely to be taken than a meal. Inevitably, chocolate, chips and 'junk food' fulfil this criterion. The working environment may not provide food which is both nutritious and satisfying, particularly some hospital canteens.

Nurses are often accused of being heavy smokers. In fact, they are only slightly more likely to smoke than their female counterparts in the rest of the community. On average, about 35% of nurses are smokers (Booth and Faulkner, 1986; Macleod Clark *et al.*, 1985). Among the reasons nurses give for smoking are stress at work, night duty and coping with death. The study by Booth and Faulkner (1986) showed that, for many nurses, smoking is a coping strategy for domestic and personal problems, just as it is for many other women. Many employers are now developing smoking policies which are, in the main, designed to restrict smoking to one area only. Employees, including nurses, are often made to feel guilty and isolated. Policies to restrict smoking or promote healthy eating should have built into them supportive measures which will enable nurses and other staff to feel that their health is of value to themselves and the workforce. For example, groups to help people discuss and cope with stress could be set up and simple measures such as ensuring that an individual nurse is not asked to extend or change her duties too often could be taken.

Working within a bureaucratic organisation such as the National Health Service can make an individual feel powerless to change the system. It therefore requires the support and guidance of managers to develop measures which will enable employees to feel that their role is of value. This involves working in a democratic way, so that the needs of the workforce can be taken into consideration.

As individuals, nurses face the same motivational and attitudinal difficulties as their patients and clients. It is feasible that nurses could apply any of the three approaches to health promotion to themselves. For example, the preventive approach can be used by nurses when they attend cervical screening clinics or have innoculations against infectious diseases before going on holiday abroad. This may involve exchange of information between nurses and the occupational health unit. The self-empowerment approach to health could be applied when nurses need to develop skills in decision-making about their own health and could be facilitated by group work or individual counselling, both of which could be provided by the occupational health unit. Finally, nurses could be much more pro-active about the health issues relevant to themselves and their patients within the working environment. This could involve campaigning for a more nutritious diet or negotiating for therapeutic massage or relaxation classes to be provided for staff.

Some of these obstacles might be overcome through the educational process. A health-based curriculum in which personal attitudes and behaviours are explored and applied to theories of health and health promotion may encourage a nurse to look at her own health positively. Project 2000 aims to achieve this. Only research which evaluates Project 2000 in terms of nurses' health outcomes will enlighten us as to the success of the programme in this respect.

In the final analysis, nurses are people who have the potential to develop, both as individuals and as professionals. Their role as health promoters may be enhanced through an educational and professional system which is supportive while assigning proper value to health. There is no doubt about the potential which nurses have to be effective in promoting health. This potential can be maximised by recognising that nurses have individual health needs, just like anyone else.

Conclusions

In conclusion, this chapter has addressed the promotion of health by looking at the concept of human potential. There are many measures by which human potential can be developed and these have been addressed using three approaches to health promotion. The first approach looked at immunisation and screening within Caplan's (1969) framework of prevention. Nurses have a very significant role to play in helping to prevent ill health by providing people with information which is relevant to their needs and being knowledgeable about the services which are available. The patients and clients in our care have different health needs and individual obstacles to overcome in order to meet those needs. By careful assessment the nurse can identify the patient's needs and use her knowledge and skill as a professional to develop and implement a nursing care plan, in partnership with the patient, which will enhance the promotion of human potential.

The second approach, self-empowerment, was illustrated by addressing the issues of diet and smoking. The underlying concept here is that individuals need to develop decision-making skills in order to make healthy choices. It is less paternalistic than the preventive approach as it assumes that individuals are autonomous beings who wish to make free choices about their lives. It has been argued that nurses can facilitate the decision-making process by providing appropriate information, helping people to clarify their attitudes and beliefs about health and by using more sophisticated skills in communication and group work to enhance decision-making. It has been suggested that the levels of skill required to apply this approach in nursing may develop with increasing experience in practice.

Finally the radical approach was discussed. This approach assumes that health problems are determined by the physical and social environment rather than individual behaviour. It was argued that by changing this environment health problems would be tackled at the 'upstream' level, making it more realistic for people to make healthy choices. For example, social deprivation was seen as an underlying determinant of alcohol abuse and depression among women. As a major workforce, nurses are seen as having a potentially significant role in influencing social policy but at the moment it appears that nurses are not very pro-active as health campaigners.

Nurses are human beings who also need opportunities to develop their potential and there may be a range of obstacles both in the work environment and in their personal lives which they need to overcome in order to achieve this. Any of the three approaches discussed may be applied to nurses themselves to promote their own health.

In conclusion, you are reminded of Seedhouse's (1986) theory of health when he says: 'Work for health is work which aims to enable and to enhance by providing the foundations for the achievement of potentials' (page 74). Clearly, nursing forms a major part of this work.

Glossary

Addiction: A state of psychic or physical dependence (or both) on a drug arising in a person following administration of that drug on a periodic or continuous basis. The characteristics of such a state will vary with the agents involved

Atherosclerosis: A narrowing and hardening of the arteries, typified by atheromatous or fatty plaques in the artery walls

Carbohydrate: A chemical compound consisting of carbon, hydrogen and oxygen which provides the most economical and the most readily digestible form of energy to the body. Carbohydrates can be *monosaccharide* (a single sugar such as glucose), *disaccharide* (containing two sugars such as sucrose) or *polysaccharide* (a complex compound containing many sugars, some of which may be digestible such as starch and others indigestible such as cellulose)

Cholesterol: A steroid found in mammalian tissue from which all other major steroids are synthesised, for example the hormone aldosterone. Cholesterol is synthesised mainly in the liver. A high plasma level of cholesterol is associated with atherosclerosis and coronary thrombosis

Demography: The social study of persons viewed collectively in regard to ethnic group, occupation or condition

Epidemic: Disease prevalent in a community for an isolated period

Epidemiology: The study of the determinants and distribution of health and disease in populations

Fatty acid: A compound which contains oxygen and a chain of carbon atoms with attached hydrogen atoms. The degree to which the carbon atoms are loaded with hydrogen determines whether they are saturated or unsaturated. A saturated fatty acid has all its carbon atoms loaded with hydrogen and there are no double bonds. Unsaturated fatty acids have double bonds to which hydrogen can be added

Immunisation: To confer immunity. Immunity is the natural reaction of the body to invading chemicals, known as antigens. The immune response to antigens results in the formation of antibodies which protect the body from future attacks. Immunity can be induced naturally (by contact with the disease itself) or artificially (by giving a **vaccine**). Artificial immunity can be *active* where the vaccine is a live or killed organism, or *passive* when an injection of prepared antibodies is given

Invasive carcinoma (cervix):   Malignant changes affecting the tissues surrounding the cervical epithelium, including the vagina, uterine body and lymph nodes

Morbidity: Relating to a disease or an abnormal or disordered condition

Mortality: The ratio of the number of deaths to the total population

Pre-invasive carcinoma (cervix):   Epithelial changes in the cervix where cells are undifferentiated and immature, known as carcinoma *in situ*

Prevalence: Number of people having a disease in a population (as opposed to incidence which refers to the number of new cases arising)

Vaccine: An agent inducing immunity. A vaccine can be *live* in that it infects, replicates and immunises in a similar way to the 'wild' strain but rarely causes the disease (for example, the measles vaccine). The vaccine may be *inactivated*, consisting of a suspension of the killed organisms (for example, the whooping cough vaccine)

References

Ashton, H. and Stepney, R. (1982). *Smoking – Psychology and Pharmacology*. Tavistock Publications, London.

Bandura, A. (1977a). *Social Learning Theory*. Prentice-Hall, Englewood Cliffs, New Jersey.

Bandura, A. (1977b). Self-efficacy: towards a unifying theory of behaviour change. *Psychological Review*, 84, 191–215.

Baric, L. (1985). The meaning of words: health promotion. *Journal of the Institute of Health Education*, 23, 1.

Becker, M. and Maiman, L. (1975). Sociobehavioural determinants of compliance with health and medical care recommendations. *Medical Care*, 13(1), 10–25.

Bedford, H. (1991). Personal communication.

Blaxter, M. (1990). *Health and Lifestyles*. Tavistock Routledge, London.

Bond, M. and Kendall, S. (1990). *Improving Your Decision Making*. Distance Learning Centre, South Bank Polytechnic, London.

Booth, K. and Faulkner, A. (1986). Links between nurses and cigarette smoking? *Nurse Education Today*, 6(4), 176–182.

British Cardiac Society. (1987). *Report of the British Cardiac Society Working Group on Coronary Disease Prevention*. British Cardiac Society, London.

Brown, G. and Harris, T. (1978). *The Social Origins of Depression: A Study of Psychiatric Disorder in Women*. Tavistock Publications, London.

Butterworth, T. (1988). Political awareness. *Nursing Times*. Community Outlook, December 1988, 20–21.

Campbell, A. (1990). Education or indoctrination? The issue of autonomy in health education. In *Ethics in Health Education*, Doxiadis, S. (ed.). John Wiley and Sons, Chichester.

Caplan, G. (1969). *An Approach to Community Mental Health*. Tavistock Publications, London.

Champion, V. (1987). The relationship of breast self examination to health belief model variables. *Research in Nursing and Health*, 10, 375–382.

Charles, N. and Kerr, M. (1986). Issues of responsibility and control in the feeding of families. In *The Politics of Health Education*, Watt, A. and Rodmell, S. (eds.). Routledge and Kegan Paul, London.

Coffey, L., Skipper, J. and Jung, F. (1988). Nurses and shift work: effects on job performance and job-related stress. *Journal of Advanced Nursing*, 13, 245–254.

Committee on Medical Aspects of Food Policy (COMA). (1984). *Diet and Cardiovascular Disease*. HMSO, London.

Datta, S.P. and Ottaway, J.H. (1976). *Biochemistry*. Baillière Tindall, London.

Dewe, P. (1988). Investigating the frequency of nursing stressors: a comparison across wards. *Social Science and Medicine*, 26(3), 375–380.

Department of Health and Social Security (1981). *Report on Avoiding Heart Attacks*. HMSO, London.

DHSS. (1983). *The Nurses', Midwives and Health Visitors Rules Approval Order*. Statutory instrument No. 873. HMSO, London.

DHSS. (1984). *Mortality Statistics: Cause, 1983*. HMSO, London.

DHSS. (1985). *Drug Mis-Use*. A Basic Briefing. HMSO, London.

DHSS. (1986). *Neighbourhood Nursing* (Chair: Julia Cumberlege). HMSO, London.

Department of Health. (1988). *Promoting Better Health*. HMSO, London.

DoH. (1989a). *Working for Patients*. HMSO, London.

DoH. (1989b). *Health and Personal Social Services Statistics for England*. HMSO, London.

DoH. (1990a). *Immunisation Against Infectious Diseases*. HMSO, London.

DoH. (1990b). *NHS and Community Care Act*. HMSO, London.

DoH. (1992). *The Nation's Health*. HMSO, London.

Doll, R. and Hill, A.B. (1952). A study of the aetiology of carcinoma of the lung. *British Medical Journal*, 2, 1271–1276.

Faulkner, A. and Ward, L. (1983). Nurses as health educators in relation to smoking. *Nursing Times*, 79(15), Occasional Papers No. 8.

French, J. and Adams, L. (1986). From analysis to synthesis. *Health Education Journal*, 45(2), 71–74.

Gott, M. and O'Brien, M. (1990). The role of the nurse in health promotion. *Health Promotion International*, 5(2), 137–143.

Graham, H. (1984). *Woman, Health and The Family*. Wheatsheaf Publications, Brighton.

Hakama, M. (1983). Cancer of the uterine cervix. In *The Epidemiology of Cancer*, Burke, G. (ed.). Croom Helm, London.

Harris, J. (1985). *The Value of Life*. Routledge and Kegan Paul, London

Health Education Authority and Sports Council. (1987). *Exercise. Why Bother?* HEA, London.

Health Education Council. (1980). *Survey of Nursing in England, Wales and Northern Ireland*. HEC, London.

Health Education Council. (1982). *Health Education in Nursing – A Workshop*. HEC, London.

King, J. (1987). Women's attitudes towards cervical smear. *Update*, 34(2), 25.

Kramsch, D., Aspen, A., Abromowitz, B., Kreimendahl, T. and Hood, W. (1981). Reduction of coronary atherosclerosis by moderate conditioning exercise in monkeys on an atherogenic diet. *New England Journal of Medicine*, 305 (25), 1483.

Maclaine, K. and Macleod Clark, J. (1991). Women's reasons for smoking in pregnancy. *Nursing Times*, 87, 22.

Macleod Clark, J., Haverty, S., Eliot, K. and Kendall, S. (1985). *Helping People to Stop Smoking – The Nurse's Role. Phase 1*. Health Education Authority, London.

Macleod Clark, J., Haverty, S. and Kendall, S. (1990). Helping people to stop smoking: a study of the nurse's role. *Journal of Advanced Nursing*, 16, 357–363.

Marmot, M., Rose, G., Shipley, N. and Thomas, B. (1981). Alcohol and mortality: a U-shaped curve. *Lancet*, 1 (8246), 580–583.

Marmot, M. (1985). Interpretation of trends in coronary heart disease mortality. *Acta Medica Scandinavica*, 701 (Supplement), 58–75.

Mattheson, J. and Marsh, A. (1983). *Attitudes, Behaviour and Smoking*. OPCS, London.

McMahon, R. and Pearson, A. (1991). *Nursing as Therapy*. Chapman and Hall, London.

Mckinlay, J.B. (1979). A case for refocusing upstream: the political economy of illness. In *Patients, Physicians and Illness*, Jaco, E. (ed.). The Free Press, New York.

Morris, J., Everitt, M., Pollard, R., Chave, S. and Semmence, A. (1980). Vigorous exercise in leisure time: protection against coronary heart disease. *Lancet*, 11 (8257), 1207–1210.

National Advisory Committee on Nutrition Education (NACNE). (1983). *Proposals for Nutritional Guidelines for Health Education in Britain*. HEC, London.

Nightingale, F. (1891). Letter to Mr Frederick Verney on the teaching of health at home. In *Buckinghamshire County Council* (1911). Reproduction of a printed report originally submitted to the Buckingham County Council in the year 1892, containing letters from Miss Nightingale on health visiting in districts, pages 17–19. Requoted from Clark, J. (1973). *A Family Visitor*, page 11. RCN, London.

Nightingale, F. (1893). Sick nursing and health nursing. A paper published at the Chicago Exhibition. In *Selected Writings of Florence Nightingale*, Seymer, L.R. (ed.), (1954). Macmillan, New York.

Office of Population Censuses and Surveys. (1982). *Mortality in England and Wales*. OPCS, London.

Office of Population Censuses and Surveys. (1990). *General Household Survey 1988*. HMSO, London.

Open University. (1985). *Caring for Health – Dilemmas and Prospects*. Open University Press, Milton Keynes.

Ottawa Charter for Health Promotion, 1986. Drafted by participants in the first international conference on health promotion, November 17–21, 1986, Ottawa, Canada. WHO, Geneva.

Parkes, K. (1985). Stressful episodes reported by first year student nurses: a descriptive account. *Social Science and Medicine*, 20(9), 945–953.

Perkins, E. (1982). *Decision Making – The Whooping Cough Dilemma*. Nottingham Practical Papers in Health Education No. 8. University of Nottingham.

Power, C., Manor, O. and Fox, J. (1991). *Health and Class: The Early Years*. Chapman and Hall, London.

Raw, M. and Heller, J. (1984). *Helping People to Stop Smoking – the Development, Role and Potential of the Support Services in the UK*. HEC, London.

Roediger, H.L., Rushton, J.P., Capaldi, E.D. and Paris, S.G. (1984). *Psychology*. Little, Brown, Boston.

Rose, G. (1987). The scale of the problem. Paper given at the first conference of Anticipatory Care Teams, York, October 2–4.

Royal College of Physicians and the British Cardiac Society. (1976). Prevention of coronary heart disease. *Journal of the Royal College of Physicians*, 10(13), 213–275.

Royal College of Physicians. (1983). *Health or Smoking?* Pitman Publishing, London.

Rubin, P.C. *et al.* (1986). Prospective survey of use of therapeutic drugs, alcohol and cigarettes during pregnancy. *British Medical Journal*, 1(2), 81–83.

Seedhouse, D. (1986). *Health – the Foundations for Achievement*. John Wiley and Sons, Chichester.

Smith, A. and Jacobson, B. (1988). *The Nation's Health*. King's Fund, London.

Smith, R. (1981). Alcohol and alcoholism: the relation between consumption and damage. *British Medical Journal*, 283, 895–898.

Sontag, S. (1978). *Illness as Metaphor*. Penguin Books, Harmondsworth.

Stamler, J. (1981). Prevention of coronary heart disease: the last 20 years. In *Eleventh Bethesda Conference, Prevention of CHD*. *American Journal of Cardiology (Supplement)*, 10–23.

Stillman, M. (1977). Women's health beliefs about breast cancer self examination. *Nursing Research*, 26(2), 121–127.

Syred, H. (1981). The abdication of health education by hospital nurses. *Journal of Advanced Nursing*, 6(1), 27–33.

Townsend, P. and Davidson, N. (eds.). (1982). *The*

Black Report. Penguin Books, Harmondsworth.

Tones, B.K. (1986). Health education and the ideology of health promotion: a review of alternative approaches. *Health Education Research*, 1(1), 3–12.

Tones, B.K., Tilford, S. and Robinson, Y. (1990). *Health Education: Effectiveness and Efficiency*. Chapman and Hall, London.

United Kingdom Central Council for Nursing, Midwifery and Health Visiting. (1986). *Project 2000 – A New Preparation for Practice*. UKCC, London.

Vartianinen, E., Viri, L., Tossavainen, K., Niskanen, E., Macalister, A. and Puska, P. (1987). Prevention of cardiovascular risk factors in youth (the North Karelia Project 1984–1988). Paper given at the 1st European Conference in Health Education, Madrid, March 25–27.

While, A. (1985). Health visiting and health experiences of infants in three areas. Unpublished PhD. thesis, University of London.

Whitehead, M. *The Health Divide* (1988). Pelican Books, London.

Williams, G. (1984). Health promotion – caring concern or slick salesmanship? *Journal of Medical Ethics*, 10, 191–195.

World Health Organisation. (1946). *Constitution*. WHO, Geneva.

WHO. (1978). *Report of the International Conference on Primary Care, Alma-Ata, USSR*. WHO, Geneva.

WHO. (1984a). *Health Promotion: A Discussion Document on Concepts and Principles*. Regional Office for Europe, Copenhagen.

WHO. (1984b). Report of a WHO meeting, October. Quoted in the *Report of the British Cardiac Society Working Group in Coronary Disease Prevention*, 1987. British Cardiac Society, London.

WHO. (1985). *Targets for Health for All*. Targets in support of the European regional strategy for health for all. Regional Office for Europe, Copenhagen.

Suggestions for further reading

Ashton, J. and Seymour, H. (1988). *The New Public Health*. Open University Press, Milton Keynes.

Broome, A. (ed.). (1989). *Health Psychology: Processes and Applications*. Chapman and Hall, London.

Coutts, L. and Hardy, L. (1985). *Teaching for Health*. Churchill Livingstone, Edinburgh.

Downie, R., Fyfe, C. and Tannahill, A. (1990). *Health Promotion – Models and Values*. Oxford University Press, Oxford.

Doxiadis, S. (1990). *Ethics in Health Education*. John Wiley and Sons, Chichester.

Ewles, L. and Simnett, I. (1985). *Promoting Health*. John Wiley and Sons, Chichester.

Health Education Council. (1984). *That's the Limit*. HEC, London.

Open University. (1985). *Studying Health and Disease*. Open University Press, Milton Keynes.

Open University. (1985). *Experiencing and Explaining Disease*. Open University Press, Milton Keynes.

Open University. (1985). *Health and Disease – a Reader*. Open University Press, Milton Keynes.

Orr, J. (1987). *Women's Health in the Community*. John Wiley and Sons, Chichester.

Seedhouse, D. (1986). *Health – the Foundations for Achievement*. John Wiley and Sons, Chichester.

Simnett, I., Wright, L. and Evans, M. (1983). *Drinking Choices*. HEC, London.

Sontag, S. (1978). *Illness as Metaphor*. Penguin Books, Harmondsworth.

Sontag, S. (1989). *AIDS and Its Metaphors*. Penguin Books, Harmondsworth.

Watt, A. and Rodmell, S. (1986). *The Politics of Health Education*. Routledge and Kegan Paul, London.

Whitehead, M. (1989). *Swimming Upstream: Trends and Prospects in Education for Health*. King's Fund, London.

4

PRIMARY HEALTH CARE

Elizabeth Raymond

This chapter explores the contribution of primary health care to the health care of the population. Primary health care is viewed as a 'frontier' service depending on flexibility, creativity and a high standard of care.

The chapter includes an account and discussion of each of the following issues:

- The nature of primary health care taking a national and international perspective
- Society's views of health and health care
- The influence on health and primary health care of political factors including the allocation of funding, social policy and health policy
- The providers of primary health care including professional carers – for example, district nurses and health visitors, practice nurses, voluntary and private services and carers within the family
- The development of the primary

health care team. The history of this care team is traced, with particular reference to general practitioners, health visitors and district nurses

- Key aspects of primary health care services in the community are highlighted: midwifery, school nursing, family practitioner services, and occupational health nursing
- Throughout the chapter, the author stresses how the partnership between members of the primary health care team and patients, carers, and the local community as a whole, is central to the quality of care

This chapter examines the concept of primary health care, considering the differing approaches of a number of different nations. Links are made between the kind of primary health care system which develops in a given country, the environmental context, and the values, attitudes and

beliefs of that society, particularly in relation to concepts of health.

It is important to establish that primary health care is a matter for every member of society, with each individual bearing his own share of responsibility. A consideration of primary health care in the UK raises several questions. Have we 'over-professionalised' primary health care to the extent that we have actually made it harder for lay individuals to share responsibility for their own health care? Are we making the best use of voluntary agencies and lay carers? How politically involved should we be in trying to influence the kind of primary health care services which are provided? What are our priorities; the treatment of illness and disease or the promotion of health and prevention of ill health?

In this chapter we focus particularly on the primary health care team and look at the historical development of the main health care professions represented in such teams. A significant proportion of the chapter is devoted to the historical development of health visiting because this professional group has a unique commitment to health promotion and the prevention of ill health. These issues have been gaining increasingly high profile and status in recent years, both internationally and in the UK. It can be argued that many of the issues and dilemmas attached to the development of health visiting have arisen precisely because of the health visitors' perspective on health. The nature of the profession is such that effective health visiting practice is not possible without a partnership in which the health visitor and her client share together in decision-making. Health visiting unequivocally seeks to foster clients' autonomy and independence, with health visitors acting as client advocates.

An implicit, and partly explicit, theme of this chapter is that of primary health care being offered in a kind of 'frontier' situation, meeting the consumer in the complex, multifaceted situation of everyday life. For primary health care services to be efficient and effective, a flexible, creative approach to the provision of care is essential. Some of the hindrances and difficulties affecting the degree of flexibility and creativity in the UK primary health care system are identified, as well as some of the strategies developed to overcome such difficulties.

With increasing emphasis on developing a needs-led service in the UK, various ways of identifying the health needs of a community have been developed, and the main approaches are reviewed briefly. The potential resources available in response are highlighted also, including private and voluntary services and alternative therapies, as, together with statutory services, they contribute to what has been termed the 'mixed economy of care' (DoH, 1989).

An overview of the major groups of medical, nursing, paramedical and social service personnel who support members of primary health care teams working in the community will also be given.

Primary health care – what is it?

The term 'primary health care' means different things to different people. In the mid 1970s, a Director of Nurse Education remarked that she had thought that primary health care was 'something to do with primary school children'. In May 1981, the Jarman Report on primary health care in London (Royal College of General Practitioners, 1981) focused almost exclusively on medical services, and concentrated particularly on the general practitioner services. The Acheson Report (London Health Planning Consortium, 1981), published at the same time as the Jarman Report, also examined primary health care in London, but as well as considering GP services, it was concerned with community nursing services, midwifery services in the community, child and school health services, and the primary health care role of accident and emergency services. In all three instances, the difficulty of definition is reflected. This is summed up in the first report from the Social Services Committee of the House of Commons on Primary Health Care (1987). This report quotes the Minister of Health as claiming that, 'One could have an endless argument about where to draw boundaries of definition'.

The Minister also acknowledged that the government definition of primary health care was a narrow one basically including only the family practitioner and community nursing services.

The flaw in the above attempts to describe primary health care is that none of them focuses on its purpose or goals. They are simply lists of groups who either receive or provide it, and they leave unanswered the question of what 'it' is.

Literature pertaining to primary health care in the UK can be divided broadly into three groups. The first group is that which envisages primary health care as being *primary in importance*. The second group is that which envisages it as being care provided at *the first point of contact* between the consumer and the health services, and the third group is that which envisages primary health care as being *non-institutional, community-based* care. In this context, 'primary health care' and 'community health care' become synonymous.

The Declaration of Alma-Ata: an international view of primary health care

At the International Conference on Primary Health Care (WHO, 1978), the Declaration of Alma-Ata included a clear statement describing primary health care as essential health care which forms the central function and main focus of a country's health system. The Declaration reiterates that primary health care is the *first level* of contact for individuals, the family and the community with the national health system, in the sense that primary health care operates as close as possible to where people live and work. It is further described as the *first element* of a continuing health care process. The Alma-Ata Declaration is echoed in a UK government Discussion Document (*Primary Health Care – an Agenda for Discussion*. DHSS, 1986a) which describes primary health care services as the front line of the health service, as including community health services, and as dealing with over nine tenths of the contacts that the public have with the health service.

The Declaration continues with a clarification of the goals of primary health care as being:

(1) Promotion of health
(2) Prevention of disease and ill health
(3) Cure and rehabilitation.

In order to achieve these goals, primary health care encompasses a range of concerns and services. The Declaration includes environmental issues such as the provision of adequate water supply and sanitation, prevention and control of locally endemic diseases, and the provision of an adequate food supply. Personal health services listed include maternal and child health care, family planning services, immunisation programmes, a pharmaceutical service, and appropriate treatment of common diseases and injuries. But it is health education that heads the list, with a concern to inform the consumer about prevailing health problems and the methods of preventing and controlling them.

The Declaration further points out that primary health care:

'reflects and evolves from the economic conditions and sociocultural and political characteristics of the country and its communities'
(WHO, 1978, page 4)

Consequently, primary health care systems develop differently in different countries, not only because the prevailing unmet health needs differ from country to country, but also because values and attitudes to health vary. Sachs (1986) describes how, in every society, each individual seeks causal explanations for ill health, and how those explanations are created in the environmental context of that individual. Explanations in each society are an integral part of the culture of that society. Because the explanations differ from society to society, the health care systems which develop as a result also differ.

In any country, the planning of an effective primary health care service requires a wide range of knowledge, including detailed knowledge of patterns of health and disease, social and cultural attitudes related to health, the prevailing economic, social and environmental conditions, the political structure, and the existing and potential resources for health care. Stephen (1979) points out that the evolution of health care is influenced by what he calls the 'mentality and philosophy' not only of consumers, but doctors also. For example, Morley (quoted in King, 1972) found that, in Nigeria at the time he was writing, three quarters of the population was rural, but three quarters of the doctors lived in the towns where three quarters of the medical resources were spent. Morley suggested that although three quarters of the people died from diseases which were preventable at low cost, three quarters of the medical budgets were spent on curative services.

Wilson (1975) and Reedy (1983) both suggest that many countries demonstrate similar imbalances. One factor which appears to contribute to such imbalances appears to be the development of medical technologies. Paine and Siem Tjam (1988) argue that such technological resources are so costly that they concentrate available finances mainly on the provision of treatment for a few, at the expense of cheaper health care facilities for many others. The authors link the dominance of medical technologies with the existence of hospital-centred health care systems. Dr Lambo, Deputy Director-General of the WHO, addressing the Expert Committee on the Role of Hospitals at the First Referral Level, which reported in 1987, described the notion of hospitals as the centre of health care systems as having dominated thinking concerning the role of hospitals until recently. Because the hospital was seen as giving leadership and guidance to all other forms of health care, the medical technology approach very much determined the shape of health systems. The WHO Expert Committee in its report (1987) proposed that a comprehensive health care system should be based on principles of primary health care, rather than hospital-centred. Paine and Siem Tjam (1988) perceive a tension between the need to provide an equitable health service to all members of a population, and the potential for 'empire-building' afforded by highly sophisticated technological medicine. They also question the extent to which the latter contributes to improved health in terms of measurable indicators such as mortality and morbidity statistics.

China is often cited as an example of a nation where political influence has run counter to the dominant pattern of health described above. The Report of an Inter-Regional Seminar organised by the WHO (1983), which considered the Chinese experience of primary health care, identified tremendous political commitment permeating all levels of government and all social and mass organisations. The report also described the participation of the people themselves in the provision of health services, in the management of the system and in mass campaigns as perhaps the most important factor in the development of the Chinese health care system. It also describes as 'appropriate technology' aspects of Chinese health care such as mass mobilisation for prevention, the development of cooperative health centres, the combined use of traditional Chinese medicine and Western medicine, and the emergence of the 'barefoot doctors'. Instead of high cost, high technology medicine for the few, barefoot doctors are the first point of contact with the health services for the many. They treat minor illnesses and have a major input in preventive health work (such as immunisation programmes) as well as being involved in health teaching and the nationwide campaign for population control. Barefoot doctors are selected and paid for locally in rural areas, as individuals whose personalities and characteristics are known to the

communities they will serve.

Finally, the health status of all the population has been improved as a result of sufficient increase in income and its equitable distribution, permitting adequate shelter, clothing and essential food at affordable prices; improvement of literacy and mass education, particularly at primary level; and environmental measures improving facilities such as water supplies and public transport.

A major thrust of primary health care as it has been described so far is the promotion of health. The way in which the primary health care system develops in any society will inevitably be influenced by the concept of health which prevails in that society (see Chapter 3).

Health in the UK – an emphasis on prevention?

Robinson (1983) suggests that it was a 'negative' model of health on which the establishment of the National Health Service was based in 1948. According to this model, health is simply the absence of disease, illness being assumed to be synonymous with the presence of disease. Successful treatment of the disease would then logically lead to restoration of health. Such a model of health would place a high premium on scientific developments and medical technology. The emphasis in this kind of health care would be on curative rather than on preventive measures.

Since it has been suggested that primary health care is significantly concerned with promotion of health and prevention of ill health, it seems likely that a society valuing Robinson's negative model of health might be one in which primary health care is relatively under-resourced.

A relationship may be seen between the prevailing concept of health within a society and the way in which individuals in that society are seen to relate to social groups and society as a whole. Phrases such as 'the British stiff upper lip', and 'an Englishman's home is his castle' suggest a society in which a premium is placed on independence and self-reliance. Such a notion appears to relate well to a concept of health as merely the absence of disease in an individual.

Three levels of prevention

In the late 1980s, health education and preventive health care measures began to gain an increasingly high profile in the UK. The proportion of peak viewing and listening time devoted to health issues appears to be increasing on television and radio, and private health facilities are advertising personal health assessments for the consumer. The new GP Contract (Health Departments of Great Britain, 1989) introduced in April 1990 required GP practices to place greater emphasis on health promotion and illness prevention, by offering 'health promotion' consultations to all patients aged 16–74 years, encouraging women patients to accept screening for breast and cervical cancer, and offering an annual home visit to all patients over 75 years, with an opportunity for a health assessment.

Preventive health care is often described as operating at three levels, as first outlined by Caplan (1969). According to him **primary prevention** means the processes involved in reducing the risk that people will fall ill. An example of primary prevention is the immunisation programme for children under five years. **Secondary prevention** he describes as the activities involved in reducing the duration of established cases of a disorder, and thereby reducing the prevalence of the disorder. The emphasis in secondary prevention is on early diagnosis and effective treatment. Screening programmes such as regular child developmental assessments and cervical screening are examples of secondary prevention. In order for a screening programme to be justified, however, the tests used need to be effective in early detection and acceptable to those being tested, and they need to be sensitive and specific enough to avoid false positive results. Furthermore, there needs to be effective and acceptable treatment available for the conditions detected through the tests. The Hall Report (1989) critically evaluates the procedures which have been used in the community for child health surveillance, and finds some of them lacking on the above criteria.

Caplan's third level, **tertiary prevention,** he describes as including rehabilitation services which aim at returning sick people as soon as possible to maximum effectiveness. Even where an individual may be suffering from a condition which cannot be cured, it is often possible to reduce the impact of the condition, and minimise or even eliminate side effects.

Health as a corporate responsibility: a concept of equilibrium

In recent years, attention has been focused on conditions which have variously been described as 'self-induced' or 'diseases of lifestyle'. These descriptions have been applied to conditions such as ischaemic heart disease, lung cancer, alcoholism and addiction, diet-related conditions, and more recently AIDS. Yet it is simplistic to imply that such conditions are the result of what individual sufferers have done to themselves without taking into account the effects of factors such as unemployment, poverty, poor housing, and social and environmental stresses over which the individual may have little or no control. For an individual to have more control over his personal health, it is necessary to recognise the responsibility of communities within society, and of society as a whole, to be involved in promoting health.

Health can be viewed as a state of dynamic equilibrium between the individual and his environment. In China, concepts of health not only emphasise the individual's responsibility, but also the collective responsibility of members of the public. Lifestyle is seen as important not only in relation to the health of the body but also in relation to healthy relationships within the social group. Burkitt (1983) asserts that traditional Chinese medicine focuses on maintaining a healthy balance in the life forces influencing the body by means of appropriate diet, rest, meditation and exercise. The political regime emphasises that the health of the body and mind are part of an individual's duty to society, and furthermore, it is the responsibility of each member of society to encourage one another in health-promoting behaviour. In traditional Chinese medicine the active participation of the patient is central. In socialist China this active participation is shown in primary health care programmes, as for example in the selection and payment of 'barefoot doctors' mentioned above, and by providing the labour for public health measures such as the draining of disease-infested swamps. According to Burkitt, China has the only health service in the world where the main emphasis is on prevention and simple technology, and the results are gratifying. Low technology health care also implies a much greater potential for active patient participation than the high technology approach of much Western medicine.

In the UK, planning for primary health care is increasingly adopting a 'needs-led' approach, which focuses on identifying the particular patterns of health needs within local populations, and the range of resources available within the health and social services, the voluntary services, and within the population itself, which can be utilised to meet the needs identified (see Community Health Profiling and Assessment of Health Needs, page 87).

Primary health care and the political dimension

In the UK, as in most countries, primary health care has its roots in voluntary and professional responses to patently unmet needs in society. The Alma-Ata Declaration (WHO, 1978) asserted unequivocally that governments have a responsibility for the health of their people. When Bob Geldof went to Ethiopia during the famine in 1985 (Geldof, 1986) he found relief efforts underfunded and hamstrung by the ideology of the Marxist government's policies. In the Sudan, with a disaster of equal proportions imminent, he found no organisation at all and a government which gave no official acknowledgement to the existence of a problem. Famine in Africa provides a vivid example of the complexity of the factors affecting health and health care. In order to resolve the health problems of Ethiopia on any long-term basis there was, and still is, a need for economic resources, political stability and an end to civil war, adequate transport systems, adequate food, water supplies and sanitation, and the knowledge and skills for putting into practice modern farming techniques which would restore rather than deplete the land. All these are in addition to the whole range of personal health services provided by what is called the primary health care team in the UK.

In any nation, the resources available to government for financing health care services are finite. Within health services as a whole there are various interests competing for funds. Institutional care is expensive for many reasons – the staffing of a 24 hour service seven days per week, the cost of high technology equipment, and the need for ancillary services such as catering and laundry. Medical research programmes are costly, and the cost of drugs is one of the largest items on the NHS bill in Britain. Nevertheless, it would seem that beliefs and values about health and health care place a greater constraint on the way in which primary health care services develop than do financial limitations. In one instance, the development of curative services may apparently take priority (as seems to have happened in Western medicine), whereas in another instance (as in China) preventive health may take priority.

A 'mixed economy of care' and the need for collaboration

In the United Kingdom, political ideology can be seen to influence primary health care in a variety of ways. For example, it has been government policy for a number of years to promote care in the community (rather than in long-term institutions) particularly with regard to the mentally ill, the handicapped and the elderly. These policies affect the workload of community staff such as district nurses and community psychiatric nurses, as well as often increasing the burden of care for relatives of patients who may then seek help from health and social service agencies.

It is difficult, if not impossible in many instances, to make a sharp distinction between the 'health care' needs and 'social care' needs of an individual, and a dominant theme in community care literature is the need for liaison, cooperation and collaboration between relevant agencies. In the White Paper *Caring for People* (DoH, 1989), which focuses on enabling the elderly, disabled, mentally ill and those with learning difficulties to live independently in their own homes wherever possible, the government envisages a 'mixed economy of care'. It becomes the responsibility of local social service authorities to promote coherent networks of local services which would include both primary health care and non-statutory services. The White Paper also recognises that most care in the community is given by family, friends and neighbours, and that practical support for such carers is a high priority. For such support to be appropriate, patients and their carers need to be consulted and involved in decisions made about the services which need to be provided.

The theme of collaboration between primary health care and social service authorities is also emphasised in the provisions of The Children Act (HMSO, 1989), particularly in the assessment of children defined as 'in need', and in the regular multi-agency review of children registered as disabled.

Housing

Housing is another area where the effects of government policy on primary health care can be seen. In inner city areas particularly, health visitors find themselves confronted by families living in damp, overcrowded, substandard accommodation, in neighbourhoods characterised by squalor and decay, and where young children are susceptible to a high incidence of respiratory tract problems, yet the health visitor knows that rehousing is impossible. There is just not enough housing available or being built. Policy trends appear to be towards the eradication of council housing, yet homes on the open market are already prohibitively expensive for first-time buyers, and media reports suggest that homelessness is on the increase.

Elaine Sheppard, in her introduction to *Bed and Breakfast: Women and Homelessness Today* (Miller, 1990) quotes Audit Commission figures published in 1989 indicating that more than 30,000 households live in temporary accommodation of various kinds. She goes on to say that this represents a rapid increase since 1982, when there were just over 5000 such families, and she also points out that most single homeless people and those who are 'intentionally homeless' are not included in these figures.

For those who do not have the means to buy their own homes or renovate the accommodation they live in, who have to share cooking and toilet facilities with uncongenial neighbours, and who are not articulate enough to promote their case to the authorities, the health care worker who is helpless to resolve these problems is likely to be seen as irrelevant.

Conflicting views on what constitutes health

Primary health care organised on a national scale is likely to develop in response to the dominant concept of health in a society. The perceptions of health held by different individuals, especially in a multicultural society such as the UK, will vary widely. For example, the family living in overcrowded, substandard housing may perceive health as related overwhelmingly to their environment. They may attribute family tensions, irritability, depression and respiratory infections all to the home environment, and see rehousing as the only solution. On the other hand the health visitor, who knows the impossibility of rehousing, may perceive better health for the family in terms of an improved ability to cope in the environment which cannot be changed. In another situation, an individual may consider himself to be perfectly healthy whilst engaging in a lifestyle generally regarded as unacceptable to society (for example, a drug abuser) or unacceptable to health care workers (for example, a heavy smoker). Furthermore, what is acceptable in one society may be totally unacceptable in another.

Consequently, one of the challenges for those delivering primary health care services is the need to reconcile the health perceptions of the health care worker and the consumer. Another challenge may be to help the consumer recognise conflicts between his own health perceptions, or those of the group to which he belongs, and those of the wider society.

Primary health care – who provides it?

Primary health care may be provided by people who are trained or untrained, by people who are paid to give care or by volunteers, and equally by carers within the family. Generally speaking, knowledge, sophisticated expertise and educational qualifications appear to be highly valued in Western societies. Emphasis is therefore placed on the quality of care given by health care *professionals*. These professionals have titles protected by statute, and only those appropriately qualified are licensed to practised. Such safeguards have been seen as essential in order to maintain some control over the quality of care given, and to protect the consumer. An alternative view is that by stressing the need for training and expertise, professional carers may actually disable potential lay carers and reduce the resources available for care. In order to protect their own status, professional groups may begin to define activities as ones which only the trained professional can perform, when in fact a lay person may be just as competent.

For a primary health care system to be as effective as possible, the issue of which activities are to be properly regarded as only the province of the appropriately trained professional carer needs to be kept under review.

Accountability or flexibility?

A further potential dilemma for the paid carer is that of accountability. To whom is he or she accountable? There are three possibilities: to the consumer, to the professional group, or to the employer. Although, in a national health system, the employer is in a sense the collective consumer, it has already been established that there may be a conflict between the perceptions of the collective consumer and the individual consumer in direct contact with the carer. Too great a commitment to the professional group may tend towards the perpetuation of practices which are more orientated towards protecting the existence of the group than to meeting the current needs of the consumer. The Community Nursing Review (Cumberlege Report, DHSS, 1986b) asserted that community nursing services in the United Kingdom are in a rut. The Review suggested that traditional working methods tend to prevail, and that district nurses and health visitors allow themselves to become set in their roles. Perhaps it is appropriate to question whether such lack of flexibility is not an inherent risk in any attempt to achieve and maintain professional status. When the level of unmet need outstrips existing resources there is a requirement for innovation and flexibility which is not best served by rigid adherence to traditional boundaries.

Acceptability to the local community

Not all trained carers are highly educated professionals. In a number of countries, acceptability to the local community has been made a criterion for selection of primary health care workers. As well as 'barefoot doctors' in China, community health workers in India have been recruited on this basis. The writer visited a Community Health Project in the Punjab in 1978, and listened to the director of the project briefing medical and health visiting staff. It was established that the community health workers recruited from the villages had credibility and were respected by the villagers, and the role of the medical and health visiting staff included supporting the lesser trained community health workers in every way possible. It is salutary

to recall that health visiting in the UK had similar beginnings when the ladies of the Sanitary Reform Association of Manchester and Salford recruited respectable working women to pay door-to-door visits to the working class poor, on the premise that because the visitors came from the working classes their advice was more likely to be heeded (Macqueen, 1962).

Partnership in caring

In considering the beliefs which underlie the structure of the NHS in the UK, Wilson (1975) seems to distinguish between the treatment of illness and disease as a task for experts, and the promotion of health as more of a partnership activity. He is concerned that too much regard for experts can rob us of the simple ways by which he says we express our mutual care for one another. Skeet (1982) echoes his views, and suggests that the nurse's role in primary health care should be to identify people's health needs, and teach and enable clients to be responsible for their own health and that of their families and their communities. She quotes Barrow (1980) as asking:

'Can nurses admit that a person or a community can be involved in their own health care and can perform urgently needed curative and preventive measures, independently of the nurses, without considering the person/community a threat to their professional standing?'

One important reason for consumer participation in primary health care is that health needs arise and exist in a social and environmental context. Since health deficits may result from factors (such as poverty or environmental pollution) which require economic, political or engineering solutions, a primary health care service operating as a totally separate and isolated entity must be doomed to failure. The primary health care worker who fails to work in partnership with the client will provide a service fit for Skeet's (1982) epitaph on 20th century medicine: 'Woefully inept in its application to those most in need'.

The nurse as the client's advocate (see also Chapter 11)

In the UK, an increasing trend in primary health care nursing, whether district nursing or health visiting, has been to stress the nurse's function as the client's advocate. This advocacy operates in three ways: by offering information and support to a client so that he can make the best decision for himself concerning his health (Kohnke, 1980), by becoming influential in upholding client decisions (Leininger, 1974), and by identifying and making available to appropriate corporate bodies data concerning wider social, economic and environmental factors and their significance for the client's health status. In this way the emphasis is on fostering as much independence and autonomy as possible on the client's part and on responding as appropriately as possible to each client as a unique individual with a unique combination of needs and health perceptions.

Widening the range of health care providers

With the introduction of the internal market into the NHS in 1991, and the separation between purchasers and providers of health services, the intention is that primary health care services of the future may be provided by a wider range of agencies than in the past. Since the NHS came into being, primary health care services have been provided mainly by local government and local health authorities, with voluntary and charitable agencies either acting on behalf of such authorities, or providing specific additional services according to the agency's particular area of concern. Purchasers of health services are now being encouraged to collaborate with voluntary agencies more closely than in the past, and to be prepared to buy services offered by private health service agencies if such agencies offer an attractive deal. An example of such private services, described in *Community Outlook* (Seymour, 1991), offers, 'comprehensive home care support within 24 hours . . . working in partnership with community nursing and social services'.

With an emphasis on tailoring local provision to local patterns of need, the combination of health care professionals and agencies providing primary health care in the future will potentially vary from one locality to another. Health service planners are increasingly making use of community health profiles to provide a database for their planning.

Community health profiling and assessment of health needs

A wide range of information exists which can help to identify priority health needs and issues locally (see Fig. 4.1), although in practice there are many difficulties to overcome if it is all to be put together in as up-to-date a state as possible, and interpreted meaningfully to form a health profile of a local community. Health and vital statistics, which have traditionally been regarded as key sources of information, suffer from several limitations. They are inevitably somewhat out-of-date by the time they have been collected and published, so that they can never reflect quickly changes which may be taking place. To date, computerised information systems, intended to speed up the processing of information, often seem to increase the delay, although the hope for the future is that increasingly efficient and user-friendly programmes will be developed. In many instances, too, health statistics relate to populations which contain a number of very different groups, and the larger the population to which they relate, the less they are likely to help clarify *local* health issues. For example, examination of data concerning patterns of housing tenure and occupational status in 1991 in Bexley Health Authority suggests quite a strong north-south socio-economic gradient in the population, so that statistical information collected for the whole health authority must inevitably have under-represented the problems of those living in the northern part and over-represented the problems of those in the south. Similar limitations apply to all statistical information which is collected.

Caseload analyses comprise one of the most up-to-date sources of information available to primary health care planners. By putting information about their caseloads into categories with common characteristics and problems, health visitors and district nurses may be amongst the first to recognise and identify newly emerging health issues. In addition to information already available from GPs about the health problems about which patients consult them, health visitors and district nurses are likely to be able to shed some light on the dimensions of what has been called the 'symptom iceberg' (Hannay, 1979); in other words, those symptoms which people experience but decide not

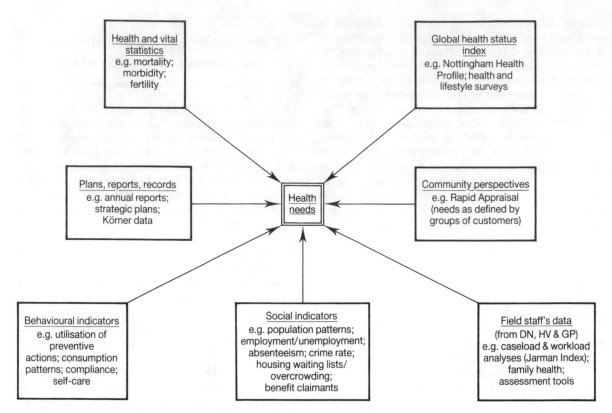

Fig. 4.1 Assessment of health needs of local populations – sources of information

to report to their GPs, and which reflect unrecognised and unmet health needs.

In recognition of the relationship between social and environmental factors and health, various deprivation indices have been devised, to identify whole populations which are in particular need and vulnerable to poor health. One of these, the Jarman Index (Royal College of General Practitioners, 1981), was based on caseload information from GPs, who identified various categories of patients who required their services more than the average. Various health authorities in recent years have developed similar approaches in seeking to establish workload implications for district nurses and health visitors based on data from activities such as family health assessments.

Further information about the health of populations can be obtained by using an assessment of the total or global health of the individuals who make up the population. Various global health status indices have been developed, and one which has been used by authorities in the UK is the Nottingham Health Profile (Hunt et al., 1981). This focuses on the replies given by individuals to questions on their state of health, and the questionnaire includes categories such as social activity, locomotion, sleep, nutrition, and family life, amongst others.

Increasingly, primary health care planners are seeking ways of developing more of a partnership approach with the local communities they are serving and trying to understand better communities' own perceptions of their priority needs. Rapid Appraisal (Annett and Rifkin, 1988) is one approach which has been used in deprived urban areas. It uses key informants from the community both to identify the health problems from that community's perspective, and to contribute to finding solutions. For example, the lollipop lady at the school crossing, the shopkeeper in the corner shop, the mothers who run the local playgroup, and the organisers of the local old people's club may all be key informants from the community. The problems seen as important by the community may not be the same as those prioritised by the authorities, so that Rapid Appraisal then involves dialogue between the community representatives and the health care agencies to reach agreement on priorities for action. In a number of urban areas, the high cost and/or lack of availability of healthy food has been highlighted as a major issue, and in at least two instances the solution has been for the local community to set up its own non-profit-making food cooperative, demonstrating that even in the most deprived areas, communities are not entirely lacking in the means to contribute to solutions to their health problems.

Primary health care services

Having established that primary health care is a matter for the whole of society, we can now focus on the primary health care services as defined by the UK Government in its Discussion Document, *Primary Health Care – An Agenda for Discussion* (DHSS, 1986a). These services include family doctors, dentists, retail pharmacists and ophthalmic services (the family practitioner services for which Family Health Services Authorities are responsible), and district nurses, midwives and health visitors, and other professions allied to medicine (the community health services). The definition is necessarily arbitrary, but is chosen so that the dominant issues concerning primary health care in the UK can be considered. In particular, detailed attention is given to the medical and nursing members of what has been called the primary health care team, since this has been described as the care team within the primary health care services. A joint working group of the Standing Medical Advisory Committee and the Standing Nursing and Midwifery Advisory Committee, reporting in May 1981, defined the membership of the primary health care team as:

> '. . . an interdependent group of general medical practitioners and secretaries and/or receptionists, health visitors, district nurses, and midwives . . .'

Secretaries/receptionists were included in the definition because of their perceived importance in facilitating communication within the team.

The primary health care team – how its membership developed

There is a continuing debate about the usefulness of primary health care teams, and part of the reason for the debate is that some are teams in name only.

A team is a group of individuals working together towards a common goal, but some primary health teams do not work together, and others do not even have common goals.

Some of the reasons for these deficits become apparent when considering how each constituent professional group has developed. Consideration of the past may help planning in the future, for the present mix of primary health care workers, their particular role descriptions, job specifications, skills, knowledge and abilities may well become outdated and irrelevant in years to come. A service which is to meet the changing needs of a changing population adequately in a changing environment must necessarily be a changing, flexible and adaptable service. Already, district nursing services are being provided increasingly by teams of nurses possessing a mix of skills and qualifications between them. The team leader will be a district nursing sister possessing a post-basic district nursing qualification, and in the future the team is likely to include post-Project 2000 first level registered nurse practitioners qualified in the care of the adult, existing registered general nurses and district enrolled nurses, and support workers. Until now the notion of skill mix in teams of health visitors has not developed to the same extent, but future teams headed by qualified health visitors may include nursery nurses, first level nurses qualified in the care of the child, and support workers. In line with the recommendations of the Cumberlege Report (DHSS, 1986b), district nurses and health visitors of the future can be expected to share a large portion of their post-basic training and subsequently develop more flexible and co-operative ways of working together.

In its Report on Proposals for the Future of Community Education and Practice (1991), the UKCC envisages a 'new discipline of community health care nursing'. This will incorporate all first level community nurses with a recordable qualification in community nursing, including community mental handicap nurses, community psychiatric nurses, district nurses, occupational health nurses, school nurses, and registered health visitors. The proposed preparation for community health care nursing for all nurses working in the community in the future will be designed to equip them with a set of core skills common to all, as well as such additional skills as are required for a specific area of practice. Whilst the UKCC is concerned to foster as flexible and integrated a service as possible, it recognises that there will still be areas of practice which require a specific preparation and entry in a particular part of the Council's Register.

The number of practice nurses employed by GPs has greatly increased in recent years, and they and community health care nurses will each need to take into account the contributions made by each group. Existing practice nurses who wish to qualify as community health care nurses will be able to undertake preparation to do so which should be modified appropriately in the light of their previous experience and education.

The emergence of the general medical practitioner

The general practitioner as we know him today began to emerge during the 19th century. His antecedents include three different types of healer. There were the herbalists, who qualified by examination to become members of the Society of Apothecaries – one of the trade guilds whose guildhall still exists in London today. Then there were the surgeons, who usually gained their skills and experience serving with the armed forces, and who were regarded as craftsmen. Finally, there were the physicians, who had long attained professional status and were graduates of university medical schools. Not surprisingly, the physicians tended to stay close to the centres of learning and were most often to be found in the larger towns. Surgeons and apothecaries provided the majority of care in rural areas.

As general practitioners emerged, they combined elements of all three groups, although surgery was a predominant influence. No initial distinction was made between specialists and general practitioners. Any registered medical practitioner could work either in hospital or in the community after the first Medical Act in 1858 established the medical register. It could be argued that, despite the trade and craftsman origins of the apothecaries and surgeons, the setting up of this register enabled their general practitioner descendants to attain full professional status.

However, as medical and scientific knowledge expanded during the latter half of the 19th century, scientific medicine became based in hospitals. Consequently those doctors who chose to specialise were increasingly likely to work in hospitals. With their high levels of knowledge and skills, they became sought after by the wealthy and acquired consultant status amongst their colleagues. Meanwhile, their generalist colleagues found themselves treating the poorer patients, unable to be selective about the kind of cases they would treat. The distinction between specialists working in hospitals and generalists working in the community remains to this day.

The growth of group practices and the primary health care team

By the early 1960s the morale of GPs had ebbed considerably. Their sense of status was low in comparison with that of their hospital colleagues, and they received comparatively low pay for work which entailed responsibility for an on-call service 24 hours each day, 365 days of the year. The Royal Commission on Medical Education (1965–8) reported:

> '. . . general practice . . . is bound to undergo great changes in the foreseeable future . . . many . . . now accept that the single-handed general practitioner and the traditional domestic or street corner consulting-room can have no place in the structure of good practice beyond the present generation.'
>
> (page 33)

The Report went on to advocate group practices able to invest in adequate administrative help and equipment to maintain efficient record-keeping and organisation of the practice. It also supported the notion of the primary health care team (although not in so many words) by arguing that GPs needed to be able to delegate a variety of tasks to colleagues in other professions, and by apparently welcoming the introduction of nurses and health visitors 'as integral members of medical practice.'

The Report was unambiguous in its view that the GP would, without question, be the leader of any team of health care professionals involved in primary care. At the time when the Report saw nurses and health visitors as becoming integral members of medical practice, student health visitors were being taught to see the same phenomenon as one of attachment of health visitors to general practices. Attached health visitors would function as practitioners in their own right, determining for themselves what was and what was not part of the health visitor's role. To this day the functioning of a primary health care team is influenced by whether its members are in a hierarchical relationship to one another or whether they are seeking to work as a partnership of equals.

The Royal Commission Report also dealt with the issue of distribution of primary health care services, suggesting that outlying rural areas could not expect the quality of facilities which would be available in urban areas, since recent medical graduates would not wish to work in areas where they would necessarily be denied access to specialised medical facilities and the constant company of other doctors, with its implications for maintaining professional competence. Ironically, the Report on Primary Health Care in Inner London (London Health Planning Consortium, 1981) found that both group practices and primary health care teams were more scarce in inner London than elsewhere. There was a disproportionately high number of elderly GPs working single-handed, normal surgery hours tended to be shorter than elsewhere, and there was considerable use of message-handling services out of surgery hours. Furthermore, it appeared that anxious patients were increasingly using Accident and Emergency Departments as a substitute for the GP service.

It would seem that the factors influencing the choice of where a GP will practise are rather more complex than the Royal Commission anticipated. Meanwhile, changes had been taking place in medical training and practice. Since 1953, all medical graduates have had to complete a further year as house officers in hospital posts before registration. Subsequently, options to train in specialties such as paediatrics, psychiatry and medicine have become available to those intending to go into general practice; so too have programmes of in-service training for practising GPs. Academic departments of general practice now exist in most medical schools, and primary health care is recognised as a legitimate field for medical research.

The status of GPs as independent contractors

Although the introduction of the internal market

into the NHS has brought with it a new emphasis on the establishment of contractual relationships between purchasers and providers of health care, GPs have had independent status and contracted their services to the NHS for many years.

This independent status had its beginnings at the turn of the century, when some GPs were paid to see patients who were members of trade unions and friendly societies. The National Insurance Act (HMSO, 1911) extended this provision to the poorest sector of the population and to all manual workers. Under the Act, GPs providing this service received a capitation fee, a system of remuneration which still continues, with the service being extended to the whole population when the NHS was established in 1948. The 1990 GP Contract introduced elements of performance-related pay, for example by setting target levels for childhood immunisations and cervical cytology. If the relevant target is not achieved, the GP will not receive the target payment. Some GP practices are employing increasing numbers of staff, including practice nurses, and the 1990 Contract requires the GP to ensure that the health professional staff employed are properly qualified for the work they do, and receive regular training. Since 1966, GPs have received reimbursement of a significant proportion of their costs incurred in employing ancillary staff and improving premises and equipment, which in theory should provide incentives to offer a high quality service to patients.

GP services may now be financed in one of two ways. Practices which are *not* fundholding receive fees, allowances and direct reimbursement of certain expenses from the Family Health Service Authority with which they have contracted to provide their services. At the discretion of the FHSA, direct reimbursement may include a proportion of the costs of employing and training staff, for example, practice nurses, and the FHSA may also pay a fee for any Health Promotion Clinics which it has approved to be run by GPs. Historically a major NHS expense has been the cost of drugs and from April 1st 1991, FHSAs acquired responsibility for allocating indicative prescribing budgets in order to contain the cost of drugs.

Practices which have successfully applied to become fundholding practices are allocated budgets by their Regional Health Authorities. These budgets enable GPs to purchase hospital and diagnostic services as they choose, within their budgets. The costs of prescribing and of employing and training staff are also covered, and an annual management fee is included. It can be argued that fundholding practices have the potential to offer patients a better service insofar as having their own budgetary control gives GPs greater freedom of choice over diagnostic treatment and referral decisions.

However GPs are financed, their contracts with FHSAs must specify whether they agree to provide contraceptive services, maternity services, child health surveillance services or minor surgery services as part of their general medical services. A major intended effect of the 1990 GP Contract appears to be to encourage the development of GP practice services in line with the general move to promote care in the community rather than in institutions wherever possible.

The health visitor: beginnings as a sanitary visitor

Whilst it may be said that the general medical practitioner emerged in the context of the rapid development of scientific medicine in the latter part of the 19th century, it could also be argued that both health visiting and district nursing emerged in the context of the social and environmental changes following in the wake of the Industrial Revolution. According to Macqueen (1962), the years from the beginnning of the 19th century to 1860 saw the development of a predominantly urban civilisation in Britain for the first time in history. Irish immigrants and workers from the British countryside flocked to the growing number of cotton factories, coal mines and iron works. Living conditions in the new towns were appalling. There was horrific overcrowding and often a total lack of sanitation. Under such conditions waterborne infections, such as typhoid and poliomyelitis, were rife. In particular, successive epidemics of cholera swept the country.

The cholera outbreaks produced a public response in a way that diseases like typhoid and typhus did not, although they were claiming thousands of lives annually. The difference was probably that, whereas the latter diseases were confined to the overcrowded urban slums where the poor lived, cholera struck impartially at rich and poor alike, in all sections of society, and its course was so rapid that the majority of victims were dead within 24 hours of the first onset of symptoms.

As the basic principles underlying the prevention of spread of infection began to be understood during the latter half of the 19th century, the fear of cholera provided the impetus for sanitary reform. Environmental measures such as piped water supply, efficient sewage disposal systems and improvements in housing conditions began to be introduced. Doctors and 'sanitary visitors' went into the homes of the poor in various parts of the country, to teach basic rules of hygiene in response to specific cholera outbreaks. They found people crowded in cellars, back-to-back houses and inner courts, all of which were dark, damp and inundated with fluid filth from ash pits or cesspools (Chadwick, 1842). There were various initiatives for visiting the homes of the poor, but the scheme introduced by the Ladies' Sanitary Reform Association of Manchester and Salford in 1862 is generally regarded as the origin of health visiting. The aims of this Association were the popularisation of knowledge about health and the physical, social, moral and religious elevation of the people (Macqueen, 1962). When distribution of pamphlets by members of the Association failed to produce results, it was decided to employ 'respectable working women' as door-to-door visitors instead. The duties laid down for these women are detailed in Table 4.1.

From the beginning, these sanitary visitors were regarded by the Association as health teachers and

Table 4.1. *Duties laid down for sanitary visitors*

Teaching of environmental hygiene and child welfare
'They must carry with them carbolic powder, explain its use, leave it where it is accepted; direct the attention of those they visit to the evils of bad smells, want of fresh air, impurities of all kinds; give hints to mothers on feeding and clothing their children.'

Social support
'Where they find sickness, assist in promoting the comfort of the invalid by personal help.'

Teaching of mental or moral health
'They must urge the importance of cleanliness, thrift, and temperance on all possible occasions.'

Later a fourth duty was added:

Group education – persuading mothers to attend meetings for talks and discussions.

(Macqueen, 1962)

social counsellors. By 1890 there were 14 such visitors on the Association's books, and in that year arrangements were made for six of them to be transferred to the employment of Manchester Public Health Department – as the first health visitors to be employed by a local authority.

Florence Nightingale (1893) was utterly convinced of the value of health visitors and she persuaded the Buckinghamshire local authority not only to employ them, but also to provide a training of 16 lectures and some practical work. The first trainees were examined in 1891 and standards were so stringent that only six of the 12 candidates were successful.

The health visitor as a well-baby nurse

The early focus of health visiting was on the health of individuals of any age, but during the early years of the 20th century the emphasis began to change. Despite the preceding public health reforms, there was public concern at rising infant mortality rates. The peak came in 1899, with a rate of 163 per 1000 (Honigsbaum, 1970). Evidence from social surveys by Booth (1890) and Rowntree (1910) began to demonstrate the effect on health of living at a bare subsistence level. In 1901–1902, 40% of army recruits were rejected as unfit on medical grounds, a situation which gave rise to national concern. By 1906 the Infant Welfare Movement was launched with prestigious support from members of the royal family as well as the Prime Minister. Health visiting became associated with the Infant Welfare Movement, and practitioners began to take on the image of 'well-baby nurses', involved from the beginning with the work of the early maternity and child welfare centres.

The 1872 Public Health Act had introduced compulsory appointment of local authority medical officers of health. Their approach to public health practice was based on epidemiological principles. From the start, health visiting combined an educative approach with a search for factors damaging to health, and as such gained strong support from medical officers of health, who became the motivating force behind the health visitors' association with the Infant Welfare Movement. At this crucial point in the development of infant welfare and public health services, the passing of the 1911 National Insurance Act effectively led to the isolation of general medical practitioners from preventive health services for mothers

and children, since the Act did not cover the dependants of insured persons. To this day, sick children are not treated in child welfare clinics.

With the increasing focus on infant and child welfare, the pattern of recruitment into health visiting began to change (Macqueen, 1962). There was an increasing tendency for qualified doctors and nurses to apply. In 1919, health visiting became formally established as a profession, with an official training scheme set up in Scotland, and a similar one for the rest of the UK set up by the new Ministry of Health and the Board of Education. Under the new schemes health visitors could qualify by three routes:

(1) One year of post-basic training for an already qualified nurse
(2) A different one-year training course for a university graduate
(3) A two-year training course for a non-nurse, non-graduate.

Because local authorities showed a strong preference for health visitors with a nursing background, the other routes to qualification eventually died out.

In 1925, midwifery was introduced as a requirement for health visiting and some form of obstetric preparation for health visiting was a requirement, until 1989. The effects of the introduction of midwifery were threefold (Macqueen, 1962). Firstly, it became impossible for several decades for men to train as health visitors. Secondly, the post-basic health visitor training course was cut to six months to accommodate the midwifery training – and this inevitably reduced the preventive and social aspects of training, a deficit which was not redressed until the 1950s, by which time health visiting was regarded as a low status, non-graduate occupation with an out-of-date training, and there was debate and uncertainty as to its future (Robinson, 1982). The third effect was to concentrate attention on the maternity and child welfare portion of the health visitor's work.

During the years before the NHS was founded, there was an outstanding decline in the infant mortality rate in England and Wales. It fell from 163 per 1000 in 1899 to 51 per 1000 in 1939, and 32 per 1000 in 1949. Although the cause of the decline was multifactorial, there was a much steeper decline in all of those European countries with services approximating to health visiting than in those without. In Scotland there was a highly significant correlation between reduction in the infant mortality rates of large burghs and the adequacy of health visitor staffing (Macqueen, 1962).

In drawing attention to the adequacy of staffing, Macqueen highlights an issue of perennial concern in health visiting, as in other health care professions. Robinson (1982) suggests that health visiting developed as a low cost method of health surveillance, and cites Ashby (1922) as demonstrating the perpetuation of this belief in the statement that it 'is a fairly cheap method and one for which a comparatively small staff suffices if the Health Visitors chosen are efficient and keen'. Although various formulae have been adopted over the years to determine the staffing establishment of health visitors in a given local authority, these formulae have only recently begun to be developed from research-based criteria and we simply do not know as yet how many health visitors is 'enough'.

The health visitor as a family visitor

With the passing of the National Health Service Act in 1946, it became the duty of all local authorities to provide a health visiting service to every family with children under five, and the health visitor's function was extended to include promotion of the health of the whole household. Under the Act, her specific responsibilities were: to give advice to expectant and nursing mothers, and to mothers and others concerned with the care of young children; to give advice on the care of persons suffering from illness, including mental illness and any injury or disability. The health visitor had evolved into a family visitor, and the inclusion of mental illness in her remit reflected changes in patterns of health and illness in society.

The Act was merely reflecting changes in the pattern of health visiting which had already begun to occur. Despite this apparent expansion in the health visitor's remit, Dingwall (1977) feels that health visiting was out of favour with the post-war Labour administration, and that after the neglect of the inter-war years health visitors were in no position to defend their work. He notes, too, how few in number they were.

The relationship between health visiting and social work

Robinson (1982) identifies specific problems in relation to the definition of the health visitor's role, and more particularly in defining the boundary between health visiting and social work, after the advent of the NHS and the passing in 1948 of the Children's Act. Since 1908, health visitors had held responsibility for child life protection, having been appointed as Infant Protection Visitors under the 1908 Children's Act. In 1948 this responsibility passed to social workers in the local authority Children's Departments specially established following the Monckton Inquiry (1945). This inquiry into the circumstances of the death of a child, Denis O'Neill, in his foster home revealed deficiencies in the system administering and supervising the placement of children in care, which the 1948 Children's Act sought to rectify. The Act also marks the beginning of a closer and more public involvement of social workers with cases of non-accidental injury to children. More than 40 years later, both health visitors and social workers have roles to play in relation to prevention, identification and intervention in the event of non-accidental injury to children. Forty years after the death of Denis O'Neill, the death of another child, Jasmine Beckford, marked yet another in a series of reports and inquiries all identifying essentially the same difficulties and failures to establish an effective system to protect children at risk.

In 1953, the Jameson Committee was set up to '. . . advise on the proper field of work, recruitment and training of health visitors in the National Health Service' (Ministry of Health, 1956; page v). The Jameson Committee saw the health visitor as the 'common factor' in family welfare, as the individual who would provide the link between an individual or family with a need and the resources (both statutory and voluntary) of the welfare state. Sidestepping the issue of the role boundary with social work, the Committee stated that the function of the health visitor should be primarily health education and social advice. The continuing blurring of this role boundary was evidenced in the Health Visiting and Social Work (Training) Act (HMSO, 1962), under which two separate Councils for the Training of Social Workers (CTSW) and of Health Visitors (CTHV) were set up, with a common chairman appointed to both Councils. In late 1964 a Joint Advisory Committee for the two Councils was established, which sought to compare and contrast health visiting and social work. The Committee came to the conclusion that, while health visitors had a responsibility to maintain regular and continuous contact with families due to their statutory position, social workers' contact with families could better be described as episodic. In the minds of many practitioners even today, this distinction seems to be translated into a focus on routine preventive work by health visitors as opposed to crisis intervention by social workers. A continuing concern of many health visitors is that regular routine preventive health care may be continually jeopardised where resources are constrained and crisis situations apparently abound.

Wilkie (1979) records that the final report of the Joint Advisory Committee in 1966 recommended that a degree of overlap between the functions of health visitors and social workers should be welcomed. At the same time, she notes, it asserted that '. . . the health visitor is a nurse and not a social worker, though her service contains an element of social work; the social worker, though not a nurse, is involved in her work in the problems of personal health'.

Historically, the major focus of role overlap between health visitors and social workers has been that of child protection. With the passing of the 1989 Children Act, there would appear to be a widening of that focus to include all children in need. Section 17(10) of the Act defines a child as being in need if:

'(a) he is unlikely to achieve or maintain, or to have the opportunity of achieving or maintaining, a reasonable standard of health or development without the provision for him of services by a local authority . . .
(b) his health or development is likely to be significantly impaired or further impaired, without the provision for him of such services, or
(c) he is disabled.'

The Act further defines a child as being disabled if he is blind, deaf or dumb or suffers from mental disorder of any kind or is substantially and permanently handicapped by illness, injury or congenital deformity.

Health visitors may be involved in the identification of children in need, collaborating with Social Service Departments in the assessment of children in need, and in the provision of support for such children when required. Local authorities have a duty to children in need, but health service authorities and trusts have a duty to cooperate and collaborate with local authorities which is discharged through activities such as those described for health visitors.

The relationship between health visiting and nursing

Elaine Wilkie (1979) points out that although the new Health Visitor Training Council had already decided that the syllabus would grow out of general nurse training and a period of obstetric or midwifery experience, in developing a formal policy for training it was unhappy with the Joint Advisory Committee's description of the health visitor as a nurse. The concern was partly due to a feeling that the public and professional stereotypes of the nurse might be detrimental to the practice of health visiting. These were the years when general practitioners were moving towards the establishment of group practices and were seeking closer working relationships with local authority nursing services. Wilkie suggests that it is not surprising that health visitors, with their nursing backgrounds, suffered from unrealistic demands made on them by general practitioners. The writer recalls discussions during the 1960s about whether or not health visitors should wear uniform. Antagonists asserted that a uniform would serve only to strengthen the association with rigid and authoritarian stereotypes of nurses in the minds of members of the public.

However, the recommendations of the Joint Advisory Committee's 1964 report were accepted, and this step led inevitably to the Health Visitor Council being incorporated into what is now the United Kingdom Central Council for Nursing, Midwifery and Health Visiting. This development was significant because the Council for the Education and Training of Health Visitors was an autonomous statutory body concerned only with health visiting interests and the regulations of health visiting. In contrast, health visiting is now only one part of the responsibility of a UKCC concerned with the regulation of every branch of nursing represented within the NHS. The assumption of the Health Visitors' Association in 1970 was that health visiting was an independent profession linked both to nursing and to social work, but separate and essentially different from both. This was supported by the CETHV itself in 1967 in its statement identifying the 'Function of the Health Visitor', and in its assertion that health visitors are practitioners in their own right, detecting cases of need on personal initiative as well as acting on referrals.

The development of principles of health visiting

A Working Group was set up by the CETHV in 1975 to examine the principles and practice of health visiting, as a necessary pre-requisite to any major curriculum revision. Ruth Schröck was invited to contribute to the Working Group, and described her view of the process which was taking place (CETHV, 1977). She seems to imply that any professional or occupational group may reach a point where internal changes call into question the whole basis for the current mode and patterns of practice. She also suggests that continuous reappraisal is a normal and necessary activity enabling any occupational group to maintain professionalism and relevance. The process includes questioning of established practices and explanations by practitioners as they realise that the established practices no longer fulfil the demands made on them by clients. Ultimately this questioning leads to the need for identification of key concepts and fundamental principles to underlie the future development of the occupation. Such a set of tentative principles was formulated by the Working Group for the health visiting profession to test and evaluate. Over a decade after the publication of those principles (CETHV, 1977), they continue to offer a challenge to traditional patterns of practice which are still very largely being pursued. The Working Group envisaged health visiting as a generalised service across the life span. One practical problem is that local authorities have a statutory responsibility to provide a health visiting service to families with children under five years of age, but there is no corresponding statutory requirement to provide a similar service to households with no under-fives.

Traditional health visiting practice lays very heavy emphasis on regular routine home visiting of families in a caseload, whereas the Working Group's principles imply a need for a more flexible approach.

The four principles of health visiting, as expressed by the Working Group, will be discussed below. They do not appear to support the notion that, while health visiting has links with both nurs-

ing and social work, it still has a clear and separate identity. The justification for health visiting is seen to rest on a belief in the value of health, so that the primary goal of health visiting is the promotion of health. Since concepts of health differ enormously, the practice of health visiting must necessarily be a negotiated activity where client and practitioner work in partnership – in order to reach agreement about the nature of the contribution the health visitor can make to the enhancement of the client's health.

The search for health needs

The first principle of health visiting is that the practitioner will *actively* search for health needs in order to promote health. The emphasis is not on waiting for health problems to manifest themselves, but on *anticipating* and wherever possible avoiding them. This principle reinforces the unique position of the health visitor as a practitioner who provides a service to the *well* population, and whose availability is not limited to situations of already existing needs or problems.

Stimulation of an awareness of health needs

The second principle of health visiting is the *stimulation* of awareness of health needs. At an individual level, for example, a client may be quite unaware of the nutritional requirements for a healthy diet, or of the potential outcomes of an inadequate one. Communities may be unaware of environmental pollutants, or social trends such as rising unemployment, with the implications these may have for health. Since health visitors are likely to be in a position to recognise changes and emerging hazards, they have a responsibility to promote public awareness of emerging needs.

Influence on policies affecting health

The third principle seems to demonstrate on the part of the Working Group an awareness which comes to all social reformers and public health protagonists sooner or later; that it is not enough to seek individual solutions to needs and problems. This principle asserts that it is part of the health visitor's responsibility to seek to influence policies affecting health. They may do this by supporting their professional bodies, and by making their knowledge and experience available both to the latter organisations and to their own NHS managers. It may on occasion be appropriate for them to act as an individual client's advocate; for example, in making representations to the local authority Housing Department or the local Electricity Board. Some health visitors may themselves serve as members of committees or working parties concerned with health-related issues.

Facilitation of health-enhancing activities

Finally, the fourth principle is that of the facilitation of health-enhancing activities. This principle has two dimensions: the individual level and the group level. At the individual client level, the health visitor may seek to enable some activity or behaviour which is desired by or of the client. At the group level, the emphasis is on being involved in the initiation or sustaining of activities within health-care related teams which will be of benefit to the client or client group.

When the Cumberlege Report (DHSS, 1986b) reflected on the way in which nurses in the community seemed to be trapped by tradition, it particularly noted the separate, traditional ways in which health visitors and district nurses appeared to work. These two occupational groups can be seen as having had quite similar beginnings, followed by widely diverging pathways and, more recently, a degree of convergence again.

The district nurse – a service for the sick poor

The beginnings of district nursing are commonly identified with the initiative of a wealthy Liverpool ship-owner, William Rathbone. His great appreciation of the nursing care given to his dying wife by a nurse trained at King's College Hospital in London made him concerned that the sick poor in Liverpool might also have the opportunity to be nursed in their own homes. Nurse training was in its infancy and schools of nursing were only just beginning to be established, so Rathbone funded the setting up of a school of nursing which would not only provide trained nurses to work in hospitals, but also staff for a home nursing scheme. Liverpool was divided into 18 sections, with one nurse in each section responsible for nursing the sick poor. Because of the localities in which these nurses worked, with the appalling conditions in

which their patients lived, accommodation was provided for them in nurses' homes. This pattern persisted into the 1960s in some areas. As a student district nurse in 1965, the writer recalls gathering for breakfast with trained colleagues and the superintendent at the head of the table in the old district nurses' home in Bermondsey – a sombre, dilapidated building which has since given way to a small shopping development.

Rathbone's scheme began in 1862, the same year as the home visiting initiative of the Ladies' Sanitary Reform Association in Manchester and Salford. Rathbone's nurses encountered the same conditions of grinding poverty, overcrowding, lack of sanitation, malnutrition and disease. In the same way that the early sanitary 'reformers' were organised by a voluntary association composed essentially of philanthropic upper class ladies, so in Liverpool the early district nurses were answerable to a voluntary ladies' committee which was instrumental in supplying 'medical comforts' and material resources such as bedding and clothing to alleviate some of the hardships of the families visited.

A number of other initiatives providing home nursing to the poor also emerged, notably in London, but it was Rathbone's approach that caught the imagination of Florence Nightingale. She felt strongly that, regardless of religion or creed, patients merited nursing care without 'strings'. She was opposed to the practice of the Biblewomen who, while they were providing nursing care, also sought to evangelise in the homes they visited. With her support, William Rathbone established the Metropolitan Nursing Association in London, following the same pattern as in Liverpool. Queen Victoria decided to give most of the Women's Jubilee Offering in 1887, a sum of £70,000, for the extension of district nursing schemes. Partly due to Florence Nightingale's advocacy, the future of the Metropolitan Nursing Association was assured. It later became the Queen's Institute of District Nursing, and continues today as the Queen's Nursing Institute. This voluntary organisation ultimately became the acknowledged body responsible for training and maintaining high standards of practice in district nursing.

Like health visiting, district nursing services developed piecemeal across the country. Prior to the inception of the NHS, services for the sick poor only were provided. Those with money paid for private nursing care. Increasing numbers of voluntary nursing associations came into being, providing district nursing services and accommodation for district nurses within local authorities. These Federations of District Nursing Associations or County Nursing Associations, as they were variously known, were affiliated to the Queen's Institute of District Nursing and as such, maintained staff who were either already district nurse trained or who were subsequently provided with Queen's Institute training by the employing association. In 1948, under the National Health Service Act, district nursing services were made available to the whole population regardless of means. The Federations and County Nursing Associations continued to provide district nursing care, but now as agents of the local authorities. Funding from then on was provided by the local authority who also employed the superintendent and her nursing staff. The Nursing Association continued to organise and administer the service and the Honorary Officer of the Association sat on the local authority health committee. In some authorities domiciliary midwives had already come under the aegis of local nursing associations, and in some areas health visitors were also included – notably in rural areas where triple duties nurses were employed.

The changing role of the Queen's Nursing Institute and introduction of mandatory district nursing training

The Queen's Institute continued to maintain its role in leading the development of district nursing, and by 1953 it had established a six-month post-registration training for the nationally recognised qualification for district nursing, the Queen's Nursing Certificate. Sadly, that year marked a watershed in the history of district nursing as a consequence of political and economic issues. The Queen's Institute failed to convince the Minister of Health of the need to maintain the six-month post-registration training, and the course was cut to four months. For the next decade the Queen's Institute fought to reverse this decision without success. In the mid-1960s it withdrew from providing district nurse training as it no longer wished to be associated with what was felt to be inadequate preparation for practice. Unlike the situation in midwifery and health visiting, district nurse training was not mandatory for practice, and

over the years the situation deteriorated until immediately prior to the introduction of mandatory district nurse training in 1981, only about 50% of practising district nurses had any post-registration training.

By this time, too, the nursing associations had relinquished their functions as local authority agents. One of the last, the East Sussex County Nursing Association, ceased its role before the re-organisation of the Health Service in 1974. However, voluntary organisations did not cease to pioneer responses to unmet need. For example, funds from the sale of property to the local authority contributed to the establishment of financial resources and care facilities for retired district nurses in East Sussex who were not eligible for an occupational pension. On a wider scale, the Macmillan Service is a voluntary initiative in response to the need for nursing care for the terminally ill.

The Queen's Nursing Institute continues to look to the future, and as long ago as 1957 was a prime agent in the establishment of one of the first integrated courses in nurse education which pioneered the way for inclusion of community nursing perspectives in basic nurse education. The proposals for nurse training and practice contained in Project 2000 (UKCC, 1986) could be seen as the logical outcome of the philosophy and vision underpinning that early experiment in integrated nurse education. Belatedly, the government of the day now seems to be reconsidering its relationship with voluntary agencies. It remains to be seen whether more fruitful and constructive partnerships can be established between voluntary groups and statutory organisations.

The changing practice of the district nurse

Patterns of district nursing practice have changed over the years. In the beginning much of their care was focused on those suffering from acute infectious diseases, with patients of any age in the life span, as well as helping to relieve material distress and providing the same kind of basic health teaching as the early health visitors. With changes in patterns of health and disease, district nurses today work with predominantly elderly patients and provide nursing care for those with chronic conditions such as rheumatoid arthritis, chronic cardiovascular and respiratory diseases, and leg ulcers. Younger patients are commonly those suffering from progressive debilitating conditions such as multiple sclerosis or those disabled in some way as a result of trauma. Contact with one patient may extend over many months or even years. Especially since the introduction of mandatory district nurse training, an increasing number of district nurses are looking beyond the nursing care of the condition which precipitated their involvement with a patient, and demonstrating a holistic approach in which they perceive preventive health care and health promotion as part of their remit. With an ageing population, it is still an issue of debate as to how the health of elderly people can best be promoted and preserved, and who has the primary responsibility for ensuring that the health needs of the elderly are met.

District nursing today and in the future

As hospital admission and discharge patterns change and technological changes increase the range of conditions which may be cared for at home, district nurses are finding themselves involved in the care of patients with more acute conditions as a result of so-called 'quicker and sicker discharges'. It is also envisaged that the recommendations of the Cumberlege Report (DHSS, 1986b) that district nursing sisters be given powers to prescribe listed items such as dressings, ointments and certain medical sprays, as well as being permitted to use their professional judgement, for example, over the timing and dosage of drugs prescribed for pain relief in terminal care, will very soon be implemented.

A further recommendation of the Cumberlege Report which may well become a future reality is the inclusion of a 'nurse practitioner' within the primary health care team. Unlike the practice nurse, who is an employee of the GP, she would be a practitioner in her own right and would be available on a sessional basis to interview patients and to diagnose and treat specific minor acute illnesses and behavioural disorders according to agreed medical protocols. Like the practice nurse she would be available on a sessional basis to give counselling and nursing advice to patients, who would either consult her directly or be referred by a GP. She would carry out health screening programmes, maintain patient care programmes, and refer patients to the community nursing team for further nursing care, but on her own initiative rather than as directed by the GP.

Midwifery care in the community

The other group of nurses listed as members of the primary health care team are the community midwives. In practice, a decreasing number of midwives remain employed in the community only. The midwifery service is organised as an integrated service. In many authorities midwives who visit mothers at home are actually based at the local maternity unit and are part of the hospital service. The decline in the domiciliary midwifery service has reflected the fall in the number of home confinements which has occurred over the last two decades. Currently about 99% of deliveries take place in hospital (National Audit Office, 1990), and it is very difficult for a midwife practising solely in the community to conduct enough deliveries to maintain competence. Ironically, whilst obstetrics has become increasingly medicalised and most midwives have lost their community base, the values of the modern midwife seem to coincide more closely with those of the health visitor than almost any other group of nurses. Midwifery stresses its concern with the care of healthy mothers and the conduct of normal deliveries. Promotion of health and health education are seen as major aspects of midwifery practice. As with health visiting, it is a matter of debate in midwifery as to whether nursing is the appropriate base for midwifery training and practice.

Generalist nurses and specialist functions

Currently, health visitors are commonly described as generalists. There is no uniform national pattern of specialisation in health visiting, but in various areas there are health visitors for the elderly, or attached to special care baby units or mother and baby units of psychiatric hospitals.

School nurses are a group of nurses whose function is essentially generalist, but who provide a service specific to one age group. Historically, their functions were carried out by health visitors, and in some areas this still happens. Recently, however, school nurses have emerged as a separate group of community nurses, holding the school nurse's certificate in addition to being registered general nurses. In the view of the Health Visitors' Association (1985), every school should have a named school nurse to whom reference can be made on any health matter concerning children at school, and to whom children can go themselves. Since school nursing has developed out of health visiting it is hardly surprising that school nursing functions include health education and health surveillance. As a result of the 1981 Education Act (HMSO, 1981), and the admission of handicapped children to ordinary schools, a developing area of school nursing is that of understanding the implications of a wide variety of disabling conditions on a child's ability to learn alongside his able-bodied peers, and to help all concerned to appreciate these.

The HVA does not advocate that with the emergence of the school nurse, health visitors should abdicate all responsibility for school age children, but rather that there should be a partnership whereby the health visitor who knows the family will be the one to make any home visits which become necessary, while the school nurse concentrates on her work with the child in school.

Amongst nurses giving specialist care in the community are some who are hospital-based and others who are community-based. These include specialists in, for example, stoma care, diabetes, continence advice, and terminal care. The other two major groups of community nurse specialists are community nurses for those with learning difficulties, and community psychiatric nurses (see Chapters 20 and 21).

Other medical, nursing and paramedical services providing primary health care

In addition to the primary health care team, primary health care services include community medical staff, family practitioner services in addition to GPs and other workers in personal and environmental health. Outside the health service, but also providing primary health care, are the occupational health services.

Community medicine

Each authority employs specialists in community medicine who are involved in advising the authority on environmental health matters, social services, and child health and school health. In child health clinics and health centres, health visitors work with clinical medical officers employed by the local authority, who carry out development assessments and child health surveillance examinations. Clinical medical officers are also involved in school medical examinations, where in addition

to monitoring the health and development of all children, they are particularly concerned with the follow-up of children with handicaps and special educational needs.

Family practitioner services

In addition to general medical practitioners, Family Health Service Authorities in each local health authority are responsible for contracts with dentists, opticians, ophthalmic medical practitioners and pharmacists to provide services to the NHS. Preventive dentistry and ophthalmic optics in particular should arguably be seen as having a closer relationship to the work of the primary health care team than is currently the case. Ophthalmic optics, for example, is concerned almost exclusively with early detection of potential problems and their avoidance. The ophthalmic optician is not concerned with pathological conditions of the eye, but with refractive errors of vision in a physically healthy eye. By correcting those refractive errors early enough, the optician seeks to prevent lowering in the standard of vision, or even total loss of vision which can occur in the absence of correction. Staff at the London Institute of Optometry, a charitable establishment where opticians train and which seeks to promote high standards of optical care, would like to see an ophthalmic optician attached to each primary health care team.

Local pharmacists are frequently undervalued and underused. Not only can they be a valuable source of advice and guidance in matters related to the use of chemotherapuetic agents, but in some areas they become a key source of local knowledge and information which can be valuable to the district nurse or health visitor in her daily practice.

The White Paper *Promoting Better Health* (DHSS, 1987) proposed to introduce an allowance for pharmacists who maintain a substantial number of records relating to medicines used by patients who are either elderly or confused and who are on long-term medication. At least one major retail pharmacy chain has gone beyond this and implemented a patient registration scheme for all customers who wish to take advantage of it. Under the scheme the local pharmacy keeps a personal record automatically updated each time a prescribed medicine is supplied, in order to guard against the risk of adverse reactions or drug interactions. Additionally, the system can be used to check whether any over-the-counter medicines purchased would react with prescribed drugs already being taken.

The Nuffield Report (1986) further recommended a renewed emphasis on the role of the pharmacist in advising patients on minor symptoms and on the most sensible and effective ways of using medicines.

Other personal health care workers

A range of community services is provided to deal with specific aspects of treatment of health problems. Many of these are clinic-based, as for example child guidance clinics, family planning clinics and speech therapy clinics. Other services also provide a domiciliary service in some areas, for example chiropody, physiotherapy and occupational therapy. Another example of a voluntary initiative in addition to those mentioned earlier is that of a voluntary society which was set up to provide mobile physiotherapists who would be based in their own homes and provide a home visiting service.

Organisation and management of nursing services in the community

In 1990, the Report of a Department of Health Working Group, entitled *Nursing in the Community* (DoH, 1990) identified five models of ways in which community nursing services were currently being managed, and these different approaches continue to exist. The five approaches are as follows:

(a) **Community Units** as 'stand-alone' community trusts act as provider agencies managing all community health services and offering them to the various purchasing agencies, such as DHAs, FHSAs and GPs. The specific mix of services would be specified and agreed in the contract with a given purchaser. Where community units are already operating in a demonstrably effective and efficient way, this model has the advantage that it enables the preservation of a good working system. One disadvantage is that getting the balance right between practice nurses and other community nurses becomes more difficult.

(b) **Locality Management/Neighbourhood Nursing**

is really an extension of the previous approach, whereby mixed teams of community staff are managed in localities either geographically or around groups of GP practices or health centres. This is in line with the recommendations of the Cumberlege Report, and offers the advantage that the detailed needs of specific communities may be addressed more appropriately because of the detailed knowledge available at the locality level. This pattern is already operating effectively in a number of places. One disadvantage is that GP practice populations may not be coterminous with locality boundaries.

(c) Under the **Expanded FHSA Model,** FHSAs become responsible for the provision of community services under an agency agreement with their DHAs. GPs continue to employ practice nurses, but can also tap into more specialised community services for any care not provided by practice nurses. According to the DoH Report, in exceptional circumstances the FHSA might directly employ staff. An advantage of expanded FHSAs is that the FHSA can take an overview across a range of community services, overcoming the problem of getting the balance right between practice nurses and other community nurses.

(d) The **Vertical Integration or Outreach** approach could take a variety of forms, but the common element is a combination of community and acute services managed within one unit. It offers the advantage of so-called 'seamless care' between acute and/or secondary care services and community services, but by the same token its major disadvantage is that it could focus on those already sick. This runs counter to the current policy of stressing health promotion and illness prevention, and could jeopardise in particular services to the 'healthy' adult population, such as well-person screening clinics.

(e) **GP-managed Primary Health Care Teams** could encompass the full range of community nursing services as appropriate locally. The teams could comprise staff all directly employed by the GP practice, community nurses other than practice nurses could work, as in the past, as attached staff, or nurses and other professionals (for example, chiropodists) could work in equal partnership with GPs. Where such a system works well it offers all the advantages of a locally-based integrated multidisciplinary team, readily accessible to practice patients. One potential disadvantage is that services available would be likely to vary from practice to practice, and would probably tend to be more limited than district-wide provision, especially in respect of specialist services.

The interface between health care and social care: needs of the mentally ill in the community

Since the 1959 Mental Health Act there has been a continuing policy of succeeding governments to locate the care of mentally ill patients in the community rather than in institutions, particularly long-stay ones. The problems which have arisen as a result lie with the continuing care of those suffering from long-term illness which prevents them from leading an independent life in the community. Tomlinson (1991) identifies two such groups: those discharged into the community after a long stay in an institution, and those whom he describes as eking out an existence in the community, vulnerable people who have not been admitted to hospital long-term. He argues that provision of community services has been based on the premise that after many years' hospital residence, the 'long-stay leavers' have poor social, domestic and self-care skills, whilst most of the other group will have retained those skills. Thus the resettlement of hospital residents has been seen as a different process from that of providing for those described by Garety (1988) as the 'never institutionalised'. The result of this belief, in Tomlinson's view, is that:

> 'longstay groups seem to be almost rewarded for their length of service in institutions with gold-plated group homes, while people in the community are reduced to applying for charity'
> (page 24)

To some extent he sees the provision for long-stay leavers as tending to replace care in large mental hospitals with asylum-like group homes in the community, still with professional staff in constant attendance. Data is beginning to accumulate which suggests that a proportion of long-stay leavers become able to manage much better in the community than has been assumed, whilst a proportion of the 'never institutionalised' need a much more supportive and sheltered environment. Ramon (1988) lists the community care services available to the long-term mentally ill as:

GP consultation/prescription on medication
Outpatient clinic appointments
Home visits by community psychiatric nurses
Day care; i.e. day hospitals/day centres
Group homes/hostels
Profit-making private residential facilities
Supportive voluntary services on the part of agencies such as MIND and the National Schizophrenia Fellowship.

However, the availability of the non-medical services in this list remains variable and patchy. Three issues seem to be of relevance:

(a)   Financial constraints are a major disincentive to the development of community services for the long-term mentally ill. Government policies have not been supported by extra government funding; indeed, there is continuing pressure on local authorities and District Health Authorities to reduce costs. Yet the House of Commons Social Services Committee concluded in 1985 that only central funding over several years would overcome the hurdle of the initial capital costs needed to develop the new facilities required. In the absence of such extra funding, no local agency has accepted responsibility for footing the bill.

(b)   Currently there is much emphasis on the need for joint planning and financing of services for the mentally ill. However, whilst health and social service authorities are struggling to meet their separate responsibilities, experience teaches that they are no more likely to cooperate in significant joint activities than they have done to date.

(c)   The will of local communities to accept more local facilities is in some doubt. Tomlinson (1991) cites examples of local residents successfully arguing against the establishment in their neighbourhoods of small homes, and in one instance a day centre, for the mentally ill.

Whilst the closing of large mental hospitals and the lack of alternative provision in the community cannot be proved to be the cause of rising numbers of mentally ill amongst the homeless and those in prison in the UK, it seems probable that it is at least a very significant factor. The House of Commons Social Services Committee (1985) suggested that a quarter to a half of the homeless in shelters or hostels at that time may have been discharged recently from psychiatric hospitals. The sad conclusion appears to be that despite a great deal of talk, and clear policy statements at national level, there is little will in the UK at present to address the needs of the mentally ill in the community, except on the part of a few voluntary and self-help agencies, and on the part of private agencies where they perceive an opportunity for developing a profitable facility.

Social care and voluntary health and social services

In April 1991, local authorities became the lead agency for community care of the elderly, mentally ill, those with learning difficulties, and the disabled. As described in the White Paper *Caring for People* (DoH, 1989), health authorities are responsible for providing health care, and local authorities are responsible for providing social care. However, one health authority chief nurse commented in a *Nursing Times* article (Fawcett-Henesy, 1989) that '. . . the White Paper has split *social* and *health* care. Yet our health care and the new social care appear synonymous to those of us engaged already in health care'.

In the future, it will be important for providers of health care in the community to be crystal clear in their definition of the terms they are using, and able to demonstrate what relationships exist between clients' needs for so-called social care and the health of those clients. For example, home help services, which provide help with daily chores like cleaning and bed-making in the home as well as shopping, can often make the difference between an elderly person being able to remain in his own home and having to be admitted for some kind of residential care. Day centres and luncheon clubs for the elderly help in a similar way, as do meals-on-wheels. Day centres can also relieve some of the pressure on relatives caring for an elderly or handicapped person, perhaps making it possible for them to cope where otherwise the burden would have been too great. Child-minders and playgroups can similarly help to relieve the stress on a young mother who feels isolated and trapped with small children in unsuitable accommodation, or child-minding and day nursery facilities may enable a single parent to go out to work. Voluntary driver and escort services in some areas may make it possible for patients to attend outpatient clinic appointments, where they might otherwise be unable to travel at all, either through lack of public transport or because of their physical disability.

Availability

A key point to be borne in mind is that not all of these services are universally available, and they are not all free at the point of use. In any locality, the would-be user needs to check on the availability, quality and costs of services provided.

A greater emphasis is being placed on collaboration with the voluntary and private sectors. Much work needs to be done in this area, and problems which have been identified in relation to statutory/voluntary collaboration include:

- Two different cultures
- Lack of understanding on both sides
- Differing priorities
- Raised expectations which may not be capable of fulfilment.

Amongst the agencies which can provide information about voluntary initiatives are the National Community Health Resource, local Councils for Voluntary Service, and local Community Health Councils.

Alternative therapies

Within the private sector an increasing range of alternative therapies is becoming available. Sachs (1986) points out that as long as people strive for survival and health, they will always look for a cure that is effective for them. In order to obtain treatment, they have to be able to communicate their personal experiences of discomfort in such a way that those they consult also regard them as ill. This is more likely to happen when the sufferer and the healer share beliefs about the causal explanations of illness. In a multicultural society such as the UK, a range of different beliefs exists, and some of these provide the underpinning for the alternative therapies on offer. Even those who have placed their faith in orthodox medicine will commonly turn to alternative therapies when they do not experience a cure by orthodox treatment. In the sense that alternative therapies may be at the first point of contact for some patients (an example would be the use of chiropractors and osteopaths by sufferers from back pain), and in the sense that most alternative therapies are offered in non-institutional settings, they qualify for consideration under the heading of primary health care. They can be classified under a number of headings, as follows:

Physical therapies

These include *naturopathy*, which is based on the premise that substances accumulating in the body as a result of wrong habits, particularly dietary ones, are the cause of all disease. Symptoms of disease are seen as the body attempting to get rid of the accumulated waste, and the aim of naturopathy treatment is to help the body to bring about a return to health. The main treatments include dietary regimes and *hydrotherapy*, which involves 'taking the waters' internally or externally. Private health clubs, hydros and spas provide saunas or Turkish baths, often with facilities for undertaking dietary treatment.

Other physical therapies include treatments such as *herbal remedies*, often seen as safe alternatives to orthodox drug treatments although this is not always the case. Closely related to herbal treatment is *aromatherapy*, which most commonly takes the form of massage using aromatic essential oils.

Homeopathy is a widely recognised system of medicine based on the principle that like cures like. In choosing a remedy, the homeopath takes a very detailed history not only of the presenting condition, but also of the patient's personality and constitution. Then the remedy prepared will be chosen to correspond to the person as well as the condition needing treatment. It will also be chosen on the basis that a substance which causes disease symptoms when present in large enough quantities can actually be used to treat the same symptoms if administered in an immensely diluted form.

Manipulative therapies available include *osteopathy* and *chiropractic*, and more recently *reflexology*. The major difference between osteopathy and chiropractic is that whilst osteopathy focuses on maintaining the normal structural integrity of the whole body, and originally osteopaths believed that their treatments were effective via the circulatory system, chiropractors focus on the spine and the role of the nervous system. Reflexology focuses on foot massage, on the principle that there are channels of energy to all parts of the body governed by specific points on the feet. Symptoms are caused by blocking of one or more channels, and relief is obtained by massage which removes the energy blocks.

The underlying thinking behind *acupuncture* is similar to reflexology, in that the aim of treatment is to restore the balance of what is called *chi* energy, by using the acupuncture needles at key points on the body.

Other physical therapies are based on movement and exercise, such as *yoga*, *t'ai chi* and *dance therapy*.

Finally, there are sensory therapies, such as *art* and *music therapies*.

Psychological therapies

A range of therapies is available which may be regarded as alternative therapies since they can be available from agencies other than orthodox psychiatric services. In the UK, particularly in the realm of *counselling* services, there has been movement towards establishing systems for recognising reputable and qualified practitioners and agencies, and trying to establish some means of quality control. *Humanistic psychology* has developed a higher profile in recent years, with an increase in the availability of therapeutic approaches, such as Rogerian therapy, gestalt therapy and transactional analysis, amongst others.

Paranormal therapies

This group of therapies is based on a belief in the existence of supernatural or psychic forces, and includes amongst others Christian healing within orthodox Christian churches, spiritualist healing within the Spiritualist movement, and therapeutic touch.

The universal characteristic of all alternative therapies is simply their failure to gain full recognition within orthodox medical practice. Some of them, particularly homeopathy, are practised alongside conventional medicine by some medical practitioners. Others are almost universally suspect to most members of health care professions. Meanwhile, as the general public has become aware of the limitations of orthodox medical treatments, there has been an increasing revival of interest in alternative therapies.

Environmental health care

Environmental health is influenced by many factors dealt with by people who have no direct involvement with primary health care services. An important example is housing and town planning. A key local authority health worker is the Environmental Health Officer, together with his team. His remit includes inspection of premises concerned with food handling, such as restaurants, bakeries and butchers. Where he is unsatisfied with the prevailing services, ultimately he has the power of closure. He is involved in the control of communicable diseases, in contact tracing, and in identifying the source of an outbreak. He also has powers to intervene where living accommodation is unfit by reason of defects such as poor repair, dampness or overcrowding. His powers alone are clearly insufficient, however, to overcome what is a perennial and serious problem in the UK: a national lack of sufficient and adequate housing for the population.

Occupational health nursing

Finally, occupational health nurses are a unique group of nurses privately employed by industrial and other organisations to provide a service to staff. The precise pattern of their work will depend on the nature of the occupation of the particular workforce they serve, but broadly speaking they are concerned with promotion of health, prevention of accidents, health screening programmes, advice on the rehabilitation of disabled staff into the work situation, and nursing duties such as wound dressing or perhaps supervision of medication.

Currently, little or no liaison exists between staff in the primary health care team and those providing occupational health care. This is regrettable, since domestic factors may be significant for health problems manifesting at work and vice versa. Occupational health nursing has much in common with health visiting, a factor also reflected in the Project 2000 Report (1986), where the UKCC asserts that the specialist nurses in health promotion in the future would be health visitors, occupational health nurses, and school nurses.

Conclusions

This chapter has considered some of the key issues concerned with the development of primary health care in the UK. An increasing emphasis is being placed on health promotion, prevention of ill health, care *in* the community, and care *by* the community. Health behaviour is targeted by na-

tional and local campaigns, such as 'healthy heart' campaigns. The 1990 GP Contract has introduced specific targets and requirements for immunisations and adult health screening. Patients are being discharged home from hospital earlier than they used to be, with all the implications this has for support services and nursing care in the community, including the needs of so-called 'informal carers' – the relatives and friends of patients at home. With the recognition by planners and health care professionals that there is a need to work in partnership with the consumers of health care services, there has also come a greater expectation that communities as well as individuals will take a greater responsibility for meeting their own health care needs.

For these changes in patterns of delivery of primary health care to be effective, even in the most disadvantaged communities, a number of factors need to be taken fully into account. These include:

(1) The variety of health-related beliefs and aspirations of individuals in a multicultural, multi-ethnic society
(2) The nature of the relationship between the health care worker and the consumer
(3) Recognition of the variation in resources and limitations existing in different groups in the community
(4) The need for an accurate and realistic assessment of the costs of meeting identified health needs in the community. Care in the community has traditionally been regarded as a cheaper option than institutional care, but it is becoming increasingly clear that this is not the case
(5) The way in which health care services are organised and delivered. The emphasis is on flexible, creative and innovative approaches to the solution of health care problems locally and nationally. However, flexibility and creativity are hampered by strict bureaucratic and hierarchical systems, and innovations often involve increased costs at the beginning
(6) The overall priorities of society. Finances are finite, so that if other areas of the economy such as national defence or technological development hold an over-riding priority, resources for effective health care may be inadequate. Furthermore, good health often seems to be an asset which is taken for granted

until it is lost, so that the state of health services may not seem to be such a high priority to healthy taxpayers.

In the last analysis, the future for primary health care does not rest on structures or organisations, or categories of health workers, but on the prevailing attitudes, values and priorities of society. As members of a service occupation, nurses encounter people from every section of society, both in sickness and in health. Consequently, preparation for nursing practice needs to include an understanding of the current health-related issues in society, and of ways in which each practising nurse can act as the clients' advocate. Nurses have a responsibility to make policy-makers aware of what they have learned at grass-roots level about their clients' health needs, and about their health-related values and attitudes. Table 4.2 lists some questions that anyone preparing for, or involved in, professional nursing practice should consider, from the points of view of both providers and consumers of health care.

Table 4.2. *Current issues of concern for nursing practice, with relation to primary health care*

(1) Whose responsibility is primary health care?
(2) How can the health promotion and prevention of ill health aspects of primary health care be made more effective?
(3) How can nurses be active in influencing health policies affecting the development of primary health care?
(4) How much control of primary health care should be in the hands of consumers?
(5) What differences in priorities and perspectives on health care exist between institutional and community-based health care professionals, private and voluntary health care agencies, practitioners of alternative health care and medicine, and lay consumers?
(6) Is hospital medicine still in danger of being practised in an 'ivory tower' separated from the realities of the everyday problems of life faced by patients before admission and after discharge?

References

Annett, H. and Rifkin, S. (1988). *Improving Urban Health – Guidelines for Rapid Appraisal to Assess Community Health Needs: A Focus on Health Improvements for Low Income Urban Areas*. WHO, Geneva.

Ashby, H.T. (1922). *Infant Mortality*. Cambridge University Press, Cambridge.

Barrow, N. (1980). Nursing; the art, science, and vocation in evolution. Cited in Skeet (1982), see below.

Booth, W. (1890). *In Darkest England and The Way Out*. The Salvation Army, London.

Burkitt, A. (1983). Health education. In *Community Health*, Clark, J. and Henderson, J. (eds.). Churchill Livingstone, Edinburgh.

Caplan, C. (1969). *An Approach to Community Mental Health*. Tavistock Publications, London.

Chadwick, E. (1842). *Report on the Sanitary Condition of the Labouring Population of Great Britain*. Edinburgh University Press, Edinburgh.

Council for the Education and Training of Health Visitors. (1977). *An Investigation into the Principles of Health Visiting*. CETHV, London.

Department of Health. (1989). *Caring for People – Community Care in the Next Decade and Beyond*. Cmnd 849. HMSO, London.

DoH. (1990). *Nursing in the Community* (The Roy Report). HMSO, London.

DHSS. (1986a). *Primary Health Care – An Agenda for Discussion*. Cmnd 9771. HMSO, London.

DHSS. (1986b). *Neighbourhood Nursing – A Focus for Care* (The Cumberlege Report). HMSO, London.

DHSS. (1987). *Promoting Better Health – The Government's Programme for Improving Primary Health Care*. Cmnd 249. HMSO, London.

Dingwall, R.W.J. (1977). Collectivism, regionalism and feminism: health visiting and British social policy, 1850–1975. *Journal of Social Policy*, 6(3), 291–315.

Fawcett-Henesy, A. (1989). Up for grabs. *Nursing Times*, 85(49), 18–19.

Garety, P.(1988). Housing. In *Community Care in Practice: Services for the Continuing Care Client*, Lavender, A. and Holloway, F. (eds.). John Wiley and Sons, Chichester.

Geldof, B. *Is That It?* Penguin Books, Harmondsworth.

Hall, D.M.B. (ed.) (1989). *Health for All Children: Report of the Joint Working Party on Child Health Surveillance*. Oxford University Press, Oxford.

Hannay, D.R. (1979). *The Symptom Iceberg: A Study of Community Health*. Routledge and Kegan Paul, London.

Health Departments of Great Britain. (1989). *General Practice in the National Health Service – The 1990 Contract*. HMSO, London.

Health Visitors Association. (1985). *Health Visiting and School Nursing – The Future*. HVA, London.

Her Majesty's Stationery Office. (1911). *National Insurance Act*. HMSO, London.

HMSO. (1948). *Childrens Act*. HMSO, London.

HMSO. (1962). *Health Visiting and Social Work (Training) Act*. HMSO, London.

HMSO. (1981). *Education Act*. HMSO, London.

HMSO. (1989). *Children Act*. HMSO, London.

Honigsbaum, F. (1970). *The Struggle for the Ministry of Health 1914 – 1919*. Occasional Papers on Social Administration, No.37. Bell, London.

Hunt, S.M., McKenna, S.P., McEwen, J., Williams, J. and Papp, E. (1981). Nottingham Health Profile: subjective health status and medical consultations. *Social Science and Medicine*, 15A, 221–229.

King, M. (1972). Medicine in red and blue. *Lancet*, 1(7752), 679.

Kohnke, M. (1980). The nurse as advocate. *American Journal of Nursing*, 80(11), 2038–2040.

Leininger, M. (1974). The leadership crisis in nursing: a critical problem and challenge. *Journal of Nursing Administration*, 4(2), 62–68.

London Health Planning Consortium. (1981). *Primary Health Care in Inner London* (The Acheson Report). London Health Planning Consortium, London.

Macqueen, I.A.G. (1962). From carbolic powder to social counsel. *Nursing Times*, 58, 866–868.

Miller, M. (1990). *Bed and Breakfast; Women and Homelessness Today*. The Women's Press, London.

Ministry of Health. (1956). *An Inquiry into Health Visiting* (The Jameson Report). HMSO, London.

Monckton, Sir W. (1945). Report on the circumstances which led to the boarding out of Denis and Terence O'Neill at Bank Farm, Minsterley, and the steps taken to supervise their welfare. Reprinted (1975) in *The Child's Generation*, Packman, J. (ed). Basil Blackwell and Martin Robinson, Oxford and London.

National Audit Office. (1990). *Maternity Services: Report by the Comptroller and Auditor General*. HMSO, London.

Nightingale, F. (1893). Sick nursing and health visiting. In *Selected Writings of Florence Nightingale*, Seymer, L.R. (ed.) (1954). Macmillan, New York.

Nuffield Foundation. (1986). *Pharmacy: The Report of a Committee of Inquiry Appointed by the Nuffield Foundation* (Chair Sir K. Clucas). The Nuffield Foundation, London.

Paine, L.H.W. and Siem Tjam, F. (1988). *Hospitals & the Health Care Revolution*. WHO, Geneva.

Ramon, S. (1988). Community care in Britain. In *Community Care in Practice: Services for the Continuing Care Client*, Lavender, A. and Holloway, F. (eds.). John Wiley and Sons, Chichester.

Reedy, B. (1983). Primary health care in Britain and abroad. In *Community Health*, Clark, J. and Henderson, J. (eds). Churchill Livingstone, Edinburgh.

Robinson, J. (1982). *An Evaluation of Health Visiting*. CETHV, London.

Robinson, K. (1983). What is health? In *Community Care*, Clark, J. and Henderson, J. (eds.). Churchill Livingstone, Edinburgh.

Rowntree, B.S. (1910). *Poverty – A Study of Town Life*. Macmillan Press, Basingstoke.

Royal College of General Practitioners. (1981). *A Survey of Primary Care in London* (The Jarman Report). RCGP, London.

Royal Commission on Medical Education (1965–8). *Report*. Cmnd 3569. HMSO, London.

Sachs, L. (1986). Health care across cultural boundaries. In *Migration & Health: Towards an Understanding of the Health Care Needs of Ethnic Minorities*, Colledge, M. *et al*. (eds.). WHO, Copenhagen.

Seymour, J. (1991). News Round-up. *Community Outlook*, 1(1), 5.

Skeet, M. (1982). A healthier life for all. *Nursing Mirror*, 155(22), 35–37.

Social Services Committee of the House of Commons. (1985). *Community Care with Special Reference to Adult Mentally Ill and Mentally Handicapped People*. HMSO, London.

Social Services Committee of the House of Commons. (1987). *Primary Health Care. First Report of the Social Services Committee, Session 1986–87*. HMSO, London.

Standing Medical Advisory Committee and Standing Nursing and Midwifery Committee. (1981). *The Primary Health Care Team: Report of a Joint Working Group*. HMSO, London.

Stephen, W.J. (1979). *An Analysis of Primary Medical Care – An International Study*. Cambridge University Press, Cambridge.

Tomlinson, D. (1991). Freedom for living. *Health Service Journal*, 101, 24–25.

United Kingdom Central Council for Nursing, Midwifery and Health Visiting. (1986). *Project 2000 – A New Preparation for Practice*. UKCC, London.

UKCC. (1991). *Report on Proposals for the Future of Community Education and Practice*. UKCC, London.

Wilkie, E. (1979). *The History of the Council for the Education and Training of Health Visitors*. CETHV/Allen and Unwin, London.

Wilson, M. (1975). *Health is for the People*. Darton, Longman and Todd, London.

World Health Organisation/United Nations Children's Fund. (1978). *Primary Health Care: Report of the International Conference on Primary Health Care, Alma-Ata, USSR, 6–12 September 1978*. WHO, Geneva.

WHO. (1983). *Primary Health Care – The Clinical Experience. Report of an Inter-Regional Seminar*. WHO, Geneva.

WHO. (1987). *Hospitals and Health for All: Report of a WHO Expert Committee on the Role of Hospitals at the First Referral Level*. Technical Report Series, No.744. WHO, Geneva.

Suggestions for further reading

Allen, N. (1990). *Making Sense of the Children Act: A Guide for the Social and Welfare Services*. Longman, Harlow.

Baly, M.E. (1987). *District Nursing* (2nd ed.). Heinemann, London.

Bayliss, E. and Logan, P. (1987) *Primary Health Care for Homeless Single People in London: A Strategic Approach*. Report of the Health Sub-group of the Joint Working Party on Single Homelessness in London. SHIL Health Sub-group, London.

Department of Health. (1991). *The Health of the Nation: A Consultative Document for Health in England*. Cmnd 1523. HMSO, London.

Green, D., Neuberger, J., Lord Young of Darlington and Burstall, M.L. (1990). *The NHS Reforms: Whatever Happened to Consumer Choice?* Health Series No. 11. IEA Health & Welfare Unit, London.

Inglis, B. and West, R. (1983). *The Alternative Health Guide*. Knopf, New York.

Leathard, A. (1990). *Health Care Provision, Past, Present and Future*. Chapman and Hall, London.

Lewith, G.T. (1985). *Alternative Therapies – A Guide to Complementary Medicine for the Health Professional*. Heinemann, London.

Luker, K. and Orr, J. (1985). *Health Visiting*. Blackwell Scientific Publications, Oxford.

McNaught, A. (1987). *Health Action and Ethnic Minorities*. National Community Health Resource/Bedford Square Press, London.

Meredith-Davies, B. (1991). *Community Health and Social Services* (5th ed.). Edward Arnold, London.

O'Donnell, O. (1989). *Mental Health Care Policy in England: Objectives, Failures and Reforms*. Discussion Paper 57. Centre for Health Economics, University of York.

Robertson, C. (1991). *Health Visiting in Practice* (2nd ed.). Churchill Livingstone, Edinburgh.

Seed, P. (ed.) (1988). *Day Services for People with Mental Handicaps: Case Studies for Practice I*. Jessica Kingsley, London.

Smith, A. and Jacobson, B. (1988). *The Nation's Health*. King's Fund, London.

Stocks, M. (1960). *A Hundred Years of District Nursing*. Allen and Unwin, London.

5

HOMEOSTASIS: THE KEY TO NORMAL FUNCTION

Dinah Gould

The purpose of this chapter is to present an overview of human physiology, identifying the mechanisms which control the internal environment and influence interaction with the external world. Nurses need to understand normal physiological processes before they can apply this knowledge when studying pathology.

The chapter will include the following topics:

- The concept of homeostasis
- Temperature control
- Negative and positive feedback mechanisms
- Common needs of living organisms
- Functions of living systems
- Major systems of the body contributing to the maintenance of homeostasis.

Homeostasis: the key to normal function

Many of the people who benefit from nursing intervention are not 'ill'. Midwives care for women throughout normal pregnancies and health visitors monitor the development of normal children. The client who has a psychiatric disorder is not 'sick' in the same way as the patient who has appendicitis.

Over the years nurses have become increasingly disenchanted with the medical model of delivering care, and as pointed out by Project 2000 (UKCC, 1986), their work is altering to meet the changing needs of society. Provision of health education and patient/client teaching are now recognised as integral parts of the nurse's role. However, before nurses can teach effectively they must have knowledge to communicate. Nurse education currently places great emphasis on social sciences and interpersonal skills, and nobody would argue that time spent teaching these is not well spent. Nevertheless, there is disturbing evidence that nurses may lack sufficient understanding of the life sciences for them to function as safe practitioners (Wilson, 1975; Gould, 1984; Akinsanya, 1985). This chapter is therefore intended as an introduction to normal *physiology* with particular emphasis on the mechanisms of homeostasis, to enable nurses better to meet the needs of their patients and clients. It is designed as an introduction to help with the understanding of structure and function described later in this book. A list of further reading is given at the end of the chapter.

The concept of homeostasis

One of the best ways to understand normal functioning is to examine the concept of *homeostasis*, first developed by the American physiologist Cannon in 1929. Homeostasis is the ability of the body to maintain internal stability despite environmental fluctuations. Adaptation according to changing need can occur because the body is able to alter its functions in a compensatory manner, even though body functions are very highly integrated.

Disease (dis-ease) can be regarded as the breakdown of homeostasis (Montague, 1981). Stress is a general term that can be used to denote any disruption in homeostasis that leads to disease. Stress could result from any physical impairment; for example, lack of oxygen supply to the *tissues*, shortage of water or essential nutrients. The concept of stress can be extended to include psychological as well as physical factors; anxiety, for example, is known to impede recovery (Wilson-Barnett, 1979) and there is a long-established body of research evidence to suggest that, by providing information and helping to alleviate unnecessary anxiety, nurses can help to promote the recovery of some patients (Hayward, 1975; Boore, 1978). The work of more recent authors supports this (Biley, 1989; Carr, 1990).

A homeostatic system consists of the basic components shown in Table 5.1. Detectors are sensory *organs* that monitor variables in the external and internal environment. Familiar examples include photoreceptors in the retina, baroreceptors monitoring blood pressure in the great vessels, and chemoreceptors which provide continual information about levels of carbon dioxide in the plasma.

Effectors are the organs that bring about the changes necessary to restore homeostasis. Muscles bring about movement, glands secrete chemicals, and many other organs, including the heart and kidneys, can be regarded as effectors because they are capable of responding to environmental changes.

Detectors and effectors communicate with one another via coordinating mechanisms which generally take the form of nervous impulses or hormones. *Hormones* are chemicals secreted by glands directly into the bloodstream, which carries them to specific target tissues, sometimes distant in the body, where they exert specific effects. Nervous coordination is swift; for example, the hand encountering a hot object will be sharply withdrawn. Hormonal control is usually slower, but its effects persist longer. Growth and development from childhood through puberty to adulthood are hormonally controlled processes. Throughout the body, millions of coordinating systems operate simultaneously, each controlled under normal circumstances so growth occurs at the appropriate time, and at the appropriate speed.

The function of the integrating centre is to receive information from the detector via nerves, hormones or both, to interpret the signal and to relay nervous or hormonal messages to the effector. In any one homeostatic system, there may be more than one detector or receptor. A great deal of integration takes place in the *hypothalamus*, a small area of the brain near the *pituitary gland*, where nervous and hormonal control systems meet. Flow of information is continuous. *Afferent* pathways conduct information to the integrating centre and *efferent* pathways carry it away. A simple homeostatic control system is shown in Fig. 5.1. The example used is temperature control, which is highly developed in mammals, including man. Average human temperature is 37°C, but some individual variation occurs and there is *circadian* variation with a peak in temperature in the evening. Females experience a slight increase (one or two degrees) just before ovulation.

Table 5.1. *Basic components of a typical homeostatic system*

Detectors	Monitor variables in the external and internal environments
Effectors	Cause changes that will restore homeostatic balance
Coordinating mechanisms	Couple the actions of detectors to effectors
Integrating centre	Receives information from detectors, interprets it and relays signals to the appropriate effectors

Temperature control

Homeostasis is achieved when thermoregulatory processes balance heat loss against heat gain. Near

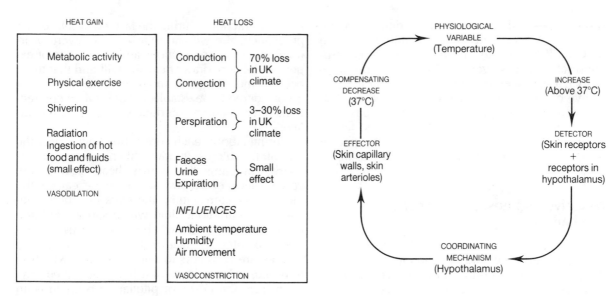

Fig. 5.1 *Temperature control*

the surface of the body, temperature can show variation on different occasions and between one place and another, but it is kept remarkably constant deep in the body (see Edholm, 1978; Marieb, 1991).

Heat is gained from *metabolic* activity, physical exercise, radiation, by ingesting hot food and fluids, and (in very cold surroundings) by shivering. Heat is lost by conduction, convection, evaporation of sweat, and to a much smaller extent in faeces, urine and expiration. Loss is influenced by ambient temperature and humidity. If the atmosphere is moisture-laden, water molecules cling to the surface of the skin and the cooling effect produced by the evaporation of water is lost. Convection currents cause sweat to evaporate rapidly and cooling takes place.

Thermoregulation is influenced by the degree of dilation or constriction of blood vessels in the *subcutaneous* tissues. When these constrict, the flow of blood to the surface of the body is reduced, so heat is retained. When they dilate, heat is lost.

The integrating centre in this system is the hypothalamus. A centre in the anterior hypothalamus controls heat loss, while another centre in the posterior hypothalamus controls heat gain. The hypothalamus operates like a thermostat, 'set' in most people at about 37°C. If the temperature of blood flowing through the hypothalamus is lower than the set point, the body will be stimulated to gen-

erate heat. The reverse will happen if the temperature of the blood is above the set point.

The detectors (thermoreceptors) are of two types: peripheral receptors in the skin which respond slowly to temperature change, and central receptors in the hypothalamus itself, which respond more rapidly. Temperature changes in the deeper tissues take place much more slowly than in the skin, but they jeopardise the health and survival chances of the individual to a much greater extent.

Physiological response to cold establishes a temperature gradient between the body core and surface. The low temperature is detected by thermoreceptors in the skin. Nervous impulses travel to the effectors represented by the skin *capillaries*. Vasoconstriction and heat conservation follow. Hairs on the skin stand on end in an attempt to trap a layer of warm air next to the body. This mechanism is of much greater importance in other mammals. The biologist Scholander (cited in Edholm, 1978) believed that man is fundamentally adapted to life in a warm climate, because heat conservation mechanisms are not highly developed in human beings.

Breakdown in homeostasis takes place when body core temperature falls to about 35°C or lower. *Hypothermia* is a major risk for elderly people, especially those who are immobile, infants, and those whose participation in outdoor sports exposes them to harsh conditions (mountaineering, fell-walking). At temperatures between 35°C and 32.2°C, the normal response is vasoconstriction and shivering. As temperature drops further, tissue metabolism is altered and the protective mechanisms of heat conservation are lost. Below approximately 24°C, heat is lost passively to the environment, followed by cardiac failure or arrest. If the victim is found in time, gradual re-warming will allow recovery without lasting ill effect.

Negative and positive feedback mechanisms

Our example of temperature control as a homeostatic mechanism draws attention to a number of key points. Firstly, it is the integrating centre which actually determines the normal value of the chemical or physical parameter under control. Secondly, the integrating centre is also responsible for interpreting this information as it is received from the detectors and for initiating the appropriate responses to be carried out by the effectors. It is important to remember that the receptors continually sample the internal and external environment for change and that feedback via the effectors is likewise a continuous process, although homeostatic change is only brought about when environmental fluctuations occur.

Most homeostatic mechanisms operate via negative feedback: an increase in the level of a product from the process under control causes it to be slowed or to cease altogether. Temperature control, like blood pressure control described on page 121, is a classic example of negative feedback.

Positive feedback is relatively uncommon. In this situation the process under control is stimulated by its product. Positive feedback generally involves events or chemical reactions which occur rather infrequently and under special circumstances, such as childbirth.

Parturition (childbirth)

Even in its non-pregnant state, the uterus is capable of spontaneous contractions. These increase as pregnancy advances because the growing fetus causes the muscular uterine wall to stretch. Contraction occurs reflexly, particularly as the hormone **oestrogen**, present in increasingly high concentration throughout pregnancy, also stimu-

lates contraction. During the last few weeks of her pregnancy, the woman will become aware of irregular uterine contractions and as the date of expected delivery draws near she will find that these become more frequent and painful, but true labour is considered to be established only when contractions have become coordinated and the cervix dilates.

During labour, each contraction begins near the top of the uterus (fundus), then sweeps downwards, pressing the baby's head against the cervix (neck of the womb). Pressure causes the membranes surrounding the fetus to rupture, releasing the amniotic fluid which surrounded and cushioned it. The baby's head now presses with renewed intensity against the cervix, stimulating its pressure receptors to initiate a reflex which in turn causes the release of a hormone called oxytocin from the posterior pituitary. Oxytocin is an extremely powerful uterine stimulant, so again the contractions become more powerful, dilating the cervix until the baby is forced into the vagina. The woman then feels an irresistible desire to push downwards so that her baby is delivered.

The ability to reproduce, culminating in parturition, is important for survival of the species as a whole, but in order for the individual to survive, a number of needs common to all living organisms must be met.

Common needs of living organisms

Water will be discussed first because it is not only essential for life but it also forms a large percentage of the body, accounting for 60% of lean body mass. The distribution of water in an average man (weighing 70kg and 1.78 metres tall) is shown in Fig. 5.2, which also demonstrates the protein, fat, carbohydrate and mineral content of the tissues.

Body fluid is named according to its location: approximately twice as much water is located inside **cells** as outside. Water inside the cells is referred to as the **intracellular** compartment; water outside cells makes up the **extracellular** compartment. Extracellular fluid can be subdivided into two further compartments: plasma, constituting the fluid portion of the blood, and **interstitial fluid** bathing the outside of the cells. Water can move from one compartment to the other, but an imbalance in the distribution of water will result in

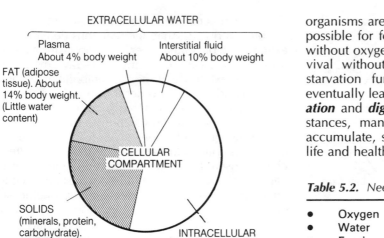

Fig. 5.2 *Fluid compartments of the body and typical composition (adults)*

homeostatic changes in an effort to restore balance. This is why the fluid intake and output of so many patients must be carefully monitored.

In 1857, Bernard (the first scientist to appreciate the phenomenon of stability in the internal environment) recognised that fluid in the extracellular compartment acts as a pool for the exchange of materials between cells and their surroundings. The extracellular pool can be regarded as a source of materials relinquished to the tissues on demand and returned when they are no longer needed. Net gain of materials into the extracellular pool is from nutrients entering via the digestive system, materials that the body has itself synthesised from these raw materials (sugars, proteins, fats), and oxygen via the lungs. Net loss from the extracellular pool occurs via urine, faeces, expired air, sweat, menstrual flow and in dead cells shed from body surfaces; the skin, lining of the gut, hair and nails. Materials can also leave the extracellular pool to be stored. A good example is the storage of fat in adipose tissue under the skin.

Homeostatic balance depends on net gain and net loss of materials, but the composition of extracellular fluid also depends on the shift of materials between different fluid compartments. Three stages are possible: negative balance (when loss exceeds gain), positive balance (when gain exceeds loss), and equilibrium (when loss and gain are equal).

The other essential requirements of all living organisms are shown in Table 5.2. Life is at least possible for four or five days without water, but without oxygen death occurs within minutes. Survival without food is possible for longer, but starvation fundamentally disturbs homeostasis, eventually leading to weakness and death. **Respiration** and **digestion** both give rise to waste substances, many rapidly becoming toxic as they accumulate, so prompt removal is mandatory for life and health.

Table 5.2. *Needs of living organisms*

- Oxygen
- Water
- Food
- Suitable range of temperature and **pH**
- Prompt removal of metabolic wastes

The needs of living organisms extend to the level of the individual cells of which they are composed and an understanding of cells helps us to comprehend the integrated functioning of the body as a whole.

The cell: the basic unit of life

Early microscope studies led two scientisits, Schlieden and Schwann, to suggest in 1836 that all living organisms are composed of individual units called cells (see also Chapter 6). Today, we know that where the body is not composed of living cells, it is made up of their products. Bone is a hard tissue in which cells are surrounded by a matrix heavily reinforced with mineral salts. The outer layer of skin covering the body surface is made of dead cells rendered tough and waterproof by the deposition of a protein called **keratin**. Both the extracellular matrix of bone and the keratinised layers of skin are the products of living cells. The structure of a typical cell is shown in Fig. 5.3. Such diagrams are of limited usefulness, however, because they give the impression that the cell is static and changeless. Nothing could be further from the truth. Cells are continually changing, taking up some materials from the extracellular compartment and releasing others. Each cell is a homeostatic unit, which in health is in a state of dynamic equilibrium with its extracellular environment.

The cell is the basic unit of life, but the cells

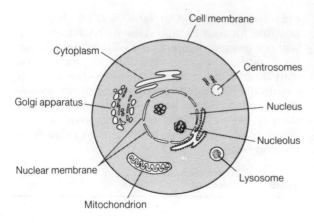

Fig. 5.3 *A typical human cell*

making up the human body are not all alike, either in structure or function, and despite their huge number and diversity, they do not operate as separate entities. Instead, groups of cells are found together as a community. Such cells, all of the same type, make up a tissue. Different tissues function together as discrete organs. In turn, organs cooperate with one another as organ systems; for example, the mouth, oesophagus, stomach and intestines collectively make up the digestive tract.

The next section is concerned with a description of the functions performed by all living systems.

Functions of living systems

All living organisms share the same common functions listed in Table 5.3, from simple *unicellular* bacteria to complex multicellular man.

Table 5.3. *Functions of living organisms*

• Metabolism	• Irritability
• Absorption	• Movement
• Respiration	• Growth
• Excretion	• Reproduction
	• Death

Metabolism

Metabolism is the name given to the millions of chemical reactions continuously taking place within living cells. *Anabolic* reactions are those in which new, big, complex molecules are made.

Catabolic reactions are those in which molecules are broken down. Anabolic reactions demand the expenditure of cellular energy, catabolism reduces it. Anabolic reactions draw their raw materials from the extracellular pool; catabolic reactions generally add to it. In order for an individual cell or a whole organism to achieve homeostatic equilibrium, anabolism and catabolism must balance. In a growing child, more anabolism than catabolism takes place. In starvation and disease states, characterised by tissue destruction, the reverse happens. In diabetes mellitus, for instance, cells are unable to absorb adequate amounts of glucose because insulin, the necessary hormone, is not present in sufficient quantities. Instead, fats and proteins are used to provide the fuel needed for metabolism and the patient loses weight.

Absorption

Actively metabolising cells must absorb molecules and ions across their membranes. Absorption is most highly developed in cells lining the gut, but it is a property shared to a greater or lesser extent by all living cells. Absorption is highly selective; the cell membrane will allow the passage of some substances much more readily than others. A third category of substances is actively pumped out by the cell. The best example from this category is sodium. The **sodium pumping** activity of cell membranes is of great clinical significance, especially during intravenous fluid replacement. The selective permeability of cell membranes accounts for the vast difference between the chemical composition of intracellular and extracellular fluid.

Again, water is of vital importance in metabolic reactions because they take place only in solution. Water is a very good solvent. Once dissolved, molecules and ions can move about freely and many collide with one another. Chemical reactions cannot occur until collision takes place. In living systems, reactions are usually promoted by **enzymes**. These are proteins able to catalyse metabolic reactions.

Life is thought to have begun in the oceans, and scientists point out that the composition of sea water and extracellular fluid is very similar.

Respiration

Man is *aerobic*: for energy to be supplied to the body, food that has been absorbed must combine with oxygen and undergo combustion. The oxidation of food to release energy, water and carbon dioxide is called respiration, and it takes place constantly in all living cells. The lungs operate like bellows, drawing in atmospheric air which contains about 20% oxygen, some of which enters the bloodstream. The air forced out of the lungs with each expiration contains less oxygen but more carbon dioxide, produced by metabolism.

Excretion

Metabolism releases waste products other than carbon dioxide which, if not removed from living cells, would rapidly accumulate, soon reaching toxic levels. The removal of waste substances is called **excretion**. In man, the chief excretory organs besides the lungs are the kidneys, which remove water-soluble wastes.

Irritability

Irritability is the ability of a living organism to respond to environmental stimuli, to move towards conditions that are favourable (warmth, food), and to withdraw (rapidly if necessary) from agents that are unpleasant or harmful. The nervous system, which is highly developed in man, permits rapid withdrawal from noxious stimuli by reflexes without involving the brain. Although the sensory organs (eyes, ears, nose, tongue and skin) rapidly detect environmental stimuli, it is necessary for these to be interpreted by the central nervous system. In addition, the capacity to learn and to remember is of immense importance in negotiating environmental hazards.

Movement

Movement is a property shared by all living cells, conferred by contractile proteins called *actin* and *myosin*, present in cell cytoplasm. Contractility is most highly developed in muscle cells. Muscles are of three different types and their function depends on the arrangement of their actin and myosin fibrils (see Fig. 5.4). In striated (voluntary) muscle, actin and myosin are arranged regularly, to form a pattern of repeating bands. Striated

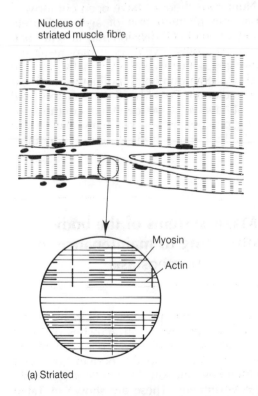

(a) Striated

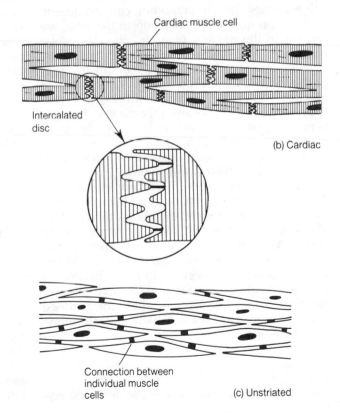

Fig. 5.4 *Striated, unstriated and cardiac muscle*

muscle is under the control of the will, and contraction (shortening) takes place when the filaments of actin and myosin slide past one another. Most striated muscles are attached to the skeleton, although there are notable exceptions, for example the muscles of the face, lips and diaphragm.

Unstriated (involuntary) muscle lacks a regular banding pattern, because the actin and myosin filaments are not highly ordered, but scattered throughout the cytoplasm. Unstriated muscle is not under conscious control, but it can remain contracted for long periods of time. It makes up the bladder, the uterus, the muscles that focus the eye, and the walls of the gut.

Cardiac muscle is in a class by itself. The cells, found only in the heart, are highly branched and striated. Cardiac muscle is not under the control of the will and is said to be inherently rhythmic. It contracts without nervous stimulation, although the nerves supplying the heart control the rate at which it beats.

Reproduction

The capacity to reproduce is vital for continuation of the species. The chromosomes, carrying genetic information from one generation to the next, are present in the nucleus of each cell. Unicellular organisms like bacteria reproduce simply by dividing into two, but this has the disadvantage of producing two identical offspring. A population of identical individuals would soon become extinct if their environment became inhospitable, because genetic variation (differences between the genes of individuals belonging to the same species) is essential for a species to adapt to fluctuating environmental conditions and survive.

In sexual reproduction, each new individual is different from its parents because it receives half its chromosomes from its mother (in the ovum or egg) and the other half from its father (in the sperm). Whether a particular chromosome comes from the ovum or sperm is purely chance. When sexual reproduction occurs, no two offspring are ever identical, except for the rare exception of identical twins. These result when one fertilised ovum splits into two at a very early stage in embryonic development.

Growth

Life for everybody begins as a single, fertilised egg, which grows to reach a critical size, then divides. Growth is an important property of living tissues, accompanied by **differentiation** – the ability of cells to undergo specialisation, thus enabling them to perform specific functions. Some cells, most notably nerve cells, become so highly differentiated that they cannot renew themselves once they become damaged. This explains why permanent, serious damage follows a spinal injury or stroke. Other cells, like the fibroblasts which give rise to connective tissue, remain relatively undifferentiated throughout the life of the individual, so repair can follow injury. Wounded skin and fractured bones heal. The ability of tissues to replace themselves persists into adulthood, although by far the most rapid growth and differentiation take place during fetal development and childhood, declining after puberty. Undifferentiated tissues tend to be found on the surfaces of the body, where exposure to damage is likely to be more frequent: highly differentiated tissue is protected deep within.

The capacity of all cells to grow and divide declines with age, so the logical conclusion to life is death. Numerous theories have been put forward to explain the phenomenon of ageing (Garrett, 1991). Cessation of cell division may be a normal, genetically controlled event, or it may result because the genes themselves eventually become damaged by environmental pollutants and exposure to radiation. Possibly all these factors, and several that have yet to be identified, contribute to the ageing process, which gradually alters functioning of all the major body systems (Eliopoulos, 1987).

Major systems of the body contributing to maintenance of homeostasis

Having discussed the principles of homeostatic control and the physiological activities of living organisms, attention will now be turned to the organ systems making up the human body and some of their key functions in maintaining a stable internal environment. These are shown in Table 5.4.

Table 5.4. *Physiological systems of the human body*

- Blood and circulatory system
- Respiratory system
- Digestive system
- Renal system
- Nervous system
- ***Endocrine*** system
- Reproductive system

Blood and circulatory system

In unicellular organisms, the entire cell surface remains in direct contact with the external environment. Molecules of oxygen and nutrients can **diffuse** across the cell membrane in sufficient quantities to sustain life, and waste substances move in the opposite direction.

Homeostasis is maintained without any need for an elaborate transport mechanism. Most of the cells making up the tissues of a multicellular organism are far away from the external environment, however, and rely on transport systems to bring oxygen and nutrients and to remove metabolites from the cellular environment. Transport is mediated by the blood which maintains links between the interior of the cell and its external environment.

If blood is allowed to stand for several hours or is spun in a centrifuge, it will separate into its component parts (see Fig. 5.5). Plasma, the fluid component, floats on top of the cells, making up 55% of the whole. Packed cell volumes or *haematocrit*, consists of red and white blood cells and **platelets**. These proportions of plasma and cells are normally maintained according to strict homeostatic control mechanisms.

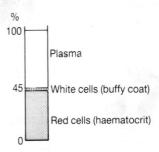

Fig. 5.5 *Composition of blood*

Tissue fluid formation and re-absorption

Adult blood volume varies between 4.5 and 5.5 litres depending on size, age and sex, but is kept constant for the individual by a series of control mechanisms operated by the renal and endocrine systems (see page 122) and at the level of the capillaries, the smallest blood vessels only one cell in thickness. It is across the walls of the capillaries that oxygen and nutrients diffuse to supply the metabolising cells, while carbon dioxide and other waste products diffuse back into the blood in the opposite direction. You will remember that between the blood vessels and the cell membranes there is a fluid which bathes the cells, and it is this interstitial fluid, often referred to as *tissue fluid*, which acts as the intermediary via which substances are transported to and from the cells. Moreover, the tissue fluid is in dynamic equilibrium and is interchangeable with plasma.

At the arterial end of the capillary, blood is under a pressure of 32 mmHg (4.3 kPa) but this drops along the length of the capillary to 25 mmHg (3.3 kPa) at its midpoint and 12 mmHg (1.6 kPa) at its venous end. The capillaries are permeable to all the constituents of plasma with the exception of plasma proteins. Thus, at the arterial end the relatively high blood pressure tends to force plasma and many of the substances it contains into the tissue spaces. Because plasma proteins are present in the blood but not in the extracellular tissue fluid, an **osmotic** gradient is set up which tends to suck fluid back into the capillary at the venous end, where blood pressure has fallen. From Fig. 5.6, you will see that these two opposing forces, blood pressure and osmotic pressure, continually force plasma out into the extracellular spaces to join tissue fluid and absorb it again as long as homeostatic balance is maintained.

Breakdown of homeostasis resulting in accumulation of excess tissue fluid (**oedema**) occurs when too much fluid escapes from the capillary or when too little is re-absorbed. The main causes of oedema are summarised in Fig. 5.7.

Haematocrit, red blood cells and haemoglobin

The red blood cells (*erythrocytes*) (see Fig. 5.8) making up the haematocrit are among the most specialised cells in the body. They are biconcave discs and their shape and lack of nuclei ensure that

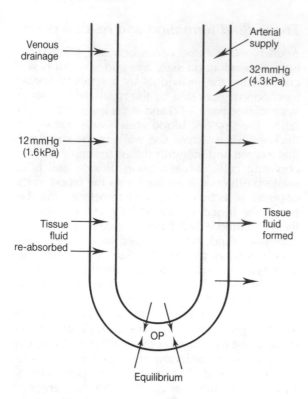

OP= osmotic pressure = 25 mmHg (3.3 kPa) exerted by plasma proteins

Fig. 5.6 *Starling's hypothesis of tissue fluid formation*

Excess tissue fluid formed as a result of raised venous pressure, due to venous obstruction caused by:	→ O ← E D E M A	Too little tissue fluid re-absorbed when osmotic pressure is reduced by deficiency in plasma proteins from:
1 Tight bandage or plaster of Paris; 2 Pressure of the baby on pelvic veins during pregnancy; 3 Right ventricular failure; 4 Varicose veins; 5 Pelvic neoplasm.		1 Malnutrition – too little protein in diet; 2 Excess protein lost by kidney (renal failure); 3 Too little plasma protein formed (liver failure).

Fig. 5.7 *Causes of oedema*

the maximum amount of space within the cytoplasm is available for carrying oxygen.

They are produced within the red bone marrow of the adult and the number present in the body is controlled according to a homeostatic mechanism involving a hormone called *erythropoietin* produced by the kidney. Under conditions where oxygen levels are low, as at high altitudes, the kidney is stimulated to release erythropoietin and the red bone marrow increases the production of erythrocytes so that more become available for the transport of oxygen. People who live at high altitudes tend to have higher levels of erythrocytes, a

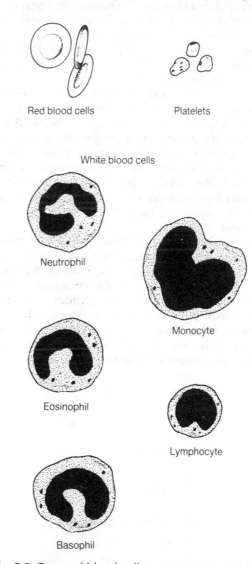

Fig. 5.8 *Types of blood cell*

physiological condition known as *polycythaemia*.

Erythrocytes contain the pigment **haemoglobin** which combines reversibly with oxygen molecules, transporting them to the tissues. Each molecule of haemoglobin contains four iron (ferrous) atoms and each of these can combine with one molecule of oxygen, so the system of carriage is highly efficient.

In health, haemoglobin level is about 12−14 g/dl. Haemoglobin levels fall if there is lack of iron in the diet, blood loss or destruction of erythrocytes, resulting in anaemia. The oxygen-carrying capacity of the blood is reduced, resulting in symptoms of tiredness, dizziness and, in severe cases, breathlessness.

White blood cells, like red cells, are manufactured in the bone marrow within the bones of the trunk and skull in the adult, but there are several different types (see Fig. 5.8) which are classified according to the size and complexity of their nucleus, and the presence or absence of granules in their cytoplasm. The granules are really packages of enzymes necessary for the destruction of invading bacteria.

Granulocytes have large lobed nuclei, and they are classified according to the colour they stain in the laboratory when chemical dyes are used to colour them for microscopy. By far the most abundant are the *neutrophils*, which stain mauve. They have the important function of engulfing and destroying bacteria (*phagocytosis*). The number of neutrophils in the blood rises sharply following an infection. These cells can leave the capillaries by squeezing through slits between the individual cells, and they are then free to wander in the tissues (see Fig. 5.9). This is called **diapedesis**. In view of their ability to exist outside the bloodstream, it is evident that any estimate of the total number of neutrophils in the body at any one time can only be approximate.

Eosinophils, which stain pink, are thought to be important in controlling infestations. For example, they destroy parasitic worms, and they contribute to the allergic response, when their numbers increase.

The *basophils*, which stain blue, appear to be important in **anaphylactic** reactions, releasing a chemical called *histamine* which produces vasodilation and hence a fall in blood pressure. Histamine raises heart rate, increases smooth muscle tone and stimulates **exocrine** secretion. Basophils can enter the tissues, where they are known as *mast cells*.

Agranulocytes have clear cytoplasm and smoothly shaped nuclei. There are two categories, *monocytes* and *lymphocytes*. Monocytes are phagocytic cells, able to enter the tissues, where they are usually referred to as *macrophages*. They are larger cells than neutrophils and can therefore engulf more bacteria. Appearing later at the scene of damage following infection or inflammation, they engulf dead cells, including any worn out neutrophils.

Lack of white blood cells disrupts homeostasis

Phagocytosis

Diapedesis

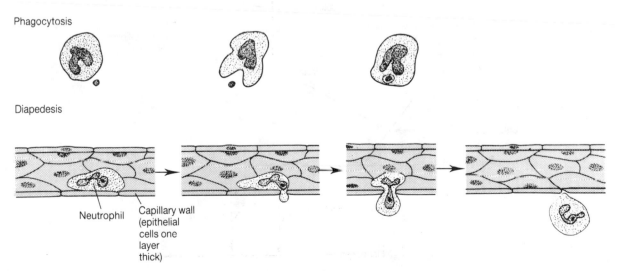

Neutrophil

Capillary wall (epithelial cells one layer thick)

Fig. 5.9 *Behaviour of neutrophils*

by reducing ability to fight infection. This is seen most clearly in rare cases where children are born unable to produce one or another of the classes of white blood cells and are unable to live unless given bone marrow transplants. Reduced white cell count is a problem accompanying certain types of chemotherapy necessary in the treatment of some malignancies. Special precautions must be taken to prevent these people developing life-threatening infections until this phase of their treatment is complete.

Platelets are tiny cellular fragments which develop from big cells in the bone marrow (*megakaryocytes*). They are vital in maintaining homeostasis because of their role in blood clotting. When a blood vessel is damaged, the platelets release a substance called *thromboplastin*. A plasma protein called *prothrombin*, normally present in the bloodstream in an inactive state, is converted by thromboplastin to the active molecule *thrombin*.

Thrombin catalyses a further reaction; another inactive plasma protein called *fibrinogen* is converted to *fibrin*. Fibrinogen is soluble, but fibrin is not. Strands of fibrin form a mesh over the damaged blood vessel. Within two minutes a clot begins to form, preventing the loss of more blood. Excessive blood loss is also prevented by vasoconstriction, especially when a major blood vessel is damaged.

The blood clotting mechanism, which provides a good example of positive feedback, is illustrated in Fig. 5.10.

Substances transported by blood

The substances transported by blood (other than the cells) are shown in Table 5.5. As you would expect, all these are under homeostatic control with the exception of drugs, which are not under normal circumstances present in the body.

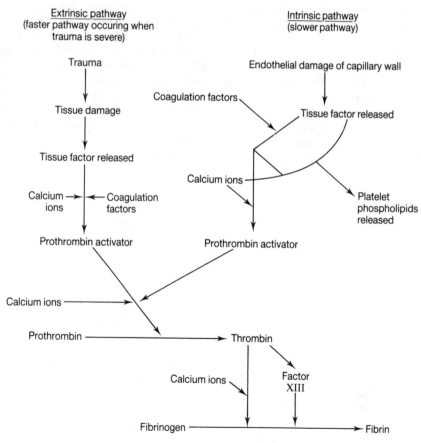

Fig. 5.10 *Blood clotting: an example of positive feedback in homeostasis*

Table 5.5. *Substances transported by the blood*

- Nutrients (glucose, amino acids, fatty acids)
- Oxygen
- Carbon dioxide
- Metabolic waste products (urea, creatinine)
- Hormones
- Enzymes
- Drugs
- Clotting factors
- Antibodies
- Heat

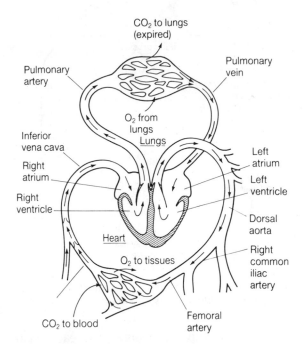

Fig. 5.11 *The heart and circulation*

Circulation

The blood is circulated by the pumping mechanism of the heart. Blood leaves the left side of the heart under very high pressure and as it travels to the tissues via the **arteries**, its pressure gradually falls until it reaches the capillaries, which are the smallest blood vessels. In between the thick-walled, muscular arteries and the capillary networks, there are small intermediate vessels called *arterioles*. The circulation has sufficient capacity to hold more blood than is actually present, so at any given time sections of it are closed down. The arterioles are important because their sphincter muscles, present at intervals along the length of each, can close, shutting down the blood supply to a particular tissue.

From the capillary networks blood returns to the heart and lungs via the **veins**. At any given time, most of the blood will be present in the veins because they are distensible and the blood, now under very low pressure, is flowing slowly. Valves present in some of the veins and the pumping action of muscles, especially in the legs, help the flow of blood against gravity, back to the heart.

An outline of the circulation and the structure of the heart is shown in Fig. 5.11. From this it should be appreciated that blood returning to the heart must first travel to the lungs to be re-oxygenated before it returns to the tissues.

Blood pressure control

Blood pressure is the hydrostatic pressure exerted by the blood on the walls of the vessels which contain it. From our discussion of tissue fluid formation (see page 117) we have already seen that every blood vessel has its own pressure. However, when we speak of measuring the patient's blood pressure we are referring to the systemic arterial blood pressure which plays the vital role of ensuring that blood flow to the metabolising tissues is adequate. If blood pressure falls too low because of severe haemorrhage, for example, supplies of oxygen and nutrients reaching the tissues decrease to a dangerously low level. An uncontrolled high blood pressure will eventually damage the delicate lining of the blood vessels. Blood pressure is therefore subject to very strict homeostatic control (see Fig. 5.12). The integrating centre (the vasomotor centre) is in the medulla, low in the brain, while the receptors are baroreceptor cells situated predominantly in the walls of the arch of the aorta and the **carotid** sinus. When blood pressure exceeds normal limits the baroreceptors fire off a rapid succession of nervous impulses received by the vasomotor centre in the medulla, which then instructs the effectors to reduce blood pressure. The effectors are the walls of the arterioles. These now dilate and the heart beats faster, so the blood can occupy a larger volume and drains away more rapidly, allowing pressure to fall. When blood pressure becomes low the arteriolar walls contract.

Blood pressure in major arteries (aorta, carotids) is determined by the rapidity with which blood is pumped into them by the heart (*cardiac output*)

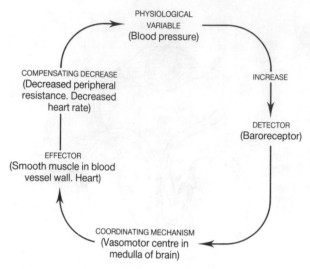

Fig. 5.12 *Role of detectors, effectors and coordinating mechanisms in blood pressure control*

and the speed with which it is able to leave via the arterioles. If the heart is pumping fast and therefore sustaining a high cardiac output, blood pressure will be high, especially if the arterioles are open, offering little *peripheral resistance* (friction encountered by blood as it flows through the blood vessels). Blood pressure is governed by the balance between cardiac output and peripheral resistance:

Blood pressure = Cardiac output × Peripheral resistance

$$BP = CO \times PR$$

Fig. 5.13 summarises the main ways in which cardiac output and therefore blood pressure is con-

trolled. A knowledge of blood pressure control is also necessary to understand the homeostatic mechanisms by which the kidney maintains fluid balance.

The renal system

The kidneys (see Fig. 5.14) not only regulate the volume of the body fluids but also control the composition of the blood and help keep pH within the very narrow range compatible with life. (Under normal circumstances, blood pH is 7.35–7.45, i.e. virtually neutral.) Hence the kidneys play a vital homeostatic role. The lungs also help to control blood pH through the excretion of carbon dioxide which is highly acidic. Respiratory control of blood pH is rapid; excretion of excess acidic or alkaline substances by the kidneys takes place more slowly.

The functional unit of the kidney is the *nephron*. Each kidney contains about a million nephrons, and in health all of them function all the time. The nephrons produce urine by a process of filtration of its bloodflow, followed by selective reabsorption of those substances the body needs to conserve.

From their dark red colour, it is evident that the kidneys must receive a good vascular supply – about 1 litre per minute at rest. Each nephron receives blood from a tuft of capillaries called the *glomerulus*. From Fig. 5.15, it is apparent that blood in the glomerulus is in intimate contact with

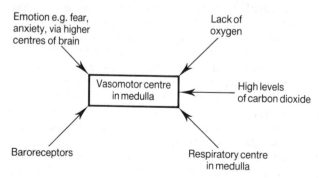

Fig. 5.13 *Factors affecting blood pressure control*

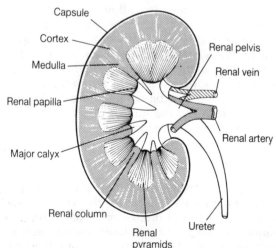

Fig. 5.14 *Longitudinal section through a kidney*

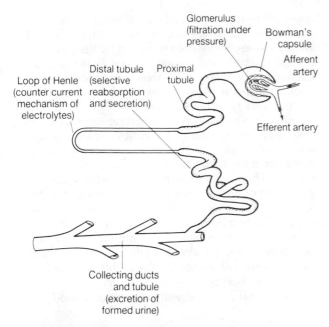

Fig. 5.15 *Structure of a nephron*

the *Bowman's capsule*, that part of the nephron which is invaginated to surround the capillaries. The single layer of cells making up both glomerulus and Bowman's capsule will allow the passage of molecules with a molecular weight of 68,000 or less. Molecules in the blood small enough to pass through the intercellular slits are forced to enter the Bowman's capsule, as a result of the pressure exerted by the blood in the capillary.

Molecules that enter the Bowman's capsule include water, urea, sugars, amino acids and ions. Blood cells, plasma proteins and other large molecules remain in the plasma. Disease and injury can destroy the ability of the glomerulus to act as a filter, so plasma proteins then enter the urine. Every minute, the glomeruli filter between 100–140 ml of plasma. This fluid flows down the proximal tubule leading to the Bowman's capsule, then into the hairpin-shaped loop of Henle dipping down into the medulla, along the distal convoluted tubule and eventually enters a collecting duct in the kidney pelvis. As the filtrate travels through the nephron, much of the water and many of the molecules and ions are re-absorbed, while others are added. Experiments have clearly demonstrated that the chemical character of the filtrate alters, and that the composition depends on the needs of the body at any given time. If, for example, the

blood contains an unusually high number of hydrogen ions (as when respiration is embarrassed in chronic bronchitis or emphysema), hydrogen ions will not be re-absorbed by the kidney tubules, and the urine will become acidic (normal range pH 5–8). A diet rich in meat tends to lead to acid production, because of the chemical structure of animal proteins. Vegetarians tend to have urine with a higher pH. Many drugs, or the breakdown products of drugs metabolised in the liver, are excreted in the urine.

Most water is re-absorbed in the proximal tubule. Sodium ions are actively pumped out to rejoin the blood, and because they are osmotically active, water follows. Although re-absorption continues in the distal tubule and collecting ducts it is more variable, depending on the needs of the tissues. Control is by two hormones: *aldosterone* from the adrenal cortex and *antidiuretic hormone* (ADH) manufactured by the hypothalamus and secreted by the posterior pituitary gland. ADH stimulates the collecting ducts to re-absorb water when the body needs to conserve fluid, resulting in the production of concentrated urine (see Fig. 5.16).

Aldosterone acts on the distal tubule, making it increase re-absorption of sodium and water via a complicated series of homeostatic control mechanisms summarised in Fig. 5.17. Secretion of pot-

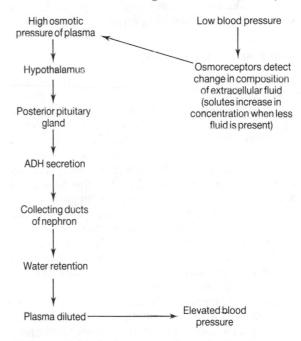

Fig. 5.16 *Role of ADH in regulating fluid balance*

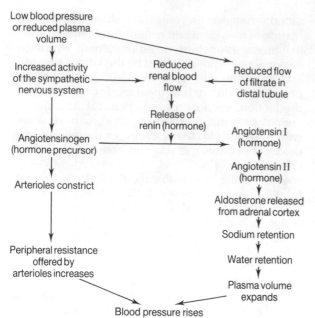

Fig. 5.17 *Role of aldosterone in salt, water and blood pressure control*

assium into the filtrate is simultaneously increased. This is one of the mechanisms by which the nephrons help to control the chemical content of the blood. Glucose is conserved by the body, but waste substances like urea remain in the filtrate.

The respiratory system

The functions of the respiratory system (see Fig. 5.18) can be summarised as: warming, filtering and humidifying inspired air, providing a continuous supply of oxygen to the tissues and continuously removing carbon dioxide. Homeostasis rapidly breaks down if these vital functions are not fulfilled. Figure 5.19 shows that the small airways eventually terminate in *alveoli* – the functional units of the lungs actively engaged in gaseous exchange. In order to fulfil their vital function, the alveoli are highly distensible. Inspiration and expiration are controlled separately by different parts of the respiratory centre in the medulla. Stretch receptors in the alveolar walls continually monitor the degree of alveolar inflation.

Control is mediated by the nervous system via the vagus nerve. Once inflation of the alveoli has reached a critical level, the respiratory centre prevents further inspiration and reflexly triggers expir-

ation, so that air is forced out of the alveoli.

Gaseous exchange occurs most efficiently and swiftly when the distance travelled by the gas molecules is kept to a minimum. To facilitate gaseous exchange, the walls of the alveoli are only one cell thick, and each is positioned next to a capillary whose wall is also only one cell thick (see Fig. 5.19). The respiratory membrane provides an enormous surface area. To achieve adequate gaseous exchange, an individual requires 1 square metre of lung tissue for every kilogram of body weight. This explains why people who suddenly gain a lot of weight experience dyspnoea (breathlessness). Respiratory problems are a major hazard among the newborn, because their lungs still have to undergo considerable development. Thirty million alveoli are present at birth, but this number increases to 300 million by the eighth year of life, to maintain homeostasis as the child grows.

The alveoli are lined with a secretion called *sur-*

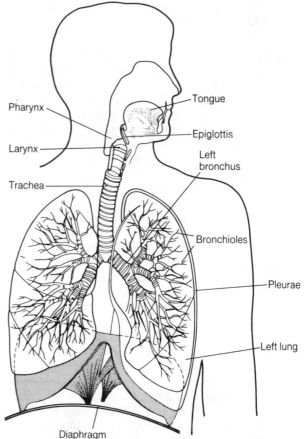

Fig. 5.18 *The respiratory system*

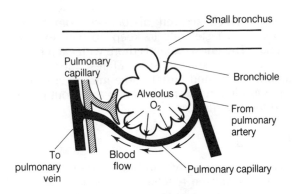

Fig. 5.19 *The respiratory membrane*

factant, which reduces surface tension, helping them to expand as well as enhancing gaseous diffusion. Babies born prematurely lack surfactant and may in consequence develop respiratory distress syndrome.

Despite the importance of the alveoli in gaseous exchange, it is usual for only the upper, better ventilated parts of the lungs to be involved in normal respiration. Only about one tenth of the blood received by each lung actually reaches the respiratory membrane.

Acquaintance with the physical laws governing the movement of gas molecules is necessary before the mechanism of gaseous exchange can be appreciated. The molecules in a gas are not attracted together as powerfully as those in a solid or liquid. Instead, they move about freely, and take up the entire space available to them at any one time. As long as temperature is constant, the volume of a gas will vary *inversely* to the pressure exerted on it; this means that if pressure is increased, the molecules will be squeezed up together and volume will decrease. This happens during expiration, when the muscles controlling respiration (the diaphragm and the external intercostal muscles between the ribs) compress the lungs. During inspiration, when the respiratory muscles relax, the alveoli are able to expand, the space available for the gas molecules is increased, and they take up the much larger space that becomes available to them as pressure falls.

The gas laws also decree that in any mixture of gases, each will behave independently, so the pressure of the mixture will be equal to the sum of the partial pressures contributed by each gas present. This is relevant to a discussion about respiration because air taken into the lungs from the

atmosphere is, of course, a mixture of gases, although only oxygen and carbon dioxide are exchanged. The proportions of atmospheric gases in inspired and expired air are compared in Table 5.6.

Table 5.6. *Gaseous composition of expired and inspired air*

	% Inspiration	% Expiration
Oxygen	21	16
Carbon dioxide	0.02	4
Nitrogen	79	80

Air that has just entered the alveoli contains more oxygen than is present in the alveolar capillary, so oxygen will diffuse from the area of higher pressure in the alveolus to the plasma. Once the plasma has become saturated with oxygen, the molecules move to areas of low tension in the red blood cells, where they combine with haemoglobin. Every gram of haemoglobin carries 1.34 ml of oxygen, so the system of transport is highly efficient. Insufficient oxygen travels in solution in the plasma to sustain life. The effect of severe iron deficiency anaemia on oxygen supply to the tissues is evident, therefore.

Blood flowing through capillaries in the tissues encounters interstitial fluid where the oxygen tensions have fallen to low levels because cells are metabolically active. First, the oxygen dissolved in the plasma diffuses into the cells. As oxygen levels in the plasma fall, oxygen separates (dissociates) from haemoglobin, diffusing into the plasma, then into the cells. The blood is never completely deoxygenated; arterial blood is about 98% saturated with oxygen, while venous blood is 70% saturated and appears darker in colour.

Carbon dioxide produced by tissue metabolism is transported by venous blood back to the lungs. Some of it is carried in simple solution in the plasma. About 25% is carried in chemical combination with haemoglobin, but by far the most is transported in the form of hydrogen carbonate ions. Red blood cells contain an enzyme called *carbonic anhydrase*, which catalyses a chemical reaction that results in the formation of hydrogen carbonate and hydrogen ions. Plasma leaving the tissues has a higher partial pressure of carbon dioxide than when it entered. When this blood returns to the lungs, carbon dioxide dissolved in the plasma diffuses into the alveoli. The carbon dioxide attached to haemoglobin separates and also enters the alveoli, and the hydrogen carbonate and hydrogen react to form carbon dioxide again. This carbon dioxide also enters the alveoli, and is voided with the next expiration.

Carbon dioxide is an acidic gas, and hydrogen ions also help to make the blood acidic. If respiration is impaired for any reason, the pH of the blood falls due to the accumulation of these substances.

During exercise, the oxygen requirements of the tissues can be increased by as much as 20% and so the tissues produce more carbon dioxide. At the cellular level, oxygen dissociates from haemoglobin at a faster rate to keep up with extra demands. The chest expands more with each breath, and the accessory muscles of respiration in the anterior neck and throat come into play; you can see muscles in the neck move, the mouth opens and the nostrils flare.

Hypoxia

Hypoxia, a breakdown in homeostasis, is defined as lack of oxygen reaching the tissues. Table 5.7 summarises some of the causes of hypoxia.

Table 5.7. *Causes of hypoxia*

Location at which disruption of respiration occurs	Cause of hypoxia	Examples of conditions resulting in hypoxia
Atmosphere	Decreased partial pressure of oxygen in the external atmosphere	High altitude or other environment, e.g. smoke-filled room, in which the partial pressure of oxygen is low
Mechanics of transporting oxygen from the atmosphere to the alveoli	Obstruction of the airways	Foreign bodies Mucus in bronchi and bronchioles, e.g. chronic bronchitis Spasm of smooth muscle of bronchioles, e.g. breakdown of alveoli – emphysema, asthma
	Increase in the volume of the potential space between the pleura, paralysis of the respiratory muscles	Pleural effusion Pneumothorax Myasthenia gravis Myopathies
	Damage to the nerves supplying the respiratory muscles	Infection, e.g. poliomyelitis, tetanus Neuropathies
	Damage to the bony support of the thorax, leading to pain on movement	Fractured ribs
Control mechanisms	Damage to the respiratory centre in the pons and medulla of the brain	Trauma Tumour
Diffusion of oxygen in the alveoli to the blood in the pulmonary capillaries	Increase in barrier to diffusion	Pulmonary oedema Absence of surfactant in neonates (respiratory distress syndrome)
Carriage of oxygen in the blood to the tissues	Inadequate pulmonary perfusion Inadequate haemoglobin	Pulmonary stenosis Right ventricular failure Anaemia
	Stasis of the systemic circulation	Left ventricular failure Haemorrhage
Diffusion of oxygen from the blood to the tissues	Increase in barrier to diffusion	Oedema
Utilisation of oxygen by the tissues	Inability of cells to utilise oxygen	Cyanide poisoning

The digestive system

Food is necessary in order to provide fuel from which the body can derive energy to drive physiological functions and remain in homeostatic balance. Food is burnt during respiration by oxygen which is carried by the red blood cells to the actively metabolising tissues. Not all the food ingested is used to provide energy; surplus carbohydrates and fats are stored to supply future needs, should supplies run low. Proteins are the structural and functional elements of the tissues. They include the enzymes that promote and control the rate of biochemical reactions, form fibrous materials like collagen that help to give tissues their shape, and together with certain specialised fats, form cell membranes. Proteins provide the fuel for cellular respiration only during starvation.

Whatever fate awaits the food we eat, it first has to be broken down into units small enough to reach the cells deep inside the body. Most foodstuffs are large, complex molecules far too big to reach the tissues unless they are broken down. This is the function of the digestive tract, a tube approximately 15 feet (5 metres) long, running from mouth to anus, with intermittent dilations specialised to perform digestive functions. Mechanical and chemical breakdown take place in the upper parts of the tract, while lower down the vast surface area of the small intestine is designed to facilitate absorption. Mechanical action of the gut (chewing in the mouth, rhythmic churning of the stomach) breaks food into smaller pieces. Chemical digestion is achieved by the action of enzymes poured from exocrine glands onto food as it passes through the gut.

Proteins

Proteins are made up of repeating units called *amino acids* (see Fig. 5.20) and the action of enzymes eventually breaks down the complex protein molecule into individual amino acids and short chains called *peptides*. Some carbohydrates are ingested as relatively simple sugars — for example glucose, sucrose, lactose in milk, and fructose in sugary fruit like grapes. Because of their chemical simplicity they are rapidly digested and absorbed. Nutritionists frown on diets with a high simple sugar content (for example, sweets, table sugar) because they supply lots of calories but no other nourishment, and do not sustain hunger

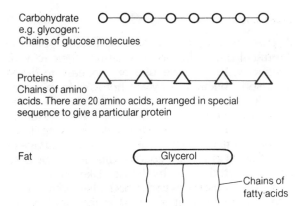

Carbohydrate e.g. glycogen: Chains of glucose molecules

Proteins Chains of amino acids. There are 20 amino acids, arranged in special sequence to give a particular protein

Fat — Glycerol — Chains of fatty acids

Fig. 5.20 *Structure of protein, carbohydrate and fat (lipid) molecules*

pangs for long, prompting further consumption. This is a recipe for obesity. Starchy foods consist of strings of simple sugar units. Plant fibres like cellulose are complex carbohydrates that man cannot digest because he lacks the necessary enzymes, so they pass through the gut unchanged, giving bulk to the faeces. Once thought to be an unimportant part of the diet, fibre is now considered to be a vital component, since it helps stimulate the muscular contractions of peristalsis that propel food along the gut. The faster the material travels down the gut, the less time it remains in contact with the gut wall. Since carcinoma of the large intestine, a common disease in Western society, is thought to be due to the presence of carcinogenic agents in highly processed food, inclusion of fibre in the diet seems to be a sound precaution.

Fats

Fat molecules are less complex. Each consists of a unit called *glycerol* attached to chains of fatty acids of variable length. Some fatty acids contain double bonds, so the molecule is flexible and the fat is soft, often liquid at room temperature. These are the unsaturated fats, mainly vegetable in origin, recommended by nutritionists. Saturated fats are solid because they contain mainly single bonds. Diets rich is saturated animal fats have been implicated as one of the many factors appearing to contribute to heart disease.

Enzymes

A class of enzymes known as *lipases* split the chemical bonds in fats, but despite their relative simplicity, these molecules are not easy to digest or absorb, because they are not soluble in water. In order for a chemical reaction to take place, the molecules must be in solution. ***Bile*** is essential here, because it acts as a detergent, breaking down fat into small droplets. Molecules on the surface of the droplets gradually go into solution one by one, and are acted upon by lipase. Like many other important substances in the body, bile is manufactured in the liver. It is stored in the gall bladder just beneath the liver. Breakdown in homeostasis occurs when bile cannot be secreted, either because there is obstruction of the common bile duct carrying bile to the duodenum (gallstone, tumour) or because the liver is damaged by a condition such as infective hepatitis (hepatitis B) and cannot manufacture bile. If failure is due to an obstruction, the bile builds up in the liver and as the body conserves and recycles bile from the bowel back to the liver via the blood, accumulation in the blood occurs. Eventually bile salts are deposited in the skin, giving the patient the characteristic yellow colour of obstructive jaundice.

Anatomical relations of the digestive tract and organs like the liver and pancreas which manufacture substances important in digestion are summarised in Fig. 5.21. The actions of the main digestive enzymes are shown in Table 5.8

Two points about enzymes need to be emphasised. Firstly, they operate only over a narrow pH range. Enzymes secreted by the stomach will not function in the duodenum, where conditions are mildly alkaline. Secondly, the active digestive enzymes are very powerful chemical substances which would damage the tissues producing them if they were allowed to remain in contact for any length of time. Most enzymes are released as inactive precursors. Conversion to the active molecule occurs only when they encounter the food to be digested. The ***epithelial*** lining of the gut is afforded the added protection of mucus, a sticky substance forming a blanket between the wall of the gut and its contents.

Fluid

Every day, digestive processes in the healthy adult result in the release of about 9 litres of fluid into the gut. All this fluid, as well as fluid taken in as part of the diet, must be re-absorbed by the intestines if the individual is to remain in water balance. Severe vomiting and diarrhoea can lead to serious dehydration. This can be fatal, especially if the victim is either very young or very old.

Remember from our discussion of the renal system that, in health, all the nephrons function all

Table 5.8. *The digestive enzymes*

Enzyme	Site of secretion	Action
* Amylase	Mouth (small amounts) Duodenum	Breaks down carbohydrates to simple sugars (disaccharides, monosaccharides)
† Pepsin	Stomach	Breaks down proteins to shorter lengths called polypeptides
* Lipase	Duodenum	Breaks fats into fatty acids and glycerol
* Carboxypeptidase	Duodenum	Continues breakdown of polypeptides to amino acids
* Trypsin	Duodenum	Continues breakdown of polypeptides to amino acids

* Works in an alkaline environment
† Works in an acid environment

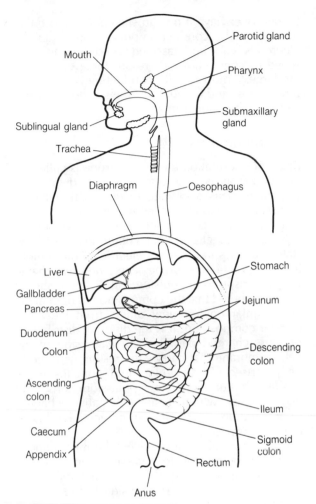

Fig. 5.21 *The digestive system*

the time. In babies and the elderly, this ideal level of functioning may not be achieved, so they are more at risk of homeostatic failure.

Paralytic ileus is a condition in which peristalsis of the gut ceases, either temporarily due to handling during surgery or through trauma. The fluid that it contains then stagnates: it cannot be reabsorbed by the intestine and returned to the homeostatic pool. In a patient experiencing paralytic ileus, no fluids or food should be given until there are signs that peristalsis is returning, usually indicated by the passage of flatus. Nasogastric aspiration helps to remove digestive fluids, which continue to be secreted, helping to alleviate some discomfort. Fluids are given intravenously to prevent dehydration.

The nervous system

The nervous system, rapid coordinator of homeostatic function, sends messages to effector organs all over the body, and constantly receives information about conditions in the internal and external environment from sensory organs. These vary in complexity from naked nerve endings in the skin to large, elaborate structures such as the eye.

Neurones

The basic unit of the nervous system is the *neurone*. Sensory neurones convey information to the integrating centre, while motor neurones convey nervous impulses in the opposite direction. Both types, and the structural differences between them, are shown in Fig. 5.22.

The neurones collectively make up the peripheral nervous system. They are bound together by sheets of connective tissue to form nerves, big enough to be clearly visible to the naked eye. The

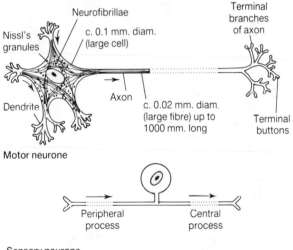

Fig. 5.22 *Sensory and motor neurones, and anatomical relationship of neurones, showing synapses*

integrating centre is represented by the brain and spinal cord, which together make up the central nervous system (CNS). *Afferent* neurones carry information to the CNS and *efferent* neurones carry information in the opposite direction. A big nerve will, however, contain neurones of both types.

The brain and spinal cord both consist of nervous tissue. The spinal cord runs from the base of the brain down to the lumbar region (see Fig. 5.23). It is important to realise that, although the cell body of the neurone is a microscopic structure, the axon that protrudes from it can be as much as a metre long. Inside the CNS, the cell bodies of the neurones are arranged together, forming the grey matter. Their axons make up the visibly paler white matter.

Nervous tissue is highly specialised; it is nourished by supporting cells, and many neurones are found in close association with the *cells of Schwann*. These cells of Schwann secrete a fatty material called *myelin*, which insulates the axon so the nervous impulse travels more swiftly. Not

all neurones have a myelin sheath, but those that do appear to conduct impulses more rapidly. Neurones can be classified according to their speed of conduction. There are three categories: the largest, most rapidly conducting A neurones, B neurones, and C neurones, the smallest in diameter, which conduct most slowly.

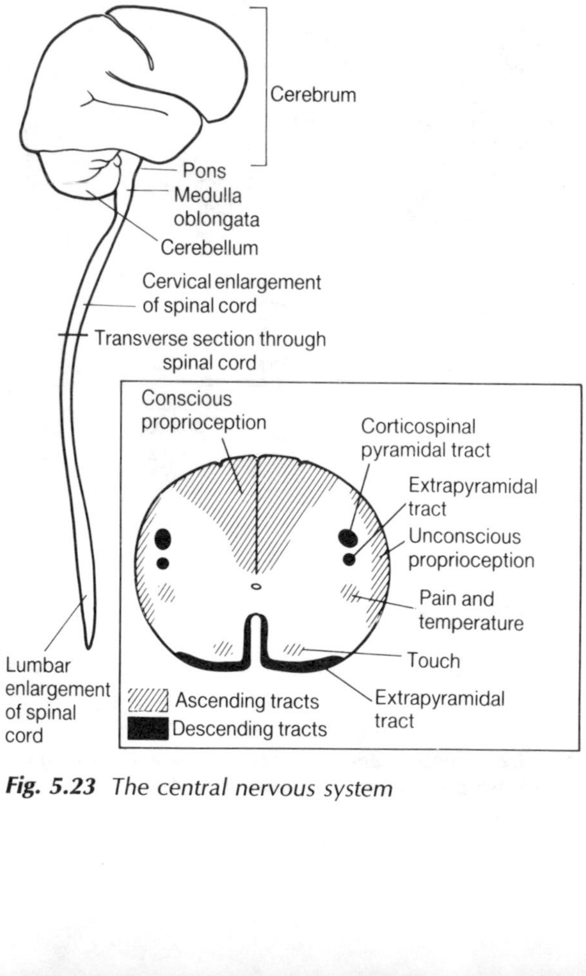

Generating impulses

Relay of information along a neurone is called an *impulse*. This is an electrical event, defined by physiologists as a change in electrical potential across the membrane of the nerve cell.

It has long been established by physiologists using micro-electrodes that a neurone in its resting state is always in a state of electrical polarisation; the inside of the membrane bears a negative charge in comparison to the outside (Fig. 5.24). It should be remembered that the composition of fluid in the extracellular environment differs from the intracellular composition. It is the different distribution of *ions* (charged particles) on each side of the cell membrane that causes the resting neurone to be polarised. Extracellular fluid contains many positive sodium ions, few potassium ions, and no proteins (which bear a negative charge). Concentration of these ions in intracellular fluid is precisely reversed.

Under normal circumstances, the membrane is extremely permeable to potassium ions, so they are free to move out of the cell, but sodium ions are actively kept out. The outside of the cell accumulates positive ions, and negative protein ions remain within. During the generation of a nervous impulse (action potential) the membrane undergoes a rapid but short-term change, so that it becomes temporarily permeable to sodium. As sodium ions enter the neurone, it depolarises. As soon as the impulse has been generated, sodium is again ejected from the cell and polarity is restored.

In order for the impulse to occur, a stimulus must be received from a receptor in contact with the neurone. Neurones make functional contact with one another and with receptors and effectors at a junction called a *synapse* (see Fig. 5.22). Synapses do not permit direct contact, however; a small gap is present. The cell body and dendrites of one neurone may have 10,000 synapses. On the axon of a motor neurone, the dendrites end in special terminal buttons. These synapse with a muscle or a gland.

Fig. 5.23 *The central nervous system*

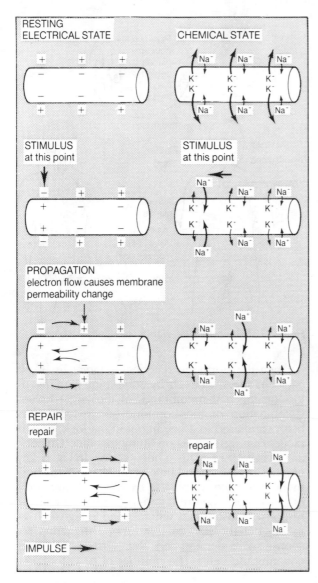

Fig. 5.24 *Resting membrane potential and action potential*

Chemical transmitters

Transmission of information across the synapse is chemical; a transmitter substance released by the dendritic endings travels across the synapse either to the next neurone in the chain, or the muscle or gland. Once transmission across the synapse has occurred, the transmitter is promptly destroyed by enzymes, otherwise its effects would be dangerously prolonged.

There are numerous different chemical transmitters in the brain and spinal cord. The most abundant are *acetylcholine* and *noradrenaline*. Poisonous gases used in chemical warfare paralyse the nervous systems of their victims by preventing the destruction of neurotransmitters once they have exerted their effects at the synapses, resulting in severe, often rapidly fatal homeostatic breakdown.

Activities of the nervous system

Activities of the nervous system can be broadly categorised according to whether or not they are under conscious control. The mechanisms permitting memory, reason and thinking are orchestrated by higher centres in the brain, but scientists are a long way from understanding how they work. Some sensory functions can be attributed to specific parts of the brain. The visual cortex, for example, is positioned in the occipital lobe, and hearing in the temporal lobe. Sight and hearing are well developed in humans, so the parts of the brain controlling them are large. Smell is less important in man and the olfactory area of the cortex is correspondingly smaller.

Human intelligence is reflected in the enormous size of the human brain. However, 'intelligence', though almost impossible to define, certainly does not appear to be related to individual brain size.

Reflex actions, like withdrawal of the hand from a hot object, involve the exchange of information between the sensory organs, the spinal cord and the effectors. Reflexes are designed for protection and can take place without the involvement of the higher centres, although information is invariably sent to the brain, which may result in pain and fear being experienced and modification of the reflex response.

Involuntary control of the viscera (heart, gut and lungs) is mediated by the autonomic nervous system. Resting functions are controlled mainly by the parasympathetic nervous system, while in stressful situations, activities of the sympathetic nervous system predominate: the heart rate increases and respirations become more frequent and deeper as we run from danger or, less usefully, as we prepare to make a speech or take an examination.

The endocrine system

The contribution of hormones to homeostatic control has been mentioned earlier. Hormones are small molecules, usually proteins or lipids called *steroids*. They are secreted from highly vascular glands called endocrine glands, and enter the bloodstream directly, not via a duct. The blood carries hormones to a target tissue, often at an anatomically distant site, where the specific effects of the hormone are mediated.

As Fig. 5.25 shows, the endocrine glands themselves are scattered. Some, like the parathyroids, which lie on the thyroid gland, and the islets of Langerhans in the pancreas, are embedded in the tissues of larger organs.

The main endocrine glands and their secretions are shown in Table 5.9. Secretion does not occur at a steady rate over each 24 hour period, but in sharp bursts occurring cyclically according to a circadian rhythm. Growth hormone from the anterior pituitary gland, for example, is released mainly at night. Synthesis of hormones takes place inside the cells of endocrine glands, where storage may also take place; secretory granules of thyroxine are clearly visible on microscopic examination of thyroid tissue.

The amount of each hormone circulating in the bloodstream is monitored by a controlling system, release usually occurring when concentration falls below a critical level. Sometimes a hormone will undergo structural alteration of its molecule to a more active compound once it has been released. This is called *peripheral conversion*. Thyroxine is converted in this way to tri-iodothyronine, which elicits a more marked response from the target tissues, but thyroxine is still a hormone in its own right, not just an inactive precursor.

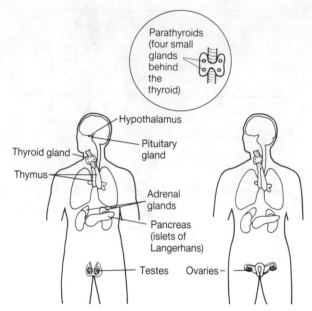

Fig. 5.25 *The endocrine glands*

Once the hormone reaches its target tissue, it exerts its specific effects by combining with receptors on the cell membranes of the target tissue. Combination of the hormone and receptor has been compared to a key fitting into a lock, or two pieces of a jigsaw puzzle fitting together (Laycock and Wise, 1983). This model, shown in Fig. 5.26, emphasises the importance of the shape of the hormone molecule; it must fit exactly into the membrane receptor before it can trigger off the cellular response. Most tissues will respond to a given hormone, but the particular hormone triggering response will depend on the surface receptors covering the cells. The number of receptors pre-

Table 5.9. *Examples of hormones and their effects (NB: Reproductive hormones are not included)*

Endocrine organ	Hormone	Effect
Thyroid gland	Thyroxine Tri-iodothyronine	Regulate metabolism
Parathyroid glands	Parathyroid hormone (PTH)	Controls levels of calcium in the blood
Adrenal cortex	Aldosterone Cortisone	Regulates sodium levels Influences protein and carbohydrate metabolism
Adrenal medulla	Adrenaline (epinephrine)	Stimulates sympathetic nervous system
Islets of Langerhans (in pancreas)	Insulin Glucagon	Allows glucose to penetrate cell membrane Promotes release of glucose from liver

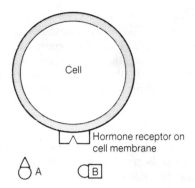

Hormone A can interact with the receptor and will therefore stimulate the cell.
Hormone B is unable to react and therefore ineffective in this particular cell.

Fig. 5.26 *Mechanisms of hormone action*

Table 5.10. *Hormones released from the anterior pituitary gland*

Pituitary hormone	Gland or tissue controlled
Human growth hormone (HGH)	Acts on hard and soft tissues to increase growth
Thyrotrophin stimulating hormone (TSH)	Thyroid
Follicle stimulating hormone (FSH)	Ovary and testis
Luteinising hormone (LH)	Ovary and testis
Adrenocorticotrophic hormone (ACTH) (corticotrophin)	Adrenal cortex
Prolactin	Breast (to initiate and maintain milk secretion)
Melanocyte stimulating hormone (MSH)	Stimulates dispersion of melanin in melanocytes in skin

sent at any one time, and the speed at which they respond, are problems physiologists are only just beginning to tackle.

Once a hormone has exerted its specific effects it is rapidly de-activated, either by the target tissue or the liver, and excreted via the kidneys.

Secretions from most of the endocrine glands are controlled by the *pituitary*, a pea-sized gland situated just beneath the brain. The pituitary consists of two lobes. The posterior lobe releases two hormones, both of which are formed in the hypothalamus: the *antidiuretic hormone* (ADH) that helps the kidneys to conserve water, and *oxytocin* which stimulates lactation and contraction of the uterus during labour. Most of the other endocrine glands are controlled by secretions from the anterior lobe of the pituitary (see Table 5.10).

Feedback

The amount of hormone present in the bloodstream is controlled by a feedback mechanism involving the pituitary. Negative feedback is the most usual form of control, and this is best illustrated with an example. Once the level of thyroxine rises above a set point, the pituitary will stop releasing thyroid stimulating hormone (TSH) and the levels of thyroxine will fall again. Negative feedback is shown in Fig. 5.27.

In recent years it has become apparent that the hypothalamus influences the function of the pituitary by the secretion of small protein hormones

called *releasing factors*. The hypothalamus lies directly above the pituitary, and the releasing factors travel to it by means of a network of blood capillaries. It is probably via the hypothalamus that hormonal control is influenced by emotional factors.

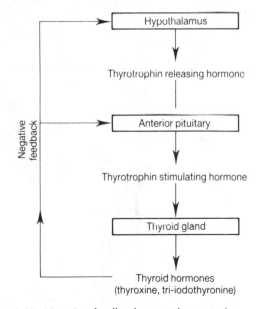

Fig. 5.27 *Negative feedback control system for hormones (example, thyroid gland)*

The reproductive system

The biological advantages of sexual reproduction and genetic variation have already been indicated. The purpose of this section is to give a brief overview of the functions of the male and female reproductive tracts. Oestrogens and progesterone are the main sex hormones in the female, while testosterone is secreted chiefly by the male.

The female reproductive system

The structure of the female reproductive system is shown in Fig. 5.28. The uterus, which houses the developing fetus, and the vagina could be considered accessory to the ovaries which are the source of ova as well as of female hormones.

Maturation of the developing ova released from the ovary at ovulation, and preparation of the uterine lining to receive a fertilised egg, are controlled by oestrogen and progesterone via two hormones from the pituitary, LH and FSH. Oestrogen, progesterone, LH and FSH are all released cyclically (up to the menopause). The menstrual cycle and more detailed physiology of the female reproductive organs will be discussed in Chapter 17, where they can be related more easily to the care of the female patient/client.

It is important to point out here that the hypothalamus appears to play a role in controlling reproductive functioning, since emotion and changes such as moving to unfamiliar surroundings (for example, leaving home) appear to have a major impact on the rhythm of the menstrual cycle.

Nutrition also appears to be an important factor, since women who are markedly underweight or overweight often do not menstruate. Improved nutrition is considered by some authorities to be the reason for the earlier *menarche* (onset of periods) experienced by young girls today.

Sex hormones

Female sex hormones are not secreted until the onset of puberty, but in the fetus, the production of male hormones is the factor which stimulates formation of the male sexual organs (Ganong, 1985). Secretion then gradually declines until puberty.

In both the male and female, sex hormones are responsible for secondary sexual characteristics, which begin to develop at the onset of puberty. In the female these include the typical curved feminine shape due to the deposition of adipose tissue on the breasts and hips, the growth of pubic and axillary hair, and enlargement of the female genitalia. Testosterone is an anabolic steroid which stimulates the growing boy to become muscular, taller, to develop thickened vocal cords so the voice breaks, and to grow hair on the face as well as in the pubic and axillary regions. The male genitalia grow and mature in response to testosterone.

The adrenal cortex in both male and female releases small amounts of testosterone, and this hormone is considered to be responsible for the sex drive in both sexes. Some authorities also believe that testosterone and the other male hormones (referred to collectively as *androgens*) play a major

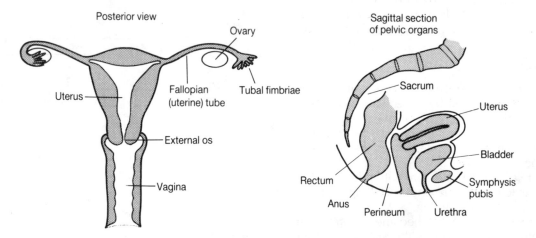

Fig. 5.28 *Female reproductive system*

role in aggression. Although this appears to be the case in experimental animals, it is not easy to generalise about human beings because aggression, like libido, is heavily influenced by psychological factors, and is at least partly under the control of the CNS.

The male reproductive system

The male reproductive system (shown in Fig. 5.29) can be likened to an elaborate plumbing system designed to manufacture sperm and deliver them into the vagina. Sperm production seems very wasteful compared to egg production. One or two mature ova are released once a month during the reproductive life of the female, but sperm are produced continuously in large numbers once the male has reached maturity. Fertility declines slowly with age, but does not cease sharply, as in the female.

The testes are made up of highly coiled seminiferous tubules, which are packed closely together. If unravelled, the seminiferous tubules from both testes would stretch for more than half a kilometre. The sperm develop from the cells of Sertoli in the walls of the tubes, and move towards the lumen as they mature, a process which takes about 70 days. Mature sperm leaving the seminiferous tubules pass through a series of ducts (*vasa efferentia*, *epididymis* and *vasa deferentia*) before travelling down the urethra. Nutrient and lubricant substances are added by glands: the paired seminal vesicles and the prostate gland, which in man completely encircles the urethra.

About 3 ml of semen are released on ejaculation, and each millilitre contains on average 100 million sperm. The body, which so carefully conserves its resources during homeostatic control, is profligate when it comes to the production of gametes, particularly sperm.

Conclusion

This chapter has provided an overview of homeostasis and normal human functioning. In the next chapter, mechanisms of disease are discussed.

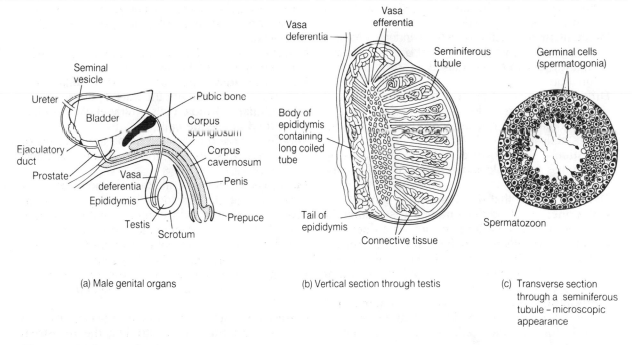

(a) Male genital organs

(b) Vertical section through testis

(c) Transverse section through a seminiferous tubule – microscopic appearance

Fig. 5.29 *Male reproductive system*

Glossary

Anaphylaxis: An exaggerated response by an individual to a foreign substance following previous sensitising exposure, e.g. hayfever (foreign substance = pollen), asthma, allergy to fur, etc. The basophils and mast cells release histamine, mediating the allergic response.

Artery: Blood vessel carrying blood away from the heart to the tissues

Bile: Secretion from the liver, stored in the gall bladder and emptying into the duodenum. Important in the digestion of fats

Capillary: Smallest blood vessel, with walls just one cell thick

Carotid: Main artery, positioned on each side of the neck. *Carotid sinus* – region where baroreceptors are situated

Cell: The smallest individual unit that can sustain life, consisting of a discrete mass of cytoplasm bounded by a plasma membrane and containing a number of subcellular organelles

Circadian rhythm: Rhythmic changes that take place in the individual according to some internally regulated mechanism, with a periodicity of about 24 hours

Diapedesis: Property of white blood cells, enabling them to squeeze through intercellular slits between cells in the blood capillary wall and gain access to the tissues

Differentiation: Ability of cells to undergo changes during embryonic development or tissue repair, so they become specialised in structure and function

Diffusion: Physical process by which gases and liquids of different densities mix when brought into contact with one another, until equilibrium is established

Digestion: Breakdown of complex foodstuffs by enzymes to simple molecules that can be absorbed

Diuretic: Drug that stimulates urine output

Endocrine: A gland that empties its secretion directly into the bloodstream, not via a duct

Enzyme: An organic catalyst, always a protein, that speeds the rate of a biochemical reaction while itself remaining unchanged at the end of the reaction

Epithelium: Tissue that covers the internal and external surfaces of the body. May be one cell thick (for example, cells lining the respiratory tract or gut) or several layers thick (for example, skin)

Excretion: Removal of waste products of metabolism from the body, either via the kidneys (water soluble wastes), skin (in sweat) or lungs (carbon dioxide)

Exocrine gland: A gland that empties its secretion onto an epithelial surface via a duct – for example, salivary glands, digestive glands

Extracellular: Outside the cell. Extracellular fluid includes the plasma and the fluid bathing the outside of the cells

Haemoglobin: Red pigment containing iron, present inside red blood cells. Haemoglobin combines reversibly with oxygen and transports it to the tissues

Homeostasis: Ability of the body to maintain internal stability despite environmental fluctuations (such as food shortage, demands of exercise)

Hormone: Secretion from an endocrine gland, entering the bloodstream directly, not via a duct, and exerting its effects in a specific target tissue often remote from the site of secretion

Hypothalamus: Area of specialised nervous tissue positioned in the brain, just above the pituitary gland. Centre of control for many body functions (for example, temperature, thirst, appetite)

Hypothermia: Fall in body temperature, taken by convention to be below 35° C

Interstitial fluid: Part of the extracellular fluid compartment, bathing the outside of the cells

Intracellular: Inside cells. Intracellular fluid is the fluid inside the cells

Keratin: Protein deposited in the upper layers of the epidermis, making the dead cells hard and waterproof

Metabolism: Sum of all the biochemical reactions taking place inside a living organism. Anabolic reactions build complex molecules from smaller ones, and demand the expenditure of cellular energy. Catabolic reactions break down complex molecules, liberating energy

Oedema: Swelling due to excess fluid in the tissues, tending to collect in dependent parts of the body, e.g. ankles

Oestrogen: Steroid hormone released by the ovary, important in controlling the menstrual

Consultant/G.P.				Surname		Hosp. no.	Sex
Ward Clinic				Forenames		Date of Birth	
Hospital Surgery				Address		Lab. no.	

	1	2	3	4	DATE COLLECTED
PENICILLIN					
ERYTHROMYCIN					
COTRIMOXAZOLE					
TRIMETHOPRIM					
AMOXYCILLIN					
TETRACYCLINE					
NITROFURANTOIN					
NALIDIXIC ACID					
CEPHALEXIN					
GENTAMICIN					
METRONIDAZOLE					
FLUCLOXACILLIN					
AUGMENTIN					
CIPROFLOXACIN					
CHLORAMPHENICOL					
CEFUROXIME					
PIPERACILLIN					
TICARCILLIN					
AZLOCILLIN					
AZTREONAM					

Date
received .... Signed ....

Date
reported ....

MICRO

Specimen and Examination Requested

Clinical Summary (inc. antibiotic therapy and site of lesion)

Doctor's signed ....

WVG 4851

cycle and in the development and maintenance of the female secondary sexual characteristics

Organ: Part of the body forming a structural and functional unit (for example, kidney, liver)

Osmosis: Passage of a dilute solution to a more concentrated one via a semipermeable membrane. In living systems, the fluid component of an osmotic solution is water. Plasma membranes are semipermeable

pH scale: Measure of the number of hydrogen ions in a solution determining its degree of acidity. The scale runs from 1 to 14. A strong acid containing large numbers of hydrogen ions will have a pH towards the lower end of the scale, for example, hydrochloric acid in the stomach has a pH of 1–2. Blood is virtually neutral with a pH of 7.35–7.45

Physiology: Study of the functioning of a biological system

Pituitary gland: Small gland situated just beneath the hypothalamus and controlled by it. The pituitary in turn controls much of the endocrine activity of the body

Platelet: Small cellular fragment derived from large megakaryocyte cells in the bone marrow. Platelets play an important part in blood clotting

Respiration: Combustion of food molecules using oxygen to release energy that will be used by the cell to fuel anabolism

Sodium pump: Enzyme system in the cell membrane actively pumping sodium ions out of the cell, into the extracellular fluid

Subcutaneous: Underneath the skin (for example, subcutaneous capillaries)

Tissue: A group of cells having the same structure and function, associated together in large numbers. The four basic tissue types include: epithelium, connective tissue, nervous tissue and muscle. In various proportions, the tissues make up organs

Unicellular: Single celled organism (for example, bacterium)

Vein: Blood vessel that carries blood back to the heart from the tissues

References

Akinsanya, J.A. (1985). Learning about life. *Senior Nurse*, 2(5), 24–25.

Biley, F.C. (1989). Nurses' perceptions of stress in preoperative patients. *Journal of Advanced Nursing*, 14, 575–581.

Boore, J. (1978). *Prescription for Recovery*. Royal College of Nursing, London.

Carr, E.C.J. (1990). Post-operative pain: expectations and experiences. *Journal of Advanced Nursing*, 15, 89–100.

Edholm, O.G. (1978). *Man – Hot and Cold*. Studies in Biology No. 97. Edward Arnold, London.

Eliopoulos, C. (1987). *The Ageing*. Clinical Nursing Diagnosis series. Williams & Wilkins, Baltimore.

Ganong, W.F. (1985). *Review of Medical Physiology*, (12th ed.). Lange Medical Publications, California.

Garrett, G. (1991). *Healthy Ageing*. Austen Cornish, London.

Gould, D.J. (1984). Equipped for the equipment. *Nursing Mirror*, 159, 21–23.

Hayward, J. (1975). *Information: A Prescription against Pain*. Royal College of Nursing, London.

Laycock, J. and Wise, P. (1983). *Essential Endocrinology* (3rd ed.). Oxford University Press, Oxford.

Marieb, E. (1991). *Human Anatomy and Physiology* (2nd ed.). Benjamin Cummings Co., California.

Montague, S.E. (1981). The contribution of biological sciences to the art of nursing. In *Nursing Science and Nursing Practice*, Smith, J. (ed.). Butterworths, London.

United Kingdom Central Council for Nursing, Midwifery and Health Visiting. (1986). *Project 2000 – A New Preparation for Practice*. UKCC, London.

Wilson, K.J.W. (1975). *The Biological Sciences in Nursing Education*. Churchill Livingstone, Edinburgh.

Wilson-Barnett, J. (1979). *Stress in Hospital*. Churchill Livingstone, Edinburgh.

Suggestions for further reading

British Medical Journal. (1988). *Basic Molecular and Cell Biology*. BMJ, London.

Closs, J. (1987). Oral temperature measurement. *Nursing Times*, 83(1), 36–38.

Drake, M. (1989). Homeostasis – normal and disturbed. In *Medical-Surgical Nursing: A Core Text*, Game, C. et al. (eds.). Churchill Livingstone, Edinburgh.

Hardy, N. (1983). *Homeostasis* (2nd ed.). Edward Arnold, London.

Hinchliff, S. and Montague, S.E. (1988). *Physiology for Nursing Practice*. Baillière Tindall, London. New edition due 1993.

Smith, K. (1980). *Fluids and Electrolytes: A Conceptual Approach*. Churchill Livingstone, Edinburgh.

Vander, A.J., Sherman, J.H. and Luciano, D.S. (1990). *Human Physiology*. McGraw-Hill, New York.

6

AN OVERVIEW OF PATHOLOGY

Anne Betts

This chapter sets out to present to readers concepts basic to an understanding of pathology in order to help them plan patients' care more effectively.

The chapter will include the following topics:

- Cell structure and protein synthesis
- Cell division
- Genetic and chromosomal abnormalities
- Acquired congenital abnormalities
- Traumatic conditions resulting from:
  - cold
  - heat
  - radiation
  - chemicals
- Inflammations and wound healing
- Immunity

- Mechanical disorders
- Metabolic and nutritional disorders
- Degenerative disorders
- Tumours
- Auto-immune diseases
- Circulatory disorders
- Shock
- Endocrine disorders
- Idiopathic disorders
- Iatrogenic disease

Pathology is the study of disease and disease processes (Thomson and Cotton, 1983).

The signs and symptoms with which patients present are manifestations of disease processes. Just as there are slight variations in the clinical picture presented by a patient so there are slight variations in the pathological changes present. Generally, a pattern of changes induced by the disease can be identified, and examination of the diseased organs, cells and tissues will reveal information about the basic nature of the disease. It is upon such knowledge that predictions as to the severity, course, possible aetiology and outcome of the disease are based. In this way pathology has become one of the foundations of modern medicine.

An understanding of pathology is important for nurses and enables them to give individualised care that meets patients' needs and achieves desired outcomes. Although the aetiology of many diseases may be unclear, most can be categorised (see Table 6.1).

Table 6.1. *The aetiology of disease – a classification*

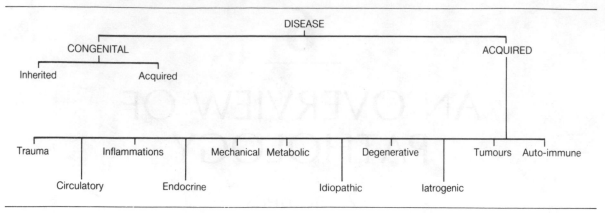

This chapter aims to provide the reader with a broad overview of pathophysiology. To aid understanding, examples are given from which the various features of a particular category can be extrapolated. However, for further information, a specialist text should be sought (see suggestions for further reading at the end of this chapter).

Congenital disorders

Congenital disorders are those present at birth which may be genetic or environmental (Jenkins, 1983).

Consider King George III who has been portrayed as 'The Mad King'. At the height of his 'attacks' he was too weak to walk or stand, and could only swallow with great difficulty. He could not sleep and suffered from excessive excitement, endless babbling, headaches, tremors, dizziness, visual disturbances and convulsions. He was repeatedly put into straitjackets while the Parliament of the day debated how to resolve the 'crisis' imposed by a 'mad' king. Recovery was spontaneous, but not permanent, and he was removed from the throne 23 years after his first attack and replaced by his son. Earlier medical records are poor but King James I was treated for 'colics' which he is said to have inherited from his mother. His urine was, he reported, 'the colour of my favourite Alicante wine.'

These characteristic features – dark red urine, hoarseness, delirium, paralysis and mental de-

rangement – are all signs and symptoms of *porphyria*, a genetic disease passed through a lengthy line of royalty and continued among George's descendants. Porphyria is an inherited disease, a genetic abnormality inherited from one or both parents and transmitted to their offspring.

Genes and chromosomes

Genes are the units of hereditary material. They carry the encoded instructions for an organism's development and function, and are located on *chromosomes* within the nucleus of each cell. The cell is the essential basic unit of the body, and an understanding of its structure and function is necessary to appreciate the nature of disease.

Under the light microscope, cells are seen to be composed of an outer membrane, some *cytoplasm*, and a *nucleus*. Under the electron microscope specialised structures known as *organelles* become visible in the cytoplasm, but every cell has the same basic structure (Fig. 6.1).

The cell membrane is a *lipoprotein*, i.e. a bilipid layer in and on which are proteins. Cell membranes are semipermeable – they maintain the integrity of a cell while allowing materials to pass in and out. Some cells which need substances to pass through rapidly have adaptations to increase the surface area, for example the microvilli of the cells of the proximal convoluted tubule of the nephron in the kidney.

The material inside the cell membrane, the *cytoplasm*, is not homogeneous but contains a complex branching network of membrane-bound cavities that are interconnected. On the outer sur-

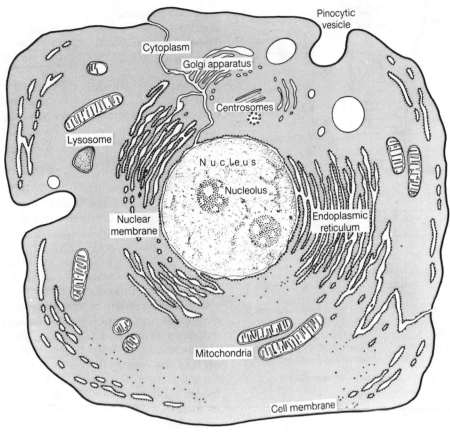

Fig. 6.1 *The cell*

face of this network are granules, known as *ribosomes*, which are the sites of protein synthesis. The network, known as *endoplasmic reticulum*, is continuous with pores in the nuclear membrane.

Enzymes, hormones and compounds such as *collagen*, *keratin* and *albumin* are all proteins. The information required for the synthesis of these proteins is stored in the genes of the cell nucleus. A carrier molecule, called mRNA (*messenger ribose nucleic acid*) conveys a coded 'message' from the nucleus to a ribosome via the endoplasmic reticulum. It is this coded message that dictates the sequence of amino acids required to synthesise a protein and it is the function of **DNA** (*deoxyribose nucleic acid*) to store the coded information. The DNA is bound and organised into strands which are folded and packaged into chromosomes. Each chromosome consists of two paired strands of DNA (Fig. 6.2) arranged in a helical shape. A length of DNA with the information necessary to make one protein is called a *gene*. Every function

of a cell depends on protein molecules. Proteins are basically long chains of amino acids. The types of amino acids and the sequence in which they occur gives each protein its own unique properties (Marieb, 1989).

There are thousands of different proteins in the human body, each with different functions, and all are made from the same amino acids but in *different combinations*.

So, if the information in the gene is incorrect then the wrong protein will be made. For example, sickle cell disease results from one change in the 287 amino acids in globin. The abnormal haemoglobin causes the red cells to become crescent-shaped when they are de-oxygenated, for example during vigorous exercise. The crescent-shaped or sickle cells are too large to pass through small blood vessels, which become clogged. The clogging promotes thrombus formation which interferes with oxygen delivery and causes pain.

Sickle cell disease only occurs in individuals

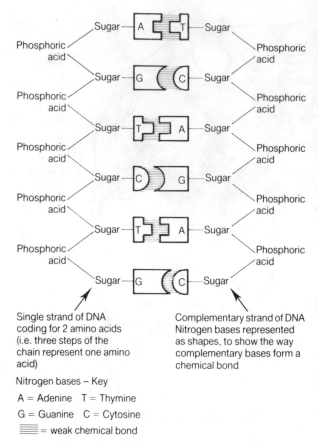

Single strand of DNA
coding for 2 amino acids
(i.e. three steps of the
chain represent one amino
acid)

Complementary strand of DNA
Nitrogen bases represented
as shapes, to show the way
complementary bases form a
chemical bond

Nitrogen bases – Key

A = Adenine   T = Thymine

G = Guanine   C = Cytosine

≡ = weak chemical bond

Fig. 6.2 *Diagrammatic representation showing coding on a single strand of DNA and the formation of complementary strands*

with two abnormal genes. Those carrying one such abnormal gene are said to have *sickle cell trait*. They do not usually display symptoms but can pass the gene on to their children (Gonick and Wheelis, 1983).

When a cell divides, the strands of DNA separate (Fig. 6.3). On each strand is formed another complementary strand, thus each original strand is replicated. When the cell divides each daughter cell will receive replicated strands and thus identical genetic information. This process, known as **mitosis**, ensures that the DNA contained in the chromosomes is divided equally between the two daughter cells after **replication** (Fig. 6.4).

The number of chromosomes per nucleus is a constant feature for each species, barring chromosomal accidents, and humans have 46 chromosomes. Careful examination of the chromosomes show that there are two sets, alike in appearance. Each pair of chromosomes that can be matched visually are known as **homologous** pairs and in man there are 22 such pairs. The other two chromosomes don't match visually and are the sex chromosomes. When a cell divides mitotically each of the new cells has the same chromosome complement as the parent cell. Sex cells, egg and sperm, undergo a reduction division known as **meiosis** in which the chromosome complement of the parent cell is halved (i.e. 23), so that when egg and sperm unite the normal (diploid) number of chromosomes (i.e. 46) is once again present (Fig. 6.5). One set of chromosomes is thus derived from

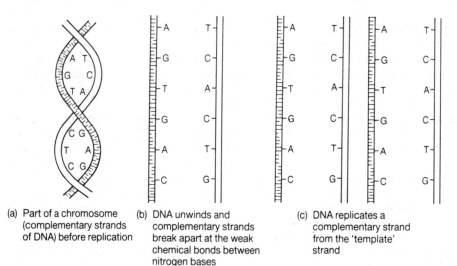

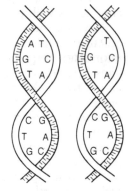

(a) Part of a chromosome (complementary strands of DNA) before replication

(b) DNA unwinds and complementary strands break apart at the weak chemical bonds between nitrogen bases

(c) DNA replicates a complementary strand from the 'template' strand

(d) DNA recoils and at cell division, one of the new identical double helices goes to each daughter cell

Fig. 6.3 *Genetic replication of cell division*

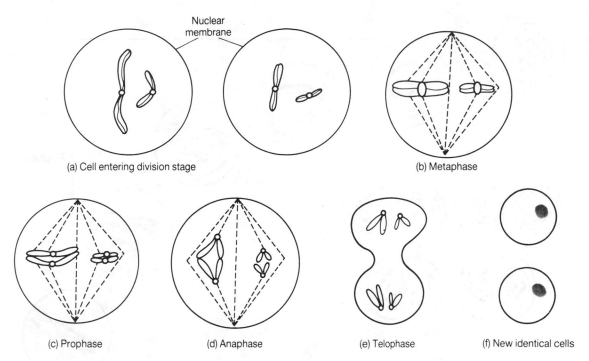

Fig. 6.4 *The stages of mitosis*

the sperm of the father and one set from the ovum of the mother.

During meiosis, the homologous pairs of chromosomes, one derived from the mother and one from the father of the previous generation, are separated; one of the pairs going to one new sperm (or ovum) the other of the pair to another sperm (or ovum). During this sharing out, 'cross overs' or **chiasmata** are formed and chromosomes may break and rejoin allowing genes of a maternal chromosome to be exchanged with those of a paternal chromosome (Fig. 6.5). Thus an infant receives one chromosome of each pair from its father, the genetic material of which may be a mixture of that of its paternal grandmother and grandfather, and the same applies for the other chromosome of each pair which comes from the infant's mother.

Genetics is the study of heredity and variation or the science that tries to explain the similarities and differences between organisms related by descent (Jenkins, 1983).

Genes are the units of hereditary material that carry the encoded instructions for an organism's development and functioning. As chromosomes are paired, all proteins will be coded by two

Table 6.2. *Demonstrating dominant and recessive inheritance*

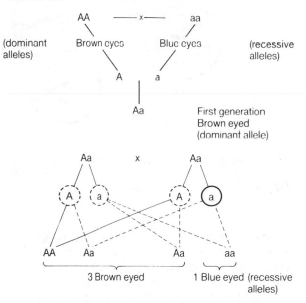

i.e. There is a 1:4 chance (probability of being blue eyed) of having recessive alleles

There is a 3:4 chance/possibility of having dominant alleles – therefore being brown eyed.

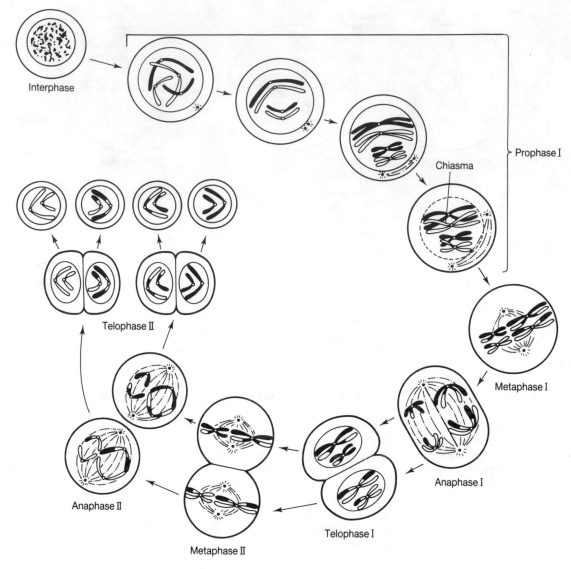

Interphase

Prophase I

Chiasma

Metaphase I

Anaphase I

Telophase I

Metaphase II

Anaphase II

Telophase II

N.B. *two pairs of homologous chromosomes are shown*

Fig. 6.5 *The stages of meiosis*

alternative forms of genes, known as **alleles**, one derived from the mother and one from the father. When alleles code for different forms of the same trait, such as eye colour, and the effects of one are masked by the other, the masking allele is said to be **dominant** (A) and the masked allele to be **recessive** (a), as shown in Table 6.2.

Genetic disorders

A monk, Gregor Mendel (1822–1884), was the first to study the results of hybridisation in plants and to discover their statistical relationships. In the past decade there has been an increasing interest shown in clinical genetics and a significant demand for genetic counselling. Indeed approximately one in 20 children admitted to hospital in the UK has a disorder that is entirely genetic in origin.

There are hundreds of diseases due to a single autosomal dominant gene – for example Huntington's chorea, osteogenesis imperfecta, polycystic kidneys, porphyria, and neurofibromatosis. Thus the mode of inheritance of genetic disorders must be understood in order to help patients and their families. It is also important for genetic counsellors to recognise varying clinical expressions of genetic disorders.

There are some 500 disorders which require both recessive alleles to be present for the condition to be expressed (see Table 6.2) – for example albinism, cystic fibrosis, galactosaemia, alkaptonuria. However, there are a number of diseases that are inherited by sex linkage, i.e. from **sex chromosomes**.

Females have two X chromosomes, one maternal and one paternal, and males have one X and one Y chromosome. Since the Y chromosome has less genetic material than the X, some genetic functions exist only on the X chromosome. The ability to make anti-haemophilic globulin is one such example. Thus if there is a deficiency of the gene a male with that defective chromosome will have haemophilia. A female with a defective X chromosome will be a 'carrier' but will not suffer haemophilia unless both X chromosomes carry the defective gene (Table 6.3).

Table 6.3. *Sex-linked inheritance*

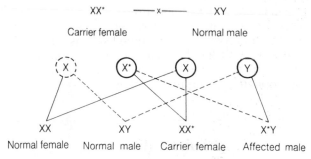

i.e. There is a 1 : 2 probability of males being affected

Not all conditions are due to 'abnormal' genes however. Some conditions are due to deletions of bits of chromosomes (for example, cri du chat and Wolf's syndrome) or to an extra **autosome** (for example, Down's syndrome in which there are three of chromosome 21, giving a total of 47 chromosomes) or to an extra sex chromosome (for example, Klinefelter's syndrome – XXY).

Genetic counselling has a considerable part to play in modern medicine and nursing. Without adequate knowledge of cell ultra-structure and the role played by chromosomes and genes, nurses would be unable to contribute effectively in supporting those individuals who may be affected or are potentially at risk.

Acquired congenital abnormalities

Some abnormalities present from birth are not inherited but *acquired* in utero. One of the most common causes of congenital heart defects is a virus infection in the mother during the first three months of pregnancy, when the fetal heart is developing. Such defects are particularly prone to develop if the infection is due to rubella (German measles).

There are three major types of congenital abnormalities of the heart and its major vessels:

(1) Stenosis in the channel of blood flow either in the heart or one of its associated vessels, for example coarctation of the aorta
(2) An abnormality that allows blood to flow from the left side of the heart or the aorta to the right side of the heart or the pulmonary artery (a left-to-right shunt), for example patent ductus arteriosus
(3) The reverse of (2), a right-to-left shunt which thus bypasses the lungs, for example tetralogy of Fallot.

During fetal life the lungs are collapsed. The factors that keep the alveoli collapsed also keep pulmonary blood vessels collapsed, so resistance to pulmonary blood flow is very high in the fetus. The blood vessels in the placenta are large and thus offer little resistance to blood flow. Hence the pressure in the fetal aorta is lower than that in the pulmonary artery. This causes almost all the pulmonary arterial blood to flow through the ductus arteriosus into the aorta rather than through the non-functioning lungs.

Similarly, much of the blood entering the right atrium flows directly through the foramen ovale into the left atrium and then into systemic circulation. This aids the ductus arteriosus in shunting blood (Fig. 6.6).

When the baby is born and inflates its lungs, the

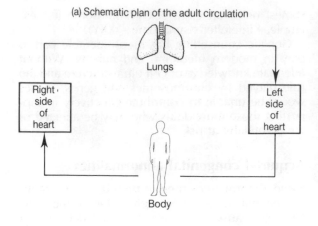

(a) Schematic plan of the adult circulation

(b) Schematic plan of the fetal circulation

Fig. 6.6 (a) Schematic plan of the adult circulation; (b) Schematic plan of the fetal circulation

alveoli fill and the resistance to blood flow through the pulmonary vessels decreases drastically. Simultaneously, the aortic pressure rises as blood no longer flows through the placenta. So pressure in the pulmonary artery falls and that in the aorta rises. As a result, forward blood flow through the ductus ceases and the ductus becomes occluded. In about one in 5000 babies the ductus fails to close.

The changes in pressure in the aorta and pulmonary artery also decrease the load on the right ventricle and increase the load on the left ventricle. Hence the right arterial pressure decreases and left arterial pressure increases. However, blood is normally prevented from flowing into the right atrium by a valve-like flap that closes over the foramen ovale.

Tetralogy of Fallot

In the tetralogy of Fallot, four abnormalities occur simultaneously. Firstly, the aorta over-rides the septum between the right and left ventricles and thus receives blood from both ventricles. Secondly, the pulmonary artery is stenosed. Thirdly, there is a ventricular septal defect which allows blood to flow into the right ventricle. Fourthly, as the right ventricle has an increased load it becomes hypertrophied.

Hypertrophy of muscle is one of the most important mechanisms by which the heart adapts to increased workloads but extreme degrees of hypertrophy can lead to heart failure. Coronary blood flow may not increase to the same extent as the muscle mass and hence coronary insufficiency can ensue.

Considering the four events of tetralogy of Fallot, it becomes obvious that blood is shunted past the lungs without being oxygenated. Indeed, as much as 75% of venous blood returning to the heart may pass directly from the right ventricle to the aorta. Hence, tetralogy of Fallot is the major cause of cyanosis in babies.

An understanding of the pathophysiology makes it easy to see why a child suffering from tetralogy of Fallot will squat when breathless. Squatting traps blood in the lower limbs and thus temporarily decreases venous return, and thus the load on the right ventricle, giving the unfortunate sufferer 'breathing space'.

With surgery to correct the defects, average life expectancy can increase from 5–10 to 50 years or more. Careful, informed nursing will make a successful prognosis even more likely as informed nurses will set specific, realistic, measurable goals from which to plan, implement and evaluate the appropriate nursing intervention.

Acquired disorders

Disorders and diseases can be acquired at any time during an individual's life. The ways in which this can happen are broadly categorised below.

Trauma

Trauma can be caused by injury or by toxicity.

Injury

Injury to the body tissues can be caused by physical agents such as heat, cold, ultraviolet light, and irradiation.

The extent to which any agent can cause cell injury or cell death is largely dependent on the intensity and duration of the exposure to the injurious agent, as well as the type of cell involved.

Injury due to mechanical forces is the result of the body impacting on another object. Tissue may be torn or crushed, bones fractured and blood flow disrupted.

Extremes of heat and cold cause damage to the cell, cell organelles and enzyme systems. For example, glucose utilisation is severely reduced during severe hypothermia (when the core temperature drops below 30°C). This impairment seems to result from inhibition of the glucose carrier systems of the cell membrane rather than from any lack of insulin.

Three temperature zones in hypothermia are of physiological significance:

(1) 35–32.2°C – vasoconstriction of skin blood vessels and shivering occurs
(2) 32.2–24°C – tissue metabolism is progressively depressed. Vasoconstriction is intense but shivering has usually ceased
(3) Below 24°C – mechanisms of heat conservation become inactive and heat is lost passively.

Acute cold injuries are of two basic types: acute freezing injury (frostbite) and non-freezing injuries (immersion foot).

Skin normally freezes at −0.53°C. Subcutaneous blood vessels are damaged and plasma leaks from the capillaries, causing blistering. The viscosity of blood increases and sludging and blockage of blood vessels occurs. Cell death seems to result from biochemical changes and disrupted enzymic activity.

Immersion foot results from prolonged exposure and the combination of cold, dependency, immobility and constriction of the limbs by shoes and clothing. Vasoconstriction, followed by raised venous pressure, sludging, blocked capillaries and thrombosis seem to be the order of events. Typically, muscle **necrosis** and nerve damage result while the skin is relatively unharmed. There is much greater venous involvement than in frostbite,

where arterial involvement predominates.

Exposure to heat, as in severe heat stroke, accelerates cell metabolism, inactivates enzymes and disrupts cell membranes. Higher temperatures (45°C+) coagulate both blood and tissue proteins.

Electromagnetic radiation is a term used to encompass a wide range of wave-propagated energies from gamma rays to radio waves. Radiation energy above the visible ultraviolet range is called *ionising radiation*. It can be divided into two main groups: *electromagnetic* radiation such as X-rays and γ rays, and *particulate* radiation consisting of particles such as α and β particles.

When X-rays or γ rays are absorbed, high energy electrons are produced in the irradiated tissue. It is these particles which can break molecular bonds and release positively or negatively charged ions; and α and β particles have the same capability. Hence the term *ionising radiation*. If DNA is affected by such ionising radiation, pieces may be 'broken off' and then the message inherent in the DNA will be altered. This occurrence is known as **mutation** (Gonick and Wheelis, 1983). If a piece of the genetic material that regulates the activity of a specific gene is affected, then unwanted activity by the gene may result. Such activity can lead to unwanted, uncoordinated cell replication or carcinogenesis, so ionising radiation can kill cells, interrupt cell division or cause a variety of mutations. Any inhibition of DNA synthesis or cell division (mitosis) will affect rapidly dividing cells – therefore, the cells of the bone marrow and gastrointestinal mucosa are very susceptible to radiation. However, because malignant cells themselves divide rapidly, radiation is used as a treatment for cancer.

Non-ionising radiation includes ultraviolet, infrared light, ultrasound, and microwaves. These all exert their effects by causing vibration and rotation of atoms and molecules, which produce heat. Hence ultraviolet light can cause sunburn, a condition in which the damaged skin cells release vasoactive and injurious chemicals resulting in the familiar erythema and blistering.

Toxicology

Toxicology is the study of the potential of chemicals to produce adverse effects in the body (Harrington and Gill, 1983).

The first principle is that *all* substances can kill if given by an inappropriate route and/or in inappropriate quantities. This is even true of water.

The adverse effects are related to the toxicity of the substance, its properties, the concentration, and length of exposure. Routes of entry may be by inhalation, ingestion or skin absorption, and once in contact with the body the effects may be local (such as irritation or allergy) or systemic.

The most common 'target organs' are the lungs, liver, nervous system, bone marrow, kidneys and the skin. The liver and kidneys are organs of metabolism and excretion and are thus likely to have to contend with the toxic substance or its metabolites.

Chemicals can cause cancer and chromosomal abnormalities, and affect normal functioning of the body organs and processes.

Whilst a nurse cannot be fully conversant with all harmful substances she should be aware of the toxicological effects of everyday substances. For example, drivers are currently being exhorted to use lead-free petrol in an effort to reduce the environmental levels. Organic lead compounds are used as anti-knock additives in petrol, but, when emitted in exhaust fumes, can accumulate in the atmosphere.

Individuals have been known to develop organic lead poisoning by using leaded petrol as a solvent when in a confined space. Cases of encephalopathy have been reported in children sniffing petrol (Waldron, 1985).

Symptoms of acute poisoning include disturbances in sleep patterns, nausea, headache, vertigo and hyperexcitability, i.e. lead affects the central nervous system. Should not we all be more aware?

Inflammations

This group includes all infections due to bacteria, viruses, parasites, worms and fungi. The tissue reaction may not be diagnostically characteristic. Response may be non-specific or it may produce a histologically significant feature such as a granuloma (i.e. a specific response). Such responses may be acute or chronic.

Acute inflammatory response

The acute inflammatory response is a reaction of living tissues to injury and is fundamentally a protective mechanism. Regardless of the cause, the basic local response is to produce heat, redness, pain and swelling with a variable degree of loss of function.

The 'injured' tissues release histamine and other chemicals which have an effect on arterioles, venules and capillaries causing vasodilation and increased permeability. This allows fluid and plasma proteins to leak into the area. Bradykinin and kallidin formed from plasma precursors increase vascular permeability and produce pain. White cells leave the bloodstream and migrate to the area. Neutrophils are the first and most numerous cells to reach the area in acute inflammation. They are amoeboid and phagocytic. Eosinophils migrate in the later stages and large numbers are often associated with parasitic infestations. Lymphocytes do not reach inflammatory areas in the initial stages but play an important part in chronic inflammation, for example tuberculosis or syphilis. The polymorphs and monocytes engulf damaged tissue and bacteria.

Phagocytic histiocytes, or *macrophages*, and giant cells, formed by the fusion of histiocytes, continue the 'clearing' process. Fibroblasts, which synthesise collagen, appear and produce fibrous scar tissue.

Monocytes and macrophages are present in various numbers in all inflammations. Polymorphonuclear leucocytes predominate in acute inflammation. Lymphocytes, plasma cells and fibroblasts predominate in chronic inflammation.

Variations in the type of inflammatory response have resulted in some differences in description. For example, inflammation of a serous membrane produces large amounts of exudate, as in a pleural effusion, and is known as *serous inflammation*; whereas the inflammation associated with profuse secretion from an epithelial surface, such as the nose, is known as *catarrhal inflammation*.

Whatever the cause, the offending agent will be more easily overcome if the reaction remains localised. The larger the number of organisms and the greater their virulence and invasiveness, the greater the chance of spread.

The outcome of any acute inflammation depends on whether the body defences or the invading organism win the battle. Complete *resolution* may occur and the area return to normal. Resolution may be incomplete and the fibrin becomes organised into scar tissue. The area may suppurate, resulting in **abscess** formation. An abscess discharging onto an epithelial surface forms a **sinus**. An abscess cavity joining two epithelialised surfaces, for example gut and abdominal surface, is known as a *fistula*.

Chronic inflammation

Sometimes, the agent producing the acute inflammatory reaction may not be effectively overcome by the inflammatory response, which may change therefore to chronic inflammation. This is characterised by infiltration of lymphocytes and plasma cells, overgrowth of fibroblasts and increased fibrosis of the area. If the local defences are totally overwhelmed, the agent may spread locally (to give *cellulitis*) or via the lymphatics (*lymphangitis*) and bloodstream (*septicaemia*).

Effects of the inflammatory process

The general effects of the inflammatory process vary considerably depending on the agent and the resistance and immunity of the host.

Pyrexia is a common sign of any inflammation and is due to the hypothalamic thermostat being 'reset' upwards by pyrogens that are released from bacteria and neutrophils as well as monocytes.

As metabolism is increased by 12.6% for every 1°C of pyrexia (Porth, 1990), prolonged pyrexia may be detrimental to recovery.

Any agent that causes an inflammatory response may also cause tissue damage.

Healing

Phagocytosis of dead cells may leave a defect, such as an ulcer, which will need to be repaired. Healing is optimal in a well-nourished, rested individual whose tissues are well oxygenated and whose immune responses are unimpaired. The process of wound healing has been described by Torrance (1986) as comprising four distinct stages (see Table 6.4) starting with an acute inflammatory reaction lasting approximately three days.

Macrophages play an essential role in the second, *destructive phase* of wound healing. They are responsible for clearing dead tissue and are also active against bacteria. They play a role in attracting fibroblasts and thus enhance collagen production. They also influence the growth of new blood vessels (*angiogenesis*).

The *proliferative phase* is characterised by ingrowth of new capillary loops into the space cleared by macrophages. The loops carry fibro-

Table 6.4. *The process of wound healing (after Torrance, 1986)*

The **acute inflammatory reaction** (0–3 days)

The **destructive phase**, involving the removal of injured tissue (1–6 days)

The **proliferative phase**, featuring angiogenesis and fibroplasia (3–24 days)

The **maturational phase** (24 days–1 year)

blasts with them and collagen synthesis begins. Fibroplasia is thus dependent upon the ingrowth of new blood vessels and vitamin C is a known stimulant of collagen synthesis (Torrance, 1986). So granulation tissue includes new capillary loops and collagen. Infection can follow inflammation and thus may result in excessive granulation.

During the *maturational phase*, the collagen fibres increase in size and become oriented along lines of tension. A scar is weaker than the surrounding tissue – which explains the incidence of incisional hernias.

Both local and systemic factors influence wound healing. Local factors include tissue perfusion, infection and the effects of dressings. Systemic factors include nutrition, age, infection and immunological function. The use of the nursing process ensures that the nurse is in the best possible position to monitor the progress of wound healing and adapt to changing conditions within the wound (Griffiths, 1991a).

Once an assessment has been undertaken, the most suitable dressing can be chosen. Johnson (1990, page 25) outlined the criteria for an ideal wound dressing. It:

(1) removes excess exudate from the wound surface
(2) maintains high humidity at the wound/dressing interface
(3) possesses high thermal insulation properties
(4) is impermeable to micro-organisms
(5) does not shed fibres or leach toxic substances
(6) allows substances to be removed from the wound without causing damage to newly formed tissue.

A moist surface encourages epidermal cell growth and mobility and induces granulation (Johnson, 1988). A drop in temperature inhibits cell division at the wound site and it may take up to four hours

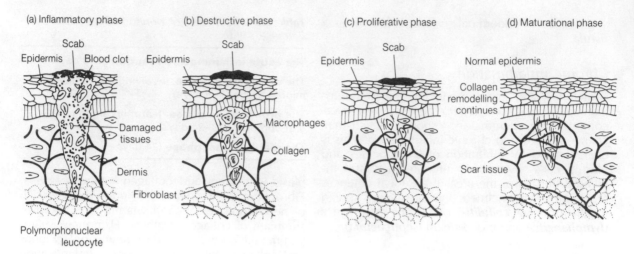

Fig. 6.7 *The stages in wound healing; (a) Inflammatory phase; (b) Destructive phase; (c) Proliferative phase; (d) Maturational phase*

for the wound to reach optimal temperature (37°C) after redressing (Morison, 1990). With a knowledge of wound healing and the properties of dressing materials such as hydrogels, hydrocolloids and alginates, nurses can make informed choices.

For example, at each stage of wound healing, various objectives should be achieved. Turner (1991) argues that nurses need to consider three questions in order to achieve objectives:

(1) At what stage is the wound (e.g. necrotic, infected, granulating, epithelialising, etc.)?
(2) What do I want the wound to do next (e.g. debride, deslough, granulate, epithelialise)?
(3) How do I achieve the goal(s) without damaging healthy tissue?

By taking such a problem-solving approach and understanding and recognising the stages of wound healing, it should be possible to make an appropriate dressing choice. All that is required is a knowledge of the performance characteristics of different dressings.

General features of various dressing types

Absorbent dressing, e.g. gauze
These dressings are absorbent and provide some insulation for the wound but may shed fibres and can adhere to the wound surface. Dressings such as 'melolin' have a non-adherent surface but, like all absorbent dressings, may still allow 'strike-through', i.e. exudate from the wound soaks through to the outside of the dressing, thus providing an access route for micro-organisms, and increases heat loss.

Film dressings, e.g. Opsite, Tegaderm
These dressings are permeable to gas and water vapour but impermeable to bacteria and water. Their transparency allows for visual inspection of the wound and they can be left in place when washing or bathing. The moist environment they produce at the wound surface promotes rapid epithelialisation (Thomas, 1990a). However, if heavily exuding wounds are dressed with semi-permeable film, exudate may accumulate under the dressing and require aspiration with a needle and syringe.

The selected dressing should completely cover the wound and overlap onto the surrounding skin, which must be clean and dry, by 3–4 cm.

Semipermeable film dressings can be applied to many different types of wound but must not be used to cover infected or deep cavity wounds (Thomas, 1990a).

Hydrocolloid dressings, e.g. Granuflex, Comfeel and Tegasorb
A 'colloid' is produced when small particles of one substance are dispersed uniformly in another. If solid particles are dispersed in liquid, a hydrophilic colloid (hydrocolloid) is produced (Thomas, 1990b). When placed on the surface of an exuding

wound, such a dressing will absorb liquid and form a gel. The gel produces a moist environment to facilitate healing but does not cause maceration of the surrounding skin.

Many hydrocolloid dressings are impermeable to both liquids and bacteria, are relatively easy to use, do not need frequent changing and do not cause trauma on removal. They also appear to promote the growth of granulation tissue (Thomas, 1990b). Currently they are mainly used for chronic wounds such as leg ulcers and should be applied so that the wound is covered completely and the dressing overlaps onto the surrounding skin by 2–3 cm. They should not be used in the treatment of infected wounds (Thomas, 1990b). However, patients should be warned that some hydrocolloids will absorb so well that they liquefy; the liquid may then have a strong smell but pain is usually reduced (Griffiths, 1991b).

Hydrogel dressings, e.g. Scherisorb
Hydrogels are jelly-like and are very efficient at debriding wounds as the necrotic tissue is rehydrated and thus softened. The dressing gel is gas and water-permeable and will absorb large amounts of exudate. They have also been found to reduce pain markedly (Griffiths, 1991b).

Alginate dressings, e.g. Kaltostat
These are highly absorbent dressings, manufactured from seaweed. They absorb exudate and in the process become jelly-like, so can be used on wounds or in cavities; indeed, alginate dressings are not recommended unless there is exudate present (Griffiths, 1991b).

Different dressings have different advantages and disadvantages. Only by understanding the process of wound healing and having a knowledge of each wound care product's performance characteristics can nurses make informed choices for the greater benefit of their patients.

Immunity

The capacity to resist organisms or toxins that tend to damage tissues or organs is known as *immunity*. Acquired immunity is the development of specific immunity against particular pathogens or toxins, and there are two basic types of acquired immunity: *humoral* and *cell mediated*.

Cell mediated immunity is promoted by T lymphocytes and humoral immunity by B lymphocytes (see Figs. 6.8 and 6.9).

In order for immunity to develop the host needs to be exposed to a foreign substance or antigen which then elicits the formation of **antibodies** (immunoglobulins). The three main varieties of immunoglobulin are known as IgG, IgM, and IgA. Two other classes are IgD and IgE.

Immunoglobulins can form a complex with an antigen and can also activate other systems such as complement (see Fig. 6.8).

IgG is the most plentiful of the immunoglobulins and is able to carry out most of the functions attributed to antibodies. IgM is important in bacterial infection. IgA is secreted onto mucosal surfaces

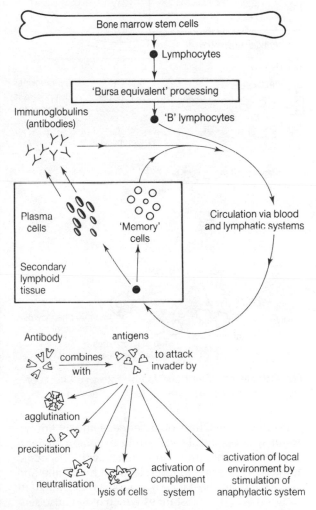

Fig. 6.8 *Development and main protective effects of the humoral immune system*

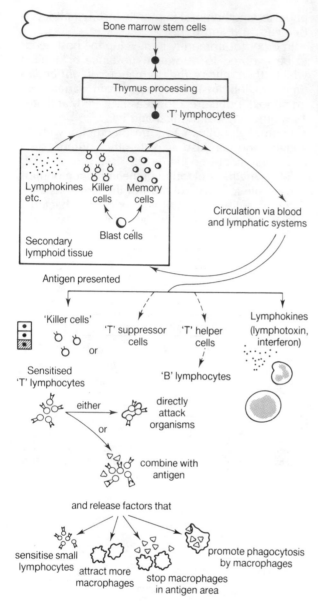

Fig. 6.9 *Development and main protective effects of the cell mediated immune system*

providing a first line of defence. Little is known about IgD but IgE binds firmly to mast cells and triggers degranulation on contact with a specific antigen. This leads to the release of histamine and slow-releasing substance of anaphylaxis (SRS-A) in addition to other substances which may cause sensitisation and allergy. IgE-mediated release of mast cell granules can be blocked by sodium cromo-glycate (Intal), hence its use in the management of asthma.

When antigen and B cell (lymphocyte) interact, the result is a plasma cell which secretes antibody. Some of the cells become memory cells, thus ensuring a faster response in future infection (see Fig. 6.8).

T cells also show antigenic specificity. When stimulated by antigen they become blast cells which differentiate into 'killer cells'. The growth, differentiation and function of cells of the immune system are controlled by small peptides known as *cytokines* (Roitt et al., 1989). They act as local chemical messengers and are secreted by and act upon the cells of the immune system. For cytokines to act, they must first bind to a specific receptor on a cell's surface. Only cells that have the correct receptor can respond.

Cytokines include the interleukins, interferons, tumour necrosis factors, and colony stimulating factors.

Interleukin 2 (IL-2) is produced by T helper cells and is essential for the maturation of T killer or T cytotoxic cells and the proliferation of B cells. It also induces the secretion of a tumour necrosis factor (TNF). IL-2 has been found to have a therapeutic effect in patients with renal cell cancer, although caution is needed as a wide variety of toxic effects can occur. Chills, fever and malaise are common, but skin rashes, arrhythmias and myocardial infarction have been reported (Moore, 1990).

The interferons have a number of biological activities including antiviral antiproliferative effects against tumour cells (see Fig. 6.9). Alpha interferon can be used for patients with myeloma (tumour of bone marrow cells), glioma (malignant tumour of glial cells in the brain), melanoma and a variety of other malignant conditions. Side effects include fever, chills, arthralgia (painful joints), myalgia (painful muscles) and headache.

'One of the most important issues in caring for patients receiving such therapy is to make sure they are well informed about their treatment, both to cope with side effects and retain realistic expectations'

(Moore, 1990, page 56)

In severe combined immune deficiency (SCID) there is an absence of both T and B cell systems. Such children have no defence against disease. In bone marrow transplantation, it is the transplanted

T killer cells that initiate **graft versus host disease**, as they attack the 'new' host.

In acquired immune deficiency syndrome (AIDS) the human immunodeficiency virus (HIV) attacks helper cells and takes over their nuclei. With a dearth of helper cells to activate T killer cells and cooperate with B lymphocytes, together with an over-abundance of suppressor cells, the patient's immune system will be seriously compromised. This leaves him vulnerable to infection and malignant conditions such as Kaposi's sarcoma. Most of the drugs now being tested are aimed at stopping the virus from replicating after it has entered the helper cell.

A large number of micro-organisms cause infections and produce the features of non-specific inflammation. Some infective agents produce a mass of granulation tissue, a *granuloma*. Mycobacterium tuberculosis is one such agent. The basic lesion is called a *tubercle*, with a central core of cheesy necrosis, known as *caseation*, surrounded by epithelioid cells, giant cells, lymphocytes and fibroblasts. The characteristic tuberculous granuloma is composed of many such tubercles. Healing is slow and is the result of progressive fibrosis. The central core may remain caseous for a considerable time and viable organisms may be reactivated at a later date. Sarcoidosis, leprosy and syphilis are also granulomatous diseases.

Nurses are in an ideal position to monitor the progress of healing and an understanding of the pathological processes involved can enhance patient care.

Mechanical disorders

This group includes all the diseases resulting from mechanical factors, such as **atelectasis**, hydronephrosis and meconium ileus which are all brought about by obstruction. This particular classification illustrates the difficulty of logical assignment of disorders to specific categories, as it includes many diseases also dealt with in other sections.

Intestinal obstruction provides a useful example from which to extrapolate various features. Blockage to the passage of intestinal contents may be classified in one of three ways.

(1) Intralumenal

Blockage of the lumen of the gut by faeces, gallstones or swallowed foreign bodies.

(2) Interlumenal

Disease processes affecting the wall of the gut which then obstructs the lumen. Examples include: tumours, particularly carcinoma; ulcerative colitis and Crohn's disease which cause scar formation and strictures; *intussusception*, i.e. invagination of one part of the bowel into another, impairing the blood supply and possibly causing necrosis.

(3) Extralumenal

Disease processes elsewhere that cause problems for the passage of gut contents – for example, tumours compressing the gut from outside; adhesions acting as elastic bands; *volvulus* (torsion of the mesentery and gut which deprives the latter of a blood supply).

The effects of such obstructions can be disastrous. Some nine litres of fluid per day are secreted by, and in the main re-absorbed by, the adult gut. The signs and symptoms will depend on the site of the obstruction, but the bowel generally empties below the obstruction. Initially, there is increased peristalsis, and even reverse peristalsis, above the obstruction. Eventually peristalsis ceases and the bowel distends with gas and fluid resulting in effortless vomiting with loss of fluid and electrolytes from the body. Gut distension compresses the blood vessels in the wall of the gut leading to **ischaemia**. Transudation of bacteria and toxins may cause peritonitis and further ischaemia may lead to necrosis and perforation.

Obstruction to the flow of urine produces similar events. Increased peristalsis in the ureters produces the pain of renal colic when a stone (*renal calculus*) is stuck in the ureter. Prolonged urinary obstruction can cause dilation of the ureters and kidney pelvis (*hydro-ureter* and *hydronephrosis*) and may lead to renal failure.

Metabolic disorders

The primary function of the digestive system is to provide the body with fluids, nutrients and electrolytes in a form that can be used at the cellular level. However, an adequate nutritional state depends on an adequate and appropriate intake, as well as its subsequent digestion and absorption.

Some diseases are due *either* to an inadequate intake of food (for example, starvation), *or* to deprivation of specific nutritional substances such as vitamins.

Inadequate intake of nutrients

The relationship between malnutrition and morbidity is well documented. Malnutrition results in weight loss, protein depletion, progressive weakness and apathy, impaired wound healing, fluid and electrolyte imbalance, skin breakdown, and depressed immune responses. Growth and health are threatened when food intake does not meet minimal requirements. Food deprivation may endanger survival.

Essential nutrients include amino acids, fatty acids, carbohydrates, minerals and vitamins. Poor nutritional status may have an adverse effect on wound healing, resistance to infection and even post-operative mortality (Goodinson, 1986). Protein, carbohydrate and fat are required for the provision of enough energy to fuel the body's activities and to supply materials to replace body tissues. A balance between energy sources and protein is needed. If an inadequate source of energy is provided by the diet then protein is broken down to supply it. Nitrogen, present in amino acids, is excreted and the patient is said to be in **negative nitrogen balance**. The amounts of nutrients needed vary according to age, size, physiological state and activity and thus expert help from dieticians may be sought.

As the first clues to the presence of malnutrition are often provided by the patient himself, nurses should be aware of the need for dietary information when taking a nursing history from the patient on admission.

It should be remembered that not only do vitamin deficiencies occur as a result of inadequate intake (see Table 6.5) but side effects of drug therapy may cause deficiency (for example, folate deficiency with methotrexate).

Excessive intakes of vitamins can also have serious consequences. Excessive intake of vitamin C has been found to result in the excretion of oxalates in the urine, which can lead to bladder stones and to increased serum *cholesterol* levels. Cholesterol is a constituent of cell membranes and is required for the manufacture of vitamin D, bile salts and steroid hormones. Although present in our diet, cholesterol can be synthesised by the liver and is eventually excreted in bile. Indeed, high levels of cholesterol in bile may lead to gallstones.

Although high levels of cholesterol are said to be 'bad for us', we all need some cholesterol for the proper functioning of our bodies. Cholesterol is insoluble in water and has to be transported in the plasma by carriers known as *lipoproteins*. The liver synthesises very low density lipoproteins (VLDLs) to carry triglycerides to adipose tissue for storage. What is left after this process are known as low density lipoproteins (LDLs). LDLs transport cholesterol in the blood to peripheral tissues for use in cell membranes and the production of steroid hormones. High density lipoproteins (HDLs) are involved in the transport of excess cholesterol to the liver for excretion in bile. Thus, the ratio of LDL to HDL is important, for raised levels of LDLs are associated with an increased risk of coronary heart disease.

Stress and smoking both increase LDL levels, whereas both aerobic and anaerobic exercise increase HDL levels. Changing one's diet can help too. Replacing saturated fatty acids such as those in butter, full fat hard cheeses and sausages with polyunsaturated fatty acids present in fish, yoghurt and branded foods labelled 'high in polyunsaturates' leads to lower LDL levels and thus a reduction in cholesterol (Lenfant, 1990). Too much cholesterol in the blood predisposes to a build-up of fatty plaques in arterial walls known as *atheroma*. Nurses should take opportunities to educate patients about the risks of an unhealthy lifestyle.

Metabolic processes

In addition to an adequate intake of appropriate nutrients, adequate metabolism is necessary for physical activity as well as for growth and repair. Foods are converted by digestion to glucose (and other simple sugars), amino acids and fatty acids. These 'simple' substances can then be used for energy. The metabolic processes result in the conversion of chemical energy from food into *adenosine triphosphate* (ATP), a high energy storage compound and the energy 'currency' of the body. This conversion is brought about by a number of different enzymes. If an enzyme is deficient, a disorder of metabolism may result (for example, phenylketonuria is caused by a deficiency of the enzyme phenylalanine hydroxylase). This results in an accumulation of phenylalanine and its metabolites which can cause severe mental retardation.

Enzymes are proteins and are therefore encoded

Table 6.5. *Vitamins: their source, function, and the effects of deficiency*

Fat soluble vitamins	Source	Function	Effect of deficiency
Vitamin A (Retinol)	Milk, eggs, fish liver oils	Needed by active body cells, including skin and eyes	Dry skin, Retinal disorder with night blindness, corneal ulceration with ultimate destruction of eye
Vitamin D	Fish, milk products (made by precursors in skin in bright sunlight)	Absorption, metabolism, of calcium, growth and maintenance of bone	Rickets in children. Osteomalacia (bone softening) in adults. Tetany (muscle spasms) if severe
Vitamin K	Green vegetables	Necessary for manufacture of blood clotting factors in liver	Rare (but found in jaundice when absorption is poor). Generalised bleeding

Water soluble vitamins	Source	Function	Effect of deficiency
Vitamin B_1	Liver, wheatgerm, nuts and yeast	Carbohydrate metabolism in all cells	Beri-beri (with heart failure), nerve disorders and confusional states
Niacin	Fish, liver, wheatgerm	Energy metabolism in all cells	Pellagra (skin rash, swollen tongue, diarrhoea and mental confusion)
Riboflavin and Pyridoxine (vitamin B_6)	Liver, kidney, milk and milk products, eggs	Energy and protein metabolism	Rare (usually part of multiple vitamin deficiency), affects skin and nerve function
Vitamin B_{12}	Meat, including liver	DNA synthesis	Pernicious (macrocytic) anaemia, spinal cord disease
Folate	Green vegetables	DNA synthesis	Anaemia, bowel disorders
Vitamin C (ascorbic acid)	Citrus fruits, other fruits, green vegetables	Formation of collagen and intercellular substance by connective tissue	Scurvy with swollen gums, bruising, weakness and failure of normal healing

on DNA. Thus many enzyme deficiencies, like phenylketonuria, are inherited conditions. In contrast, gout is an inflammatory type of arthritis caused by deposits of sodium urate crystals in and around joints. Primary gout results from errors in purine metabolism that lead to excessive uric acid levels. An attack of gout can result from the high uric acid levels that are a consequence of taking antineoplastic (i.e. *cytotoxic*) drugs or eating purine rich foods (such as red meat, anchovies, and leguminous vegetables) together with low uric acid excretion via the kidney.

Whatever the cause of the illness, all patients need sufficient food of the right type. Deficiencies lead to essential metabolic requirements being met out of the body stores, which may not be adequate.

Degenerative disorders

Changes occurring in cells in degenerative conditions are indicative of cell dysfunction but not of total cell death. Most of the changes are reversible, if the initiating cause is removed, but if they are prolonged or severe they may result in cell necrosis (Thomson and Cotton, 1983). Microscopically, *hydropic degeneration* is characterised by water accumulation in a cell. Normally the osmotic pressure of intracellular fluid is maintained by the 'sodium pump'. If this fails, the osmotic pressure rises and water enters the cell. Severe electrolyte disturbances, such as depletion of potassium following burns, are examples of causes of such degenerative change.

Another degenerative condition is *fatty change*, in which fat accumulates within the cytoplasm, because of cell damage. Such 'fatty change' is reversible but if the cause (be it infections or toxic agents such as excess alcohol or carbon tetrachloride) is not removed, then such change may progress to necrosis or cell death.

Alcohol is the most important drug of dependence and in Europe and North America, the incidence of alcoholism is about 5% of the adult population (Gillies *et al.*, 1986). Ninety five percent of ingested alcohol is metabolised in the liver and the rest excreted in expired air, sweat and urine. Enlargement of the liver is due to fatty infiltration in 70–80% of alcoholics (Gillies *et al.*, 1986). How alcohol leads to cirrhosis of the liver is not yet clear, but intakes above 36 units/week in women and 51 units/week in men are highly likely to lead to cirrhosis. The average rate of elimination of alcohol from the body is 8 g/hour, i.e. 1 unit.

1 unit = ½ pint beer
   = 1 glass wine
   = 1 glass of sherry
   = 1 measure of spirits

Women have more subcutaneous fat and usually less muscle tissue than men, so given the distribution of alcohol into lean body tissues, women will achieve higher blood levels than men – drink for drink. For this reason, the recommended intakes for men are no more than 21 units/week and for women 14 units/week or less.

Chronic alcoholism can seriously affect the central nervous system, cause peptic ulceration and pancreatitis, depress the immune response and damage the liver. Indeed, life expectancy in alcoholics is reduced by some 10%.

There are two basic types of necrosis: *coagulative necrosis*, commonly seen following deprivation of the blood supply as in myocardial infarction, and *colliquative necrosis*. The latter implies rapid liquefaction of dead cells and occurs particularly in the central nervous system. The term *gangrene* is applied to the necrosis of tissue in bulk.

It is important to understand that such change is initially reversible. Often, the nurse is ideally placed to provide appropriate health education, for example, to those in hazardous industries or those at risk for other reasons such as alcoholic excess combined with an inadequate diet.

Tumours

Dysplasia is the term given to alteration in the size, shape and orientation of epithelial cells, which is commonly associated with chronic inflammation or irritation (Thomson and Cotton, 1983). It is usually a reversible change, particularly if the chronic inflammation/irritation is treated. However, the changes may persist and progress to malignancy (*neoplasia*).

Neoplasia, new growth, tumour and cancer are all words used to describe a disease which is unlike any other. It can affect any body organ, be curable or rapidly fatal.

Cancer is an ancient disease and evokes many fears and phobias. Nurses need to understand the many facets of this disease in order to meet their patients' needs, and to dispel fears and misconceptions. Cancer is one of the major health problems of our time. It is the second major cause of death in the UK, and statistically one in four of all infants born in the UK will develop cancer at some time in their life.

A *neoplasm* is an abnormal mass of new tissue. The word *tumour* is a term that includes any swelling or enlargement. Tumours are qualified as being *benign* or *malignant* and are generally named according to the tissue from which they originate.

Carcinomas are malignant tumours of epithelial origin and *sarcomas* are malignant tumours of connective tissue. Hence we refer to *carcinoma of the stomach* (an epithelial lining) but *osteosarcoma* – a malignant bone (connective tissue) tumour. It may not be possible to determine the origin of the tumour cells and these cases are referred to as *undifferentiated* or *anaplastic* carcinomas or sarcomas.

Benign and malignant tumour characteristics are very different (see Table 6.6).

A *metastasis* is a secondary tumour separate from the primary growth. Such spread can occur via the circulatory system or lymphatics, by direct seeding into a serous cavity (such as the pleural or peritoneal cavity), or by implantation during surgery or biopsy.

Table 6.6. *Benign and malignant tumour characteristics*

Benign tumours	Malignant tumours
Resemble tissue of origin	Often undifferentiated
Grow by expansion and often a capsule is formed	Extend by invasion and infiltration
Slow growing, may stop and even regress	Growth erratic but often rapid
Never metastasise	All can metastasise
Often harmless except in an 'awkward' place such as the brain or the endocrine system	Fatal due to invasiveness

All possible signs and symptoms can be produced by malignant tumours. Patients may have obvious complaints such as a cough or haematuria, or general complaints such as fatigue, weight loss, fever or pain.

It has been estimated that the survival rate from cancer could be improved by up to 50% with early detection. Researchers have found no single cause for cancer but some authorities believe that some 70% of cancers are environmentally related (Krol, 1984). This includes those resulting from personal habits such as diet and smoking as well as external environmental influence (see Table 6.7).

It is estimated that there are some 14 million adult smokers in the UK (OPCS, 1990). Tobacco smoke is made up of 'mainstream smoke' – from the mouth end of the cigarette – and 'sidestream

Table 6.7. *Contributory and predisposing factors to the development of a cancer*

Factor	Example
(1) Chronic irritation	Sunlight (over half of all skin cancers occur in Australia and Florida)
(2) Chemicals	Tar, soot, asbestos, vinyl chloride, cigarette smoke
(3) Irradiation	High incidence in radiologist pioneers and Hiroshima victims
(4) Nutritional	Some artificial colourants and other additives are known to be harmful

smoke' which comes from the burning tip. Almost 85% of the smoke in a room is sidestream smoke which is high in toxic substances. Four thousand chemicals are present in cigarette smoke, 55 of which are known carcinogens (Royal College of Physicians, 1978). Britain has a high rate of lung cancer with 40,000 cases a year – 90% of them are smokers (OPCS, 1990).

The substances most detrimental to health are tar, nicotine and carbon monoxide. Tar produces *ciliostasis* (paralysis of the ciliated epithelium that lines the respiratory tract) and an increased production of mucus. So mucus pools, providing an excellent environment for bacterial growth. Repeated infections lead to inflammatory changes, fibrosis and chronic obstructive airways disease. The irritant effects of tar and all the carcinogens present in it may induce mutation and carcinogenesis (see page 147). Nicotine is an *alkaloid* and a powerful drug, causing addiction in the same way as heroin and alcohol. Carbon monoxide attaches itself to the haemoglobin in red cells and reduces their oxygenation. The heart has to work harder as a result.

Additionally, smoking increases cholesterol levels and platelet stickiness, giving an increased tendency to thrombosis. Some studies have suggested that passive smokers (inhalers of 'secondhand' smoke from contaminated air) may be inhaling the equivalent of three cigarettes a day, and that passive smoking affects adult lung function, increases the risk of respiratory and cardiovascular symptoms and ischaemic heart disease (Hole *et al.*, 1989) and increases the risk of lung cancer (Wald *et al.*, 1986). The children of parents who smoke are more likely to have chronic coughs, persistent wheeze, tonsillitis, bronchitis and pneumonia and have an increased risk of glue ear (Chen *et al.*, 1986).

So smokers' (and passive smokers') health is likely to suffer as a result of inhaling tobacco smoke, but how does cancer start?

Although the cause is not understood, it is likely that disruption of the control of gene expression is at the root of the problem. Some regulatory change allows a cancerous cell to proliferate unimpeded and research is currently focusing on the cell membrane. Substances on the cell surface, controlled by genes, normally provide signals to cells to slow down or stop dividing. The regulatory function of these substances depends on contact with neighbouring cells (contact inhibition). If a cell loses its contact inhibitory properties, it is free to divide unchecked, and there are some indications that cancer cells have lost some of the regulatory substances and gained new substances that enable them to escape being attacked by the body's immune system.

Grading and staging

After a tumour has been determined to be malignant, two other processes will assist medical staff in selecting appropriate treatment.

Grading is carried out on tissue obtained by biopsy and is an indication of the 'aggressiveness' of the tumour. For example, Grade I tumours are well differentiated and slowly growing. Grade IV tumours are undifferentiated, or anaplastic, and usually rapidly growing.

Staging describes the extent of the disease in a patient. Information is classified according to the *TNM system* of the International Union against Cancer, where T = the extent of the primary tumour, N = involvement of lymph nodes and M = absence or presence of metastases. This basic classification is then further subdivided to indicate size and infiltration of the tumour, extent of lymph node spread and the degree of metastatic spread (Sepion, 1990). Nurses with an understanding of the system can more fully appreciate the implications for patients at different stages of disease. For example the treatment and prognosis of a patient with T1, N0, M0 carcinoma of the urinary bladder where the tumour is confined to the urinary mucosa is very different to T3, N0, M0, where the tumour has infiltrated *paravesical* tissues (those surrounding the bladder). Note that only T has changed.

In the first example treatment may be **endoscopic** with or without cytotoxic drugs, whereas in the second example radical radiotherapy and *cystectomy* (removal of the bladder) is likely.

The label 'cancer' is often the beginning of an overwhelming fear, so informed nurses may be in a unique position to reduce the fear of the disease in the minds of patients, their relatives and the public, and thus to facilitate early detection.

Autoimmune disease

In *autoimmune disease* the host destroys its own tissue as a result of immune responses to 'self'. Both B and T lymphocytes are implicated (see page 151), but the causation is not well understood and there are several possible theories. Auto-antibodies may be produced in response to destruction of tissue from other disease processes or as a result of chronic or persistent viral infection (for example, the appearance of smooth muscle antibodies during infection with the hepatitis B virus). The elderly are particularly likely to develop auto-immune diseases and this can be due to gradual failure of the normal mechanisms which suppress T cells reacting to 'self'.

The possibility that genetically determined immune responses are involved is supported by the relationships shown to exist between the HL-A system of antigens and certain diseases, for example HL-A B27 and **ankylosing spondylitis**. The name *human leucocyte locus A* was originally given to the system when early research concentrated on white cells. Although the system now deals with a broader scope of antigens the name has stuck, with the addition of letters and numbers (such as HLA-B27).

Hashimoto's disease is an autoimmune disorder that is often present in people with other auto-immune disorders such as pernicious (macrocytic) anaemia or rheumatoid arthritis. Women between the ages of 30 and 50 have the highest incidence of the disease which is characterised by thyroid enlargement, circulating antithyroid antibodies and eventual myxoedema if untreated.

Although the exact mechanisms of autoimmune disease have yet to be classified, the genetic background of an individual is undoubtedly important.

Circulatory disorders

This is a large group of disorders which includes all diseases of the heart, blood vessels and blood, together with all the disorders of circulation such as oedema and thrombosis.

Congestion is an increase in the amount of blood present in the tissues which may be due to obstruction of the venous return locally, as in deep vein thrombosis, or generally, as in heart failure.

Oedema is the excessive accumulation of extracellular fluid in the tissues. *Osmosis* refers to the passage of water from a solution of low concentration (i.e. with a large number of water molecules) to a solution of high concentration across a semipermeable membrane. Solutes which

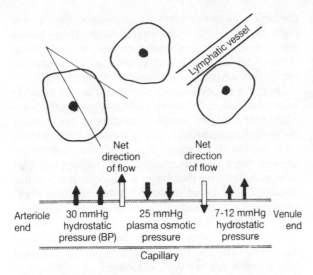

Net direction of flow   Net direction of flow

Arteriole end   30 mmHg hydrostatic pressure (BP)   25 mmHg plasma osmotic pressure   7-12 mmHg hydrostatic pressure   Venule end

Capillary

Fig. 6.10 *The passage of fluid across the capillary wall*

are large particles and which result in the passage of water by osmosis are said to exert an *osmotic pressure*. Blood exerts an osmotic pressure within the capillaries (semipermeable membranes) of approximately 25 mmHg. This osmotic pressure is largely contributed by plasma proteins, particularly albumin, and thus plasma proteins tend to draw water into capillaries (see Fig 6.10). The pressure of capillary blood (hydrostatic pressure) is approximately 30 mmHg at the arterial end, and only 7–12 mmHg at the venous end. The net effect is an outflow of tissue fluid at the arterial end (where hydrostatic pressure exceeds osmotic pressure) and a net inflow at the venous end (where osmotic pressure exceeds hydrostatic pressure). Any excess can be drained via local lymphatic vessels. These factors ensure a constant circulation of tissue fluid together with nutrients. In oedema, one or more factors is altered. For example, in nephrotic syndrome, large quantities of albumin are excreted in the urine, thus the osmotic pressure of blood falls and the fluid normally drawn into capillaries remains in the tissues. Other causes of oedema include: increased venous pressure as in heart failure, lymphatic removal by surgery, lymphatic obstruction, or increased capillary permeability as in burns.

Shock

A reduction in the *effective* circulating blood volume is known as *shock*. This may be due to a

decrease in the cardiac output resulting from inadequate pumping, or a decrease in blood returning to the heart (venous return). Such a decrease in venous return may be a direct result of diminished blood volume (*hypovolaemia*) or decreased *vasomotor tone* (i.e. pooling of blood in the periphery). Initially, compensatory mechanisms are brought into action. Heart rate and peripheral resistance are both increased, helping to maintain blood pressure. As a result the patient has a tachycardia and appears pale. In hypovolaemic shock, if blood loss continues, the normal physiological mechanisms cannot compensate and progressive shock ensues. A decreased blood volume leads to a diminished venous return and hence a poor cardiac output.

The cardiac muscle itself becomes deprived of blood, further depressing cardiac output. Poor flow to and through organs leads to the build-up of toxic waste products and stasis of blood, causing disseminated intravascular coagulation (DIC). This process uses up clotting factors, and bleeding continues and may become more profuse. DIC may affect lung blood vessels, leading to a reduction in blood oxygenation. A reduction of oxygen reaching the heart will further affect the myocardium and the cardiac output continues to fall. Unless this downward spiral can be stopped, shock will become irreversible as other organs become irretrievably damaged due to lack of oxygenated blood, and the patient will die.

So the effects of shock vary according to the severity and duration of the condition and nurses need to understand the compensatory mechanisms, as well as the progression of the condition, in order to nurse patients effectively.

Infarction

Approximately 10% of all patients with an acute myocardial infarction have severe enough 'pump' failure to die of circulatory shock before physiological compensatory mechanisms come into play. The commonest cause of myocardial infarction is *coronary thrombosis*. A thrombosis is a solid mass formed from the constituents of the blood during life (Thomson and Cotton, 1983). There are three major predisposing factors:

(1) Changes in the wall of the vessel that predispose to platelet deposition (for example, *atheroma*)

(2) Changes in composition of blood (viscosity) –

as in *polycythaemia*, dehydration, or **macro-globulinaemia**

(3) Changes in blood flow such as stasis or turbulence.

Outcomes of thrombosis include: a thrombus becoming occlusive and completely blocking a blood vessel; organisation of fibroblasts leading to a fibrous area being produced which may become calcified or recanalised to restore some continuity of blood flow; or a portion of the thrombosis becoming detached and forming an embolus.

Embolism is the impaction in some part of the vascular system of any undissolved or particulate material brought there by the bloodstream. This includes fat globules, gas bubbles, tumour fragments and parasites and the effects depend on the site of impaction and the size of the embolus, as well as the availability of a collateral circulation. Embolic occlusion of a vessel, in the absence of an adequate collateral circulation, will result in death of the affected tissue, i.e. infarction.

Infarction occurs more commonly, therefore, in tissues with so-called 'end arteries' (such as the kidney or heart). Organs with a rich collateral circulation (such as the liver or skin) are rarely the site of infarction. In all tissues, except the central nervous system, the cells of an infarct undergo coagulative necrosis. The usual end result is phagocytosis of dead tissue and healing by organisation (fibrous tissue) leaving a scar at the site of the infarct – a scar that is weaker than the surrounding tissue.

Heart disease

Coronary heart disease was responsible for 153,084 deaths in England and Wales in 1988 – equivalent to 27% of all deaths (NEA, 1990).

It has been stated elsewhere (see page 154) that blood cholesterol plays an important part in the development of coronary heart disease. Narrowing of the coronary arteries by atheroma predisposes to thrombus formation. The fatty plaques of atheroma contain lipids, including cholesterol and carbohydrates.

There is evidence that vigorous lowering of cholesterol slows progression and starts regression of atheroma (Lenfant, 1990). Current recommendations are for a blood cholesterol of less than 5.2 mmol/l (Morgan, 1988).

Hypertension is the second major risk factor in the aetiology of coronary heart disease; the third is cigarette smoking. Prolonged untreated high blood pressure causes weakening of the arterial lining (*intima*) and increases its permeability to cholesterol. This assists the formation of atheroma.

Defining hypertension is difficult as there is no firm consensus, although almost all authorities agree that a resting systolic pressure of 160 mmHg denotes hypertension. So although risk factors such as family history, age and sex cannot be altered, there are a number of risk factors that can be controlled and that have a major impact on the prevention of heart disease. These include cigarette smoking, blood cholesterol levels, hypertension, obesity, lack of exercise, and stress. Nurses are in an excellent position with regard to promoting healthy lifestyles in their patients, provided they themselves are well informed.

Endocrine disorders

The endocrine and nervous systems both perform the same general functions of communication, control and integration. Indeed, the ability of man to adapt and respond to changes in his environment is mainly the result of the coordination of these two systems.

Endocrine disorders can sometimes be difficult to diagnose and treat because of their complex interrelationships, and nurses need a good understanding of normal and disordered function in order to meet patients' needs.

The most common endocrine disorders result from over- or undersecretion of a particular hormone. Consider *thyrotoxicosis*, which results from overproduction of thyroxine and/or tri-iodothyronine. These thyroid hormones are essential for a normal rate of cell metabolism. An increase in the level of circulating thyroid hormones will give rise to an increase in the patient's metabolic rate which will have a complex effect on most body tissues and will affect physical and mental health.

Metabolic rate can increase 60–100% above normal leading to an increase in the rate of food utilisation. Protein catabolism and fat metabolism are thus enhanced. The increased metabolism leads to greater heat production and hence decreased tolerance to heat and a warm, moist skin. Heart rate is increased, as are respirations. The rate of secretion of digestive juices is increased, as is the motility of the gut which may lead to diarrhoea.

There is an increased sensitivity of neuronal synapses and muscles react with vigour. The increased rate of cerebral activity, together with muscle tremor, means that relaxation and sleeping are difficult. An appreciation of the action of the hormones can help the nurse understand and thus explain the patient's condition. Knowledge of the synthesis of the hormones aids understanding of treatment and planning of care.

Iodine and the amino acid tyrosine are required for the synthesis of tri-iodothyronine (T3) and thyroxine (T4). Iodine from the diet (we need some 50 mg per year) is converted to iodide and then 'trapped' by the follicle cells of the thyroid gland. The iodide is converted to an oxidised form by intracellular enzymes and then bound to tyrosine. Tyrosine is first iodised to mono-iodotyrosine (MIT) and then to di-iodotyrosine (DIT). Subsequent combination of MIT and DIT form the active tri-iodothyronine (T3) and tetra-iodothyronine (T4 or thyroxine).

Antithyroid drugs such as the thiocyanates and perchlorates decrease the iodide 'trap', causing a decline in levels of T3 and T4. Carbimazole inhibits the formation of MIT and DIT as well as their coupling to form T3 and T4.

Understanding that changes in behaviour are characteristic of either excessive or deficient production of thyroid hormones is important too. Simple questions may elicit unexpected emotional responses because of emotional lability.

Such lability may be elicited for an entirely different reason. In women between the ages of 40–55 years, the ovaries begin to lose their ability to produce oestrogen. It is this lack of oestrogen that causes the symptoms associated with the *climacteric*, referred to by many as the 'menopause'.

Symptoms can be divided into three main groups:

(1) Vasomotor: e.g. hot flushes and palpitations
(2) Urinogenital: e.g. loss of tone and elasticity in muscles and mucous membranes of the uterus, vagina and urethra; loss of lubrication in the vagina which may lead to painful intercourse (*dyspareunia*); increased vaginal susceptibility to infection; stress incontinence
(3) Psychological: e.g. tiredness, headaches, insomnia, depression, irritability, dizziness, fatigue.

The fall in oestrogen levels affects bone-producing cell (*osteoblast*) activity and bone mass is lost, leading to *osteoporosis* (softened, crumbly bone). As a result, fractures are more common and one in four women over the age of 60 will suffer an osteoporotic fracture (Ottaway, 1990).

To prevent osteoporosis, women require an adequate intake of calcium (recommended daily allowance = 500 mg), regular exercise and oestrogen for osteoblasts to utilise the calcium efficiently.

Oestrogen also affects the ratio of HDLs to LDLs (see page 154) and helps to maintain low serum cholesterol levels. With lowering levels of oestrogen, serum cholesterol levels rise. In women before the menopause the incidence of coronary heart disease (CHD) is five times lower than in men (Ottaway, 1990). After the age of 55 years, generally women's cholesterol levels become higher than those of men and the incidence of CHD becomes equal. In the USA, some 40% of women are on hormone replacement therapy (HRT) (Ottaway, 1990) and it has been postulated that the falling rate of CHD in the USA is in part due to the number of women protected by HRT.

The most obvious treatment for menopausal symptoms is oestrogen replacement. However, there is considerable discussion at present as to whether HRT can cause breast cancer. Nurses need to be able to present all the facts to their patients who will then be in a position to make a decision having weighed all the advantages and disadvantages.

Idiopathic disorders

Idiopathic diseases are those with no known cause, given the present state of knowledge. This is a miscellaneous group and includes such diverse disorders as anorexia nervosa, ulcerative colitis and Guillain-Barré syndrome.

A good example of a modern medical mystery is *myalgic encephalomyelitis* or chronic fatigue syndrome. People with this condition suffer from a variety of unexplained symptoms which include low grade pyrexia, sore throat, tender lymph nodes, muscle pain, muscle weakness, headache, joint pain without swelling, sleep disorders, neurological problems such as memory loss, visual disturbances, difficulty concentrating, and extreme fatigue. Mood swings are common, as is a very low grade dementia (Ramsay, 1988). Occasionally *alopecia* (loss of hair) is reported. The writer developed ME four years ago and has suffered, and sometimes still does, from all of these symptoms. Diagnosis is largely a matter of ruling out other disease, but there is as yet no treatment available.

However, the outlook is changing (Ramsay, 1988). Mounting evidence suggests that ME is an immune system disorder in which the body works hard but inefficiently to control common viral infections. Neurological evidence is also accumulating (Ramsay, 1988). Scans of ME patients show abnormal blood flow to one of the two temporal lobes and the hippocampus (Cowley *et al.*, 1990). The latter plays a central role in the formation of memories.

Nurses must try to adopt a non-judgemental approach when dealing with patients for whom doctors cannot find a diagnosis. Telling people they are not ill is an easy way out when an illness doesn't conform to current disease labels or respond to conventional treatment.

Iatrogenic disease

Iatrogenic diseases are those resulting from treatment of existing conditions. This is due to several factors which may exist in the elderly: declining physiological function such as reduced renal clearance, multiple treatments for multiple pathology and hence greater potential for drug interactions, and non-compliance on the part of the patient (Cartwright and Smith, 1988).

Seventy-five per cent of people aged more than 75 years receive some kind of drug. Two thirds of these people receive between one and three drugs and the other third are taking between four and five drugs at the same time (Bliss, 1981; cited by Wade and Bowling, 1986). Nurses caring for the elderly need to be familiar with the absorption, distribution, metabolism, detoxification and excretion of drugs and be alert to possible problems.

Drug regimes should be simple and prescribed according to the patient's history and pharmacodynamics. To be useful, a drug must enter the body in a reliable way, reach the site of action, and be eliminated within a reasonable time. Simplicity,

risk, appropriateness and lifestyle must be taken into consideration. Changes in homeostatic mechanisms mean that central nervous system activity and/or blood pressure are easily affected and can lead to confusional states. Drug-induced nutrient deficiencies can also occur, even in the presence of an 'adequate' diet. For example, prednisone, phenobarbitone, phenytoin and glutethimide all interfere with calcium absorption and may accelerate osteoporosis.

Drugs can provide relief from suffering and an improved quality of life for the elderly and nurses can have an important influence on drug prescription, administration and compliance. All that is necessary is the application of knowledge and skill to avoid drug-induced problems which may be as injurious as the original problem being treated.

Conclusions

This chapter has not set out to explain pathophysiology in detail but rather to help the reader to appreciate the importance of a sound understanding of disordered function. A brief overview of the causation of disease has been put forward in the hope that the reader will feel better equipped to approach more detailed texts when setting out to plan rational care to meet patients' needs arising from their disease processes.

Useful addresses

(for leaflets and information about the menopause, HRT, etc.)

The Amarant Trust	National Osteoporosis
14 Lord North Street	Society
London SW1P 3LD	Barton Meade House
	PO Box 10
	Radstock
	Bath BA3 3YB

Glossary

Abscess: A localised collection of pus within an organ or tissue

Alleles: Alternative forms of a gene, occupying

the same place on the chromosome and affecting the same character but in different ways

Angiogenesis: Formation of new capillary loops in 'granulation tissue'

Ankylosing spondylitis: An erosive inflammatory form of arthritis, affecting the sacroiliac joints and the spine, which produces an increasingly rigid spine

Antibodies: Proteins (immunoglobins) formed in response to an antigen which react with that antigen or one closely related to it

Atelectasis: A failure of aeration of a part of the lung due to blocking of the air passages, for example by a plug of mucus

Autosome: Ordinary chromosomes, i.e. the chromosomes which are not sex chromosomes (22 pairs in humans)

Cellulitis: A rapidly spreading inflammation within tissues – often due to β haemolytic streptococci

Chiasma (*plural*, **Chiasmata**): Region(s) of contact where crossing over occurs between chromosomes

Chromosome: Thread-like structure in the nucleus visible at cell division formed of DNA and protein

Cytoplasm: The contents of a cell inside the cell membrane excluding the nucleus

DNA: Deoxyribonucleic acid – the chemical whose molecular form determines hereditary characteristics

Dominant (gene): Gene which is expressed in the presence of a contrasting gene or allele

Endoscopy: Examination of the interior of the body by a lighted optical instrument often via a natural orifice, for example cystoscopy is examination of the bladder (urinary)

Fistula: A track connecting two epithelial surfaces, for example the skin and the gut

Gene: Unit of genetic information on a chromosome

Graft versus host disease: When lymphoid cells are transferred from a donor to a recipient the donor cells may establish themselves but 'reject'

this new host. This can result in death

Homologous chromosomes: Chromosomes that are identical in their content of genes

Hypertrophy: An increase in the size of tissues due to an increase in individual cell size

Ischaemia: Deprivation of oxygen or other metabolic necessities

Lymphangitis: Inflammation of lymphatic vessels

Macroglobulinaemia: A neoplastic disorder (lymphoma) which results in an accumulation of macroglobulin (an IgM) in the blood

Meiosis: Nuclear division in which the chromosome number is halved (haploid)

Mitosis: Nuclear division in which cells retain diploid number of chromosomes (i.e. a complete set). In humans the diploid number is 46

Mutation: Spontaneous change in a chromosome or gene

Necrosis: Cell death

Negative nitrogen balance: Nitrogenous excretion exceeds intake leading to protein breakdown, muscle wasting, poor wound healing

Nucleus: A highly specialised region containing the chromosomes

Polycythaemia: An increase above normal of the red blood cell count and/or haemoglobin level

Recessive (gene): Gene which, in the presence of its contrasting allele, is not expressed

Recombination: Combination of genes in the offspring, not present in either parent

Replication: Reproduction of DNA and chromosomes

Sex chromosomes: The X or Y chromosomes. The human female has 44 autosomes and two X chromosomes. The human male has 44 autosomes, one X and one Y chromosome

Septicaemia: Invasion of the bloodstream by actively multiplying micro-organisms

Sinus: A track connecting a cavity (for example, an abscess cavity) to an epithelial surface (for example, the skin)

References

Cartwright, A. and Smith, C. (1988). *Elderly People, Their Medicine and Their Doctors*. Routledge, London.

Chen, Y., Wanxian, L. and Shunzhang, Y. (1986). The influence of passive smoking on admissions for respiratory illness in early childhood. *British Medical Journal*, 293, 303–306.

Cowley, G., Hoger, M. and Joseph, N. (1990). Chronic fatigue syndrome. *Newsweek*, November 12, 34–40.

Gillies, H.C., Rogers, H.J., Spector, R.G. and Trounce, J.R. (1986). *A Textbook of Clinical Pharmacology* (2nd ed.). Edward Arnold, London.

Gonick, L. and Wheelis, M. (1983). *The Cartoon Guide to Genetics*. Barnes and Noble, New York.

Goodinson, S.M. (1986). Assessment of nutritional status. *Nursing*, 3(7), 252–258.

Griffiths, A. (1991a). Wound care: can the nursing process help? *Professional Nurse*, January, 208–212.

Griffiths, G. (1991b). Choosing a dressing. *Journal of Wound Care Nursing* in *Nursing Times*, 87(36), 84–90.

Harrington, J.M. and Gill, F.S. (1983). *Occupational Health*. Blackwell Scientific Publications, Oxford.

Hole, D., Chopra, C., Gillies, C. and Hawthorne, V. (1989). Passive smoking and cardio-respiratory health in a general population in the west of Scotland. *British Medical Journal*, 229, 432–437.

Jenkins, J. (1983). *Human Genetics*. Benjamin Cummings Co., California.

Johnson, A. (1988). Wound management: are you getting it right? *Professional Nurse*, May, 306–309.

Johnson, A. (1990). Does the perfect dressing exist? *Nursing Standard*, 49, 25–27.

Krol, M.A. (1984). The patient with cancer. In *The Clinical Practice of Medical-Surgical Nursing*, Beyers, M. and Dudas, S. (eds.). Little, Brown and Co., Boston.

Lenfant, C. (1990). The cholesterol facts. *American Association of Occupational Health Nurses Journal*, 38(5), 209–210.

Marieb, E. (1989). *Human Anatomy and Physiology*. Benjamin Cummings Co., California.

Moore, J. (1990). Biological therapies. *Nursing Standard*, 4(46), 53–56.

Morgan, B. (1988). Screening and coronary heart disease. *Practice Nurse*, 1(8), 351–352 and 359.

Morison, M. (1990). Wound cleansing – which solution? *Nursing Standard* (supplement), 4(52), 4–6.

Office of Population Censuses and Surveys Monitor. (1990). *Cigarette Smoking 1972–1988*. OPCS, London.

Ottaway, E. (1990). Hormone replacement therapy. *Nursing Standard*, 4(47), 28–30.

Porth, C. (1990). *Pathophysiology: Concepts of Altered Health States* (3rd ed.). Lippincott, New York.

Ramsay, A.M. (1988). *Myalgic Encephalomyelitis and Post-Viral Fatigue States: The Saga of Royal Free Disease* (2nd ed.). ME Association/Gower Publishing, London.

Roitt, I., Brotaff, J. and Male, D. (1989). *Immunology* (2nd ed.). Churchill Livingstone, Edinburgh.

Royal College of Physicians. (1978). *Smoking or Health?* RCP/Pitman, London.

Sepion, B. (1990). Investigations, staging and diagnosis: implications for nurses. In *The Child with Cancer: Nursing Care*, Thompson, J. (ed.). Scutari Press, London.

Thomas, S. (1990a). Semi-permeable film dressings. *Nursing Times*, 86(10), 49–51.

Thomas, S. (1990b). Hydrocolloid dressings. *Nursing Times*, 86(45), 36–38.

Thomson, A.D. and Cotton, R.E. (1983). *Lecture Notes on Pathology*. Blackwell Scientific Publications, Oxford.

Torrance, C. (1986). The physiology of wound healing. *Nursing*, 3(5), 162–168.

Turner, V. (1991). Standardisation of wound care. *Nursing Standard*, 5(19), 25–28.

Wade, B. and Bowling, A. (1986). Appropriate use of drugs by elderly people. *Journal of Advanced Nursing*, 11, 47–55.

Wald, N., Nanchahal, K., Thompson, S. and Cuckle, H. (1986). Does breathing other people's tobacco smoke cause cancer? *British Medical Journal*, 293, 1217–1221.

Waldron, H.A. (1985). *Lecture Notes on Occupational Medicine* (3rd ed.). Blackwell Scientific Publications, Oxford.

Suggestions for further reading

Behan, P.O., Goldberg, D.P. and Mowbray, J.F. (eds.). (1991). *Postviral Fatigue Syndrome*. Churchill Livingstone/British Council, Edinburgh.

Boore, J.R.P., Champion, R. and Ferguson, M.C. (eds.). (1987). *Nursing the Physically Ill Adult*. Churchill Livingstone, Edinburgh.

Brewis, R.A.L. (1991). *Lecture Notes on Respiratory Disease*. Blackwell Scientific Publications, Oxford.

David, J. (1986). *Wound Management*. Martin Dunitz, London.

Fallowfield, L. and Clark, A. (1991). *Breast Cancer*. Tavistock/Routledge, London.

Fletcher, R.F. (1987). *Lecture Notes on Endocrinology* (4th ed.). Blackwell Scientific Publications, Oxford.

Heller, T., Bailey, L., Gott, M. and Howes, M. (1987). *Coronary Heart Disease: Reducing the Risk*. Open University/John Wiley and Sons, Chichester.

Mackenna, B.R. and Callander, R. (1990). *Illustrated Physiology* (5th ed.). Churchill Livingstone, Edinburgh.

Shanson, D.C. (1989). *Microbiology in Clinical Practice* (2nd ed.). Wright, London.

Weinberger, S.E. (1986). *Principles of Pulmonary Medicine*. W.B. Saunders, Philadelphia.

Westaby, S. (1985). *Wound Care*. Heinemann, London.

7

PSYCHOLOGY AND HEALTH CARE

Alan Myles

The main aim of this chapter is to explore how a knowledge of psychology can inform and enhance professional practice in health and nursing care. A feature of the chapter is the direct application to practice alongside a critical appaisal of the various concepts and theories.

The following key areas are addressed:

- Learning
  —from a behavioural perspective
  —from a cognitive perspective
  —from a social learning perspective

- Information processing
  —sensation
  —attention
  —perception
  —remembering
  —forgetting

- Motivation
  —from an energiser perspective

  —from a channeller perspective
  —from a maintenance perspective

- Personality
  —psychoanalytic, type, and trait approaches
  —self-concept
  —attitudes, values and beliefs
  —person perception

- Social interaction
  —exchange theory
  —social skill model
  —dramaturgical model

What is psychology?

Wade and Tavris (1990) define psychology as 'the scientific study of behaviour and mental processes and how they are affected by an organism's physical state, mental state, and external environment'. It can be argued that psychology has a way of 'outgrowing' its definitions, but Wade and Tavris' definition does take into account the reciprocal effect between the individual and the environment, and therefore seems to be most appropriate for the study of psychology in the context of health care.

What are the goals of psychology?

According to Wade and Tavris, the main goals of psychology are straightforward. They are to:

- describe
- understand
- predict
- control/modify

$\left.\right\}$ behaviour/mental processes

In the context of health care, psychology can provide frameworks for describing the behaviour, thoughts and feelings of health care professionals and their respective client groups alike. For example, what is meant by a low self-esteem, and why do many people suffer from a low self-esteem? A knowledge of psychology can enable us to make relatively confident predictions about how some things can be modified. For example, if we know that certain actions tend to lower a person's self-esteem whereas other actions tend to enhance it, we can use this knowledge effectively in professional practice in a range of different contexts.

What do psychologists do?

There are several fields in which psychologists can specialise. Those which are likely to be of most interest to health care professionals are briefly summarised in Table 7.1. As the table suggests, psychology has much to offer the work of health care professionals, e.g. clinical nurses, nurse teachers, nurse managers, and nurse researchers.

Table 7.1. *Specialisms within psychology*

Clinical	Concerned with emotional and behavioural problems and mental health
Educational	Concerned with teaching and learning, educational testing and ***curriculum*** development
Industrial	Concerned with ***ergonomics***, skills-analysis and job-training, and human relations in the work setting
Experimental	Applies scientific research methods in the study of human and animal behaviour

The key areas shown in Fig. 7.1 will now be successively addressed.

Learning

The nature of human learning is of obvious concern to all nurses in terms of their own education and with respect to teaching patients. Learning has been the subject of much investigation by psychologists, especially educational and experimental psychologists. In this part of the chapter, learning will be examined from both a behavioural and a

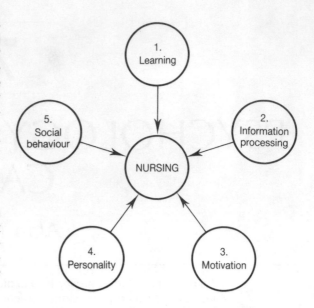

Fig. 7.1 *Key concepts in psychology applied to nursing*

cognitive perspective. Examples of the application of principles from each standpoint will be given in the context of nursing practice, nurse education, and nursing management.

Learning from a behavioural perspective

James (1970) defines learning as 'any more or less permanent change in behaviour as a result of prior experience.' Although James is not a behaviourist his definition has a behavioural tone, as will become evident in this section. The origins and major tenets of behaviourist psychology will be summarised below, preceded by a résumé of the factors which led to its inception.

Wilhelm Wundt (1832–1920) was responsible for setting up the first psychological laboratory. Wundt wanted to explore the mind in a less abstruse way than philosophers and to duplicate the progress being made in the physical sciences. He hoped to discover the structure of conscious sensory experience by analysing its elements. Wundt and his students studied vision, hearing, perception, attention, feelings and other elements of conscious experience using a technique called ***introspection***. This technique involved a rigorous training in the reporting of immediate experiences under precisely controlled laboratory conditions. In the physical sciences, for example chemistry, complex compounds can be reduced to their elements with a consensus of viewpoint. The most troublesome aspect of Wundt's work was that his introspectionists frequently disagreed. This is hardly surprising, especially since much is now known about the *subjective* nature of human perception (which will be explored later in the chapter). **Behaviourism**, which arose as a reaction to the subjective nature of introspectionism, subsequently dominated psychological research for decades. John B. Watson (1878–1958), known as the 'father' of behaviourism, argued against introspection and proclaimed that psychology could only become truly objective and scientific if it limited itself to studying behaviour which is overt, as opposed to the former which is covert. The three key tenets on which behaviourist psychology is based are contiguity, classical conditioning and operant conditioning.

Contiguity

Erwin Guthrie (1886–1959) taught psychology at the University of Washington after a period of study based largely on philosophy. His behaviourist theory of learning is based on one general principle, that of simultaneous contiguous conditioning, which simply means that if two events occur together repeatedly, they will become associated. Later, when only one event is present, the other will also be remembered. This is called contiguity learning and is the basis for such practices as mathematics and language drills. Many of us have had the experience of learning basic facts in school through the repetitive pairing of a stimulus and a correct response, for example arithmetic tables, rules of spelling such as 'i before

e except after c', and capital cities in geography. The application of the principle of contiguity in nursing education and nursing practice could be as follows:

(1) Whenever possible, students should be encouraged to practise pairing desired responses with the appropriate stimuli; for example, when teaching a junior colleague a **psychomotor skill** such as the use of a particular lifting technique, the correct sequence should be observed.
(2) The repetition of inappropriate responses should be prevented – for example, if a patient has not learned how to use a salbutamol inhaler properly, he needs further tuition.

The main criticism of Guthrie's theory of learning is that he pays little attention to the concept of **reinforcement**. However, the significance of his concept of contiguity should not be overlooked. He does emphasise the overall significance of presenting stimuli in a planned way. This is important when nurses are involved in teaching colleagues or patients psychomotor skills and will be taken up in more detail later in the chapter.

Classical conditioning

Ivan Pavlov (1849–1936) was a Russian physiologist who developed an extensive theory of **conditioned reflexes**. His experiments involved inducing salivation in dogs as a response to the sound of a bell by repeatedly pairing the two stimuli. His theory of **classical conditioning** can be illustrated as shown in Fig. 7.2.

Some of the principles underlying behavioural

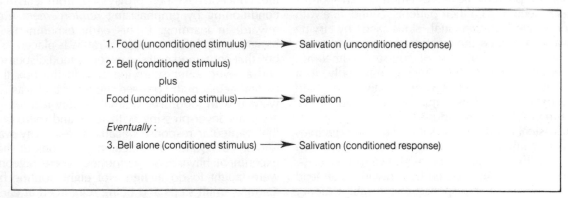

Fig. 7.2 *Classical conditioning (after Pavlov)*

therapy, particularly the treatment of **monophobic states**, are based on classical conditioning. Watson and Reyner (1920) were able to demonstrate the acquisition of a conditioned emotional response such as fear in their famous 'Little Albert' experiment (cited in Coon, 1986).

In this experiment, a nine month old child called Albert was observed in the presence of a white rat, a rabbit, and a dog. He showed no fear and often reached out to touch the animals. However, if Albert was presented with a sudden loud noise, the reader will not be surprised to hear that this did elicit a fear response. Watson started to pair the loud noise to the subsequent presentation of the white rabbit until it alone elicited the fear response. In Pavlov's terms the white rabbit had become the *conditioned stimulus* for the *conditioned response* of fear and anxiety as demonstrated in Fig. 7.3. In later experiments, children who also demonstrated fear responses to animals were *desensitised* by associating the feared object with a pleasurable stimulus such as sweets. It was often necessary to proceed slowly by introducing only the phobic stimulus, for example a dog, at some 'safe' distance from the child. Eventually the child could tolerate the presence of the once feared animal. This process of systematic desensitisation has been used extensively in treating a range of **neuroses** such as **agoraphobia**, **arachnophobia**, and fear of the dark. In the context of paediatric and adult nursing, pain could be regarded as the unconditioned stimulus for the unconditioned response of fear, anxiety and possibly hypertension. Patients may learn to become *very* anxious and even physically sick at the thought of some nursing procedure such as an aseptic dressing if previous procedures have led to inordinate discomfort. In order to prevent negative emotional responses nurses need to gain their patients' confidence with appropriate interpersonal skills and by trying always to reduce their patients' discomfort to an absolute minimum. This of course is sometimes extremely difficult to achieve, especially if a patient's wound is in a very sensitive area, and **prophylactic analgesia** may be required before commencing the procedure.

Classical conditioning is based on the principles of contiguity and contingency; in other words, an 'if' . . . 'then' relationship as shown in Fig. 7.3 – if there is a bang followed by a rabbit – can lead to a reflexive fear response to the rabbit alone. However the relatively automatic learning by

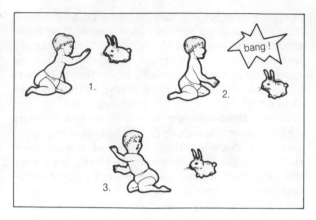

Fig. 7.3 *Conditioned emotional response*

classical conditioning calls for no deliberate action on behalf of the learner and clearly not much learning occurs via this process. Advertisers try to make some use of this principle by pairing a brand of perfume or aftershave cologne with attractive members of the opposite sex so that prospective customers will think that they will become desirable if they use the product. This is known as *higher order conditioning*. Most people are of course actively involved in the learning process, constantly taking purposive actions which can have both positive and negative results. Operant conditioning is the behavioural learning process that involves these purposive actions.

Operant conditioning

Edward Thorndike (1874–1949) established the basis for **operant conditioning** but Brian F. Skinner is generally regarded as the person who developed the concept. Skinner progressed from classical conditioning by emphasising *reinforcement* (i.e. reward) in learning. In his early experiments a hungry animal (for example, a rat) was placed in a box that contained nothing except a food dispenser and a lever. After scurrying around the box the animal accidentally pressed the lever and was rewarded with food. The animal rapidly learned to associate lever-pressing with food and increased that particular response because the activity was reinforced. Quite sophisticated variations of that experiment have been performed where pigeons were taught to do a 'figure of eight' routine by learning small steps and being reinforced at each stage. The dolphins at Disneyworld have been taught by operant conditioning to leap out of the aquarium through hoops to entertain the spectators.

The principles of operant conditioning have been applied extensively, both in education and in therapy. Readers may have learned factual material using programmed texts but these have been largely superseded by Computer Assisted Learning (CAL). The basic requirements are usually: a cathode-ray tube display terminal (TV screen), a teletypewriter (keyboard), a single or twin disk drive unit, a print-out unit, a range of software (floppy and hard disks).

The computer presents problems or questions to which the student must respond by typing the response or writing on the display screen with a special pen. Depending on the level of sophistication of the software, the computer can do several things. For example, if a student was working on a drug calculation the feedback may be:

- 'Wrong – please try again'
- Printing out the error
- Giving remedial teaching
- Asking the student to call for a teacher
- Giving the right answer and presenting another problem.

If the student gives the correct response she may be rewarded with a word of praise and encouragement.

It can be seen that this type of learning is based on Skinner's principles of operant conditioning. However, software in nursing education is becoming much more sophisticated, and this is especially true of that which incorporates interactive video and requires a problem-solving approach to learning which is more cognitive. The cognitive approach to learning will be explored later in the chapter.

In summary, behaviour can be considered as being sandwiched between two sets of environmental influences, i.e. those that precede it (its antecedents) and those that follow it (its consequences). Logically, therefore, if behaviour can be influenced by its antecedents and consequences, then it can be altered by some change in the antecedents, the consequences, or both. The relationship between antecedents, behaviour and consequences can be seen in Fig. 7.4.

Antecedents provide information about which behaviours are appropriate in a given situation – in other words, which behaviours lead to positive

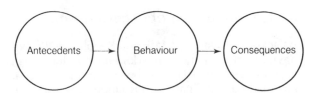

Fig. 7.4 *Relationship between antecedents, behaviour and consequences*

consequences and which ones lead to negative consequences. Showing junior colleagues or patients how to perform a particular skill – such as drawing up an injection or self-administering insulin – gives you the opportunity to reinforce accomplishments and increase the likelihood of that behaviour occurring in the future in similar circumstances. In psychological research much more work has been done in studying the effects of consequences rather than antecedents, since according to the behavioural view, the consequences have a great influence on determining whether the person will repeat the action in the future. In clinical practice, for example, a treatment for clients suffering from anorexia nervosa is based on principles of operant conditioning. After establishing a rapport with the client, an explicit hierarchy of rewards is scheduled in return for weight gain. Only after specific mutually agreed gains in weight is the client allowed visitors and permitted to get up and visit the occupational therapy department. The strict manipulation of these reinforcers by the nursing staff is designed to ensure life-saving weight gain and needs to be accompanied at every stage by supportive contact with the client.

Behaviour modification programmes have been used with varying degrees of success for a range of other problems such as ***childhood autism***, ***hyperactivity*** in childhood, and mental handicap.

Behaviourist psychology has been harshly criticised for its mechanistic approach to learning, and indeed if a 'pure' behaviourist stance were adopted those criticisms would be justified. Learning is much more complex than a series of stimulus-response links. However, the contribution of behaviourist psychology to education and clinical practice is acknowledged.

Critical discussion of behaviourism

As acknowledged by Clark and Keeble (1990), behaviourism remained the dominant influence in psychology from 1913 until well into the 1960s. It has made a significant contribution to health care and education.

Wade and Tavris (1990) suggest that classical conditioning may account for the acquisition of positive feelings as well as fears and phobias. This is clearly of much relevance for the work of health care professionals in a range of settings, as previously described. The behaviour of drug addicts has also been explained with reference to contiguity and classical conditioning. Siegel (1983) (cited by Wade and Tavris, 1990) argues that habitual drug users learn to respond to cues, such as the presence of needles, in a compensatory way; an example of contiguity. Habitual drug users also develop a **tolerance** for the substance and subsequently need more of the drug to produce the same effects.

Operant learning principles have been used in many settings with success, e.g. behaviour modification, motor skill acquisition, and programmed learning as described earlier. However, problems can arise from this approach with a dependence on extrinsic reinforcers undermining intrinsic motivation. For example, a student may rely too much on reinforcement from her teacher rather than on self-reinforcement.

Behaviourist psychology also exerted an influence on the genesis of **behavioural objectives** in education, their use causing controversy and debate which still rages to this day. One criticism of behavioural objectives is that they are too prescriptive and can trivialise the educational process. A counter argument is that they provide direction for both teachers and students.

The limitations of behaviourist psychology are now widely acknowledged. Behaviourism is founded on experiments in objectively measured overt behaviour, usually on animals (Clancy, 1981). Its tenets are essentially environmentalistic, with both overt and covert behaviour explained as responses to stimuli. It is too mechanistic, and pays little attention to the study of mental processes which must occur between a stimulus and an individual's response to it. The term 'black box' was introduced to acknowledge the existence of **intervening variables** between the stimulus and the response.

The 'black box' will now be 'opened' and its 'contents' examined for the remainder of the chapter, starting with an exploration of learning from a cognitive perspective.

Learning from a cognitive perspective

Cognitive psychologists argue that we are not merely passive receptors of stimuli from the environment, but that we actively process the data we receive and transform it into new forms and categories. The concept of a *cognitive field* was initiated by Max Wertheimer (1880–1941) and other *gestalt* psychologists such as Köhler and Koffka. Gestalt is a German word meaning form, pattern, structure or configuration. It refers to integrated wholes, not merely the summation of units or parts. In the Canary Islands, Köhler used chimpanzees as subjects in learning experiments which involved the use of thought-out strategies to obtain reward. The chimpanzees needed to join two sticks together or form a platform from scattered boxes to reach a banana as shown in Fig. 7.5. Köhler inferred that the chimpanzees made use of internal cognitive processes, re-structuring the situation to solve the problem. Cognitive learning forms the basis for effective problem-solving and, according to Fox (1975), includes seven sequential steps (see Fig. 7.6).

Following on from this, it now seems appropriate to consider a more cognitive definition of learning. Woolfolk and Nicolich (1984) define learning as *an internal change* in a person, the *formation* of new associations, or the *potential* for new responses; in short, a relatively permanent change in a person's capabilities. Cognition then refers to those mental processes that perceive the sensory input in various ways, encode it, store it in memory, and retrieve it for later use. Perception and information processing will be covered in some detail later in the chapter following a review of social learning theory.

Social learning theory

Arguably, social learning theory has particular significance for nursing education and nursing practice in particular. Biehler and Snowman (1982) define it as 'a form of behavioural learning theory attributing changes in behaviour to observation and imitation'. Essentially, it is a theory derived from both behavioural and cognitive theories of

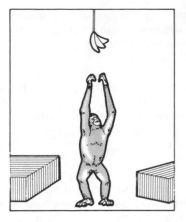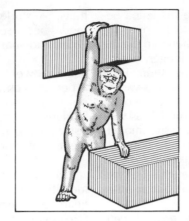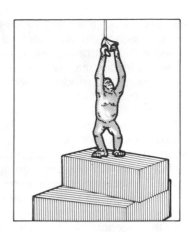

Fig. 7.5 *Problem-solving experiment*

learning applied to personal, social and professional behaviour. Social learning theory emphasises the reciprocal interaction between behaviour and the environment. It differs from a strict behaviourist position by stressing the importance of cognitive processes. Social learning theorists consider that an individual's reactions are governed to a large extent by anticipated consequences; for example nurses learn to observe the correct procedure for administering prescribed drugs because the consequences of a drug error can be catastrophic for both the patients and the nurse. The three main tenets of social learning theory are **vic-**

```
            (1) Recognition of the problem
                (cannot reach fruit)

(2) Data collection ──────► (3) Hypothesis formulation
    (boxes in room)             (stacked boxes will allow
                                 fruit to be reached)

(4) Select plan for ──────► (5) Test hypothesis
    hypothesis testing          (climb on top of boxes)
    (stack boxes end-on)

        (6) Interpretation of results
            (fruit reached successfully)

        (7) Evaluation of the hypothesis

Termination                  Modification
```

Fig. 7.6 *Cognitive learning as the basis for effective problem solving*

arious learning, identification with role models and **self-regulatory processes**, each of which will now be discussed.

Vicarious learning

Atkinson *et al.* (1990) define vicarious learning as 'learning by observing the behaviour of others and noting the consequences of that behaviour'. Emotions can also be learned vicariously by watching the emotional responses of others as they undergo pleasant or unpleasant experiences, for example two student nurses receiving praise and reproof respectively from the ward sister for certain aspects of nursing care.

Albert Bandura is one of the main social psychologists associated with this theory. He began his career as an enthusiastic advocate of operant conditioning. Later he realised, however, that it is not always essential for someone actually to make responses and be reinforced, but that identification with models can influence behaviour strongly. Three early experiments by Bandura and two associates aroused a great deal of interest in observational learning and stimulated many other psychologists to analyse the impact of modelling and imitation on behaviour. In the first experiment (Bandura, Ross and Ross, 1963) a child was seated at a table and encouraged to play with a toy that was provided. The model sat at a nearby table and either played quietly with Tinker Toys for ten minutes or played with the Tinker Toys for one minute and then played aggressively (punching, kicking, sitting on, hitting with a hammer) with an inflatable clown for several minutes. After watching one or the other of these modelled behaviours each child was allowed to become engrossed with an attractive toy and then told that he or she could not play with it any longer, a condition thought to produce mild frustration. Each child was then led to a room containing a variety of toys including those played with by the model. Children who did not observe the model, as well as those who observed a non-aggressive model, displayed little imitative aggression. By contrast, children who had observed an aggressive model engaged in considerably more aggressive behaviour in response to the clown doll and to other toys.

In the second study, similar results were obtained in response to viewing a film of either an adult or an adult dressed as a cartoon character engaging in aggressive behaviour. The third study attempted to determine what effect rewarding the model for aggressive behaviour would have on children's imitative behaviour. In general, children were more aggressive when they had seen a model positively reinforced than when the model was punished. With reference to social learning theory, it is suggested that the increase in violent crime and sexual offences is attributed to more explicit violence and sex on television and video which are negative outcomes. However, on a more positive note, models can be chosen for more appropriate reasons.

Identification with role models in nursing

Secord and Backman (1964) define identification as 'a process accounting for the choice of one model rather than another'. They cite several principles which account for the choice. Some of these will now be discussed in the context of nursing practice.

Vicarious reinforcement
A person is chosen as a model because she receives rewards that are experienced vicariously; in other words the observer feels as though she were experiencing the rewards herself in lieu of the model. If a student nurse is praised by a patient for making him comfortable, a colleague may adopt that particular modelled behaviour.

Similarity
A person is chosen as a model because the observer perceives that they share similar personality traits. A student may choose a colleague as a model because she believes that they are both outgoing and share similar tastes in music.

Social power
A person is chosen as a model because she has the *power* to reward (but does not necessarily reward). Students may model themselves on their ward sister for this reason – and for the reverse reason, the fear of reproof.

Identification is no doubt multi-determined in nearly all everyday situations. However, a literature review reveals that the key attributes of the most popular role models are that they are warm and genuine, good communicators, and have status within the organisation where they are employed.

The final tenet of social learning theory is that of self-regulatory processes.

Self-regulation

There are two main sources of reinforcement, as shown in Fig. 7.7, i.e. *internal* (evaluation by self) and *external* (evaluation by others). It should be noted that the external source of reinforcement need not be direct since it can also be vicarious. The reinforcement from either source can range from positive to negative.

Four examples should clarify the model. A student nurse may conduct an aspect of nursing care (such as the application of an aseptic dressing) which produces an external outcome (a comfortable patient with a non-infected wound). This is accompanied by a self-evaluative reaction, for example professional pride. If the patient expressed his gratitude then this situation could be located

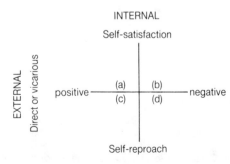

Fig. 7.7 *Self-regulatory processes*

conceptually in the top left hand corner of the model (position a). The reader may wish to consider situations in nursing practice which could be conceptually located in positions *b, c* and *d*, before comparing them with the following scenarios.

In position *b*, a student nurse may feel pleased that she has spent a very worthwhile period talking to and reassuring her patients, but at the same time she attracts reproof from her staff nurse for spending too much time at the bedside and not completing other duties. In position *c*, a student nurse may receive some form of praise from a colleague for rapidly completing the patient's dressings, but reproach herself because her technique was of a less than satisfactory standard. In position *d* a psychiatric nurse may receive criticism from a colleague about the way he facilitated an encounter group which he also feels did not go well.

Erickson (1983) contends that social learning theory is a paradigm for nursing. In other words student nurses are strongly influenced by the colleagues with whom they interact, especially the ward sister (Fretwell, 1982).

Another example of social learning theory applied to nursing is standard-setting. Students can learn to improve their standard of care by vicarious learning in the practice setting by watching their colleagues assess the effectiveness of care provided, e.g. in pain control. Vicarious learning can also occur in different primary health care settings while nurses on their common foundation programmes observe community nurses providing care in different contexts, e.g. in doctors' surgeries or patients' homes.

Two recommendations arise from the discussion above. These are firstly, that you maintain high professional standards, and secondly, that you model those behaviours you would wish your colleagues to emulate by showing enthusiasm for nursing and striving for excellence.

At this point readers may regard social learning theory as only moderately behaviouristic because of the influence of cognitive processes. These cognitive processes enable an individual to foresee the probable consequences of a course of action and to alter behaviour accordingly. In the context of nursing practice, nurse education, nursing management and nursing research, self-reinforcement arising from professional behaviour based on one's own standards of conduct provides important motivational control.

Critical discussion of social learning theory

Social learning theorists emphasise the reciprocal relationship between the individual and the environment. In other words, the focus is on:

(a) individual characteristics, e.g. of a nurse
(b) aspects of the environment, e.g. of a hospital ward
(c) interaction between (a) and (b) and vice versa

Vicarious learning is an important mode of learning in the context of health care. However, critics of this approach suggest that it does not distinguish between the causes of actions and their consequences (Wade and Tavris, 1990). For example, a nurse may be observed communicating with a distressed client in a particular way and being effective in reducing the client's anxiety. However, the reasoning behind that nurse's course of action and the reason why her actions were effective are not fully explained by social learning.

The importance of good role models has been emphasised. However, role models may be chosen by nurses for the 'wrong' reasons, for example fear of censure. Nevertheless, it is imperative that those health care professionals who are in a position to be chosen as role models, for example primary nurses, discharge their roles and responsibilities in a warm, caring and professional manner.

Whereas strict behavioural approaches to learning emphasise extrinsic reinforcement, the concept of intrinsic reinforcement features in the self-regulatory processes of social learning theory. For example, intrinsic motivation can sustain the actions described for positions (a) and (b) in Fig 7.7, i.e. maintaining an aseptic technique and relieving anxiety respectively. Problems of **cognitive dissonance** may arise when the pressure to conform becomes intense. This is another example of social learning theory not sufficiently explaining causality.

In conclusion, the cognitive perspective of social learning theory is a welcome shift from the strict behaviourist stance. The contribution to our understanding of some key aspects of health care made by the processes of vicarious learning, role modelling and self-regulation is acknowledged.

Attention will now be turned to other 'riches' to be found inside the 'black box', i.e. those associated with the way we process information.

Information processing

Information processing theorists study the ways in which stimuli from the environment are perceived, transformed into meaningful information, stored in memory, recalled for use, and translated into observable behaviour (Lindsay and Norman, 1977). It is important, for a variety of reasons, that nurses develop an understanding of how information is processed. In this part of the chapter, research on sensation, attention, perception and memory will be explored in relation to clinical nursing and in terms of the nurse as an educator.

Sensation

Sensation is said to occur when any sense organ receives a stimulus from the external or internal environment. This frequently occurs without our conscious awareness, for example pressure from clothing. Figure 7.8 shows the sensory pathways for touch and pressure and how they are linked by

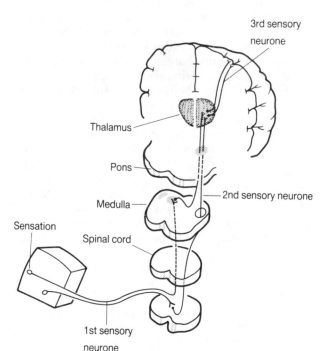

Fig. 7.8 *Sensory pathways for touch and pressure from receptors in the brain*

a chain of three neurones with the parietal lobes in the brain. The ascending sensory neurones not only run to the thalamus, sensory cortex and cerebellum, but in addition collaterals are sent to the reticular formation which extends throughout the brain stem from the medulla to the thalamus. Destruction of the reticular formation leads to deep sleep and insensibility to sensory stimuli. There seems to be an optimal level of sensory excitation which is modulated by the ascending reticular activating system. Studies have shown that adverse effects occur if optimum levels of sensory excitation are transcended (Ashworth, 1979; Child, 1986). They found that patients in quiet single hospital rooms became disorientated due to sensory deprivation. Other situations where this can happen are when patients lie in bed less than fully conscious because of drugs or illness with the constant hiss of oxygen or the hum of equipment, accompanied by a low level of background voices from which no words can be distinguished. This has obvious implications for care and nurses need to be alert to patients who are especially at risk from sensory deprivation – for example those in isolation, intensive care units, and the elderly. Patients in intensive therapy units are also at risk from sensory overload and problems of disorientation, especially if frequently 'disturbed' by nursing interventions such as monitoring blood pressure, tracheal suction and postural changes. Nurses should aim for the optimum level of stimulation which means protecting patients from both sensory deprivation and sensory overload.

Attention

The ability of human beings to process some of the incoming sensations and to ignore everything else is known as *attention*. Both the observer and the stimulus possess characteristics which are likely to influence attention. The following are likely to be of relevance to nurses and can be conveniently divided into internal and external factors.

Internal factors

(1) *Interest* or lack of it is likely to influence attention, so when planning to teach a junior colleague about a nursing topic it is important to gain the individual's interest by explaining the relevance of the topic in question.
(2) *Fatigue* can be of a general nature (due to lack

of sleep or a long and busy period of ward work) or it can be more specific. An example of more specific fatigue may occur when we are 'swamped' with information. It is important, therefore, not to overload junior colleagues or patients with information when explaining things to them.

(3) *Personality* has been shown to have a bearing on how long different people can pay attention and it would seem that extraverts need more voluntary rest pauses in comparison with introverts.

External factors

(1) *Variability* of the stimulus is likely to affect attention. An example of such a variation is a change in vocal intonation to emphasise key points in a ward report session. Posters and wall-charts ought to be regularly changed if attention to their message is to be gained as we readily adapt to unchanging stimuli.

(2) *Novelty* is always likely to influence attention so if you are asked to give a talk on a topic in the College of Nursing or on the ward, it is advisable to vary the presentation with the use of colourful visual aids and to provide additional stimuli by fostering audience participation.

(3) *Cueing* by saying 'watch this' and 'note that' will draw attention to phenomena, for example when demonstrating to a colleague the presence of pitting oedema in a patient with congestive cardiac failure, or the rise and fall of fluid in an underwater seal drainage bottle during inspiration and expiration in a patient with a pneumothorax.

It is thus argued that a knowledge of the internal and external factors that influence attention is important for the nurse in terms of both her clinical and educational roles. There are several other factors which influence attention and additional reading will be recommended at the end of the chapter.

Perception

Coon (1986) defines perception as the process of meaningfully organising sensation. Human perception can be regarded as an active hypothesis-testing process influenced by context, set and past experience. Clarke (1980) feels that the importance of this for nursing is that if perception is a process of forming hypotheses, then it is possible to form both accurate and inaccurate hypotheses. Before a consideration of some of the possible problems of misperception in clinical practice and nursing education, the importance of context, set and experience will be discussed.

Refer to Fig. 7.9 and see how *context* alters the meaning of the middle figure. Although exactly the same image appears on the retina, readers are likely to perceive it as the figure thirteen in the transverse row of numbers, but as the letter 'B' in the longitudinal column of letters.

$$\begin{array}{c} A \\ 12 \; 13 \; 14 \\ C \end{array}$$

Fig. 7.9 *Context and perceptual meaning*

Set can also influence human perception strongly. Set refers to the response system that predisposes an individual to view and approach a problem in a pre-determined manner (de Tornyay and Thompson, 1987). Have a look now at Fig. 7.10 and imagine you are at a circus. It is quite probable that you have perceived a trainer and a

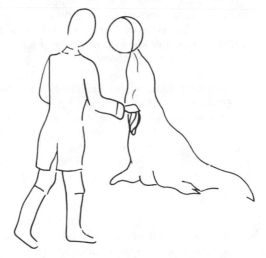

Fig. 7.10 *The influence of set on perception*

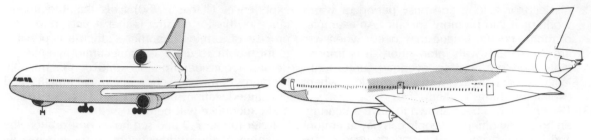

Fig. 7.11 *Experience and perceptual meaning*

seal balancing a ball on its nose. However if you had been asked to consider Fig. 7.10 as though it were a costume ball it is more likely that you would have seen a man and a woman with the man graciously asking the lady for a dance.

Past *experience* also influences human perception; for example, have a look at Fig. 7.11 and identify the two aircraft. Both aircraft are big, wide-bodied passenger jetliners with three engines that look quite similar on first glance. However, past experience (and interest) would enable an individual to differentiate the Tristar on the left from the DC10 on the right.

Perceptual problems and the nurse

As indicated above, it is possible to form both accurate and inaccurate perceptions as a result of context, set and past experience. Some of those instances will now be highlighted.

(1) A patient on a medical ward complains of abdominal pain, and in fact needs an appendicectomy. Because of the context, this is not diagnosed as quickly as it might be if a patient on a surgical ward demonstrated the same symptoms.
(2) Hyland and Donaldson (1989) explain how patients can reject information if it is perceived as threatening. Thus, a negative set is created which can lead to misperception of the prognosis.
(3) James (1970) conveniently subdivides the processes involved in perception into *organisation and utilisation*.

Organisation refers to the way in which the brain transforms the multitude of scattered nerve impulses it receives into a meaningful picture of what they represent (*percept formation*). A patient

recovering from a general anaesthetic is likely to perceive the sound of nurses' voices, the pressure of bedclothes, the smell of antiseptic and the position of his body from **proprioceptors**.

Utilisation refers to the way in which different individuals respond to the percept. Two patients could return to the ward following almost identical surgery but respond quite differently. One patient is thankful that the operation was successful and just wants to go back to sleep, whereas the other patient is quite disturbed, possibly due to a previous bad experience following surgery.

There are several other reasons why information from the environment is misperceived, especially when the perceiver expects a different sensation from the one she actually receives. If you see a notice in an area of town that says 'Polite Notice No Parking' it is probable that you would see this as 'Police Notice No Parking' because that would be something you would expect to see. This phenomenon could have very serious consequences in the context of being confronted with drugs of similar names when conducting a medicine round. It is easy to confuse *prednisone* with *prednisolone* and administer the wrong drug. Drug errors can be catastrophic for both patients and nurse for different reasons, ending at worst in a fatality. It is possible that a nurse may select *Dipyridamole* from the drug trolley instead of *Disopyramide* because she expects to see Disopyramide and subsequently administers a drug which reduces platelet stickiness instead of a drug prescribed for **ventricular arrhythmias**.

The use of language can also lead to several misunderstandings. For example the term **'peristaltic tumour'** is used to describe the wave of peristalsis following a test-feed for a child with congenital hypertrophic **pyloric stenosis**. A parent could misinterpret this to mean that their child has a malignant disease, with obvious implications.

It can be argued, then, that a knowledge of sensation, attention, and perception is of considerable importance to all nurses, especially those primarily involved in clinical practice. A brief account of the processes involved in remembering and forgetting will now follow.

Remembering

The scientist and science fiction writer Isaac Asimov estimates that the human brain records over one quadrillion separate bits of information in a lifetime. The three main processes involved in remembering are *encoding, storage* and *retrieval* (Child, 1986). Encoding is the process of assimilating information into meaningful forms (putting into memory) and is clearly influenced by perception. Storage is the commitment of information into memory (maintaining in memory) and is influenced by the way the data is organised and related to existing memories. Retrieval refers to the reproduction of information when required (recovering from memory) and is influenced by internal and external cues, as will be subsequently discussed.

Five types of remembering have been described by psychologists. These are: recall, recognition, relearning, redintegration and eidetic imagery. Each in turn will now be discussed with reference to some of the research findings.

Recall

Recall refers to remembering or reproducing facts and information without explicit cues from the environment – as one does, for example, when sitting an examination where the questions have not been previously seen.

Recognition

Recognition refers to remembering information based on explicit cues from the environment – as when sitting a test based on multiple choice objective questions where subjects are required to select the answer from four or five alternatives. Haber (1970) showed subjects 2560 slides in one of his experiments, one slide every 10 seconds. The subjects were then shown 280 pairs of photographs comprising some from the original set and others of a new but similar type. Haber's subjects could tell with 85–95% accuracy the ones they had seen from the original 2560. The suggestion is that rec-

ognition is a far more economical process than 'pure' recall, and has implications for the use of visual aids when teaching patients. Police 'line-ups' which attempt to identify criminal suspects are based on the process of recognition.

Relearning

Relearning means exactly what it implies: the learning again of material that an individual has learned previously, but perhaps has some difficulty in recalling. However, in some of the experimental work an individual need not necessarily have 'learned' the material. Burtt (1941) described an experiment where a Greek passage was read to a 15 month old child every day until he was three years old. At eight years of age the child showed no evidence of recall. The child was asked to read passages from other Greek texts and selections from the original passage, but indicated no recognition of any of the material. The child was then asked to memorise the original passage plus several others of equal difficulty and was able to memorise the original passage 25% faster than the other passages. The implications are that it is a worthwhile exercise to revise previously learned material at regular intervals and that it will probably be a less demanding exercise than the original learning task – as can be seen by referring to the saving score formula (Fig. 7.12).

$$\frac{\text{Original trials minus Relearning trials}}{\text{Original trials}} \times 100$$

For example, if it takes 5 trials to learn about the process of glomerular filtration and only 2 trials to relearn the process after an interval, the saving score is 60% because

$$\frac{5-2}{5} \times 100 = 60$$

Fig. 7.12 *The Saving Score formula*

Redintegration

Redintegration refers to the reconstruction of an entire past experience from one small recollection (for example, the perfume or aftershave of a former lover). The BBC *Crimewatch* programme shows

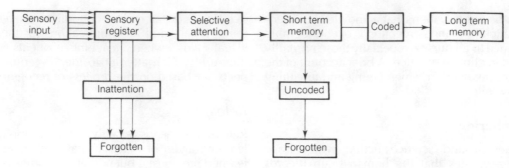

Fig. 7.13 *An information processing model of memory*

reconstructed crimes in the hope that witnesses will recall vital information from one cue. The implications of this when taking examinations are that the recollection of a patient for whom you have cared can bring back to mind several aspects of nursing care and medical management.

Eidetic imagery

Eidetic imagery refers to photographic memory and has been the subject of quite extensive research. It is most often observed in childhood where some children can recall pictures in striking detail after only a short exposure. However, most eidetic skills disappear during adolescence and eidetic children do not have a better long term memory than non-eidetic children.

Attention will now be directed to the three stages of memory that have been described. Data must pass through all three stages if it is to be stored for a long time and this is represented in Fig. 7.13.

Sensory register

The sensory register is also called *sensory memory* or *super short term memory*. It holds an exact copy of what it has seen for half a second or less. If you close your eyes for one minute with your hand in front of your face and then blink rapidly, you should see the after-image of your hand for a split second after closing your eyes. The sensory register is the bridge between *percept organisation* (receiving information) and memory (storing information).

Short term memory

The short term memory only holds information for short periods lasting from about four seconds up to twenty minutes. If data is not coded while in the short term memory it will be permanently lost, which saves our minds from being cluttered with trivia. Short term memory is our working memory, for example when doing addition and looking up telephone numbers. The average short term memory can hold seven digits, plus or minus two, but the short term memory trace rapidly decays after 18 seconds without rehearsal.

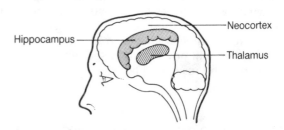

Fig. 7.14 *Lateral view of brain to show hippocampus*

When new information is received from the sense organs, it is routed via the *thalamus* to the *hippocampus* which has a special role in the storage of new information. If any new information has any connection with long term memory already in the *neocortex* then the hippocampus becomes much more sensitised to it. If no connection can be found it is in danger of being forgotten. This means that, when teaching a patient or a colleague about something new, it is important to try and ascertain what they already know first and then proceed from that standpoint. For example, if a patient has some knowledge of food values, that knowledge can be linked to a teaching session about diet and health and is more likely to be remembered. If information is quite new, the hippocampus needs longer to become sensitised to it.

Readers may have experienced this when studying. After 20 minutes or so, new material starts to 'sink in' (and in a sense it is sinking into the neocortex). The point here is that you need to persevere at a learning task, with frequent rehearsal, for networks to be laid down in the neocortex.

Long term memory

The long term memory permanently records information that has been successfully coded and has practically unlimited storage capacity. It can be considered as a network of meaningful interconnections covering the neocortex like a fine piece of lace. The facility for recall from long term memory is related to the way information has been coded and stored in the first place. People who have good memories excel at organising information and making it meaningful. The relevance of this for nursing students (or indeed any student) is to have well-organised study habits.

The long term memory then acts as an encyclopaedia or huge 'warehouse' for storing information. Long term memories are repeatedly revised as new information is received.

Forgetting

The four causes of forgetting and their implications will be discussed below.

Decay

Neural trace decay appears to be true of short term memory which operates like a 'leaky bucket'. New information is being poured in but being replaced by still newer information. The implications for teaching are that if you are involved in giving a talk in the College of Nursing, the provision of supplementary holding mechanisms such as colourful visual aids are likely to help people rehearse the information whilst it remains in their short term memory. Decay is much less likely from long term memory. Some unused memories may fade while others remain for life – as found in elderly people who often have vivid recollections of their distant past.

Interference

Interference is a very important cause of forgetting and has been researched in terms of *retro-active* and *pro-active inhibition*. Retro-active inhibition refers to the tendency for new learning to interfere with the retrieval of old learning (Coon, 1986). Pro-active inhibition occurs when prior learning interferes with later learning. Each type of interference was studied by Postman (1969) who gave the subjects in his experiments lists of words to learn.

The results of Postman's experiments are given in Table 7.2.

Table 7.2. *The effects of retro-active and pro-active inhibition*

Retro-active inhibition

Experimental group:	learn list A then learn list B then test A
Control group:	learn list A then rest then test A

The experimental group remembers less from list A than the control group because list B has interfered 'backwards' with list A

Pro-active inhibition

Experimental group:	learn list A then learn list B then test B
Control group:	rest then learn list B then test B

Again the experimental group remembered less because list A has interfered 'forwards' with list B.

The implications for studying are to avoid 'cramming' similar subjects when studying, especially during the same evening.

Cue-dependent forgetting

Quite often memories are available but not readily accessible. This is sometimes known as the 'tip of the tongue phenomenon'. The answer to a question is known but the relevant cue is missing. When teaching a group of colleagues or patients, try and provide cues to help people answer questions. It is likely that your colleagues and patients will gain more satisfaction from answering questions with gentle cueing rather than being told the answer.

Emotional factors

Acute anxiety can affect memory and can affect confidence before an important examination. This may lead to signs of panic when reading the question paper.

The relationship between arousal and performance can be seen in Fig. 7.15 and has been described as the Yerkes-Dodson effect after the two psychologists who studied the phenomenon. The implications of this are considerable for nursing education and clinical practice. It is important to be thoroughly prepared for examinations, and to avoid retro-active and pro-active inhibition, by systematic study and frequent revision.

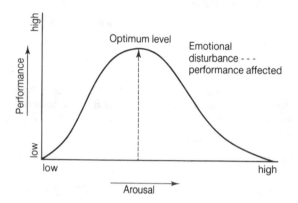

Fig. 7.15 *The Yerkes-Dodson effect*

If you still tend to panic in the examination try some positive coping statements to counteract negative self-statements (see Fig. 7.16). Such posi-

---

Exam preparations:

• I have studied hard for this exam

• I will read the paper carefully and not rush into question selection

• If I get nervous I will take four deep breaths and pause for a moment

At the start of the exam:

• Relax now, I deserve to pass this

• Stay organised, formulate essay plans, and focus on each question

---

Fig. 7.16 *Coping strategies for examinations*

tive coping statements can shift your state of arousal to the left of the curve, whereas negative statements such as 'I can't do this' and 'I don't know anything' can shift you too far to the right and affect performance.

After a doctor's ward round nurses often have to return to the patient's bedside to go over again something that has been explained by the doctor. The patient may have been too anxious to take it all in at the first account.

Critical discussion of information processing

In this section of the chapter, the physiological basis of sensation has been outlined briefly. Some of the main internal and external factors which influence attention have been explained and are of particular significance in the educational role of the nurse.

Several factors which influence perception have been addressed and are clearly important in the day-to-day practice of the nurse as some misperceptions can have dire consequences.

The remaining part of this section was devoted to human memory, broadly defined by Clancy (1981) as the faculty which enables an individual to reproduce information which has been learned, to repeat learned behaviour, or to re-experience in the mind past experiences. He goes on to say that remembering is the process of reproducing or re-experiencing previously learned material or past experiences and that forgetting is a failure in that process. Four theories of forgetting were explained. The *decay* theory is characterised by the notion that forgetting is due to a lapse in time and a subsequent weakening of the neural trace. But as Clancy points out, this simple model does not account for why we sometimes remember material that was previously thought to be forgotten.

The *interference* theory is said to take place retro-actively when recently learned material interferes with the ability to remember previously learned material, and pro-actively when previously stored material interferes with the ability to remember more recently learned material. The importance of this explanation is only evident when the two sets of information are of a similar nature and therefore this theory cannot be regarded as comprehensive.

Cue dependent forgetting occurs when an individual is unable to retrieve information because of insufficient internally or externally generated cues. It is regarded as a convincing theory, along with the *emotional factor* theory, although in the latter a distinction needs to be made between forgetting due to an over-aroused state, as in an examination situation, and motivated forgetting because of conscious or unconscious desires to eliminate awareness of painful or unpleasant experiences.

It can be stated with confidence that a knowledge of the host of influences on remembering and forgetting is of major importance to the role of the nurse, both as a care-giver and student with her own learning needs.

Attention will now be given to the concept of motivation.

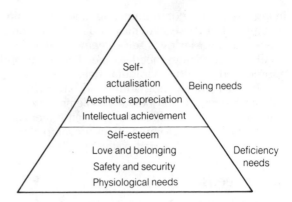

Fig. 7.17 *Maslow's hierarchy of human needs (adapted from Maslow, 1970)*

Motivation

Atkinson *et al.* (1990) regard motivation as a general term referring to the regulation of need-satisfying and goal-seeking behaviour. A need is any deficiency a person has, be it biological or psychological. As patients' and clients' needs are affected by problems of physical and/or mental health, it can be seen that a knowledge of motivational theory is crucial for nurses working in a range of specialisms.

There are a number of different theories of motivation which, according to Hamner and Organ (1978), can be classified under the following headings:

- energiser theories
- channeller/director theories
- maintenance theories

Energiser theories attempt to explain what energises or initiates behaviour. Channeller/director theories distinguish what directs or channels behaviour towards a particular goal, and maintenance theories explain the factors which sustain behaviour once initiated.

An energiser approach to motivation

Maslow (1970) is the best known proponent of this approach to motivation. He has suggested that there is a hierarchy of human needs which

comprises both deficiency and being needs (Fig. 7.17).

Deficiency needs

When deficiency needs are not met, motivation increases to find ways of satisfying them and is likely to decrease to some extent when they are met. Maslow views the most basic needs of all human beings as those for food, water and oxygen. In terms of patient care, Maslow's physiological needs can be linked to activities of daily living – such as eating, drinking, eliminating and breathing – and are clearly the concern of every nurse in the delivery of care. Maslow's safety and security needs primarily address physical safety – such as the need to feel out of danger from the physical environment. The specificity of these needs vary. The toddler who is expanding his physical world needs to explore the environment which is stabilised by his parents. The adult has a greater need to live by societal conventions and rules. In any event, the activity of daily living 'maintaining a safe environment' would seem to equate with Maslow's theory here.

The need for love and affiliative relationships dominates Maslow's third deficiency need. This need is present from birth from maternal bonding to relating with other members of the immediate family, progressing through a range of different relationships with friends of both sexes throughout the seven epochs of the human life, namely: infancy, childhood, adolescence, young, middle and late adulthood, and the senilium (old age). Affiliative needs encompass other activities of daily living, such as communicating and expressing sexuality, but these activities could also be considered under Maslow's self-esteem needs.

All human beings need to feel important and appreciated and this particular need is of special significance from young adulthood onwards. Clients who have mental health problems may have a negative self-image linked to low self-esteem and it is the nurses' role to help clients develop a more positive self-image as part of therapy.

Being needs

When being needs are met, a person's motivation may well increase to seek further fulfilment of the same needs. Intellectual achievement and aesthetic appreciation are self-explanatory but self-actualisation merits further explanations. Self-actualisation refers to the fulfilment of one's potential and can be summed up in the assertion, 'What a person can be, he or she ought to be'. If this occurs then the person has met all the other needs, is content, and has developed an equilibrium within and with the environment.

Maslow's theory is useful to the nurse because it can be used as a framework for planning individualised care. Imagine a 30-year-old woman admitted for a hysterectomy. Following surgery she will need her airway maintained and hydration via an intravenous infusion until she can breathe spontaneously and is able to eat and drink normally (physiological needs). The nurse will be responsible for this aspect of care to ensure that her patient's physiological needs are met. She will also need to position her patient properly so as to prevent injury from hospital equipment and the development of pressure sores while on bed-rest (safety needs). Affiliative needs can be met to some extent by the nurse adopting a friendly and supportive manner when interacting with her patient and ensuring that there is minimal disturbance during visiting by significant others in the patient's life. Webb and Wilson-Barnett (1983) conducted a descriptive study of recovery from hysterectomy. In their literature review they found that the social support given to or withheld from women having a hysterectomy is a potential influence on their subsequent adjustment. In some cultures and religions the concept of wholeness as a woman and ability to bear children are especially highly valued and the uterus is a symbol of femininity. Following hysterectomy some women may suffer depression

and feelings of inadequacy (esteem needs). Nurses need to be sensitive to this aspect of care and give advice, information and encouragement as appropriate. Because of the role of social support in promoting recovery, partners and families should be included in joint counselling. Webb and Wilson-Barnett go on to recommend that these aspects should be integrated into patient care at all stages: pre-operatively, during recovery, and following discharge. Nurses need extensive training in the skills of information-giving and counselling so that they can more ably satisfy their patients' deficiency and being needs.

A channeller/director approach to motivation

Locke (1976) is one of the chief proponents of this approach to motivation, stating that motivation is channelled so that individuals attain satisfaction from their actions. His research demonstrated that the setting of specific goals leads to more effective performance than general goals such as, 'I will give of my best'. This theory can be regarded as underpinning *management by objectives* or MBO for short. MBO is an approach to management where the objectives for the job are discussed and agreed by superior and subordinate. The criteria for successful achievement of the job are agreed and both parties meet periodically to review progress.

The similarities between MBO and the process of contract learning can be drawn here. A *learning contract* can be defined as a teaching/learning strategy where a student negotiates with his or her facilitator the objectives, methods for achieving the objectives, and criteria for evaluating his or her achievement of those objectives (Myles, 1991). The contracts can range from informal verbal to formal written agreements between the parties and serve to channel/direct behaviour.

A maintenance approach to motivation

Herzberg (1966) is the main proponent of this approach to motivation. He proposed a 'motivation-hygiene' theory to describe, explain and predict motivation related to work performance. He interviewed a range of people from different occupations, including nurses, to ascertain what gave them satisfaction at work and what caused them to work harder.

He found that a number of factors caused dissatisfaction if they were inadequate, which are also relevant in the context of a practice area. Those factors may include:

- Salary
- Job security
- Status
- Ward policy
- Working conditions
- Professional relationships.

Herzberg described these as *hygiene* factors, i.e. if the factors were adequate they would prevent dissatisfaction but not necessarily satisfy. The public health analogy is that good sanitation can prevent some diseases but not make an individual healthy (Payne, 1983).

The factors which Herzberg's respondents said made them happy are called *motivators*. Applied to a clinical setting they can be described as:

- Interesting nature of work
- Feelings of significant achievement in patient care
- Being recognised as an individual
- Being given appropriate responsibility for patient care
- Opportunities for personal growth

Herzberg claimed that the motivators were the more powerful of the factors. They are of much importance in maintaining motivation in health care settings and could be used as part of the framework for a clinical audit.

Critical discussion of approaches to motivation

Maslow's energiser theory has been criticised on several accounts. People do not always behave as the theory might suggest. Some people deny themselves safety or friendship to focus on the higher-level needs for knowledge and understanding. His concept of self-actualisation is also problematic in terms of its verification. However, the basic premise of prepotency of need is useful. *Prepotency* refers to the notion that unless needs lower in Maslow's hierarchy have been at least partially met, it is likely to be difficult to address higher needs. For example, in an educational context, a student's desire to satisfy deficiency needs

(e.g. security) may compete with the teacher's desire for her to achieve being needs (e.g. knowledge and understanding). When you are involved in teaching patients and/or junior colleagues, it is important to try and put them at their ease so that they can more readily learn.

Locke's channeller theory can be recommended for its emphasis on goal-setting and intrinsic motivation. For Locke, it is the process of goal-setting and the efforts to achieve those goals which direct motivation rather than the 'rewards' that accrue when successful, i.e. extrinsic motivation. While supporting Locke's premise, it is suggested that outcomes are important. For example, in the context of a cardiac rehabilitation programme, it is important that the person who is overweight and hypertensive following a myocardial infarction achieves weight loss and normotension through diet, graduated exercise and compliance with an anti-hypertensive drug as prescribed.

Herzberg's maintenance theory can be criticised on methodological grounds. Cooper and Makin (1983) suggest that the evidence used by Herzberg to differentiate between his hygiene factors and motivators is less than clear. Nevertheless, his theory is useful when considering the quality of working life.

Attention will now be turned to the nature of human personality and associated psychological studies of relevance to health care professionals.

Personality

What is it? One often hears statements such as, 'She has lots of personality but he hasn't any at all. I can't understand what she sees in him!' This is taken to mean that the lady in question is cheerful and outgoing but her boyfriend is rather dull. This implies that personality is something you have a 'quantity' of, with some having more than others. This is not how psychologists regard personality, which they would generally define as:

'a distinctive and relatively stable pattern of thoughts, feelings and behaviour patterns in response to the internal and external environment which characterise an individual'
(adapted from Wade and Tavris, 1990)

Three different approaches to the study of personality will be explored in this section of the chapter, starting with Freud's psychodynamic theory.

Psychodynamic theory

Freudian and neo-Freudian theory is called *psychodynamic* because of its focus on the psychic energy within the person. For Freud, the personality is made up of three interacting systems: the *id*, *ego* and *superego*.

The id

The id is that part of the personality which contains inherited psychological energy, particularly sexual and aggressive instincts. The id demands immediate gratification and is totally selfish, motivated purely by hedonism.

The ego

The ego is that part of the personality which represents reason and good sense, restraining the hedonistic demands of the id.

The superego

The superego is that part of the personality which represents morality and social standards. It is often seen as our conscience.

According to psychoanalytic theory, the healthy personality has to keep a balance between the three systems. A person who is id-orientated tends to be selfish and impulsive. A person who is superego-orientated tends to be rigid, moralistic and somewhat authoritarian. Both extreme types are seen as maladjusted. A person who has a strong ego (as distinct from being *egocentric*) is able to balance the hedonistic demands of the id and the harsh demands of the superego for perennial restraint. This sort of person is seen as well-adjusted according to psychoanalytic theory.

If someone feels threatened, that individual can utilise *ego defence mechanisms*. These act like a 'mental anaesthetic', unconsciously distorting or denying reality. Several varieties of mental defence have been described in the literature (Child, 1986; Atkinson *et al.*, 1990). A selected few will be addressed here for their relevance to health care.

(1) In *denial*, an individual simply refuses to admit that something terrible has happened. For example, if someone's husband dies in intensive care, she may deny that her husband has died and goes on planning for his discharge home.

(2) In *projection*, an individual's unacceptable feelings about himself/herself are projected onto someone else. For example, a patient who is dissatisfied with the way he is rehabilitating may blame the nursing staff for his lack of progress. A student who has not done well in a course assignment may blame her teacher.

(3) In *reaction formation*, an individual deals with unconscious anxiety by transforming it into its opposite. For example, a highly anxious patient may behave in an overconfident way on admission to hospital and needs more help to relax than his outward persona would suggest.

(4) In *regression*, an individual reverts to an earlier life-stage. This can be seen in a children's ward when a normally continent child reverts to bedwetting due to the trauma of hospitalisation.

Type theories of personality

Friedman and Rosenman's (1974) type theory of personality is of relevance to health care because of the link with illness. They describe type A people as very success-orientated, impatient, and always in a hurry. They tend to be irritable, lead highly stressed lives, and are susceptible to myocardial infarctions and other cardiovascular disorders such as angina pectoris.

Type B people have lower serum cholesterol and betalipoprotein levels and are much more phlegmatic than type A people. They have a lower incidence of hypertension and coronary heart disease, as might be expected.

It is asserted that type A people are more likely to be admitted to coronary care units with a myocardial infarction and may continue their type A behaviour during their hospitalisation. This can impede their recovery, requiring the nursing and medical staff to encourage those patients to modify their outlook on life.

Trait theories of personality

Rather than classifying people into discrete types, trait theories consider that a person can best be

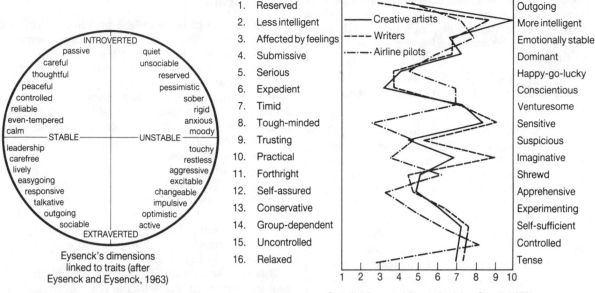

1.	Reserved — Outgoing
2.	Less intelligent — More intelligent
3.	Affected by feelings — Emotionally stable
4.	Submissive — Dominant
5.	Serious — Happy-go-lucky
6.	Expedient — Conscientious
7.	Timid — Venturesome
8.	Tough-minded — Sensitive
9.	Trusting — Suspicious
10.	Practical — Imaginative
11.	Forthright — Shrewd
12.	Self-assured — Apprehensive
13.	Conservative — Experimenting
14.	Group-dependent — Self-sufficient
15.	Uncontrolled — Controlled
16.	Relaxed — Tense

Eysenck's dimensions
linked to traits (after
Eysenck and Eysenck, 1963)

Cattell's sixteen source traits (after Cattell, 1973)

Fig. 7.18 *Trait approaches to personality*

described by measuring their scores on a number of traits.

Traits are relatively permanent and enduring qualities that an individual shows in most situations. For example, if you are normally optimistic and phlegmatic, these qualities can be considered as stable traits of your personality.

Contemporary personality theories within psychology have taken either a trait or type approach and there are a number of personality tests which aim to measure an individual's personality in a scientific way. Eysenck (1963) and Cattell (1973) are two well-known psychologists whose tests have been used extensively in nursing in this country and the USA, and overviews of their trait approach can be seen in Fig 7.18. Both tests require subjects to answer a series of questions. Their answers are calculated using a complex statistical procedure called factor-analysis and both tests are known for their high reliability in depicting accurately an individual's personality.

Another test, the Minnesota Multiphasic Personality Inventory (MMPI), is used to measure 'normality', depression and schizophrenia (see Fig. 7.19). The MMPI is composed of 550 items to which subjects must respond and their responses are converted into a standard score. Standard scores are conversions to a scale of measurement and again are calculated using statistical pro-

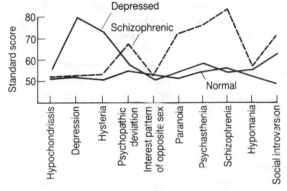

1. **Hypochondriasis:** reflects exaggerated concern about one's physical health
2. **Depression:** high scorers are marked by feelings of worthlessness, hopelessness, and pessimism
3. **Hysteria:** reflects somatic complaints related to psychological disturbances (psychosomatic problems)
4. **Psychopathic deviancy:** shows a disregard for social and moral standards and emotional shallowness in relationships
5. **Masculinity/femininity:** indicates degree of traditional 'masculine' aggressiveness or 'feminine' sensitivity
6. **Paranoia:** Disproportionate suspiciousness, jealousy or mistrust.
7. **Psychasthenia:** suggests presence of irrational fears (phobias) and compulsive (ritualistic) actions
8. **Schizophrenia:** reflects withdrawal, unusual and bizarre thinking or actions
9. **Hypomania:** suggests emotional excitability, manic moods or behaviour, and excessive activity
10. **Social introversion:** high score indicates a tendency to be socially withdrawn

Fig. 7.19 *MMPI profile*

cedures. The MMPI measures ten major aspects of personality and by comparing a client's profile with that of normal adults, various mental health problems can be identified and used as the basis for therapy.

Critical discussion of approaches to personality

Psychoanalytic approaches to personality have been the subject of much criticism in psychology, notably from devotees of the scientific research paradigm (Wade and Tavris, 1990). They claim that many of the ideas are based on untestable hypotheses and subjective interpretation. The counter argument to that criticism could be made by those subscribing to a more naturalistic research paradigm, in that subjective interpretation is a 'respectable' aspect of the research process, provided certain procedures are followed. Another criticism of this approach is based on the generalisation of findings from client groups in therapy to the population at large. Nevertheless, the psychoanalytic approach to personality has made a useful contribution to our understanding of human behaviour, particularly the study of mental defence mechanisms.

The main criticism of type theories of personality is their oversimplification. For example, we can no doubt all think of people who fit the description of a type A or type B person, but we can think of many more who do not really slot into either category. Another problem of this approach is *stereotyping*, described later in the chapter. However, Cooper and Makin (1983) feel that type theories can be useful so long as the variation between people of different types is larger than the variation between people of the same type. The studies on type and risk of coronary heart disease have also made a useful contribution to the nurse's role in health education/promotion.

Critics of trait approaches claim that they overemphasise the importance of inherited genetic factors as the basis of personality. Social learning theorists argue that insufficient attention has been paid to the reciprocal effect of the environment on the person's manifestation of their traits, which can account for inconsistencies in behaviour. They go on to state that many personality tests measure the stability of the self-concept rather than the stability of traits, the focus of the next section of the chapter.

Self-concept

The self-concept is described by Burns (1982) as having a descriptive and an evaluative element. The descriptive element is often termed the self-picture or self-image, i.e. what people see when they look at themselves. For example, a young woman might describe her figure as good but lacking in muscle tone. The evaluative element is often termed self-esteem, self-worth or self-acceptance, and refers to how people feel about themselves. For example, the young woman just referred to might feel that she needs to tone up her muscles to feel better about herself. This leads to behavioural options; for example, the young woman might take up aerobic classes and light weight training. However, the self-concept is affected by much more than physical attributes, as represented in Fig. 7.20.

It can be seen from Fig. 7.20 that there are several influences on the self-concept. Successful experiences in school are no guarantee of a positive academic self-concept, but they increase the possibility that such will be the case. The extent to which people have rewarding jobs is likely to exert an influence on the self-concept as often demonstrated by the lack of self-esteem of people who have been unemployed for some time. Nurses working in the field of mental health will find that much of their work will be concerned with helping their clients to develop a more positive social and emotional self-concept. Related to this is the effect that disfiguring surgery can have on the self-concept; for example, patients with a stoma or a mastectomy. It can be seen that a knowledge of the self-concept and ways of enhancing a negative self-concept is of prime importance to all health care professionals.

Attention will now be focused on attitudes.

Attitudes

The effects of attitudes are intimately woven into the way a person perceives the world and acts towards it. Our tastes in music, clothes, sport and leisure activities are all touched by our attitudes, as are the types of people whom we prefer for our friends. Attitudes, values and beliefs are related and overlapping **constructs** and their conceptual differences will now be examined.

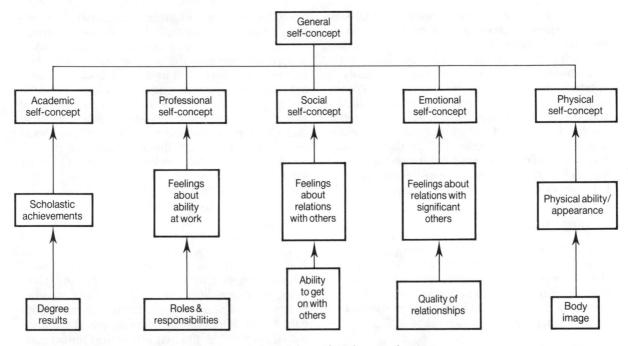

Fig. 7.20 *Organisation of the self-concept (adapted from Shavelson et al. 1976)*

Beliefs

Beliefs are assumptions about the probability that an object exists, possesses certain characteristics, and relates in specific ways to other objects (Scheibe, 1970). They serve as behaviour guides, with or without sensory data to confirm them. They are largely *cognitive* in nature, i.e. pertaining to thinking, knowing and understanding. An example of a belief is, 'Certain micro-organisms can cause meningitis'. There is sensory data to confirm this belief as can be found in any pathology department.

Values

A person's beliefs tell us what he thinks is true, or at least probably true, whereas a person's values tell us what he desires to be true. Values are largely *affective* in nature, i.e. pertaining to emotions or feelings. Allport *et al.* (1960) define a value as a hypothetical construct which tends to stress concepts of ultimately desirable goals or end-states, for example true friendship, individualised patient care, self-determination and freedom of choice. By and large values tend to have an enduring quality.

Attitudes

Gagné (1977) defines an attitude as an internal state that influences the choices of personal action made by an individual. They can have a significant effect on behaviour and tend to be fairly consistent. Figure 7.21 illustrates the three aspects of attitudes and their relationship to beliefs and values.

Although there is much disagreement about the nature of attitudes, it is generally accepted that they exhibit three different aspects. The cognitive component is linked to a person's beliefs, while the affective component is linked to a person's values. Some attitudes rest almost entirely on the cognitive

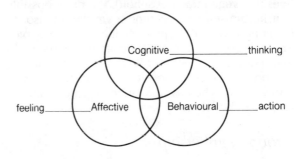

Fig. 7.21 *Three components of attitudes*

component and are based on sound factual arguments, whereas others are based mainly on the affective component and carry emotional impact. The behavioural component is interesting in that an individual's attitudes may not necessarily be inferred correctly from his behaviour. For example, an individual may hold an anti-pollution attitude and yet drive to work daily. The individual knows that exhaust fumes contribute to atmospheric pollution but uses the car daily because it is convenient. Therefore the immediate consequences of our actions can explain discrepancies between our attitudes and our behaviour.

Attitude formation

Reflect for a moment on your own personal attitudes to the following: extra-marital sex; vegetarian diets; ethnic minority groups; soul music. How do you think that you formed those particular attitudes? It is likely that it was due to some of the following six reasons.

Direct contact

Direct contact with the attitude object can be strongly influential in the formation of attitudes. You could develop a strong negative attitude to a particular political party if you have an unpleasant encounter with one or more of the party's members. The relevance for nursing practice is that this could affect a nurse's feelings and actions to patients/clients who belong to any group with whom previous bad experiences are associated.

Interaction with others

Interaction with others, especially people who are held in high regard, is potentially a strong influence on attitude development. If an individual lives in a vegetarian household, it is quite possible that he himself will become a vegetarian also. In the context of nursing practice it is possible to 'pick up' both positive and negative attitudes from one's peer groups and senior colleagues. An example of the former would be a positive attitude to research-mindedness whereas task-oriented care is an example of the latter.

Group membership

An interesting experiment by Schacter (1951) dem-

onstrates the effect of group membership on attitude formation. Schacter formed discussion groups to consider the case of a juvenile delinquent. Most group members took the position that what the boy needed was love, kindness and understanding. Schacter then introduced a 'deviant' into the group. The deviant was in fact a colleague of Schacter, whose role was to adopt a tangential attitudinal position to the majority of the group members and advocate the use of corporal punishment for the juvenile under discussion. Consider for a moment how the group members reacted to the deviant. At first they directed all their comments to him to try to change his attitude to those of the group. If the deviant complied he was gradually accepted by the group, but if he stuck to his original position he was almost totally excluded. The implications of this experiment could be quite far-reaching in a variety of nursing contexts. Consider, for example, the impact of a new member of staff on the ward whose attitudes to nurse education and democratic leadership are at variance with those held by the majority of the clinical staff.

Child-rearing

Parental influence is very powerful in the formation of attitudes. Studies have shown that if both parents belong to the same political party, the chances are that offspring will eventually support the same party. Sadly, though, those who have been victims of child abuse may become abusers of their own children, adopting similar attitudes to those of their parents.

Mass media

Even with over 3 million people currently unemployed, most homes own a television. The government has expressed much concern over the effect of programmes which contain explicit sex and violence on the attitudes of viewers, especially those who are impressionable. Patients and clients may come to departments with attitudes to nurses which have been shaped by television programmes.

Chance conditioning

People often develop strong attitudes toward cities, restaurants, and ethnic groups on the basis of one or two unusually good or bad experiences. Nurses can develop strong attitudes to different special-isms based on either very good or very traumatic experiences during their allocation.

Functions of attitudes

A great deal of experimental and survey data indicates that attitudes are closely interwoven with a person's perceived needs, helping that person towards desired goals (Rosenberg, 1960). Different approaches have been used to categorise attitudinal function; for example Katz's (1960) approach which is given here.

Instrumental function

The instrumental function is linked to social learning theory in that the utility of attitudes lies in obtaining rewards and avoiding punishments. For example, a nurse's attitudes towards her patients will be influenced by working with other nurses, as previously mentioned. The nurse who accepts the norms and values of the group is likely to increase her chances of gaining professional approval, and of being liked and accepted by her colleagues.

Knowledge function

This is based on an individual's need to impose a stable, organised and meaningful structure on the world. Katz proposes that each individual has a need to give adequate structure to the universe, providing a sufficient basis for interpreting much of what is perceived as important for that individual. For example, a nurse will learn about different nursing models and develop both positive and negative attitudes about different models on the basis of a cognitive perspective alone. Those attitudes may change when the nurse has the opportunity to 'test' the different models in action.

Value-expressive function

The value-expressive function is one in which the individual derives satisfaction from expressing attitudes appropriate to personal values. For example, a nurse may openly express humanistic attitudes to AIDS sufferers which gives a positive expression to the central values she holds about nursing. Those values are likely to be based on beneficence

(doing good) and non-maleficence (not doing harm).

Ego-defensive function

The final function of attitudes is ego-defensive, and refers to ways in which attitudes defend our self-image. Menzies (1970) suggested that nurses as a social group use defensive techniques in order to alleviate the anxiety that is engendered by their close contact with suffering. Nurses learn to 'distance' themselves emotionally from patients because the need to protect themselves from more anxiety is high.

Attitudes and clinical practice

It is important both for nurses and for their clients to recognise their existing attitudes about issues which are relevant to them. This can be done by personal reflection and by discussing those attitudes with friends or colleagues. For example, the author suggests that regular ward-based discussions should take place between all grades of medical and nursing staff about the policies that guide practice in that setting.

Nurses should also be aware of the different attitudes that may be held by different ethnic groups. For example, Chinese Americans and also Filipinos tend to view mental illness as a stigma on the family name and may only seek professional help when the family can no longer cope with the problem.

Inappropriate attitudes can militate against the delivery of effective care. For example, the nurse who adopts a moralistic, judgemental attitude to clients who have been admitted with alcohol or drug abuse problems might have difficulty understanding how individual factors have contributed to the client's behaviour. Nurses need to assess the client's and his family's attitudes towards the substance abuse problem so that appropriate treatment can be implemented on an individual basis. Readers are reminded of the potency of social learning theory discussed above, and should model those attitudes that are appropriate for delivery of care on an individualised, non-judgemental basis. It is highly desirable that nurses develop attitudes which will assist them to gain the cooperation and trust of their patients, and which will ensure that they conduct their professional work with responsibility.

Person perception

Many psychologists argue that social behaviour is determined more by the situation in which a person finds himself than by the relatively enduring traits/characteristics of that individual. Another polarised view purports that behaviour arises predominantly from structured dispositions (traits) within the individual. Proponents of the two viewpoints have been able to muster a significant amount of evidence to support their respective positions but careful reflection is likely to suggest that there is merit in the reconciliation of both (as with the behavioural and cognitive views of learning discussed earlier). Reconciliation allows for both predispositional and situational variables to account for behaviour in social situations. The way a patient behaves in hospital is going to be influenced by his personality and his past experiences of hospitals, and this will have an effect on the nurse's impressions of him and vice versa. This leads on to a consideration of what person perception actually is, the factors that influence our judgements, and the reasons for inaccuracies in person perception.

Person perception focuses on the process by which impressions, opinions or feelings about other people are formed. In other words, it is the forming of judgements about people which influences a person's thoughts, feelings and actions towards the person perceived. It includes subjective judgements that go beyond direct sensory. When admitting a patient or interacting with a client for the first (and indeed subsequent) time, nurses will make both static and dynamic judgements about that person. *Static judgements* refer to the relatively enduring or continuous aspects of the person – for example, their ethnic background, socio-economic status, political orientation, intelligence, and personality traits. *Dynamic judgements* refer to the relatively transitory aspects of a person that can change readily and rapidly in response to stimuli from the environment – for example, facial expression, speech and body position. The kinds of judgements that are made can elicit certain responses and affect the judgements made about the nurse. This is known in social psychology as the *reciprocal effect*. Modes of perception will vary between individuals and be influenced further by the amount of information available, the degree of interaction, and the extent to which the relationship between them is well-established or not, as the case may be.

Secord and Backman (1964) describe in detail the factors that influence our judgements, of which some will now be outlined.

Assimilation effect

This refers to the tendency to regard other people's opinions as more like our own than they really are. It can be compared with the *contrast effect* which is the tendency to regard other people's opinions as less like our own than they actually are.

Primacy effect

This is the tendency to make judgements on the basis of first impressions and more or less avoid changing those first impressions. This has implications when admitting patients or interviewing clients in the community for the first time. It should of course be remembered that the first impressions made by nursing staff will also be subject to the primacy effect in the minds of patients and clients.

Concern with particular traits

As individuals we tend to value some traits more highly than others – for example warmth, cleanliness and honesty. The tendency is then to judge others on the extent to which those individuals possess those traits. This has important implications in the context of nursing management when staff are being assessed on their performance. A corollary of this is the *halo effect*, which is the tendency to bias our perception of another person in the direction of one particular trait that we particularly like or dislike.

Stereotyping

This is the tendency to assign certain traits to particular groups in society and to assume that all members of that group share those traits. For example, studies have shown that Italians are more likely to express pain vocally than most white Americans. A nurse who is responsible for the care of a patient of Italian background might conclude that if the patient is silent he is not feeling any pain, but such a stereotype may bear no resemblance to reality (Potter and Perry, 1985).

This short discussion about some of the factors that influence the judgements we make about people leads on to a brief consideration about inaccuracies in person perception. Research from the field of social psychology suggests that our interpersonal perceptions are often erroneous, especially when we are forming judgements about people who are different from ourselves. The reasons are multifarious and some will now receive brief attention.

Unexpressive people

If there is little data on which to make a judgement, perhaps it is more likely that perceivers will 'fall victim' to the points already made, for example assimilation, contrast and primacy effects, coupled with implicit personality theory. This is important in any practice setting but perhaps especially so in the fields of mental and community health.

Inconsistent behaviour

Evaluation and prediction can become difficult if people vary their behaviour widely in different settings. Again with mental health and the community in mind, clients can adopt inconsistent behaviour, especially if they seek acceptance from diverse groups – adolescent substance abusers, for example.

Concreteness in perception

Individuals who tend to perceive situations in simplistic/dualistic terms (for example, good/bad) tend to transfer this to social perception. It is worth considering the 'shades of grey' that occur across a range of situations and being more reflective when making judgements about people.

Mental defence mechanisms

Mental defence mechanisms, referred to earlier, are techniques used to avoid, deny, or distort sources of anxiety (Coon, 1986). If nurses feel guilty about their dislike of a colleague or patient they may in fact complain that it is they who are the subject of dislike. The fact that these attitudes are projected onto others may in turn affect their behaviour in reciprocity.

Assumed similarity

This is the tendency to see other people as 'one of us'. The corollary is that we then think that those individuals will think and act like us. This can lead to problems in relationships when in fact they act contrary to our expectations.

As nurses are constantly required to assess patients/clients in a variety of contexts, both institutional and community, it is proposed that a knowledge of personality, attitudes and person perception will inform their judgements about people. Communication is likely to proceed more smoothly and effectively if perceptions of others are more consonant with reality.

We will now make an examination of the relationship between studies in social interaction and therapeutic behaviour in nursing practice and health care.

Social interaction

It is suggested that the process of assessing, planning, implementing and evaluating individualised care in a variety of practice settings requires at least the following: problem-solving skills, a sound knowledge base, and skills in social interaction. A problem-solving model has been described earlier in the section on learning from a cognitive perspective.

It is the responsibility of every nurse to ensure that she has an up-to-date knowledge of subject matter, especially that which is pertinent to her particular specialism.

With the advent of a more individualised approach to care, the importance of skills in social interaction cannot be overemphasised.

Social interaction is not a clearly defined area in social psychology, and has been researched from several different perspectives. In the following discussion, social interaction will presume verbal and non-verbal communication in the context of therapeutic behaviour. Three different models of social interaction will be examined, and their relevance for nursing practice and health care assessed.

Exchange theory

In their formulation of exchange theory as a model of social interaction, Thibaut and Kelley (1959) emphasise the reinforcement value of social behaviour. An individual's social behaviour is not merely seen as the stimulus for another's response, but is directed towards achieving self-reinforcement. Exchange theory focuses on the rewards to be gained during interaction. Interaction viewed in this manner can be represented as an exchange matrix (for example, Fig. 7.22 portrays a hypothetical matrix for a nurse-client interaction). At any one stage in a nurse-client interaction it is assumed that there is a repertoire of possible behaviours in which each can engage. The repertoire of behaviours is likely to offer differing degrees of satisfaction or reinforcement to the nurse and client respectively, and is represented numerically as *reward units* in the matrix. These reward units or satisfactions include psychological reinforcements such as feelings of security and increased self-esteem. If Fig. 7.22 is used to represent a health visitor interacting with a mother in the community who is worried about child-rearing, the nurse's and client's possible repertoire of behaviours are represented as N1, N2, C1 and C2. It can be seen from the matrix that the exchange N2 + C1 offers the highest degree of mutual satisfaction with 11 and 12 reward units respectively. That particular exchange could be characterised by the mother being encouraged to air her worries and concerns about child care, without being made to feel silly and incompetent. The client is reinforced by being reassured and gaining additional information. The nurse can in turn gain satisfaction from the manner in which she facilitated the interaction and from the opportunity to use her knowledge and expertise. It is important to note that each person's rewards depend not only on what that person does, but also on what the other person does at the same time. It can be seen from exchange N1 + C2 that the exchange was less rewarding for both participants, as they gained only five and three reward units respectively. Perhaps in that instance the nurse was more directive and less facilitative, and the mother more inhibited in her response. Reward units are therefore *mutually contingent*, dependent on each other.

Exchange matrices are used by social psychologists to conceptualise and analyse the characteristics of an encounter. Readers may wish to reflect for a moment on recent exchanges with clients and colleagues, and consider the degree of satisfaction obtained by each participant in terms of an exchange matrix.

Exchange matrices reveal not only the likely outcome of an encounter (for example, the nurse/client satisfaction or dissatisfaction) but also something about the relationship between the participants. They can indicate whether there is a conflict of interests and which of the two is in the position of greater social power.

The most useful feature of the exchange theory approach is that it draws attention to the rewarding qualities which one person's behaviour may have for another. Several nurse researchers have shown how the provision of adequate information can result in a reduction of patient anxiety (Boore, 1978; Webb and Wilson-Barnett, 1983) and lower level of dependence on post-operative analgesia (Hayward, 1975). The exchange theory perspective suggests that the giving and receiving of information is rewarding for both nurse and client. The resultant reduction in anxiety is also mutually rewarding – psychologically for the nurse and both psychologically and physiologically for the client.

The social skill model

This model compares the development of skills in social interaction with the development of proficiency in psychomotor skills. Argyle (1972) extended a five-characteristic model of a motor skill to encompass the more complex interactive processes involved in a social encounter.

Argyle is the most prominent British social psychologist associated with the social skill model (Argyle, 1972; 1973; 1987). However, Fitts and Posner's (1967) three stage model of motor skill acquisition can also be adapted to learning and developing skills in social interaction.

Nurse's possible actions

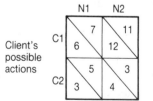

Possible exchanges:

N1 + C1 = 7 + 6 Reward Units
N1 + C2 = 5 + 3   *"*   *"*
N2 + C1 = 11 + 12 *"*   *"*
N2 + C2 = 3 + 4   *"*   *"*

Fig. 7.22 *Nurse–client exchange matrix*

Fitts and Posner's model comprises three stages: the cognitive phase, the associative phase, and the autonomous phase. During the cognitive phase, a person grasps the nature of the skill and establishes a plan by identifying and sequencing motor sub-routines. For example, to take and record a patient's blood pressure a nurse needs to know the order of sub-routines (position the cuff correctly on the arm; locate the pulse in the ante-cubital fossa; blow up the cuff, etc.). In terms of developing skills in social interaction, a nurse needs to learn sets of responses appropriate to different situations; for example, a district nurse in the community is likely to be involved in a chain of exposition, pausing, asking and fielding questions when explaining to a diabetic patient how to balance diet, exercise and insulin. During the associative phase of motor skill acquisition, the nurse practises her skills (for example, taking blood pressures, gaining feed-

back, and developing motor coordination). When developing social skills, too, it is important to practise and, through feedback, to develop interactive coordination, when taking patient histories for example.

During the autonomous phase of motor skill action the nurse becomes proficient at that particular skill. For example, she can perform the task with smoothness, timing, precision, dexterity and economy of action. In the context of social skills, a nurse who has reached the autonomous phase will be able to interact with *perceptual sensitivity* (i.e. with a consciousness of verbal and non-verbal cues), in a rewarding manner (i.e. with warmth), with sensitive use of appropriate vocabulary, and with poise. The acquisition of motor skills is compared with the development of social skills using Fitts and Posner's model in Fig. 7.23.

The social skill model as a way of concep-

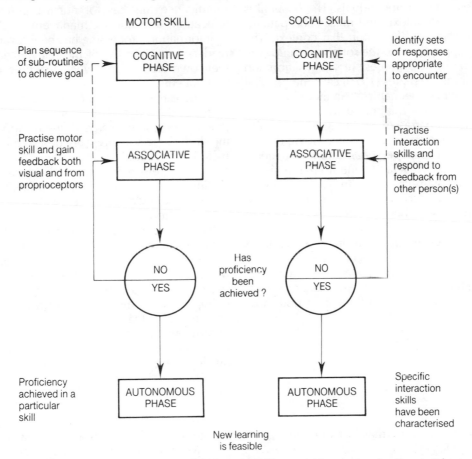

Fig. 7.23 *Application of Fitts and Posner's model of motor skill acquisition to developing social interaction skills (adapted from Myles, 1987)*

tualising the process of social interaction is compatible with exchange theory in spite of the differences. Exchange theory focuses on rewards and relationships whereas the social skill model provides us with a 'conceptual map' of social behaviour (Argyle, 1972). Argyle's model has led to the development of training techniques to improve individuals' social skills, and he is responsible for the setting up of the social skills training unit at Littlemore Hospital, Oxford.

The dramaturgical approach

Several theorists have drawn an analogy between social interaction and theatrical drama (Goffman, 1971; Milgram, 1974). This particular approach focuses on the way people define the situation in which they find themselves. It draws attention to the context of the social interaction and the role relationships between individuals. The hospital is an example of a context, and nurses and patients have a role relationship within that context. The behaviours appropriate to the roles we occupy are learned as part of the process of socialisation and specific training. Menzies (1970) calls the hospital culture a 'defence mechanism', in that close contact with patients is minimised to safeguard the nurse against embarrassment. She gives examples of warm, humane social interaction being denied by task allocation, ***depersonalisation*** of patients and nurses, and a detachment from emotional stress caused by relations with patients. Every nurse then has a responsibility to ensure that the sort of culture described by Menzies is not pervasive today.

The dramaturgical approach draws attention to the context of social interaction, and it is argued that often two-way communication should exist between all those involved in health care provision for therapeutic behaviour to flourish in both hospital and community settings.

Conclusions

In this chapter the origins and nature of psychological enquiry have been explored briefly. Reference has been made to some of the specialisms within psychology, including clinical, educational and social psychology, which should be of particular interest to nurses. The scope of psychological research is now vast and therefore it has been possible to select only some of those areas for discussion, but the areas covered in this chapter have been chosen for their particular relevance to nursing practice. The nature of learning has been explored from a behaviourist, cognitive and social learning perspective. Readers are reminded of the potency of reinforcement by role models and the significance this has for nursing practice, nurse education, and nursing management. The nature of information processing has been examined and readers are reminded of the relevance of this for their own studies and when teaching colleagues and patients.

Three different approaches to motivation were then considered and their relevance for nursing practice explored. Three different approaches to the study of personality were described which also included an examination of the self-concept, attitudes, and person perception. This is an important section since health care is about people, and an increased knowledge of the psychology of personality can inform and enhance the process of caring. The chapter concluded with an exploration of how different models of social interaction provide frameworks for discussing communication between the providers of health care and their clients.

Theory can both inform and enrich practice. It is hoped that some of the issues covered in this chapter will at least partially achieve the objective of providing readers with an overview of the ways in which psychology can inform and enrich nursing practice and health care.

Glossary

Agoraphobia: An abnormal fear of open spaces or public places

Arachnophobia: An abnormal fear of spiders

Behavioural objectives: Clear and unambiguous statements about what a student will be able to do following a learning experience

Behaviourism: The school of psychology that emphasises the study of overt behaviour

Childhood autism: A severe childhood disorder characterised by mute behaviour, tantrums, self-absorption, fantasy, and a disregard of external reality

Classical conditioning: Reflexive responses are attached to new stimuli by pairing the new stimuli with stimuli that naturally elicit the response

Cognitive dissonance: A state of disequilibrium which occurs when a person's beliefs/values are inconsistent with their behaviour

Conditioned reflex: In classical conditioning, this is a learned response that becomes attached to a conditioned stimulus

Construct: An explanatory concept not directly observable but inferred from observable events

Curriculum: A course of study to be followed

Depersonalisation: Individual differences between people are denied – for example, in a hospital culture characterised by depersonalisation, patients are referred to in impersonal terms

Ergonomics: The study of the relationship between workers and their working environment

Hyperactive: Extremely or abnormally active

Intervening variable: Any characteristic, quality or attribute which may affect postulated causal relationships between other variables

Introspection: A psychological technique used to examine one's own conscious experience through the exploration of personal thoughts, feelings and sensations

Monophobic states: States of fear evoked by specific circumstances (for example, fear of dogs, fear of cats)

Neuroses: Behaviour disturbances primarily characterised by excessive anxiety and subjective discomfort

Operant conditioning: The strengthening of a response by a reinforcing stimulus if, and only if, that response occurs

Peristaltic tumour: A visible gastric peristalsis following ingestion – in someone suffering from *pyloric stenosis*

Prophylactic analgesia: Pain-killing drugs given in anticipation of a painful experience

Proprioceptors: Receptors located on muscle spindles, tendons, joints, and in the vestibular apparatus which give awareness and information as to the position and movement of a joint or part of the body

Psychomotor skills: Manipulative skills that require the coordination of sensory stimuli to effect purposeful movements

Pyloric stenosis: Narrowing of the pyloric sphincter

Reinforcement: Any stimulus that brings about learning or increases the frequency of a response; a reward

Self-regulatory processes: In social learning theory, these refer to self-imposed standards and rules adopted by individuals for regulating their behaviour, comprising self-administered rewards and sanctions for success and failure respectively

Tolerance: The increasing resistance to a drug's effects that occurs with continued use

Ventricular arrhythmias: Disturbances in the ventricular action of the heart

Vicarious learning: In social learning theory, this refers to learning by observing the behaviour of others and noting the consequences of that behaviour

References

Allport, G.W. (1960). *Manual. Study of Values* (3rd ed.). Houghton Mifflin, Boston.

Argyle, M. (1972). *The Psychology of Interpersonal Behaviour* (2nd ed.). Penguin Books, Harmondsworth.

Argyle, M. (1973). *Social Encounters*. Penguin Books, Harmondsworth.

Argyle, M. (1987). *The Psychology of Interpersonal Behaviour* (4th ed.). Penguin Books, Harmondsworth.

Ashworth, P. (1979). Sensory input and altered consciousness. *Nursing*, 1(8), 350.

Atkinson, R.L., Atkinson, R.C., Smith, E.E., Bem, D.J. and Hilgard, E. (1990). *Introduction to Psychology* (10th ed.). Harcourt Brace Jovanovich, San Diego.

Bandura, A., Ross, D. and Ross, S.A. (1963). Vicarious reinforcement and imitative learning. *Journal of Abnormal and Social Psychology*, 67, 601–607.

Biehler, R.F. and Snowman, J. (1982). *Psychology Applied to Teaching*. Houghton Mifflin, Boston.

Boore, J.R.P. (1978). *Prescription for Recovery*. RCN, London.

Burns, R. (1982). *Self-Concept Development and Education*. Holt, London.

Burtt, H.E. (1941). An experimental study of early childhood memory. *Journal of General Psychology*, 58, 435–439.

Cattell, R.B. (1973). Personality pinned down. *Psychology Today*, 7, 40–46.

Child, D. (1986). *Psychology and the Teacher* (4th ed.). Cassell, London.

Clancy, L. (1981). *Essays in the Psychology and Sociology of Education*. New Horizon, Bognor Regis.

Clark, E. and Keeble, S. (1990). *Introduction to Psychology*. Distance Learning Centre, South Bank Polytechnic, London.

Clarke, M. (1980). A sense of perception. *Nursing Mirror*, June 12, 41–43.

Coon, D. (1986). *Introduction to Psychology* (4th ed.). West, St Paul.

Cooper, L. and Makin, P. (1983). *Psychology for Managers*. Macmillan, Basingstoke.

de Tornyay, R. and Thompson, M.A. (1987). *Strategies for Teaching Nursing* (3rd ed.). John Wiley and Sons, New York.

Erickson, H.C. (1983). *Modeling and Role Modeling: A Theory and Paradigm for Nursing*. Prentice-Hall International, New Jersey.

Eysenck, H.J. and Eysenck, S.B.G. (1963). *The Eysenck Personality Inventory*. University of London Press, London.

Fitts, P.M. and Posner, M.I. (1967). *Human Performance*. Prentice-Hall International, New Jersey.

Fox, D.J. (1975). *Fundamentals of Research in Nursing* (4th ed.). Appleton Century Crofts, New York.

Fretwell, J.E. (1982). *Ward Teaching and Learning: Sister and The Learning Environment*. RCN, London.

Friedman, M.D. and Rosenman, R.H. (1974). *Type A Behaviour and Your Heart*. Knopf, New York.

Gagné, R. (1977). *The Conditions of Learning* (3rd ed.). Holt Rinehart and Winston, New York.

Goffman, E. (1971). *Relations in Public*. Allen Lane, London.

Haber, R.N. (1970). How we remember what we see. *Scientific American*, May, 104–112.

Hamner, W.C. and Organ, D.W. (1978). *Organisational Behaviour: An Applied Psychological Approach*. Business Publications Inc., Dallas.

Hayward, J. (1975). *Information – A Prescription Against Pain*. RCN, London.

Herzberg, F. (1966). *Work and The Nature of Man*. World Publishing, Cleveland.

Hyland, M.E. and Donaldson, M. (1989). *Psychological Care in Nursing Practice*. Scutari, Harrow.

James, D.E. (1970). *Introduction to Psychology*. Panther, St Albans.

Katz, D. (1960). The functional approach to the study of attitudes. *Public Opinion Quarterly*, 24, 163–204.

Lindsay, P.H. and Norman, D.A. (1977). *Human Information Processing* (2nd ed.). Academic Press, New York.

Locke, E.A. (1976). The nature and causes of job satisfaction. In *Handbook of Industrial and Organisational Psychology*, Dunnette, M.D. (ed.). Rand McNally, Chicago.

Maslow, A. (1970). *Motivation and Personality* (2nd ed.). Harper and Row, New York.

Menzies, I. (1970). *Defence Systems as Control Against Anxiety*. Tavistock Publications, London.

Milgram, S. (1974). *Obedience to Authority: An Experimental View*. Tavistock Publications, London.

Myles, A.P. (1987). Psychology. In *The Curriculum in Nursing Education*, Allen, P. and Jolley, M. (eds.). Croom Helm, Kent.

Myles, A.P. (1991). Curriculum pathways to Project 2000. In *Nursing: A Knowledge Base for Practice*. Perry, A. and Jolley, M. (eds.). Edward Arnold, London.

Payne, R. (1983). Organisational behaviour. In Cooper and Makin (1983), above.

Postman, L. (1969). Experimental analysis of learning to learn. In *The Psychology of Learning and Motivation*, Bower, G.H. and Spence, J.T. (eds.). Academic Press, New York.

Potter, P.A. and Perry, A.G. (1985). *Fundamentals of Nursing*. Mosby, St Louis.

Rosenberg, M.J. (1960). An analysis of affective-cognitive consistency. In *Attitude Organisation and Change*, Rosenberg, I. and Rosenberg, M.J. (eds.). Yale University Press, New Haven.

Schacter, S. (1951). Deviation, rejection and communication. *Journal of Abnormal and Social Psychology*, 46, 190–207.

Scheibe, K.E. (1970). *Beliefs and Values*. Holt Rinehart and Winston, New York.

Secord, P.F. and Backman, C.W. (1964). *Social Psychology*. McGraw-Hill, Tokyo.

Shavelson, R.J., Hubner, J.J. and Stanton, G.C. (1976). Self-concept: validation of construct interpretation. *Review of Educational Research*, 46, 407–442.

Thibaut, J.W. and Kelley, H.H. (1959). *The Social Psychology of Groups*, John Wiley and Sons, New York.

Wade, C. and Tavris, C. (1990). *Psychology* (2nd ed.). Harper and Row, New York.

Webb, C. and Wilson-Barnett, J. (1983). Hysterectomy: a study in coping with recovery. *Journal of Advanced Nursing*, 8, 311–319.

Woolfolk, A.E. and Nicolich, M.L. (1984). *Educational Psychology for Teachers* (2nd ed.). Prentice-Hall International, New Jersey.

Suggestions for further reading

Broome, A. (ed.) (1989). *Health Psychology: Processes and Applications*. Chapman and Hall, London.

Burnard, P. (1990). *Learning Human Skills: A Guide for Nurses* (2nd ed.). Heinemann, London.

The Open University Press. *D305, Blocks 10 and 12*. (Very good coverage of attitudes and social interaction respectively.)

Kagan, C.M. (1985). *Interpersonal Skills in Nursing*. Croom Helm, Kent.

Sundeen, S.J., Stuart, G., Rankin, E. and Cohen, S. (1989). *Nurse-Client Interaction: Implementing the Nursing Process* (4th ed.). Mosby, St Louis.

8

COMMUNICATING FOR HEALTH

Paul Barber

'I fall far short of achieving real communication – person-to-person – all the time, but moving in this direction makes life for me a warm, exciting, upsetting, troubling, satisfying, enriching, and above all a worthwhile venture'

(Rogers *et al.*, 1967; page 275)

This chapter constitutes a philosophical and practical exploration of the following themes:

- How the individual, their attitudes and emotional presence manifest themselves in communication

- Health, what this means and how it informs care communication

- The relationship of personal development to the 'art of communication'

- Intervention analysis, and how we might set about indentifying our own communication style

- Professional supervision, and how this can be structured to develop further your ability to demonstrate care through communication

Periodically throughout this chapter I offer a critique of professional practice and have set activities entitled 'reflections' to stimulate you into questioning your own clinical practice and professional traditions.

'What is wrong is not the great discoveries of science – information is always better than ignorance, no matter what information or what ignorance. What is wrong is the belief behind the information, the belief that information will change the world. It won't. Information without human understanding is like an answer without a question – meaningless. And human understanding is only possible through the arts. It is the work of art that creates the human perspective in which information turns to truth . . .'

(Archbishop MacLeish; quoted in BBC radio broadcast, 1991)

This chapter is not about how to communicate. It does not attempt to change you and I doubt if I can teach you anything new. What I am attempting to do is to share with you, to inform you how I view the world and to ask you to consider how my understanding might add to yours. My information is the creation of all those I have known, bits of values and perceptions we created together which have since stuck to me. In each new relationship I discover a new part of me. As I have frequented the company of carers for some 20 odd years, much has stuck. In sharing my information here, I hope you will now run with it, shift it around a bit, throw out the parts you can't use and create something worthwhile from the bits you can.

In this chapter I attempt to say a little about what for me makes for good communication. As I believe we communicate who and what we are in all we do, and because I see the world largely through humanistic spectacles, I emphasise the part personal development plays in communication. Having been bored to death by books that try to reduce communication to a science, I emphasise the 'art' of communication and the role intuition plays in this, In order to provide a framework for self-appraisal, I have also included something on intervention analysis which is less a science than a means of self-assessment and a clarifier of communicative intention, along with occasional activities called 'reflections' so that you can apply insights from this chapter to yourself and to clinical practice. Lastly, I have included a little on supervision as an example of how you might further develop your ability to demonstrate care through communication.

Where possible, I also offer a critique of nursing practice and professionalism so as to heighten your own questioning of what you do:

'Traditions are a splendid thing; but we should create traditions, not live by them'
(Franz Marc, in Rogers *et al.*, 1967; page 115)

Demonstrate that you can share of yourself, show understanding of your own internal processes and show that you are able to communicate this to others, and as long as you have ability to ask for and receive care yourself, I will have little doubt in your skills to communicate care for others.

Communication: core qualities and definitions

'Knowledge is a function of being. When there is a change in the being of the knower, there is a corresponding change in the nature and amount of knowledge'
(Aldous Huxley, in Goldberg, 1989; page 135)

Professional development and personal development rest one upon the other. Because care com-munication is an expression of self, professional helpers need to stay alert as to how they as individuals offer support to their clients and value the human condition. In short, how they practise the caring arts. At the last analysis the carer's therapeutic use of self underpins care communication.

In essence, I believe nursing care is about creating a relationship with the client whereby they begin to heal themselves. For this to happen within the nurse-client relationship, contact, change and communication must be related.

Contact involves the direction of attention, perception, receptivity and empathy towards another. This requires us to let go of our preconceptions and open up ourselves to the enquiry of others. In short, we need to clear and clean the psychological window through which we view the world. Good contact occurs when two people are able to explore each other's reality, see the other and listen to the whole of them – while engaging in turn with the whole of themselves. In the Chinese character that represents 'listening', the heart is also portrayed. When I am fully attuned to another, it is as if I meditate upon them while allowing my mind, senses, feelings and intuitions to form an integral 'sense' of them. My listening, to be effective, must have heart.

Change concerns letting go of the past, exploring the present and risking the future. It involves treating life experimentally and having courage, courage to face up to what does not work in your life and to let old patterns go. As Kierkegaard remarks:

'Life can only be understood backwards; but it must be lived forwards'
(Kierkegaard, in Rogers *et al.*, 1967; page 167)

For us to live our life in a forward way and to engage the reality of that continuum we call 'health', we must learn to make 'change' a friend, for change is essential to health. Health is not an absence of physical or of mental dis-ease, nor the experience of continuous physical and mental well-being. It is rather all of these; an ability to move fluidly from one state of being to another. Health is thus an endless flow of changes (Young, 1990).

Communication is about sharing and self-understanding. If we have not yet begun to understand ourselves – what of ourselves can we share? Practice is important to communicate efficiently;

being aware of those complicated experiences that resonate in our inner world and finding words to express this is essential if communication is to have effect:

> 'I reject any organized pretence to an objective knowledge of man. I know only what I sweat from my own personal struggle to stay alive. Psychotherapy is not a professional routine. It is a personal venture. The client is "like me". I reject any professional boundary between us. I "make it" as a person or I fail'
> (Richard Johnson, in Rogers *et al.*, 1967; page 67)

Good communication, I find, is able to transmit the intimate reality of one person to another, develops a channel along which trust and understanding flow, is relevant to what is happening now, and evokes the creative energy of those involved.

Besides being core ingredients of the care relationship, contact, change and communication are the goals of nurse-client interaction and criteria of health.

Health: a definition

> 'He [the infant] would laugh at our concern over values, if he could understand it. How could anyone fail to know what he liked or disliked, what was good for him and what was not?'
> (Barry Stevens, in Rogers *et al.*, 1967; page 29)

Health, in this chapter, is regarded as a positive quality of well-being, the ability to move in the direction of self-actualisation, to take creative risks and trust in yourself. It is seen to require personal and interpersonal competency. Health is thus an adventure, a state of mind where problems are seen as challenges, symptoms are guides to our lifestyle, and emotions are energies we engage through the act of living. Health is thus the search after our own fullness of being and our ability to relate this to others. In this context, pre-occupation with health is not healthy. Health is not a medicated condition nor the building of sanitised defences against the world – this is nearer a fight for survival. Health is an ability to adapt, risk, and to welcome change, rather than a concept to be defined. Health is dynamic; to hold it still long enough for definition is to kill it.

Simply, health is for the joy of it – the creative energy underpinning our ability to grow.

Personally, I feel much of health education has remained all too mechanical and tended towards:

- servicing the body machine;
- knowing the best foods to feed it;
- knowing how best to keep it clean;
- preventing bad habits or curing ill health.

This cognitive, task-orientated approach to health leaves little room for emotional, intuitive or spiritual components of care. The individual's potential for 'personal growth' has all too often played but a little part in modern care practices.

Generally, health education has looked at the tasks but missed the processes. The caring professions often echo this, controlling the care environment rather than enriching the individual's potential. Concentration upon disfunction by carers has tended to lead to client care being seen as problematic. It is not by accident that nursing models which emphasise systematic problem solving and task performance have displaced models which attend more centrally to the therapeutic relationship. This is a comment on our professional times and their bias towards a pseudo-scientific rationale.

Communicating with the self: the role of personal growth

> 'The only dimension of life over which you have limited control is the length. By putting your attention on what you do to extend your life, you can utilize the potential you have for its duration. But be aware that every day you control the depth and width of your experience, your life'
> (Benares, 1985; page 64)

Much of nursing care, though it may be task-centred, involves intuitive nurturing and a good deal of self-investment. Because care has more to do with quality than quantity, i.e. what transpires being generally more important than how often it happens, care communication depends more than anything else upon the nature of the nurse-client relationship. Because it is primarily an art, care communication may all too often be professionally labelled as unscientific and undefinable. When they step out from their role of a 'hands-on' practitioner into the cold light of professional assessment alongside other professionals, many expert nursing practitioners find it difficult to convey what they do.

Traditionally, nurses were not taught the appropriate language to decode interpersonal behaviour – much of which is intuitive – into intellectual terms. The essence of what constitutes care in professional communication has thus tended to be lost.

Although Project 2000 has recommended an injection of a good deal of science and cognition into care practice in order to remedy role insecurity, the expressive arts of care, which are hard to reference, have tended to remain in the hearts of expert carers. Theories can be taught; attitudes need to be experienced and lived.

When a person moves more fluidly between the external universe and the internal one within themselves, they acquire increased self-understanding and are better equipped to communicate and liberate insight in others.

Personally, I view myself as an evolving organism who, by application of will and consciousness, has the potential to grow in any direction. This potential I see as limited by the choices I allow myself, by what I decide are the fixed boundaries of my behaviour, and by the cultural reality I personally ascribe to. I increase or decrease myself via the tightness of these symbolic boundaries I impose upon myself.

This is expressed figuratively in the box opposite.

When I start to explore, question and define 'who I am', 'what I do' and 'where I am going', I begin to draw boundaries around myself. The wider I draw these boundaries, the more options I allow myself. The wider I draw my personal boundaries, the richer my potential life experience and personal range.

'Personal growth' can now be seen as an extra, formed from and upon the evolving edge of experience. It is what we gain when we push our boundaries of self a little further out, risk stepping beyond convention – without causing harm to ourselves or others – and when we allow ourselves to experience a little growing pain.

WHO I AM

I   My individual self, a continually moving, evolving and changing sense of identity which I invest in my personality, an individually created persona through which I express my consciousness.

↓

WHAT I DO

Culture   The medium through which I relate to others, a source of containment and safety, a boundary and provider of language and social reality, the media through which I express myself.

↓

WHERE I AM GOING

Personal growth   The positive dovetailing of myself with my social reality so as to maximise my integration with the whole, my relationship with life, my joyful expression of health, spiritual aspirations and acceptance of universal laws: the seasons, birth, a time to live and a time to die.

Developing the self so as to enhance communication

'What's to say? I have a feeling that everybody knows everything so far as human interaction goes, and that we only choose to ignore or to forget'

(Shlien, in Rogers *et al.*, 1967; page 275)

I believe at the last analysis it is the quality of the person, rather than their skills, that elevates professional communication to excellence of care. Such qualities of person do not arise spontaneously from within; they are rather the product of a good deal of uncovering, self-exploration, personal reflection and intrapersonal development. Personal growth and professional development here go hand in hand.

Care communication does not really concern itself with training, nor with moulding or teaching the client what to do nor how to do it. This is nearer propaganda. A truly proficient care communicator would never dream of imposing their process upon a client or inducing them towards imitation of themselves. Care communication is more to do with unfolding. It is directed towards enabling a client to recover themselves so that they may further self-explore with a view to knowing themselves better.

When we turn to Carl Rogers (1983) for guidance as to what we need in order to be more appreciative, self-aware, socially sensitive and valuing of others as communicators of care, he suggests that we need to move away from:

- facades, pretence and putting up a front;
- rigid concepts of 'what ought to be';
- meeting the expectations of others for the sake of 'having to please';
- pretence and the hiding of feelings;

And that we should seek within to gain greater:

- self-direction;
- positive feelings towards oneself;
- sensitivity to external events;
- openness with regard to our inner reactions and feelings.

I have observed that when we acquire these qualities in ourselves, other subtle effects emerge which in turn affect others. We have less need to defend our routines or impose our beliefs, and develop greater tolerance towards the failings of those around us. As we become sensitive to our own inner (intrapersonal) process, we find we can better listen and attend to the inner world of those around us. Good contact and communication with others we find to be nourishing, and in realising this begin to value deep, honest and communicative relationships the more. At this stage superficial relations are no longer satisfying and we begin to move even further in the direction of sharing our emotions and inner experiences. This is essential for carers; if you are unable to share or honour your own emotional life or experiential depth, how can you value the same in others let alone help them acquire health? Movement in the direction suggested describes 'personal growth' and this, I suggest, is indicative of psychological health.

Overconformity often blinds us and stills our questioning, suffocating our potential for growth. Almost as a reflex we may find ourselves – as care professionals – blindly conforming to what appears to be 'the one right way'; nothing kills personal potential or growth as quickly as this. Compulsive behaviour tends towards rigidity, is repetitive and largely unaware. It is the antithesis of growth.

Many of us feel overburdened and clogged up with a host of 'shoulds' and 'musts' picked up in childhood. Professional education all too often adds more to the list. Eventually, if we aren't careful, we spend more time nursing institutional systems rather than our clients.

Changing prevailing patterns of doing things is not easy. Sometimes we come to believe, rather irrationally, that if we step out of line we will be cast out and denied love. This fear of rejection – a relic of the child within us – does much to keep us chained. We forget that by the act of being alive we have the right to be seen, to be heard, to be free, to be loved and respected; these need not be earned.

I know that I experience 'growth' when I step outside the tried and tested, the known parts of me, out beyond my usual personal boundaries, when I risk feeling uncomfortable, embarrassed and shy. Personal growth is comparable to a behavioural spiral which forever strives to conquer more of our experienced reality.

In order for us to 'grow', what is necessary, I would suggest, is an ability to move beyond our present world view, to see things differently and to extend our own personal boundaries. This requires us to forsake the 'known', to step beyond our usual behaviour patterns and engage an unfamiliar world.

Consider, for example, phases of the experiential learning cycle in the model below:

Unconscious incompetence

At this phase of the learning cycle, we are unaware of what it is we don't know; here ignorance is bliss and we have little incentive to engage in new activity and learning.

During this stage we might say to ourselves: 'I'm fine as I am. Why change things? It would not be me if I were to do things differently'. Often we need to be confronted with our blindness by others, if we are to move beyond this point.

Conscious incompetence

At this stage we become aware of a deficit, a skill we as yet lack and must practise to achieve.

During this stage we recognise that though we attempt to do something, we do not yet have the hang of it. Here we may say to ourselves: 'I'm trying but it doesn't feel like me doing it; I still feel very uncomfortable'. We need support and encouragement at this time.

Conscious competence

With practice, our competence grows, we begin to recognise those gains we make and no longer feel deficient.

At this stage our skill grows but we need to concentrate to maintain it. Here we may say to ourselves: 'I can do this now, I can own this skill as my own'. We need to be trusted to monitor ourselves at this time and to make our mistakes without criticism.

Unconscious competence

In time our skill may become automatic, so much so that we lose awareness of what it is we do.

At this stage, we may say to ourselves: 'I know I can do this but I'm not sure how, it just comes naturally'. At this stage we need help to unpack what it is we do so we may refine the process all over again.

Placing the above in its dynamic whole, it begins to resemble a moving spiral (Fig. 8.1).

Letting go of what we know to conquer something new, confronting ourselves with our resistance to learn, risking failure by letting go of the tried and trusted are all part of learning. In this context, shyness and embarrassment are growing pains and part and parcel of the process.

Reflection

Pause here to reflect upon the following questions and your own growth as a professional carer:

Who am I as a care giver: how does my role infuse itself with my identity?

Where have I come from professionally: what am I exploring at this stage of my professional career?

Where am I going: what is my potential, the direction and purpose I am engaged with, and towards what professional goal does my vision guide me?

What professionally frustrates me: what are the blocks, constraints and obstacles I see before me?

How might I better progress: what steps do I need to take, what plans do I need to make, how might I prepare myself?

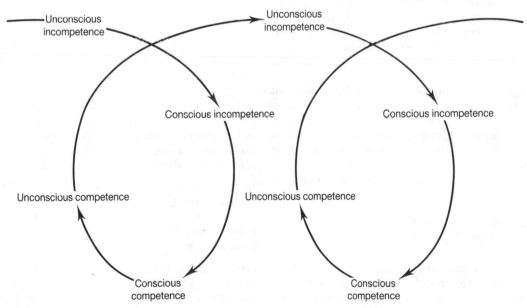

Fig. 8.1

Who or what might help me: what resources are available to me, what skills do I need to develop, who might assist me?

What will it be like when I get there: my imaginative construction of what awaits me, the emotions and energies it elicits, my motivations to continue along my present path?

Consider what you have discovered about yourself through the above.

Becoming a self-creating person: the first duty of a care communicator

'To become aware of what is happening, I must pay attention with an open mind. I must set aside my personal prejudices or bias. Prejudiced people only see what fits these prejudices'
(*I Ching*, 1951; page 345)

The emotional part of ourselves never really grows up. We develop many ways to contain our emotions, to understand and express them, but at root, feelings are ageless. Within us a part has remained unchanged since we were first born. We meet this part of ourselves again when we are infused with emotional energies, such as when we grieve, laugh, experience joy or excitement. A very real part of self-care comes from taking time to listen to the child within us, to hear it, and meet its needs.

Growth in this context describes the process of self-discovery whereby an individual learns to accept themselves and explores what it is to be a fully functioning human, while moving towards *self-actualisation*. This latter term requires further consideration.

Maslow (1970) equated the self-actualised person with:

● being that self which I truly am;
● being all that I have it in me to be.

The self-actualised person was further envisaged as being able to approach life in a fresh and excited way; to view the world through the eyes of a child – with wonder and awe; to be resistant to cultural expectation – though not rebelliously so; to take a philosophical long term view of their life; and as having a good sense of humour. Simply, they appeared to be well integrated within themselves and able to make direct contact with reality.

Evidence from research into how the self develops (Loevinger, 1976) suggests that individuals some way along the road towards self-actualisation, who are beginning to realise their personal potential and become more integrated, tend to be better able to exhibit the following:

● tolerance of ambiguity;
● respect for autonomy;
● an ability to express feelings;
● flexibility;
● creativity;
● courage to face internal conflicts.

Such persons are well on the way to becoming what Heron (1989) describes as self-creating persons:

'Autonomous behaviour now becomes reflexive. The person becomes self-determining about the emergence of their self-determination. They consciously take in hand methods of personal and interpersonal development which enhance their capacity for voluntary choice, for becoming more intentional within all domains of experience and action'
(page 20)

Three core intrapersonal processes are ongoing in the self-creating person, according to Heron (1990);

Unravelling: where the individual actively works on restrictions that emanate from their past, such as childhood traumas and social conditioning, undoing compulsive behaviours and raising to consciousness reflexive conventional habits.

Receptivity: where the person attempts to become more aware about the exercise of personal choice and power, their intuition, and generally contemplates with enhanced attention what goes on around them.

Relationship: where attention is focused upon self in relation to others, and the person recognises that personal autonomy only emerges fully in aware relationships with other autonomous persons.

Perhaps now we are approaching an understanding of what might be called 'super-health' and where our personal potential can lead. Communicating our own 'health' by example, while helping others to uncover and develop their own human potential, is the prime goal of care communication. But how do we communicate the whole of ourselves, keeping our unravelling, receptivity and relationship to the fore while facilitating another towards our vision of health? For this a model is necessary, a conceptual framework with which to gauge where we are and what we do.

The 'how' of communication: intervention analysis

'I will not let you – or me – make me dishonest, insincere, emotionally tied up or constricted, or artificially nice and social, if I can help it'
(Gendlin, in Rogers *et al.*, 1967; page 275)

Six Category Intervention Analysis, a device for identifying interpersonal behaviour developed by John Heron (1986), has been taught in the Human Potential Resource Group within Surrey University for two decades, refined in numerous workshops there, and widely applied to nursing (Burnard and Morrison, 1987; Barber, 1991a; Morrison and Burnard, 1988 and 1989) and the supervision of carers (Barber, 1991b).

Simply, Six Category Intervention Analysis describes six interventions grouped under two sub headings:

3 *Authoritative Interventions*: Prescriptive; Informative; Confronting.
3 *Facilitative Interventions*: Cathartic; Catalytic; Supportive.

A more thorough overview of these is given in Chapter 14 (Table 14.1) of this book.

In a study by Morrison and Burnard (1989) of 84 general trainees at various points in their 3-year training, findings suggested that students saw themselves most skilled in Prescriptive, Informative and Supportive interventions, and least skilled in Confronting, Cathartic and Catalytic ones. That nurses would benefit from more familiarity with facilitative interventions has been repeatedly suggested in the professional literature (Yura and Walsh, 1978; Marriner, 1979; McFarlane and Castledine, 1982; Barber 1991a).

Professional helpers, when they come to act as guardians of their discipline and its formalised systems, have a tendency to behave in a manner reminiscent of critical and/or controlling parents, by using degenerative forms of authority to:

'prescribe' what should happen;
'inform' clients of their decision; and
'confront' the client when they wish to control their behaviour.

Authoritative interventions, when sensitively used and underpinned with support, help to set the scene and define the context in which we relate. Used in an authoritarian rather than an appropriate and supportive person-respecting manner, they feel punitive.

Sometimes, when practitioners take it upon themselves to act as the guardians of a ward or their professional discipline, they overuse authoritative interventions.

Authoritative interventions, when used in a therapeutic way, can set safe boundaries and complement care; when used in the defensive form described in the passage above, they undergo therapeutic degeneration, to manipulate rather than help the client.

Prescriptive or Directive interventions are relevant to the delegation of responsibilities and tasks; they are necessary in climates where a good deal of direction takes place and in times of crisis. They are intended to influence and direct the behaviour of another.

Here, a practitioner may seek to advise, propose or instruct a client to perform certain tasks:

'Would you fill in this form for me, please?';
'You should raise this in the meeting later';
'Take your medication now, please'.

If overdone, such interventions cause a client to be practitioner-directed rather than self-directed and prevent the growth of self-determination, breed institutionalisation – that is, cause dependence upon systems external to the self, such as the ward and its routines – and undermine initiative and experimentation.

Informative interventions may be used to increase awareness, develop new insight and to transfer specialist knowledge. A practitioner employing these seeks to impart new information. A carer uses this kind of intervention as the primary mode of communication when they say:

'Your next appointment is for 10 o'clock, Friday next';
'Smokers tend to produce less healthy babies more susceptible to disease';
'It is common to find your sex drive reduced while taking tranquillisers'.

If overdone, such interventions may blunt self-direction and enquiry, but if left undone a client may feel at the mercy of the clinical environment and a pawn in a medico-professional game.

Confronting interventions help to identify restrictive attitudes and to bring to mind denied aspects of behaviour; for example, when you inform another of the stress they generate within you when they behave in a specific way. These interventions challenge the restrictive attitudes, beliefs and behaviours of a client, and bring to attention unseen or avoided awarenesses; in this, they serve a consciousness-raising function. Because these interventions – though informative – are to some degree shock-inducing and communicate uncomfortable truths, they need to be well timed and especially respectful of the client. Examples of such interventions are provided below:

'As a drug injector you have a high risk of becoming HIV positive';
'You were ill advised not to come sooner; X-rays reveal a growth in your lungs';
'You knew what you were saying was false; why did you deceive me?'.

If overdone, confronting interventions may give rise to a loss of confidence and security. They can also be perceived as punitive and attacking. If left unsaid, they foster collusion and abet denial – causing a loss of appreciation of differences and personal boundaries, and induce a sense of false security built upon avoidance of the real issues.

We must be alert to the attachment of moral correctness and/or judgemental opinions of right or wrong to authoritative interventions. They should be used in a value-free way to reap the maximum benefit. Tone of voice, posture and presence all play a part here.

Though authoritative interventions are common to professional care, facilitative ones, which honour person-centred care and the authority of the individual client, are a good deal more rare. Cathartic, catalytic and supportive interventions release emotional tensions, liberate awareness and enhance self-esteem.

Cathartic interventions encourage the release of pent-up feelings; they allow for the expressive needs of others. They encourage clients to express painful emotion and discharge bottled-up distress related to, for example, earlier anger or grief. These interventions aim to give the client permission to share and express their pent-up emotional energies. It is important that the practitioner pitches their interventions at a level the client is ready for and able to cope with. The nurse or midwife needs to have confidence in their own ability to act as an emotional container if they are to function successfully in this area. I offer examples of cathartic interventions below:

'It's fine to feel sad right now – give yourself permission to feel more';
'You look angry – do you have something you want to say to me?';
'Follow your body – let it express what it wants to do'.

Cathartic interventions need to be followed by a period of reflection, as catharsis often liberates a good deal of new insight. When pent-up emotions are released, energy is usually freed and new solutions can come rapidly to mind. Heron (1990) makes the point that culturally we are not very well prepared for the exercise of cathartic interventions, emotional control rather than release being the preferred social option in Western society. This I believe is as true of professional preparation, in that emotional energies are pushed underground in clients and carers alike, and emotional release – even in psychiatry – is seemingly viewed with suspicion and a degree of fear.

Catalytic interventions encourage self-reflection and initiate client-centred problem solving. They are used to facilitate independence, self-discovery and self-direction. For example:

'How might you change your lifestyle to reduce your present stress?';

'In what way can you modify your diet to reduce carbohydrate intake?';
'How might you take better care of yourself?'.

Catalytic interventions are at heart educational, educating especially the client's ability to manage and change themselves through self-generated insight. In this, catalytic interventions facilitate client-directed activity and independence and are especially appropriate before discharge from formal care, in the resolution phase of the therapeutic relationship.

Supportive interventions confirm to an individual their intrinsic worth and value. They affirm a client's self-image, attitudes and beliefs, actions and creations, and offer unconditional positive regard. They do not collude with a client's rigidities or defences, but rather convey intimate and authentic caring. A carer makes use of such interventions in the following ways:

'I feel concerned for you':
'I feel very touched by the way you show your appreciation';
'I enjoy the communication we share together'.

Sharing yourself with another, honestly saying how you feel, these are part and parcel of supportive interventions; all these undo professional distance, put the person back in the frame and honour the human condition.

Reflection

Imagine three catalytic and three cathartic interventions you could make to a client who complains of feeling distressed.

Imagine three supportive interventions you might make to a junior member of staff you find in tears after the death of a client they nursed.

A senior colleague demands that you break off from attending to a distressed relative and orders you to help with a new admission. Reflect upon three confronting and three informative interventions you could make.

List three prescriptive interventions you might make to an insensitive doctor who has just caused undue distress to a newly admitted client.

Which interventions do you find come easily to you; which are more difficult to construct?

For each of the six categories of interventions described, list non-verbal ways, such as touch, posture, tone of voice, attitude and manner, in which these interventions might be reinforced/portrayed; e.g. placing a hand gently on a client's shoulder to enable crying (catharsis); staying with a client when they are experiencing pain or giving your full attention to a client who is experiencing fear (supportive).

You either win or you learn: learning from mistakes

'The only thing that makes life possible is permanent intolerable uncertainty: the joy of not knowing what comes next'
(Ursula Le Guin, quoted by Hayward and Cohan, 1990)

For every positive and well-timed intervention, there is a series of potentially degenerative ones. Heron (1986) identifies four basic kinds of degenerative response which can affect the six categories described. Such interventions have the characteristics of being:

- unsolicited;
- manipulative;
- compulsive;
- unskilled.

Unsolicited interventions may occur in relationships where there is no therapeutic contract; that is, where no formal practitioner-client relationship is established. Here a person make take it upon themselves to inform, confront or advise another inappropriately. This has the likelihood of being intrusive to and disrespectful of the person; at its most invasive it may be aggressive or stereotypic. For example, a practitioner may say to a complaining client:

'You have no right to complain, this residence has a fine reputation';

'You've no one to blame but yourself for your illness'; or
'Don't be silly, you're just down in the dumps, you'll feel better later'.

Manipulative interventions are ones motivated by self-interest and tend to disregard the client's position. These are essentially political and abusive in nature, and involve a good deal of power-play. A more subtle form is when the practitioner manoeuvres the client into saying or doing things that fit the professional belief system in which they work; as when a medical rationale is used to explain away discontent:

'You're only angry because your hormones are disturbed';
'It's normal to be a little depressed and grumpy following childbirth'.

Manipulative interventions are largely deliberate, have a tendency to be calculated and geared to a specific outcome. Clients are especially susceptible to manipulative interventions:

- when they are newly admitted to a clinical area;
- in times of crisis when dependent upon the practitioner and their skills;
- when ignorant of the professional and/or clinical rationale employed;
- when regressed and disorientated through pain or anxiety.

Students new to the clinical area – who need to feel secure and experience a sense of belonging if they are to learn and professionally survive – are naturally enough prone to be vulnerable to manipulative interventions. As a student myself, I remember receiving manipulative interventions of the following order:

'If you don't do things as I want them I'll have you moved';
'Don't argue with me, I'm in charge, just do it'.

Compulsive interventions are more a symptom of subconscious distress than a deliberate ploy: for example, when a practitioner unconsciously acts out their own stress and frustration to others. Obsessional doing and needless business just for the sake of keeping active so as not to dwell upon internal anxiety and fears are examples of this.

Compulsive behaviours I find commonplace in the helping professions, especially in those areas where routine and set ways of performance are favoured. Interventions such as these include the acts of the compulsive helper, the overconformist practitioner who fears rejection and obsessionally conforms unquestioningly to routine, the unassertive nurse and midwife who, through their own emotional incompetence, mismanage and/or damage their clients. Burn-out can contribute to this. Unexpressed and repressed guilt or shame likewise can drive practitioners onto this self-punishing treadmill.

Interventions here may have the effect of punishing, overlooking and abusing others:

'I haven't got time to listen to you now';
'You're making far more fuss than is warranted';
'You can't be in pain, you had your pain-killers two hours ago'.

They may also take the form of colluding with the client:

'You're right, what's the point of stopping now when the damage is done'.

Compulsive interventions can only be undone through a practitioner's work upon themselves. Supervision, attendance at assertiveness workshops, becoming a member of a personal growth group or seeking out counselling can all be of help here. Heron observes:

> 'There appears to be one golden rule for all would-be practitioners: never become a helper until you have worked on how angry you feel at your parents' and teachers' mismanagement of you in the interests of making you good'
> (Heron, 1990; page 147)

Unskilled interventions are simply ones of an incompetent nature. These tend to occur when a practitioner has too few interactive options to mind, is unable to self-assess or evaluate, lacks practice, has received insufficient guidance or supervision, or has had a scarcity of role models to learn from. A general lack of timing, appreciation or sense of occasion characterise such interventions.

All the above examples of degenerative interventions fail to hear or attend to the client, have a defensive or belittling edge, deny the client's reality, and lack the essential ingredient of being at root supportive of the client's worth. Given that degenerative interventions increase stress and illustrate the need for further training and/or quality supervision, their frequency is a valuable guide to the state of health of a ward or care team.

Reflection

How common are those degenerative interventions listed below in the clinical field where you work?

	Very common	Common	Infrequent	Rare
Unsolicited				
Manipulative				
Compulsive				
Unskilled				

Which of the above degenerative interventions – if any – do you have a tendency to use?

Supervision: care communication by example

'When I feel smashed or trapped or bound or pushed, it is helpful to me to ask myself, "What illusion is fouling me up now?". The illusion is what I think about something. The facts just are. I know this most clearly through reflecting on what happens in emergencies when "there is no time to think"'

(Stevens, in Rogers *et al.*, 1967; page 69)

Hinshelwood (1987) observes that staff individually and as a team take the brunt of desperate demands for relief and reassurance. It is a truism, and a sad indictment of the caring professions and their management, that the staff of caring communities do not experience a sense of being cared for themselves.

Much of communication is symbolic; individuals respond to unique meanings derived from their earlier life events, and negotiate new values via social interaction with others (Blumer, 1969).

For instance, the degree of emotional warmth or distance a client perceives in a nurse may be influenced as much by previous exposure to nurture, gender issues or those personal meanings they attach to dependency and care. What transpires within the nurse-client relationship may similarly affect their attitude to the clinical setting and care service as a whole.

Hidden emotional hurts all too easily arise to complicate practitioner–client communication. Practitioners and clients, though they meet as strangers, are propelled into levels of intimacy rarely found in other relationships. This relationship, where 'intimacy' and 'strangers' combine, demands unconditional trust from clients and their relatives, and puts enormous psychological pressure upon the carer to act responsibly, give generously of themselves, and in part play out the role of a perfect nurturing parent. Interestingly, anything less than perfection is rarely tolerated by next of kin or unit managers alike.

Thus, coupled with the managerial stress of the job, professional helpers must also survive those projections – emotional labels – that relatives put their way. To be treated as a 'symbol' and related to as an 'all-knowing' or 'all-giving' provider, to act out the label of the 'perfect parent' is depersonalising, for it reinforces the 'role' rather than the 'person'. The individual within the professional uniform may end up feeling very lonely indeed. It is little wonder carers often report feeling drained, not knowing if they are coming or going, or feel lost even to themselves.

It is a tall order to ask nurses to attend to the hidden agenda attached to communication; it is far better if they are exposed to professional preparation where their interactions are examined, and to clinical supervision of a kind which feeds back to them 'how they are perceived' when they relate.

When carers are left to deal by themselves with the discomforts which emanate from the job, they are ill prepared to learn from their mistakes. Professional guidance, in the form of supervision, seeks to shape uncomfortable and stressful events so as to enhance future skills. Without this, the faults which arise in practice are perpetuated.

Tangled relationships and interpersonal communication in climates where supervision is absent have a tendency to become unnecessarily traumatic.

Nurses, who are thrown together with their clients in situations where anxiety over illness or the prospect of death is to the fore, risk having their own fears evoked. Caring is intimate and can be terrifying, especially when you are there for others (the clients) and there is no one to support you. Unconscious mental defences naturally arise at such times.

Defence mechanisms – coping strategies which give respite from anxiety and protect the self by enabling an individual to deny or distort a stressful event, so as to restrict his or her awareness and emotional involvement with it – give short term respite, but in the long term restrict performance and cripple adaptation.

Clarifying and unblocking communication is a salient task of care. It is what carers need to address in client care, and what supervisors must attempt to address with their supervisees. It is therefore useful for carers to acquaint themselves with the more common unconscious defence mechanisms that block or misdirect communication.

Opposite, examples are given of a number of mental defences; these in turn are related to their psychological root and social use (modified from Kroeber, 1963 in Barber, 1991b).

I find these mechanisms as common in the staff team as in the client population, and see them as forming a basis for much professional behaviour. Their protracted presence and/or overuse I see as diagnostic of burn-out and the need for clinical supervision. They are also natural enough occurrences in professional environments where people spend little time listening to or caring for each other.

Reflection

Which defences, if any, of those described are found in your clinical area?

Which are you most prone to?

Professional carers have a duty to care for themselves, for if they can't receive care themselves they have no business forcing care on others. Nurses who don't care for themselves all too often give out 'dead lifeless care'. Care such as this is damaging and more akin to duty. Though dutiful caring rarely kills anyone, it is, at core, insensitive and robs the therapeutic relationship of love.

Though helping professionals may operate from a basis of care, the culture they have evolved does

Table 8.1. *Mental defence mechanisms*

Psychological root	In normal coping	As a defence
Impulse restraint or emotional control	→ Appropriate suppression: holding back disruptive impulses, e.g. sexual feelings towards clients	→ REPRESSION: uncomfortable emotions pushed out of awareness; purposeful forgetting
Selective awareness or tuning in to what interests us	→ Concentration: focusing our attention	→ DENIAL: refusal to face up to or recognise undesirable material; arguing black is white
Role modelling or copying the actions of others	→ Socialisation: learning social norms and values	→ IDENTIFICATION: submerging your own identity within another person or group; forever playing 'nurse'
Sensitivity or opening ourselves to others	→ Empathy: identifying similarities between ourselves and others	→ PROJECTION: to project unwanted qualities in oneself onto others; seeing what is really your own anger in another
Impulse diversion or holding onto and releasing emotional energies elsewhere	→ Sublimation: expressing anger harmlessly in sport	→ DISPLACEMENT: to take an emotion from its site of origin and to express it elsewhere; when a senior makes you angry, you then vent your discontent upon a student/client
Time reversal or reliving and/or enacting earlier behaviours	→ Playfulness: letting go of our controls to allow for creative spontaneity	→ REGRESSION: to regress back to an earlier functional and/or emotional level; to be overdependent upon ward routines

not, it seems, permit them to show kindness to one another.

Professional carers readily become habituated to their clinical world so that they no longer see its faults – indeed, they have a vested interest in not doing so if they are to belong. Accepting everything that their practice throws at them and devoid of quality counselling or supervision, unconsciously they take on high levels of stress and all too easily come to see stress-induced responses – symptoms of burn-out – as relatively normal:

(1) Inability to concentrate upon the job at hand;
(2) Impulsive acting out of feelings;
(3) Excessive smoking and/or drinking;
(4) Loss of energy;
(5) Pre-occupation with work;
(6) Inability to relax;
(7) Absenteeism and sickness;
(8) A chronically disturbed sleep pattern;
(9) Irritability;
(10) Rapid swings between emotional highs and lows;
(11) Memory disturbances;
(12) The sense that life is a fight rather than something to be enjoyed.

This syndrome of stress may in time become a culture of stress; stressed nurses in turn communicate stress to clients so that before long high levels of anxiety permeate the organisation at all levels. When this occurs, staff can no more recognise stress than a fish can recognise water. Stress now is seen to be a natural feature of the clinical work. Nurses so affected are not without insight; it is rather that they are bereft of the necessary skills to detach themselves from the institutional and professional traditions they live by.

Reflection

Reviewing symptoms of burn-out described below, tick on the scale provided their frequency within yourself:

	Common	Occasional	Rare	Never
Inability to concentrate				
Impulsively acting from feelings				
Excessive smoking and/or drinking				
Loss of energy				
Pre-occupation with work				
Inability to relax				
Absenteeism and sickness				
Disturbed sleep				
Irritability				
Mood swings				
Memory disturbances				
Life more a fight than enjoyment				

Two or more ticks in the common column and you would be wise to slow down, seek counsel or support, and reorganise the balance of your life.

In the light of this exercise, pause to reflect how healthy you consider yourself and the culture of your workplace to be.

How does stress in your workplace affect client care?

In order to enhance care communication and interpersonal understanding, I suggest a three-pronged approach to supervision, where attention is paid to:

● unpacking the effects of organisational dynamics, professional collusions and personal defences which breed stress;

- using the unfolding relationship between the supervisor and supervisee as an action guide to what occurs in care communication, the phases of therapeutic engagement, and as a setting where interventions may be practised and new ways of engagement explored;

- developing the potential of the supervisee to grow as a person, glean new insight into self, their relationships with others and their professional role.

Essentially this approach to supervision is experiential, reflective upon the social and personal psychodynamics, and approaches the 'self' and communication experimentally.

In terms of a definition, we can now say that supervision is the engagement of a relationship where an experienced and hopefully skilled practitioner meets with a less experienced individual to appraise, explore, and systematically analyse what makes for good care communication and facilitation, while sharing in a relationship which enacts 'caring for carers'.

Within this relationship, four functions are able to be performed:

(1) Education in the necessary knowledge, skills and research-mindedness the job requires; here the nurse explores the skill base they require.

(2) Orientation to the clinical area and maintenance of a balance between an 'individual's level of skill' and the 'nature of the work' they are assigned; here, clinical induction occurs and an appropriate mix of personal skill to professional responsibility is established.

(3) Support and counsel via the enactment of a therapeutic relationship which nurtures and offers care to the supervisee; here, the developmental phases of the therapeutic relationship are engaged, unconditional regard and value for the person of the supervisee expressed, and the formation of a caring relationship experienced by the supervisee at first hand.

(4) Facilitation of self and interpersonal awareness via experiential exploration, rehearsal and/or analysis of the developing supervisor–supervisee relationship; here, interactions are analysed, emotional responses explored and new social skills synthesised from experience to inform the supervisee's future clinical practice.

It is not always easy to distinguish between when someone is caring for you or attempting to control you. Carers do not always realise which of these they seek to do themselves.

Supervision needs to untie the social and intrapersonal knots clinical encounters produce, so that new ways of responding and/or ways of being may be liberated and fresh insights emerge for future practice. In this sense, clinical life itself is approached experimentally, what works is retained, and what produces conflict or is deemed to be non-therapeutic is explored in order to illuminate further learning.

Reflection

What manner of supervision have you received during your professional life? Which of the four functions of supervision described above did it include? Indicate the degree of this on the scale provided:

(1) Education in the necessary knowledge, skills and research-mindedness the job requires.
     Lots Some Little None

(2) Orientation to the clinical area and maintenance of a balance between an 'individual's level of skill' and the 'nature of the work' he/she is assigned.
     Lots Some Little None

(3) Support and counsel via the enactment of a therapeutic relationship which nurtures and offers care to the supervisee.
     Lots Some Little None

(4) Facilitation of self and interpersonal awareness via experiential exploration and analysis of the developing supervisor-supervisee relationship.
     Lots Some Little None

What might you be able to offer if you were to perform as a supervisor within your clinical setting? Relate your answer to the four areas described above.

Epilogue

'The mad are persecuted because so many find it hard to love them. As for madness itself, it is the feeling that we can't love until we have time. Until we love we never have the time'

(Benares, 1985; page 65)

In this chapter I have tried to get at the soul of care communication rather than its mechanics, and share some of my thoughts and intuitions as to what this might be. As I glance through the text and reflect on what I have said, I feel a need to make one last statement, one which will somehow integrate the whole. This is it:

Love has to be at the heart of all care communication: love for self — without which we cannot love others — and love for the adventure of life itself — without which there is no such thing as health to self-explore and communicate more fully what it is to be human.

References

Barber, P. (1991a). Caring — the nature of a therapeutic relationship. In *Nursing: A Knowledge Base for Practice*, Perry, A. and Jolley, M. (eds.). Edward Arnold, London.

Barber, P. (1991b). *Who Cares for the Carers?* Distance Learning Centre, South Bank Polytechnic, London.

Benares, C. (1985). *Zen without Zen Masters*. Falcon Press, Phoenix, Arizona.

Blumer, H. (1969). *Symbolic Interactionism: Perspective and Method*. Prentice-Hall, New Jersey.

Burnard, P. and Morrison, P. (1987). Nurses' perceptions of their interpersonal skills. *Nursing Times*, 83(42), 59.

Goldberg, P. (1989). *The Intuitive Edge*. Aquarian Press, Wellingborough.

Hayward, S. and Cohan, M. (1990). *Bag of Jewels*. Intune Books. Australia.

Heron, J. (1986). *Six Category Intervention Analysis*. Human Potential Resource Group, University of Surrey, Guildford.

Heron, J. (1989). *The Facilitator's Handbook*. Kogan Page, London.

Heron, J. (1990). *Helping the Client*. Sage, London.

Hinshelwood, R.D. (1987). *What Happens in Groups*. Free Association Books, London.

I Ching (Wilhelm translation). (1951). Routledge and Kegan Paul, London.

Kroeber, T. (1963). The coping functions of the ego mechanisms. In *The Study of Lives*, White, R. (ed.). Atherton Press, New York.

Loevinger, J. (1976). *Ego Development*. Jossey-Bass, San Francisco.

Marriner, A. (1979). *The Nursing Process*. Mosby, St Louis.

Maslow, A.H. (1970). *Motivation and Personality*. Harper and Row, New York.

McFarlane, J.K. and Castledine, G. (1982). *A Guide to the Practice of Nursing Using the Nursing Process*. Mosby, St Louis.

Morrison, P. and Burnard, P. (1988). Student nurses' interpersonal skills. *Nursing Times*, 84(12), 69.

Morrison, P. and Burnard, P. (1989). Students' and trained nurses' perceptions of their own interpersonal skills: a report and comparison. *Journal of Advanced Nursing*, 14, 321–329.

Rogers, C. (1983). *Freedom to Learn in the Eighties*. Merrill, Columbus, Ohio.

Rogers, C.R., Stevens, B., Gendlin, E.T., Shlien, J.M. and Dusen, W.V. (1967). *Person to Person: The Problem of Being Human*. Condor Books, Souvenir Press, London.

Young, P. (1990). *The Art of Polarity Therapy*. Prism Press, Bridport.

Yura, H. and Walsh, M.B. (1978). *Human Needs and the Nursing Process: Philosophy, Theory, Concept, Process*. Appleton Century Crofts, New York.

9

THE NATURE OF STRESS AND ITS IMPLICATIONS FOR NURSING PRACTICE

Elisabeth Clark and Susan Montague

The aim of this chapter is to explore the nature of stress, its causes and effects and its relationship to the development of ill health.

The chapter includes the following topics:

- Theoretical approaches to studying and understanding stress
- Sources of stress in health and illness with particular emphasis on how such information impinges on nursing practice

- The nature and function of biological and psychological stress responses and the relationship between them
- Evidence on how stress might be implicated in the development of ill health

---

Introduction

Stress is an inextricable part of life. It is, according to the eminent stress physiologist Hans Selye (1976), 'essentially reflected by the rate of all the wear and tear caused by life'.

These introductory remarks beg many questions about the nature, causes and effects of stress. We hope to answer these – and hopefully, to provoke more – within the pages of this chapter.

Despite a huge volume of research and interest in the subject, stress remains a somewhat elusive phenomenon. Nonetheless, the development, in this century, of the concept of stress has contrib-

uted significantly to current understanding of health and illness. The existence of a relationship between stress and illness has grown to near acceptance in the scientific world (Kline Leidy, 1989) and according to Fletcher (1991), few now doubt that psychological factors play an important role in mental health and physical disease.

For all these reasons, we consider it crucial that nurses have a clear understanding of stress, both in everyday life and in relation to ill health. Because of their prolonged day-to-day professional contact with people, nurses are perhaps the best placed of all members of the health care team to take action to prevent unnecessary stress and to minimise and alleviate prolonged stress. If nurses lack such understanding they may be less able to manage their own lives effectively, to work efficiently, and may unwittingly increase their clients' experience of stress. The nature of nursing varies widely but is such that the job can and does cause severe stress in its participants. It is therefore immensely important for nurses to be sensitive to and to recognise signs of stress in themselves and in their colleagues and to take appropriate steps to alleviate this. It is important to remember here that people are not always able consciously to recognise either the signs of stress in themselves and others, or that they are experiencing stress, or to identify its causes. In other words, they may not be able to articulate their distress clearly. Rather, stress may manifest itself indirectly in high rates of absenteeism from work, turnover and wastage. Despite the high level of interest in occupational stress and its effects, reflected in the ever-increasing literature on the subject, there remains a need in some quarters to challenge the belief that professional workers should be able to cope with difficult situations and that to admit to stress is a sign of failure or weakness.

Understanding stress is, we believe, the key to its prevention and alleviation – and the whole subject assumes even greater importance in circumstances where there are cutbacks in resources, staff shortages and uncertainties created by organisational restructuring (Sutherland and Cooper, 1990).

Despite its apparent familiarity and common usage, the term 'stress' is not easy to define and is often used to mean several different things. For instance, it is frequently used to describe subjective feelings experienced when we are under great pressure in our lives, as in 'I'm feeling really stressed at the moment'. It can also be used to refer to those conditions which trigger the negative feelings; for example, 'Things at work are pretty stressful'. If you read a number of books and articles about stress, you will find that various different definitions of the term are used. In trying to make sense of these definitions, it is helpful to understand the main approaches that have been adopted in studying the subject (see next section) since these influence how stress is defined.

Finally, you will notice that stress is generally thought of and expressed in a negative sense, as illustrated in the above two examples. It is important to realise, however, that stress should not always be construed as negative, unpleasant and potentially harmful. Indeed, as Selye pointed out, positive and pleasurable experiences, such as playing competitive sports and, to quote Selye himself (1976, page 1) 'the ecstasy of fulfilment', contribute to the wear and tear of life. Indeed, in such instances, stress can be considered to be the 'spice of life'. Thus stress can be associated with both positive and negative experience. Selye referred to 'eustress' and 'distress' to distinguish between the two. 'Eustress' is the amount of stress necessary for an active, healthy life, whereas when increasing levels of stress become maladaptive (exceeding the person's adaptive capacity to cope) and thus potentially harmful, this is 'distress'. In the remainder of this chapter our focus will be on maladaptive stress since it is this which produces most distress and dis-ease.

Approaches to studying stress

A number of different approaches have been used when studying stress. One approach views stress as a stimulus – an event or a set of circumstances or conditions which threaten a person's well-being and give rise to a stress reaction. Because of the possible confusion, the term 'stressor' is sometimes used to describe the stimulus in order to differentiate it from the stress response. When someone talks about the 'stress of overwork', they are referring to stress as a stimulus. This idea of stress as a stimulus originated from engineering and the finding that material eventually weakens if unequal pressures are placed upon it. Those working within this tradition aim to identify the particular characteristics of a situation or event that make it stressful.

A second perspective focuses on the set of responses – physiological and/or psychological – that occur when an animal or human is faced with a threatening or demanding situation. This response-based approach has been particularly important in the development of biological concepts of stress. The work of the Canadian physiologist Hans Selye is an example of such an approach to the study of stress. In 1956, Selye published his first major book on the subject, entitled *The Stress of Life* (a second edition was published in 1976). Selye's important ideas about stress are discussed in detail in the section on the biological responses to stress (page 222).

Both of these approaches, however, fail to take account of the meaning of events. This important realisation provided the basis of a third perspective which is known as the *interactionist* or *transactional* model of stress. It assumes that stress reflects the relationship (or transaction) between a person and his environment. According to this approach, stress should not simply be seen as either a stimulus or response, but as the product of a person's interpretation of the significance of a threatening event (the stimulus) and of their resources to cope with it (the response).

Demand→Perception→Response

This perspective is derived from the work of Cox and his colleagues at Nottingham University during the 1970s. Cox (1978) describes stress as 'part of a complex and dynamic system of transaction between the person and his environment' (page 18). He goes on to suggest that 'Stress may be said to arise when there is an imbalance between the perceived demand and the person's perception of his capability to meet that demand' (page 18). For the remainder of this chapter, stress will be considered essentially from this transactional viewpoint.

Although we shall be focusing on damaging or harmful stress, it is important to recognise that human beings require some degree of stress in order to function effectively. As already discussed, stress is a necessary part of life and cannot be avoided: it provides the necessary drive and challenge required to maintain life. There comes a point, however, when increasing levels of stress become harmful and the demands exceed a person's adaptive capacity and thus their ability to cope, at which point stress becomes dysfunctional. Figure 9.1 shows the relationship between performance and demand. From this you can see that performance is relatively poor at low levels of demand, but improves steadily as the level of demand increases until optimal performance is reached at moderate levels of demand. As demand levels increase further, so performance begins to deteriorate progressively. Welford (1973) claimed that stress occurs whenever the demand departs from moderate levels and this helps to explain why people working on a monotonous production line often find their work stressful. Low levels of demand can be as stressful as high levels, and produce similar effects on performance.

So when thinking about stress, it is important to acknowledge that it is not simply something negative 'out there' in the environment, but that it depends on an individual's cognitive appraisal of the situation and of the available resources to deal with it. It is not, therefore, possible to identify certain situations as 'stressful' and others as 'not stressful'. Rather, stress must be viewed on a more individualised basis as a function of the interaction between a person and his environment. Faced with similar demands, two people may well react quite differently, with one person viewing the situation as a challenge, whilst the other may exhibit symptoms of anxiety and distress. From this it should be apparent that such an approach acknowledges important individual differences and that it fits well within a philosophy of individualised care.

On a methodological note, Cox (1978) points out that the research that is associated with each of the three approaches tends to differ in its emphasis. The response model typically treats stress as a dependent variable, describing it in terms of people's responses to threatening stimuli. Meanwhile, researchers who view stress in terms of the characteristics of the stressor (the stimulus) usually treat it as an independent variable, the effects of which can be systematically studied. Finally, those working within the interactionist model usually investigate stress as an intervening variable between stimulus and response.

Sources of stress

If you were asked to reflect for a moment on the sources of stress in your life at the present time you would probably, like me, come up with a fairly long list. My list includes adjusting to a new job, tight writing deadlines, work pressures, having to travel daily on the M25 motorway, and trying to

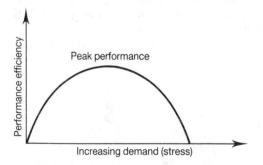

Fig. 9.1 *The relationship between performance and demand*

arrange for renovations to be carried out on the old house in which I am presently living. These and other stressors are likely to be familiar to you.

When thinking about stressors it is important to remember that the majority – with the exception of a disaster (such as a hurricane or flood) or traumatic events (such as a car crash, rape or a life-threatening illness) – should be thought of as potential rather than actual sources of stress. Consider the taste for loud music of some teenagers; whilst this may feature in your own list of stressors now, it may not always have done so. Meanwhile, for some the absence of music might be considered to be a source of stress. Likewise, a parachute jump is likely to be viewed rather differently depending on the individual concerned. Factors such as age, personality and previous experience are likely to affect whether or not a particular stimulus is regarded as stressful by a specific individual.

Returning briefly to disasters and traumatic events, it is important to recognise that they can have a long-lasting effect on the individual(s) concerned. As a result, certain people go on to develop what has come to be known as post-traumatic stress disorder (PTSD). The main symptoms include a pervading sense of numbness and estrangement, phobias, nightmares reliving the trauma, and anxiety which may present as major sleep disturbances, lack of concentration or being overly alert (Figley, 1986). It is essential for anyone working with individuals suffering from PTSD to have a good working knowledge of bereavement processes since the issue of mortality (one's own and that of other people) often has to be confronted, and terrible, vivid images of death and destruction may be imprinted on people's minds (Clegg, 1988).

Work-related stress

Your list of stressors may have included a number of work-related sources of stress. Occupational stress appears to occur most frequently in occupations such as nursing, where the physical and psychological demands are high whilst autonomy is relatively low (Lees and Ellis, 1990). Research undertaken in both the United Kingdom and the United States has identified some of the sources of stress reported by nurses at differing points in their career.

In their systematic study of stress in nurse man-

agers, Hingley and Cooper (1986) found that potential stressors could be grouped into nine main categories:

- Workload
- Working relationships with more senior colleagues
- Role conflict and ambiguity
- Dealing with death and bereavement
- The conflict between home and work
- Lack of career prospects
- Interpersonal relationships with patients/clients, relatives and colleagues
- Lack of resources
- Keeping up with changes.

Although Hingley and Cooper's study focused on nurse managers, research undertaken with other groups of nurses have identified similar stressors (Marshall, 1980). Perhaps not surprisingly, studies of student nurses have also found that coping with death and dying is frequently listed as a stressor (see, for example, Birch, 1979; Parkes, 1985; Arnold, 1989; Lindop, 1991). Similarly, relationships with colleagues and patients/clients have also been identified (Parkes, 1985; Arnold, 1989; Lees and Ellis, 1990; Lindop, 1991), as has work overload (Parkes, 1985; Lindop, 1991) and coping with changes such as moving wards (Birch, 1979; Price, 1985). In addition, lack of confidence and anxieties about carrying out certain clinical procedures (Parkes, 1985; Lees and Ellis, 1990), carrying out tasks in front of others (Kushnir, 1986), and differences between ward-based and theoretical aspects of training (Melia, 1987; Lindop, 1991) are also cited as stressors.

Research by Lees and Ellis (1990) has identified a wide variety of stressors in nursing. As you can see from Table 9.1, no fewer than 26 categories emerged. Fifty-three subjects took part in the study: 20 trained staff, 20 students and 13 ex-students who had left their training programmes before the end. Several of the stressors, such as dealing with death and dying and conflict with doctors, featured in all three groups, whilst others were found to affect some groups more than others, and some were restricted to one group only. The stressors that affected only one group were specifically associated with that group's role (e.g. only trained staff allocate the off-duty roster).

Lees and Ellis also asked respondents to state which incidents and/or situations they found to be

Table 9.1. *The 26 categories of stressor identified by Lees and Ellis (1990). For each stressor, the percentage of each group, and of the total group of 53 subjects, citing it as a stressor is given (reproduced with permission from Journal of Advanced Nursing)*

Stressor	Trained	Student	Leaver	Total
Understaffing	75	25	23	43
Dealing with death and dying	25	55	46	41
Conflict with nurses	35	25	46	34
Overwork	25	30	15	25
Conflict with doctors	40	15	8	23
Hours	10	10	39	17
Cardiac arrests	5	30	8	15
Responsibility/accountability	25	5	8	13
Training junior staff	25	0	0	9
Dealing with relatives	15	5	8	9
Lack of resources (beds/equipment)	20	0	0	8
Aggressive patients	10	5	0	6
Study/exams	0	15	0	6
Carrying out certain nursing procedures	5	5	0	4
Feeling inadequate to carry out procedures	0	10	0	4
Seeing patients in distress	0	5	8	4
Staff rough to patients	0	0	15	4
Conflict with 'others' (porters/admin.)	5	0	0	2
Child abuse	5	0	0	2
Dealing with overdose patients	5	0	0	2
Living in nurses home	0	0	8	2
Open visiting	5	0	0	2
Doing the off-duty	5	0	0	2
Disorganisation of workload on the wards	0	0	8	2
Being in a new situation for the first time	0	5	0	2
Heat in hospital	0	0	8	2

the most stressful. For the trained staff, the major stressors were understaffing (35% of the group of trained staff), followed by conflict with doctors (25%). For the student nurses and the student leavers, the main stressor was dealing with death and dying (30% and 31% respectively).

Some units or particular areas of work have also been reported to be more stressful than others. For example, the Special Care Baby Unit (Thornton, 1984), the Intensive Care Unit (Bailey et al., 1980; Bishop, 1981) and the Accident and Emergency department (Thompson, 1983; Brunt, 1984). You will notice that the workload in each of these areas tends to be unpredictable and involves the use of high technology equipment.

The negative effects of stress may be at least partly responsible for the high attrition rate from nurse training. For example, Birch (1979) reported that 66% of the sample he studied left because they could not cope with the stress, whilst Beck (1984) found that 20% of students failed to reach

their final year at a major teaching hospital because of stress. Other effects include high rates of absenteeism (Campbell, 1985; Price, 1985) and exhaustion (Albrecht, 1982; Lindop, 1991). It should be noted that all these results derive from nurse training schemes in existence before Project 2000 courses started.

If you are interested in assessing the amount of stress currently in your working life, you should turn to the Appendix where the Professional Life Stress Scale is reprinted. The purpose of this scale is to help you to think about your working life. Fontana (1989) emphasises the importance of treating it as a useful but rough guide to your stress level, rather than as a precise measurement tool.

So far we have focused largely on work-related stress, but it is important to acknowledge that stress is not restricted to work and that aspects of our personal lives may also be stressful and affect our work. Many of the changes which occur period- ically in our lives, such as moving house or pregnancy, can be a source of stress, since any change – even one that is desired and joyful – requires some form of adjustment. Throughout life, therefore, each of us experiences the need to adapt to new circumstances.

Researchers have spent many years investigating the effects of both positive and negative life events such as moving away from your family home, suffering from a severe illness, marriage, the birth of a child, the death of someone close to you, divorce, or promotion at work.

Life changes

In 1967, Holmes and Rahe published a scale, derived from clinical experience, which attempted to measure the impact of such life events. This scale, containing 43 items, was developed by examining the case histories of about 5000 individuals and identifying those life events which regularly preceded the onset of illness. They assumed that stress could be induced by a variety of different life events – both positive and negative – which require some kind of adjustment in a person's life. They also assumed that specific stressors could be added up and used to indicate the total amount of stress a person had been under during a specified period of time. So, for instance, if I had experienced 14 of the 43 listed life events over the previous year, then my overall stress score would be 14.

However, implicit in their original scale was a further assumption which Holmes and Rahe were themselves unhappy about: an assumption of equal weighting given to different life events of varying seriousness. Intuitively, a minor traffic offence would seem relatively insignificant when compared with the death of a loved one. They therefore modified the instrument by assigning differential weights to specific life events, using a magnitude estimation procedure. To do this, 394 subjects were informed that the life event of 'marriage' had been assigned an arbitrary value of 50 and they were asked to rate each of the remaining 42 events proportionately as requiring more or less adjustment than marriage. The mean (average) value assigned to each life event was calculated and then divided by ten to give a specific number of life change units (LCU) for each item. Table 9.2 shows the 43 items included in the Social Readjustment Rating Scale (SRRS) which may be used to determine the total amount of life change a person

has experienced over a fixed period of time.

When looking at Table 9.2, you might like to reflect on how many of the 43 life events are the concern of the nurse or midwife in relation to her clients. Let us consider for a moment the likely score of a woman who has just returned to work after maternity leave. Her score will certainly include: pregnancy (40), gain of new family member (39), wife begins or stops work (26), change in sleeping habits (16), and may also include change' in financial state (38), revision of personal habits (24) and change in eating habits (15). The total number of life change units could, therefore, be as high as 198. The possible addition of other events (such as death of close family member or close friend, sexual difficulties, trouble with in-laws), over which she has little or no control, would increase her score to even higher levels. Thus, knowledge of life events may help you to appreciate the range of stressors which an individual is facing. It should, however, be noted that general life event scales such as the SRRS may not be entirely appropriate for use with specific client groups, such as pregnant women, since they do not include many items relevant to that particular group. Barnett *et al.* (1983) report the development of life event scales for use with primiparous and multiparous women which include high-ranking items from existing general life event scales, together with items that are relevant only to pregnant women.

An extensive review of the literature on maternal stress by Levin and DeFrank (1988) found stress to be a health risk for both mothers and babies: life change stress was predictive of antenatal complications and of premature labour. As a result, they suggest that those responsible for caring for pregnant women should find out what stressors women are exposed to and offer their support to mothers under stress, and also refer them to appropriate support groups.

In addition to a person's overall stress score, it is important to remember that a number of other factors may influence how someone perceives and reacts to their situation. These include personal factors such as individual appraisal of the situation, self-esteem and coping skills, and situational factors such as the amount of support available, the predictability of the stressor and the amount of control that may be exerted over its duration. If, for example, the occurrence of a potentially stressful event can be predicted, this may allow individuals to prepare themselves. Conversely, uncertainty

Table 9.2. *The Social Readjustment Rating Scale (Holmes and Rahe, 1967)*

Rank	Life Event	Mean Value
1	Death of spouse	100
2	Divorce	73
3	Marital separation	65
4	Jail term	63
5	Death of close family member	63
6	Personal injury or illness	53
7	Marriage	50
8	Fired at work	47
9	Marital reconciliation	45
10	Retirement	45
11	Change in health of family member	44
12	Pregnancy	40
13	Sex difficulties	39
14	Gain of new family member	39
15	Business readjustment	39
16	Change in financial state	38
17	Death of close friend	37
18	Change to different line of work	36
19	Change in number of arguments with spouse	35
20	Mortgage over $10,000*	31
21	Foreclosure of mortgage or loan	30
22	Change in responsibilities at work	29
23	Son or daughter leaving home	29
24	Trouble with in-laws	29
25	Outstanding personal achievement	28
26	Wife begins or stops work	26
27	Begin or end school	26
28	Change in living conditions	25
29	Revision of personal habits	24
30	Trouble with boss	23
31	Change in work hours or conditions	20
32	Change in residence	20
33	Change in schools	20
34	Change in recreation	19
35	Change in church activities	19
36	Change in social activities	18
37	Mortgage or loan less than $10,000*	17
38	Changing in sleeping habits	16
39	Change in number of family get-togethers	15
40	Change in eating habits	15
41	Vacation	13
42	Christmas	12
43	Minor violations of the law	11

Interpretation of total score:

- a total score of up to 149 describes no life crisis
- a score between 150 and 199 describes a mild life crisis
- a score between 200 and 299 describes a moderate life crisis
- a score over 300 describes a major life crisis.

If your score is high, you might like to consider whether it is possible to postpone any events requiring further adjustments in your life over which you may have some control, such as moving house, to prevent your score rising further.

* Please note that in 1967, $10,000 constituted a substantial financial burden. This figure would need to be considerably increased to be equivalent in 1993.

may make it very difficult to deal with a stressful event. Those who have cared for a person with cancer may already be aware that, for many, it is the uncertainty about whether or not the treatment will be successful that is particularly hard to cope with – the uncertainty of not knowing – rather than the disease itself. Different ways of coping with stress and the issue of control will be considered later.

Moreover, when thinking about a specific patient/client/colleague, it is important to gauge the amount of social support that they have. A major life event (such as a life-threatening illness, the death of a baby, child or partner, or divorce) is almost certainly more bearable if social and emotional support is available (Cohen and Wills, 1985). Stress may also be easier to bear if an opportunity is provided to talk with others who have experienced a similar stressor. To meet this need, a number of national organisations and local groups provide specialist support (e.g. the Stillbirth and Neonatal Death Association, the Gay Bereavement Project and the National Association for Staff Support – the latter provides support for health care workers).

In the light of earlier discussions which have emphasised the importance of the subjective experience of stress, you may have been surprised that the SRRS, which has been widely employed in stress research, uses standardised weightings. This remains an unresolved, controversial issue. Certainly, some studies have shown cultural differences and also, perhaps not surprisingly, some age differences. For instance, Ruch and Holmes (1971) found that a group of adolescents rated sexual difficulties as the fifth most stressful item, whilst older adults rated this item thirteenth. Yet even this kind of approach overlooks the issue of individual differences in the perception and subjective experience of potentially stressful events. Despite such reservations concerning the SRRS, overall stress scores have been used in a number of prospective studies to predict the likelihood of adverse changes in health of large numbers of subjects (see, for example, Rahe, 1974; Rahe and Arthur, 1977). Since Rahe was a captain in the United States Navy, many of the subjects were naval personnel. Small but statistically significant relationships have been reported between the number and intensity of life events and the incidence of illness (as indicated in medical records) whilst living in similar conditions on board ship. Most people, however, appear to cope with life changes without becoming ill. Moreover, correlational data needs to be interpreted with care. Any increased susceptibility to illness may not result from the direct effects of the stressful events themselves, but from other associated factors which are difficult to separate from the effects of stress; for instance, a person who has recently been bereaved may not be eating or sleeping properly. Alternatively, poor health may increase the likelihood of experiencing stress-related events such as work difficulties, changes in sleeping habits or marital difficulties; that is to say, early stages of the illness prior to the onset of specific life events may have caused the stressful life events to happen rather than the other way round. Certainly, Hudgens (1974) argued that 29 of the 43 events included in the SRRS are often the symptoms or consequences of illness. Finally, it is also possible that both stress and illness are due to some other, as yet unidentified, variable (such as personality), and that the correlation between the two is spurious.

Two further methodological points may also be important. Firstly, some of the research is retrospective and relies on people's ability to recall incidence of either stressful events or of illness. Consequently, the data may be unreliable in that it may reflect people's failure to recall accurately and their tendency to be selective. Secondly, the experience of stress may encourage people to become more aware of their health, take more notice of symptoms they might otherwise ignore, and consult their doctor: the experience of stress may change how people behave in relation to their

health. Thus, it would seem reasonable to regard stress associated with life events as a possible predisposing factor in the development of illness. The evidence certainly does not enable us to identify stress as a sufficient causal factor.

One further assumption made by Holmes and Rahe has also been challenged; namely, that any change – whether good or bad – requires adjustment and is therefore stressful. Individuals have consequently been asked to evaluate specific events as 'good' or 'bad' and estimate the impact on their lives. Using this approach, Sarason *et al.* (1978) found that people who had experienced a number of negative events were more likely to report either physical or emotional problems within six months. Suls and Mullen (1981) argue that the weight of evidence suggests that undesirable events are potentially more stressful than desirable ones, even though both require some form of adjustment. Since an individual's perception of the situation is crucial, one might expect negative experiences to produce more severe effects than positive ones.

The daily hassles of life

If you think back to the SRRS, you will appreciate that the life events included are fairly major, compared with the numerous minor irritations that most of us experience on a daily basis – irritations such as losing one's purse or having an argument with a friend or colleague. DeLongis *et al.* (1982) investigated whether these more minor events were also related to health. They asked 100 men and women aged between 45 and 64 to complete checklists and questionnaires and record on a daily basis both irritating things ('hassles') and pleasant things ('uplifts') that occurred over a 12 month period. They found that overall the accumulation of daily hassles was a better predictor of psychological symptoms and health than were the more major life events identified by Holmes and Rahe. The two are almost certainly related, however. For instance, a major life event such as divorce may create a number of more minor hassles, such as arranging childcare facilities or attending school functions without the support of a partner.

Further research is clearly needed to investigate the obviously complex relationship between major life events, minor frequent irritations and the onset of illness, especially since individual variation has been reported in the way people react. DeLongis *et al.* (1988) found that while most individuals became more anxious as the number of minor hassles in their lives increased, this was not the case for about 30% of people who reported improved levels of coping and more positive mood. This latter group were found to have higher levels of self-esteem and better networks of social/emotional support than those who did not cope as well.

In addition to coping with specific life events and daily hassles, it is also important to be aware that patients may well experience stress in relation to the care they receive.

The stress of hospitalisation

For those working in a hospital environment which has become totally familiar, it is important not to lose sight of those aspects of the environment and the routine which may be a source of stress for individual patients and clients. There is now considerable evidence that hospitalisation is a stressful experience (see, for example, Franklin, 1974; Wilson-Barnett, 1986). A number of studies undertaken in the past 20 or so years have identified specific stressors, measured stress responses and evaluated attempts to alleviate stress (e.g. Langer *et al.*, 1975; Wilson-Barnett and Carrigy, 1978; Johnson, 1983; Wilson-Barnett, 1984). It is clearly essential for health care professionals to be aware of sources of stress for individual patients so that they may attempt to prevent, or at least reduce, the stress and thereby promote improved physical and psychological well-being in those being cared for.

In this context, it is important to note that many of the physical and behavioural changes associated with stress (such as insomnia, irritability and changes in eating habits) may inappropriately be associated with the primary diagnosis, and other possible causes may be overlooked. Work by Volicer and Volicer (1978) and Wilson-Barnett (1979) and others has shown that the hospital environment is strange and may be associated with unhappy memories. Many patients feel that they lack information or are provided with conflicting information and do not have opportunities to discuss any concerns that they might have. Some resent being made to feel dependent and the loss of control over their own situation and their own bodies. Greater insight into the source(s) of stress for individual patients may be obtained by using the Hospital Stress Rating Scale which was created by

Volicer and Bohannon (1975) to assess the degree of stress associated with different aspects of care (see Table 9.3).

Biological responses to stress

The concept of the internal environment and homeostasis

In the early part of this century, the French physiologist Claude Bernard (1927) taught that one of the most characteristic features of multicellular organisms is their ability to maintain the physical and chemical composition of the immediate fluid environment of their cells within a narrow range of values, within which cellular function is optimal. Organisms are able to do this despite wide fluctuations in their external surroundings.

Bernard was the first to conceptualise the extracellular interstitial fluid as this thermostatically controlled and chemically stable 'milieu intérnale' (internal environment) for our cells.

Cannon (1932) recognised that the composition of the internal environment of the cells is repeatedly disturbed by the metabolic activities of the organism. He called the process by which the organism attempts to maintain the relative constancy of its internal environment, 'homeostasis'. The term 'homeostasis' refers to the continual tendency of the internal fluid environment to return towards a steady state after each fluctuation. It does this through a system of negative feedback mechanisms. These 'homeostatic mechanisms' operate via the specialised systems which communicate directly with the external environment (respiratory, gastro-intestinal and renal) and are controlled and coordinated by the specialised cells of the nervous and endocrine systems. There are a huge number of homeostatic mechanisms which maintain life and health and the function of these makes up a large part of the subject matter of physiology (Williams and Montague, 1988).

Many health problems can be understood as being the result of a breakdown in homeostasis. As we shall see later, stress can be viewed as a set of physiological responses to demand in homeostatic systems.

As well his work on homeostasis, Cannon (1929 and 1935) also carried out research on the function

Table 9.3. Hospital Stress Rating Scale

Factor	Stress Scale Events	Assigned rank	Mean rank score
1. Unfamiliarity of surroundings	Having strangers sleep in the same room with you	01	13.9
	Having to sleep in a strange bed	03	15.9
	Having strange machines around	05	16.8
	Being awakened in the night by the nurse	06	16.9
	Being aware of unusual smells around you	11	19.4
	Being in a room that is too cold or too hot	16	21.7
	Having to eat cold or tasteless food	21	23.2
	Being cared for by an unfamiliar doctor	23	23.4
2. Loss of independence	Having to eat at different times than you usually do	02	15.4
	Having to wear a hospital gown	04	16.0
	Having to be assisted with bathing	07	17.0
	Not being able to get newspapers, radio or TV when you want them	08	17.7
	Having a roommate who has too many visitors	09	18.1
	Having to stay in bed or the same room all day	10	19.1
	Having to be assisted with a bedpan	13	21.5
	Not having your call light answered	35	27.3
	Being fed through tubes	39	29.2
	Thinking you may lose your sight	49	40.6
3. Separation from spouse	Worrying about your spouse being away from you	20	22.7
	Missing your spouse	38	28.4
4. Financial problems	Thinking about losing income because of your illness	27	25.9
	Not having enough insurance to pay for your hospitalisation	36	27.4
5. Isolation from other people	Having a roommate who is seriously ill or cannot talk with you	12	21.2
	Having a roommate who is unfriendly	14	21.6
	Not having friends visit you	15	21.7
	Not being able to call family or friends on the phone	22	23.3
	Having the staff be in too much of a hurry	26	24.5
	Thinking you might lose your hearing	45	34.5
6. Lack of information	Thinking you might have pain because of surgery or test procedures	19	22.4
	Not knowing when to expect things will be done to you	25	24.2
	Having nurses or doctors talk too fast or use words you can't understand	29	26.4
	Not having your questions answered by the staff	37	27.6
	Not knowing the results or reasons for your treatments	41	31.9
	Not knowing for sure what illnesses you have	43	34.0
	Not being told what your diagnosis is	44	34.1
7. Threat of severe illness	Thinking your appearance might be changed after your hospitalisation	17	22.1
	Being put in the hospital because of an accident	24	26.9
	Knowing you have to have an operation	32	26.9
	Having a sudden hospitalisation you weren't planning to have	34	27.2
	Knowing you have a serious illness	46	34.6
	Thinking you might lose a kidney or some other organ	47	35.6
	Thinking you might have cancer	48	39.2
8. Separation from family	Being in the hospital during holidays or special family occasions	18	22.3
	Not having family visit you	31	26.5
	Being hospitalised far away from home	33	27.1
9. Problems with medications	Having medications cause you discomfort	28	26.0
	Feeling you are getting dependent on medications	30	26.4
	Not getting relief from pain medications	40	31.2
	Not getting pain medication when you need it	42	32.4

of the autonomic nervous system and adrenal medulla. Working with laboratory animals and humans subjected to conditions of cold, lack of oxygen and loss of blood, he described the 'fight or flight' response which prepares the body to react to a threat or danger (see also section on 'acute stress') and described his subjects as being 'under stress'.

Hans Selye's theory of stress

Selye's pioneering concepts, research and developing theory of stress are founded in the classical ideas of Bernard and grew in parallel with the work of Cannon.

In the 1920s, Selye, then a medical student, reflected on the mechanisms that might underlie what he later called 'the syndrome of just being sick'. This syndrome is composed of a collection of diagnostically unimportant signs and symptoms such as a coated tongue, fatigue, diffuse aches and pains, feeling and looking ill. In other words these features are non-specific and not characteristic of any one disease.

A decade later, Selye was involved in research where rats were injected with extracts of glands of varying degrees of purity in order to identify ovarian hormones and their functions. To his surprise, when he examined the rats' bodies he found the following changes irrespective of the preparation to which the rats had been subjected:

- Atrophy (wasting) of the thymus and lymph nodes;
- Bleeding ulcers in the stomach and duodenum;
- Enlargement and hyperactivity of the adrenal cortex.

Selye found that this syndrome, which he called the general adaptation syndrome (GAS), was produced by any noxious agent he tried. It seemed to be a pattern of response to the fact of trauma rather than to any specific stimulus or demand – and perhaps an experimental replica of the syndrome of 'just being sick'.

Selye found that it was possible to divide the physiological responses associated with the GAS into three quite distinct phases which occur over time (Fig. 9.2). He called the initial response the 'alarm reaction'. In this stage, stores of hormone in the adrenal cortex were depleted by increased secretion into the blood. Selye also observed that the blood became more concentrated and that the

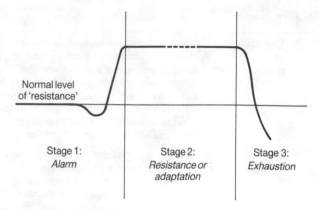

Fig. 9.2 *The three phases of the general adaptation syndrome (GAS) (Selye, 1976)*

animal lost weight. No animal could remain in this state for long. It either returned to normal, passed into the next stage of adaptation (or resistance), or died. Progress depended on the intensity and duration of the demand. Selye viewed the alarm stage of the GAS as the expression of a generalised 'call to arms' of the defensive forces of the body.

In the second stage of the GAS, the animal successfully adapted to (or resisted) the effects of the agent (demand) to which it had been exposed. Observed physiological characteristics were quite different to those of the alarm stage. The animal regained weight, blood concentration returned to normal and the adrenal cortex accumulated reserves of hormones.

An animal eventually entered the third phase of the GAS, that of exhaustion, if the effects of the agent continued unabated. Symptoms of exhaustion were essentially similar to those of alarm and the animal died as a result.

Significance of the general adaptation syndrome

Selye called the general adaptation syndrome 'general' because it was produced only by agents which had a general effect on the body; he called it 'adaptive' because it produced a state of habituation and stimulated defence or resistance and survival in response to demand. The GAS was a syndrome because its various components were interdependent and coordinated. Selye (1946) postulated that the syndrome was produced by 'non-specific stress' and later (1976, page 64) defined stress as 'the state manifested by a specific syndrome which consists of all non-specifically induced changes within a biologic system'. Selye emphasised that the state of stress is manifested only by the appearance of the GAS and defined the 'stressor' as any agent that elicits this syndrome.

By 'non-specifically induced changes', Selye means those changes that are produced by many agents, as opposed to changes elicited by only one. For example, the characteristic and diagnostic skin rash is a specific effect of infection by the measles virus, whereas a non-specific effect is the inflammatory response which may also be produced by other irritants. It is important to distinguish local inflammation (termed local adaptation syndromes (LAS) by Selye, 1976) from the GAS, which is produced only by agents which have a general effect on the body. Generalised inflammation could therefore activate the GAS.

Selye's very broad concept of stress has been extremely influential and is still used by both biological and human scientists. He was one of the first research workers to claim that inappropriate stress responses can produce physical diseases and named many disorders, including conditions of inflammatory and immunological origin, as being stress-induced 'diseases of adaptation' (Selye, 1946). Research which has developed these early ideas of Selye is discussed in the final section of this chapter.

Selye's description of the specific features of the general adaptation syndrome was, of course, limited by the state of the physiological knowledge and the investigatory techniques available at the time of his original research. Further research, building on that of Selye, has produced more detail of the physiological changes which occur in response to stressors. These responses, their functions and their relationship with psychological responses in stress are discussed in the next section.

Research has also produced evidence, contrary to Selye's theory, that noxious agents do *not* always produce the GAS (Mason, 1971). There is also evidence that the response to stress does not always follow the specific pattern described by Selye. It has been shown (Mason *et al.*, 1976; Terman *et al.*, 1984) that the components of the response can vary with the characteristics of the stressor, between species and between individuals. People exhibit characteristic, possibly familial patterns of response to stress. For example,

one person may have gastro-intestinal symptoms as the most obvious feature of stress, whilst for another, changes in heart rate, blood pressure and breathing pattern may predominate. Selye's (1976) discussion of 'conditioning factors' goes some way towards making the above evidence compatible with his theory. Conditioning factors may be internal or external to the body and affect the reaction of tissues to stressor agents. External conditioning factors may be concurrent psychological events, for example, whereas internal conditioning factors include inherited characteristics and the effects of past experiences, especially those of coping with that stressor. Despite such discussion, Selye's stress theory is grounded in biology and the body's physiological response to stressors and largely ignores psychological processes or the scope for individual variation in the experience of stress.

The stress response

The stress response has both physiological and psychological components and both these represent attempts at coping with, that is, reducing or removing, the source of stress. The mental and behavioural strategies that make up the psychological component of the stress response (see next section) are called 'coping mechanisms'. These are the responses of the person, which he then appraises as being successful or unsuccessful in altering the demand in the desired direction. Such mental and behavioural responses are almost always, if not always, accompanied by a physiological response to the demand. The function of this physiological response is to facilitate survival and mental and behavioural attempts at coping. As such, the physiological stress response can itself be viewed as a form of coping mechanism.

Physiological coping occurs at an unconscious, reflex level, although it can certainly be influenced by consciously apprehended events (Mason, 1971; Frankenhauser, 1975). In contrast, it can be argued that although some aspects of psychological coping may be instinctive in origin, for example, freezing, fighting, fleeing, responses are largely based on learning and hence subject to social and cultural influences.

The entire stress response is usually functional and adaptive, in that it leads to physiological, mental and behavioural adjustments which enable a person to cope with the demand upon him. If coping is successful the person is likely to learn from the experience and so have an even greater capacity to cope in similar situations in the future. However, if coping is ineffective and demand does not abate, the person will continue to experience stress and in time this may lead to structural and functional damage, ill health, exhaustion and, in extreme cases, death.

Physiological responses to stress

Control mechanisms

Physiological responses to stress are regulated by the hypothalamus which is a small area of the brain lying, as its name suggests, below the thalamus in the floor of the third ventricle in the brain stem. The hypothalamus controls autonomic nervous activity and hence a number of homeostatic mechanisms, for example, temperature regulation. Through its nervous and vascular connections with the pituitary gland, which lies just below it, the hypothalamus also plays a major role in controlling the secretion of hormones.

The hypothalamus also forms part of the limbic system of the brain. The limbic system is the part of the brain involved in the interpretation of emotion (Hilton, 1981; Ganong, 1991) and has connections with the reticular formation which controls the level of arousal. As well as the hypothalamus having many nervous connections within the limbic system, there are also known pathways between it and the cerebral cortex. These latter pathways are likely to be the ones via which conscious appreciation of events by the cerebral cortex has an effect on physiological function. In other words, the existence of these nerve pathways between the limbic system and the cortex explains how mental events can influence physical response. Stimulation of the limbic system produces the experience of emotions such as anxiety, fear, anger, sorrow and via the hypothalamus, physiological stress responses. For example, a patient who sees another patient suffer a cardiac arrest may experience both acute anxiety and physiological stress responses. Figure 9.3 summarises the major components in the activation of the stress response. Feedback to the hypothalamus occurs by a number of routes, depending on the nature of the stressor. In stress it may be that the incoming stressor stimuli over-ride normal homeostatic negative feedback mechanisms, thus allowing

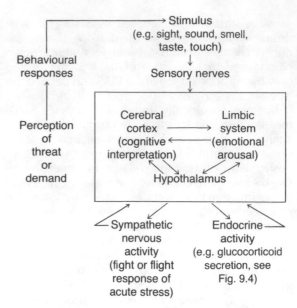

Fig. 9.3 *The major components in the activation of the stress response*

physiological functioning to take place at levels outside the usual 'normal' range (Hilton, 1981).

Acute stress

The physiological changes that occur in the alarm stage of the GAS are short term responses to cope with acute stress. These responses occur mainly as a result of increased sympathetic nervous activity and the resultant secretion of catecholamines (adrenaline and noradrenaline) from the adrenal medulla. Increased secretion of other hormones such as glucocorticoids, aldosterone, antidiuretic hormone, thyroxine and glucagon also begin. This state of arousal cannot be maintained for long because the physiological changes associated with it disrupt homeostasis and are not compatible, in the long term, with life. If the need for adaptation is very intense and the demand (stressor) not removed, the affected person will become exhausted and die. For example, the physiological stress response to a sudden, severe haemorrhage functions to maintain sufficient blood pressure to preserve blood supply and prevent ischaemic damage to vital organs such as the heart and brain. This maintenance of supply occurs at the expense of the gastro-intestinal organs and kidneys. If the response has to be maintained, these latter organs can be damaged, sometimes irreversibly, by hypoxia. Rapid replacement of the blood lost is essential in these circumstances and reduces the stressor demand and hence the degree of physiological stress experienced.

The function of the sympathetic nervous system in stress

The sympathetic nervous system is part of the autonomic or involuntary nervous system which controls the activity of smooth muscle, cardiac muscle and the secretion of exocrine glands, for example, digestive glands and sweat glands. Activation of the sympathetic nervous system via the hypothalamus brings about those physiological changes which were first described by Cannon (1929) as the 'fight or flight' response. This response is adaptive in that it increases the chances of survival in situations which involve either physical injury and/or physical activity.

Nervous activity produces changes which are rapid and specific. Most post-ganglionic sympathetic fibres produce noradrenaline as their chemical transmitter at tissue receptor sites (that is, they are *adrenergic fibres*). The sympathetic neurones which supply blood vessels in skeletal muscle and sweat glands are exceptional in that they are *cholinergic* (they produce acetylcholine as the chemical transmitter at receptor sites). Cholinergic post-ganglionic sympathetic fibres bring about vasodilation when stimulated (Ganong, 1991).

The adrenal medulla secretes the hormones adrenaline and noradrenaline into the blood. In humans, about four times as much adrenaline as noradrenaline is secreted. The medulla is stimulated to secrete its hormones by activation of a long, cholinergic, pre-ganglionic sympathetic fibre. Hormones also act by combining with tissue-based adrenergic receptors and produce a longer lasting and more widespread effect than nervous activity.

When the catecholamines are released into the blood it has been observed that adrenaline and noradrenaline are secreted together. However, research also indicates differential secretion in these hormones (Asterita, 1985). Stimuli which induce increased arousal, anxiety and apprehension are associated with increased secretion of adrenaline. Such conditions also increase cortisol secretion whereas increased secretion of noradrenaline occurs following stimuli that induce increased effort and exercise (Frankenhauser, 1975).

It is possible that the relative proportions of adrenaline and noradrenaline secreted in stress may partially explain whether the emotion experienced is one of anger or fear. Over 30 years ago, Funkenstein (1955) introduced evidence that marginally less adrenal activity occurs when anger is experienced than when the emotion is fear or anxiety. There is further evidence that the secretion of noradrenaline is related to aggressive behaviour and adrenaline secretion to fearful behaviour (flight) in animals. Predatory animals, such as lions, predominantly secrete noradrenaline while prey animals, such as rabbits, secrete more adrenaline. Such evidence suggests that the primary behavioural response to threat of primitive man was 'flight' rather than 'fight'. Nowadays a variety of learnt social and cultural factors may modify such responses.

Tissue-based adrenergic receptors have been subdivided according to their function into alpha (α) and beta (β) receptors (Ganong, 1991). α receptors are found in smooth muscle in the walls of blood vessels in the viscera, skin and in the radial muscle of the iris of the eye. Their stimulation produces contraction of the smooth muscle and hence vasoconstriction in the gut and skin and dilation of the pupil of the eye.

β_1 receptors are located in the cardiac muscle. Their stimulation produces an increased conduction velocity and decreased refractory period of the muscle fibres and hence their increased contractility. The spontaneous rate of depolarisation of the sino-atrial node is increased.

β_2 receptors occur in smooth muscle in the walls of the airways, bladder and uterus and in blood vessels supplying skeletal muscle. Their stimulation produces relaxation of smooth muscle and dilation of affected blood vessels and airways.

Noradrenaline predominantly combines with α receptors and adrenaline combines with both α and β. This difference in function explains the various therapeutic uses of the catecholamines. For example, noradrenaline is mainly used to raise blood pressure because of its α effects on blood vessels and slight β effect on cardiac muscle, whereas adrenaline is useful in asthma (β effect on bronchioles) and in anaphylactic shock (β effect on the heart and bronchi, α and β on peripheral blood vessels).

Signs and symptoms of acute stress

The majority of the signs and symptoms of acute stress are the direct result of sympathetic nervous arousal. They are summarised in Table 9.4. Symptoms are subjectively experienced and may be communicated to a sympathetic nurse, whereas physical signs may be observed by the nurse herself. Recognition is the key to prevention and alleviation.

Long term (chronic) stress

The physiological responses in chronic stress are predominantly the result of increased glucocorticoid secretion from the adrenal cortex, although the secretion of many other hormones is also altered (Mason, 1968). The length of time an individual can remain in the stage of adaptation (resistance) depends on the intensity of the stressor and the adaptive capacity of that individual. If the stressor is not removed, exhaustion will eventually occur when the adrenal cortex can no longer main-

Table 9.4. *Physical signs (including common clinical measurements) and symptoms which may occur in acute stress*

Site	Physiological basis	Physical signs and common clinical measurements	Physical symptoms
Cardiovascular system	Increased cardiac rate and output	Tachycardia Pulse of full volume Raised blood pressure	Pounding heart Palpitations Chest pain Headache
Respiratory system	CNS arousal If the hyperventilation is not in response to physiological need, low pp CO_2 results and leads to vasodilation, fall in blood pressure and, in extreme cases, tetany	Increased rate and depth of ventilation Tetany in extreme cases	Dizziness, faintness, panic (in extreme cases) Tingling in the extremities Muscle spasm (in extreme cases)
Gastro-intestinal system	Reduced blood supply to and reduced secretion in gastro-intestinal tract		Dry mouth Indigestion/dyspepsia
	Decreased or increased motility of tract	Vomiting Diarrhoea Constipation Anorexia or overeating	Nausea Diarrhoea (often frequent) Constipation Anorexia or overeating
Skin	Contraction of pilomotor muscles Cholinergic sweating Reduced blood supply	Erection of hair Sweating Pallor	Clammy palms
Eye	Contraction of radial muscle	Dilated pupils	Blurred vision
Muscle	CNS arousal	Muscle tension, tremor Muscle spasm in severe cases Lack of coordination	Headache Muscle tension, tremor, twitching Lack of coordination Back pain
General	CNS arousal	Insomnia Restlessness	Insomnia Restlessness Fatigue/weakness
	Increased metabolic rate	Low grade pyrexia	Feeling hot or cold

Reproduced with permission from Boore, J. R. P., Champion, R. and Ferguson, M. C. (eds.) (1987). **Nursing the Physically Ill Adult.** *Churchill Livingstone, Edinburgh.*

tain its glucocorticoid secretion. Selye (1976) used the term 'adaptation energy' to describe the energy consumed during stress. He postulated that such energy is determined genetically and is finite, so that when it is used up, exhaustion and death occur. The *stress theory of ageing* has developed from this idea. One important aspect of this theory is the assertion that exposure to stressors accelerates ageing – that is, the greater the 'wear and tear' of life, the faster adaptation energy is consumed. Evidence for the role of stress in the ageing process remains inconclusive. However, the proposition that genetically programmed events may be influenced by life experience of stress is both logical and appealing.

Adrenocorticoid activity in stress

The adrenal cortex is quite distinct, in both structure and function, from the adrenal medulla, despite their close proximity to one another. Unlike the medulla, the secretion of the adrenal cortex is not directly controlled by the nervous system but by the action of other hormones in the blood. Figure 9.4 summarises the negative feedback control of glucocorticoid secretion. Note that, as described earlier, the stressor effect may overcome the negative feedback mechanism. Ramsey (1982) states that animal studies have produced evidence that the feedback loop may function at a higher set point in long term stress, so that a higher steroid hormone level must be reached before negative feedback occurs.

The adrenal cortex secretes three groups of steroid hormones:

- *Glucocorticoids* which have a general regulatory effect on metabolic processes. Cortisol (hydrocortisone) is the major glucocorticoid in humans. In physiology, increased secretion of this hormone is practically synonymous with the presence of stress. The characteristics of the GAS originally described by Selye in the 1930s are largely the result of the increased glucocorticoid secretion which occurs in stress.
- *Mineralocorticoids* which regulate salt and water balance. The major mineralocorticoid is aldosterone.
- Small amounts of *sex hormones*.

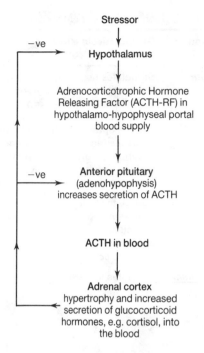

Fig. 9.4 The control of glucocorticoid secretion

The physiological effects of glucocorticoids

The main actions of the glucocorticoids are on the metabolism of carbohydrates, proteins and fats (Table 9.5). Most changes are catabolic in nature; that is, they break down larger molecules and are sparing of glucose. In most tissues many of these actions are antagonistic to those of insulin and so lead to a rise in blood glucose level. Glucocorticoids are, however, relatively inactive in the heart and brain so allowing extra glucose to be available to the cells of these organs. In addition to their direct effects, glucocorticoids also have some 'permissive' actions; that is, they must be present to allow some other hormones to affect metabolic reactions. For example, the catecholamines, adrenaline and noradrenaline, require the presence of cortisol in order to influence some metabolic pathways.

Cortisol's anti-inflammatory activity has meant that it and other glucocorticoids can be used therapeutically (steroid therapy) to suppress inflammation in many conditions such as rheumatoid arthritis. However, inflammation is an essential stage in the process of wound healing and if this

Table 9.5. *Physiological effects of glucocorticoid (cortisol) secretion in acute and chronic stress*

Body function or site	Glucocorticoid effect	Short term physiological effects	Additional long term physiological effects
Carbohydrate metabolism	Stimulates hepatic gluconeogenesis	Increased plasma glucose	
	Enhances elevation of blood glucose produced by other hormones e.g., adrenaline, glucagon		
	Inhibits uptake of glucose by most tissues (not brain) by antagonising peripheral effects of insulin	*Glycosuria (if renal threshold exceeded)	
	Inhibits activity of glycolytic enzyme hexokinase	(Steroid diabetes)	
Protein metabolism	Stimulates breakdown of body protein and depresses protein synthesis	Increased plasma levels of amino acids	*Muscle wasting
		Increased nitrogen content of urine	*Thinning of the skin
	Stimulates hepatic deamination of amino acids	Negative nitrogen balance	*Loss of hair
			*Depression of the immune response
Lipid metabolism	Promotes lipolysis	Increased plasma levels of fatty acids and cholesterol	*Redistribution of adipose tissue from periphery to head and trunk
		Increased ketone body production and ketonuria	
Calcium metabolism	*Antagonises vitamin D metabolites and so reduces calcium absorption from the gut		*Osteoporosis
	Increases renal excretion of calcium		Kidney stones
Vascular reactivity	Permissive for noradrenaline to induce vasoconstriction	*Prevents stress-induced hypotension	
	Reduces capillary permeability		
Inflammatory response	*Stabilises membranes of cellular lysosomes (inhibiting their rupture)	*Inhibition of inflammation	*Gastric ulceration
	*Suppresses phagocytosis		
	*Reduces multiplication of fibroblasts in connective tissue and hence decreases production of collagen fibres	*Decreased formation of granulation tissue	*Reduced rate of wound healing
	*Inhibits formation and release of histamine and bradykinin	*Reduced allergic response	
Immune response	*Reduced immunoglobulin synthesis	*Decreased white blood cell count	
	*Decreased levels of lymphocytes, basophils and eosinophils	*Immunosuppression and decreased resistance to infection	
	*Atrophy of lymphoid tissue		
Water and electrolyte balance	Enhances sodium ion and water reabsorption in distal tubules and collecting ducts of renal nephrons	Increased extracellular fluid volume	
	Reciprocal potassium and hydrogen ion excretion (mineralocorticoid effect)		

Body function or site	Glucocorticoid effect	Short term physiological effects	Additional long term physiological effects
Blood	*Enhances coagulability *Reduces levels of lymphocytes, basophils and eosinophils *Increases levels of erythrocytes, platelets and neutrophils	*Reduced blood clotting time *Decreased white blood cell count *Haemoconcentration (increased viscosity)	
Central nervous system	*Emotional changes (in excess or deficiency) May facilitate learning and memory (ACTH may independently facilitate learning and memory)	*Emotional changes Increased rate of learning Enhanced learning	

*These physiological effects occur only when high plasma levels of glucocorticoids, similar to those found during steroid therapy, are present.

Reproduced with permission from Boore, J. R. P., Champion, R. and Ferguson, M. C. (eds.) (1987). Nursing the Physically Ill Adult. *Churchill Livingstone, Edinburgh.*

inflammation is reduced by corticosteroid therapy, wound healing will be delayed. Glucocorticoids are also used for their immunosuppressive effect in reducing rejection in grafting and transplantation. However, high levels of these hormones also reduce white blood cell count and antibody formation, so reducing resistance to infection.

The physiological effects of high plasma levels of glucocorticoids collectively produce Cushing's syndrome. This syndrome can occur pathologically or be due to clinical therapy using the hormones. According to Hilton (1981) there is evidence that plasma levels of glucocorticoids of severely stressed people are as high as those found in patients with Cushing's disease. Such levels have been found, for example, in post-operative patients, students following oral examinations and people in anxiety states.

The function of other hormones in stress

Research evidence suggests that the secretion of nearly every hormone is altered in stress (Asterita, 1985). The secretion and major effects in stress of hormones other than catecholamines and cortisol are summarised in Table 9.6. The major hormones whose secretion is increased in stress (catecholamines, cortisol, glucagon, thyroxine and growth hormone) all have a predominantly catabolic effect on metabolism and there are numerous instances of facilitating interactions between them, some of which are noted in Table 9.6.

The adaptive nature of the stress response

The contents of Tables 9.4, 9.5 and 9.6 summarise the nervous and hormonally induced changes that together constitute the physiological stress response. The physiological changes of acute stress occur in response to threatening signals and are adaptive insofar as they facilitate effective coping and survival in situations requiring physical activity and in which injury may occur. The acute stress response varies hardly at all between species and it is likely that such responses developed early in vertebrate evolution (Hilton, 1981).

The characteristics of the response may be summarised as follows. Central nervous arousal occurs and skeletal muscles tense. The defensive behaviour of freezing and 'playing dead' is a manifestation of extreme muscle tension. The pupil of the eye dilates, enlarging the visual field. Erection of hair increases the apparent size of the animal (although this response is of little significance in man, it is functional in small furry mammals).

Nutrients are mobilised in anticipation of a period of fasting and exercise. They are circulated to organs such as the heart and skeletal muscle whose efficient function is crucial to fight and flight. Such organs are supplied at the expense of those whose function is non-essential in the short term, such as the gastro-intestinal tract and kidney.

Extracellular fluid volume and blood coagulability increase — adaptive responses in case of

Table 9.6. *The secretion and effects of other hormones in stress*

Hormone	Endocrine gland of origin	Physiological functions	Effect of stressor on secretion	Physiological effects in stress
Somatostatin	Hypothalamus	Inhibits secretion of growth hormone and thyroid stimulating hormone Suppresses output of insulin and glucagon	Inhibited	Secretion of growth hormone and thyroid stimulating hormone facilitated Secretion of insulin and glucagon increased
Antidiuretic hormone	Hypothalamus and posterior pituitary	Increased water reabsorption from the distal tubule and collecting duct of renal nephrons May also influence learning by direct action on the brain	Increased	Increased extracellular fluid volume Enhanced learning
Growth hormone	Anterior pituitary	Reinforces carbohydrate and lipid mobilising effects and insulin antagonism of catecholamines and cortisol May stimulate uptake of amino acids by injured tissue, but unable to counteract catabolic effect of cortisol on body protein	Increased in acute stress Cortisol suppresses release, so decreased in chronic stress	Promotes gluconeogenesis and elevation in blood glucose Facilitates tissue growth and repair Retarded growth in chronic stress
Thyroid stimulating hormone, Thyroxine and Tri-iodothyronine	Anterior pituitary Thyroid	Raised metabolic rate Acts synergistically with catecholamines	Increased in acute stress but secretion suppressed by cortisol in chronic stress	Potentiation of catecholamine effects in acute stress
Aldosterone	Adrenal cortex	Increased sodium ion reabsorption from distal tubule and collecting duct of nephron	Increased	Increased extracellular fluid volume
Glucagon	Pancreas (α-cells)	Promotes glycolysis and gluconeogenesis Presence of cortisol permissive for these actions	Hypoglycaemia is major stimulus for secretion but large increases in secretion also occur in response to other stressors, such as cold exposure, exercise and acute anxiety	Raised plasma glucose
Insulin	Pancreas (β-cells)	Promotes entry of glucose into most body cells	Catecholamines suppress release	Actions inhibited

Hormone	Endocrine gland of origin	Physiological functions	Effect of stressor on secretion	Physiological effects in stress
		Anabolic effect on lipid and protein metabolism	Cortisol and growth hormone antagonise peripheral effects	
Gonadotrophins (follicle stimulating and luteinising hormones)	Anterior pituitary	Secretion of gonadal steroids reduced	Inhibited	Irregularity or cessation of menstrual cycle Failure of ovulation Infertility

Reproduced with permission from Boore, J. R. P., Champion, R. and Ferguson, M. C. (eds.) (1987). Nursing the Physically III Adult. *Churchill Livingstone, Edinburgh.*

blood loss – and amino acids become available for immediate tissue repair.

It is easy to see that in animal and early human societies, this emergency response to physical threat must often have had survival value. Even today, each time we take exercise or suffer accidental or surgical injury, our ability to produce an acute stress response facilitates survival. As discussed earlier, prompt relief of stress minimises the risk of tissue damage.

Individuals who for some reason are unable to produce an efficient stress response are less able to survive trauma and disease. Loss of adrenomedullary function is not fatal, as sympathetic nervous activity parallels most of the actions of circulating adrenaline and noradrenaline. However, loss of adrenocortical secretion quite rapidly causes death through hypotension, hypoglycaemia and concomitant brain dysfunction.

People suffering from undersecretion of glucocorticoids (Addison's disease) are particularly susceptible to stressors. They may be unable to survive (cope with) quite minor life events, for example, dental extraction, unless they are given artificial hormone. People who take glucocorticoids therapeutically and so have artificially high plasma levels of the hormone may also require hormone cover in such situations, because their normal mechanisms of secretion are suppressed.

The maladaptive potential of the response

Today, human stressors are frequently of psychosocial origin and as has been explained in this section, can also trigger the physiological stress response. If appropriate coping responses do not involve physical exercise and/or injury (as is the case more often than not!) then the physiological stress responses are inappropriate because the resources that are mobilised are not used. In such circumstances sympathetic arousal produces distressing symptoms (see Table 9.4) and in the longer term tissue damage may also occur.

Stress relief

In such circumstances stress can be relieved either by reducing the perceived demand on the individual or by increasing the individual's perceived ability to cope with the demand, for example, by education. Learning a technique such as meditation or muscle relaxation can be helpful, since successful use of such techniques induces a state that is the opposite of sympathetic arousal (Wallace and Benson, 1972). Taking exercise is another effective means of stress relief since physical activity utilises the physiological response appropriately. Techniques such as biofeedback systematically train the stressed individual to exercise control over some aspect of his stress response.

Tranquillising drugs, alcohol and tobacco relieve stress by temporarily suppressing the person's perception of the demand upon him. Their use is associated with other health risks but may be justified in the short term if they help the person to cope until the problem resolves or more effective coping methods are found.

The suggestions for further reading at the end of this chapter include texts which describe techniques for stress relief in more detail.

Adrenal reserves of glucocorticoids vary both between individuals and over time for any one person. If a person experiences long term stress, these reserves are diminished and in very severe cases may become exhausted. This is the parallel of the stage of exhaustion of the general adaptation syndrome. It may also be the physiological reflection of 'burn-out'. Signs and symptoms of impending glucocorticoid exhaustion include feelings of weakness, lightheadedness, extreme fatigue, unease and irritability, gastro-intestinal disturbance, low blood pressure, hypoglycaemia and abnormal sensitivity to change in environmental temperature. Clearly the best action is to recognise and help the person to cope with his stress before such a situation occurs. If, however, a person experiences these symptoms, rest and relief from stress are imperative. In some circumstances artificial glucocorticoid cover may be necessary.

The similarities between the pharmacological effects of the catecholamines and cortisol and the pathological changes associated with many 'diseases of civilisation' have lead to stress being implicated in the aetiology of these diseases. Although it is known that plasma levels of glucocorticoids as high as those in Cushing's syndrome can induce pathological change, for example, gastric ulceration, the long term ability of lower plasma levels of these hormones to produce disease has not yet been proved.

Evidence for the role of distress in the aetiology of disease is discussed in the last section of this chapter.

Psychological responses to stress

Despite the limitations of Selye's early research, it stimulated a lasting interest in the subject and much research. This research aimed to discover whether the observation of a characteristic set of physiological reactions to a variety of environmental stressors – the GAS – could be generalised to include the reactions of humans exposed to a range of stressors in their everyday lives. Indeed, Selye's ideas about non-specific responses to stress continued to be influential for a number of years until evidence became available which suggested that some unpleasant conditions did not lead to GAS (e.g. Mason, 1971), and that physiological responses may differ according to the nature of the stressor (see, for example, Mason *et al.*, 1976; Terman *et al.*, 1984). Selye's research, therefore, laid the foundations for later studies concerned with the possible influence of psychological processes.

It is now apparent that cognitive and emotional factors intervening between stimulus and response may help to account for observed differences in the endocrine response to stress. For instance, Mason *et al.* (1976) found that humans will produce catecholamines initially when exposed to strong aversive stressors such as heat or noise, but if subjective feelings of competitiveness are minimal, they will not produce the expected increase in cortisol secretion. The absence of cortisol is significant, given the role it is believed to play in inhibiting the immune response. Similar findings have been reported for children admitted to hospital for tonsillectomy (Knight *et al.*, 1979) and for women undergoing breast biopsy for possible malignancy (Katz *et al.*, 1970). Physiological reactions to aversive stimuli appear to be linked to variations in how people perceive the threatening event. This possibility highlights the importance of taking subjective reactions and feelings into account.

As long as people feel able to meet the demands that are made upon them, they are likely to view stress positively as a challenge. As soon as this situation changes, however, and their ability to cope in relation to the demand decreases, then the all too familiar negative responses to stress occur.

You will almost certainly have experienced a range of feelings associated with the negative experience of 'being under stress'. This may include emotions such as anxiety, fear, guilt, tension, anger, aggression, irritability, depression, tiredness, a feeling of worthlessness, apathy, hopelessness and frustration. Lazarus (1976) refers to these negative emotions which occur as a result of stress as 'stress emotions'. In addition to these negative emotions, stress may impair cognitive ability (Hebb, 1972). You may have experienced this first-hand when you have been unable to concentrate or organise your thoughts logically when sitting an important examination.

According to Lazarus, stress emotions can serve a useful purpose in that they often trigger a variety of behaviours which are attempts to deal with the stressful situation, i.e. most of us are motivated to reduce the unpleasant feelings associated with stress. The way in which we do this has been called 'coping'. We also owe this concept to Lazarus (1966) who suggested that the term 'coping' refers to 'strategies for dealing with threat' (page 151). Cox (1978) suggests that coping is the key to understanding psychological responses to stress.

Lazarus and Folkman (1984) suggest that two rather different kinds of processes may be involved in coping with stress:

- problem-focused coping
- emotion-focused coping.

In the first of these, the individual deals directly with the problem: after evaluating the situation, the individual does something either to change it or avoid it. The alternative process, emotion-focused coping, is a more indirect means of coping, concerned more with reducing anxiety than with dealing with the situation responsible for producing the anxiety.

Problem-focused coping

This means of coping involves conscious action and can take several forms. If a potential cause of stress can be anticipated, one may take steps to reduce the harm when it does occur. The provision of information to reduce fear of the unknown is an excellent example of helping to produce this kind of coping. Janis, an American social psychologist, was one of the first people to investigate stress in patients awaiting surgery, and the benefits of giving accurate prior information and reassurance about post-operative discomfort (see Janis, 1971, or Langer *et al.*, 1975). The often cited research of nurse researchers such as Hayward (1975) and Boore (1978) provides further evidence of the benefits of reduced post-operative anxiety levels in patients when they have been given information about what to expect before the operation.

Another example of problem-focused coping is provided by the person who decides to develop new skills (for instance, by doing an assertiveness training course) to deal with colleagues more effectively.

Two further means of problem-focused coping are aggression and escape, which are behavioural responses associated with the physiological responses of 'fight' and 'flight'. Although each may be effective in the short term, neither allows one

to come to terms with the threat, and each may be responsible for difficulties, such as anxiety, in the longer term. You may either vent your aggression directly on the perceived source of the frustration (for example, in the case of course-related stress, on the college in which you are studying) or you may vent your anger on some more readily available target (such as throwing a plate or arguing with a friend). For similar reasons, it is not uncommon for patients to become angry with those responsible for caring for them.

Alternatively, the feelings associated with stress may motivate a person to escape from the stressful situation; in this case they might decide, if work or studying was the stressor, to leave their job or the course. Under normal circumstances, one might argue that escape is more appropriate for physically threatening rather than psychologically threatening events.

Emotion-focused coping

Palliative strategies, such as alcohol, drugs (sedatives and tranquillisers) or relaxation techniques, may be used to moderate the distress frequently associated with a stressful experience by reducing its psychophysiological effects. Psychological mechanisms which distort reality may also be used to moderate distress. When studying the unconscious, Anna Freud (1946) identified a number of psychological ways, known as *defence mechanisms*, by which a person could deceive himself about the presence of a threat by distorting reality in some way.

Lazarus (1976) suggested that a number of defence mechanisms might be used to reduce the perception of threat, including:

- denial
- identification
- displacement
- repression
- reaction formation
- projection
- intellectualisation.

You may already be familiar with several of these defence mechanisms. For instance, you may have cared for someone who has a life-threatening disease, but who refuses to accept that he is ill (denial) and thus discounts what he is told about the prognosis. Similarly, intellectualisation may be used by health care professionals to enable them to become emotionally detached from a situation which might otherwise be threatening or intolerable. Professional people may only be able to control their own feelings by not identifying too closely with the suffering of particular patients. Most psychology textbooks will provide a more detailed description of defence mechanisms (see, for example, Chapter 15 in Atkinson *et al.*, 1990).

Although originally used by Freud to describe unconscious mechanisms, Cox (1978) suggests that we may deliberately employ one or other of these defence mechanisms as a means of coping with a stressful situation. Cox also reminds us that such concepts are difficult to evaluate scientifically since they are rather loosely defined (as are many of the concepts deriving from psychoanalytic theory), and they are descriptive rather than predictive. However, he goes on to say:

> 'Despite this they have, like most psychoanalytic concepts, had some impact on psychological thought and the practice of psychology'
>
> (page 84)

People probably use both types of coping strategy. Whilst it might appear that problem-focused coping is the more effective approach to adopt, it is important to remember that some problems simply cannot be solved or at least not immediately. For instance, when someone who is close to you dies, you may need some means of emotion-focused coping to reduce the emotional distress in the short term, until you feel ready to face up to the loss and its consequences, and can subsequently seek out more effective methods of coping.

It is now recognised that the success of coping strategies may partly depend on the extent to which people believe that they can control their situation. Seligman's theory of learned helplessness originated from a series of studies carried out with dogs (Seligman, 1975). He found that dogs readily learned to escape a mild electric shock by jumping away from the source, and that if a light was switched on briefly before the shock was administered, the dogs learned to avoid the shocks altogether by escaping into the 'safe' area. However, dogs who had previously experienced electric shocks which they had been unable to avoid continued to endure the shocks and sat passively: they did not learn to escape, or the appropriate avoidance response, even when a new situation allowed them to do so. Moreover, Seligman found that this kind of learned helplessness was very difficult to overcome.

Although this model of learned helplessness in animals is far too simple to explain human behaviour, our ability to cope with stress is likely to be affected by the feeling that we have a certain amount of control over our lives. Certainly, Glass and Singer (1972) found that the belief that an aversive event could be controlled was sufficient to reduce anxiety, even if that belief turned out to be false, or if the control was never exercised. According to Rotter (1966), people differ in their belief about the degree of control they can exert: some individuals have a greater sense of being in control of their lives than others which may in its turn affect their coping ability.

If people believe they cannot influence the situation in which they find themselves, then feelings of helplessness are likely to develop and lead to inactivity, as a result of what Lazarus (1976) calls the hopelessness of their situation. In order to help such people, it would be necessary to assist them in re-establishing control over their situation by suggesting possible ways of coping. In this context, it is interesting to note the results of a field experiment undertaken in a nursing home by Langer and Rodin (1976) in which the residents' perception of control was manipulated. The reported benefits of perceived control included increased sociability and activity levels of the residents and improved health ratings. These improvements were still found in an 18-month follow-up study (Rodin and Langer, 1977).

Many health care professionals learn to cope with the demands of their work, with or without some form of external support, and continue to function effectively. Those who experience difficulties in coping with work-related stressors whilst remaining in the working environment are likely to become exhausted, may suffer from burn-out, and may leave the profession or drop out of their education programme. The following statement made by a Nursing Officer summarises many of the key issues:

> 'The stereotyped image of the qualified nurse is that she is committed totally to her patients, is skilled, fit and strong, and gives care as opposed to needing it. But of course . . . it just is not true. Nurses need help and support . . . just as much

as our students and our patients. Unfortunately this does not seem to be recognised by the public, the organisation or indeed, the profession itself'
(Hingley and Cooper, 1986)

Concern about recruitment, retention and wastage means that far more emphasis needs to be placed on stress management and support groups so that individuals are not left to cope alone. There are a number of ways, besides alcohol and medication, that may be used to reduce stress, including relaxation training, biofeedback, meditation, stress innoculation, physical exercise, assertiveness training, counselling and sharing the problem with others through support schemes.

The list of further reading at the end of this chapter includes a number of useful resources to help you to deal more effectively with stress. In particular, you are recommended to look at:

- Bond, M. (1986). *Stress and Self Awareness: A Guide for Nurses.* Heinemann, London.
- Burnard, P. (1991). *Coping with Stress in the Health Professions: A Practical Guide.* Chapman and Hall, London.
- Fontana, D. (1989). *Managing Stress.* British Psychological Society/Routledge, London.
- Gillespie, C. (1987). Stress reducing strategies. *Nursing Times,* 83 (39), 30–32.

Stress and illness

As long ago as 1932, Cannon suggested that vital body organs could be damaged if the activity of the autonomic nervous system is maintained in a highly aroused state as a result of prolonged exposure to stress. In this section, we shall briefly examine some of the evidence concerning the relationship between physical illness and stress-related factors.

Behavioural medicine has become a recognised interdisciplinary field of study that aims to understand how psychological, physiological and social variables interact to cause illness, and also to identify ways in which health can be promoted. What are your beliefs about a possible relationship between a person's psychological and emotional state and susceptibility to illness? Think for a moment about the following four questions.

Do you believe that:

(1) a person is more likely to develop an illness, such as 'flu, when feeling under pressure?
(2) a person's personality can affect the likelihood that he will suffer from coronary heart disease?
(3) stress is a causal factor in cancer?
(4) psychiatric illness is associated with changes in immune status?

Whatever your beliefs, it is interesting to note that these and similar assumptions can be traced back to some of the earliest medical thinkers and predate the relatively recent growth of interest in this subject (Harvey, 1988).

It is certainly well established that physical illness may be produced in laboratory animals exposed to severe and prolonged environmental stress. Weiss (1972), for example, reported that healthy rats who were able to escape from electric shocks showed fewer gastric lesions than those who were helpless and could not escape. Control rats who received no electric shocks showed no ulceration of the stomach. Similarly, Sklar and Anisman (1979) induced tumours in mice by implanting cancerous tissue and then studied the impact of stress on the rate of growth of these tumours. The tumours of the mice who were exposed to electric shocks grew faster than those of the control mice, and they died sooner.

One cannot simply generalise from animals to humans, and ethical constraints obviously preclude researchers carrying out similar experiments with human subjects. Considerable research has, however, been carried out in relation to people being exposed to respiratory viruses. For example, in a carefully controlled trial undertaken at the (now disbanded) Common Cold Unit run by the Medical Research Council, 394 healthy volunteers were exposed to nasal drops containing one of five respiratory viruses or saline (the control condition). They found a positive correlation between respiratory infection rates and the degree of the subject's psychological stress, even after controlling for other possible contributory factors such as age, gender, season of the year, personality traits, smoking and amount of exercise taken (Cohen et al., 1991). In this type of experimental research, the investigator is able to exert a considerable amount of control over the study and determine which individuals are allocated to specific experimental conditions.

In this field, however, researchers are unable to undertake many highly controlled studies because of ethical and practical constraints. Rather, they are forced to undertake studies which compare the effects of naturally occurring differences in the variable of interest, such as the effects of different levels of stress on the development of illness. So, for instance, a researcher may choose to compare people with high stress/anxiety levels with those with low stress/anxiety levels. This type of research is known as quasi-experimental and does not allow the researcher to identify causal factors. When considering the evidence from a quasi-experimental study, it is necessary to remember that while stress may be identified as a possible contributory factor in the development of illness, illness itself is likely to be a source of stress, thus making it impossible to identify causal relationships unequivocally.

As we shall see, many of the claims that specific illnesses are associated with particular aspects of social behaviour, including stress, have either not been systematically tested, or, if they have been tested, the emerging evidence has often been conflicting. One exception to this is the assertion that particular patterns of behaviour predispose people to develop coronary heart disease (CHD).

Stress and CHD

Heart disease is a major cause of death in many countries, including the United Kingdom (Julian and Marley, 1991). Epidemiological data has identified a series of traditional risk factors including family history, a person's sex, high systolic blood pressure, heavy cigarette smoking and raised levels of cholesterol in the blood. Even when looked at together, however, these factors only account for about half the variation in CHD. It would appear that other psychosocial factors play a part.

After observing the behaviour of their patients, two American cardiologists identified the major behavioural characteristics of the male who is prone to develop CHD (Friedman and Rosenman, 1959). Their list included highly competitive behaviour, overcommitment to work, high achieving, impatience, restlessness, hostility, an exaggerated sense of the urgency of passing time and the need to do everything in a hurry – all of which have become more common in 20th century industrialised, urban society. These behaviour characteristics are referred to collectively as the 'Type A' pattern of behaviour. Although this behaviour pattern may resemble a personality type, it is important to remember that the researchers were investigating the relationship between specific behaviours and the incidence of CHD, not personality. There is, as yet, no evidence that a particular type of personality is more prone to develop CHD. The 'Type B' behaviour pattern, on the other hand, is characterised by more relaxed behaviours.

A double-blind prospective epidemiological study – the Western Collaborative Group Study – confirmed the predictive validity of a Type A behaviour pattern. In this study, 3524 American men aged between 35 and 59, who were well at the start, were followed up over eight and a half years. During this time, the drop-out rate was remarkably low and 3154 completed the study. Individuals exhibiting Type A behaviour patterns were found to be 2.37 times as likely to develop CHD as were the Type B men. Even when traditional risk factors were controlled for, men exhibiting Type A behaviours were still about twice as likely to develop CHD. In addition, Type A men were five times more likely to suffer a second myocardial infarction than other men with CHD (Rosenman et al., 1975). Similar findings have been reported in other studies (e.g. Steptoe, 1985), including long term prospective studies (Haynes et al., 1980).

Attempts have been made to explain these findings. It has been suggested that in response to stress, Type A individuals have higher noradrenaline levels in the blood and that this may lead to heart lesions and damage to the arteries, and may also increase the extent to which platelets aggregate, making thrombosis formation more likely.

It remains to be seen whether Type A behaviour characteristics are consistently found to predict CHD reliably, and also whether a similar relationship is found in women. One idea that is currently being investigated is whether any of the specific characteristics (such as achievement, aggression or time consciousness) might be better predictors of CHD than the overall combination of the Type A behavioural pattern. Indeed, it has been suggested by Barefoot et al. (1989) that level of hostility may be a better predictor of CHD than Type A behaviours overall. It also remains to be seen whether it is possible to modify successfully the behaviour of Type A individuals who have suffered a heart attack and thus decrease the risk of recurrent attacks (Cooper, 1989).

Stress and cancer

Another disease which has received a considerable amount of attention in recent years is cancer: in particular, the idea that stress may be a causal factor in its aetiology. It is clearly important that any empirical evidence is evaluated carefully so that patients are not 'blamed' for their illness. An excellent review of some of the early evidence relating specific aspects of stress to cancer is provided by Temoshok and Heller (1984). They highlight the difficulty of drawing firm conclusions given the diversity of studies that have been carried out. They conclude that the incidence of major life events (such as those measured by the SRRS) appears to be a less important factor than the way in which such events are handled. They also suggest that there is a growing amount of evidence to support the idea that cancers are most frequently found in individuals who do not express their emotions and who react in a hopeless manner to difficult situations. At the present time, however, it must be emphasised that the empirical evidence is largely suggestive rather than conclusive and it is important not to overstate the case.

Stress and the immune system

Following on from the study of specific diseases, researchers have also been trying to find out how stress may exert its effect. Those working in this rapidly developing field of psychoimmunology are trying to uncover ways in which the brain and the immune system interact to affect our susceptibility to disease. The immune system provides a complex means by which the human body is able to protect itself against disease. The immune response is triggered by antigens which produce an increase in both lymphocytes and antibodies that either contain or destroy the antigen. There are three different types of lymphocyte, each with different functions:

- T helper cells which help to produce antibodies
- T cytotoxic and natural killer cells which are able to destroy cells
- T suppressor cells which are able to modify the activity of other cells or antibodies.

A number of research studies have studied the effects of stressful life events on the immune system by either counting the numbers of lymphocytes and other types of cell and/or measuring the reactivity of lymphocytes. Evidence is now accumulating that suggests that stress may affect the immune system's ability to protect the body from the effects of invading substances such as viruses. One of the earliest studies was carried out in Australia and arose out of the well-known fact that people who have recently been bereaved are far more likely to become ill or even die when compared with matched non-bereaved people. For example, Bartrop et al. (1977) reported depressed lymphocyte function in 26 people whose spouses had died six weeks earlier, compared with those who had not suffered a recent bereavement. Schliefer et al. (1982) also found a similar drop in the number of lymphocytes and in their reactivity in a group of men during the first two months following the death of their wife from breast cancer. In some of the men, lymphocytes were affected for up to one year following bereavement.

Kiecolt-Glaser et al. (1984) took blood samples from 75 first-year medical students one month before their exams (to provide a baseline) and again during exam week; these students were also asked to complete the SRRS. They found that activity of the natural killer cells (large white blood cells that destroy foreign cells) decreased significantly overall from the first to the second blood samples, suggesting greater susceptibility to illness during this stressful period. Moreover, those students who had high stress scores on the SRRS had lower natural killer cell activity than those with lower stress scores. It is important to note, however, that it is not possible to rule out the possibility that the observed changes in natural killer cell activity found in this study were mediated by other factors, such as use of drugs, increased alcohol consumption, not eating enough or changes in sleep pattern.

In another study, Kiecolt-Glaser et al. (1987) compared the immune functioning of a group of women who had been divorced within the previous six years with that of another group of married women who were matched on a number of social and demographic variables. Overall, they found significantly lower immune functioning in the divorced group than the group of married women. Moreover, they also found differences within the divorced group, in that those who had been divorced for one year or less showed reduced immune functioning compared with those who had been divorced for longer.

Arnetz *et al.* (1987) studied a group of 25 Swedish women, of whom 17 had been unemployed for one year (the experimental group) and eight were employed (the control group). Of those who were unemployed, nine received standard financial benefits and the remaining eight received a support programme in addition. Although the researchers found no significant differences in the actual number of lymphocytes between the three groups, they did find that the reactivity of the lymphocytes was significantly greater in the experimental group who received the psychosocial support, compared with the unemployed women who merely received standard benefits.

Immune system activity may also be compromised in people with severe depression. Stein *et al.* (1985) measured the reactivity of lymphocytes in a group of severely depressed patients and found it to be significantly lower than that of a carefully matched group of non-depressed control subjects. The numbers of T cells were also significantly reduced. It is interesting to note that similar changes were not found in patients hospitalised for a major physical disorder, patients with schizophrenia, or those suffering from less severe depression.

It would appear from current evidence that the activity of the central nervous system and the neuro-endocrine system are closely associated with emotional activity. The sheer complexity of the immune system and its relationship with other physiological systems, however, makes it inappropriate to do anything more than speculate about the nature of the relationship between stress and immune responses (Martin, 1987). This is an area of research that should yield important new findings in the future. If you are interested in this area, you should look out for the latest information published in scientific and medical journals such as *New Scientist, Nature* and the *British Medical Journal.* For the present, it is unclear whether the relationship between stressful life events and the incidence of physical illness may be due to actual changes in health mediated by the immune system, or to lowered ability to cope with disease already present. On the other hand, to overlook stress as a possible factor contributing to the disease process and its treatment is likely to be an important omission.

Finally, when one considers the possibility of a relationship between high levels of occupational stress and specific diseases, it is important to remember that certain kinds of people may choose stressful jobs in the first place and therefore the disposition and temperament of such individuals is a confounding variable.

Now that we have examined some of the evidence concerning the relationship between stress and illness, we shall return to the four questions set out at the beginning of this section. Available evidence seems to suggest that individuals are more likely to develop an illness when they are feeling under pressure (Question 1). Whilst there is evidence that specific behaviour patterns – namely Type A behaviours – affect the likelihood that a person will suffer from coronary heart disease, this has not, as yet, been related to personality *per se* (Question 2). Question 3 about stress being a causal factor in cancer is not supported by the available data: stress may well be a contributory factor, but correlational data does not enable claims to be made about causal factors. Lastly, there is no evidence that psychiatric illness *per se* is associated with changes in immune status (Question 4); people with severe depression have, however, been found to have fewer T cells and reduced lymphocyte reactivity.

The answers to these questions highlight the care needed when analysing available evidence and the danger of making unwarranted assertions or generalising the findings too widely. You will notice that at best we can only talk about 'the likelihood' of something occurring or a high correlation between two factors. Individual variation in the experience of stress is certainly evident when one looks at the relationship between stress and health/illness. Although correlational data may enable us to predict the likelihood of a person who exhibits Type A behaviours developing CHD, it is important to remember that many people who fall into that category do not develop the disease. Moreover, reactions to stressful life events cannot be understood without taking account of factors which mediate their effect, such as degree of anticipation and control over the occurrence of an event. Further research is needed to extend our understanding of the highly complex relationship between stress-related factors and the likely onset of specific illnesses.

Conclusion

In the preceding pages we have discussed the nature of and sources of stress and have viewed stress as a phenomenon which is the reflection of an imbalance between the demand made upon a person and that person's perceived ability to cope with that demand. Physiological and psychological stress responses, their function in coping and their relevance in relation to health care have been described in some detail and an outline given of the evidence for linking stress with ill health as well as methodological problems associated with such research. It is important to recognise that the synthesis of research findings on stress given in this chapter represents only an outline of current understanding in what is a major area of ongoing research.

That stress is an all-pervasive phenomenon in health care is clear. It is equally clear that there is no easy means of tackling the problem. Certainly, the first step is to understand the nature of stress and that it can be, to quote Cox (1978), 'a threat to the quality of life and to physical and psychological well-being'. Next comes the need to develop the skills to recognise stress when it occurs, both in oneself and in others. For most people, dealing successfully with stress is likely to involve quite significant changes in behaviour and lifestyle. One of the major remaining challenges for those involved in health care is to develop creative ways of dealing sensitively and effectively with the inevitable sources of stress associated with their work.

Appendix – Professional Life Stress Scale

The following instructions are provided by Fontana (1989):

'Complete it [the scale] quickly, and don't think too hard before responding to each question. Your first response is often the most accurate one. As with any stress scale, it isn't difficult to spot what is the "low stress" answer to each question. Don't be tempted to give this answer if it isn't the accurate one. Nothing is at stake. *You are as stressed as you are.* Your score on the scale doesn't change that, one way or the other. The purpose of the scale is simply to help you clarify some of your thinking about your own life.'

Use the key on page 242 to assess your results.

1. Two people who know you well are discussing you. Which of the following statements would they be most likely to use?
   (a) 'X is very together. Nothing much seems to bother him/her.'
   (b) 'X is great. But you have to be careful what you say to him/her at times.'
   (c) 'Something always seems to be going wrong with X's life.'
   (d) 'I find X very moody and unpredictable.'
   (e) 'The less I see of X the better!'

2. Are any of the following common features of your life?
   - Feeling you can seldom do anything right
   - Feelings of being hounded or trapped or cornered
   - Indigestion
   - Poor appetite
   - Difficulty in getting to sleep at night
   - Dizzy spells or palpitations
   - Sweating without exertion or high air temperature
   - Panic feelings when in crowds or in confined spaces
   - Tiredness and lack of energy
   - Feelings of hopelessness ('what's the use of anything?')
   - Faintness or nausea sensations without any physical cause
   - Extreme irritation over small things
   - Inability to unwind in the evenings
   - Waking regularly at night or early in the mornings
   - Difficulty in taking decisions
   - Inability to stop thinking about problems or the day's events
   - Tearfulness
   - Convictions that you just can't cope
   - Lack of enthusiasm even for cherished interests
   - Reluctance to meet new people and attempt new experiences
   - Inability to say 'no' when asked to do something

- Having more responsibility than you can handle.
3. Are you *more* or *less* optimistic than you used to be (or about the same)?
4. Do you enjoy *watching* sport?
5. Can you get up late at weekends if you want to without feeling guilty?
6. Within reasonable professional and personal limits, can you speak your mind to: a) your boss? b) your colleagues? c) members of your family?
7. Who usually seems to be responsible for making the important decisions in your life: a) yourself? b) someone else?
8. When criticised by superiors at work, are you usually: a) very upset? b) moderately upset? c) mildly upset?
9. Do you finish the working day feeling satisfied with what you have achieved: a) often? b) sometimes? c) only occasionally?
10. Do you feel most of the time that you have unsettled conflicts with colleagues?
11. Does the amount of work you have to do exceed the amount of time available: a) habitually? b) sometimes? c) only very occasionally?
12. Have you a clear picture of what is expected of you professionally: a) mostly? b) sometimes? c) hardly ever?
13. Would you say that generally you have enough time to spend on yourself?
14. If you want to discuss your problems with someone, can you usually find a sympathetic ear?
15. Are you reasonably on course towards achieving your major objectives in life?
16. Are you bored at work: a) often? b) sometimes? c) very rarely?
17. Do you look forward to going into work: a) most days? b) some days? c) hardly ever?
18. Do you feel adequately *valued* for your abilities and commitment at work?
19. Do you feel adequately *rewarded* (in terms of status and promotion) for your abilities and commitment at work?
20. Do you feel your superiors: a) actively *hinder* you in your work? b) actively *help* you in your work?
21. If ten years ago you had been able to see yourself professionally as you are now, would you have seen yourself as: a) exceeding your expectations? b) fulfilling your expectations? c) falling short of your expectations?

22. If you had to rate how much you like yourself on a scale from 5 (most like) to 1 (least like), what would your rating be?

Key for Professional Life Stress Scale

1. a) 0, b) 1, c) 2, d) 3, e)4.
2. Score 1 for each 'yes' response
3. Score 0 for *more optimistic*, 1 for *about the same*, 2 for *less optimistic*
4. Score 0 for 'yes', 1 for 'no'
5. Score 0 for 'yes', 1 for 'no'
6. Score 0 for each 'yes' response, 1 for each 'no' response
7. Score 0 for 'yourself', 1 for 'someone else'
8. Score 2 for 'very upset', 1 for 'moderately upset', 0 for 'mildly upset'
9. Score 0 for 'often', 1 for 'sometimes', 2 for 'only occasionally'
10. Score 0 for 'no', 1 for 'yes'
11. Score 2 for 'habitually', 1 for 'sometimes', 0 for 'only very occasionally'
12. Score 0 for 'mostly', 1 for 'sometimes', 2 for 'hardly ever'
13. Score 0 for 'yes', 1 for 'no'
14. Score 0 for 'yes', 1 for 'no'
15. Score 0 for 'yes', 1 for 'no'
16. Score 2 for 'often', 1 for 'sometimes', 0 for 'very rarely'
17. Score 0 for 'most days', 1 for 'some days', 2 for 'hardly ever'
18. Score 0 for 'yes', 1 for 'no'
19. Score 0 for 'yes', 1 for 'no'
20. Score 1 for a), 0 for b)
21. Score 0 for 'exceeding your expectations', 1 for 'fulfilling your expectations', 2 for 'falling short of your expectations'
22. Score 0 for '5', 1 for '4' and so on down to 4 for '1'

INTERPRETING YOUR SCORE

Scores on stress scales must be interpreted cautiously. There are so many variables which lie outside the scope of these scales but which influence the way in which we perceive and handle our stress that two people with the same scores may experience themselves as under quite different levels of strain. Nevertheless, taken as no more than a guide, these scales can give us some useful information.

0–15 Stress isn't a problem in your life. This doesn't mean you have insufficient stress to keep yourself occupied and fulfilled.

The scale is only designed to assess undesirable responses to stress.

16–30 This is a moderate range of stress for a busy professional person. It's nevertheless well worth looking at how it can reasonably be reduced.

31–45 Stress is clearly a problem, and the need for remedial action is apparent. The longer you work under this level of stress, the harder it often is to do something about it. There is a strong case for looking carefully at your professional life.

46–60 At these levels stress is a major problem, and something must be done without delay. You may be nearing the stage of exhaustion in the general adaptability syndrome. The pressure must be eased.

References

Albrecht, T.L. (1982). What job stress means for the staff nurse. *Nursing Administration Quarterly*, 7(1), 1–11.

Arnetz, B.B., Wasserman, J. and Pettrini, B. (1987). Immune function in unemployed women. *Psychosomatic Medicine*, 49, 3–12.

Arnold, J. (1989). Experiences and attitudes of learner nurses during their first year of training, Unpublished Report of Manchester School of Management, University of Manchester Institute of Science and Technology.

Asterita, M.F. (1985). *The Physiology of Stress*. Human Sciences Press Inc., New York.

Atkinson, R.L., Atkinson, R.C., Smith, E.E., Bem, D.J. and Hilgard, E.R. (1990). *Introduction to Psychology* (10th ed.). Harcourt Brace Jovanovich, San Diego.

Bailey, J.T., Steffen, S.M. and Grout, J.W. (1980). The stress audit: identifying the stressors of ICU nursing. *Journal of Nursing Education*, 19(6), 15–25.

Barefoot, J.C., Dodge, K.A., Peterson, B.L., Dahlstrom, W.G. and Williams, R.B. (1989). The Cook-Medley hostility scale; item content and ability to predict survival. *Psychosomatic Medicine*, 51, 46–57.

Barnett, B.E., Hanna, B. and Parker, G. (1983). Life event scales for obstetric groups. *Journal of Psychosomatic Research*, 27(4), 313–320.

Bartrop, R.W., Luckhurst, E., Lazarus, L., Kicoh, L. and Penny, R. (1977). Depressed lymphocyte function after bereavement. *Lancet*, 1, 834–836.

Beck, J. (1984). Nurses have needs too II: take time to care for yourselves. *Nursing Times*, 80(41), 31–32.

Bernard, C. (1927). *Introduction to the Study of Experimental Medicine* (trans. H.C. Green). Macmillan Press, New York.

Birch, J. (1979). The anxious learners. *Nursing Mirror*, 148(1), 17–22.

Bishop, V. (1981). This is the age of the strain. *Nursing Mirror*, 153(6), 18–19.

Boore, J.R.P. (1978). *Prescription for Recovery*. RCN, London.

Brunt, C. (1984). Assessing anxiety levels. *Nursing Times*, 80(7), 37–38.

Campbell, C. (1985). Disturbing findings. *Nursing Mirror*, 160(26), 16–19.

Cannon, W.B. (1929). *Bodily Changes in Pain, Hunger, Fear and Rage* (2nd ed.). Appleton Century Crofts, New York.

Cannon, W.B. (1932). *The Wisdom of the Body*. Appleton Century Crofts, New York.

Cannon, W.B. (1935). Stresses and strains of homeostasis. *American Journal of Medical Science*, 189, 1–9.

Clegg, F. (1988). Disasters: Can psychologists help the survivors? *The Psychologist*, 1(4), 134–135.

Cohen, S. and Wills, T.A. (1985). Stress, social support, and the buffering hypothesis. *Psychological Bulletin*, 98, 310–337.

Cohen, S., Tyrell, D.A.J. and Smith, A.P. (1991). Psychological stress and susceptibility to the common cold. *New England Journal of Medicine*, 325(9), 606–612.

Cooper, C. (1989). Are Type As prone to heart attacks? *The Psychologist*, 2(1), 19.

Cox, T. (1978). *Stress*. Macmillan Press, London

DeLongis, A., Coyne, J.C., Dakof, G., Folkman, S. and Lazarus, R.S. (1982). Relationship of daily hassles, uplifts and major life events to health status. *Health Psychology*, 1, 119–136.

DeLongis, A., Folkman, S. and Lazarus, R.S. (1988). The impact of daily stress on health and mood: psychological and social resources as mediators. *Journal of Personality and Social Psychology*, 54, 486–495.

Figley, C. (1986). *Trauma and Its Wake* (Vol. 2). Brunner Mazel, New York.

Fletcher, B. (1991). *Work, Stress, Disease and Life Expectancy*. John Wiley and Sons, London.

Fontana, D. (1989). *Managing Stress*. British Psychological Society/Routledge, London.

Frankenhauser, M. (1975). Experimental approaches to the study of catecholamines and emotion. In *Emotions: Their Parameters and Measurement*, Levi, L. (ed.). Raven Press, New York.

Franklin, B.L. (1974). *Patient Anxiety on Admission to Hospital*. RCN, London.

Friedman, M. and Rosenman, R.H. (1959). Association of specific overt behaviour patterns with blood and cardiovascular findings. *Journal of the American Medical Association*, 169, 1286–1296.

Freud, A. (1946). *The Ego and the Mechanisms of Defence*. International Universities Press, New York.

Funkenstein, D.H. (1955). The physiology of fear and anger. *Scientific American*, 192, 74–80.

Ganong, W.F. (1991). *Review of Medical Physiology* (13th ed.). Large Medical Publications, Los Altos.

Glass, D.C. and Singer, J.E. (1972). *Urban Stress: Experiments on Noise and Social Stressors*. Academic Press, New York.

Harvey, P. (1988). Stress and health. In *Health Psychology: Process and Application*, Broome, A. (ed.). Chapman and Hall, London.

Haynes, S.G., Feinleib, M. and Kannel, W.B. (1980). The relationship of psychosocial factors to coronary heart disease in the Framingham Study Part 3: eight-year incidence of coronary heart disease. *American Journal of Epidemiology*, 111(1), 37–58.

Hayward, J. (1975). *Information: A Prescription against Pain*. RCN, London.

Hebb, D.O. (1972). *Textbook of Psychology* (3rd ed.). W.B. Saunders, Philadelphia.

Hilton, S.M. (1981). The physiology of stress – emotion. In *The Principles and Practice of Human Physiology*, Edholm, O.G. and Weiner, J.S. (eds.). Academic Press, London.

Hingley, P. and Cooper, C.L. (1986). *Stress and the Nurse Manager*. John Wiley and Sons, Chichester.

Holmes, T.H. and Rahe, R.H. (1967). The social adjustment rating scale. *Journal of Psychosomatic Research*, 11, 213–218.

Hudgens, R.W. (1974). Personal catastrophe and depression: a consideration of the subject with respect to medically ill adolescents, and a requiem for retrospective life-event studies. In *Stressful Life Events: Their Nature and Effects*, Dohrenwend, B.S. and Dohrenwend, B.P. (eds.). John Wiley and Sons, New York.

Janis, I.L. (1971). *Stress and Frustration*. Harcourt Brace Jovanovich, New York.

Johnson, J.E. (1983). Preparing patients to cope with stress while hospitalized. In *Patient Teaching*, Wilson-Barnett, J. (ed.). Churchill Livingstone, Edinburgh.

Julian, D. and Marley, C. (1991). *Coronary Heart Disease: The Facts*. Oxford Medical Press, Oxford.

Katz, J.L., Weiner, H., Gallagher, T.F. and Hellman, L. (1970). Stress, distress and ego defenses: psychoendocrine response to impending tumor biopsy. *Archives of General Psychiatry*, 23, 131–142.

Kiecolt-Glaser, J.K., Garner, W., Speicher, C., Penn, G., Holliday, J. and Glaser, R. (1984). Psychosocial modifiers of immunocompetence in medical students. *Psychosomatic Medicine*, 46, 7–14.

Kiecolt-Glaser, J.K., Fisher, L.D. and Ogrocki, P. (1987). Marital quality, marital disruption and immune function. *Psychosomatic Medicine*, 49, 13–34.

Kline Leidy, N. (1989). A physiologic analysis of stress and chronic illness. *Journal of Advanced Nursing*, 14, 868–876.

Knight, R.B., Atkins, A., Eagle, C.J., Evans, N., Finkelstein, J.W., Fukushima, D., Katz, J.L. and Weiner, H. (1979). Psychological stress, ego defenses and cortisol production in children hospitalized for elective surgery. *Psychosomatic Medicine*, 41, 40–49.

Kushnir, T. (1986). Stress and social facilitation: the effects of the presence of an instructor on student nurses' behaviour. *Journal of Advanced Nursing*, 11, 13–19.

Langer, E., Janis, I.L. and Wolfer, J.A. (1975). Reduction of psychological stress in surgical patients. *Journal of Experimental Social Psychology*, 11, 155–165.

Langer, E.J. and Rodin, J. (1976). The effects of choice and enhanced personal responsibility for the aged: a field experiment in an institutional setting. *Journal of Personality and Social Psychology*, 34(2), 191–198.

Lazarus, R.S. (1966). *Psychological Stress and the Coping Process*. McGraw-Hill, New York.

Lazarus, R.S. (1976). *Patterns of Adjustment*. McGraw-Hill, New York.

Lazarus, R.S. and Folkman, S. (1984). *Stress, Appraisal and Coping*. Springer, New York.

Lees, S. and Ellis, N. (1990). The design of a stress-management programme for nursing personnel. *Journal of Advanced Nursing*, 15, 946–961.

Levin, J.S. and DeFrank, R.S. (1988). Maternal stress and pregnancy outcomes: a review of the psychosocial literature. *Journal of Psychosomatic Obstetrics and Gynaecology*, 9(1), 3–16.

Lindop, E. (1991). Individual stress among nurses in training: why some leave whilst others stay. *Nurse Education Today*, 11(2), 110–120.

Marshall, J. (1980). Stress among nurses. In *White Collar and Professional Stress*, Cooper, C.L. and Marshall, J. (eds.). John Wiley and Sons, Chichester.

Martin, P. (1987). Psychology and the immune system. *New Scientist*, April 9, 46–50.

Mason, J.W. (1968). A review of psychoendocrine research on the pituitary adrenocortical system. *Journal of Advanced Medicine*, 30, 567–607.

Mason, J.W. (1971). A re-evaluation of the concept of 'nonspecificity' in stress theory. *Journal of Psychiatric Research*, 8, 323–333.

Mason, J.W., Maher, J.J., Hartley, L.H., Mougey, G.H., Perlow, H.J. and Jones, L.G. (1976). Selectivity of corticosteroid and catecholamine responses to various natural stimuli. In *Psychopathology of Human Adaptation*, Serban, G. (ed.). Plenum, New York.

Melia, K.M. (1987). *Learning and Working: The Occupational Socialization of Nurses*. Tavistock Publications, London.

Parkes, K. (1985). Stressful episodes reported by first-year student nurses: A descriptive account. *Social Sci-*

ence and Medicine, 20(9), 945–953.

Price, B. (1985). Moving wards: How do student nurses cope? *Nursing Times*, 81(9), 32–35.

Rahe, R.H. (1974). The pathway between subjects' recent life changes and their near-future illness reports: representative results and methodological issues. In *Stressful Life Events: Their Nature and Effects*, Dohrenwend, B.S. and Dohrenwend, B.P. (eds.). John Wiley and Sons, New York.

Rahe, R.H. and Arthur, R.J. (1977). Life-change patterns surrounding illness experience. In *Stress and Coping*, Monat, A. and Lazarus, R.S. (eds.). Columbia University Press, New York.

Ramsey, J.M. (1982). *Basic Pathophysiology, Modern Stress and the Disease Process*. Addison Wesley, London.

Rodin, J. and Langer, E.J. (1977). Long-term effects of a control-relevant intervention with the institutionalized aged. *Journal of Personality and Social Psychology*, 35(12), 897–902.

Rosenman, R.H., Brand, R.J., Jenkins, C.D., Friedman, M., Strauss, R. and Wurm, M. (1975). Coronary heart disease in the Western Collaborative Group Study: final follow-up experience of 8½ years. *Journal of the American Medical Association*, 233, 872–877.

Rotter, J.B. (1966). Generalized expectancies for internal versus external control of reinforcement. *Psychological Monographs*, 80, 1.

Ruch, L.O. and Holmes, T.H. (1971). Scaling of life change: comparison of direct and indirect methods. *Journal of Psychosomatic Research*, 15, 221–227.

Sarason, I.G., Johnson, J.H. and Siegel, J.M. (1978). Assessing the impact of life changes: development of the life experiences survey. *Journal of Consulting and Clinical Psychology*, 46, 932–946.

Schliefer, S.J., Keller, S.E. and Camerino, M. (1982). Suppression of lymphocyte stimulation following bereavement. *Journal of the American Medical Association*, 250, 374.

Seligman, M.E.P. (1975). *Helplessness: On Depression, Development and Death*. W.H. Freeman, San Francisco.

Selye, H. (1946). The general adaptation syndrome and the diseases of adaptation. *Journal of Clinical Endocrinology*, 6, 117–128.

Selye, H. (1976). *The Stress of Life* (2nd ed.). McGraw-Hill, New York.

Sklar, L.A. and Anisman, H. (1979). Stress and coping factors influence tumour growth. *Science*, 205, 513–515.

Stein, M., Keller, S.E. and Schliefer, S.J. (1985). Stress and immunomodulation: the role of depression and neuroendocrine function. *Journal of Immunology*, 135, 827–833.

Steptoe, A. (1985). Type-A coronary prone behaviour. *British Journal of Hospital Medicine*, 33, 257–260.

Suls, J. and Mullen, B. (1981). Life events, perceived control and illness: the role of uncertainty. *Journal of Human Stress*, 7, 30–34.

Sutherland, V.J. and Cooper, C.L. (1990). *Understanding Stress: A Psychological Perspective for Health Professionals*. Chapman and Hall, London.

Temoshok, L. and Heller, B.W. (1984). On comparing apples, oranges and fruit salad: a methodological overview of medical outcome studies in psychosocial oncology. In *Psychosocial Stress and Cancer*, Cooper, C.L. (ed.). John Wiley and Sons, Chichester.

Terman, G.W., Shavit, Y., Lewis, J.W., Cannon, J.T. and Liebeskind, J.C. (1984). Intrinsic mechanisms of pain inhibition: activation by stress. *Science*, 226, 1270–1277.

Thompson, J. (1983). Call Sister: stress in the A&E department. *Nursing Times*, 79(31), 23–27.

Thornton, S. (1984). Caring for special babies III: stress in the neonatal intensive care unit. *Nursing Times*, 80(5), 35–37.

Volicer, B.J. and Bohannon, M.W. (1975). A hospital stress rating scale. *Nursing Research*, 24(5), 352–359.

Volicer, B.J. and Volicer, L. (1978). Cardiovascular changes associated with stress during hospitalisation. *Journal of Psychosomatic Research*, 22, 159–168.

Wallace, R.K. and Benson, H.B. (1972). The physiology of meditation. In *Readings from the Scientific American* (1976) *Human Physiology and the Environment in Health and Disease*. Part IV, Responses to Psychosocial Stress. W.H. Freeman, San Francisco.

Weiss, J.M. (1972). Psychological factors in stress and disease. *Scientific American*, 226(6), 104–113.

Welford, A.T. (1973). Stress and performance. *Ergonomics*, 16, 567.

Williams, C. and Montague, S.E. (1988). The characteristics of living matter. In *Physiology for Nursing Practice*, Hinchliff, S.M. and Montague, S.E. (eds.). Baillière Tindall, London.

Wilson-Barnett, J. (1979). *Stress in Hospital*. Churchill Livingstone, Edinburgh.

Wilson-Barnett, J. (1984). Interventions to alleviate patients' stress: a review. *Journal of Psychosomatic Research*, 28(1), 63–72.

Wilson-Barnett, J. (1986). Reducing stress in hospital. In *Clinical Nursing Practice: Recent Advances in Nursing 14*, Tierney, A. (ed.). Churchill Livingstone, Edinburgh.

Wilson-Barnett, J. and Carrigy, A. (1978). Factors affecting patients' responses to hospitalisation. *Journal of Advanced Nursing*, 3(3), 221–228.

Suggestions for further reading

Asterita, M.F. (1985). *The Physiology of Stress*. Human Sciences Press, New York.

Atkinson, R.L., Atkinson, R.C., Smith, E.E., Bem, D.J. and Hilgard, E.R. (1990). *Introduction to Psychology* (10th ed.). Harcourt Brace Jovanovich, San Diego.

Bailey, R. and Clarke, M. (1989). *Stress and Coping in Nursing*. Chapman and Hall, London.

Bamber, M. (1988). Slant on stress. *Nursing Times*, 84(11), 61–63.

Bond, M. (1986). *Stress and Self Awareness: A Guide for Nurses*. Heinemann, London.

Burnard, P. (1991). *Coping with Stress in the Health Professions: A Practical Guide*. Chapman and Hall, London.

Clarke, M. (1984). Stress and coping: constructs for nursing. *Journal of Advanced Nursing*, 9, 3–13.

Clarke, M. (1984). The constructs 'stress' and 'coping' as a rationale for nursing activities. *Journal of Advanced Nursing*, 9, 267–275.

Cooper, C. (1989). Are Type As prone to heart attacks? *The Psychologist*, 2(1), 19.

Cooper, C.L., Cooper, R.D. and Eaker, L. (1988). *Living with Stress*. John Wiley and Sons, Chichester.

Copp, G. (1988). The reality behind stress. *Nursing Times*, 84(45), 50–53.

Cox, T. (1978). *Stress*. Macmillan Press, London.

Crawley, P. (1988). Coping with stress: CHAT for nurses in adversity. *Nursing Times*, 84(36), 27–28.

Dewe, P.J. (1987). Identifying strategies nurses use to cope with work stress. *Journal of Advanced Nursing*, 12, 489–492.

Elkind, A.K. (1988). Do nurses smoke because of stress?. *Journal of Advanced Nursing*, 13, 733–745.

Fletcher, B.C. (1991). *Work, Stress, Disease and Life Expectancy*. John Wiley and Sons, Chichester.

Fontana, D. (1989). *Managing Stress*. British Psychological Society/Routledge, London.

Fromant, P. (1988). Coping with stress: helping each other. *Nursing Times*, 84(36), 30–32.

Gillespie, C. (1987). Stress reducing strategies. *Nursing Times*, 83(39), 30–32.

Health Education Authority. (1988). *Stress in the Public Sector: Nurses, Police, Social Workers and Teachers*. HEA, London.

Hingley, P. and Harris, P. (1986). Burn-out at senior level. *Nursing Times*, 82(31), 28–29.

Hingley, P. and Harris, P. (1986). Lowering the tension. *Nursing Times*, 82(32), 52–53.

Hughes, J. (1990). Stress: scourge or stimulant? *Nursing Standard*, 5(4), 30–33.

Hyde, J. and Taylor, J. (1989). Stress for beginners. *Nursing Standard*, 3(46), 38–39.

Johnston, D.W. (1989). Will stress management prevent coronary heart disease? *The Psychologist*, 2(7), 275–288.

Kline Leidy, N. (1989). A physiologic analysis of stress and chronic illness. *Journal of Advanced Nursing*, 14, 868–876.

Kunkler, J. and Whittick, J. (1991). Stress management groups for nurses: practical problems and possible solutions. *Journal of Advanced Nursing*, 16, 172–176.

Lindop, E. (1991). Individual stress amongst nurses in training: why some leave while others stay. *Nurse Education Today*, 11(2), 110–120.

Martin, P. (1987). Psychology and the immune system. *New Scientist*, April 9, 46–50.

McGrath, A., Reid, N. and Boore, J.R. (1989). Occupational stress in nursing. *International Journal of Nursing Studies*, 16(4), 343–358.

Milne, D. and Watkins, F. (1986). An evaluation of the effects of shift rotation on nurses' stress, coping and strain. *International Journal of Nursing Studies*, 23(2), 139–146.

Murgatroyd, S. and Woolfe, R. (1982). *Coping with Crisis: Understanding and Helping People in Need*. Harper and Row, London.

Nolan, M.R., Grant, G. and Ellis, N.C. (1990). Stress is in the eye of the beholder: reconceptualizing the measurement of carer burden. *Journal of Advanced Nursing*, 15, 544–555.

Ostell, A. (1991). Coping, problem solving and stress: a framework for intervention strategies. *British Journal of Medical Psychology*, 64, 11–24.

Selye, H. (1976). *The Stress of Life*. McGraw-Hill, New York.

Shipley, P. (1989). Stress and coping in working mothers. *Nursing Times*, 85(13), 54.

Sutherland, V.J. and Cooper, C.L. (1990). *Understanding Stress: A Psychological Perspective for Health Professionals*. Chapman and Hall, London.

Swaffield, L. (1988). Coping with stress: sharing the load. *Nursing Times*, 84(36), 24–26.

Tyler, M. (1990). Stress management: 'the group approach'. *Nursing Standard*, 4(20), 22–23.

Wilson-Barnett, J. (1986). Reducing stress in hospital. In *Clinical Nursing Practice: Recent Advances in Nursing 14*, Tierney, A. (ed.). Churchill Livingstone, Edinburgh.

Some of the ideas in this chapter have previously been published in *Nursing the Physically Ill Adult* by Boore, Champion and Ferguson, published by Churchill Livingstone, 1987.

10

THE PATIENT AS A CONSUMER OF HEALTH CARE

Rosemary Rogers

This chapter explores the concept of the patient as a consumer of health care. It examines how the person becomes a patient and his role within the health care system.

It will consider the following aspects:

- The growth of a consumer ideology within the health service, with a discussion on whether this is appropriate to health care

- The process of becoming a patient, describing access to health care in hospital and the community, and changes in care settings

- The growth of private health care

- The development of complementary medicine

- Patient choice within the health care system, discussed with particular reference to the NHS and Community Care Act (1990)

- Health education and health promotion, with discussion on individual and state responsibility for health

- The different categories of care patients may require

- The relationship between the patient and his carers, with particular reference to partnership and involvement in care

- Patients' rights as individuals and in law

- The patient as a consumer and his rights to information and representation

- The complaints procedure, including complaints by patients or relatives and complaints by staff

Just as travellers on British Rail recently may have been bemused to hear themselves referred to on the public address system as 'customers' instead of 'passengers', so patients may be surprised to find that they can be considered to be 'consumers' of health care.

In private health care, the term may gain more ready acceptance. Here, after all, the patient can usually exercise some choice over the timing of treatment, the personnel who care for him and the place where treatment is carried out. Yet almost everyone at some time during their lives will become a patient. As such they will be a consumer of health care, in whatever setting – the private hospital, the NHS hospital, the GP's surgery or the homeopath's clinic.

While the language of consumerism is relatively new in the National Health Service, the concept of the patient as an active 'consumer' rather than a passive 'patient' has gained much ground over the past decade. It is reflected in the new organisation of the NHS – as a market place where services which are priced competitively and presented attractively will attract more patients and more resources; where 'consumer satisfaction surveys' are increasingly used and where quality is monitored and audited.

It is also increasingly reflected in patterns of patient care. Patients are becoming more involved in decisions over their treatment and care, given more information, and allowed to exercise some choice. Increasingly, their individual rights are respected, as are those of consumers of any other service.

The growth of a consumer ideology in the NHS has its roots in the management changes of the early 1980s when, as a result of the Griffiths Report (DHSS, 1983), consensus-style management was replaced with executive management. General managers replaced multidisciplinary management teams at unit, district and regional level. On short term contracts, they were expected to perform as their counterparts in private business – to work to 'targets', to achieve 'efficiency savings' and value for money. Many of these new managers came, as did Roy Griffiths himself, from the private business sector.

Local firms are now encouraged to advertise their services on health care premises, or even lease space to operate from health care premises. Wards, beds, even nurses' uniforms, it has been suggested, could carry sponsorship logos (Willis, 1989). As part of the much wider sea change in political ideology that the United Kingdom witnessed in the 1980s, the NHS is, more and more, expected to operate as a cost-effective business, providing a quality service within rigorously enforced cash limits.

At the same time there is increasing emphasis on monitoring and auditing the quality of services provided by the health service, with new management posts established in 'customer services' and 'quality assurance', many of them held by nurses. The term quality assurance has become a familiar part of NHS vocabulary, accompanied by patient satisfaction surveys, quality circles and nursing and medical audit.

Staff such as porters and receptionists have in some centres been given training in dealing with people, encouraged to smile and be friendly and polite, in a campaign similar to the 'guest relations programs' in the United States, described by Leppanen-Montgomery (1988). In the customer services campaigns run by many US hospitals, she states, nurses and all employees are encouraged to smile at their 'customers' under all circumstances, to avoid seeming 'in a hurry'. Posters proclaiming 'the customer is always right' adorn the walls and patients are actively encouraged to contact the administrators if they have any complaints.

Patients in Britain are now encouraged to 'shop around' for health care – the NHS and Community Care Act (HMSO, 1990a) makes it easier to change your GP. Opticians are now allowed to advertise their services and there were suggestions (since dropped) that dentists and GPs should be allowed to do the same. GPs are required to list the services they offer to help people choose which practice they join.

The process in the UK reached its zenith with the NHS and Community Care Act 1990, in which the NHS was restructured to create an internal market. Health authorities are purchasers of care, hospitals and community services are providers. Based on the health needs of its local population, the health authority 'purchases' care according to the best deal offered by local health care providers. Under the system, increasing numbers of hospitals have been allowed to become self-governing trusts, funded purely on the basis of the deals they strike with district health authorities. Using a similar principle, GP practices may hold their own budgets, buying from provider units the best care available for their patients in terms of its cost and availability.

In the government White Paper *Working for Patients* (DoH, 1989a) which preceded the legislation, the changes were presented on the basis of their benefits to the consumer. Money would follow patients, it argued. Consumer choice would be improved because services would be bought on the basis of which providers offered the best deal

– not just the cheapest but that with the shortest waiting list and the best quality services, detailed in contract specifications drawn up by the purchaser. Included in the changes are arrangements for auditing the medical services available and for questioning consumers on the quality of the services they receive.

Later in this chapter, we shall look at how much scope for choice the patient has as a consumer of health care, and at whether or not that has been improved by the recent changes. Firstly it is necessary to ask how comfortably the language and the techniques of consumerism sit within the health sector, particularly the publicly funded health sector.

As Buchan (1990) points out, patients are not always voluntarily making use of the services provided. They may even be uncooperative and downright hostile. Neither can they enter or leave the health care market at will. They are constrained by the availability of services.

But while the concept of the health service as a market place, in which aggressive customer care techniques are permissible, may be arguable, the idea of the patient as a consumer is more apt. For the concept of consumerism carries with it the concept of patients' rights. The consumer is empowered by his status; he has legal rights, and rights as an individual, to choice, self-determination, information and involvement in his treatment and care.

Becoming a patient

Patient care and treatment takes many forms and occurs in many settings. Almost everyone will be a patient at some point in their lives, whether in the primary or secondary health care setting, in NHS or private health care, through conventional or complementary medicine.

People consult their doctor on average four times a year and there are more than half a million consultations with family doctors each working day. Each year over 30 million courses of dental treatment are carried out and over 11 million sight tests (DoH, 1989b).

The GP refers about 10% of his or her patients to hospital consultants, with over 37 million NHS outpatient visits each year. Almost 1 million patients are treated in NHS hospitals as day patients and between 1987 and 1988, there were 6.62 million inpatients treated in the NHS (DoH, 1989b). Some patients first attend hospital as an emergency and in the same year, Accident and Emergency departments had nearly 14 million attendances.

In the primary health care sector, health visitors visit some 4 million people at home each year, while between 1987 and 1988 there were over 8 million visits to child health clinics. In the same year, over 4 million pupils were seen by school nurses, there were almost 3 million attendances at family planning clinics and 3.5 million people were treated by district nurses (DoH, 1989b).

While hospitals have traditionally received the largest share of NHS resources, efforts have been made to shift more funds to community services, as patients have been discharged home earlier and services for the mentally ill and mentally handicapped have been moved from hospital to community. The average length of hospital stay fell from 13.3 days in 1979 to 10.7 days in 1985 (DoH, 1989b). From just under 10,000 places in hostels and homes for the mentally handicapped in 1977, a decade later over 16,000 places were available in the community.

Meanwhile the population is living longer and also surviving previously life-threatening diseases, resulting in an increase in the need for long term care or support for the chronically ill or the dependent patient.

These changing patterns are reflected in changing staffing roles. Training curricula for health care professionals, especially nurses, are far more community-oriented than before. Diplomates from Project 2000 courses (UKCC, 1986) will have spent time in their training in schools, factories, GP surgeries and health clinics as well as on the wards. The number of practice nurses employed by GPs has risen dramatically as GPs have realised their value in carrying out a range of procedures previously undertaken by medical staff.

Community psychiatric nursing services have developed and there are now 50 paediatric community nursing services in the country, compared with only four a decade ago (Whiting, 1990). The development of the clinical nurse specialist role in areas such as paediatrics, intravenous therapy, diabetes and nutrition has provided a bridge between hospital and home, allowing a growing number of patients to avoid previously inevitable hospital visits.

Private health care

Private health care is a significant alternative to the NHS and there has been rapid growth in the provision of private sector care over recent years.

The number of private acute beds rose from just over 6000 in 1979/80 to just over 10,000 by 1988/89 (Appleby, 1989). By 1986 the private health care sector was providing 7% of all non-psychiatric and non-maternity inpatient stays in England and Wales, and 11% of all day case episodes (Nicholl et al., 1989). The value of the independent acute hospital market rose by 15% from £492 million in 1987/88 to £556 million in 1988/9 (Health Care Information Services, 1990).

Most of the caseload of the private sector is routine, elective surgery and the largest element of its clinical activity, some 19%, is in the termination of pregnancy – 70,000 out of a total of just over 500,000 cases treated as inpatients and day cases in 1986 (Nicholl et al., 1989). An estimated 28% of all hip replacements are done privately and 20% of all inguinal hernia repairs.

The private sector treats proportionately fewer children and older people and tends to avoid complicated 'high tech' operations. There is also a marked regional imbalance, with six times as many private beds per head of population in the Thames regions as in the Northern regions (Nicholl et al., 1989). Thus although it has grown considerably, the private sector still provides treatment for only a limited range of conditions and a limited group of people in limited areas (Goldacre, 1989).

Private hospital treatment is funded mainly from insurance schemes, subscribed to either privately or provided as an employment 'perk'. Its attractions are mainly that it offers the patient more control over the timing of treatment and a way of avoiding long hospital waiting lists – hence the predominance in the private sector of operations such as hip replacement and varicose vein ligation, where NHS waiting lists are long. Some health authorities have done deals with private health care companies to allow certain operations to take place in private hospitals in order to cut waiting lists and the recent changes in the NHS offers greater scope for such arrangements.

In 1989, the government tried to encourage the further use of the private sector by giving tax relief on private health care insurance to the over-60s. It is doubtful whether this has significantly affected take-up, however.

The other rapid area of growth in the private sector has been in the number of private and residential nursing homes, which has risen fivefold since 1979 – a growth stimulated by changes in supplementary benefit regulations. At the beginning of the 1980s, local authorities provided 70% of all residential places for people aged 65 or over. By the end of the decade they provided less than half (Hudson, 1990).

Complementary medicine

Alternative or – as it is more properly called – complementary medicine is also undergoing a rapid expansion as people look for alternatives or complements to conventional systems of health care. A 1986 Which? survey showed that one in seven people had visited a complementary practitioner within the past year, while the Handbook of Complementary Medicine (Fulder, 1984) estimates that there are 30,373 complementary therapists in the UK, of whom at least 2209 are medically qualified.

Most of the medical profession remain sceptical about its value, largely on the grounds that it is not 'scientific' (BMA, 1986). Nevertheless, many doctors do refer their patients to alternative practitioners – over 10% of consultations with osteopaths, hypnotherapists, chiropractors and acupuncturists follow doctors' referrals, according to one study (Moore et al., 1985).

People turn to alternative or complementary medicine for a variety of reasons. They may feel conventional medicine has failed, having had varied and repeated orthodox treatments which have brought little relief. They may fear the direct or indirect effects of increasingly complex and technologically sophisticated treatments. Patients from different ethnic backgrounds may be accustomed to using different forms of therapy.

Alternative therapies have also traditionally used a more holistic approach to an individual's problem than does conventional medicine, often questioning a patient exhaustively on diet and lifestyle before attempting to apply any treatment or remedy. This approach can seem increasingly attractive when GP consultation times are much shorter.

The Which? survey showed that the most

common types of practitioner consulted were osteopaths, homeopaths, acupuncturists, chiropractors and herbalists. Furnham and Smith (1988) found no evidence that people were from any one social class or age group, while Sharma (1991) found that all the patients she interviewed had consulted conventional practitioners on their condition before turning to alternative practitioners. All said they would continue to consult their GP for any new health problems that occurred.

Complementary medicine is most commonly used for chronic conditions for which orthodox medicine offers only limited relief; for example, back pain, allergic conditions, migraine, depression, tiredness, arthritis (Moore *et al.*, 1985), although patients suffering from life-threatening diseases such as cancer also turn to it, either in addition to or instead of conventional medicine.

As Sharma concludes: 'Patients of alternative medicine usually continue to be users of conventional medicine but they are more likely to be critical of the treatment they receive and are prepared to go elsewhere to seek treatment which is satisfactory to their own criteria. They have added other forms of therapy to their battery of resources in dealing with ill health, rather than abandoned orthodox medicine' (Sharma, 1991, page 51).

The nurse's responsibility is to respect the right of the patient to choose.

Patient choice

We have looked at where people are cared for in the health care system, whether in the public or private sector, through conventional or alternative models of care, through acute, chronic or long-term illnesses, and in cases of physical or mental ill health or handicap.

But what choice do people have in the health care they are given? When Roy Griffiths, a Sainsbury's executive, was appointed to chair the 1983 NHS Management Inquiry (DHSS, 1983), jokes, headlines and cartoons on the subject of 'supermarket health care' abounded. But can the philosophy of the supermarket really be transposed onto the health care system? Can people expect to exercise the same degree of choice over their operations as over their oranges?

The answer, of course, is no – or at least, not entirely. As already discussed, patients do not necessarily enter the health care system willingly. They do not choose to be ill in the same way that

they decide they need more groceries. Even private sector patients, who may be able to choose the timing of an elective operation, have little control over a road traffic accident or a burst appendix, when they will enter the health care system as an emergency.

Within the NHS, a person has a right, within certain geographical constraints, to choose his own GP, or rather to apply to be accepted onto a GP's list – the GP can refuse. But at that point, any influence over where and by whom the patient is treated should he require any other form of treatment or care effectively ends.

This is not so in the private sector, of course, or with alternative medicine, which is not publicly funded. Here the only constraints on the patient are price and geographical location. Yet even patients in the private sector have limited influence over which hospital they are treated in and which medical or nursing staff manage their treatment and care.

During the 1980s, the government sought to introduce greater patient choice into the health care market. Allowing tax relief on private health care insurance for the over-60s offered people greater opportunity to choose to go private. GPs have been required to make public the services they offer, as a way of helping people decide which practice to join. Opticians are now allowed to advertise their services and there was talk in the early 1980s of extending this facility to GPs, although the proposal was quietly dropped.

The White Paper *Working for Patients* (DoH, 1989a), which heralded the organisational changes in 1990, declared its stated objective was 'to give patients, wherever they live in the UK, better health care and *greater choice of the services available*' (my emphasis).

The principle of the NHS reforms was to introduce the concept of the internal market into the NHS by effectively requiring hospitals and community services to tender for contracts to provide clinical services with the health authorities (purchasers), in the same way that cleaning, catering and laundry services had already been put out to tender.

The effect, the government claimed, would be to increase responsiveness to consumer needs because 'money would follow patients'. Purchasing health authorities, and GPs if they chose to be budget-holding practices, would have the freedom to place their contracts for hernia repairs, hip replacements, hysterectomies and so on with who-ever was perceived to be offering the best deal. Hospitals would be paid according to how many patients they treated – or, in the philosophy of the re-organisation, how much business they attracted.

Many professionals and consumer organisations argue, however, that far from increasing patient choice, the changes have in fact restricted it. Patients are referred for treatment according to local contractual arrangements, rather than per-sonal preferences. What limited choice previously existed, it is argued – for example, a smaller hos-pital closer to home in preference to the district general hospital 25 miles away – has disappeared, with GPs having to send the patient where the contract has been placed.

Likewise the doctor's freedom to refer a par-ticular patient on professional grounds to a par-ticular consultant has gone. Patients can no longer be referred elsewhere for treatment if the treatment they require (for example, in-vitro fertilisation) is not available in their own health authority, or be sent to a particular consultant practising in a dif-ferent part of the country because he or she has some particularly specialised expertise that may be able to help them.

The government argued that by separating health authorities from the delivery of care, their role could become much more purely the advocates of the community they represent. The new struc-tures, it is argued, require health authorities to de-termine the real health care needs of the local population and to commission services accord-ingly. Equally, provider units can be required by purchasers to set up effective systems for moni-toring and acting on consumer satisfaction with the services they provide. In this respect, and used correctly, the changes could hugely enhance the degree to which the services available match existing need.

Yet at the same time the provision for direct con-sumer representation within the new system has been reduced. Prior to the changes, health authori-ties had between four and six members appointed by the relevant local authority, giving them some representative function. Under the new arrange-ments, they have five executive and five non-executive members, all appointed by the regional health authority, which in turn is appointed by the Secretary of State.

The role of the Community Health Councils,

meanwhile (discussed in more detail on page 260), has been frozen rather than expanded. During the consultation process leading up to the changes, the CHCs fought for tougher watchdog powers within the changed NHS. Yet, although retaining most of their previous rights, such as observer status at health authority meetings and the right to be consulted over changes in health care provision such as hospital closures, they have no formal role in monitoring contracts for services.

Neuberger (1990) points out the illogicality of trying to bring the principles of the market place into the NHS yet excluding the actual consumer from the decision-making process. She suggests:

'In order for a market to work adequately, the purchaser of the service has to be the same, or barely distinct from, the user (as in the case of parents buying clothes for their children, for in-stance). The problem comes when the purchaser of services is not the consumer. The purchaser, in this case, is the District Health Authority, in whose interests it clearly is to get services as cheaply and as efficiently as possible. But the consumer who is not paying for services may have other priorities, such as the services being within easy reach of home, or of a particular type'

(page 18)

Health and illness

Concepts of health and illness vary between dif-ferent societies and different individuals (see also Chapters 1 and 2). As Sarson points out in an earlier edition of this book (Sarson, 1989), whether a health problem is perceived as such usually de-pends on how the individual determines health or illness and to what extent it alters or disrupts their lifestyle.

The World Health Organisation (1978) describes health as: 'A state of complete physical, mental and social well-being and not merely the absence of disease or infirmity'. This definition recognises that health is determined not simply by disease but by much wider social, environmental, economic and political considerations.

The WHO set targets for health in 1978 in its 'Alma Ata' declaration, with the slogan 'Health for all by the year 2000', inviting each of its regions to identify appropriate targets for their own areas

(WHO, 1978). The European region responded with 38 targets for health, published in 1985 (WHO, 1985).

Health is affected by our lifestyle, for example tobacco and alcohol intake, physical exercise, stress, and by our environment, through the housing we inhabit and the quality of the air we breathe and the water we drink. Certain diseases can be linked to particular age or cultural groups, others are more prevalent in particular geographical areas or different socio-economic classes. The link between poverty and ill health has been shown many times, perhaps most notably by Sir Douglas Black in the Black Report of 1980 (DHSS, 1980).

How far are we as individuals responsible for the state of our own health, or should government intervene forcefully in encouraging a more healthy lifestyle? For example, the government can choose simply to educate the public about the dangers of tobacco smoking and alcohol, or it can levy high enough taxes on tobacco and alcohol to act as a powerful deterrent. It can simply warn people that they are more likely to survive a car accident if wearing a seat belt, or make wearing rear and front seat belts mandatory. It can educate the public on the importance of having their children immunised against preventable diseases or it can choose to make immunisation programmes mandatory. It can tackle the link between poverty and ill health by providing better housing and increasing state benefits, or encourage wealth creation by controlling public expenditure and keeping inflation low, arguing that a healthy economy will promote a healthy population.

For the past decade the UK has tended to follow the less interventionist route. That is not to say it has been inactive. The government has funded several costly public information campaigns, covering issues such as drink-driving, AIDS and HIV, drug abuse, road safety, and immunisation. It has tried actively to improve health screening of the population, most notably through the new GP contract introduced in 1990 (DoH/Welsh Office, 1990). GPs are now required to invite patients to attend for a consultation as soon as they register with a new doctor to undergo a basic examination and to be offered advice on lifestyle. Further examinations should be offered at three-yearly intervals and at one-yearly intervals for the over-75s. Payments for immunisations will only be made once a pre-set target has been reached.

However, this activity is not strictly health promotion, defined by WHO (1978) as 'the process of *enabling* people to increase control over and thereby improve their health' (my emphasis). There is no evidence that public information campaigns alone influence people to change their habits, while researchers have found that screening programmes can have adverse effects by creating an unwarranted belief in the value of such a service (Anderson, 1983). Small (1990) believes they may create a false sense of security: 'A "human MOT" may even be seen by some patients as a kind of life insurance policy to reassure them that the old, ingrained, "harmful" health habits have, after all, done little damage'.

Although a signatory to the 1978 WHO Alma Ata declaration, the government has not endorsed the European targets published in 1985. And while Wales, Scotland and Northern Ireland have all published national health promotion strategies, the Department of Health in England did not produce its own targets for improving health until 1990, with the publication of the Green Paper *The Health of the Nation* (DoH, 1991a) and the White Paper of the same name in 1992.

The paper identifies three main health challenges:

- People still die prematurely or suffer ill health from largely preventable conditions;
- There are significant geographic, ethnic, social and occupational variations in health;
- There are still marked variations in the quantity and quality of health care in different parts of the country.

The paper calls on health authorities to:

- identify key areas which are of the greatest concern and where there is the greatest opportunity for improvement;
- set objectives for improvement of health;
- monitor the results.

The document has been widely welcomed as exciting, politically daring and long-awaited. Yet critics argue that it continues to over-emphasise individual responsibility for ill health, focusing on particular diseases and habits instead of on particular groups within the population and their habits, or on the social causes of disease.

On being a patient

Once a health problem is perceived and help sought, the transition begins from person to patient. Yet help is sought and care given in a variety of settings, mostly outside the formal health care setting.

The categories of care

The Committee of the Royal Commission of the NHS (1979) identified four categories or gradations of care which the individual might need. They are:

(1) The care which a healthy person will exercise for himself so that he remains healthy.

This includes adopting as healthy a lifestyle as possible, undergoing health checks such as blood pressure monitoring and breast and cervical screening, and taking advantage of whatever immunisations and vaccinations are available. The number of cervical smears examined almost doubled from 2.24 million in 1977 to 4.09 million in 1987/8 (DoH, 1989b) while uptake rates for vaccinations and immunisations also rose over the same period, most dramatically for pertussis immunisation (see Table 10.1).

Table 10.1. *Vaccination and immunisation rates. A ten-year comparison (DoH, 1989b)*

	1977	**1987/8**
Diphtheria	78%	87%
Tetanus	78%	87%
Polio	78%	87%
Pertussis	41%	73%
Measles	50%	76%
Rubella	69%	86%

(2) The self-care which the slightly ill person will exercise, which may involve medication and treatment

People receive their information on health from a wide variety of sources – from family, friends, newspapers, magazines and agony columns, and TV and radio programmes, including educational programmes, soaps and phone-ins.

Most problems are initially – and often com-pletely – self-treated, sometimes with help from a High Street chemist, especially for medication. Less than one complaint in four is actually taken to a doctor. A survey by a GP found that some attempt at self-treatment had been undertaken by 95% of his patients before he was visited (Elliott-Binns, 1973).

Help may be provided by an occupational health service or by the school nursing service. Another important source of advice and practical help is the many hundreds of self-help groups, often founded on the impetus of a lack of shared information and support for a particular condition. The most common among these are listed at the end of this chapter.

(3) The care provided by a person's family and by health and social services available outside hospital.

A huge amount of care takes place informally in the community by family, friends and volunteers, with widely varying degrees of support from health and social services. As people live to greater ages and as the number of people surviving chronic or long term illnesses increase, this aspect of care will become more and more significant. Gray (1983) showed how hospital and professional community care provided less care than informal care and self-care.

In a government survey in 1985, 14% of people over the age of 16 said they were looking after or providing some regular service for someone who was sick, elderly or handicapped (OPCS, 1988). Almost one in five households contained at least one person looking after someone living with them and 5% included a carer who was devoting at least 20 hours a week to caring for a sick or dependent person. The report estimated there were approximately 6 million carers overall in Great Britain, 3.5 million of them women, 2.5 million men.

These informal carers are enormously significant, as the alternative would usually be institutional care. The support provided by health and social services depends on the degree of illness, disability and dependence, but the services that are available include home helps, meals on wheels, day centres, district nursing visits, physiotherapy and occupational therapy. If the individual is dependent on a carer who is not employed by the health or social services, respite care facilities are available to give the carer some time off.

New arrangements for the provision of community care are currently in the pipeline, born of the Department of Health White Paper *Caring for People*, published in 1989 (DoH, 1989d). Planned for full implementation in April 1993, social services will be responsible for assessing the total needs of people being cared for in the community. Based on that assessment, they will design and plan a suitable package of care drawn from all the relevant agencies, including health services. This should help relieve the problems that can arise when care is required from several agencies but coordinated by no single body. As a result it can be fragmented and patchy, with too many people slipping through the net.

Again, self-help and support groups play an important role in the community, with groups existing for virtually every condition. They range from the long-established and well-known such as Age Concern, Mencap, MIND and the British Diabetic Association, to those run literally from someone's sitting room, helping the family and victims of some rare and little-known condition.

Councils for Voluntary Service, local non-governmental organisations, act as umbrella groups for local voluntary organisations, helping to promote voluntary activity and acting as links between voluntary organisations and statutory authorities.

(4) The care which can only be provided in hospital or other residential institutions.

This type of care is usually the most significant for a patient as it is in this setting that the transition from person to patient becomes complete. The person is away from home and to a large extent away from family and friends. He loses much of the status that he holds in his community, much of the choice about his daily diet, clothing and activity. He has to submit to the routine of the institution and restrictions imposed by the care and treatment he is given.

The patient's role

Once a person is admitted to hospital it is easy for them to become subsumed into the identity, routines and regulations of that institution, and for staff to see them more in terms of their physical condition than the whole person they are.

The patient will automatically be at a disadvantage. He usually will be unfamiliar with the layout of the ward and with the ward routine, and will be uncertain of what is expected of him. Removing his clothes and putting on nightwear reduces his dignity and sense of personal identity. Simple physical arrangements – lying or sitting on the bed while the confident, knowledgeable staff remain standing – may increase his sense of helplessness and loss of control.

At the same time the patient may be feeling ill and will certainly be anxious. He is handing over control of his illness and his body to another group of people. They hold information about himself and his condition of which he may be unaware. They will usually have the benefit of a greater understanding of that information.

To the ward staff, undergoing the routine of 'admitting a patient' for the hundredth time, it is easy to fail to understand and make allowances for these feelings. Yet the person who becomes a patient still retains rights as an individual and it is important that these are respected. Given the patient's acute vulnerability at this stage, they should even be over-emphasised.

Most important is the right to information – about the patient's condition but also on the more mundane level of the practical details of what is going to happen, when and why; explanation about hospital routines, procedures and treatments, all of which will reduce anxiety and increase the patient's confidence, morale and sense of control and of partnership in his care (Wilson-Barnett, 1979).

Providing this information has become a very important part of the nurse's role. It should be considered part of the total nursing care of the patient (Wilson-Barnett, 1983).

Assuming the sick role

The concept of the sick role was first defined by the American sociologist Talcott Parsons (1951). A patient is expected to assume the role of the sick person and conform to certain expectations society then has of him.

He has certain rights – being exempt from normal activities and from work, and the right to expect help from others, family, friends and health professionals. But he also has obligations – to want to get well and to resume normal or near normal activities as soon as possible, and secondly to do all that is possible to get well, cooperating with those helping him and complying with treatment regimes.

However, society's expectations of the patient may not always conform with what the patient himself wants. A further debilitating course of chemotherapy, for example, which medical staff agree will prolong life but not achieve remission or cure, may be what his family and society expect him to undergo but not what the patient himself wants or what is in his best interests.

The patient and his carers

Our society has always tended to believe that the doctor knows best and that decisions about our health care are best left in the hands of the professionals. As medical care has become more complex and sophisticated and as new boundaries of 'curing' are broken every year, respect for what medical practitioners can achieve has grown. They are seen as remote from and somehow 'above' their patients. Patients on the other hand are expected to do what they are told, obey the rules and more fool them if they don't.

Nursing, however, particularly over the past decade, has started to develop a different course – that of partnership with and advocacy for their patients. For years, nurses fulfilled the 'doctor's handmaiden' image (Salvage, 1985), caring for their patients according to how the doctor, rather than the nurse or the patient, saw fit.

The introduction of the nursing process and the development in the 1980s of models of nursing care (Kershaw and Salvage, 1986) redefined the nursing role and emphasised how care should be negotiated between nurse and patient. Developments such as primary nursing (Wright, 1990), nursing-controlled beds (Pearson et al., 1988) and research into the therapeutic effects of good nursing care (Pearson, 1989) have strengthened the potential of the nurse's role, redressed the balance in the partnership between patient and nurse and enhanced the nurse's ability to act as the patient's advocate (see also Chapter 12).

Most nursing care is now planned on the basis of one or other model of care which is tailored to be appropriate to the setting in which it is given. With the help of nursing models, it should be possible to draw up an individual care plan for each patient, taking into account his physical, psychological and social needs. In doing this, the nurse must not make value judgements about a patient's lifestyle or culture.

The relationship between the patient and his ca-rers will be influenced by the type and severity of the illness and by the setting in which care has been given. Sarson (1989) cites the studies carried out on the interaction between patients and carers in different settings, including their own homes (McIntosh, 1981), intensive care units (Ashworth, 1980), wards caring for elderly people (Wells, 1980), and on different groups of patients, including stroke patients (Kratz, 1978), cancer patients (Bond, 1978) and antenatal patients (McIntyre, 1978).

Involving the patient in decisions about his care becomes more difficult the more sick or vulnerable the patient is, particularly with elderly people and those who are mentally ill or who have learning difficulties.

Recent studies in day centres, for example, showed wide discrepancies in the views of what staff thought best for those attending and what the clients themselves wanted. McCarthy et al. (1986) found that the living skills rated as most essential by staff, including buying meals, reading, writing and using public amenities, were often considered unimportant by the attenders. They considered meeting other people, getting out of the house, and the availability of a cooked meal as more important than the programme of activities offered (Davis, 1986).

Renshaw (1987) describes how users can be involved in shaping mental health services at four levels of delivery – the individual programme plan, allowing groups of service users to contribute their views and wishes, at the level of service planning, and finally in helping to achieve a shift in public attitudes.

The chief advantage the professional carer has over the patient is information, and studies have shown that the lack of information is one of the greatest sources of dissatisfaction among patients.

In a survey of patients who had been in coronary care units, Wallace et al. (1985) found huge discrepancies between the information patients wanted and what they received. Ninety percent wanted information on the cause of their illness and only 40% reported being told about it; 90% wanted to know their diagnosis and only 70% reported being told it; 90% wanted to know how long recovery would be, while 40% reported being told; 80% wanted information about their medical treatment and only 40% reported being told. 'Most people know their diagnosis but feel uninformed about its cause, the process of recovery and treatment,' the authors concluded.

Information on discharge is just as important as on admission. Back in 1970, Skeet (1970) found that 37% of patients were discharged with less than 24 hours notice; 19% needed practical help at home and often did not know how this would be met; while 59% received no advice on discharge other than 'look after yourself'.

More recent research shows the situation has not really improved and in 1989 the Department of Health recommended hospital units should draw up discharge procedures, with planning and preparation for discharge beginning on admission (DoH, 1989c). In a small-scale study into discharge procedures for elderly patients, Vydelingum (1989) found both patients and carers felt they had not been sufficiently involved in preparation for discharge. The length of notice of discharge ranged from 24 hours to one week, while meals on wheels services took between five and ten days to materialise from the time the patient arrived home, and home help services between ten and 14 days.

In a study into the problems surgical patients faced after discharge, Vaughan and Taylor (1988) concluded that many people experienced difficulties that could have been removed or alleviated by giving them better information at the time of discharge. Twenty nine percent were unsure when they could safely bath or shower and 26% were unsure if their diet was appropriate to aiding recovery. Only one out of a sample of 64 was given any advice on sexual activity following their operation and only two were advised when they could start driving again.

Wilson-Barnett (1979) showed how stress and anxiety are reduced with explanations about hospital procedures, routines and treatment, while Hayward (1975) showed how patients who had received pre-operative information on anaesthesia, operative techniques and post-operative sensations reported less pain and required less analgesia than those who had not been given the same information.

Providing the information that patients need and educating them about their condition should be included in the total nursing care of the patient (Wilson-Barnett, 1983). Children, the elderly, those with learning difficulties or those who do not speak English as a first language will require special attention.

The psychological and emotional support that nurses need to give to patients is increasingly recognised in curricula for nurse education. Some subjects, such as death and dying, disablement and mental illness are extremely difficult to discuss with a patient without prior education, training and experience. Similarly, in investing more in a patient's emotional well-being, the nurse herself can become over-involved in her patients and risk stress and burn-out.

Nevertheless, the quality of the relationship between nurse and patient is a vital factor in patient satisfaction, in turn affecting compliance in treatment and improving the outcome (see also Chapter 8). Patients must be allowed to share in decisions about their care and treatment and must be given the information and advice to empower them to do this.

The rights of the patient

The patient has certain rights, both as an individual and in law. As a result of the Patient's Charter (DoH, 1991b), he now has rights specifically as a user of the National Health Service.

The charter is not enshrined in any legislation but it can be used as a standard against which care can be measured and as a basis for any complaint. It sets out seven existing rights within the NHS and affirms three new rights (Tables 10.2 and 10.3). It also sets national and local standards which health authorities should adopt (Tables 10.4 and 10.5).

The patient's rights as an individual may be summarised as follows:

(1) *The right to individualised care*. The patient is, first and foremost, a person and this should be recognised by providing him with individualised care (as discussed above). In doing so the nurse must accept that a patient's behaviour is influenced by previous experience, by background and culture, and by his or her illness. The nurse must therefore avoid making value judgements about lifestyle or behaviour, based on her own values and background.

(2) *The right to holistic care*. The patient has the right to have his total care needs — physical, psychological and social — taken into account, bearing in mind that they are inter-related.

(3) *Cultural needs*. Britain is a multicultural society and this is strongly reflected in the mix of

Table 10.2. *A citizen's existing rights within the National Health Service (DOH, 1991b)*

(1) To receive health care on the basis of clinical need, regardless of ability to pay
(2) To be registered with a GP
(3) To receive emergency medical care at any time
(4) To be referred to a consultant, acceptable to the patient, when the GP thinks it necessary and to be referred for a second opinion
(5) To be given a clear explanation of any treatment proposed, including any risks and any alternatives
(6) To have access to health records and for them to be treated confidentially
(7) To choose whether or not to take part in medical research or medical student training.

Table 10.3.   Three new rights (DOH, 1991b)

(1) To be given detailed information on local health services, including quality standards and maximum waiting time
(2) To be guaranteed admission for virtually all treatments within two years of being placed on a waiting list
(3) To have any complaint about NHS services investigated and to receive a full and prompt reply from the chief executive of the health authority or general manager of the hospital. If the patient is still unhappy, the case can be taken to the Health Service Commissioner

Table 10.4. *National standards (DoH, 1991b)*

- Respect for privacy, dignity and religious beliefs
- Arrangements for people with special needs
- Information to be given to relatives and friends about the progress of treatment, subject to the patient's wishes
- An emergency ambulance should arrive within 14 minutes in an urban area, or 19 minutes in a rural area
- Outpatient clinics to give specific appointment times and patients to be seen within 30 minutes of it
- Operations not to be cancelled on the day of arrival. If an operation is postponed twice, the patient will be admitted within one month
- A named, qualified nurse, midwife or health visitor to be responsible for nursing or midwifery care
- A decision should be made about any continuing health or social care needs before discharge

Table 10.5. *Local standards (DoH, 1991b)*

Health authorities should set and publicise local standards including:

- First outpatient appointments
- Waiting times in Accident and Emergency departments
- Waiting times for being taken home after treatment where transport is required
- Better signposting around the hospital
- Ensuring staff wear name badges

people who seek health care. Patients from different ethnic groups have different lifestyles, family patterns, religious beliefs, dietary habits and attitudes to health and illness which must be understood, respected and, as far as possible, catered for while they are receiving health care.

Patients from these groups may be more socially disadvantaged than others and many will have problems with language and communication. As a result they will find it harder to get the information they need to get the best from health care services.

Health information, particularly in areas where ethnic minority groups are concentrated, must be available in different and relevant languages. Visiting arrangements may need to be more flexible to take account of an extended family structure or religious restrictions on travel on certain days. Hygiene and dietary habits must be respected when planning care and nutritional needs.

(4)   *The right to maintaining links with home and family.* This is especially important for children, for whom the trauma of separation from family can be far worse than that caused by events in hospital. Since the Platt Report (Ministry of Health, 1959) highlighted the damage that could be caused by such separation, visiting arrangements for children have been completely relaxed in most hospitals, with one or both parents usually allowed to stay. Far from being the encumbrances they were once viewed as, parents in many centres are now actively involved in their child's care while in hospital, often carrying out complex procedures with the supervision and support of nursing staff.

Many more children with chronic and life-threatening conditions are now nursed at home with the help of paediatric community nursing staff. This drastically reduces the need for hospital visits and means that as near normal a family life as possible can be maintained (Whiting, 1990).

Open and flexible visiting arrangements are equally important for adults. The involvement of the family in a patient's care should also be encouraged as they may have to take on important aspects of the care once the patient goes home.

Newspapers, library services, mobile telephones, radios and televisions are all important links with the outside world. Patients who have been in hospital for several weeks may be encouraged to go home for one or more weekends before they are ready to be discharged completely. This is an important indication to patient, family and staff as to how ready the patient is for discharge, as well as allowing the patient to begin to pick up his life outside a hospital or institution again.

Patients and family will need as much information as possible on discharge, including advice on lifestyle, medication, how to obtain any equipment and supplies they will require, and what services and support will be available to them. They will also need as much notice of discharge as possible in case any particular arrangements have to be made.

Armitage (1991) stresses the importance of planned discharge to help prepare the patient for going home. Many hospitals now employ clinical nurse specialists in areas such as stoma care, kidney disease, nutrition or diabetes. These nurses can act as a bridge between hospital and home, helping to prepare the patient for discharge and visiting him once home.

Legal rights

The patient has the legal right to decide whether or not to accept treatment – to *informed consent*. The onus is on medical staff to explain the implications of treatment and surgery to him, and a signed consent form must be obtained for every surgical procedure or invasive investigation that is carried out.

For a person to make appropriate decisions regarding his health care and treatment, he needs as much information as possible. In practice, the quality of information given to the patient varies and until recently, patients had no legal right to information concerning their case. Since November 1991, patients have had the legal right to see their medical records, even though doctors will still be able, at their discretion, to withhold certain facts. Doctors will be obliged, however, to make

their medical notes more easily understandable to the lay person (HMSO, 1990b).

The situation becomes more complicated in the case of children or people who are not in a position to make a decision regarding their care. They may be unconscious or they may have some degree of learning difficulty. In such cases, responsibility for informed consent falls upon the parents, guardian or next of kin. If the person acting on the patient's behalf does not agree with the medical staff, however, the case could be decided in court.

Children under the age of 16 are increasingly being recognised as being able to make a valid contribution to informed consent. The Gillick case in 1987 established the legal principle whereby a doctor could administer treatment, in this case contraceptive pills, against the wishes of the parent.

There are certain exceptions whereby a patient can be treated without consent, however. They are:

(1) If a person has a notifiable disease or is carrying an organism capable of causing one.
(2) If a person has been detained under the provisions of the Mental Health Act (1983), the Mental Health Amendment Act (Scotland, 1983) or the Mental Health Act (Northern Ireland, 1961).

Adult patients, except those in the categories listed above, are free to discharge themselves from hospital, even if medical or nursing staff wish them to stay. They will usually have to sign an undertaking that they are doing so against medical advice and accept personal responsibility for any consequences.

The patient under most circumstances, therefore, has the legal right to refuse treatment, but does he have the legal right to insist on treatment? This issue was raised in 1988 when a heart operation due to be carried out on a baby boy was cancelled because no beds were available. The boy's parents took Birmingham Health Authority to court, arguing that he was legally entitled to the operation. They lost their case, however, the judge ruling that such decisions lay within the discretion of the health authority's management and medical staff.

The patient as a consumer

In recent years there has been an unprecedented increase in the interest and participation of people in their own health care. It is this factor that marks the difference between the *patient* and the *consumer* – the former implying a passive role as a recipient of health care, the latter an active role where the person is informed, involved and empowered.

Information

The National Consumer Council, in its document *Patients' Rights* (1983), states that patients will 'get the best from the health service only when they know what is reasonable to expect from it, what their rights and responsibilities are, and when they have the confidence and skill to exercise them. Patients clearly need more and better information about what services are available and how to gain access to them; what choice they have in terms of doctors and services; how they can influence decision-making in the health service; and how they can make a complaint when something goes wrong.'

The population is generally better informed about health and health care provision than ever before. Documentary programmes show sickness and curing, operative techniques and medical emergencies in unsparing close-up. Programmes such as *Jimmy's* and *Hospital Watch* chronicle actual hospital events as they occur. Television soaps find health problems a fertile ground for new story-lines but also make a serious attempt to treat such problems in a responsible and informative way.

Meanwhile, health and the NHS are rarely off the political agenda and consequently feature regularly in news and current affairs programmes. Radio programmes such as *Does he take sugar?* deal with patients' rights as consumers of health care, while newspapers and magazines carry regular features and problem pages on health.

As a result, the patient enters the health care system not only better informed than ever before but also with high expectations of what it is able to deliver. News reports of a 'miracle new cure' for cancer or of a life-saving transplant for a child can be misleading and raise patients' expectations to an unrealistically high level.

While information about health is readily available, information about the health service and how to use it is less easy to come by. The patient's right to such information is now enshrined in the Patient's Charter (DOH, 1991b), however, and patients are entitled to complain if they cannot gain access to it.

Community Health Councils (see below) are one important source. They are able to advise patients on health provision in their area and on complaints procedures. CHCs are also increasingly involved in health promotion.

Patient support and self-help groups are another source of information. Organisations such as the National Childbirth Trust will frankly advise members on which hospitals are more likely to encourage 'natural' childbirth, for example, or advise women on how to arrange for a home birth. The British Association of Cancer United Patients (BACUP) has a phone-in cancer information service and also produces information booklets and audio-visual materials.

The College of Health, established in 1983, has published several consumer guides to using the health service, on subjects such as alternative medicine, homes for elderly people, obtaining second opinions, and hospital waiting lists. The College also operates a telephone information line giving advice on waiting lists.

Representation

Specific consumer representation in the NHS was first introduced in 1974 with the establishment of Community Health Councils (CHCs), defined as 'bodies to represent the views of the consumer' (HMSO, 1973).

Each district health authority has a CHC, whose functions are to represent the local community's interests in local health services provision to those responsible for managing it. They have an observer role at HA meetings, they visit NHS premises, comment on health authority plans and on proposals for changes in local health care provision. They advise on and take up patients' complaints and monitor the number and type of complaints as a measure of public satisfaction.

Although these functions were largely retained in the changes brought about by the NHS and Community Care Act (1990), CHCs have no powers to monitor the purchasing decisions made by GP fundholders as opposed to health authorities, and they cannot follow patients from their boundaries if contracts are made with hospitals in different health authorities.

Patients are increasingly able to express their views through quality assurance schemes and consumer satisfaction surveys, first introduced following the Griffiths NHS Management Inquiry (DHSS, 1983). This principle was again emphasised in the White Paper *Working for Patients* (DoH, 1989a) and the Department of Health has issued guidance on the conduct of consumer surveys and other patient relations activities (Carr-Hill *et al.*, 1989).

Pressure groups such as the National Association for the Welfare of Children in Hospital (NAWCH), the National Childbirth Trust (NCT), Age Concern, MIND and Mencap campaign to achieve better standards of care and provide another source of consumer representation in health care.

NAWCH, renamed Action for Sick Children in November 1991, draws its membership equally from parents and professionals. It has produced a charter for children which sets standards of care for children in hospital and can be used as a tool to monitor quality. Age Concern also has a charter of rights for elderly people.

At the 1986 national conference of MIND, the organisation which campaigns on behalf of people with mental illness, almost half the participants were or had been recipients of mental health services (Renshaw, 1987). NCT members are drawn almost entirely from parents or women and their partners who are expecting a child.

The Patient's Charter (DoH, 1991b) is also intended to strengthen the consumer's voice in health care and re-affirm his rights. As well as setting out patients' rights within the NHS, it sets national and local standards on subjects such as waiting times for an ambulance, within Accident and Emergency and outpatient departments, and for transport home after treatment when necessary.

Patient complaints

The right to make a complaint about any aspect of treatment or care is an important part of the patient's rights as a consumer of health care and it has been enshrined in the Patient's Charter (DoH, 1991b).

This states that the patient has the right 'to have any complaint about NHS services – whoever provides them – investigated, and to receive a full and prompt written reply from the chief executive of (the patient's) health authority or general manager of (the patient's) hospital. If (the patient is) still unhappy, (he) will be able to take the case up with the Health Service Commissioner' (DoH, 1991b).

A formal complaint is usually made in the first instance to the hospital or community service involved, either verbally or in writing, and it should immediately be reported to the senior manager who is responsible for investigating it. The patient and any staff involved should be kept informed of any steps that are being taken.

Clinical complaints should be referred to the consultant in charge of the case who will discuss how it is to be handled with the senior manager.

Most complaints can be satisfactorily dealt with at local level. Often all the patient will require is an assurance that his voice has been heard and that action will be taken. When a complaint is likely to involve litigation, the health authority will seek legal advice and the staff concerned should be made aware of the help that is available to them through their professional association or trade union.

Cases which appear to involve professional misconduct by a doctor or a nurse will first be examined by the hospital or community services management before a decision is taken as to whether to refer the case to the General Medical Council or, for nursing, to the National Boards in England, Scotland, Wales and Northern Ireland. They in turn decide whether a case should be referred to the Professional Conduct Committee of the UK Central Council for Nursing, Midwifery and Health Visiting.

The Health Service Commissioner, or Health Ombudsman as he is also called, is brought in when a patient feels a case has not been dealt with satisfactorily by the health authority. He is not entitled to examine clinical cases, although he can investigate the way clinical complaints are handled. The Health Service Commissioner publishes an annual report. His office investigated 990 complaints in 1990/91, the highest number since the office was established in 1973 (Health Service Commissioner, 1991).

Staff complaints about patient care

Patients may for various reasons be either unwilling or unable to complain about their care. Nurses, by virtue of their close and continuous contact with patients, are arguably in the best position both to recognise that care falls short of the standards patients have a right to expect, and to complain about it.

According to the Code of Professional Conduct (UKCC, 1992), it is part of the nurse's professional responsibility to do so:

> 'As a registered nurse, midwife or health visitor, you are personally accountable for your practice, and, in the exercise of your professional accountability, must:
>
> (1) Act always in such a way as to promote and safeguard the well-being and interests of patients/clients.
> (2) Ensure that no action or omission on your part, or within your sphere of responsibility, is detrimental to the interests, conditions or safety of patients and clients.'

This could involve witnessing an infringement of a patient's rights by another colleague. Beardshaw (1981) uses the term 'conscientious objectors' for staff who speak out against such abuses and includes a checklist for 'whistle-blowers' who contemplate making such a complaint.

McCarthy (1986), cited in Sarson (1989), describes five categories of patient abuse:

(1) Physical abuse – from rough handling to punching, slapping, kicking or worse
(2) Sexual abuse – forcing or promoting unwelcome sexual attentions or practices
(3) Psychological abuse – causing emotional distress by verbal means such as badgering, demeaning, coercing, provoking or frightening, or by making someone undertake or witness acts which are personally distasteful
(4) Neglect/deprivation – deliberately withholding basic rights and comforts such as food, light, heat, personal hygiene and contact with others
(5) Misappropriation of personal effects – stealing money, valuables, articles with sentimental attachments or any other personal belongings.

Making such a complaint can be extremely difficult and the staff member may face victimisation from colleagues and management. There can be no doubt that many cases go unreported for these reasons.

Other types of 'whistle-blowers' include staff who complain that adequate standards of patient care cannot be maintained because of inadequate staffing levels or resources. Pyne (1987) makes it clear that the Code of Conduct should equally support nurses in these circumstances and the Royal College of Nursing has recently invited nurses confidentially to report inadequate standards of patient care. Nurses who complain openly to management may again face problems, as demonstrated by the case of Graham Pink, who eventually lost his job after consistent complaints that the low nurse staffing levels at his hospital constituted a danger to patients (Robinson, 1990).

Conclusion

Patients are no different from people. They become patients by virtue of a process of illness or dependence that could happen to anyone at any time. As patients, however, they have to adjust to a new role and to temporary or long term dependence on others.

They become users of the health care system and as such it is fitting to consider them as consumers. The term implies that the individual has some control, that he is entitled to choice, to information, to participation, and to have his voice heard. It implies that the patient is autonomous and has rights and beliefs that must be respected. He should be treated as a partner in his care, fully involved in and informed of any decisions taken.

This is not always easy, as the control has in the past been firmly with the health care professionals. It is often far easier to make decisions on another's behalf, especially when they are sick and vulnerable. But it is precisely because people who enter the health care sector are vulnerable that the balance needs to be redressed.

References

Anderson, R. (1983). Public attitudes to and experience of medical check-ups. *Community Medicine*, 5, 11–20.

Appleby, J. (1989). Private acute care. NAHA Health Care Data Briefing. *Health Service Journal*, 99, 523.

Armitage, S. (1991). *Continuity of Care*. Scutari, Harrow.

Ashworth, P. (1980). *Care to Communicate: An Investigation into Problems of Communication between Patients and Nurses in Intensive Therapy Units*. RCN, London.

Beardshaw, V. (1981). *Conscientious Objectors at Work*. Social Audit, London.

Bond, S. (1978). Processes of communication about cancer in a radiotherapy department. Unpublished PhD thesis, University of Edinburgh.

British Medical Association. (1986). *Report by the Board of Science and Education of the BMA on Alternative Therapy*. BMA, London.

Buchan, J. (1990). Caring for the consumer. *Nursing Standard*, 4(18), 46.

Carr-Hill, I., McIver, S. and Dixon, P. (1989). *The NHS and Its Customers*. York University Centre for Health Economics, York.

Davis, A. (1986). Who wants day care? *Community Care*, May 8.

Department of Health. (1989a). *Working for Patients*. HMSO, London.

DoH. (1989b). *Health and Personal Social Services Statistics for England, 1989*. HMSO, London.

DoH. (1989c). *Discharge of Patients from Hospital*, HC(89)5. HMSO, London.

DoH. (1989d). *Caring for People*. HMSO, London.

DoH/Welsh Office. (1990). *Statement of Fees and Allowances for General Medical Services, 1990*. HMSO, London.

DoH. (1991a). *The Health of the Nation: A Consultative Document for Health in England*. HMSO, London.

DoH. (1991b). *The Patient's Charter*. HMSO, London.

DoH. (1992). *The Health of the Nation*. HMSO, London.

DHSS. (1980). *Inequalities in Health* (The Black Report). HMSO, London.

DHSS. (1983). *NHS Management Inquiry Report* (The Griffiths Report). HMSO, London.

Elliott-Binns, C. (1973). An analysis of lay medicine. *Journal of the Royal College of General Practitioners*, 23, 255–264.

Fulder, S. (1984). *The Handbook of Complementary Medicine*. Coronet Books, London.

Furnham, A. and Smith, C. (1988). Choosing alternative medicine: a comparison of the beliefs of patients visiting a general practitioner and a homeopath. *Social Science and Medicine*, 26(7), 685–689.

Goldacre, M. (1989). The rise in private health care. *British Medical Journal*, 298, 202–203.

Gray, M. (1983). Four box health care: development in a time of zero growth. *Lancet*, 2, 1185–1186.

Hayward, J. (1975). *Information: A Prescription against Pain*. RCN, London.

Health Care Information Services. (1990). *The Fitzhugh Directory of Independent Healthcare Financial Information – Acute Sector 1990–91*. HCIS, London.

Health Service Commissioner's Annual Report for Session 1990/91. (1991). HMSO, London.

HMSO. (1973). *NHS Reorganisation Act*. HMSO, London.

HMSO. (1990a). *NHS and Community Care Act 1990*. HMSO, London.

HMSO. (1990b). *Access to Health Records Act 1990*. HMSO, London.

Hudson, B. (1990). The rise and rise of private care. *Health Service Journal*, 100, 1520–1521.

Kershaw, B. and Salvage, J. (eds.). (1986). *Models for Nursing*. John Wiley and Sons, Chichester.

Kratz, C. (1978). *Care of the Long-Term Sick in the Community, Particularly Patients with Stroke*. Churchill Livingstone, Edinburgh.

Leppanen-Montgomery, C. (1988). Patients are more than customers. *American Journal of Nursing*, 88(9), 1257–1258.

McCarthy, B., Benson, J. and Brown, C. (1986). Task motivation and problem appraisal in long-term psychiatric patients. *Psychological Medicine*, 16, 431–438.

McCarthy, D. (1986). Blowing the whistle. *Nursing Times*, 82(11), 123.

McIntosh, J. (1981). *Communication and Awareness in a Cancer Ward*. Croom Helm, London.

McIntyre, S. (1978). Obstetric routines in ante-natal care. In *Relationships between Doctors and Patients*, Davis, A. (ed.). Saxton House, London.

Ministry of Health. (1959). *The Welfare of Children in Hospital* (The Platt Report). HMSO, London.

Moore, J., Phipps, K. and Marcer, D. (1985). Why do some people seek treatment by alternative medicine? *British Medical Journal*, 290, 28–29.

National Consumer Council. (1983). *Patients' Rights: A Guide for NHS Patients and Doctors*. NCC, London.

Neuberger, J. (1990). A consumer's view. In *The NHS Reforms: Whatever Happened to Consumer Choice?*, Green, D. (ed.). Institute of Economic Affairs Health and Welfare Unit, London.

Nicholl, J., Beeby, N. and Williams, B. (1989). Role of the private sector in elective surgery in England and Wales, 1986. *British Medical Journal*, 298, 243–247.

Office of Population Censuses and Surveys. (1988). *General Household Survey 1985: Informal Carers*. HMSO, London.

Parsons, T. (1951). *The Social System*. Routledge and Kegan Paul, London.

Pearson, A. (1989). Therapeutic nursing – transforming models and theories into action. In *Theories and Models of Nursing*, Akinsanya, J. (ed.). Churchill Livingstone, Edinburgh.

Pearson, A., Durand, I. and Punton, S. (1988). The feasibility and effectiveness of nursing beds. *Nursing Times*, 86(47), 48–50.

Pyne, R. (1987). The UKCC Code of Conduct. *Nursing*, 3(14), 510–511.

Renshaw, J. (1987). The challenge of enabling the client to be a consumer. *Social Work Today*, 18, 10–11.

Robinson, J. (1990). Think Pink. *Nursing Standard*, 5(8), 43.

Royal Commission on the National Health Service. (1979). *The Merrison Report*. Cmnd 7615. HMSO, London.

Salvage, J. (1985). *The Politics of Nursing*. Heinemann, London.

Sarson, B. (1989). On being a patient. In *Nursing Practice and Health Care* (1st ed.), Hinchliff, S., Norman S. and Schober, J. (eds.). Edward Arnold, London.

Sharma, U. (1991). Using 'alternative' medicine. *Health Visitor*, 64(2), 50–51.

Skeet, M. (1970). *Home from Hospital*. Dan Mason Nursing Research Committee, London.

Smail, S. (1990). Health promotion and the new GP contract. *Practice Nurse*, 2(9), 391–392.

United Kingdom Central Council for Nursing, Midwifery and Health Visiting. (1992). *Code of Professional Conduct for the Nurse, Midwife and Health Visitor* (3rd ed.). UKCC, London.

UKCC. (1986). *Project 2000: A New Preparation for Practice*. UKCC, London.

Vaughan, B. and Taylor, K. (1988). Homeward bound. *Nursing Times*, 84(15), 28–31.

Vydelingum, V. (1989). Discharge of the elderly. *Nursing Times*, 85(35), 50.

Wallace, L., Wingett, C., Joshi, M. and Spellman, D. (1985). Heart to heart. *Nursing Times*, 81, 45–47.

Wells, T. (1980). *Problems in Geriatric Nursing Care. A Study of Nurses' Problems in Care of Old People*. Churchill Livingstone, Edinburgh.

Which? (1986). Magic or medicine? *Which?* October.

Whiting, M. (1990). Home care for children. *Nursing Standard*, 4, 52–53.

Willis, J. (1989). The hard sell. *Nursing Times*, 85, 22–23.

Wilson-Barnett, J. (1979). *Stress in Hospital*. Churchill Livingstone, Edinburgh.

Wilson-Barnett, J. (1983). *Patient Teaching*. Churchill Livingstone, Edinburgh.

World Health Organisation. (1978). *Report of the International Conference on Primary Care, Alma-Ata, USSR.*, WHO, Geneva.

World Health Organisation Regional Office for Europe. (1985). *Targets for Health for All*. WHO, Copenhagen.

Wright, S.G. (1990). *My Patient, My Nurse: A Guide to Primary Nursing*. Scutari Press, Harrow.

Useful addresses

Age Concern England
Astral House, 1268 London Road, Norbury, London SW16.
Tel. 081 679 8000

Association of Community Health Councils for England and Wales
Mark Lemon Suite, Barclays Bank Chambers, 254 Seven Sisters Road, London N4 2HZ.
Tel. 081 272 5459

BACUP (British Association of Cancer United Patients)
121/3 Charterhouse Street, London EC1M 6AA.
Tel. 071 608 1661

College of Health
18 Victoria Park Square, London E2 9PF.
Tel. 071 980 6263

Commission for Racial Equality
Elliott House, 10/12 Allington Street, London SW1E 5EH.
Tel. 071 828 7022

Contact a Family
16 Strutton Ground, London SW1P 2HP.
Tel. 071 222 2695

Disabled Living Foundation
380/384 Harrow Road, London W9 2HU.
Tel. 071 289 6111

Mencap
117/123 Golden Lane, London EC1V ORT.
Tel. 071 253 9433

MIND: National Association for Mental Health
22 Harley Street, London W1N 2ED.
Tel. 071 637 0741

National Association for the Welfare of Children in Hospital (NAWCH) (Now: Action for Sick Children)
Argyle House, 29/31 Euston Road, London NW1 2SD.
Tel. 071 833 2041

National Children's Bureau
8 Wakley Street, London EC1V 7QE.
Tel. 071 278 9441

National Consumer Council
20 Grosvenor Gardens, London W1 ODH.
Tel. 071 730 3469

National Council for Voluntary Organisations
26 Bedford Square, London WC1B 3HU
Tel. 071 636 4066

Royal National Institute for the Blind
224/228 Great Portland Street, London W1N 6AA.
Tel. 071 388 1266

Royal National Institute for the Deaf
105 Gower Street, London WC2 8NJ.
Tel. 071 240 0806

The Health Service Commissioner for England
Church House, Great Smith Street, London SW1P 3BW.

The Health Service Commissioner for Scotland
Second Floor, 11 Melville Crescent, Edinburgh EH3 7LU.

The Health Service Commissioner for Wales
Fourth Floor, Pearl Assurance House, Grey Friars Road, Cardiff CF1 3AG.

11

MANAGING HEALTH CARE DELIVERY

Tom Keighley

This chapter goes beyond discussion aspects of managing care in clinical areas by addressing political, professional and social issues which influence effective management.

The chapter includes reference to and discussion of:

- Notions of care in relation to culture, patients' rights and expectations, and their choices within a health care system

- Management in relation to nursing, with particular reference to leadership and change

- Philosophy, beliefs, values and expectations, as they relate to management

- The place of information within management

- The use and allocation of governmental, financial and people resources

- Professional issues, such as accountability and effective decision-making

- Quality in health care with particular reference to quality assurance

- Professional politics and future trends as they affect nursing management

To write about management is to be presented with a choice. Either one can describe the tasks involved and the skills required to undertake them, or one can move to another plane which assumes that the books on tasks and skill acquisition have already been written by those who understand these things in great detail, and that to consider management should be to consider both the people who are managing and those who are managed.

In deliberating about the processes of management within the NHS, it is necessary to understand the people involved in those processes, and to ex-plain some of the notions of care that underlie those processes. The importance of having a mechanism to establish common beliefs and underlying values is emphasised throughout the chapter. So often internal conflicts and possible obstructions to the delivery of service, which so bedevil the management of health care, result from conflict of values.

Also, it is necessary to emphasise the importance of management as an interpersonal skill – and one where success rests primarily on the ability to effect change.

Notions of care

Whatever care is, it is clearly a very personal thing. To ask patients whether they have been 'well cared for' can often lead to total miscommunication.

The experience of care

Patients who have inadvertently received the wrong care (for example, those who have been dispensed the wrong tablets or given the wrong injection) may well offer the response that they have been looked after extremely well. Conversely, a patient who has been admitted as an emergency to the Accident and Emergency department, who has undergone massive life-saving treatment and been the subject of a number of technical interventions from a variety of expert health care professionals may exhibit negative feelings about the care received. Such patients will often indicate that there has been poor communication, that staff have not had time to talk to them, and that the nurses have appeared uncaring.

To any health care professional, but perhaps particularly to a nurse, the comments from these patients can be mystifying. It is clear, therefore, that the experience of being cared for is surrounded by individual beliefs and perceptions. Sadly, there is an accumulating body of evidence to suggest that nurses' aptitude for caring, as perceived by the recipient of care, is decreasing (see, for example, Moores and Thompson, 1986; Audit Commission, 1991; Barr and Rogers, 1991), while our own professional assessment of performance suggests that we are getting better (Wilson-Barnett, 1984; Anderson, 1986; Reid, 1988).

Cultural aspects of care

One of the major determinants of care is culture. Culture is one term which is subject to a multitude of misinterpretations and has a variety of meanings. In this context, culture refers to those observably common traits found in groups of individuals, which act as prompts to behaviour but which are only occasionally part of the verbal explanations of that behaviour. Good examples that can be seen regularly are the clothes that people wear, the food that they eat and the nature of the extended relationships which they maintain (Argyle and Trower, 1979). One major error is to behave as if only the colour of the skin or the nature of the language spoken can determine a particular culture.

In many areas of health care, the response to multicultural care has been simply to appoint translators and issue a list of surnames that the health care professionals are likely to encounter in their daily work. More recently, health authorities have tried to adapt the nature of the food which they offer in an attempt to meet the dietary requirements of particular groups of individuals. However, although the requirements of a halal diet can now be met within most hospitals, vegans are likely to have immense problems eating appropriately.

There are also major cultural influences which determine the expectations individuals may have about care. Many nurses will be aware of the need that some people have to cry, and indeed to wail, in the presence of extreme emotion or pain. This can be very embarrassing for those brought up to believe in the stiff upper lip and the existence of pain thresholds (see Chapter 15). Further, there are expectations about the need for rest, the appropriateness of particular types of food, indeed, even the relationship between a particular age and a particular illness. In the UK where early mobilisation and rapid discharge from hospital are part of our own health culture (Audit Commission, 1986), the expectations of individuals from different cultures (including West European cultures) can be in conflict with the prevailing behaviours and standards set within the organisations to which they come for their health care. Such a dichotomy has to be responded to and understood.

The third aspect of culture in health has already been referred to; it is the culture which exists among health care professionals delivering care. In this country, the culture of nursing has spent well over 400 years maturing into its modern form. By continuing to evolve, it remains an important element in the nature of health care provision and, indeed, its management (Abel-Smith, 1960). Recognising the nature of the local culture of an organisation, as well as the overall culture of the profession, and where that fits into the society from which nursing arises is an important aspect of nursing provision and management.

An example of a major change in the culture of nursing was the compulsory introduction of the different facets of the nursing process into the syllabus of training (General Nursing Council, 1977). Concerns were expressed about the forms that nurses had to use, the amount of time that the nursing process took, the difficulty of its application to the ward or department in which particular groups of nurses were working and the sideways comments about it being an 'American import'. What was important about this change was that it posed a massive challenge to the culture of nursing. The very existence of several phrases to describe the one phenomenon, e.g. 'systematic approach to care', or 'an individualised care programme' indicates the difficulty the profession had in assimilating the change. It challenged the intuition on which care processes were so often based. It denied the validity of 'standing next to Nellie' as a way of acquiring professional skills, and demanded that nurses be able to communicate what they claimed they were doing for the patient. The fact that the profession did not leap at this opportunity to demonstrate its expertise and ability, and still presents the most whimsical explanations for its failure to implement the nursing process in every care area, suggests that there is something very fundamental about the nature of this challenge.

Rights and expectations

It has been argued that the fundamental challenge in implementing the nursing process is not simply to acquire the recording skills or even to develop the knowledge which would allow a rational basis for the delivery of care to be demonstrated, but rather that the nursing process has both humanistic and existentialist elements. This means that the process is based on the individual, the human being, around whom care centres, and demands that every nurse consider first and foremost the needs of the individual patient/client. This demand brings in the existentialist element. No health care professional can meet the needs of an individual without consulting with that individual or with that individual's significant other(s) who is his representative or advocate. Such consultation is a two-way process. Having asked someone what their needs are, one is not (except in a *totalitarian state*) entitled to impose one's own views on the individual, and even less to undertake particular activities on or about that individual without his consent. This is a devastating challenge to a group of professionals who for many hundreds of years have imposed nursing care on the individuals wishing to receive it in an *autocratic* manner.

The cultural challenge of the nursing process is such that it demands that nurses refocus their approach to care in a way that hands control of the care process to the recipient of care rather than the giver. Increasingly, the challenge is being addressed through the evolution of primary nursing. This provides new opportunities to develop new models of care and new profiles of service delivery (Malby, 1991). Importantly, this approach addresses the issue of personal accountability for care delivery within a wider organisational system. It provides greater clarity in the management of care and identifies who is responsible for ensuring that professionally determined needs meet the patient's expectations.

Patients or clients have rights and expectations. In an era when there have been a number of instances of nurses demanding their rights (as, indeed, they have every right to), there have been numerous instances of patients not having their rights respected (see, for example, DHSS, 1978). However, no right exists without a concomitant duty. Some would argue that patients, particularly in the mental health and mental handicap services, suffer the rigours of society's judgements about their duties rather more than is appropriate. This emphasis on the right of patients to choose the care that they shall receive, and the right to continue to have care options offered to them even when they reject what the nurse might consider to be the most appropriate of those health care options, is crucial to the health service that will be developing during and beyond the final decade of this century. This is recognised in the development of the Citizen's Charter (HMSO, 1991) and the Patient's Charter (DoH, 1991b).

Further, the process of education about health and illness has occurred at a remarkable rate over the last decade and individuals are now far more aware of the alternatives they might have as well as what they can expect from the system (Boyd and Sellars, 1982: Welsh Consumer Council, 1988; Davies, 1989). Going are the days when everybody in a ward sat there overly grateful for the little they had received. In many areas, particularly in the community, midwifery, mental health and mental handicap care, patients and clients are much more demanding and far better able to express their expectations (see any of the Reports of

National Development Team, Mental Health Act Commissioners, Hospital Advisory Service). This requires a totally different approach to health care delivery from nurses, and indeed from all health care professionals working with patients and clients.

Personal potential and freedom of choice

In terms of managing care, an awareness of these changes demands two things from nurses. First, there is the need to develop the ability to interact with patients in such a way that they have a full and informed choice. There is little point in giving people options if they are not equipped to judge between them. The ability to educate patients to make such judgements and to be aware of the consequences of different judgements is an important step towards giving back to patients the control of their illness, and control of their lives.

Second, it is necessary to recognise that recipients of care have enormous personal potential. It has long been recommended that all new entrants to nursing should undergo a compulsory admission to hospital for some minor aspect of care in order to understand what actually happens to people once they come into the health service. For many years encounters with GPs have been criticised as being technically adequate but, from the patient's point of view, personally unfulfilling (Ritchie *et al.*, 1981) although this is now changing with the wide uptake of GP training programmes. This is as nothing when compared to the experience of patients on admission to hospital. Studies have shown how otherwise intelligent and insightful individuals are seemingly reduced to gabbling, head nodding, unduly grateful recipients of the service, particularly in the first 48 hours or so (Raphael, 1962; Goffman, 1968a). These studies have been replicated regularly since then, and it appears that patients continue to have similar experiences (Farrant, 1983; Bohlin and Larsson, 1986; Christenson, 1990; Mains *et al.*, 1991).

This is simply because they cannot comprehend or relate to the system in which they are being cared for. While there is a natural dependency which develops whenever somebody is ill or when they are exposed to a new institution, it is essential to enable patients to be both appropriately dependent but also independent in the areas in which they would normally expect to be independent and are still capable of being so (Goffman, 1968b).

Examples of factors which reduce independence include compulsory mealtimes and the enforced wearing of night attire 24 hours a day. The demand that individuals stay in bed when they would normally be out of bed and could well prefer to be so, the nature of the curt communications which vary from a social, 'How are you today?' through to detailed – and often public – enquiries about the activities of bladders and bowels, are further examples. These illustrate a lack of any notion of what might be considered to be socially acceptable to that individual.

While the environment in which patients are cared for does not always enhance the independence of the patient, nursing has rarely used the opportunities offered in a creative manner. By doing so, there would be the option of increasing the independence of the patients as well as maintaining their self-regard, respect and individuality (Wolfensberger, 1969).

Such an approach would ensure that not only would individuals know of their rights and options prior to admission, but that it would be possible to enhance the potential of the patient to achieve much earlier adaptation and development in relation to the problem that has brought them into the health care system.

Caring – the core of nursing

The discussion so far has concentrated on the nurse and it has been assumed that the terms 'nurse' and 'carer' are synonymous. While this is the case in many dictionaries and lexicons, it is not in reality. Others too deliver care, but the constant equating of nursing with caring emphasises the fact that caring is absolutely central to the nature of nursing (see also Chapter 12). Also, the general public holds nurses in high regard. This is not always beneficial to nursing, especially when massive inadequacies in practice can be demonstrated. Society has expectations about the nurse's role and performance, and assumes that the delivery of nursing care is the reason for her existence.

Nursing: art or science?

One of the ongoing debates in nursing is whether nursing is an art or a science. The point of this debate is twofold. First, it seems important to many individuals (nurse researchers, for example) to be able to categorise nursing under one of these headings in order to enable them to understand what it is that nurses do. To describe the activity of nurses as caring does not seem to be sufficient. For instance, while the medical profession acknowledges its background as originating from subjects known as 'The Arts' in the medieval universities, it now describes itself very firmly as a science. The implication here is that, as a profession, the practitioners of medicine have moved away from those nebulous, indefinable and unprovable notions which are prevalent in the arts, over to a rational, empirically demonstrable base which is associated with the sciences.

The second reason why this debate is ongoing is that there are occasions when it is easier to attract resources if a subject is seen to rest in one camp or another. Currently there is much more political support for subjects that are seen to be scientific (and, by implication, practical and down-to-earth) rather than the arts which in some way may be seen to be intangible. Professor Prophit has addressed this issue on a number of occasions and demonstrated it to be a quite inappropriate and unnecessary distinction (Prophit, 1986). Nursing could well be the creative combination of both an art and a science, drawing on the strengths of both in order to meet the needs of the recipients of care. The artistic side is represented by the deep personal caring, the emphasis on the individual, and the regard for fellow practitioners in a way that is very human. On the other hand, the sciences can offer a rational base for performance and activity, the opportunity to investigate practice, and to structure those investigations in such a way that others can understand them, evaluate them, and come to appreciate their significance. Perhaps the real issue in terms of managing care is not to engage in the either/or debate but to promote actively the perception of nursing as both an art and a science (Watson, 1979).

Defining management

In attempting to describe the relationship between caring and nursing, there is equally a need to address the position or notion of management within nursing. Management may be described in three ways. First, it is often portrayed within a framework of *decision-making*. For example, the principal rationale for implementing changes in the NHS in 1984 was to do away with the consensus form of decision-making and bring in a chief executive

system to sharpen up both the process and the way in which decisions were made within the service. By contrast, management may be described in terms of *administration*, a process by which decisions are implemented. Administrators are less concerned with the business of change than managers and in that sense are undervalued within the organisation of health care. Their role is seen much more in terms of maintenance and process. The third notion about management is that of *leadership*. Leadership may be described in terms of vision and of seeing beyond the horizon. It is often suggested that there are very few leaders or that there are very few people with leadership skills.

It is not always helpful to stick rigidly with these three separate notions of decision-maker, administrator and leader but to have a concept of management which incorporates all three, and requires the individual who is the manager, at whatever level in an organisation, to be visionary, to make decisions and to maintain the organisation. Such a unifying view not only gives value to all three aspects of management but also values the individuals who specialise in different aspects of it.

Managing nursing

To understand the management of nursing, it is necessary to be clear about two major aspects of care. These are the dispensing of care prescribed by others and the dispensing of care determined by nurses. Both have major consequences in terms of resources but it is rare for both to be assessed and practised together. Too often, the medical presumption determines the nature and duration of care, rather than the decision about the patient's care needs being a joint one (Downe, 1990; Robinson, 1991). To manage nursing care effectively, it is necessary to be able to distinguish between the two forms of prescription and represent both adequately in decision-making fora. If this is not done, decisions about service provision are made which ignore the nursing care component, and patients suffer (Stephenson, 1990; Fraser, 1990).

Similarly, there is a need to avoid being overprotective about care. The management of nursing care is not just the management of the care prescribed by doctors or the care prescribed by nurses and other health care professions. There is a very large area of work that takes the form of shared care (Plank, 1982). In this context care is delivered to the patient either jointly by the nurse and a relative or significant other, or a relative or significant other has been taught to undertake care and does it under the supervision of the nurse. By sharing care and managing such shared care, nursing is integrating itself fully into the processes that surround individuals within society. In the past, the profession has been far too isolationist and parochial and has often implied that only nurses can understand what it is they do. While caring is central to nursing, as pointed out earlier, caring is not exclusively undertaken by nurses, and though others may acquire some skills, the nurse is still perceived as the expert. There is no need for nurses to be defensive about the amount of nursing that others undertake; indeed, there is an increasing need for nurses to acquire advanced skills and techniques.

Venue of care

For too long nursing practice has been seen as something that occurs within special buildings known as hospitals, undertaken with a sense of magic ritual determined by procedure books, something for which special clothes and preparation are required.

Clearly, these notions are outdated. The need for individualised care, the understanding of what is truly meant by primary care, and the changes that are already afoot in society suggest that there is need for greater flexibility and awareness of the options that will be available for the profession in the future. It seems a good rule of thumb to work from the premise that care is best delivered in the home or as near to the recipient's home as is possible. This idea will be explored in some depth later in the chapter. It could be argued that one has to be very fit to survive the experience. Florence Nightingale's (1859) maxim about first doing the patient no harm is best followed by ensuring that hospitals are places that individuals only come to in an emergency or when technical expertise is unavailable at the bedside in their own home. The opportunities for professional development, if this maxim is pursued, are immense. It effectively redefines what is meant by the management of care.

The reforms within the NHS have moved this up the agenda. The implementation of the GP contract (Lowe, 1990; Potrykus, 1991; Bain, 1991a; Bain 1991b), the rapid and unplanned expansion of the number of practice nurses, and the creation of GP fundholders have all effected major changes in the way in which care is delivered. The best management of these changes is still evolving but will be dependent upon good local health needs definition, and education and training of an appropriate form and to an appropriate level for all concerned.

Notions of management

As has already been pointed out, there is a distinction between administration, management and leadership. Management is best conceived of as a combination of all three with one or other predominating as a form of activity. The usefulness of this tripartite approach is that it provides a reflective framework to review the activities of individuals in management positions, as well as providing a model by which individuals presented with problems can review approaches open to them.

A number of writers have gone to great lengths to identify the numerous factors which can be found among each of the three types of activity (Bennes and Slater, 1968; Benveniste, 1974). Good nursing management is a combination of all these factors and needs to be seen as such if the essence of nursing management is to be effectively established in the current structures of the health service. The important point is the nature of the nursing outcomes. Weak management rarely gives emphasis to evaluation of its decisions or to the establishment of outcomes by which those decisions can be seen to be implemented. It requires a combination of leadership, management and administration both to determine the outcomes and to evaluate them. The greater use of evaluation and the establishment of measurable outcomes would strengthen the process of nursing management and enable both the profession and those outside it to appreciate its value to an organisation.

Perhaps one of the greatest weaknesses in nursing management is that described by Jones and Rogers (1976). Their study showed not only that staff did not know what the nursing officers did, but also that the nursing officers themselves seemed very uncertain about their roles. This was manifested during the 1984/1985 re-organisation, when numerous authors in the health service and from the nursing profession suggested that the abolition of the nursing officer grade would be a major benefit following the Griffiths proposals (Rowden, 1986).

Leadership

It is true that nurse managers have not always represented either themselves or their work in the best possible, or most understandable, light. However, behind what appears to be a gross disregard for the process of management is the question of whether or not the profession at large wishes to have any leadership. Leadership can take many forms, but managerially, it is impossible to lead any organisation or part of an organisation that rejects the notion of leadership. The forces required to impose leadership against the will of large numbers of people do not exist in a free society. Clearly there has been great reticence to adopt nurse managers as nurse leaders. However, there has not been similar reticence in undermining their position or denying them the credibility which they require in order to undertake their work. Further, the roles they have been expected to undertake have become increasingly distant from that originally described in the Salmon Report (Ministry of Health, 1966). Without a consensus in the profession, nursing management and nursing leadership will not, and cannot, exist.

Change agents

The most important, but perhaps the most difficult role of the nurse leader who is appointed to a management position is to act as change agent. Such a leader is not required to be a senior nurse, but is often a G grade ward sister or charge nurse who, in effect, is being given the management responsibility for a single unit of care. This unit of care may be encompassed by four walls, but increasingly in the future it will be simply an extended caseload made up of numerous types of patients in various locations such as community units, patients' houses and hospitals. The style of leadership needed in this situation will be one that creates an atmosphere in which a particular quality of care is delivered and where the nature of that care will be continuously evolving as individuals' needs change.

This care will only be delivered intermittently by the sister/charge nurse and, therefore, she will have to be able to lead others into working in ways which enable the goals and objectives set to be achieved.

The notion of the nurse manager as leader and change agent is not one that is readily perceived. Far more often, the nurse manager is seen as a glorified administrator with all the prejudiced connotations of that term, or as the agent of another more senior manager. The profession requires leadership, and senior nurses, be they managers or educationalists, are the people best equipped to provide it.

Values and competencies

The budding manager also needs to value and demonstrate competence. This in reality is competence in a wide range of activities other than the managerial responsibilities she is appointed to fulfil. However, the phenomenon of actually needing to have direct 'hands-on' responsibility for care as a passport to being accepted in any position is one that radically weakens the profession rather than strengthening it.

The fact of non-acceptance because of diminishing clinical skills is one problem; another is the difficulty in acquiring competence in managerial skills. While the profession has developed an increasing number of qualifications for nurse educators and practising nurses (Rogers, 1983), there has been a very slow growth in the amount of management education and training available, though there is clearly a number of very good managers who have had little in the form of training but have significant skills in other fields. Competence, however, has to be demonstrated and demonstrated early in the role undertaken.

Interpersonal skills

Successful managers and leaders have highly developed interpersonal skills which leave everybody feeling special (Peters and Waterman, 1982). It is a form of communication which is direct and personal without intruding into the privacy of individuals or leaving them overwhelmed or undermined. It enables people to feel as if they are growing with their manager and their leader, while at the same time achieving, both personally and organisationally, in ways that might have been previously undreamed of.

Such interpersonal skills are a highly developed form of social behaviour which enables everybody to live and work together while ensuring the personal representation of self in the daily life of the organisation. This necessitates insight about oneself (see Chapter 14) combined with a readiness to apply that knowledge to achieving objectives. Such an approach leads to the demystification of leadership as a notion. It suggests that leadership is an activity at a higher level to both administrative processes and decision-making. Rather, it is an activity in which the humaneness of the people involved is recognised and used in a considered and considerate manner in order to achieve goals and objectives which they themselves share and are committed to. This is a manifestation of a humane organisation and is an approach to management which is based on managing human beings rather than managing machinery (Christopher, 1985).

Confidence and control

Management in nursing requires that individuals have confidence in themselves, physical energy to undertake the work, and what might be known as 'stickability' when the going gets tough. Confidence must not amount to being overly self-assured and energy should be utilised in a way that recognises that it is not boundless or limitless. The stickability notion is one that arises from a determination to get things done, but has within it the implication that there is a time to recognise when something is no longer possible and it is appropriate to determine another way forward.

The other, often remarked upon, feature of successful managers is their degree of self-control. Often, this is manifested by the presence of a highly developed sense of self-discipline both in terms of the volume of work undertaken and, perhaps more especially, in terms of emotional control. Truly effective managers and leaders demonstrate that they are hardly ever (and usually never) overwhelmed by anxiety at the size or nature of the task to be undertaken.

Practical theory and management

Other features of management include the ability to plan for the future, to organise the present, to delegate appropriately, to give direction without being commanding, to guide rather than to dictate and to effect a degree and type of coordination which is almost *gestalt* in its effect (i.e. the whole appears far greater than the sum of its parts). Such features require a deep understanding of management theories to account for the appropriateness of the action that is being proposed, but this knowledge is very practical and is acquired in order to be applied, primarily to the process of decision-making. Such qualities lead very often to a process known as reality re-definition (Stewart, 1985). Good managers and leaders have the ability to re-focus the direction that their units are moving in. They do this by negotiating a different future to the one that was being worked for and in that sense re-define the reality of the environment and time within which work can be undertaken. This is a very important skill because within the NHS, such ideas as a five-year strategic plan are now less and less credible, as the funding base and objectives for health care change almost annually and the service seems set to be put through yet more re-organisations in the next decade.

Nursing has demonstrated a great facility in producing managers and leaders. It needs to build on past experiences in a positive and creative way to ensure that management as an essential component of all nursing practice is both valued and developed. Individuals with special talents need to be nurtured and directed to undertake work appropriately. Failure to do this in the last 15 years has been a major weakness in nursing managers. It is one that the profession now has an opportunity to address and correct.

Determining a philosophy

To many people, management is the art of getting things done, rather than considering whether there is a framework or purpose which ties together the actions that individual members of an organisation might be asked to undertake. When considering the disparate nature of the multidisciplinary approach to health care which is increasingly being adopted in the UK, it is difficult to see how a cohesive approach to the task in hand can be achieved without the determination of a ***philosophy***.

Philosophy, beliefs and expectations

It has long been established that, within any individual, there will exist a number of different philosophies (Schrock, 1977). Clearly, there is the personal philosophy which has developed as part of the maturing process of the individual, an amalgam of those beliefs, understandings and expectations which have been acquired within the family, through education and through life experiences. It is expressed in behaviour, both in terms of stated attitudes and characteristic responses in the presence of particular stimulants.

The second major philosophy that is likely to exist is the professional philosophy which has been acquired through the process of education and training and working in the discipline of nursing. Many writers (for example, Bevis, 1983) have identified the complexity of the philosophies that any individual nurse may carry around with her, and processes exist for determining which of those particular philosophies may be leading to particular types of behaviour. Therefore, conflicts may arise from the wide range of professional philosophies that individuals hold.

The third group of philosophies are managerial. Such philosophies vary in origin from personal values held about the people with whom the manager works, through to the impetus which may be driving a particular manager to undertake any task in hand. Amalgamating the vast range of philosophies that many individual nurse managers experience presents a complex pattern of influences, both internal and external, which affect the way in which a manager operates.

Professional values versus managerial values

A manifestation of this conflict is the debate which often springs up in the professional press about the tension between professional values and managerial values (for example, Slack, 1985). It is suggested that individual professionals have the right to operate in particular ways because their values and philosophies indicate that they should. The refusal of managers to acquiesce to individuals being lead purely by professional values is often seen as a demonstration of a lack of understanding about the issue in hand, a lack of sensitivity to the individual attempting to pursue such a mode of operation, or very often as the manager lacking credibility in the field in which the management decision is being made. Occasionally, there are instances of individuals experiencing what they describe as professional and managerial conflict

in their own role (Blackford, 1982). It is a major problem, so often arising from naivety on the part of professionals who believe that the values and philosophies that lead them can exist **autonomously** without any recognition of the relationship between their actions and the actions of anyone else.

In the broader field of pure philosophy, it has long been established that the rights of any individual are always curtailed when the rights of another individual are being affronted in some way (Warnock, 1960). This leads to an interesting debate about rights not existing without concomitant duties. The question to be posed to many professionals who believe that their professional judgement should reign supreme is to query at what point they will no longer insist on their own judgement being the only one that they will accept. Certainly in nursing, it is unlikely that the profession will ever enjoy the autonomy that would permit individual judgements to rule supreme. The individual who is experiencing an internal conflict between professional values and managerial values will need to determine whether it would be possible to exercise professional judgements in a situation where a course of action is based on managerial values.

Another area of conflict is highlighted in the debate about whether individual clients' needs should be the chief determinant of any unit management's objectives. The philosophies can be very different indeed. The unit management could be solely engaged in attempting to continue the services they are responsible for within the resources allocated to them. The individual client, and/or the client's advocates, may be far more concerned about seeing individual needs fully met.

The debate on the nature of needs is sketched out in Chapter 12. However, the pursuit of the resources to meet a client's needs can conflict very actively with the short timescales of management objectives and the limitations under which many management teams feel they exist. Very often, members of a management team may wish to act as advocates for individual client groups and while this is right and proper, it can produce even greater conflict for the individual concerned, given the emphasis on corporate management. It is not easy to advise in this situation but it should be recognised that, certainly within the NHS, for those experiencing it this is a conflict which will become harsher as time goes by and the rate of change becomes ever greater.

A clarification process

The team which wishes to work cohesively, and to understand the position that each individual holds in that team, needs to go through the process of determining a philosophy (Fig. 11.1). This can be done most simply by the establishment of those common beliefs, values and social expectations which each member of the team holds. It is necessary to be sure that the language used has a common meaning, as so often there is a tendency for different groups to use terms differently, leading to confusion when it is discovered that a word does not have a shared meaning.

A good example is the term 'patient'. It seems almost a caricature to suggest it, but to a doctor, the patient very often is somebody who comes to him in the guise of a supplicant seeking his advice and guidance, and willing to receive the treatment at almost any personal cost and without question. In contrast, nurses will use the term 'patient' to mean an individual for whom they have a responsibility. It is interesting to observe how an increasing number of nurses refer to the people to whom they are offering a service as 'clients', so indicating yet another state of autonomy that might be exhibited by a 'patient'. Many nurses are prepared to nego-

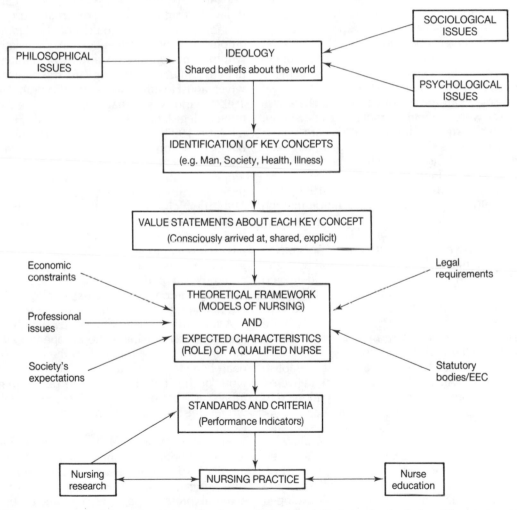

Fig. 11.1 *Determining a philosophy (From RCN Research Society,* Submission to the Judge Commission 1984. *Reproduced with permission)*

tiate and educate the patient in a way that leaves him in control of the care process and, therefore, not at all the supplicant but more the determiner of treatment. It is clear, therefore, that without exploring these important differences, even the use of the common term 'patient' can lead to a great deal of confusion and misunderstanding.

Going on to consider pure nursing, it is important to determine what are the key or essential concepts which direct the work of the nurse in any particular area. Again, the problem here is one of definition, as there is often rapid agreement as to what are the essential concepts that guide and direct the role and function of a nurse without agreement about what it is that nurses do. The great advantage of clarifying the key concepts is not only achieving a unanimity of position within the team, but enabling team members to express to others what they believe to be important.

At the next stage in this process, it is possible to determine frameworks of care within which the individuals will be operating. One of the great weaknesses about the nursing process debate was that nurses were taught to adopt a process without having any particular framework of care within which that process existed. Of late, there has been an increasing debate about which models of care nurses should adopt (Whittington and Boore, 1988; Biley, 1990; Chalmers et al., 1990; McKenna, 1990). This can delay recognition that the model itself is simply an attempt to project a particular framework within which questions can be asked and answers sought. It is quite possible to determine frameworks of care within almost any environment in which care is being delivered which, while being an amalgam of many published models, may not actually be a total representation of any one. This is probably wise because it is rare that any model meets all the needs of any particular care group.

The need primarily is for the team to establish the framework within which care can be delivered and to understand the processes being adopted to deliver care (Sines and Bicknell, 1985).

One of the other major advantages of determining a framework of care is that it allows a much greater degree of specificity to be achieved in the roles of individuals within that framework. From a management point of view, clarification of role enables an understanding to be developed about what can be achieved by individuals or groups of individuals. It also ensures that training

is modified, adapted and developed in order to prepare people for roles that they will be undertaking. Further, it permits debate to occur about the change of role and how such change fits into the overall performance of individuals. This has rarely been done well in nursing, and so often is the root cause of the dissatisfaction and frustration experienced by dedicated and highly trained individuals.

External influences

It is worth remembering that frameworks of care, role determination and the setting of objectives are not internal professional issues. They can all be influenced significantly by external sources which cannot, and indeed should not, be ignored. Examples of such influences are legislative and within common law. Examples of statutes which directly influence nursing are the Nurses, Midwives and Health Visitors Act (HMSO, 1979 and 1992), various National Health Service Acts, and related legislation like the Mental Health Act (HMSO, 1983b). Other Acts of Parliament have a direct effect on role and function but are apparently almost tangential to the nursing role. Examples of this are the Registered Homes Act (HMSO, 1984a), the Data Protection Act (HMSO, 1984b) which influences the way in which confidentiality is handled by all the professions, and the Police and Criminal Evidence Act (HMSO, 1984c) which has a number of sections indicating the way in which nurses should act with regard to drugs and rape in particular. Outside legislation (but within common law) is the expectation that nurses are first and foremost citizens of the realm.

A more distant legislative body which has a direct effect on nursing is the European Parliament, through which are established the common European Directives for Nursing. Also influential is the work of the statutory bodies in determining such things as professional codes and establishing written instructions for both practice and education.

At a more local level, there is the influence of local authorities, voluntary organisations, community health councils and a whole host of pressure groups. It is only by being very aware of the external pressures and responding to them that nursing is able to continue to determine the frameworks within which roles can be described. The previous tradition of ignoring such external pressures is a recipe for dodo-like extinction.

Standards

The recognition of these external factors and their influence on frameworks and roles enables realistic standards to be established, which will be acceptable to the society in which any particular group of nurses is working. The determination of a philosophy, of a framework of care, of roles and of standards, also determines the place of advice within a decision-making framework.

This has been an attempt to explain the importance and position of determining a philosophy within any particular group and in particular within groups of nurses. The outcomes can be immensely rewarding and prevent, or indeed resolve, a number of the difficulties that seem such a 'bugbear' to many in organisations at the current time. It is a forerunner and prerequisite of good management practice.

The need for information

Perhaps the cry heard most frequently from managers in any organisation when confronted with a problem, or a decision to be made, is that there is not enough information to make a decision. So often, the truth of the matter is that not only does the information exist, but also the decision-makers have had access to the information. The important point is that the information must be geared to enable decision-making to occur.

It is a failure not to recognise that the value of information is determined by the parameters within which it is perceived and understood. For instance, judgements about how many nurses are needed are very different when bed occupancy is low in a unit and when bed occupancy is high. Information about staffing levels is always available in the sense that an organisation knows how many people it is paying. However, it is not always available in a decision-making format that relates the numbers of staff available to the needs of dependent patients. The framework of the decision and of the organisation in which that decision is being made will determine the relevance, significance and usefulness of information. It has long

been recognised in the field of social sciences that no fact or piece of information is value-free (Durkheim, 1897) and that the values as discussed earlier in this chapter will largely determine the nature of information and the role it plays in an organisation.

A rational base for decision-making

Implicit in seeking information is the assertion that there should be a rational and accountable base for the decisions reached. This may seem so obvious that it does not need to be stated, but day-to-day experience will remind individuals of the numerous instances where a decision was clearly based on intestinal judgement or some combination of myth, mystery and magic which it is almost impossible to explain. Often, the lack of a rational base for decision-making leads the decision-maker to assert that his decisions are professional – i.e. based on the innate understandings to which his professional background has given rise. This is clearly unsatisfactory, particularly in the profession of nursing where public **accountability** is a crucial element of the individual practitioner's life.

The question of available information is matched by another question about sources of information. The will of the profession to establish itself as an independent entity has often led individuals to foreclose on sources of information because they were not nurse-generated.

In any rational decision-making process, data sources and information bases should be widely accessed. Clearly, there comes a point when it is no longer viable to seek for sources of information and the need arises for a decision to be taken. It is necessary also to understand the background and nature of these sources in order to integrate them into the decision-making arena. However, other members of the decision-making team may not credit sources in the way that perhaps a nurse may. The validity of certain sources of information is very often determined by the previous experience in academic and developmental terms that an individual has had. It is necessary within the management arena to negotiate and establish the credibility of sources of information before then using information from that source. This relates to the earlier references to values and underlines once more the need for appropriate values clarification. Further, it emphasises another point made earlier about timeliness and relevance. Having knowledge and information is useless if the appropriate time cannot be chosen to integrate that information into the decision-making process.

Information and outcomes

The integration of information into the decision-making process hinges very much on being able to link the nature and use of a particular source of information to particular outcomes. Those new to management seem to experience greatest difficulty in relating what they know to the nature of the decision to be taken. The solution to this is to develop an understanding of the decision-making process that is being adopted and to work within the established values of the organisation. This leads to an understanding of how information can be used and when it is best to use it. An example of how the same information can be used differently is the relaying of what is known about pressure sores. Administrators and finance officers will always be interested in both the cost of treating pressure sores and the need to change practice in terms of how the cost of running the organisation will be beneficially affected. In contrast, clinicians like nurses and doctors tend to be far more interested in individual patient outcomes and take a more altruistic approach to consideration of the issue (Wickens, 1983).

Neither is particularly right or wrong but in crude terms, this demonstrates how one single source of information can be presented differently to make the same point, i.e. that practice may need to change. Information can also be used to determine outcomes. It is a current problem in general management that so much nursing information does not facilitate the determination of health care outcomes (Altschul, 1982). Therefore, the nature of information influences decision-making.

Since 1979, within the NHS, there has been an attempt to structure the information that is available for decision-making. This was based on the realisation that most of the information systems available were created in order to answer Parliamentary questions placed by MPs and peers. Once the information had been sought, it was common for the Department of Health to request that information should be gathered regularly. Prior to 1979, the routine returns of information were geared mainly to a need at the centre of the health service to be able to deal with questions placed by external sources. The decision to set up the review in 1980 under the chairmanship of Edith Körner resulted in a change of thinking. It was decided that information supplied to the DHSS would only be collected if it was required at local levels for decision-making. This has almost become a principle and the information strategies that are currently being developed within the NHS are based on providing information that will be relevant and timely for local managers to use in their decision-making processes. The aggregation of such information is then collated and forwarded for central use. As a result of the Körner Reports, a number of major information systems have been developed and April 1988 saw the initiation of routine and widespread data collection within the NHS in a way that has never occurred in the past. Some of the systems developed are particularly strong but still dependent on the way they are implemented. In some areas of care (the community, for example) there was such a lack of information that it has been a massive exercise to determine information needs and develop appropriate systems for data collection and presentation. The next decade will see a continuous process of evolution in the collection and presentation of information and will underline the assertion made above that decisions should be made from a rational basis.

The late 1980s saw the development of a number of Information Technology (IT) exercises linked to resource management. This is currently being evaluated (Clough, 1990; Morrison, 1990; Millar, 1991) but has already achieved two things. First, recognition that those most directly involved in service delivery are best placed to generate the relevant data. Second, that there must be a continuous stream of information which ties service delivery to management decision-making. This has had real impact on nurses at all levels. Practitioners have had to learn new skills related to the technology, and structure their work both to deliver care and record it more fully. Managers have had greater access to nurse-generated data and have had to learn new interpretive skills. Finally the gaps in the data and information base have been exposed and have had to be addressed. These IT initiatives have created new dynamism in the service as organisations have competed to be involved, and have started a process which has spread over into many other areas of work in health care.

Application of information

One of the difficulties affecting managers faced with this sudden influx of information is the tendency to be distracted by material that is not directly relevant but which looks interesting. An analysis of what information is needed for specified purposes depends on managers understanding what those purposes are. There is some usefulness in reviewing information that becomes available as part of the collection exercise, even if it is not needed directly.

One area of disappointment is the way in which nursing research has failed to provide information in a timely manner to influence the development of information systems in the health service. The challenge facing the profession over the next decade is the generation of research-based information which will be relevant and applicable in terms of the information systems that managers are using. This has been given new impetus by the appointment of a Director of Research and Development to the NHS Management Executive.

Another area of concern is the paucity of information about the quality of care. There is the very real possibility that the major debate about the quality of care will be determined without the significant contribution that the nursing profession can make, simply because the framework that is generating nursing research is itself neither relevant nor timely. The creation of a Research and Development role on the NHS Management Executive may help to address this lack of framework. There is a real need for an extensive development of the nursing research resource so that more nurses researching at post-doctoral level exist and the profession is less dependent on pre-doctoral research studies for its research base.

Patients and information

Through the 1970s and early 1980s, nursing research was a major stimulant to practice development in this area of care. Now a whole host of specialist reports and expert papers being generated by generic research units, very often attached to or placed within universities, are replacing the previous source of expertise. They vary in relevance but very often provide the stimulus which enables local management to address particular issues. Another major source is the specialist material that individual client groups produce, e.g.

MIND and Mencap, which, because they are focused in a certain way, enable staff to review their own performance within the expectations of such client groups. Indicators for practice can be determined very quickly from such reports.

This leads us on to the very necessary point that the recipient of care is often the best source of information. Failure of adequate consultation with this source produces a service that professionals may be very happy with but that leaves the users completely dissatisfied.

Consideration of the health care recipient as a source of information raises a number of issues about confidentiality (see also Chapter 13). Concerns about confidentiality have come to a head because of the enactment of the Data Protection Bill (HMSO, 1984). The profession has been moving towards a position where the health care recipient should have full and open access to all information (Vousden, 1987). This position has not been supported by the more senior of medical personnel but the principle has been understood and is beginning to be integrated in practice. It is necessary to be clear that confidentiality exists to ensure that the rest of the world does not find out about what is communicated between patients and health care professionals. This raises difficult questions — for example, about what (if anything) a patient's relatives should be told before the patient himself, or with whom in the health care team information can be shared. This is especially topical as not all health professionals have their own statutory body (social workers and psychologists do not, for example). The need for confidentiality remains paramount but to date many health care professionals have not demonstrated their understanding of the need for it nor its place within modern practice.

This problem has been further addressed by the passing into law of the Access to Health Records Act (1990). From November 1991 this gave access to all handwritten health care records written after that date (Allsopp, 1991). The importance of this is not so much that it extends individual rights and freedoms but that it lays new responsibility on all health care professionals to share their working methods and conclusions more systematically with patients and clients. Managers should see this as a major quality opportunity.

In conclusion, the integration of information in the decision-making process and its use and application are skills that managers need to develop. It is still, and will remain, necessary for the generation of information to be related to management's need to make decisions. Processes will evolve for the patient or client to be central to the generation of information and the outcomes of the decisions made.

It will be important to make data collection for management purposes relevant to those (such as ward-based and community nurses) who are responsible for input of data. If they lack motivation, data accuracy will be affected. They will need feedback relevant to them and their work to continue to do this data collection effectively.

The distribution and use of resources

The great weakness in recent times has been to discuss the delivery of health care in terms of cost rather than in terms of what people can do in the service. This has in part been due to the ways in which financial activity can be evaluated. Also, it is due to individuals failing in their responsibility for the workforce and for explaining clearly that finance, along with personnel and administration, is a support function to enable a workforce to serve the health care recipients.

The allocation of resources by government

The allocation of resources is based on a process which, with modification, has been long established. The Treasury reviews the proposed spending of government departments during the summer and early autumn. Departmental heads in government (i.e. Secretaries of State) are then allocated a sum of money for the next year to achieve particular priorities that have been agreed. The upward consultation processes from the organisations they run enables them to develop some idea of what the appropriate priorities are, and how much they will cost.

However, there is also the external political agenda which affects the allocation of resources. In health care terms, this has led to community care, care of people with mental health needs, care of people with a mental handicap, elderly people and children being given priority over the acute services of general hospitals. The status of these

priorities is now unclear as the current central government funding priority rests within the implementation of the NHS reforms. Following the allocation of resources at government level to government departments, the NHS hears details about its allocation in the early part of the year and this is relayed to regional health authorities. They in turn, having been exposed to upward pressures to determine priorities, make allocation of those resources to their district health authorities. This enables health authorities to allocate resources within their own units of management around the beginning of April.

This process appears comparatively drawn out until one considers the complexity of the organisation that is being run. The total figures are in excess of a million people, so it is indeed a large and complex organisation to manage. Within the system, there are a number of new processes at all levels to try and ensure that the resources are spent appropriately (DHSS, 1983). This does not mean that resources can only be used on previously agreed objectives but that priority must be given to the work that has been previously agreed.

At government level, the public expenditure review committees and the Auditor General's office look frequently at both the total and more particular aspects of NHS spending. The Department of Health itself, under the leadership of the Minister of Health, reviews regional health authorities, who in their turn review the district health authorities. This is an attempt to ensure a unity of purpose as well as being part of the process of public accountability.

One of the great weaknesses of resource allocation is that it is based on traditional patterns of usage. This means that if some units have very high or very low throughput, they are more likely to attract or lose resources. Therefore, there is difficulty in generating or liberating resources to address newer priorities. Another factor is that resource allocation is very often based on heads of population. In the main, this is often inappropriate and ignores the degree of deprivation that any group within the population may experience. It also ignores the supplementary support that organisations, also working in the health care field, may be giving. In particular, this means that the local authority, which has its own agenda of spending and resource allocation, can make a significant difference to the health needs of the population, a process which will be addressed as the work on

The Health of the Nation (DoH, 1991a) Green Paper progresses.

Workforce, finance, estates

Within the health service generally, but particularly in Directly Managed Units (DMUs) or trusts, it is useful to consider resources under three headings. Workforce has already been mentioned, as has finance, but the third major resource is that of the estate on which health care is delivered. These three elements do not exist in isolation. Good managers demonstrate the ability to manipulate and vary the three resource components in such a way as to maximise the impact and effect of the service. So often the difficulty is that individuals responsible for each of these resources defend their corners and are judged by their colleagues as to their success or failure on the basis of whether or not they can acquire more of the resource that they manage. An example of how inappropriate this can be is the Estates Manager who may be seen by colleagues to be a failure because of sale of land and property when other elements of the organisation may be completely dependent on those sales in order to develop new and more appropriate services. Hospital closures are not, in themselves, disasters. A cool and reflective review of what is happening often reveals that the closure of a hospital follows the re-provision of those resources on another site and/or the relocation of those resources into another area of health care (Wagstaff, 1987)

The balancing of the different resource issues is an example of how managers need to be open-minded and not defensive, to recognise that there will never be enough resources and that the challenge is to get the best out of the resources that are available.

Evaluation of resource allocation

One problem is that resource allocation decisions, because they are made within a particular year, are rarely evaluated before the resource picture changes. This has become more difficult with frequent changes in the management structure in the health service in recent years and it would be one of the major benefits of a period of slower, and locally led, change in structure. Little is known about the full impact of resource allocation decisions. A good example of this is that the decision-making around the development of a new health care unit can take upwards of five years from the first formal agreement through to the first health care recipients walking through the door.

It can then take a period of two or three years after that to establish the firm running of the organisation and to evaluate fully what has been achieved. At this point there has been a time lapse of some eight years and a great deal can change in any social group during that time – both in terms of the population to be served and those providing the service. Evaluation of such change is therefore not a simple matter. However, this lack of evaluation has meant that the assessment of performance by acquisition of resources has held sway, which needs to be replaced by a principle of only allocating resources where they can be used. Nursing could well be embarrassed over the next few years as budgets allocated for the nursing workforce become underspent due to demographic changes (UKCC, 1986). It will take great courage to be able to debate this and to decide appropriate use of those resources to enhance the delivery of nursing care without them necessarily being spent directly on the nursing workforce.

There is a need to match local competence to higher political objectives, one of the major priorities for the NHS Management Executive. It is an ability which needs to be developed in all components of the health service and in so doing will enable the rivalries and parochialism to be broken down. An example of the complexity of this is the management of medical consultants in the NHS. While their contracts rest with regional health authorities, it is the DMUs and trusts which have to make the decisions about the resources the consultants are using. There is a higher political intent to control resource usage and clearly there is failure here in terms of linking intent to the ability to achieve.

Another example is the debate on skill mix. This concerns what skill mix of nurses should be utilised in any health care environment. Despite a major departmental review (DHSS, 1986), there has been a limited development in terms of what can be done. At a local level, few nurse managers are equipped to handle skill mix issues appropriately. It is still very difficult to determine the balance of trained to untrained nurses to learners in any particular health care arena, and there is little objective work available to link staffing levels to patient dependency (Macguire, 1986).

Developments in resourcing: clinical budgeting and ward budgeting

Clinical budgeting has proved very difficult to implement (Bryan, 1985) as it means relating allocation of resources to the activity of particular doctors and their teams and is often seen as an infringement of clinical freedom. There have been some successful examples of clinical budgeting where doctors have realised that their use of resources limits the ability of their own colleagues to perform. By and large, however, it has been difficult to enable clinical budgeting to be introduced without a major revolution in the understanding by doctors of their use of resources. In contrast, very successful work has been done on ward budgeting (Plant, 1985; Darley, 1990; Shafer, 1991). This is a process whereby ward sisters or their equivalent in other areas of care are responsible for the budget that is spent within the areas they control. This has resulted in much more effective use of resources at a local level, and is a bright light on the horizon in terms of enabling nurses to be fully responsible for their actions, and the resources they utilise.

Intraprofessional issues

Numerous texts and, indeed, general discussion within nursing tend to describe the profession as dividing into four areas:

(1) Service
(2) Education
(3) Research
(4) Management

Service refers to those individuals who have responsibility for direct, hands-on care. *Education* incorporates all those who are responsible for teaching. *Research* includes all those establishing the profession's knowledge base. Perhaps, naively, it needs to be stated that *management* refers to those nurses responsible for managing the service.

This superficial synopsis is crude. Any detailed analysis of the structure of the profession reveals that individuals in all four areas are undertaking all four types of task and usually in such an interrelated manner that it is difficult to distinguish one

from the other. Instead of simply being a useful framework for analysis, the notion of a fourway divide in the profession has become almost a mythical belief that nursing is reluctant to discard. In considering a number of roles, for example the ward sister, the district nurse and the health visitor, it is very often impossible to distinguish whether they are primarily service givers, teachers, researchers or managers, as they seem to have to be able to combine all four of these activities at any one time.

Another area of debate is the specialist/generalist divide. A number of people have argued that the major change in nursing, particularly since 1945, has been the increasing development of specialisms within the profession at the cost of the roles that were previously considered to be generalist (White, 1985). However, the development of specialisms may be an attempt to enhance the credibility and power base of particular groups at the expense of others and, therefore, not necessarily beneficial either to individual nurses or the patients to whom they are responsible (White, 1985). On the other hand, the emergence of specialists has made a significant contribution to standards of care and education.

A further problem has been the uncertainty surrounding the role of the *senior nurse*. The role of the nursing officer was described in the Salmon Report (Ministry of Health, 1966) as a senior member of staff who combines the managerial experience of a ward sister with the advanced knowledge of a clinical specialist. In the 1984 reorganisation of the NHS, the role was once more redefined with the two elements of management and clinical practice very often being separated out. It is not clear at this point whether this will benefit the service or not, but the very fact that it happened indicated that after some 16 years there was still a sufficient degree of uncertainty in the profession about the place of such posts to fail to justify them continuing. This is particularly sad at a time when patient care requires greater skills and expertise than at any point in the past, and when there is evidence that good nurse managers are outstanding if they can be found (Hutt, 1987).

Management as an activity

The very negative view of the profession about nursing management is part of a wider disbelief in the credibility of, or need for, managers above the level of ward sister. The development of ward budgeting has brought home to many individuals at ward level the reality of site management in various forms. However, there is still a tendency for management to be seen as an add-on to the more important business of care rather than as an integrated activity in the total role. Control over the profession of nursing could well depend on whether the profession itself gives management any credibility.

It has often been argued that only nurses can manage nursing. The emphasis is on the phrase 'manage nursing'. That assertion is justifiable. The wider assertion – that only nurses can manage nurses – is clearly untrue. The whole history of the nursing profession, particularly in the UK, is littered with examples of nurses being very successfully managed by non-nurses. It seems unlikely that in the future nurses will be the only people managing nurses and further, that nurses will be expected to manage far more than simply nurses and nursing. This latter notion would not have been at all strange to Nightingale whose belief in a tripartite management of care (the doctor, the hospital secretary and the nurse) was more closely achieved in the 1984 re-organisation than at any point since the establishment of those institutions that she fostered in the latter part of the 19th century.

The position of nurses in management has changed again with the NHS reforms. The establishment of a board position on the trusts for a nurse confirms the need for nursing management at the highest levels. Further, it demonstrates the capacity of nurses to play major corporate roles in the management of the service. It confirms the re-emergence of nursing as a process requiring the attention of the 'top of the house' in any health service organisation.

The question that then arises is about the resources that are required for management. The primary resource is time. It is clear in all that has been said so far about the role and function of any individual, particularly the ward sister, that a significant change in role is foreseen. Individuals will have to acquire the skills to prioritise their work in a way which enables them to take a clinical lead, guide the team they are responsible for, and also act as the on-site manager for all the resources utilised. The recognition that time is a major resource is not always present and to use time constructively is both a skill and an art. At

one extreme an individual can appear to be an imitation of the Mad Hatter, constantly rushing around while achieving little, and at the other extreme so laid back that there is a real danger that the chair will tip over. Various techniques and personal presentations can be affected but the real art is in relating the use of time to objectives and the skill is in utilising time to maximum benefit in terms of the number of things that can be done (McGee-Cooper, 1984).

Accountability

The understanding of accountability is a comparatively recent development in the profession. One of the major outcomes of the Nurses, Midwives and Health Visitors Act (1992) has been the establishment of a Code of Conduct, now in its third edition (UKCC, 1992a; see also Chapters 13 and 14). This, in conjunction with *The Scope of Professional Practice* (UKCC, 1992b), covers all significant aspects of nursing practice, and specialist addenda have been published on the giving of medicines, advertising and confidentiality. Such developments have emphasised the need to:

'safeguard and promote the interests of individual patients and clients; serve the interests of society; justify public trust and confidence, and uphold and enhance the good standing of the professions'
(UKCC, 1992b)

The emphasis is on personal accountability for action, be it acts of omission or commission. There is a need for professional development, and to act within established knowledge and skill bases. The value of a team approach to care, and the place of the customs, values and spiritual beliefs of health care recipients is recognised, including processes for conscientious objection.

The establishment of these principles leads to further explicit statements within the Code about regard for privileged relationships, confidentiality, relating resources to actions, protecting junior staff from excess workloads, the development of professional competence in others, and inappropriate use of professional qualifications. The existence of the Code can be seen as merely the public statement which incorporates the good practice that the profession has been pursuing over many years. More importantly, it establishes the criteria by which any nurse can be considered acceptable by both the profession and society at large. It is the principal tool of the statutory body (i.e. the UKCC) when it comes to retaining nurses on, or removing them from, the Register and determining whether or not they are fit to practise. It is now necessary to remain registered for practice and not to practise without registering.

These details of professional accountability may change over time. The astute professional not only makes herself aware of the guidance issued by statutory bodies and professional organisations about professional accountability, but also establishes her own code of practice for the area in which she is working. The changes in professional practice and management structure all necessitate nurses taking the general principles and devising specific criteria for practice which ensure a linkage between the code and individual roles and functions. Such an approach protects against individuals being overtaken by changes in both practice and organisational structure. This enables specific training needs to be spelt out during the performance review process, and for personal and professional developments to be maintained.

Accountability, therefore, is clearly a dynamic process. Creative use of the process will help produce the next generation of nurse leaders.

Management resources

There is much that individuals with a training in administration can teach nurses who are acquiring management skills, particularly as resources are so limited. It needs to be recognised that in this country, outside the private sector, the NHS has the lowest management costs of any health service in Europe or North America (HMSO, 1986). This fact alone should be a warning to all working in the NHS that the resources available for management are very limited indeed and that, therefore, the process of management is much more part of the active role that individuals play both as clinicians and as teachers than other health services would normally anticipate.

Evidence is accumulating that the lack of this resource could well be one of the reasons for difficulties in effecting change in the health service (King Edward's Hospital Fund, 1985). The possibility exists, therefore, that processes of management will only maintain systems rather than change them (Bevan and Ingram, 1987; Rawles, 1989).

This can lead to internal organisational conflict as the priorities of care change and different groups within the profession attempt to achieve those priorities whilst other groups obstruct them, simply because there is not the management resource to effect the change. An example of this is the difficulty that an acute general hospital has in doing anything other than meeting the very urgent and massive demands placed upon it. At the same time, those with foresight can see ways of making that unit operate differently in order to facilitate the greater move of resources into the community. While there is little management resource available, there is limited opportunity for such an acute unit to change.

Finally, one of the most straightforward ways of addressing these intraprofessional issues is through the development of the interpersonal skills that managers need. So often, training is about how to administer the flow of information and communication in an organisation. Rarely is sufficient time given to the development of those personal skills which are required in order to effect that communication and to take on the very important leadership role that nurse managers require (see also Chapter 14).

It was suggested earlier that leadership is the most obvious demonstration of interpersonal skills and the ability to control emotions, to be sensitive, to encourage and support individuals, to withhold pressure, and to work under pressure. All these facets, along with time management, need to be developed constructively and deliberately as the major resources individuals have at their disposal.

Interprofessional issues

This section looks at some of the areas in which conflict or potential conflict exists between nursing and other health care professionals.

Handmaids or colleagues?

The debate about nurses as doctors' handmaids, or at the other extreme as mini-doctors, is commonly an issue for discussion (Bishop, 1983; Stilwell, 1988; Hogg, 1989). Clearly, what needs to be achieved is a health care team made up of a number of health care professionals, each being clear about their own role and the role that their colleagues undertake. Similarly, there needs to be a consideration of how roles overlap and that this is not necessarily a bad thing. An illustration of this in mechanistic terms is the pattern of slating that can be seen on a roof. The slates are not laid side by side, but overlap to a considerable degree in order to ensure that the building is waterproof. So it needs to be with the roles of health care professionals. The overlap in skills and roles ensures continuity of service delivery.

Professional language

Language does not exist in a vacuum and the same words can have very different meanings for different people. Those meanings are determined by the situation in which people are working and the sort of training and experiences they have had. It is clear, therefore, that meanings need to be negotiated. One cannot be like Lewis Carroll's Humpty Dumpty who said that words meant whatever he insisted they meant (Carroll, 1872).

A further complication is that nurses use certain terms with a particular technical meaning and do not always explain that meaning. Examples of such words would be 'professional', 'accountable' and 'responsible'. The clarification of these terms is an important process in avoiding interprofessional conflict.

This is of great benefit as it means that nurses have the opportunity to respond to individuals and groups who wish to develop a greater understanding of the practice of nursing and the roles that individual nurses are attempting to fulfil. However, this requires an openness of mind on the part of nurses and the ability to justify what they are doing.

There is much research completed, dating back at least to the work of Isabel Menzies (1960), to show that nurses have been very slow to develop an understanding of why they undertake the tasks they do and so demonstrate real weakness in terms of being able to explain the rationale behind their activities to people other than nurses.

Interprofessional rationality

This inability to negotiate on behalf of nursing care runs parallel with a disregard for the intellectual and, on occasions, for the rational in nursing. Too much nursing practice is based on the myth, mystery and magic of generations of previous practice. The way that nurses who have studied in universities and other institutions outside the NHS have had to struggle in order to fulfil the criteria of training and subsequently be taken into practice has been reported frequently (Luker, 1984). It is ironic that nurses coming in with degrees are staying at the bedside often three times longer than those with more traditional forms of preparation for practice (RCN, 1985). Further, there is frequent mention in the nursing press of the profession's failure to utilise the research that is available and to incorporate appropriately within the staffing structures of the NHS those nurses with research skills who would be able to provide the rational base for practice which is urgently required (Barnett, 1981; Chapman, 1989; Waterworth, 1990).

This disregard for the intellectual and the rational is a major weakness when in nearly all other professions advancement is based on acquiring those rational, cognitive skills which are so often associated with further academic attainment and with research. This clearly is a major area of conflict which is weakening the profession's position, both in terms of health care delivery and in terms of its position within the overall team of health carers.

Further, there is an urgent need for consensus when any management change is to be effected and active direction given to the nature of the service. The need for consensus and the concomitant need for negotiation to achieve that consensus is a clear manifestation of real general management skills.

However, the need to work towards agreed objectives and priorities, and the recognition that it is only possible to achieve those objectives and priorities by team effort, is ensuring an appreciation for the need for consensus and team work. Nurses need to integrate themselves into teams in a way which will enable the greatest possible contribution to be made from within the nursing framework.

Personal power

The need to be able to relate to non-nurse general managers remains. So often, this is a function of personality on both sides rather than a problem of interdisciplinary conflict. Part of the issue is the recognition of what is sometimes known as *per-*

sonal power (Argyle, 1969). This is that power which is *other* than the authority invested in an individual because of the post that he holds. Everybody has personal power. What differs is the ability of individuals to utilise it in an effective way. It is not about the acquisition of further power or the ability to dominate and control, but rather the exercise of ability and the making of the appropriate and necessary contributions.

In the future it will not be possible to define simply and in traditional terms the roles and functions of groups of health care professionals. The history of the development of health care professionals reveals not only how things have changed but also the pace of that change (Baly, 1980). There is no evidence that the pace will slow down, rather the converse, that it will speed up (Toffler, 1981). This speeding up of change needs to be handled consciously and sensitively.

The development of roles can be the most exciting and challenging element of a person's career. Failure to appreciate how it will improve the service can lead to the changing of roles being the most devastating and destructive experience of a person's career. It is only by addressing the process consciously, and within the framework of the notion of a community of carers, that it will be possible to integrate all health care professionals to form a cohesive team with individual data bases and skill areas.

Decision-making and change

For many people, decision-making is the principal component of any leadership activity. The ability to create an environment in which decisions are taken, the skills to lead others to reach a decision and the ability to enact the consequences of the decision are all part of that leadership. Too often, decisions are taken without consideration of the period of preparation and the processes which ensure the fulfilment of the decision. Further, decision-making is not always about changing things. It can simply be a decision to retain the *status quo*. To consider decision-making and change, therefore, is actually the consideration of two totally different processes.

Leadership and change

After decision-making, the creation of a change culture is probably the second major component of any leadership activity. Change can be reversion to what existed before, or it can be the choosing of something new.

A change culture requires an organisational ethos which values change. It probably also requires a higher degree of bravery than is normally attributed to members of an organisation, in that they can be appointed to undertake one particular activity and, because they act as change agents, they develop the organisation in such a way that it is something other than what it was when they arrived. Some would argue that nurses have not been brave enough to do this and have preferred to allow evolutionary change (Salvage, 1985). Such an argument can sometimes seem to be a coward's charter and a form of assertion that it is impossible to do things other than within the existing frameworks. This is unacceptable when working in an organisation that determines objectives and priorities and seeks to address the problems that arise within the organisational process. To consider continuously that change will evolve suggests that, externally, there is some greater force that cannot be influenced and which will itself determine that change. In analytical terms, change is charted by events and the choice is to allow the events to emerge, or to create them by considering various problems that can be addressed.

The process of problem identification needs to be carried out organisationally through the processes identified earlier in this chapter. The problems will emerge as the objectives and purposes of the organisation and will be identified in terms which have a common meaning, ensuring that there is a unified team approach to the solution. The danger is to attempt to address problems without having identified them in a way that achieves that unity of assent. Failure to do so results in people feeling undermined, devalued and ***marginalised*** within an organisation. If change is to occur as a process, then it is necessary to take the vast majority of people along with the change agent.

Barriers to change

The fear of change and the fear of decision-making are very real in organisations because there is often security in the continuity of things as they are. However, for creative individuals with a mission to improve an organisation and, in particular, in nursing and the NHS, there can be a real fear of no change. Having identified the current weaknesses, inadequacies and failings of the system and feeling that there is a professional, personal accountability issue here, allowing something that is less than the best that can be provided to persist is unacceptable and inappropriate. Such individuals who attempt to address this can perhaps be described as 'positive deviants' in that they are seeking not to destroy but to improve and to change rather than to negate.

Decision-making processes

A number of writers have identified different decision-making processes and the model described by Allison (1971) offers a framework to analyse both decisions that have been taken and possible decision-making pathways that can be explored given the presence of certain problems or options. Three major processes appear to exist. The first is described as a *rational decision-making process*. This works on the basis that when a problem arises, the decision-maker (or decision-makers):

(1) agree a definition of the problem;
(2) discover all the possible solutions;
(3) match the problem with the resource implications;
(4) choose a solution that best matches the problem;
(5) implement the solution.

The second decision-making process is known as the *organisational process*. This suggests that in organisations, particular individuals or departments are established to handle particular issues. Once the problem is identified, the problem is referred to the responsible person and existing processes are used to produce a solution. This is a very bureaucratic approach. It maintains the routine operations of an organisation but tends to work on the basis of precedent and internal consultation.

The third decision-making process is the *political decision-making process*. This is based on two fundamental tenets. It acknowledges that there are some people in organisations with so much power that they can railroad through their own personal decisions as no single individual or group

of individuals can put together sufficient resources to stop them. The second tenet is that if an individual is not powerful enough to railroad through his decisions, then he can negotiate and bargain in order to achieve what he wishes to see happen. This has elements of power but also of dealing and trading.

Given the existence of these three different processes, it is clear that all three exist within the NHS and that, given different sorts of problems and different types of decisions, different processes are appropriate. The rational decision-making model is probably best used when new problems, new challenges and new types of decisions have to be made (see also Chapter 12). The organisational process is one that excels when dealing with routine issues. The political process is probably best utilised when there is a decision to be made that crosses boundaries or challenges, at a fundamental level, the traditions of an organisation. Clearly, in an ideal world where time and resources were never limited, the rational approach would be preferred, but it is necessary to be pragmatic and to acknowledge that different processes have different benefits as well as different weaknesses. The important thing is to try and be conscious of the processes being adopted and to utilise those that will achieve the best results.

Disjunctive incrementalism – muddling through

Some writers in this field have suggested that there are major weaknesses in any decision-making process that works to fixed goals or objectives (for example, Lindblom, 1959; see also Chapter 12). The notion of **disjunctive incrementalism** suggests that though a goal or objective may be determined, the nature of life is such that even in very short time spans, things change and the goal can very quickly become inappropriate or not as totally appropriate as it was originally (Lindblom, 1959). This results in either the goal itself being slightly modified, or the process that was being used to achieve it being changed, or both. Again, this is not necessarily a bad thing, as organisations like the NHS are dynamic organisms in so much as they are made up far more of the people that work in them and the people who are cared for than they are of fixed structures which can very rapidly become outmoded and inappropriate.

This process of disjunctive incrementalism is

matched by a concern about when a decision is not a decision (Parry and Morriss, 1974). Certainly, decisions can be considered under three headings. A decision to make a decision, a decision to do something, even if it is to leave things alone, and thirdly, a decision not to take a decision. This three-way consideration will often reveal that when approaching a decision, decision-makers will avoid making a decision and choose to make no decision at all. The real weakness in organisational terms is not to recognise that one of the three processes is underway and to be left wondering, at the end of what was supposed to be a decision-making process, precisely what has been achieved.

Another analytical technique is to consider actively the internal and external factors that are leading to a decision being made. Within the health service, it is often quite possible to be able to distinguish between the external decision-making forces (i.e. changes in social structure, dictates of central government, and the workings of a local authority) and the internal pressures which can take the form of professional advice from health care professionals, changes in the resource allocation or even something quite straightforward such as part of a building becoming unusable. Being clear about what the pressures are to make a decision contributes to a greater understanding of possible solutions.

Decision-making as action

A partial solution to carrying out decisions is always to link decisions to a particular end or objective. Such an approach means that, when decisions have to be amended or changed, it is possible to be honest and open because not just the decision but the objective and the process were already extant. This takes the nature of change into an arena of conscious consideration and makes it part of everyone's life rather than it merely being something in which others further up the hierarchy engage.

The nature of decision-making and change is complex and in both theory and practice is poorly understood. It is only by constantly working at the understanding of the processes associated with decision-making and change that it will become a more natural part of the health service in the future than it is today.

Quality in health care: a decision-making case study

The debate on quality in the NHS was triggered to a large extent by the Griffiths Report (DHSS, 1983) which said:

> 'Whether the NHS is meeting the needs of the patient and the community and can prove that it is doing so is open to question'
> (Paragraph 2, page 10)

> 'The driving force behind our advice is the concern to secure the best deal for patients in the community within available resources; the best value for the tax payer; and the best motivation for staff. As a caring, quality service, the NHS has to balance the interests of the patient, the community, the tax payer and the employee'
> (Paragraph 3, page 11)

Clearly, therefore, the message to general managers from the Griffiths Report was to seek some way of assuring that the service they were responsible for was being delivered at an appropriate level of quality.

There is great difficulty in determining the meaning of quality. Quality can be said to be customer satisfaction. It is necessary to be clear that the answer to the question of what is quality will be determined by certain central components, for example, health care, service, treatment, outcome, and patient/client.

Often it is asserted that quality is free because it is said to be more concerned with the attitudes of staff in the service than with anything else. The NHS shows us how quality will always cost. For example, complaints about waiting lists can only be resolved by putting more money into dealing with waiting lists. It is essential to consider the quality–cost scale and to recognise that every service can be assessed at a particular level of quality and that, by the judicious manipulation of resources (all of which will have a financial element), the quality standard can be moved either upwards or downwards.

The perception of quality is a separate issue. One recipient may be perfectly satisfied with a comparatively poor service whereas another recipient may be dissatisfied with a comparatively high quality, high cost service. These perceptions are so often based on expectations of what the service can deliver. Equally, it is important to recognise that people within the service need to be satisfied if they are to perceive themselves as working in a high quality service. For example, the ward sister who cannot get an adequate service out of the laundry will not believe that she is working in a high quality service.

A definition of quality which leads to an interesting approach to care is that elicited from industry, where so often the quality criterion is fitness for purpose. This is primarily to do with a degree of reliability. For example, open-toed sandals are perfectly adequate and reliable for walking along the beach, but they would be considered as low quality walking shoes if used to scale Ben Nevis. At the moment, there is an urgent need to agree a definition of quality which is workable amongst those employed in the health service but primarily is acceptable to the recipients of health care.

The history of quality assurance

A number of posts exist within the health service under the title of Director of Quality Assurance or Director of Patient Services. These give emphasis to the management of quality. The notion of quality assurance dates from the First World War where the large munitions factories operated mainly with unskilled female workforces. There was a need for constant review of the technical functions they were undertaking. To do this, the customer (i.e. the Ministry of Munitions) sent inspectors in. The notion of quality assurance originates, therefore, from *customer* inspection.

As industry developed after 1918, the notion of customer inspection remained central to quality assurance and the next development was that the inspection was not undertaken by customers but internally, by the company involved in the production of any particular item. The real weakness of this was that the internal pressures of the system would often prevent internally determined standards from being achieved.

The next major change originated in Japan and was a process of total quality management in which the emphasis was placed on enabling the individuals to do what they should do before being concerned about the product. The motto adopted was, 'First we make people and then we make things'.

The NHS is some way from this position. Cur-

rently, it combines customer inspection in the form of bodies such as Community Health Councils, the Health Advisory Service, the Health and Safety Executive and the Mental Health Act Commissioners, and the use of internal inspection methods, for example, *Monitor*, *Qualpacs* and the occasional *patient survey*. While Monitor, Qualpacs and patient surveys are useful in terms of quality audits, they do not assure the quality of the process being provided.

The importance of quality

The measurement of the quality of a service is now becoming easier than ever before. The data base which is emerging through the contract-setting process is providing more information for decision-making in the health service. However, measures arising from the Körner reporting system are essentially *activity levels*, *efficiency*, *effectiveness* and the *economy* of the service. Butt and Palmer (1985) give several measures that indicate value for money and these include activity, efficiency, effectiveness, economy and measures of appropriateness, awareness, accessibility and acceptability. It is, perhaps, a true observation to suggest that organisations which do not have a profit motive are better judged by these latter four measures.

How to measure quality

A possible approach to the measurement of quality is illustrated in Fig. 11.2. This purposely does not use the Donabedien (1966) approach of structure, process and outcome – while these three headings are useful at one level, they are not directly relevant to the health service in the UK. Firstly, the structures of health services vary from health authority to health authority and, in fact, should do if they are to be responsive to individual consumers' and groups of consumers' needs. Secondly, there is great difficulty in agreeing what the process of the health service truly is. Is it, for example, the passage of a number of people through beds, or the number of dressings performed, or the incidence of particular infections? Or can these, of themselves, be seen as outcomes of particular processes? Further, there are very few pure outcomes of the health service. Currently, the only one that is readily available is the number of people going through the service, but even this is quite actively manipulated as individuals experience double ad-

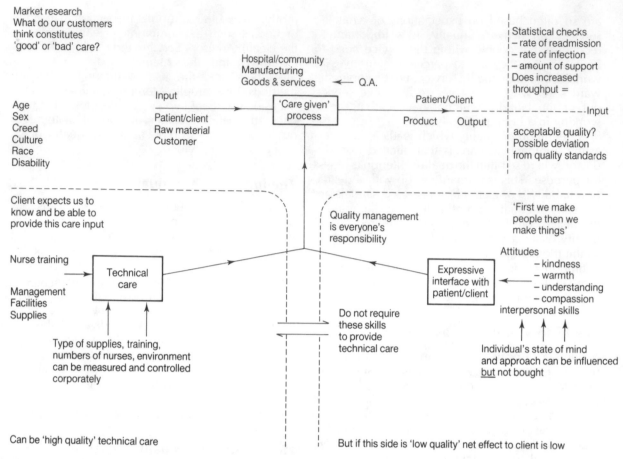

Fig. 11.2 *Developments in quality assurance*

missions or the number of deaths or discharges is added up together and not separately. However, as a model which enables systems to be interrogated and understood, the Donabedien approach has some usefulness.

The approach described here works from within established data bases. It also recognises that the NHS is highly labour-intensive and that it is the most junior members of staff who interact most frequently with the recipients of health care. Further, there is the recognition that if a higher quality of service is to be achieved, it is primarily to these groups of staff that the service must look to implement quality systems. It becomes necessary to identify and measure the key aspects of performance.

Two aspects of the process of care are identified: the technical and the expressive. These were described by Buswell (1986) in a study of the York-

shire Bank and have been adapted to apply in the health service. The technical aspects of care are controllable inputs and the client expects these to be known and to be appropriately provided during care. This includes staff who have been trained appropriately, the provision of necessary and appropriate management, the availability of an acceptable range of facilities, and the provision of appropriate supplies. These aspects can be controlled corporately and will result in a high quality of technical care.

The second component is expressive care and relates to the interface between patients and clients and the staff who care for them. This is a measurement of the kindness of staff and the warmth of staff in the attitudes that they demonstrate to the patient. The patient will perceive a degree of understanding and compassion, which provides a measure of the interpersonal skills that the individual staff members have. These interpersonal skills will be heavily influenced by the individual state of mind and the approach can be influenced but not bought. This borders on the Japanese notion of making the people before making the things, and on the idea that quality management is everybody's responsibility.

Clearly, technical skills without expressive skills result in low quality care, and vice versa. The two combined result in a process of care giving. It is possible to identify clearly inputs into that box in terms of who or what the patient or client is and expects. The use of market research and the identification of what potential customers think of as good or bad, and such details as, for example, patients' age, gender, creed, culture, race and disability are all recorded routinely on admission. Once they leave the process, various statistical checks exist – for example, the rate of re-admission, the rate of infection, the amount of support that is required. Such information enables questions to be asked about whether increasing throughput results in a lowering of the quality of care that individuals will accept.

Total quality management

The adoption of total quality management (TQM) is one of the changes associated with many of the leading-edge components of the NHS. It is a generic term which covers a number of 'whole organisation' approaches to quality. The characteristic feature is that change to achieve a higher quality of service occurs at all levels of the organisation (Shafer, 1991). It requires a number of elements to be present in the organisation. They are:

(1) clear and obvious leadership from the top of the organisation;
(2) high levels of training to improve the quality of the service;
(3) systems like quality circles to ensure that improvement and problem-solving are done by those most involved in the service;
(4) systematic appraisal of performance;
(5) consumer orientation.

The NHS has taken two major steps forward with the introduction of general management and the implementation of the reforms, which enable this approach to quality to be delivered. Firstly, general managers are adapting the Management by Walking Around (MBWA) characteristics to TQM approaches. This form of management is more akin to leadership, and the exposure to staff and service users that results is having a profound influence on the amount and extent of training that such managers commission.

Secondly, a number of provider organisations have purchased consumer orientation packages for their staff and commissioned regular market surveys to ensure that they and their staff have regular feedback on service users' views about and expectations of the service being offered. This will be an increasingly important part of the material considered by health purchasers and providers as the health market becomes increasingly competitive.

The market orientation is occurring at a time when standard setting among all groups of health care professionals is becoming an integral component of the role. The government recognised this by making audit an essential element of the reformed NHS. Not only is medical, nursing and associated health care professions audit underway, external auditors have been commissioned to provide an external eye on the audit processes. In conjunction with the developments in the resource management and information technology fields, this suggests that clinical audit (the generic term) will be an important part of the health care professional's role in the future and provide a major assurance of quality in the service delivery.

Professional politics

A decade ago it would have been barely possible to talk about the politics of nursing in this country. In the intervening period there has been the most exciting development of awareness and ability in both the process of politics and in the creation of an agenda which will need to be resolved politically. In a chapter on the management of care it may seem strange to be considering professional politics, but the nature of the politics of nursing is such that nursing has been increasingly concerned about the processes of care – rather than about the status and position of nurses themselves, although this too is a major political issue. It is also necessary to accept that politics is a life-giving business. Without processes for negotiation and debate, organisations (including those surrounding nursing) deny themselves renewal and regeneration.

Political agendas

In the main, the political agenda of nursing is handled by professional organisations. These organisations include the Royal College of Nursing (RCN), the Royal College of Midwives (RCM) and the Health Visitors' Association (HVA). These are professional organisations that have taken on trade union activities. In contrast, there are two major trade unions involved which have some professional input; the Confederation of Health Service Employees (COHSE) and the National Union of Public Employees (NUPE), which are due to merge in 1993.

The standard advice to anybody entering the profession is, whatever you do, join an organisation. New entrants to the profession are bound to ask why, and as careers progress, the reason for joining such organisations has much less to do with trade union defensiveness and far more to do with the need to have a voice within the political debate about where the profession is going.

To enter that debate, it is necessary to be clear about the external political agenda, i.e. that agenda with which a nursing organisation would confront the rest of the world, and the agenda that is being pursued internally within an organisation as that organisation itself changes and develops.

An example of this can be seen at the annual representative body meeting of any of the organisations. At such meetings there is a very clear distinction between the agenda items which relate to the structure and running of the organisation and those items that are concerned with nursing and care.

The political agenda which is worked up by such organisations is influenced by a number of different sources. An example of this is the International Council of Nurses (ICN) which is the worldwide body representing national nursing associations at global level. Its great strength is in leading nursing in countries where it is developing. Perhaps its greatest weakness is that it only includes one nursing association from each country. In the UK, where there is a multiplicity of nursing associations, there is a fear that the ICN cannot be properly influenced. However, the professional agenda to which the ICN works can have a massive effect – even in this country – and with the publications on, for example, ethics (ICN, 1973) and

research (ICN, 1986), the council has given a lead worldwide.

A second body that influences the professional agenda is the World Health Organisation (WHO). In recent years the nursing component of WHO has been strengthened. The work that WHO does is at government level and, through its subsidiary branches in each continent, it has had a major effect upon the course of nursing. Perhaps the most obvious example from the last decade is the way in which WHO in Europe has promoted the implementation of the nursing process and a massive development in nursing research across the whole of Europe.

Rather closer to home, but still a massive influence, are the Departments of Health in all four home countries. Here is a major resource of nurses working directly to government ministers. Their awareness of the political agenda that ministers, and indeed all MPs and peers, are working to enables them to have a major influence on the formation of policy. The interaction between the government departments where nursing exists and the professional organisations occurs constantly and is a major source of professional political activity in all organisations.

To someone just entering the profession, or to a nurse who is only just developing an interest in professional politics, the different positions and types of activity engaged in by the RCN, the RCM and the HVA can appear very confusing. This is a particular challenge for any nurse who could belong to more than one of the organisations. The issue is made more complex by the existence of the two trade unions, COHSE and NUPE. Many in the profession have dreamed of some type of unification of all these organisations so that there would be just one nursing association. This in broader political terms would be a massive advantage in that the government in direct negotiation with the profession would not be able in any sense to divide and rule.

The Joint Committee of Professional Nursing, Midwifery and Health Visiting Associations, which meets regularly with the department, represents over 20 groups, many of them with tiny memberships. Often sources of pressure like the Joint Committee can be given equal weight with, say, an organisation like the Royal College of Nursing representing over a quarter of a million people.

An advantage of having many different organisations is that it enables a higher level of specialisation to develop and the very competition sharpens up the activities of some of the larger organisations. It has been argued, for example, that the existence of the Association of Radical Midwives has been a major stimulus for change within the RCM.

Of decreasing significance in recent years has been the role played by trade unions like COHSE and NUPE. Their total membership of qualified nurses has fallen and they lack, at the most senior levels, the expertise and knowledge that major nursing organisations have in terms of representing the professional political agenda. The development of a trade union facility within the major nursing organisations has alleviated the concern that many felt in the early 1970s about organisations like the RCN and the RCM becoming trade unions. Also their performance in recent years has been much stronger on the labour relations front.

Another major determinant of the professional political agenda are the statutory bodies. These include the national boards for all four home countries and the United Kingdom Central Council for Nursing, Midwifery and Health Visiting (UKCC). The statutory bodies are charged in law to direct the training and education of nurses as well as determining the standards to which these nurses will work. This has resulted in the publication of a Code of Conduct referred to above (and reproduced in full on page 336) and the implementation of radically different training processes within the profession.

External political pressures

Other influences on the professional political agenda are a group of external bodies which serve different functions but whose contribution is very significant. One example is the National Association of Health Authorities and Trusts (NAHAT) which in many respects acts as the professional body for health authorities and trusts. By constant review of the concerns of their members, and on occasions surveying health authorities' performances in particular areas, these bodies have been able to create political debate and concern about certain issues. Current examples are the need to reform nurse education and the demographic problems that are beginning to affect the NHS as

the supply of individuals to be employed begins to dry up (UKCC, 1986).

Another type of group are those organisations which represent powerful groups of other professionals in the NHS. Perhaps the best known of these is the British Medical Association (BMA) but others which are significant are the Institute of Health Service Managers (IHSM) and the Chartered Institute of Public Finance and Accountancy (CIPFA). These organisations representing doctors, managers, administrators and finance officers are interested in areas where there is overlap in terms of both practice and outcomes. For instance, the BMA expressed very active concerns about the implementation of the nursing process while the IHSM has continued to pursue certain issues that relate to the implementation of the general management around nursing. Such organisations can operate in tandem with the nursing organisations or, on occasions, can appear to be in conflict. The skilled negotiator looks for allies rather than generating enemies and, therefore, it is significant that the private contacts between the organisations have resulted in very few public disagreements.

Another form of influence comes from external sources of expertise. Perhaps the most prominent at the moment is the King Edward's Hospital Fund for London, known as the King's Fund. This is a health services development agency which promotes improvements in health and social care. Not only through its teaching programmes and consultative work with organisations but also through the presence on its staff of a number of highly experienced and skilled individuals, it has been able to lead the health care debate in many areas. Some would argue, for example, that the whole issue of general management emerged from within the King's Fund.

Other sources that can influence the profession are specialist units like the Health Service Economics Unit at York, which, by generating a particular form of economic analysis of the health service, have forced change into the system.

Finally, another group of bodies which can influence the professional political agenda are those more powerful organisations which represent particular patient/client interests. Two examples which have gained and retained prominence are the National Association for the Welfare of Children in Hospital (NAWCH) and Mencap, an organisation concerned with the care of people who have a mental handicap. These organisations are based on very extensive local activity and, therefore, local knowledge. By specialising in particular areas, they have been able to influence government and the professional organisations in particular ways, so ensuring that the clients on whose behalf they advocate are properly cared for, and that the quality of care offered improves.

Determining the professional agenda

With all this external influence and the constant internal processes within organisations, the question that arises is, 'How is the professional agenda determined?'. Clearly, a number of factors influence this but there are three primary ones. The first is how much time an organisation has to commit to a particular issue. The second is the amount of resources – financial, administrative and even sometimes in terms of buildings – which are available. Finally, but perhaps most importantly, it all depends on how close an issue is to the current perception of the main interests of the organisation. It is necessary to be aware that professional organisations have clear objectives and priorities themselves and the relationship between those objectives and priorities and any particular item will usually determine whether or not a particular issue is picked up and dealt with. This approach may appear to be very pragmatic and in many instances it is.

On occasions, particular issues get on the agenda because of the sponsorship or advocacy of a particular individual but usually they are there because their presence enables the organisation to achieve something it has been pursuing for some time. It is very difficult to get new items on to the agenda simply because the agenda is always so full and success seems to rest with those individuals or groups who can tie new issues to ones that are already around. The danger of this is that the agenda items become so extensive that it is impossible to work with them. However, the process of redefinition and the opportunity to re-address issues enables progress to be made.

A major influence here is the input that is received from the more senior members of the profession who can provide the organisations with continual updating on the current state of play in the NHS and what the forthcoming agenda for the service may be. Their role is crucial.

Two examples of how professional organisations have effected movement in the profession through the development of particular agenda items is the work on standards of care (RCN, 1980, 1981; Kitson *et al.*, 1990) and the debate on education (RCN, 1985). Both of these arose from within professional organisations at a time when there was no other major resource to address these issues and it was becoming difficult to change practices and beliefs. The handling of these issues has demonstrated that the organisations with greatest resources tend to get further in terms of effecting an active political influence, but the primary concern throughout must be that the political professional agenda concerns the delivery of care and those who deliver it. It is the public way of combining concerns about both issues that makes the agenda life-giving and a vital part of every nurse's professional life.

The future

In concluding this chapter on the management of care, it is necessary to consider the future of health care in this country. Two major elements are leading to a fundamental restructuring of health services worldwide. These two elements are at work in the UK. The first is the ever-increasing cost of the delivery of health services. The second is a redefinition of what is meant by a Health Service.

Health culture in society

Work on controlling costs has demonstrated that while it may be possible to achieve a higher level of efficiency (i.e. in terms of throughput), it is unlikely that there will be any straightforward way of limiting the increase in costs over the next two decades. Rather, this is an era when the increasing technical skills of health care professionals mean that even where it is cheaper to treat some conditions, at the other end of the continuum, conditions that were previously untreatable are receiving a lot of attention. It is interesting, too, that the untreatable conditions from the past tend also to be the high cost treatments of the present (Donley, 1984).

The concerns about the notion of a health service are unresolved, but they hinge on a wish to create a service which deals with people's health rather than people's illnesses. Many of the conditions that people are treated for are in some senses self-inflicted in that they arise from smoking or other elements of adopted lifestyle (Marsh, 1985). This whole debate about cost and the nature of health will take a considerable period of time to work through but will be the prime motivator in determining the health services of the future.

Elements of social change

Nursing is a product of society and one of the major constituents of any change in nursing is change within that society. Perhaps the three most important elements of change within our society in the foreseeable future are:

(1) the economic status of individuals;
(2) the ethnic mix of our population;
(3) the nature of relationships between individuals.

Since 1979 this country has been engaged in a major restructuring of the national economy. Clearly this process will continue well into the 1990s and, as a result of it, individuals are engaged in a far higher level of personal choice than they ever were in the past. This may or may not be desirable but it is obvious in our society. Changes in the processes of education (NATFHE, 1988), in the operations of local authorities (Child Poverty Action Group, 1987), the water authority (HMSO, 1983a) and other household services, as well as the increasing number of people taking out private health insurance (OHE, 1987), all suggest that the concept of personal choice through economic position will continue at a substantial rate. Such a change challenges the philosophy of equal shares, a belief that seems to underlie the health service. This necessitates a refocusing of the service in order to meet the increasing self-choice element that the economic change produces.

Similarly, as the culture of society changes, so the NHS will need to adapt to the demands of different ethnic groups. To date, failure to do so has resulted in limited provision of ethnic health care. Meeting the health needs of different ethnic and cultural groups would act as a source of positive enrichment to our society, and could act as a major stimulant in the development of new caring skills for many groups of health care professionals. This applies in particular to nurses.

The third element is the change in the nature of the personal relationships which exist in our society. For a long time commentators have noted the breakdown of the extended family (Young and Wilmott, 1962). By and large, this has been recorded in comparatively negative terms.

Recently, however, some historians have begun to think more positively about the changes in our society which reflect in effect the third great revolution after the agricultural and industrial revolutions (Wood, 1986). It is now suggested that with the technological revolution experienced since the Second World War, previous patterns of family structure in this country are no longer appropriate and that the current rates of divorce and single parent families are not something to be overly concerned about in any negative sense but to be recognised, rather, as the pattern of the future. However, if this is to be the case, the demands on the health service will change substantially as there will be fewer and fewer individuals with families who can care for them. This will make increasingly necessary the provision of a health service which is geared to the individual alone, rather than within the context of a broader family.

Demography and need

Not unrelated to such speculation are the changes in demography which will result in a very different profession. When shown in a graph the incidence of births in this country takes on a wave form, rising and falling every 15 to 20 years or so. Terms like 'baby boom' referred to the number of babies born in the immediate post-war period. This was matched by a second boom some 20 years later as these individuals themselves began families. What is interesting at the moment is that society has hit very low levels of reproduction and having done so, does not appear to be climbing from that low level at anything like the rate which has been seen when the level has fallen in the past. This clearly means that the society which has been responsible for producing nurses can no longer do so at the levels of the past. Nursing can no longer rely on an ever-continuous stream of female eighteen-year-olds coming in through training schools and, as a result, needs to do some very active and extensive work to change the roles nurses will undertake in order to be able to recruit and retain staff (Brown, 1988).

From the above, it is clear that there will be a major redefinition of health needs and health provision. The trend undoubtedly will be towards individuals becoming much more informed and taking a far more active role in both the prevention of illness and the treatment of disease when it is present. This will give nurses a more consultative role, that of technical experts when more sophisticated care is required than can be delivered by friends, relatives and individuals themselves. Similarly, the central provision of the service by the government will change as the level of the gross national product changes, reflecting the number of people working in the country.

Neither is it impossible to envisage a situation where the large general hospitals are considered to be less necessary and the service is geared round very extensive community services and much smaller local units of interim care. Further, increasing links with Europe make credible the idea of a unified European Health Service with common standards of training for all health care pro-

fessionals and a common level of service provision. The recognition that these are ways forward in terms of managing care will be slow to develop but will certainly be on the agenda.

Conclusions

The management of care in the 1990s will see periods of quite massive structural change matched by equally massive change in nursing role. It is exciting and positive; those entering the profession at this point can be promised a future which will challenge both their intellect and their commitment. Also, they can be promised entry to a profession which will always be exciting and rewarding. The objective of all managers must be both to adapt and develop the service to meet the needs of the people they are there to serve and to enable those who are providing the service to develop in such a way as to experience satisfaction and pleasure in the service they offer.

Glossary

Accountability: The process by which responsibility is publicly addressed and reported on

Autocracy: Government by one person

Autonomy: The power or right of total self-determination

Disjunctive incrementalism: A process in policy analysis which identifies the deviations and breaks in the process of decision-making

Gestalt: A belief that the organised whole is greater than the sum of the parts constituting it

Marginalise: To remove from the centre, to render unimportant and secondary

Philosophy: A term with many meanings but essentially concerned with the nature of knowledge, causes, laws, principles and reasoning

Totalitarian state: A form of government which controls everything and tolerates no opposition

References

Abel-Smith, B. (1960). *A History of the Nursing Profession*. Heinemann, London.

Allison, G. (1971). *Essence of Decision: Explaining the Cuban Missile Crisis*. Little, Brown, Boston.

Allsopp, K. (1991). Access to Health Records Act 1990. *Journal of the Medical Defence Union*, 2, 26.

Altschul, A. (1982). *The Consumer's Voice: Nursing Implications*. RCN, London.

Anderson, P. (1986). The Delphi Technique in practice. *Australian Journal of Advanced Nursing*, 3 (2), 22–32.

Argyle, M. (1969). *Social Interaction*. Tavistock Publications, London.

Argyle, M. and Trower, P. (1979). *Person to Person: Ways of Communicating*, Harper and Row, London.

Audit Commission for Local Authorities in England and Wales. (1986). *Making a Reality of Community Care*. HMSO, London.

Audit Commission. (1991). *Measuring the Quality – The Patient's View of Day Surgery*. HMSO, London.

Bain, J. (1991a). General practice and the new Contract.

I Reactions and impact. *British Medical Journal*, 302 (6786) 1183–1186.

Bain, J. (1991b). General practice and the new Contract. II Future directions. *British Medical Journal*, 302 (6787) 1247–1249.

Baly, M.G. (1980). *Nursing and Social Change* (2nd ed.). Heinemann, London.

Barnett, D. (1981). Do nurses read? *Nursing Times*, 77 (49), 2131–2134.

Barr, L. and Rogers, S. (1991). Evaluating health care services. *Journal of Health Services Management*, 87 (1), 30–32.

Bennes, W. and Slater, P. (1968). *The Temporary Society*. Harper and Row, New York.

Benveniste, G. (1974). *Bureaucracy*. Boyd and Fraser, New York.

Bevan, G. and Ingram, R. (1987). Reviewing RAWP. *British Medical Journal*, 295 (6605), 1039–1042.

Bevis, E.O. (1983). *Curriculum Building in Nursing – A Process* (3rd ed.). Mosby, St Louis.

Biley, F. (1990). How to analyse nursing models. *Nursing*, 4 (12), 8–10.

Bishop, V. (1983). Colleagues, collaborators or hand maidens? *Nursing Mirror*, 156 (25), 31–33.

Blackford, N. (1982). Report accuses and Walsh replies. *Nursing Mirror*, 155 (13), 11–12.

Bohlin, A. and Larsson, G.(1986) Early identification of infants at risk for institutionalised care. *Journal of Advanced Nursing*, 11 (5), 493–497.

Boyd, C. and Sellars, L. (1982). *The British Way of Birth*. Pan Books, London.

Brown, P. (1988). Will you not come back again? *Nursing Times*, 84 (7), 44–45.

Bryans, W. (1985). Controlling the purse strings. *Nursing Times*, 81 (16), 30–31.

Bushwell, D. (1986). The development of a quality measurement system for a UK bank. In *Are they Being Served: Quality Consciousness in Service Industries*, Moores B. (ed.). P. Allan, London.

Butt, H. and Palmer, B. (1985). *Value for Money in the Public Sector: The Decision Makers Circle*. Basil Blackwell, Oxford.

Carroll, L. (1872). *Through the Looking Glass*. Reprinted (1982) in *The Complete Illustrated Works of Lewis Carroll*, Chancellor Press, London.

Chalmers, H., Kershaw, B., Melia, K. and Kendrich, M. (1990). Nursing models: enhancing or inhibiting practice? *Nursing Standard*, 5(11), 34–40.

Chapman, C. (1989). Research for action, the way forward. *Senior Nurse*, 9(6), 16–18.

Child Poverty Action Group. (1987). No presentations without taxation. *Poverty*, 68, 6–8.

Christenson, M.A. (1990). Adaptations of the physical environment to compensate for sensory changes. *Physical and Occupational Therapy in Geriatrics*, 8(3/4), 3–30.

Christopher, K. (1985). Striving for excellence. *Dimensions in Health Service*, 62, 3.

Clough, K. (1990). Guest Editorial. *British Journal of Health Care Computing*, 7(6), 5.

Darley, M. (1990). Clinical practice budgeting. *Nursing Standard*, 4(46), 47–49.

Davies, P. (1989). The NHS goes to the opinion polls. *Health Services Journal*, 99(5156), 750–751.

Department of Health. (1991a). *The Health of the Nation*. HMSO, London.

DoH. (1991b). *The Patient's Charter – Raising the Standard*. HMSO, London.

Department of Health and Social Security. (1978). *Report of the Committee of Inquiry into Normansfield Hospital*. HMSO, London.

DHSS. (1983). *Recommendations on the Effective Use of Manpower and Related Resources. Report of the NHS Management Inquiry Team (The Griffiths Report)*. DHSS, London.

DHSS. (1986). *Mix and Match – A Review of Nursing Skill Mix*. DHSS, London.

Donabedien, A. (1966). Evaluating the quality of medical care. *Millbank Memorial Fund Quarterly*, 44, 166–206.

Donley, F.R. (1984). The effect of changing health care policy on cancer nursing. *Oncology Nursing Forum*, 11(4), 64–66.

Downe, S. (1990). Conflict of interests. *Nursing Times*, 86(47), 14.

Durkheim, E. (1897; reissued 1950). *Rules of Sociological Method*. Free Press, New York.

Farrant, E. (1983). The vital spark. *Nursing Times*, 79(19), 50–51.

Fraser, R.A. (1990). Pain after day-care tubal ligation. *Nursing Times*, 86(28), 56–57.

General Nursing Council for England and Wales. (1977). *Training Syllabus, General Register of Nursing*. GNC, London.

Goffman, E. (1968a). *Stigma*. Penguin Books, Harmondsworth.

Goffman, E. (1968b). *Asylums*. Penguin Books, Harmondsworth.

Her Majesty's Stationery Office. (1979). *Nurses, Midwives and Health Visitors Act*. HMSO, London.

HMSO. (1983a). *Water Act*. HMSO, London.

HMSO. (1983b). *Mental Health Act*. HMSO, London.

HMSO. (1984a). *Registered Homes Act*. HMSO, London.

HMSO. (1984b). *Data Protection Act*. HMSO, London.

HMSO. (1984c). *Police and Criminal Evidence Act*. HMSO, London.

HMSO. (1986). *The Government Expenditure Plans, 1986–7 to 1988–9*. HMSO, London.

HMSO. (1991). *The Citizens Charter – Raising the Standard*. HMSO, London.

HMSO. (1992). *Nurses, Midwives and Health Visitors Act*. HMSO, London.

Hogg, P. (1989). Extended role of the nurse. *Radiography Today*, 55(628), 33.

Hutt, R. (1987). *Chief Officer Career Profiles*. Brighton Institute of Manpower Studies, University of Sussex.

International Council of Nursing. (1973). *Code for Nurses; Ethical Concepts Applied to Nursing*. ICN, Geneva.

ICN. (1986). *Report on the Regulation of Nursing*. ICN, Geneva.

Jones, D. and Rogers, A. (1976). *Nursing Staff Appraisal in the Health Service. Final Report to the National Staff Committee for Nurses and Midwives*. Polytechnic of Central London, London.

King Edward's Hospital Fund. (1985). *Evaluation of Management Advisory Service and Performance Review Trials in the NHS*. Kings Fund, London.

Kitson, A.L., Hyndman, S., Harvey, G. and Yerrell, P. (1990). *Quality Patient Care – The Dynamic Standard Setting System*. Scutari Press, Harrow.

Lindblom, C.E. (1959). The science of muddling through. *Public Administration Review*, 19, 79–99.

Lowe, R. (1990). Primary health care: the GP contractor, defending your territory. *Nursing Standard*, 4(13), 50–51.

Luker, K.A. (1984). Reading nursing: the burden of being different. *International Journal of Nursing Studies*, 21(1), 1–7.

Macguire, J. (1986). Not a prescription. *Senior Nurse*, 5(4), 10–11.

Mains, S., McBride, A.B. and Austin, J.K. (1991). Patient and staff perceptions of a psychiatric ward environment. *Issues in Mental Health Nursing*, 12(2), 149–157.

Malby, R. (1991). Audit ability. *Nursing Times*, 87(19), 35–37.

Marsh, A. (1985). Smoking and illness: what smokers really believe. *Health Trends*, 17(1), 7–12.

McGee-Cooper, A. (1984). Time management. *Acorn Journal*, 44(2), 180–183.

McKenna, H. (1990). Which model? *Nursing Times*, 86(25), 50–52.

Menzies, I. (1960). A case study in the functioning of social systems as a defence against anxiety. *Human Relations*, 13, 95–121.

Millar, B. (1991). Good tools, good workers. *Health Service Journal*, 101(5267), 32–33.

Ministry of Health and Scottish Home and Health Department. (1966). *Report of the Committee on Senior Nursing Staff Structures (The Salmon Report)*. HMSO, London.

Moores, B. and Thompson, A.G.H. (1986). What 1357 hospital in-patients think about aspects of their stay in British acute hospitals (questionnaire survey). *Journal of Advanced Nursing*, 11(1), 87–102.

Morrison, T. (1990). End piece. *British Journal of Health Care Computing*, 7(6), 40.

National Association of Teachers in Further and Higher Education. (1988). Kenneth Baker's revolution. *NATFHE Journal Extra*, NATFHE, London.

Nightingale, F. (1859). *Notes on Nursing: What It Is and What It Is Not*. Harrison, London.

Office of Health Economics. (1987). *Compendium of Health Statistics* (6th ed.). OHE, London.

Parry, G. and Morriss, P. (1974). When is a decision not a decision? In *British Sociology Yearbook Vol.1: Elites in Western Democracy*, Crewe, L. (ed.). Croom Helm, London.

Peters, T.J. and Waterman, R.H. (1982). *In Search of Excellence*. Harper and Row, New York.

Plank, M. (1982). *Teams for Mentally Handicapped People*. Campaign for Mentally Handicapped People, London.

Plant, J. (1985). In sole charge of the ward. *Health and Social Services Journal*, 95, 1198–1199.

Potrykus, C. (1991). GP Contract; a salaried service for family doctors. *Health Visitors Journal*, 64(7), 216.

Prophit, P. (1986). *The Art and Science of Nursing*. Keynote address to RCN Research Society Conference, Reading University.

Raphael, W. (1962). Do we know what patients think? *International Journal of Nursing*, 4, 209–223.

Rawles, J. (1989). Castigating QALYs. *Journal of Medical Ethics*, 15(3), 143–147.

Reid, N. (1988). The Delphi Technique: its contribution to the evaluation of professional practice. In *Professional Competence and Quality Assurance in the Caring Professions*, Ellis, R. (ed.). Chapman and Hall, New York.

Ritchie, J., Jacoby, A. and Bone, M. (1981). *Access to Primary Health Care*. Office of Population Censuses and Surveys, London.

Robinson, J. (1991). Working with doctors. *Nursing Times*, 87(10), 28–31.

Rogers, J. (1983). *Career Patterns of Nurses Who Have Completed a JBCNS Certificate. Report of the Follow-up Study, Vol.1*. DHSS, London.

Rowden, R. (1986). The management of nursing: Nightingale to Griffiths. *Nursing*, 3(7), 77–79.

Royal College of Nursing. (1980). *Standards of Nursing Care*. RCN, London.

RCN. (1981). *Towards Standards*. RCN, London.

RCN. (1985). *The Education of Nurses: A New Dispensation. Report of the Commission on Education (The Judge Report)*. RCN, London.

Salvage, J. (1985). *The Politics of Nursing*. Heinemann, London.

Schrock, R.A. (1977). On political consciousness in nurses. *Journal of Advanced Nursing*, 2(1), 41–50.

Shafer, W. (1991). Managing a budget at ward level. *Professional Nurse*, 6(11), 677–680.

Sines, D. and Bicknell, J. (1985). *Caring for Mentally Handicapped People in the Community*. Harper and Row, London.

Slack, P. (1985). Why nurses are missing out. *Nursing Times*, 81(5), 12–14.

Stephenson, M.E. (1990). Discharge criteria in day surgery. *Journal of Advanced Nursing*, 15(5), 601–613.

Stewart, R. (1985). *The Reality of Management* (2nd ed.). Heinemann, London.

Stilwell, B. (1988). Patient attitudes to a highly developed extended role. *Recent Advances in Nursing*, 21, 82–100.

Toffler, A.C. (1981). *The Third Wave*. Pan Books, London.

United Kingdom Central Council for Nursing, Midwifery and Health Visiting (1986). *Project 2000. A New Preparation for Practice*. UKCC, London.

UKCC. (1991). *Handbook of Midwives Rules*. UKCC, London.

UKCC. (1992a). *Code of Professional Conduct* (3rd ed.). UKCC, London.

UKCC. (1992b). *The Scope of Professional Practice*. UKCC, London.

Vousden, M. (1987). Do you really need to know? *Nursing Times*, 83(49), 28–30.

Wagstaff, A. (1987). *Econometric Studies in Health Economics: A Survey of British Literature, Discussion Paper 32*. Centre for Health Economics, University of York.

Warnock, M. (1960). *Ethics Since 1900*. Oxford University Press, Oxford.

Waterworth, S. (1990). Basing practice on research. *Nursing Standard*, 5(11), 30–33.

Watson, J. (1979). *Nursing – The Philosophy and Science of Caring*. Little, Brown, Boston.

Welsh Consumer Council. (1988). *Getting to Out-Patient Clinics*. Welsh and National Consumer Councils, Cardiff.

White, R. (1985). *The Effects of the NHS on the Nursing Profession 1948–61*. King's Fund, London.

Wickens, I. (1983). *Effective Unit Management*. King's Fund, London.

Wilson-Barnett, J. (1984). *Key Functions in Nursing; 4th Kathleen Raven Lecture*. RCN, London.

Whittington, D. and Boore, J. (1988). Competence in nursing. In *Professional Competence and Quality Assurance in the Caring Professions*, Ellis, R. (ed.). Chapman and Hall, New York.

Wolfensberger, W. (1969). The origin and nature of our institutional models. In *Changing Patterns in Residential Services for the Mentally Retarded*, Krugel, R.B. and Wolfensberger, W. (eds.). President's Panel on Mental Retardation, Washington DC.

Wood, M. (1986). *Domesday: A Search for the Roots of England*. BBC Publications, London.

Young, M. and Wilmott, P. (1962). *Family and Kinship in East London*. Penguin Books, Harmondsworth.

12

FRAMEWORKS FOR NURSING PRACTICE

Jane Schober

The detailed aims of this chapter are expressed fully at the bottom of this page and on page 301.

The chapter includes the following topics:

- The nature of individuality
- The nursing process as a process for decision-making
- Nursing activities and the proper task of the nurse
- The nurse and the demand for health care
- Understanding nursing as a personal service
- Communication – a key to a personal service
- Nurses and the concept of care
- Attitudes, values, beliefs and their influence on nursing

- Patient participation and nursing care
- Nursing theory and nursing knowledge
- Nursing theory and nursing models
- Approaches to nursing care planning based on a nursing model
- A consideration of some models of nursing including those of:
  - Peplau
  - Roy
  - Orem
  - Johnson
  - Roper, Logan and Tierney

This chapter is an exploration of factors which are important to the quality of nursing care. It is intended that it will contribute to a greater understanding and appreciation of the influence all nurses have over their own practice, and hence the power and control nurses have over the health of people in need of nursing care. The chapter brings together a number of important issues perti- nent to the delivery of nursing care in today's health service.

The chapter aims to explore the nature of indi- vidualised patient care and approaches to nursing practice. It discusses factors influencing the interpretation of nursing activities and considers key health care demands for the role of the nurse. The idea of nursing as a personal service is discussed, as is the influence of effective communication. The concept of care is explored and consideration given to the influence of attitudes, values and beliefs on nursing.

The chapter goes on to examine the importance of patient participation in care, to discuss the relationship between nursing theory and nursing practice, and to identify frameworks for nursing practice which may be incorporated into care planning.

When you as a nurse come to read this chapter, you do so having made decisions to devote time, energy, interest and, perhaps, a career to nursing. Above all, you have made a commitment to nursing based on a choice to offer a service to people in various states of health. Whatever you do and say to people in your care depends on the quality of your helping skills and your understanding of their needs. The way you give care is central to the quality of nursing and your influence over this should never be underestimated.

One of the most significant developments in nursing in recent years has been the move to promote individualised patient care, which is reflected, for example, in the development of nursing theory and primary nursing in the United Kingdom.

The nature of individuality

Carl Rogers (1967) defined the individual as having:

> 'One basic tendency and striving – to actualise, maintain and enhance the experiencing organism. . . . The organism woven through struggle and pain towards enhancement and growth'

The individual (or organism) is a whole being characterised by biological, psychological and intellectual components. These factors influence the internal dynamics of the individual and the way day-to-day situations and stimuli arising from the internal and external environment are processed. Rogers emphasises that nothing is static and everyone faces ever-changing situations. The motivation to grow, develop and enhance oneself is a fundamental drive and it depends on situations or an environment characterised by trust, respect and acceptance. Relationships which bear these characteristics allow those involved to participate and share in decisions and take responsibility for

actions which will occur. This may be described as a 'healthy' environment. Conversely, an environment which is threatening and stressful, or where people feel undervalued, may result in much of their energy being used to adapt, cope and indeed survive the circumstances they face.

Nurses face stressful circumstances all the time. Tragedy, despair and grief are never far removed from the nurse's daily work. Though good may ultimately come from these life events, the processes resulting in positive outcomes depend to a large extent on the ways people come together, support each other, share the events and accept each other. These are as important for patients and families as for the nurse.

Some of the research referred to in this chapter will highlight instances where nurses appear to reject some of their caring responsibilities by failing to accept or cope with particularly demanding circumstances; for example, people who are dying whose questions may be seen as 'awkward' by the nurse. It is important that the reader considers these findings not as a criticism of nurses, but as reflections of reality requiring attention to help nurses develop skills which will enable them to cope appropriately in the future.

The nursing process as a process for decision-making

When the nursing process was introduced into the UK in the 1970s much attention was given to the management and delivery of nursing care. Today it is widely acknowledged that the effective management of care depends on systematic holistic care which promotes shared decision-making and the independence of patients and clients (Vaughan and Pillmoor, 1989).

WHO and the nursing process

The World Health Organisation definition encapsulates the features of the nursing process by emphasising that many of the characteristics referred to rely on intellectual activities and effective problem-solving and decision-making. These contribute to assessing, planning, implementing and evaluating care in a systematic manner.

The WHO (1977) definition states:

'The nursing process is a term applied to a system of characteristic nursing interventions in the health of individuals, families and/or communities. In detail it involves the use of scientific methods for identifying the health needs of the patient/client/family or community and for using these to select those which can most effectively be met by nursing care; it also includes planning to meet these needs, provide the care and evaluate the results. The nurse in collaboration with other members of the health care team and the individual or groups being served, defines objectives, sets priorities, identifies care to be given and mobilises resources. He/she then provides the nursing services either directly or indirectly. Subsequently, he/she evaluates the outcome. The information feedback from evaluation of outcome should initiate desirable changes in subsequent interventions in similar nursing care situations. In this way, nursing becomes a dynamic process lending itself to adaptation and improvement'

By implication, any process suggests that there is an identifiable purpose and a system for organising and achieving the purpose. Key features of the process also include inspiration, creativity and productivity. It is the merging of decision-making skills bearing these characteristics with caring activities which is central to the meaning of nursing process.

By applying this to nursing it is clear that nurses have the potential for original creative decision-making based on the application of sound knowledge and expertise to care situations.

The Comprehensive Rational Model

The nursing process can be likened to the Comprehensive Rational Model of decision-making based on the work of H.A. Simon (1950).

The model contains the following elements:

(1) Goal-setting
(2) Identifying ways to achieve goals
(3) Evaluating each option
(4) Selecting the optimum solution
(5) Acting on or implementing the plan
(6) Reviewing outcome(s).

The similarities with the assessment, planning, implementation and evaluation activities of the nursing process are clear. The model makes a key assumption that the decision-maker will take into consideration all possible options and consequences in the light of a thorough understanding of a situation.

However, in practice this approach will be influenced by time constraints, by habits and routine, and by the current precedent. It is also true that in practice decisions often occur when the first satisfactory outcome or solution is found. So when making decisions about care with, or on behalf of, patients, awareness of choices being influenced by what may be the quickest or easiest, rather than the best, solution relies on expert judgement.

The Incrementalist Model

Another model of decision-making, the Incrementalist Model (Lindblom, 1959), offers a step-by-step approach to decision-making. Change is gradual but continuous. The decisions are usually influenced by bargaining processes and a narrower range of options is considered before decisions are reached. By implication those with the greatest power are likely to have the greatest influence. Within the nurse–patient relationship, the nurse holds expert power as she would usually know more about care and treatment. Thus, the sharing of knowledge is a key way of allowing patients to be part of the decision-making process. This step-by-step approach to decision-making may be characteristic of how many decisions are made about care and is more in tune with, for example, short term goal-setting. It would be useful also to consider how a more 'rational' approach would enhance the quality of decision-making.

It is important for nurses to consider how their decisions about care are reached and the factors influencing them. This is particularly important in relation to:

(1) identifying a philosophy of care for the ward/unit;
(2) the process of assessment which is the key to effective care planning;
(3) the beliefs and attitudes of members of the care team which may influence the way care is prioritised – these are usually reflected in the philosophy of care;
(4) how the nurse shares her power with the patient in relation to information-giving, relationship-building and the development of a therapeutic partnership for care;

(5) the way the nurse involves the patient (and his family) in the care process, and the appropriateness of this involvement for all concerned;

(6) the motivation and bias of the care team in the light of previous care decisions;

(7) how solutions are reached – whether the nurse is prepared to try alternatives, innovate and initiate as appropriate, or be content with the status quo.

The nursing process should be viewed as a way of making decisions about the care of an individual or a group. However, it does not inform the nurse as to what to assess, what to aim for in care or how to implement care. It is through the development and understanding of frameworks for assessment and care planning that this emerges. Thus, insight into the nursing needs of those requiring care is essential. A means to this end comes from the ability to select and analyse approaches to nursing care which ultimately helps the nurse to plan care to promote the health of the individual. This demands a holistic approach to nursing care where physiological, psychological, social, spiritual and cultural needs are considered. Such approaches to care may be found in a number of nursing models which will be considered later in this chapter.

This introductory section has raised some of the important issues facing nurses. The reference to individuality aims to emphasise not only some of the implications of approaching nursing as a process of individualised patient care, but also that an adherence to these principles as a means of supporting nursing staff is essential for a healthy, caring climate in which both nurses and patients are trusted, accepted and supported. In many situations this ideal may not be achieved, but striving towards it will provide the motivation for improved practice.

Already some key responsibilities of nurses are being emphasised. Indeed, they are spelt out clearly in many professional documents – such as the Code of Professional Conduct (UKCC, 1992) and in terms of employment, contracts and role descriptions. It is because the responsibilities of the nurse and nursing are so vast that this chapter aims to examine and discuss factors influencing the ways in which nurses give care.

Nursing activities and the proper task of the nurse

Consideration of what nurses do demands careful consideration of the term 'proper task'. The Oxford English Dictionary offers these definitions for the word *task*: a 'piece of work imposed', activities 'voluntarily undertaken', 'assigned as a definite duty' and 'a piece of work that has to be done'. 'Proper' also has perspectives worthy of consideration. The word is described as meaning 'belonging or relating exclusively or distinctly', then 'in conformity with demands of society, decent, respectable.'

Rather than suggesting an answer to what constitutes the proper task, current factors impinging on the work imposed on and belonging to nurses will be discussed and will take into consideration the demands of society. This will automatically cause the discussion to consider issues relating to the role of the nurse, as 'role' may be seen as a set of task expectations (Tajfel and Fraser, 1978).

It is widely accepted that nurses have a responsibility to provide a quality caring service (The Nurses, Midwives and Heath Visitors Act, 1979; Kitson, 1989). Inevitably, the nature of the service is influenced both by those who provide it and by those who receive it. Historically it may be seen that nurses have been greatly influenced by decisions over which they appear to have had little or no control (even if this is by their own choice). Examples of such influence include the grouping of patients according to their medical or disease label, and the traditional view that nurses are there to carry out doctors' orders (Salvage, 1985).

The influence of the medical model as interpreted by nurses should not be underestimated – particularly as nursing knowledge has depended on medical science for the greater part of this century. As a group, nurses may have been backward in coming forward to make decisions about the service they provide. This was further manifested by the division of labour and tasks according to their status within a hierarchical organisation (for example, the nurse 'in charge' carries the keys). Never have the conflicts of the way nurses value their roles been so apparent as they have been over the past 25 years. The work of Menzies (1960) revealed how skilfully nurses nurture a social system to defend themselves against the anxiety of complex and demanding interpersonal relationships. Stockwell (1972) identified ways in which nurses reward patients who are cooperative, cheerful, know the nurse's name, and avoid asking awkward questions, by giving them more time and attention. Roberts (1984) found that nurses 'like' patients whom *they* find interesting, and who are cheerful despite undergoing surgery. He also found that they 'disliked' demanding, 'selfish' and 'critical' patients.

It would therefore appear that, even though *care* is the central feature of the nurse's function, some nurses appear to contradict this by their inability to cope with the patients who appear to be the most vulnerable by being unaware of personal needs, fears and the vulnerability caused by ill health (Barber, 1991).

Guidelines

Today there exist guidelines in the Nurses, Midwives and Health Visitors Act (1979, 1992), the Code of Professional Conduct (UKCC, 1992) and from professional organisations (such as the Royal College of Nursing) which advocate that nurses should promote health and prevent illness, be competent in the total planning of care, and use knowledge from the behavioural sciences, physical sciences and nursing research to develop the knowledge, skills and attitudes to provide individualised patient care.

So far the discussion has considered the nurse's perspective. It is important now to examine trends in the pattern of health care delivery and to include perspectives from the patients or consumers who use the service.

The nurse and the demand for health care

In 1974 the British Medical Association (BMA) stated:

> 'As society's needs and demands have increased, available resources have not grown sufficiently to meet them, and everywhere there is scarcity of the personnel required to promote the health of the community'

This statement suggests trends that are as pertinent today as they were in 1974. The emphasis on health promotion and sickness prevention is further reinforced by the overwhelming role the media is playing in communicating knowledge of health matters to the public at large. The BMA saw the nurse as part of the health care team and in possession of qualities which could extend to include preventive, curative, assessment and counselling responsibilities. Therefore, further demands are made on nurses as they are expected to meet growing needs, extend their caring function and meet the health care requirements of patients. Though this appears to exert considerable pressure on the way nurses function, it may be suggested that nurses possess considerable potential in the choices that are made about the nature of their role and they may also exert a great deal of power and control over the environment in which nursing and health care takes place.

It is the way the nurse perceives the needs of patients and their health care demands which broadly determines the nature of her function.

Examining historical perspectives about the aims of nursing, there seem to be key themes in common – the promotion of health, and the promotion of individualised care (Henderson, 1966; Orem, 1990) – but definitions of nursing do not necessarily relate to what nurses are actually doing. So alongside developments in nursing education, for example, the introduction of Project 2000, and nursing management in relation to role preparation, for example the Post Registration Education and Practice Project (UKCC, 1990), it is left to each individual nurse to determine her function and control standards.

Studies of patients' perceptions of nurses have revealed that patients approve of nurses who are alert to their needs, provide emotional support and are kind and sympathetic (Brietung, 1980; Benner and Wruebel, 1989). It is recognised that the nature of need may take differing forms; for example, functional needs (Maslow, 1970; Faulkner, 1985; Roper *et al.*, 1990), adaptation needs (Roy, 1984), self-care needs (Orem, 1985), and interpersonal and information needs (Peplau, 1988). The way nurses value the significance of these needs, learn to recognise them, plan care to meet them, and evaluate whether needs have been met, rests with the nature of the relationship between the nurse and the patient.

It is necessary to acknowledge that, even though this is perhaps the work which belongs to nurses, nurses will be unable to judge the efficiency and cost-effectiveness of their actions without monitoring and evaluating the quality and outcomes of the care process. There is evidence emerging in the UK which provides insight into the quality of the care process and also provides indicators of nursing actions which are essential under defined clinical circumstances (Kitson, 1987). It appears that here is the opportunity for nurses to answer the question of what their proper task is within the context in which they work. The use of evaluative systems which gather information about the quality of the care process, and the outcome of their actions, will contribute to a greater understanding of the effectiveness of nursing (Kitson, 1987; DoH, 1989).

Understanding nursing

From the outset, the personal nature of the nurse's work is a key feature. Indeed, the intimate contact between nurses and patients becomes a daily occurrence not simply in the physical sense (though this for many requiring care is the most invasive of all experiences) but also in the social and emotional sense. Elements of oneself, which are usually concealed and the preserve only of family and friends, are made public. Feeling ill, needing an operation and being in pain may be frightening and alienating events and they require professional help. However, these events for health workers are everyday occurrences, they are part of the culture. There is a risk therefore of nurses failing to acknowledge the significance of an individual's health state on his usual functioning.

Henderson (1979) suggests that the nurse who values nursing and its 'personal, individualised and human character' gives 'holistic rather than disease-centred care.' This is not to assume that health care based on a medical model is not individualised, nor that care which focuses on the disease and excludes attention to psychosocial reactions and manifestations is ignoring the individual's unique combination of characteristics and responses. This at times will need to be the priority for determining interventions. However, nurses hold a privileged position in the health care service. They hold the key to entering caring relationships at a time when people who are not experiencing optimum health may be at their most vulnerable.

Communication: a key to a personal service

An effective interpersonal relationship between nurse and patient depends largely on communication which is therapeutic and demonstrates respect, concern and care (see also Chapter 8).

However, communication problems – and, more specifically, poor information-giving – dominate complaints about the interaction between health care workers and the public (Ley, 1988; Dimond, 1990). Despite complaints procedures, the Health Service Commissioner, and increased general awareness of the problem, there appears to be no evidence that the number of complaints is decreasing (Health Service Commissioner, 1991). The examination of the nature of complaints is certainly a useful indicator of patient satisfaction. However, in this country, their investigation depends on health authority definitions of what constitutes a complaint and attitudes to complaints procedures. Also, investigations tend to focus on specific issues such as lost property, lack of supervision and accidents, rather than details of the interaction between patients, their doctors and nurses (see also Chapter 10).

Deficiencies within the relationships between doctors and patients appear to be at the root of the complaints about the impersonal nature of the service (Maguire *et al.*, 1980). Korch (1968) found that doctors failed to enquire systematically about how patients and relatives adapt socially and psychologically to the disease process. Maguire's (1980) study revealed further perceptual difficulties, as doctors failed to assess the full extent of pain, disability and side effects of cytotoxic therapy in over 50% of a group of women following mastectomy. It may be suggested that not only does the orientation towards the medical/disease model distort the attention of doctors, but also doctors in this study failed to make links between clinical manifestations and individual responses and hence underestimated their significance for the person concerned.

It would be inappropriate to use these findings as generalisations but it is clear that they indicate issues which should be of concern to nurses, particularly as evidence regarding patient satisfaction reveals that anxiety is reduced when open and honest interaction occurs between doctors and patients (Ley, 1977; Parkes, 1980). Though these studies do not reveal the long term benefits of such interaction, they do correlate with the findings of Engstrom (1984) who found dissatisfaction associated with lack of information regarding prognosis, medical examination, progress and medication dominating patients' concerns. These would all affect short term reactions to their health situation. Increasing attention is being given to the development of communication skills among doctors and nurses which confirms the growing awareness within these professions of the need for all the benefits of such education.

Interaction between nurses and patients

Over a hundred years ago Nightingale (1860) recognised the need for nurses to use social skills, to demonstrate their interest in patients and to avoid impersonal activities. However, despite this clear recommendation, it appears that nurses may have been influenced more by their own expectations of patients.

Stockwell (1972) demonstrated that nurses may be highly selective in their communication with patients. Nurses rewarded patients who knew the nurses' names, cooperated in their care and communicated willingly, by spending more time with them. The 'unpopular patients' in this study were those who complained, were demanding or demonstrated more discomfort than the nurse thought appropriate to the situation. This stereotyped attitude towards patients goes against the ideals of individualised care and the desire to give more time to patients. Menzies (1960) revealed that though nurses perceive personal fears of patients, they may adopt defensive behaviours such as avoiding patients' questions, providing negative responses and changing the subject. Faulkner (1984) suggested that this behaviour may be affected by poor communication skills. Feelings of inadequacy and inability to cope in certain care situations are not uncommon and should not be ignored, rather they should be acknowledged so as to encourage a supportive environment for both patients and nurses.

It is important to recognise from these findings that while patients' needs are not being met, nor necessarily are nurses' needs. In her analysis of nurse-patient interaction, Chapman (1976) suggests that the goals and needs of both patients and nurses need to be acknowledged, as they influence the nature of the interaction. Her model of interaction (Fig. 12.1), which is based on social exchange theory (Homans, 1961), contains elements which influence the balance in the relationship between nurses and patients. The plus and minus signs indicate that there is an imbalance and that the patient is 'in debt' to the nurse. However, as Chapman acknowledges, there is no indication of the strength or depth of any of the elements. They should alert the reader to the significance of the potential power of nurses and their personal needs over patients made vulnerable by their health state, changes in their environment and their dependency. Restoring the imbalance demands that nurses recognise the importance of sharing information and decision-making with patients. However, nurses need positive feedback, rewards, gratitude and support and it is not enough to rely on or expect this from patients. Indeed, attention should be given to appropriate ways of creating a caring climate in which all members of the health care team are valued and experience a sense of worth, where their contribution is acknowledged, and where personal development is part of the culture.

So far the discussion has been concerned with factors affecting the relationships between two groups of health care workers (i.e. doctors and nurses) and patients. There are obvious features in common, not least the need of both groups to continue the development of educational programmes to support staff, to promote the perception and assessment of psychological and information needs and to plan opportunities for staff to examine openly stressful situations. Calnan (1983) suggests that:

'It is the duty of the doctor and nurse not to conceal reality, not to cause social disruption, and not to prevent understanding. Failure in any one of these is grievous social harm'

This perhaps summarises a significant area of mutual concern which, if realised, would in itself reduce much of the current dissatisfaction with communication with doctors and nurses.

Nurses and the concept of care

One of the most influential statements about nursing is that famous one by Virginia Henderson:

NURSE		PATIENT
+ Knowledge		− Physical needs
Technical		Disability
Organisational		Disease
Medical		Physical dependency
+ Skill		− Psychological needs
	Interaction	
Caring techniques	? Balancing	Information
Ability to relieve	situation	Ego maintenance
discomfort		Security
+ Power		+ Gratitude
−		
Ability to control life		
of others by ability		+ Personality
to provide or withhold		−
information or services		
+ Need to 'help'		+ Dependency
−		−
'To be wanted' (compassion)		Loss of power over life
		or decision-making
− Need to gain experience/learn		

Affected by:	
Culture	Age
Professionalisation	Occupation
Medical Science	Culture
Organisation	Diagnosis

KEY: + = areas of surplus − available to 'make-up' deficiencies elsewhere

    − = areas that need to be 'made-up'

From: Chapman, C. (1976). The use of sociological theories and models in nursing. *Journal of Advanced Nursing*, I,111 − 127. Reproduced with kind permission of the author and publisher.

Fig. 12.1 *Model of the nurse-patient interaction process and the maintenance of equilibrium*

'The unique function of the nurse is to assist the individual sick or well in the performance of those activities contributing to health or its recovery (or to a peaceful death) that he would perform un-aided if he had the necessary strength, will, or knowledge. And to do this in such a way as to help him gain independence as rapidly as possible'

(Henderson, 1966)

This definition of nursing has been recognised all over the world as capturing the essence of what nurses do. It makes explicit the need to value holistic elements of care through helping, promoting independence and combining artistic and scientific activities. Henderson's definition of the unique function of the nurse skilfully incorporates her interpretation of the 'intrinsic nature of nursing', particularly when considered along with her belief that nursing 'will never be seen as anything less than essential to the human race' (Henderson, 1979).

The Department of Health and Social Security (DHSS, 1977) also referred to care being at the heart of nursing by stating that:

'whatever changes may occur at the perimeter of the nurse's professional role, caring for people remains the essence of her profession'

Care is used here as a specific quality underlying practice but only refers to activities which are the responsibility of nurses rather than the value system underlying their execution. The concept of care has far-reaching implications. Griffin (1983) sees care as 'a fundamental concept both in the philosophy of human nature and that of personal relationships with others'. Therefore, in seeking an understanding of care, it is necessary to acknowledge the possible meanings associated with it and relate these to settings associated with the caring professions. Griffin identifies 'interest, concern, guidance, protection and serving' as being on a continuum with 'inclination or liking of a person, attachment or wanting to be near someone'. Therefore there is more to the concept of care than the skills or actions associated with it. Campbell (1984) views caring as a form of loving characterised particularly by the nature of the companionship between the nurse and patient. He regards companionship as:

'a closeness which is not sexually stereotyped; it implies movement and change; it expresses mutuality; and it requires commitment. . . . The good companion is someone who shares freely, but does not impose, allowing others to make their own journey'

(page 49)

It is necessary to consider also that though a nurse may value some if not all of these aspects of care, she may not display them. There may be many reasons for this but there is certainly an inter-relationship between the way a nurse values and prioritises these nursing qualities and the way her care is practised (Harrison, 1990).

Central to this is a moral aspect of caring. Schröck (1981) examines philosophical aspects of nursing without suggesting specific values for nursing. She suggests that through the analysis of moral concepts the nurse's own beliefs may be explored, so enhancing self-knowledge. She sets forth a selection of concepts here; they include 'telling the truth, respecting physical and emotional privacy, safeguarding adult rights, using but not abusing professional power and preventing incompetent practices'. These examples are essentially patient-centred. Perhaps nurses also need to consider and explore these and other concepts associated with themselves – for example, feelings of fear, embarrassment, revulsion and despair. All these issues imply that the nurse may be influenced by her own interests, therefore the caring activities could be influenced accordingly. Also, Schröck's

examples are associated with everyday nursing activities and need to be discussed openly by nurses as they develop their own philosophy for nursing practice. These may then help nurses explore the nature of care, the social impact of nursing, and the influence of the care environment, which Johns (1989) suggests are important features of a philosophy of nursing. The uncertainty associated with these issues has perhaps resulted in nurses ignoring their potential impact on subsequent decision-making and the nature of the relationship with the patient. All these factors may influence the content, quality, tone and priorities of an interaction and thus how care is demonstrated.

Attitudes, values and beliefs and their influence on nursing

It is important to begin by differentiating between values, attitudes and beliefs. Steele and Harmon (1979) suggest that:

Values are 'an affective disposition towards a person, object or idea, they give direction to life'

Attitudes are 'dispositions or feelings towards a person, object or idea'

Beliefs are 'a special class of attitudes in which the cognitive component is based more on faith than fact'

Therefore values and attitudes are difficult to differentiate but Clarke (1981) suggests that 'values are usually defined as systems of attitudes towards a class of (usually) abstract concepts. Thus an individual may have an attitude towards abortion but the value system of which that attitude is a part is centred around the issue of sanctity of human life or the importance of women's rights'. Therefore, focusing on value systems may be seen as a means of exploring priorities within individuals, groups and society. Also, values are ordered and part of a hierarchy (Steele and Harmon, 1979), therefore it is easy to see that conflicts are possible considering the number of variables which exist in any nurse-patient situation (social background, age, customs, knowledge of current situations, and personality, to name but a few).

Nurses face possible conflicts in other areas associated with care delivery, for example between professional and organisational recommendations and between the values of the social system and the service ideology. The effects of this type of incompatibility on decision-making may not be in the best interests of the patients or the nurse. Therefore if the nurse is to promote a personal service, it is necessary to maximise opportunities for value clarification among nurses and across the disciplines associated with health care. This would contribute to and facilitate more effective decision-making. Initially it would be important for nurses to realise the potential effects of conflicting values on themselves and their practice. Steele and Harmon (1979) suggest ways which may contribute to self-examination of values and understanding of their influences and which may, in turn, contribute to self-knowledge and the increase in the choices available for applied decision-making.

Raths *et al.* (1976) describe the process of values clarification as examining, choosing and acting on beliefs. This process may be used as a means of being in touch with one's values which enhances the helping relationship. By selecting specific issues essential to or related to the provision of a personal service, the development of the nurse's own insight into such matters may be applied to interactions with patients to support them in their decision-making.

This whole process demands not only expert facilitation and a supportive environment for nurses to explore their attitudes and values, but also skill in the selection of issues appropriate to the experience of the nurse.

It is suggested that the aspects of care raised by Schröck (1981) — telling the truth and respecting emotional and physical privacy — are concepts which underpin the quality of an interaction between all health care workers and patients. Because in practice, dilemmas may arise from these, it is necessary to find ways of helping staff to clarify them. Values associated with other aspects of care may be more specific in character but are as susceptible to conflict. These include the assessment of pain, maintaining confidentiality and talking about sexual needs. These examples relate to individuals and/or groups of patients but illustrate issues which should be addressed as part of the preparation of nurses for a particular clinical allocation. This could then be followed up during and after the experience, through the use of specific examples from practice and the analysis of critical incidents.

Personal values and attitudes have a significant effect on problem-solving and decision-making, indeed they influence the way needs are identified and prioritised. There is much to be learnt from the exploration of attitudes and values in nursing; they influence both the developments of nurse–patient relationships and the way care is planned and carried out.

Patient participation and nursing care

The notion of patient participation suggests involving the patient in planning his care and is seen as complementary to the concept of individualised care (Brearley, 1990). Patient participation depends on a supportive climate in which problem-orientated, spontaneous, empathic and mutual decision-making occurs (McMahon and Pearson, 1991) The values of nurses which would contribute to these qualities of communication are summarised by Sundeen *et al.* (1985) who state:

'In an environment of respect and acceptance the individual directs his energies towards self-definition, constructive relationships with others and positive control over his life and destiny'

Individualised care is the fundamental principle which enables the achievement of this aim but allowances should be made for those patients who choose not to participate to this extent. In 1987, the Royal College of Nursing stated that:

'Each patient has a right to be a partner in his own care planning and receive relevant information, support and encouragement from the nurse which will permit him to make informed choices and become involved in his own care'

(RCN, 1987)

This could be further determined through the identification and application of appropriate aims for care. The use of a nursing model based on the identified needs of the patient and goals for care which reflect the priorities for intervention from the patient's and nurse's perspective may all encourage patient participation. This is further emphasised by Dicken (1978) who identified mutual goal-setting as the key motivational factor for patients to participate in their own care and suggests it is necessary to:

'involve the patient . . . set attainable goals . . . spell out the method . . . describe the expected results . . . and . . . set a target date'

(Dicken, 1978)

These factors all contribute to a greater understanding of the needs of the patient and the roles of both the nurse and the patient in a particular situation. Though participation in mutual decision-making may be affected by the physical and psychological state of the patient, there may be opportunities to involve the family. These principles could then be applied effectively to partners, family members and friends, who may be eager to participate actively in care, or where it may be necessary that this is encouraged (for example, in the care of a child, a lover or a spouse). However, the nurse should assess and explore the appropriateness of pursuing this strategy with individuals to limit any additional stress which may result.

Nursing as a therapeutic activity

So far in this chapter, brief reference has been made to nursing as a therapeutic process, particularly in relation to the nature of the nurse—patient relationship and thus the partnership which develops between them. The notion that nursing has the potential to heal is acknowledged by Hockey (1991) who suggests that:

> 'Therapeutic nursing can now be explained as the practice of those nursing activities which have a healing effect or those which result in a movement towards health or wellness. It is important to emphasise that both "healing" and "health" must be regarded as multidimensional, and should include physical, emotional, spiritual, mental and environmental considerations'

This chapter has also considered a number of factors important to the care process, and how the personal attributes of the nurse influence her actions and the quality of the nurse—patient relationship. It is important now to consider the resources nurses can draw on to help with the wide variety of care demanded of them.

A major source of support to help nurses cope with the realities of practice comes through learning. The understanding and use of new knowledge comes from the study of nursing practice and the application of knowledge from other disciplines, such as psychology, sociology and physiology, to nursing and health care.

Nursing theory and nursing knowledge

Nursing is essentially a practice discipline, but the quality of the practice depends on attitudes, knowledge and abilities for effective care. The way nurses use knowledge and apply theory will influence their approach to nursing; sound decision-making depends on using knowledge expertly.

By implication, there appears to be more to the relationship between theory and practice than simply an understanding of what is done and why. In order to discuss the relevance of theory in nursing practice, it is necessary to examine two main relationships. Firstly, the relationship between knowledge and nursing practice and secondly, the relationship between the presence of theory, its interpretation, and its relevance to practice. Nurses know how to act but whether they have understanding of their actions is debatable. The Oxford English Dictionary defines knowledge as 'theoretical or practical understanding', being 'well informed', and 'familiarity gained by experience'. These definitions imply that knowledge may be acquired *without* theoretical input.

Benner (1984) considered the differences between practical and theoretical knowledge in detail and suggested that those who acquire practical skills may not be able to account theoretically for their actions. She goes on to suggest that knowledge development occurs by extending 'know-how'.

The extension of 'know-how' appears to form a major part of knowledge development in nursing this century. Consider the way nurses have responded to the demands of developments in technology, treatments and patterns of health care; and consider too the way that nurses have inherited procedures once carried out by doctors.

Rather than research into nursing practice developing, nurses found themselves taking on medical and technical tasks as medical know-how expanded and developed. Therefore, it may be suggested that the recognition of the relevance of theory was distorted by the pre-occupation with watered down medical know-how.

Today the picture is changing. The growing body of nursing research and knowledge is reflected in nursing texts, nursing journals and in the opportunities for nurses to study nursing and health-related subjects at centres of higher education. Using theory in practice is regarded as an effective means of introducing change (Wright, 1989) and research-mindedness as a way of questioning, testing, developing and ultimately generating nursing knowledge.

However, there are two other perspectives which deserve mentioning here, namely knowledge embedded in expertise and the notion that there are complementary areas of practical knowledge. It would be a mistake to assume that just because some practical knowledge may lack theoretical ground, it lacks validity. Benner (1984) suggests that know-how may be acquired through experience, hence leading to expertise, and states that 'adequate description of practical knowledge is essential to the development and extension of nursing theory'.

This conclusion gives clear direction to the way practice may serve the development of knowledge. However, in the United Kingdom, it is recognised that the use of nursing research as a means of developing and transmitting knowledge has been very limited – especially before 1960 (Hunt, 1981) – and those who publish research studies tend to be nurse leaders and teachers rather than those working in clinical areas. It appears that during this period nurses did not value the potential contribution of nursing to health care and also failed to recognise the potential wealth of knowledge at their fingertips.

In an American study by Smoyak (1976) into the theoretical content of nursing textbooks, it was found that graduate nurses who were asked to identify theoretical content, identified:

'very little theory – some facts (although some were outdated or questionable and better classified as Myths) and lots and lots of principles for practice. . . . Such principles are rarely based on research findings; they evolve from the pragmatics of having to get the work done expeditiously. They tend to solidify, rock-like, with each passing day and it is difficult to question them'

(Smoyak, 1976)

There seem to be marked similarities between the limited value placed on research in this study and the UK experience. Perhaps the problems are self-perpetuating if the quality of nursing literature fails to represent reality as perceived by those functioning within it. However, the recognition of principles is an important issue. The Concise Oxford Dictionary (1979) defines principle as a 'fundamental source', a 'fundamental truth as a basis of reasoning', 'a general law', 'personal code'. This poses the question as to whether the nurses in this study were able to identify theory defined by the same authority as 'a system of ideas based on general principles'.

The Smoyak study therefore suggests that nurses are in fact using theory and questioning its value but at the same time recognising that research is the means of validating it. It is now necessary to explore the nature and purpose of theory and its use in practice.

Nursing theory and nursing practice

Chinn and Jacobs (1991) define theory as 'a systematic abstraction of reality that serves some purpose' and which describes, controls and predicts the events that are of concern to the particular discipline. In the light of this, theory of nursing could contribute towards resolving ambiguity by showing what is happening and serving as a predictor of nursing actions.

If theories are able to describe on the one hand and predict on the other, there exists a range of potential in terms of their use and development. It is necessary, therefore, to examine the sources and types of theory – particularly since traditionally the use of theory has been limited. Nurses possess a range of personalised theories demonstrated by the range which exists in some approaches to practice; for example, the prevention and treatment of pressure sores, giving mouth care and pre-operative information-giving.

Nurses may view the presence of formal theory with suspicion, particularly as so little practical nursing is carried out by qualified nurses. If theory is unrecorded, not only may it go unquestioned and untested, but it may be generating irregular practices. The importance of theory for practice must be to support practice if its relevance is to be acknowledged.

The need, then, is to encourage the development of *inductive* theory, i.e. the development of theory from the study and scrutiny of nursing practice.

This section has examined the relevance of theory to nursing by examining nursing knowledge, the development of theory and the use of theory. There is no doubt that the value placed on the use of theory in practice has been variable, but it remains that nursing theory depends not only on knowledge shared with other disciplines but also on the nurse's ability to identify with theory and to generate and use it. However, its relevance may not be fully realised until nurses value the meaning and the purpose of assessing, planning, implementing and evaluating care.

The challenge is enormous and as Fawcett (1989) states, 'the time has come for knowledge to be validated by research into the primary determinant of nursing practice. Only when this goal is realised will nursing be able to declare its independence'.

Nursing theory and nursing models

Nursing is a complex activity and may be demonstrated in a wide variety of ways. Models help to make sense of the range of approaches to care by offering a representation of an aspect of reality. The model itself is not real but 'frequently abstract' . . . and 'contains many or most of the features of reality' (Chapman, 1985).

Models are essential to the growth of nursing theory and nursing knowledge as they contain the elements of the theory which may or may not be directly amenable to practice.

Models may also contain the ideas and experiences of nurses and it could be said that all nurses have their own model of nursing which is usually demonstrated through their actions, attitudes and expertise – that is to say, essentially through their practice. These models should be scrutinised and subjected to empirical study.

Nurses who have applied themselves to a greater understanding of nursing through the formulation of a model have usually taken their ideas and their experiences about nursing, health, man and society and sought to explain the inter-relationship between them.

The features of nursing models

Contemporary nursing models have key features in common as a result of this process. These may be summarised as follows:

(1) Priority is given to the integrity of the individual
(2) Assessment of the health needs of the individual is the foundation for all decision-making and problem-solving activities concerned with care
(3) Value is placed on the promotion of optimum

health for the individual throughout the period of care
(4) Each model offers a theme or approach to nursing which provides a means of focusing on the needs of the individual – for example, self-care, adaptation. Therefore the model is the guide to the decision-making process.

For clinical nursing practice a model:

> 'gives direction for the assessment process and provides a systematic approach to patient care. It shows the nurse what to look for and how to provide nursing care'
>
> (Rambo, 1984; page 5)

Choosing a model of nursing

The choice of a nursing model and approach to nursing care may follow one of two general perspectives. The choice may be influenced by the *needs of the individual patient* and may be chosen following a comprehensive assessment and an understanding of the care priorities. Alternatively, the choice may depend on *broader criteria* and take into consideration not only the *needs of a larger group of patients*, but also factors associated with the health care team, the care environment and resources. This is particularly pertinent where the clinical environment is being used for basic or post-basic education and where one model is used it not only facilitates good care but also effective oral and written communication between staff.

It is important to emphasise here that care plan design may inhibit or facilitate care. This is particularly so in a clinical learning environment where well-designed records not only allow the features of the model to be made explicit but also prompt the inexperienced user towards comprehensive assessment and record-keeping.

Assessing patients using a nursing model

The aims of patient assessment and history-taking are as follows:

(1) To ascertain initially whether the patient is at risk and to intervene (in an emergency) to maintain life
(2) To establish a rapport and begin the process of building a trusting relationship
(3) To collect information and data which will be used to plan care

(4) To review and interpret the patient's current health state and to decide what his needs and problems are

(5) To gather information regarding the patient's previous health state, to establish a baseline which may be used as a means of judging progress and recovery or degrees of deterioration

(6) To identify the level of understanding of the current situation of patients, their partners and families.

Most documented models of nursing offer an assessment format to guide the gathering of patient information. Unless the nurse is very familiar with the model, or the records are designed around the model, using different formats may not be practical.

Marjory Gordon (1985) offers an assessment format which has been designed as a way of gathering information which then allows the nurse to choose the most suitable approach or model of nursing (see Fig. 12.2). This is based on an assessment of functional health patterns.

This comprehensive tool for assessment prompts the nurse to consider biological, physical, social, psychological, spiritual and cultural aspects of need. Therefore it may be applied in any setting. That is not to say that all patients warrant such a detailed assessment (it might not be appropriate, for example, for a patient being admitted as a day case). However, it is imperative that the nurse considers how an individual's health needs and problems may affect his behaviour, his lifestyle, his relationships, and his self-image. She should *then* conduct her nursing assessment accordingly.

Other factors which are significant to the assessment process are:

(1) the acute or chronic nature of the presenting health needs
(2) the age of the patient
(3) the probable length of time needed for care
(4) the ability of the patient to participate in care
(5) past experience of care.

These factors, which affect care in the long and short term, guide the nurse and indicate areas where greater or lesser amounts of detail are necessary for effective care planning. At all times assessment data should serve to maximise the safety and comfort of patients, as they need to feel secure, at ease, and confident about what is happening to them and around them.

Assessment is not a one-off activity, it is continuous. It is essential that information-giving and a sharing of what is happening are part of the process. It may mean that the nurse has to admit she does not know the answers to some questions, and there is nothing wrong with this. Indeed, it is appropriate for the nurse to judge the times when either seeking the answer or acknowledging and accepting a response is the appropriate intervention, rather than always feeling she has to give an 'answer'.

The prerequisites for effective assessment are given in Table 12.1.

Table 12.1. *Effective assessment: a summary*

Effective assessment depends on:

- The nurse knowing the general intention of an interaction
- Social skills which are used to establish a rapport and a relationship which may then develop during the period of care
- Interviewing skills which are used to gather and give information and to clarify the purpose and intentions of both parties
- Problem-solving and decision-making abilities being applied to the available information
- Observing and using verbal and non-verbal cues
- Learning and listening to what is said and implied – questioning to explore and clarify what is said
- Attending to verbal and non-verbal responses and checking whether they appear to contradict each other
- Using language which is understood and explaining new terms
- Receiving, reflecting on and summarising the points made to check the accuracy of perception and understanding
- Recording what is factual, observable and whenever possible involving the patient with this

Approaches to nursing: care planning based on a nursing model

Nursing models may be classified in a number of ways according to their themes and aims. Classification also helps to identify specific theories associated with the model. When learning about models of nursing and seeking out what may be gained from them for practice, it is important to consider a number of factors which will contribute to a full understanding of the model (Fig. 12.3).

Fig. 12.2 *Assessment of functional health patterns*

1. Health perception / Health management	Assessment of general health, ways patient keeps healthy, past experience of treatments, hospital, fears/worries, current perception of health, smoking/drinking habits
2. Nutrition	Daily food and fluid intake Likes and dislikes Appetite, weight, dental history
3. Elimination	Bowel and urinary elimination pattern Any excess sweating
4. Activity and exercise	Perception of energy, ability and desire to exercise-type and frequency, leisure activities/play activities

Perceived ability for: (code level — see Functional Level Code below)

Feeding	Dressing	Home maintenance
Bathing	Grooming	Toileting
Mobility	Bed mobility	Cooking

Functional Level Code

Level 0:	Full self-care
Level I:	Requires use of equipment or device
Level II:	Requires assistance/supervision from another person
Level III:	Requires assistance/supervision from another person, equipment or device
Level IV:	Is dependent and does not participate

5. Sleep and rest	Sleep and rest pattern, effects of sleep Factors influencing rest and sleep
6. Cognitive – perceptual ability	Hearing, sight, change in memory Learning ability, whether information is needed Pain, discomfort, site/nature of pain, frequency, what helps
7. Self-perception	Self-image, self-esteem in relation to health state, what may be causing anger, fear, anxiety
8. Roles and relationships	Home situation which may influence health Next of kin, partner, sources of support People who need contacting, able to visit Family commitments and dependants
9. Sexuality and reproduction	Sexual needs, changes relating to health state and effects on partner Females – menstrual cycles Contraceptive requirements Questions, anxieties, fears about sexuality relating to health care and current health state
10. Coping — stress — tolerance pattern	Effects of life events in recent past Coping abilities, what helps when anxieties arise What and who is helping in this situation
11. Values and beliefs	Spiritual needs, religious persuasion and practices. Cultural factors and their current influence
12. Other	Any other factors or issues relevant to the individual

Adapted from: Gordon, M. (1985). *Manual of Nursing Diagnosis 1984–1985*. McGraw Hill. Reproduced with permission from the publisher.

The background of the model

Consider the origins of the model, when and where was it devised and how the author developed the model. Answers to these questions will alert the reader to the context of the work and what the original intentions of the model were.

The aims of the model

Examine the aims of the model. These may be expressed as aims of nursing. These will reveal the focus of the model and usually tell the reader whether the approach to nursing extends from the nurse–patient relationship and/or whether nursing aims to respond to states of health. Further understanding of the model will be gained from consideration of any assumptions the author makes about nursing, health, man or society.

Definitions and meanings

Identify what the author means by *Health, Nursing, Man, and Society*. These concepts will provide an image of the model. They should reveal how the author sees the relationship between a definition of health and how nursing may respond to people with associated health needs in a particular social setting.

Theories associated with the model

Identify any theories or research referred to by the author. This will provide useful insight into how, for example, certain work from the behavioural and social sciences has been applied to nursing through the formulation of the model. It is useful to refer to the original source of these theories for a full appreciation of the work.

Application of the model to clinical practice

Though the author may not offer specific examples of how the model has been used in clinical practice, it should be possible to find examples in the literature of how some models have been applied in both British and American health care settings. (The further reading list at the end of this chapter contains useful examples from British literature.) By considering these examples it is possible to see how models may be interpreted and applied in a variety of ways.

Evaluating a model of nursing

Making judgements about the potential value and use of a model of nursing depends not only on an understanding of the model but also full appreciation of what the model means to those concerned with the delivery of care. While the models referred to here are models of nursing, the approaches to care found in each of them have implications for the way health needs are identified, prioritised and the way care is planned and delivered. Therefore, it may be said that as a guide for planning nursing care, the choice of model is a reflection of the beliefs and values held by those delivering care and may also be a reflection of the expertise and skills available.

Examples of work by prominent nurse theorists are given below. In each section one model is described in detail.

Nursing to promote nurse/patient interaction and interpersonal relationships

---

These models include the approaches developed by Hildegard E. Peplau (interpersonal relationships), Joan P. Riehl (symbolic interactionalism), and Imogen King (the theory of goal attainment).

The work of Hildegard Peplau: a theory of interpersonal relationships and psychodynamic nursing

Peplau's approach to nursing developed from her work with the mentally ill. Her major work was published in the 1950s but the reader should not be deterred by its age. The work grew from her insights into how the nurse–patient relationship is, in itself, a therapeutic tool. She states:

'Psychodynamic nursing is being able to understand one's own behaviour to help others identify felt difficulties and to apply principles of human relations to the problems that arise at all levels of experience'

(Peplau, 1952)

Fig. 12.3 *Analysing models of nursing*

The aims of the model

The aim of the model is to use the nurse—patient relationship to help patients explore and understand the meaning of their feelings in a way which ultimately offers the patient the opportunity to identify with what is happening and to be involved in care. Peplau describes four phases of the interpersonal relationship:

(1) Orientation
(2) Identification
(3) Exploitation
(4) Resolution.

These phases provide a framework for the development of a relationship and should be viewed as overlapping stages made unique by each nurse—patient relationship.

Orientation

Orientation occurs at the beginning of the relationship, and is a period during which the nurse and patient can begin to get to know each other. It is a time for the nurse to help the patient recognise his needs and for the nurse to be generous with herself, to help the patient understand her role and explain her involvement in care.

Identification

Feelings are explored to ascertain the nature of need. The nurse uses positive feedback to support, encourage and help the person gain insight into the nature of his behaviour. This is a time for the nurse to promote a trusting relationship and to strengthen bonds which contribute to the person gaining confidence.

This phase may be likened to a period of assessment where needs are explored and identified and goals begin to emerge.

Exploitation

This is the time for the nurse to build on the features and qualities of the relationship so far as to help the person take responsibility for identifying further goals.

Resolution

New goals replace the old and the nurse helps the person prepare for ending the relationship and to be secure away from the support of the relationship with the nurse.

Definitions and meanings

Peplau offers the following definitions.
Health is defined as:

> 'a word symbol that implies forward movement of personality and other ongoing human processes in the direction of creative, constructive, productive, personal and community living.'
>
> (Peplau, 1952)

Nursing is defined as a:

> 'human relationship between an individual who is sick or in need of health services, and a nurse especially educated to recognise and to respond to the need for help'
>
> (Peplau, 1988)

Society is not defined but Peplau encourages the nurse to consider the person in relation to his cultural background and the environment in which he finds himself. This is particularly important when the person is facing changes.

The nurse's role and the nurse—patient relationship

Peplau describes six roles associated with stages of the relationship:

(1) *Stranger* – this is the first role. The nurse and patient meet as strangers. The nurse should aim to extend social skills and establish an atmosphere of acceptance
(2) *Resource* – the nurse offers information. She clarifies and encourages patient involvement and patient understanding
(3) *Teacher* – the nurse gives information; she guides and facilitates
(4) *Leader* – the nurse leads the process of identification and goal-setting
(5) *Surrogate* – the nurse represents people relevant to the patient to help the patient recall feelings and experiences
(6) *Counsellor* – the nurse helps the person reflect,

recognise, accept, and come to terms with the aspects of experience and feelings.

Theories associated with the model

Peplau refers to psychological and psychoanalytical theories and to theories of motivation, personality, psychotherapy and social learning.

Although this work has grown out of caring for the mentally ill, Peplau suggests that the principles may be applied to any other setting if an interpersonal relationship exists.

This approach to the formulation and establishment of an interpersonal relationship deserves continued attention and the importance of this work should be valued in all aspects of nursing.

Nursing to promote patient adaptation

The key name in the promotion of patient adaptation is that of Callista Roy.

Roy's work began in the early 1960s at Mount St Mary's College in California. Her ideas about nursing developed from observation of patients and the way they used to adapt to their health states. Much of her early work was with children and she observed their ability to cope with change and adapt to both physical and psychological changes.

The aims of Roy's model

The focus of the model is the concept of adaptation. Roy sees nursing as a means of promoting adaptation in people requiring health care.

Definitions and meanings

Roy's interpretation of health is based on her idea that adaptation is a state of physiological and social integrity. She defines health as 'a state and a process of being and becoming integrated and whole' (Roy, 1989).

Nursing is defined as a theoretical system of knowledge which prescribes a process of analysis and action related to the care of the ill or potentially ill person (Roy, 1984).

Man is defined as a person who is a 'biopsychosocial being in constant interaction with a changing environment' (Roy, 1984).

Rather than a definition of society, Roy defines the environment as 'all the conditions, circumstances and influences surrounding and affecting the development and behaviour of persons or groups' (Roy, 1984).

The concept of adaptation

Roy's study of the meaning of adaptation led her to describe adaptation in relation to nursing and health needs. She suggests that a person responds to different health states according to his level of adaptation. Where a person is unable to adapt unaided to a particular health problem, the nurse intervenes and assesses the nature of the problem. Roy identifies four modes of adaptation which represent her understanding of how people behave and respond (see Table 12.2).

Table 12.2. *The four modes of adaptation identified by Roy*

Physiological	Responses to physiological and biological demands
Self-concept	Responses to beliefs and feelings about oneself
Role function	Responses to role function in relation to one's role set
Interdependence	Responses to relationships with people and other sources of comfort and support

First level assessment

Roy suggests that states of health may affect one or more of these modes (see the examples in Fig. 12.4). She stresses that each mode is inter-related with the other; for example, a person with a newly formed colostomy may not only need help to cope with the pain following surgery but also experience feelings of embarrassment about how he looks (self-concept), anxiety about how he is going to cope at home and on return to work (role mastery), and how his partner is going to react to him when shown the colostomy (interdependence). These four modes form the basis of assessment which is

		Examples of common adaptation problems
Physiological		
Exercise and rest	PHYSIOLOGICAL	Insomnia
Nutrition	MODE	Nausea
Elimination		Incontinence
Fluid and electrolytes		Hypovolaemia
Oxygenation and circulation		Dyspnoea
Regulation of temperature, senses and the endocrine system		Pyrexia
Self-concept		
Physical self	SELF-CONCEPT	Loss of libido
Personal self	MODE	Guilt, poor self-image
Role function		
Primary roles	ROLE FUNCTION	Role conflict
Secondary roles	MODE	Role failure
Tertiary roles		Role distance
Interdependence		
Interdependence on others	INTERDEPENDENCE MODE	Loneliness
With others		Isolation

Fig. 12.4 First level assessment

divided into two parts – the first level assessment and the second level assessment.

Each mode is used to guide assessment. The nurse identifies whether the person is adapting or exhibiting problems. Needs or 'maladaptive behaviours' identified from the first level assessment are then assessed more closely to discover more information which will help the nurse to plan care with a greater understanding of the stressors affecting the patient.

Second level assessment

The person who is found to be having problems with one or more aspects of his health is said to be unable to adapt unaided to certain stimuli in the *internal* environment (for example, stressors such as infection, immobility, fear, and inability to communicate) as well as in the *external* environment (for example, stressors such as living alone, bacteria and viruses, and lack of information).

Each need or problem is explored to reveal the stimuli affecting them. These are classified as shown in Fig. 12.5.

The inter-relationship between these details illustrates how an understanding of the patient's beliefs would help the nurse plan care specific to the actual problems and, in this situation, the beliefs of the person. It should be noted that not all focal stimuli have an obvious contextual or residual stimulus. Time spent with the patient and continuous assessment will do much to help and sup-

Focal	The causative stimulus, the main reason for the problems
Contextual	All other stimuli which may influence the focal stimuli
Residual	The beliefs, feelings, attitudes relating to the situation as expressed by the person

Example: Based on one problem of a woman with a malignant breast tumour

FOCAL	CONTEXTUAL	RESIDUAL
Pain from right breast following lumpectomy	Presence of a wound infection	Believes that if the pain does not go away the cancer will return

Fig. 12.5 Second level assessment

port the patient, allowing more details to emerge.

The use of this model demands that the nurse develops a trusting relationship and is able to maintain her contact with the person.

Theories associated with the model

Roy refers to the work of Harry Helson (1964) who developed a theory of adaptation. Other work, including that by Hans Selye (1978), is used to refine the concept of adaptation.

Roy's adaptation model offers nurses an approach to care which applies equal attention to physiological, psychological and social aspects of the response to stimuli – whether these be generated from within the person or from the environment. The model also offers useful insights into how knowledge of a patient's adaptation level, coping abilities, and associated life experience and beliefs provide a comprehensive base from which to plan care. Thus goals and interventions are orientated to the promotion of the patient's adaptation level, the nurse acting on his behalf as necessary.

This model may be considered where people need help in coming to terms with chronic illness, changes in body image, or are found to be having difficulty coping and adapting.

Nursing to promote self-care

The work of Dorothea Orem has been particularly influential in the context of encouraging the patient to be a partner in his own care.

Orem's self-care model

Orem first published her work about self-care nursing in 1971, at a time when consumerism was gaining momentum and the American public appeared to be seeking value for money for their health care as well as looking beyond conventional medically dominated health care services. The concept of self-care is explained in detail in Orem's (1990) work and is open to a number of interpretations.

Often 'self-caring' appears on British care plans, particularly where people appear to be able to look after themselves. The reality may be that the patient receives little or no care at all.

It is important to challenge this notion of 'do it yourself care'. This model offers an opportunity to explore the implications of self-care nursing, not only for the patient but also for the nurse. Self-care nursing is essentially about shifting responsibility for decision-making and caring activities *appropriately* from nurses to patients. It means allowing people to hold on to the control they would normally have over their lives, as they experience the health care and treatment they need.

The aims of the model

The aim of the model comes from Orem's notion of self-care, which she sees as, 'The practice of activities that individuals initiate and perform on their own behalf in maintaining life, health and well-being' (Orem, 1985).

The model provides a means of enabling this to be achieved for people who need interventions, support, teaching and guidance from nurses.

Definitions and meanings

Orem suggests that health depends on a person's ability to be self-caring, and is therefore a balance between initiating self-care and being able to undertake self-care activities to meet personal needs. She describes individual needs as 'universal self-care requisites' which need to be met in order to maintain health. These are listed in Table 12.3.

The requirements are common to everyone and form the basis of the assessment process. Orem suggests that an individual who is unable to be

Table 12.3. *Orem's universal self-care requisites*

- The maintenance of air intake

- The maintenance of food and water intake

- The maintenance of elimination

- The balance between activity and rest

- The balance between solitude and social activity

- The prevention of hazards to oneself

- 'Being normal'

self-caring or be in control of one or more of these areas of need, who needs help or support, is in a state of ill health and requires health care which restores him to a position from which he will once again be as self-caring as possible.

Orem also describes 'developmental self-care requisites' which relate to the experience and maturation of the person. She suggests that people have needs relating to their stage of growth, development and life experiences which should be considered when support is needed for them to be self-caring.

The third area of self-care requisites relates to the effect of disease, trauma, injury and illness on self-care and is called 'health deviation self-care requisites'. Included here is the notion that when a person becomes dependent and needs support, he will often demonstrate self-care actions when seeking information and help.

These three categories form the basis of the nursing assessment which aims to identify the self-care requisites or the actions necessary for the person to be self-caring.

Care planning using Orem's model

Nursing is seen as a system in which the promotion of self-care is therapeutic for the patient. Care planning depends on: the *assessment* of universal self-care requisites, developmental self-care requisites, and health deviation self-care requisites, in order to *identify* the person's self-care demands or needs in relation to each requisite, self-care ability, self-care deficits, and potential for self-care.

An example of care planning using Orem's model, based on one need of a young man who incurred facial injuries following a road traffic accident, is given in Fig 12.6.

Orem describes three systems or approaches to nursing.

Wholly compensatory nursing. The nurse takes responsibility for the total care of a person who is unable to carry out any self-care activities.

Partly compensatory nursing. The nurse undertakes aspects of care that the person is unable to do independently or without help.

Supportive—educative nursing. The nurse supports and guides the person to carry out self-care which as yet he is unable to do without knowledge, skill, practice or assistance.

Care planning using this model depends on the nurse adopting one or more of these approaches to care depending on the needs and skills of the person, his willingness to undertake self-care activities, and the ability of the nurse to guide, support, teach or compensate for changes that have occurred in a person's ability to be self-caring. During a period of care, one or all of the systems may be applied as changes in health and dependency occur.

Theories associated with the model

Orem's ideas about nursing and self-care have been, by and large, a product of her nursing experiences and her understanding of health care requirements. However, she does refer to other nurse theorists (for example, Imogen King and Virginia Henderson) as well as to sociologists and psychologists.

The self-care concept in health care is not attributable to nursing alone. Orem (1984) states:

Universal self-care requisites	Self-care demand	Self-care ability	Self-care deficit	Potential for self-care
Maintenance of food intake	Well balanced diet	Unable to tolerate solid food Manages puréed food and prefers to use a straw	Motivation deficit Finds eating a great effort Knowledge deficit relating to the detail of a well balanced diet	Long term self-care Short term depends on healing and pain control and return of appetite

Fig. 12.6 *Care planning using Orem's model*

'The self-care theory component of the general theory of nursing is common to the health professions and to all members of social groups. Physicians as well as paramedical groups help people with aspects of self-care and with development of capabilities to engage in self-care. Persons helped may or may not be in need of nursing or may or may not be under nursing care'

It is easy to see that the promotion of self-care may be closely associated with approaches to health education and prevention of illness as well as being pertinent to the involvement of people in their health care. These ideas about nursing and self-care should encourage nurses to consider the implications of their actions and their relationships with people needing care. To be self-caring people need information, appropriate support, assistance and help. The nurse also needs to be able to judge with the person whether they are willing, able and prepared to participate in this way. There may be patients who are not interested or who are unwilling to undertake self-care activities, so offering the opportunity and information for this is vital.

Now is the time for nurses to think more about giving people the choice to participate actively in their own care and to undertake self-care activities as a way of contributing more actively to the maintenance of their own health.

Nursing to promote an understanding of the whole person

This approach to nursing is often associated with systems theory. Systems models of nursing offer an approach to nursing which considers how an individual's internal activities interact and are influenced by external activities. A system is any activity which is organised; therefore it can be said that man is a system and is subject to change and stresses.

Other familiar examples include transport systems and the telephone system. All have inputs, throughputs and outputs – for example, a transport system is characterised by people catching a flight (input), taking a journey (throughput) and reaching a destination (output). This simple principle may be applied to nursing whereby the internal activities of a person are considered in relation to ex-

ternal events or stimuli. Attention is paid to how the interaction between them affects the person. Using this approach, ill health occurs if the inputs (i.e. stresses, such as viral infections, trauma or bereavement) result in outputs (for example pyrexia, injury or depressive illness) which are more than the person can cope with unaided.

Nursing models based on systems theory include the work of Dorothy E. Johnson (behavioural systems model), and Betty Neuman (systems model). Roy's adaptation model may also be classified as a systems model.

The work of Dorothy Johnson

Johnson's behavioural systems model of nursing was developed in the late 1950s. She regards man as a behavioural system and therefore the observation and analysis of the behaviours, which are the outcome of the interaction between internal and external activities, are the concern of nursing.

The aims of the model

Johnson sees nursing as a means of guiding and facilitating effective behaviour for people in a state of health. The model is applicable for health maintenance as well as for supporting those experiencing ill health.

Definitions and meanings

Johnson offers explanations of health, nursing, the person and the environment. Health is dependent upon the interaction between personal achievement, relationships with others, defensive responses, dependency on others, elimination, ingestion and pleasurable responses, sexual and caring responses.

These seven aspects of behaviour are important for health and are regarded as drives or motivators. Johnson (1989) calls them 'behavioural subsystems', and sees health as a 'purposeful, adaptive response, physically, mentally, emotionally and socially, to internal and external stimuli in order to maintain stability and comfort'.

Nursing is seen as a way of preserving the person's behaviour by helping the person to achieve an equilibrium by providing care and resources while one or more of the subsystems are under stress. Nursing is regarded as complementary to medical activities.

Table 12.4. Johnson's 'behavioural subsystems'

- Personal achievement
- Relationships with others
- Defensive responses
- Dependency on others
- Elimination
- Ingestion and pleasurable responses
- Sexual and caring responses

Johnson sees man as a behavioural system, an integrated whole using energy to restore and maintain a balance between different behaviours.

The environment is seen as everything which is not part of a person's behavioural system. The person relies on a stable environment and is influenced by environmental factors which threaten, are disturbing and are in excess of a person's tolerance.

Care planning using Johnson's model of nursing

Assessment in Johnson's model of nursing has two stages.

The first stage assessment

Each subsystem is considered in order to identify whether a problem exists.

The nurse should also identify whether a problem in one subsystem is having, or is likely to have, an effect on another.

The second stage assessment

From the problems identified, the nurse differentiates between problems which are *structural* and problems which are *functional*, as each subsystem has structural and functional requirements. This helps to clarify the nature of the problem. The nurse plans care to influence and change the *goal*, *action* and *choice* in each structural problem and to regulate the amount of *protection, nurture* and *stimulation* in each functional problem.

Intervention

The nurse acts to restore equilibrium with or on behalf of the person. The nurse may act as facilitator, guide, protector and assistant.

Evaluation

The nurse considers and judges changes in behaviour using the goals for care and involving the person in the process.

Theories associated with the model

Johnson refers to Nightingale's work as well as to work of behavioural scientists. She also refers to work relating to motivation, social learning theory, learning, adaptation and behavioural modification.

Johnson's model of nursing offers nurses an approach to care which emphasises the importance of considering the reasons for change in a person's behaviour. Assessment using the seven subsystems guides this process and, though they do not appear to include all behavioural activities, they should be considered from a biological, psychological and sociological perspective. Also, although the model appears to focus on the individual, Johnson acknowledges that it may be applied to the care of groups — for example, families.

Nursing to promote and maintain independence

The work of the British nurses Nancy Roper, Winifred Logan and Alison Tierney is concerned with everyday activities necessary to us all.

The activities of daily living

This work developed from research undertaken by Nancy Roper in the 1970s. Using insights gained from the study of psychology and sociology, she devised a *model of living* before the model for nursing emerged. She identified the *activities of daily living* (see Table 12.5) as activities essential to life and the quality of life. Dying is seen as the final act of living.

Each activity of daily living is related to two continua. The first relates to life span (conception–death); the second relates to level of indepen-

Table 12.5. *The activities of daily living*

- Maintaining a safe environment
- Communicating
- Breathing
- Eating and drinking
- Eliminating
- Personal cleansing and dressing
- Control of body temperature
- Working and playing
- Mobilising
- Sleeping
- Learning
- Expressing sexuality
- Procreating
- Dying

dence (independence–dependence). These aspects provide a useful way of considering how each activity of daily living is influenced by the age and maturity of the person and level of dependence or independence. These elements of the model of living are present in the model for nursing.

Definition and meanings

Roper *et al.* (1990) offer ideas about health which emphasise the importance of considering factors such as age, culture, education and environment as well as psychological and social factors, all of which influence health and an individual's potential for health. They define nursing as follows:

> 'Within the context of a health care system and in a variety of combinations, nursing is helping a person towards his personal independent pole of the continuum for each activity of living, helping him to remain there; helping him to cope with any movement towards the dependent pole or poles, in some instances encouraging him to move towards the dependent pole or poles; and because man is finite, helping him to die with dignity'

Man is viewed as unique and – particularly in relation to his knowledge, attitude and ability – associated with each activity of living. This will

contribute to an understanding of the person as well as his health state.

Roper *et al.* emphasise the importance of understanding a person within his social context. They suggest that details of social background, living conditions, lifestyle and social relationships contribute to this.

Following refinements to the model of living, the model for nursing developed, based on assessing and planning care relating to twelve activities of living (Table 12.6).

Table 12.6. *The activities of living*

- Maintaining a safe environment
- Communicating
- Breathing
- Eating and drinking
- Eliminating
- Personal cleansing and dressing
- Controlling body temperature
- Mobilising
- Working and playing
- Expressing sexuality
- Sleeping
- Dying

Care planning using the activities of living model

Each person is assessed to clarify his independence in relation to each activity of living, the reasons for the level of independence, the type of help and support needed and how appropriate activities and behaviours can be maintained. A thorough assessment will enable goals and interventions to be planned.

Assessment

Each activity of living is considered in order to assess how the person's state of health may be influencing his level of independence. The person's usual ability is also assessed. By considering how independent the person was prior to this period of care, the nurse has a useful record of what may be achievable following care, and of how the person has been affected over a period of time.

The degree of independence may therefore be influenced by:

(1) physical, psychological and social environments;
(2) disability and disturbed physiology — either congenital or acquired;
(3) tissue changes — which can be pathological or degenerative;
(4) accident;
(5) infection.

Assessment is not a once-only event. Rather it is a continuous process whereby information about the person is added to that already gained, to clarify the understanding of the person's needs and to refine records.

The nurse needs to assess:

(1) previous routines;
(2) what the patient can do for himself;
(3) what the patient cannot do for himself;
(4) problems;
(5) discomforts.

Goals and interventions

Nursing goals and interventions stem from according priority to the needs and problems identified during assessment. The nurse plans care to help support the person, to minimise deterioration, and to prevent him from becoming inappropriately dependent.

Theories associated with the model

Roper *et al.* (1990) draw on sociological and psychological work including the work of Maslow, particularly in relation to the model of living.

Models of nursing: a summary

The models of nursing described in this chapter offer just a few examples of work available to enhance the understanding and practice of nursing care.

It should be emphasised that this work offers nurses insight into a variety of approaches to care and as such is a resource to guide and facilitate the care process. The models should be used not as rigid ways of understanding and communicating knowledge of patients, their needs and their problems. Models of nursing need to be tried and tested in different settings and the themes they offer studied and researched. This will contribute even more to the developing knowledge and understanding of nursing.

We must look forward to a time when nurses regard people in need, not as passive recipients of care but as potentially active participants in decisions about care. An understanding of different approaches to care offers nurses the potential and choice to do this.

A final area which deserves attention is that of *reflective practice*, i.e. developing ways of learning from experience which may help to modify and change approaches to practice.

Making effective judgements about care is a constant challenge to nurses but is central to the quality of care. For nurses to develop skills to enable them to be reflective practitioners is a key part of this process. Reflection is a way for practitioners to analyse experiences in order to develop new insights and understandings. This may involve changes in attitudes and values, skills and knowledge as the interpretations of experiences and events are evaluated and reassessed.

Ultimately, reflective practice is a way of taking stock of events, experiences and outcomes and can be a means of learning from past actions and current situations.

Reflection is described by Bolt (1991) as a process which involves:

Actions — being aware of, learning from and evaluating previous actions

Critical thought — being able to provide rationales for the way judgements and interpretations about experiences are made

The self — recognising and being aware of the effects of experiences on emotions, senses, feelings and behaviour.

As reflective practitioners, nurses may have the means by which they can grow and develop both as professional practitioners and individuals.

Reflection is a process which may benefit individuals and groups and be part of professional development programmes such as the English National Board Higher Award, Individual Performance Review (IPR), and educational programmes as part of self-assessment and quality assurance.

Bolt (1991) concludes:

'Reflective practice seems to involve becoming aware of and questioning the taken-for-granted assumptions and our habitual ways of seeing and behaving, in order to establish their relevance and validity in the present'

(page 68)

Conclusions

This chapter has addressed many issues relating to the quality of nursing care and how care may be approached. Elsewhere in this book you will discover additional ideas about health (Chapters 1, 2 and 3), managing care (Chapter 11), and managing yourself (Chapter 14), all of which play a significant part in determining the optimum approach to nursing care in a wide range of ever changing circumstances.

This chapter closes with some thoughts and ideas for you to consider. In an attempt to understand your potential contribution to nursing and health care, it is necessary to consider your place in a much larger scheme of things. Remember, and try to accept, the enormous part you play in the lives of those you care for. You have the power to involve and be involved with those who are vulnerable, in need, and often fearful and ignorant of what is happening to them and around them. These feelings are true for nurses too; they need to be acknowledged, accepted and worked with, so as to allow greater understanding of the realities of caring. Continue to learn and be receptive to the teaching and skills of others. Use resources like this book, the research undertaken by others and theoretical sources to enhance your own ideas, expertise and practice. Go on learning from those around you – especially the people you care for. They offer the greatest insight into the approach to care they need. The rest is up to you.

References

Barber, P. (1991). Caring; the nature of a therapeutic relationship. In *Nursing: A Knowledge Base for Practice*, Perry, A. and Jolley, M. (eds.). Edward Arnold, London.

Benner, P. (1984). *From Novice to Expert: Excellence and Power in Clinical Nursing Practice*. Addison-Wesley, New York.

Benner, P. and Wruebel, J. (1989). *The Primacy of Caring: Stress and Coping in Health and Illness*. Addison-Wesley, New York.

Bolt, E. (1991). *Becoming Reflective*. Distance Learning Centre, South Bank Polytechnic, London.

Brearley, S. (1990). *Patient Participation: The Literature*. Scutari Press, Harrow.

Brietung, A. (1980). What patients remember about their nurses. *Journal of Practical Nursing*, 30(2), 19–20.

Calnan, J. (1983). *Talking with Patients*. Heinemann, London.

Campbell, V. (1984). *Moderated Love*. SPCK, London.

Chapman, C. (1976). The use of sociological theories and models in nursing. *Journal of Advanced Nursing*, 1, 111–127.

Chapman, C. (1985). *Theory of Nursing: Practical Applications*. Harper and Row, London.

Chinn, P.L. and Jacobs, M.K. (1991). *Theory and Nursing: A Systematic Approach* (3rd ed.). Mosby, St Louis.

Clarke, M. (1981). Two aspects of psychology and their application to nursing. In *Nursing Science in Practice*, Smith, J.P. (ed.). Butterworths, London.

Department of Health. (1989). *A Strategy for Nursing*. DoH, London.

Department of Health and Social Security. (1977). *The Extended Role of the Nurse*. HC(77)22. HMSO, London.

Dicken, A. (1978). Why patients should plan their own recovery. *Registered Nurse*, March, 52–55.

Dimond, B. (1990). *Legal Aspects of Nursing*. Prentice Hall, London.

Engstrom, J. (1984). The patient's need for information during hospital stay. *International Journal of Nursing Studies*, 21(2), 113–130.

Faulkner, A. (1984). *Recent Advances in Nursing 7: Communication*. Churchill Livingstone, Edinburgh.

Faulkner, A. (1985). *Nursing: A Creative Approach*. Baillière Tindall, Eastbourne.

Fawcett, J. (1989). *Analysis and Conceptual Models of Nursing* (2nd ed.). F.A. Davis, Philadelphia.

Gordon, M. (1985). *Manual of Nursing Diagnosis 1984–1985*. McGraw-Hill, New York.

Griffin, A.P. (1983). Philosophy and nursing. *Journal of Advanced Nursing* 5, 261–272.

Harrison, L.C. (1990). Maintaining the ethic of caring in nursing. *Journal of Advanced Nursing*, 15, 125–127.

Health Service Commissioner. (1991). *Annual Report for Session 1990/91.* HMSO, London.

Helson, H. (1964). *Adaptation Level Theory: An Experimental and Systematic Approach to Behaviour.* Harper and Row, New York.

Henderson, V. (1966). *The Nature of Nursing: A Definition and Its Implications for Practice, Research and Education.* Macmillan, New York.

Henderson, V. (1979). Preserving the essence of nursing in a technological age. *Nursing Times*, 75(20), 12.

Hockey, L.E. (1991). Foreword. In *Nursing as Therapy*, McMahon, R. and Pearson, A. (eds.). Chapman and Hall, London.

Homans, T. (1961). *The Human Group.* Routledge and Kegan Paul, London.

Hunt, J. (1981). Indications for nursing practice; the use of research findings. *Journal of Advanced Nursing*, 6, 189–194.

Johns, C. (1989). Developing a philosophy. *Nursing Practice*, 3(1), 2–4.

Johnson, D.E. (1989). The behavioural system model for nursing. In *Conceptual Models for Nursing Practice* (3rd ed.), Riehl, J.P. and Roy, C. (eds.). Appleton Century Crofts, New York.

Kitson, A. (1987). Raising standards of clinical practice: the fundamental issue of effective nursing practice. *Journal of Advanced Nursing*, 12, 321–329.

Kitson, A. (1989). *A Framework for Quality: A Patient Centred Approach to Quality Assurance in Health Care.* Scutari Press, Harrow.

Korch, B. (1968). Gaps in doctor-patient communication. *Paediatrics*, 42, 855–871.

Ley, P. (1977). Psychological studies of doctor-patient communications. In *Rachman's Contributions to Medical Psychology*, Rachman, S.J. (ed.). Oxford University Press, Oxford.

Ley, P. (1988). *Communicating with Patients.* Croom Helm, London.

Lindblom, C. (1959). *The Science of Muddling Through.* Open University Press, Milton Keynes.

Maguire, P., Tait, A. and Brooke, M. (1980). Emotional aspects of mastectomy. *Nursing Mirror*, 150(2), 17–19.

Maslow, A. (1970). *Motivation and Personality.* Harper and Row, Philadelphia.

McMahon, R. and Pearson, A. (eds.). (1991). *Nursing as Therapy.* Chapman and Hall, London.

Menzies, I. (1960). *Social Systems as a Defence against Anxiety.* Tavistock Publications, London.

Nightingale, F. (1860). *Notes on Nursing: What It Is and What It Is Not.* Dover Publications, New York.

Nurses, Midwives and Health Visitors Act (1979). HMSO, London.

Orem, D. (1984). Personal correspondence. In *Nursing Theorists and Their Work*, Marriner, A. (ed.). Mosby, St Louis.

Orem, D. (1985). *Nursing: Concepts of Practice* (3rd ed.). McGraw-Hill, New York.

Orem, D. (1990). *Nursing: Concepts of Practice* (4th ed.). Mosby, St Louis.

Parkes, C.M. (1980). Bereavement counselling. *British Medical Journal*, 281, 3–6.

Peplau, H.E. (1952). *Interpersonal Relations in Nursing.* Putnams, New York.

Peplau, H.E. (1988). *Interpersonal Relations in Nursing* (2nd ed.). Putnams, New York.

Rambo, B.J. (1984). *Adaptation Nursing: Assessment and Intervention.* W.B. Saunders, Philadelphia.

Raths, L., Harman, M. and Simons, S. (1976). *Values and Teaching.* Macmillan, New York.

Roberts, D. (1984). Non-verbal communication: popular and unpopular patients. In *Recent Advances in Nursing 7: Communication*, Faulkner, A. (ed.). Churchill Livingstone, Edinburgh.

Rogers, C. (1967). *On Becoming a Person.* Constable, London.

Roper, N., Logan, W.W. and Tierney, A.J. (1990). *The Elements of Nursing* (3rd ed.). Churchill Livingstone, Edinburgh.

Roy, C. (1984). *Introduction to Nursing: An Adaptation Model* (2nd ed.). Prentice Hall, New Jersey.

Roy, C. (1989). Adaptation models. In *Nursing Theorists and Their Work*, Marriner, A. (ed.). Mosby, St Louis.

Royal College of Nursing. (1987). *A Position Statement on Nursing.* RCN, London.

Salvage, J. (1985). *The Politics of Nursing.* Heinemann, London.

Schröck, R. (1981). Philosophical issues. In *Current Issues in Nursing*, Hockey, L. (ed.). Churchill Livingstone, Edinburgh.

Selye, H. (1978). *The Stress of Life.* McGraw-Hill, New York.

Simon, H.A. (1950). *Administrative Behaviour.* Macmillan, New York.

Smoyak, S.A. (1976). Is practice responding to research? *American Journal of Nursing*, 76, 1146–1150.

Steele, S.M. and Harmon, V.M. (1979). *Values Clarification in Nursing.* Appleton Century Crofts, New York.

Stockwell, F. (1972). *The Unpopular Patient.* RCN, London.

Sundeen, S.J., Stuart, G., Rankin, E. and Cohen, S. (1985). *Nurse–Client Interaction* (3rd ed.). Mosby, St Louis.

Tajfel, H. and Fraser, C. (1978). *Introducing Psychology.* Penguin Books, Harmondsworth.

United Kingdom Central Council for Nursing, Midwifery and Health Visiting. (1992). *Code of Professional Conduct for the Nurse, Midwife and Health Visitor* (3rd ed.). UKCC, London.

UKCC. (1990). *Report of the Post Registration Education and Practice Project*. UKCC, London.

Vaughan, B. and Pillmoor, M. (1989). *Managing Nursing Work*. Scutari Press, Harrow.

World Health Organisation. (1977). *The Nursing Process. Report on the First Meeting of a Technical Advisory Group*. WHO, Geneva.

Suggestions for further reading

Barber, P. (1987). *Using Nursing Models: Mental Handicap Nursing*. Hodder and Stoughton, Sevenoaks.

Chalmers, H. (1988). *Using Nursing Models: Choosing a Model*. Edward Arnold, London.

Collister, B. (1988). *Using Nursing Models: Psychiatric Nursing*. Edward Arnold, London.

Easterbrook, J. (1987). *Using Nursing Models: Elderly Care*. Hodder and Stoughton, Sevenoaks.

Jolley, M. and Brykczyńska, G. (1992). *Nursing: The Challenge to Change*. Edward Arnold, Sevenoaks.

Marriner, A. (1989). *Nursing Theorists and Their Work* (2nd ed.). Mosby, St Louis.

McGilloway, O. and Myco, F. (1985). *Nursing and Spiritual Care*. Harper and Row, Philadelphia.

McMahon, R. and Pearson, A. (eds.). (1991). *Nursing as Therapy*. Chapman and Hall, London.

Perry, A. and Jolley, M. (eds.). (1991). *Nursing: A Knowledge Base for Practice*. Edward Arnold, London.

Styles, M.M. (1982). *On Nursing: Towards a New Endowment*. Mosby, St Louis.

Webb, C. (1987). *Using Nursing Models: Women's Health*. Hodder and Stoughton, Sevenoaks.

Willis, L.D. and Linwood, M.R. (1984) *Recent Advances in Nursing 10: Measuring the Quality of Care*. Churchill Livingstone, Edinburgh.

13

ETHICS, MORALITY AND NURSING

Verena Tschudin

This chapter offers the reader the opportunity to explore principles and theories about ethics and morality. The chapter aims to lead the reader from an exploration of the relation between personal attributes, attitudes and ways of thinking to making ethical decisions.

The chapter includes discussion of:

- Ways of determining values, attitudes and beliefs, including nursing values

- Ethical models such as deontology, teleology and response ethics, and ethical principles such as the value of life, goodness, justice, truth and individual freedom

- Codes of practice, including the Code of Professional Conduct (UKCC, 1992)

- Ways of making ethical decisions. Examples relating to nursing are

included to illustrate the application of theories and principles

- Ethical issues concerning patients and nurses. Included here is reference to informed consent, confidentiality, trials and conscientious objection

- Professional values, including accountability and autonomy, are briefly explored in the latter part of the chapter

Ethics and morality are concerned with good and right, and being good and doing right. The theoretical study of ethics and morality is therefore *what* and *who* is good and right, who says so, and on what basis.

Morality tends to be the domain of the *personal* good and right, and ethics of the *social* good and right. These two aspects necessarily overlap and complement each other.

One way of expressing the personal experience

of good and right has traditionally been through the practice of virtue (e.g. prudence, courage, cleanliness, constancy). The more common expression nowadays would be holding certain values (e.g. values of creativity, experience and attitudes). Whichever language or concept a person prefers, what is involved is something chosen and acquired, held as relevant, and acted upon. Because of such values or virtues, a person is able to relate to another, at a level which is nurturing and helpful. A person without virtues or values tends to be unstable, shifty, rebellious, 'unprincipled' or 'phoney'.

To be good personally and do right is not enough. Down the ages, philosophers such as Socrates, Kant and Mill have wrestled with the problem of what *does* hold society together, and what *should* hold it together. Is it possible to legislate for morality? For example, a person's sexual morality may lead to illness; does the state then pick up the bill without question? How a child is brought up may be a couple's personal choice, but how does society deal with such problems as parental abuse, neglect and inadequacy?

The study of ethics is not only for those with time and the opportunity to speculate. It is acutely relevant to those, like nurses, with a 'hands-on' job and often little time to make life and death decisions. The challenge and difficulty of ethics is that it demands reason and reasoning against a setting of human frailty and vulnerability, of feelings and relationships which are stronger than will and mind. It is not in overlooking or avoiding one or other aspect that a decision can be reached or a stance taken. It is through listening, empathy and personal experience of conflict that we come to a decision, a sense of meaning and a capacity to help.

Beliefs, attitudes and values

Not only do different societies hold different values; each person holds unique values which differ from other people's. To know our own values means that we are more able to live with other people's values, and not expect them to conform to ours.

Belief

Belief is the most basic of the values a person holds. It is based more on faith than fact. A person believes that people are basically honest; that the earth is good to live on; that the economy will come right; that the NHS will survive. There is evidence against all these, but nevertheless the belief survives and drives a person to act according to that basic belief.

Attitudes

Out of belief come the attitudes which we hold about ourselves and others. The person who believes that people are basically honest treats all others as honest people and is honest with them. One of that person's attitudes may be to promote honesty. An attitude is not only something of the mind, but something which shows itself in action, particularly in the attitude to those who surround us.

Values

Our values are less fixed and more dynamic than either beliefs or attitudes. There is generally an element of motivation or goal in our values. A child's highest value may be play, an adolescent's, peer relationships. Young adults may be concerned with security in partnerships and work. The 'mid-life crisis' is characterised by often drastic changes of values.

Society, background, upbringing and training all shape our values. Our temperament shapes our values too. An extravert will want to be with people, to be the centre of attraction, and is happiest in a large ward with plenty going on around. An introvert gets most energy from being alone, will shun parties, and in hospital will probably keep very much to themselves.

The psychologist C.G. Jung (1964) recognised four different 'functions' by which people orient themselves through experience. '*Sensation* (i.e. sense perception) tells you that something exists; *thinking* tells you what it is; *feeling* tells you whether it is agreeable or not; and *intuition* tells you whence it comes and where it is going.' A person who is more sense-oriented values facts and experiences, is practical and down-to-earth. A person who is attuned to intuition, on the other hand, lives in anticipation, will see possibilities, and functions best with imagination and ingenuity. A thinking type of person prefers to make decisions on the basis of principles and analysis and will therefore often be a good judge, but may come across as cold and calculating. A feeling person will often work in a caring profession, and be working towards harmony, be devoted to people and look for humane and workable solutions.

Keirsey and Bates (1984) recognised another area where temperaments differ; that of judging and perceiving. 'Do I prefer endings and the settling of things or do I prefer to keep options open and fluid?' Given a deadline, a judging person (the words refer more to 'being orderly' than to making judgements) will 'get the show on the road', whereas a perceiving person tends to 'wait and see'.

This thumbnail sketch of different temperament types will give an idea of the vastness of possible values held by different people. Being of a certain temperament does not mean that a person cannot change; on the contrary, personal growth demands that we become at home in all the functions. This is one area where values change and vision is expanded.

Another way of knowing and learning the values which we hold is through experience. Frankl (1962) speaks of three types of values:

(1) *Creative* values, which we discover through what we do, particularly helping others

(2) *Experiential* values are those which we discover through appreciating people, events and artistic and natural beauty

(3) *Attitudinal* values are discovered through our reactions to circumstances over which we have no control, such as our own and other people's sufferings (see Table 13.1)

Table 13.1. *Values*

We *have* different values because of our different temperaments: Extravert – Introvert Sensing – Intuiting Thinking – Feeling Judging – Perceiving
We *discover* different values by: Doing a deed (creative values) Experiencing the value (experiential values) Suffering (attitudinal values)

Frankl is specific on two more points: we do not create our values, but we *discover* them; and values do not *push* us, but they *pull* us.

Nursing values

The basic personal and temperamental values are expressed through the work or profession someone chooses. Someone with strong person-oriented values is more likely to go into nursing than someone attracted by history and battles, or botany and the outdoor life.

The over-riding value in nursing must be care: the giving and receiving of caring.

The Canadian nurse-philosopher M. Simone Roach (1987) has distilled her thinking on caring into five component parts (Table 13.2). She believes that 'Caring is the human mode of being', that to be truly human is to care. A sick person is restored to health through care; and someone desperately needy is often restored to a sense of well-being by caring for someone yet more unfortunate.

Table 13.2. *The 'Five Cs' of caring*

Compassion
Competence
Confidence
Conscience
Commitment

The component parts of caring all start with the letter C. Compassion is the act of meeting the other where she or he is, and where it hurts. It is a kind of standing alongside, 'being there', not explaining and not identifying but allowing oneself to be touched by one's own vulnerability. This requires listening and hearing what a person is saying, in order to act compassionately, i.e. 'with passion'.

To act compassionately, and correctly, a person has to be competent. A nurse has to be skilled, but more than that. Giving an injection or doing a dressing can be done quite mechanically; doing it in such a way that the patient feels valued as a person is what competence is.

That sort of competence instils confidence. Caring is only effective when it is rooted in a relationship which is trusting, respecting and creative. Caring is not arbitrary, but is itself guided by human values. Conscience is the expression of relationships and responsibilities. Conscience is the moral awareness of responsibilities to self and others.

None of this would be possible without a commitment to the person, task or cause in question. This is highlighted very strongly in primary nursing (see Chapter 4). The nurse has made a commitment to the patient, and the patient or client is now in a relationship with the nurse which is based on a kind of contract, but also on the nurse's compassion, confidence and conscience.

This highlights another aspect of ethics which is often disregarded: the importance of feelings. Ethics tends to be seen as logical, rational and perhaps even detached acting. The more intangible aspects of feelings and relationships have tended to be seen as obstacles and interfering with logical decision-making. Yet this is what nurses are in touch with when they care for someone. These aspects bring another dimension to ethics: that of *holistic* relating.

Ethical models

Many nurses argue that ethics has little to do with them. 'Better to get on with the job than to crack one's head over theories,' they say. And while they rush to a patient whose intravenous infusion has stopped, another patient calls for a bedpan. Who gets their attention first? An ethical decision will have been made, but on what basis?

With more holistic and patient-centred care, nurses are rightly drawn into case discussions and their views are considered and valued. It is important in such situations to see the issues clearly, to listen carefully to all sides, and to combine reason – rational, theoretical arguments – with emotion – feelings, intuitions and compassion.

Traditionally two overall models of ethical theory have been described: *deontology* and *teleology*. Each theory stands logically on its own, but it is often not possible to follow one theory strictly, and many ethicists go above or beyond narrow theories.

Deontology

The word *deontology* comes from the Greek *deontos* meaning duty. This theory argues that there are basic duties and obligations with which people should conform. An action is not judged by its consequences, but is either right or wrong depending on whether it agrees with a moral principle or goes against it. Our actions are morally valid if we follow those rules and principles. The main question for deontologists is, 'What *ought* to be done in this situation?'

In 1987 the media made much of the case of a mentally handicapped 18-year-old girl, where the dilemma was whether or not she should be sterilised for her own protection. The deontological argument is to judge the action *itself*. Is it right to sterilise this person now? The answer according to this theory would probably be 'no', because there is no health reason for the operation. The risks accompanying operations, the girl's inability to understand what is happening and why, and the interference with her basic human rights argue against sterilisation from this standpoint.

Teleology

Teleology (from the Greek *telos*, end, result) considers an action in view of its consequences. Utilitarianism is a form of teleology which is based on the principle that an action is right if it brings the greatest happiness to the greatest number of people. An action is therefore morally right if its goal is what matters. A historical duty or obligation has no influence in this theory. The main questions are: 'What is the goal?' and 'Is the outcome good?'.

Viewed in this light, the 18-year-old girl should be sterilised if it means that her life will be made easier and better and that suffering will be prevented, both for her, her mother and a future unwanted child.

The concept of the NHS rests largely on utilitarian principles: to provide health care and treatment for all at the time of need is more desirable than to provide it only for those who can pay, or deserve it.

Other approaches

With these two theories largely cancelling each other out, it is not surprising that other approaches have been established. *Natural law ethics* is one such theory, which takes as its starting point the human rights: the right to life, liberty, happiness, etc. Any interference with bodily functioning is considered a violation of natural law. *Situation ethics* was popular in the 1960s and 1970s. This postulates a person-centred approach rather than a principle-centred ethic, and the main thrust is to enhance human creativity, encouraging all that contributes to personal life and freedom (Fletcher, 1967). A further notion, that of a *response ethic*, has been put forward by Niebuhr (1963). This approach stresses the meaning of responsibility. The main question posed by this method is not what ought to be done, or what is the goal, but, 'What is happening?'. The answer given – the response made – is based on the responsibility each party has to the other.

This theory rests on the premise that what we have in common is our humanity. In order to stay human (personally) and within humanity (socially) we have to act humanly. How we interpret that humanity colours our actions. Niebuhr stresses that we are creative and responsive human beings, and to remain human we have to be creative and responsive within a framework of freedom and fidelity. Roach's 'Five Cs' of caring fit particularly well into this approach to ethics.

Five ethical principles

The above theoretical models are wide-ranging and somewhat abstract. To use them on a day-to-day basis would involve a much deeper knowledge of their intricacies. In order to make these theories accessible, people have established *principles* which need to be considered when making ethical decisions. One such set of principles was established by Thiroux (1980) and they are outlined in Table 13.3. These principles are applicable to all walks of life but they can be adapted to suit particular spheres, such as nursing.

The Principle of the Value of Life

Thiroux starts with the Principle of the Value of Life. What we all have in common is life; without life there would be no 'goodness or badness, justice or injustice, honesty or dishonesty, freedom or lack of it' (Thiroux, 1980). Although we all have life, we each experience it in a way that is unique. This principle is analogous to the notion of the 'respect for persons' in other systems (Campbell, 1984; Gillon, 1986). Whenever such terms or concepts are used, one has to ask further: 'What do we mean by life, by respect, by personhood?'. It is immediately obvious that there are no black-and-white answers. It also becomes obvious that because of our individuality we all experience these concepts differently and use and apply them differently. When talking with colleagues and patients, we should therefore be wary of assuming that they use the term in the same way as we do. We see this immediately when we look at only one infringement of this principle: abortion.

A person's experience and values will influence

Table 13.3. *Principles of ethics*

The Principle of the Value of Life
Human beings should revere life and accept death

The Principle of Goodness or Rightness
We should strive to be 'good' human beings and attempt to perform 'right' actions

The Principles of Justice or Fairness
Attempts must be made to distribute the benefits from being good and doing right

The Principle of Truth Telling or Honesty
Meaningful communication – an absolute necessity in any moral system and any moral relationship – depends on truthfulness and honesty

The Principle of Individual Freedom
Individuals, with individual differences, must have the freedom to choose their own ways and means of being moral *within the framework of the first four basic principles*

his or her view of this subject. One person may see abortion as killing and murder, and wrong without any doubt. Another may argue that a fetus who is not capable of independent life is not a person, or at least not yet. 'Respect for the person' may not only mean that we do not take life, or do not interfere with another's life, but that we do not impose our views on another. Thus we see that this principle of the value of life is the basis not only for decisions about abortion, euthanasia, war, suicide and capital punishment, but also for such concepts as patient advocacy, responsibility and accountability.

By 'life' is not meant 'life at any cost'. In revering life, and the person who has life, we also accept that this life must someday end. With the ever-increasing debate about euthanasia, nurses will be confronted more and more with debates about and requests for active and passive euthanasia. On what grounds, then, does a nurse decide what to say and do? We need to have insight and awareness of our own values, feelings and an understanding of the facts to be able to argue a case.

The Principle of Goodness or Rightness

Morality and ethics are concerned with what is good and right, and what is bad and wrong. But *what* is good or acceptable when one person holds one set of values and another person holds others?

The emphasis which has been put on differing values is reflected in this dilemma. The American Declaration of Independence lists three such 'goods': 'life, liberty and the pursuit of happiness'. Some people may argue that the pursuit of happiness is egoistical, and that a greater good would be the pursuit of truth (or knowledge or peace or creativity). 'Good' cannot simply apply to abstract terms. Any good or right that we do is 'good' or 'right' in the context of human experience and in human relationships.

It can be argued that good and right are ideals, and that in daily life there are many times when we fall short of the ideal. This has been recognised particularly in medicine, where it is impossible only ever to do good. For many reasons, treatments and care are often second or even third best. In acknowledging this, medicine has established the principle of non-maleficence (i.e. doing no harm). This may seem a negative approach, but it is one that accepts the frailty of human beings and their systems (see the Principle of Justice or Fairness, below). Gillon (1986) suggests that 'we seem to have . . . a perfect duty to all other people not to harm them. On the other hand, we do not have a duty to benefit all other people'.

If goodness and rightness are ideals to strive for, then they can also be seen as calling forth the practice of virtue. Such practice of virtue leads not to smug self-satisfaction, but to creativity, harmony and integration in and between people.

The Principle of Justice or Fairness

Good and right do not stand alone; they have to be put into practice. Where there is harmony and integrity between people, there is also justice. What happens between two people should also happen between societies and nations. It is often argued that if those with a lot of money (their good) would give it to the poor, they (the poor) would become happy because they would also then be rich (the greatest good for the greatest number). It can be seen clearly, however, that this is not the case, because the values of both parties differ fundamentally.

Within health care, the Principle of Justice or Fairness is perhaps the most often quoted principle, as well as the most often violated and idealised. The concept of the NHS is that everybody who needs care or treatment gets it at the time of need. The assumption is that the government, the

health authorities and all with influence on the purse-strings of health care should ensure that this ideal is upheld. In the present climate of cut-backs, savings and rationalisation, this principle gets quickly distorted or disregarded. It becomes a case of fighting for and saving what one can, and priorities are decided not on the basis of who deserves something most but who can shout loudest. This may sound somewhat stark; however, in recent years there have been several cases where patients only got what they needed by appealing to the national press.

The philosopher Kant (1772–1804) is perhaps best known for his dictum, 'Treat every rational being, including yourself, always as an end and never as a mere means'. This implies respect for all human beings; it implies that good and right are done; it implies, above all, that justice is recognised as a basic way of life.

The Principle of Truth Telling or Honesty

This principle is probably the most difficult one to maintain or uphold. Human relationships are delicate, and to protect our vulnerability we have built up defences against exposing ourselves to others.

Many patients say that they can cope with bad news or difficult prognoses; what they cannot cope with is uncertainty and deception. Most patients do not need nurses and doctors to tell them the really bad news: they need nurses and doctors who listen to them while they express their feelings, fears and anger, regrets and hopes about what they have come to suspect. Such listening is not easy, because it involves the listener deeply, probably exposing her or his own inadequacies, and fear of saying and doing the wrong things. This is the underlying reason for the injunction not to 'tell' a particular patient. Patients have been driven to incredible feats in order to find out what their diagnosis and prognosis are.

If one has to give a patient an answer to a particularly difficult question, or to impart unasked-for news, the skill lies in the way the information is given. Respecting the patient, valuing him or her as a person, keeping in mind the good, and trying at least not to do harm, all this helps us to be aware of how such a conversation should be carried out. The challenge is not in how often one has to give bad news but in how often one has listened, and heard what that person said. We have a truth to give, but more importantly, we have a truth to hear and respect.

The Principle of Individual Freedom

Thiroux (1980) makes the point strongly that individual moral freedom is limited by the other four principles; that there is a necessity to protect and revere life, do good and prevent bad, treat human beings justly, tell the truth and be honest. In view of the astonishing variety of human values, needs, wants and concerns, this necessity is indeed powerful. We have individual freedom only so long as we do not harm someone in a serious way. A rapist cannot simply apply this principle to himself: the other four principles apply too, and in the light of all these, this 'freedom' of his is not legitimate.

Gillon (1986) makes a distinction between freedom, liberty, licence and doing what one wants to do, and acting autonomously, on the basis of thought or reasoning. A good act may become a virtuous act by the fact of having chosen freely to perform it in a particular way (autonomy as a nursing issue will be examined later).

Inglesby (1988) describes how one nurse respected a patient's beliefs and individuality:

'While working in a geriatric ward I often looked after a man from Jamaica with motor neurone disease. He refused to have his face washed every morning because the wind blowing through the doorway was in fact "a spirit who put dust in the water". He did not want the dust to go into his eyes and so refused to have water on his face.

At first I thought he was developing senility because for me this situation and his belief was unacceptable. I don't believe there are spirits in the air, nor harmful dust placed in the water by spirits, but I realised that the man, brought up in Jamaican culture, did genuinely believe in spirits. This particular spirit was a bad one and his dust could blind.

I could have dismissed the patient's fears and washed his face anyway, because I don't believe in invisible spirits. Alternatively, I could have respected his wishes and left his face alone. But on most mornings his face would need washing, because he could not feed himself very well, and breakfast cereal would stick around his mouth and chin.

I found that he and I could come to an agreement: he let me wash his face as long as I kept the water from his eyes. Sometimes, though, his eyes did need cleaning, and I did this after the matter was discussed with the patient.

We chose a time when the spirit was not in the vicinity!'

Freedom – liberty, autonomy – is 'built into' the human structure in the same way as life is. And like life, freedom is not an absolute: it functions only in relation to other people and other concepts.

These principles are not absolutes either, but they can serve as maps on a journey: guiding and directing the decision-making process.

Rights and responsibility

As a society we are more and more conscious these days of our rights. 'Consumer rights' has become a 'growth industry'. As citizens we expect to have the right to clean air and water, access to wholesome food, civil and criminal protection, education, and health care. These rights are on the whole universal.

Other rights, such as freedom of belief, speech and expression, freedom to organise, freedom from 'state violence', are not nearly as common, certainly not under repressive or totalitarian regimes.

Within these broad rights we hear more subtle rights expressed. In nursing and medicine we hear of the right for care, a child's right to love, the right to be heard, the right to refuse treatment, the right of the unborn child – among many other such rights.

One person's rights are another person's duties or responsibilities. What one person enjoys as a right depends on another person's performance of a specific duty. The patient's 'right to care' depends on the nurse's ability and skill, but more still on her willingness to perform her task in a humane, 'caring' way. Thus, 'the association of rights and duties is not a logical relationship but a moral one' (Chapman, 1980).

In a caring and professional relationship it is expected that the patient's interests must come first. This statement takes us into areas where it could be argued that doctors and nurses should then *not* treat a patient who attempted suicide, or that they should collude with requests for euthanasia. It is precisely in respecting the patient's freedom and requests that the responsibility to him lies. The responsible carer does not shrug her shoulders and walk off; rather, she hears the words of the request itself, and *in addition*, she hears what lies behind them. It is this 'extra', this willingness to respect the whole person, which is part of the special role and responsibility of nurses and carers.

In the present economic climate of health care where staff shortages are common, time is at a premium. Where time is scarce, good communication is even more scarce, because it takes time to say and hear what really matters.

Rights born out of frustration are not, however, 'real' rights. The person who has been kept waiting for hours in an outpatients department and claims his right to see the doctor on time; the patient who has had a series of operations and is still in pain; the nurse who asked for help with her workload and is dismissed: all these can claim a right to be heard, cared for, taken seriously. But these rights are temporary and correspond more to a want than a real fundamental need. It means that someone somewhere has not taken seriously his or her responsibility towards a fellow human being.

If one is concerned with 'logical' approaches only, then everyone will be out to get as much as they can; everyone will be concerned with their own rights. But the relationship between rights and responsibilities is not logical; rather, it is based on morality. We are not born ethical beings, but we become so. We have no intrinsic rights (apart from life and liberty) except those given to us by those who choose to act responsibly. The one who says, 'I have a right to . . .' depends on the one who says, 'I give . . .'. That giving, caring, sharing of what one has, is what makes a person moral, a 'human being'.

Codes of practice

The Code for Nurses, first issued by the International Council of Nurses in 1953 and revised twice, has stood unaltered since 1973. It declares that 'the fundamental responsibility of the nurse is fourfold: to promote health, to prevent illness, to restore health, and to alleviate suffering'. The international flavour of that Code is evident in its emphasis on health promotion and the nurse's 'responsibility for initiating and supporting action to meet the health and social needs of the public'.

The publication in 1983 of the first Code of Professional Conduct for the Nurse, Midwife and Health Visitor by the United Kingdom Central Council was a significant step forward for nursing in Britain. Wide discussions took place and many suggestions were made by nurses and incorporated into the second edition of the Code in 1984 and 1992 (UKCC, 1992; see Table 13.4).

A code of practice is not a legal document, but it gives direction and cohesion to the body for which it has been designed. The UKCC Code of Professional Conduct was drawn up at a time when difficulties were becoming more and more evident within nursing and within the NHS.

Such a code has to be wide enough to include many possibilities for action, but also specific enough to enable a nurse to apply it to her particular work. Ideally it should be a distillation of ethical theories and principles, put into a practical framework for action. When an ethical decision has to be made, a nurse should be able to follow the code and decide in which direction it points her or him.

Some of the more obvious areas of ethical concern for a society or profession (such as confidentiality, safety aspects, use and abuse of privilege, refusal of gifts and the use of qualifications for advertising) are expected to be covered in any code of practice. The areas in the UKCC Code which have caused the most concern and debate are the acknowledgement of any limitations of competence (Clause 4), regard to the environment of care (Clause 11) and regard to the workload of colleagues (Clause 13). With ever greater pressure on resources both of people and material, these clauses are significant.

The story related below is an example of what could happen anywhere in nursing, and of the various clauses of the Code which are infringed.

Two nurses on duty at night in a children's ward happened also to be very good friends. One of them had found one of the children, who was diabetic, to be sweating and looking very pale. After a quick blood sugar test which confirmed a hypoglycaemic coma, the child was transferred to the intensive care unit. The nurse was puzzled, and turned to her friend and colleague. This one grudgingly owned up to having given the child too much insulin earlier by mistake. She was not going to report it, fearing an inquiry and trouble, and expecting her friend not to report it either but to keep confidence

(Carlisle, 1991)

Table 13.4. *Code of Professional Conduct for the Nurse, Midwife and Health Visitor (UKCC, 1992. Reprinted with permission of the UKCC)*

Each registered nurse, midwife and health visitor shall act, at all times, in such a manner as to:

- **safeguard and promote the interests of individual patients and clients;**

- **serve the interests of society;**

- **justify public trust and confidence and**

- **uphold and enhance the good standing and reputation of the professions.**

As a registered nurse, midwife or health visitor, you are personally accountable for your practice and, in the exercise of your professional accountability, must:

(1)   Act always in such a manner as to promote and safeguard the interests and well-being of patients/clients

(2)   Ensure that no action or omission on your part or within your sphere of responsibility is detrimental to the interests, condition or safety of patients/clients

(3)   Maintain and improve your professional knowledge and competence

(4)   Acknowledge any limitations in your knowledge and competence and decline any duties or responsibilities unless able to perform them in a safe and skilled manner

(5)   Work in an open and co-operative manner with patients, clients and their families, foster their independence and recognise and respect their involvement in the planning and delivery of care

(6)   Work in a collaborative and co-operative manner with health care professionals and others involved in providing care, and recognise and respect their particular contributions within the care team

(7)   Recognise and respect the uniqueness and dignity of each patient and client, and respond to their need for care, irrespective of their ethnic origin, religious beliefs, personal attributes, the nature of their health problems or any other factor

(8)   Report to an appropriate person or authority, at the earliest possible time, any conscientious objection which may be relevant to your professional practice

(9)   Avoid any abuse of your privileged relationship with patients and clients and of the privileged access allowed to their person, property, residence or workplace

(10)   Protect all confidential information concerning patients and clients obtained in the course of professional practice and make disclosures only with consent, where required by the order of a court or where you can justify disclosure in the wider public interest

(11)   Report to an appropriate person or authority, having regard to the physical, psychological and social effects on patients and clients, any circumstances in the environment of care which could jeopardise standards of practice

(12)   Report to an appropriate person or authority any circumstances in which safe and appropriate care for patients and clients cannot be provided

(13)   Report to an appropriate person or authority where it appears that the health or safety of colleagues is at risk, as such circumstances may compromise standards of practice and care

(14)   Assist professional colleagues, in the context of your own knowledge, experience and sphere of responsibility, to develop their professional competence, and assist others in the care team, including informal carers, to contribute safely and to a degree appropriate to their roles

(15)   Refuse any gift, favour or hospitality from patients or clients currently in your care which might be interpreted as seeking to exert influence to obtain preferential consideration and

(16)   Ensure that your registration status is not used in the promotion of commercial products or services, declare any financial or other interests in relevant organisations providing such goods or services and ensure that your professional judgement is not influenced by any commercial considerations

Safeguarding the interests of patients and clients is and must be the nurse's main duty. But there is no mention in the Code of safeguarding the interests of best friends and senior colleagues. Neither can the Code be used as a document for defence when things have gone wrong.

In addition to and supplementing the Code, the UKCC has published a number of *Advisory Documents*: on Advertising (1985), Administration of Medicines (1986), Confidentiality (1987), Exercising Accountability (1989) and *The Scope of Professional Practice*. These documents elaborate the relevant clauses in the Code of Professional Conduct and aim to give more specific guidelines than is possible in the Code itself.

Making ethical decisions

It seems that the difference between a problem and a dilemma is that a problem can be solved, but a dilemma is a choice between two or more equally impossible positions. In ethics we are often in such impossible situations. We can think particularly of the case of a mother with several children already and pregnant again. Should she have an abortion or not? Or a newborn baby with Down's syndrome and other abnormalities. Should the child be operated on or not? A choice is almost impossible.

Although in many instances time is of the essence for reaching a decision, it is often not so urgent that good and thorough discussion cannot take place. Then again, this may be difficult because the persons concerned are understandably anxious and perhaps not able to be as objective as might be desired. It is therefore the more imperative that those such as nurses, who help a patient to come to a decision, are able to be clear and matter of fact, *and* empathic.

Any decision reached will have gone through a process. Nurses are familiar with the four steps of the nursing process, and these same steps can apply to making ethical decisions.

For a decision to be reached, all the alternatives have to be examined; each alternative has to be seen in terms of possible solutions; a decision will have to be reached and carried out; and eventually an evaluation of this will also need to take place.

Let us look at these steps of the decision-making process in the light of the example given in Fig.13.1. Imagine that the staff nurse takes Mr James to a quiet place and systematically works through the four steps of the decision-making process with him.

Mrs Annie James, aged 49, has been getting progressively weaker following a mastectomy 18 months earlier. She had had several episodes in hospital following pathological fractures and also hypercalcaemia. Each time, she was very low but rallied remarkably. This time, though, she seemed not to respond well, and her husband was particularly upset to see her with drips and tubes. They had not exactly talked about her dying but had concentrated more on living. Mrs James was now not really able to hold a conversation, but her expression had something of a plea which Mr James interpreted as 'I've had enough'. He asked a staff nurse, with whom he had formed a good relationship, if he should ask the doctor that the drip be removed and that his wife be left to die peacefully and without 'heroics'. The staff nurse was not surprised by this question, and she could see how he was in two minds, as his wife had always rallied before. She cannot make the decision for him, but she can help him to come to a decision himself.

Fig. 13.1 *Profile: Mrs Annie James*

Step one: assessment

— Mr James is unsure, in two minds, but would like the nurse to help him to make a decision.
— The issue is whether he should ask the doctor to remove the drip and stop treatments for his wife or whether to continue. At this stage he is asking the nurse to help him make up his mind about the next step. (It is important to hear clearly what is asked, as only this will lead to appropriate responses. The implication is that Mr James is asking for euthanasia for his wife; this may be the next step, and will have to be considered as it will colour the decision to see the doctor or not.)
— What are the main reasons for Mr James asking the nurse to help him make up his mind?
— What does Mr James feel in the pit of his stomach as he talks to his wife? to the nurse now? to his friends and family?
— Can he say all he wants to say, i.e. does he trust the nurse enough?
— Are there relevant things he wants or needs to say now, even if they seem out of place, or trivial?
— What does he feel his relationship with his wife is now?
— Does he or the nurse feel they are trespassing on any laws or values, or religious precepts?
— Does he feel he himself can live with his decision?

— Who might support him — now and in the future?
— Is a drip considered overtreatment, or inappropriate treatment?
— What other treatments are involved, and to what extent?
— Has the problem become urgent recently, or is it a long-standing problem?
— If no decision is taken either way, how long might it take until Mrs James either recovers or dies?
— Would this time be considered reasonable and could Mr James cope with it?
— How does Mr James interpret his wife's expression?
— Are there other signs which might lead him to think he is correct?
— What does he think his wife *feels*?
— Has Mrs James talked to any nurses about her condition? What did she say? What did they *hear*?
— Who else is involved: children, family, friends?
— What is the role of the nurses and doctors perceived to be?
— Who is considered to be the key person in making a decision? (Mr James hinted that it might be the doctor.)
— How would all the various people be involved? What would they have to do?
— Could any aspect of a decision be made easier? How?
— Have any of the people involved been in a similar situation before? What can they contribute from their experience?
— What is different in this situation from others known?
— Are there any other factors to be considered which have not yet been mentioned?

Step two: planning

— What are the possible solutions?
— Could anything else be changed now, or later?
— Who would be helped most by either solution, or outcome?
— Does Mr James need more time to think and talk through the issues, or is a decision urgent?
— Which of the ethical principles is particularly questioned: the value of life; goodness; justice; truth; freedom?
— Is it important to know this for allaying future guilt and misunderstanding?

— Is there any professional responsibility questioned or involved?
— Do the values which nurses and doctors hold clash or interfere with those of Mr and/or Mrs James?
— Is a compromise called for?
— Is anyone going to be hurt by a particular decision? Who? In what way? Who is going to be hurt least? Most?
— Are there other possibilities and decisions which have not yet been clarified?
— What is the goal of all these careful deliberations?
— Which is the best solution?

Step three: implementation

— Who has to take what action?
— Is that person now ready to take that action? (It may mean doing nothing, but having to live with that decision *is* an action too.)

Step four: evaluation

— Has the decision solved the problem?
— If not, why not?
— Were the predicted outcomes realistic?
— If not, why not?
— Does the problem still stand? How? Where is it?
— Which particular issues are or were crucial?
— How do the people involved now feel?
— Was this an isolated problem, or is it a common one?
— If it occurs regularly, what can be learnt from this situation?
— What should or could be changed in similar situations?
— Who should make changes?
— What are they?
— How realistic are they?

It must be clear that in most situations where ethical decisions have to be made, it is impossible to go through this process in this way. The point of outlining such a process is that it can be a stimulus or an *aide-memoire* for a nurse when in such a situation, helping her to be aware that there *is* a process a person goes through, and that the nurse can help to make this easier by asking a few relevant questions rather than making assumptions or imposing her own value system.

This basic model can apply in any process where ethical decisions have to be made. It can be seen that for such decisions to be reached, there needs to be:

(1) both rational thinking and empathy to understand the feelings involved;
(2) good communication, based on truth and honesty;
(3) a sense that the outcome should be good, and that harm has been avoided;
(4) respect to be shown for the individuals' lives;
(5) respect for the individuals' freedom, values and beliefs;
(6) evaluation of an outcome, so that justice should be more readily applicable in similar situations.

Thus it is possible to see how all the theory so far mentioned is relevant to nursing, and to the process of making ethical decisions.

Some ethical issues concerning patients

The advances in medicine in recent years have not been wholly beneficial. Every new treatment or discovery has also brought new questions and new concerns.

It is often claimed that nurses (and doctors and the public) do not recognise ethical situations when they meet them. It is possible to say that anything which infringes any one of the ethical principles is therefore an ethical situation. Some issues have, however, been particularly evident in recent years.

Informed consent

In her book *Whose Body Is It?*, Carolyn Faulder (1985) takes the whole notion of consent to pieces. In her view, informed consent consists first of all of *the right to know*, but then also of *the right to say no*.

It is a reflection both of communication and memory that many patients do not know what they are actually signing in a consent form for operation. Byrne, Napier and Cuschieri (1988) asked 100 consecutive patients (with an average age of 55 years) having operations in a Scottish surgical unit, '2–5 days post-operatively, what had been done to which organ. 27 did not know which organ had been operated on, and 44 did not know what procedure had been performed. Those who did not know were 12–13 years older (average age 63 years) than those who did know'.

When the consent of the patient or client is not sought for any treatment or intervention, that person's life is devalued. A paternalistic stance is taken; truth telling or honesty is compromised; trust is lost; individual freedom cannot be exercised: in other words, harm is done. This may not be blatantly obvious at first, but the slow erosion of confidence is more damaging than a frank admission of uncertainty over the outcome of a treatment.

It is difficult to measure consent, and the degree to which it is really informed. In an effort to clarify the meaning of the word 'consent', not only has the adjective 'informed' been used, but also 'true', 'educated', 'responsible'. This shows the real concern that underlies this area of care.

It is sometimes argued that it is impossible to give a patient or client *all* the facts needed to make an informed or educated decision, as really only the expert has all the accompanying facts. It can equally be argued that the information *given* will help the patient to decide as the doctor or nurse desires, for if the information which is *withheld* were also given, the patient may decide not to cooperate.

Informed consent does not only cover medical information. It also covers nursing information, and increasingly also information about alternative and complementary therapies.

Confidentiality

The notion of confidentiality rests on trust. The principle of the value of life (respect for the person) and individual freedom come particularly into play here, as do the principles of truth telling and goodness or rightness. With greater emphasis on the counselling role of the nurse has also come a greater responsibility to respect and guard the information gained in this way.

The question is, 'What is confidentiality?' and, 'What is confidential material?'.

The purely legal aspects of confidentiality concern particularly the patient's case notes and the forms signed before anaesthetic and operation. The UKCC advisory document on Confidentiality (1987) lists four categories under which information may be disclosed:

(a) with the consent of the patient/client;
(b) without the consent of the patient/client when the disclosure is required by law or order of a court;
(c) by accident;
(d) without the consent of the patient/client when the disclosure is considered necessary in the public interest.

This last category will present most difficulty, as it covers issues such as child abuse, drug use or trafficking or other illegal acts perpetrated by patients/clients.

Confidentiality is a complex issue which is easily overlooked and easily breached. It is an issue over which nurses are often in conflict with doctors. Nurses are not meant to be spies, but they also need to be on their guard that patients' rights are neither infringed nor taken for granted (Tschudin, 1992).

New treatments

Ethical issues only arise at the fringes of care and treatment, when the new is not (yet) integrated. Thus it can be said that operations and anaesthetics were once on the borderline but have now become established practice. At present, certain transplants are on the borderline, such as the recent innovation of using fetal tissue transplants for Parkinson's disease which has presented medicine with a new challenge. This is very good news for the patients concerned, but it has brought with it new ethical questions. How is a fetus obtained? Is the mother aware of – let alone consenting to – the use of the fetal tissue?

The use of so-called 'spare-part surgery' is equally debatable; how far can or should it be pursued?

The accompanying concern to advances is usually that of economics: can we (the country through taxes or the health authority through allocation and charging fees) afford it? Does it mean that one person is expensively kept alive where others only benefit from cheaper treatments?

There will never be clear-cut lines drawn and decisions will rest with individual patients, nurses, doctors and administrators. Nurses are, however, in a strong position to influence such decision-making.

Clinical trials

Much has been written and said about clinical trials: how they ought to be done; who can do them; what their aim is.

Nurses will inevitably be asked in the course of their work to take part in trials of many kinds. This is right and good, but they should have a healthy suspicion, and not agree to take part before they have assured themselves of certain points. Among these are:

(1) What sort of a trial is it: historical or randomised?
(2) Is the trial really necessary?
(3) Has the trial been approved by an ethics committee?
(4) Does the hospital/health authority have an ethics committee to which the nurse can refer her concerns in case of doubt or difficulty? The Department of Health has issued a booklet entitled *Local Research Ethics Committees* (1991) which lays a duty on district health authorities to establish Local Research Ethics Committees (LRECs) which 'should have eight to twelve members . . . drawn from both sexes and from a wide age group, (and) should include hospital medical staff, nursing staff, general practitioners, (and) two or more lay persons' (HSG(91)5).
(5) Who will benefit (the patient or some statistician)?
(6) Are the patients informed about the trial? If so, how?
(7) How much of the nurse's time and skill is involved?
(8) Could it bring the nurse into situations of conflict over loyalty to her patients?

These are some of the basic issues involved. Each trial brings with it its own questions. To be professional, nurses need to question what is being done to patients in the name of science and research. Only by doing this can they ensure that the best care is given.

Some ethical issues concerning nurses

Many of the ethical issues which concern nurses have already been mentioned, and again only a few can be touched upon here. For some nurses some issues are not a problem, while for others many more issues are real problems. Individuality is not a handicap, but a stimulus to greater creativity. These issues can be seen to relate particularly to rights and responsibilities.

Conscientious objection

An act of conscientious objection or civil disobedience is non-cooperation with the law. In nursing this applies at present only to abortion. The Abortion Act 1967 has a 'conscience clause' on which objection can be officially based. The UKCC Code of Professional Conduct (1992) (Clause 8) makes it a duty for the nurse to declare such objections.

Abortion is not a 'treatment' in law and that is why a nurse can object to taking part. However, she has no grounds in law to withhold legitimate *treatment* from any patient based on the patient's lifestyle, race, sex, age, political or social status, and her objection to any of them. A nurse cannot object legally to assisting in electro-convulsive therapy, nor to caring for patients with HIV or AIDS, nor to giving medically prescribed treatments to a dying patient, even though she has personal, religious or emotional objections.

Yet caring effectively for patients often means standing at the boundary of the possible and the impossible. Many changes in care have come about because nurses broke through the boundary and risked their security, reputation and even promotion. Those who do object to treatments for whatever reason must weigh up their decisions carefully. The outcome may be satisfaction, but then again it may not.

Advocacy

An advocate is one who pleads the cause of another. This implies that the other cannot do this for himself or herself. It is therefore particularly important to be clear why and how a patient cannot speak for himself. This is really only the case in severe physical or mental illness. But people who are unassertive or ignorant of facts need help with *that* first.

To be able truly to be an advocate, argues Walsh (1985), nurses would need to be independent. As soon as sides are taken, a split in loyalty arises. Like Walsh, Webb (1987) sees advocacy ideally as self-advocacy, in that the role of the nurse is 'to inform the client and then to support him in whatever decision he makes'. In the example of Mrs Annie James, the husband can be seen as her advocate, and the nurse as the advocate of Mr James.

The areas in which nurses can act as advocates on behalf of patients concern:

(a) the quality of care corresponding to the principles of the value of life and of goodness or rightness;
(b) the access to care by patients, corresponding to the principle of justice;
(c) the information regarding care received by patients, corresponding to the principle of truth telling or honesty;
(d) any alternatives to care open to patients corresponding to the principle of individual freedom.

In order to be effective advocates, nurses need to be good communicators. To be advocates, they need to be well versed in a variety of disciplines, in particular ethics, and also know where their limits are so that they know when they overstep them positively or negatively.

Accountability

Accountability is often linked with economy and saving money, but this is rather too narrow a view of the term.

Accountability arises directly out of responsibility. To be able to be accountable, a nurse must have an authority to act. This can be an authority based on conscience and ethical values (moral accountability) or that based on professional competence (legal accountability). In either case there must be a basis in knowledge, which can be explained and defended (Binnie, 1984). In making ethical decisions – being accountable for oneself and responsible to others – it can be seen that it isn't enough to say, 'I just feel that something is right/wrong'.

Accountability is not only having an answer

when something goes wrong, but it is a continuous process of monitoring of personal and professional values. Self-knowledge is therefore a basic requirement, not only for self-growth and self-improvement, but also to be put at the service of those who require care. Personal responsibility is expressed in professional accountability.

Professional autonomy

Nursing can probably never become an independent profession because it cannot function apart from medicine, physiotherapy, dietetics and many other disciplines. By establishing its own research basis, however, it has gained a large measure of independence. This can only be good – for patients, for nurses, and for the profession. The more that nurses can contribute themselves to their own working conditions and environment, the more they will also be satisfied with their work.

Autonomy is inevitably linked with power: who has the last word; where does the buck stop? It is not power *over* others that should be aimed at, but power *with* others. Professional autonomy which dominates cannot be respected; autonomy which is shared and is fair and just should be a task for nurses on an intellectual and practical level (Jameton, 1984).

With the increasing use of primary nursing and key workers, nurses are taking upon themselves a degree of autonomy which may still be alien to many of them. Used correctly and effectively, primary nurses do not have any more 'power' than other nurses, but they share their knowledge and skills with their patients in a partnership. Thus the ideal of an ethic of nursing, based on caring and relationship, is enhanced. In this way also, ethical decisions are not taken in splendid isolation, with the nurse carrying all the responsibility: more personal caring will mean more discussion, more listening, more empathy – and more open and shared decision-making.

Two current issues

Limited resources

The media are often quick to highlight how much or how little Britain spends on health care. It seems that most other industrialised countries spend more. It seems also that however much is spent, it will never be enough.

The present economic system places great emphasis on efficient and effective use of resources and cost reductions where possible. This, as nurses know to their cost, can sometimes go too far. Mistakes may be made, people may feel too pressured and become ill, and care may be reduced to essentials only. A vicious circle then starts when more care is needed more often with ever less means.

Private health care

The economic system has created more personal wealth and so, the argument goes, people should now pay for their health care. Taking more responsibility for one's own health is therefore encouraged.

The perception is that private health care helps to relieve the long waiting lists in hospitals. People get more individual attention and, because they are better informed, better cared for, and take more interest in their health when they pay for it, patients stay in private hospitals for shorter periods and recover more quickly.

These are just two issues which concern every nurse and doctor, and every patient and potential patient. Is there an answer to the problem? Is it even a problem which can be seen in terms of a solution?

Conclusions

Looking back over this chapter and over the points raised, we may come to some conclusions, if not solutions.

An introduction to philosophy was given on the basis of values. Ethics and morality are based on what is good and right. But that may not be enough, and 'excellence' (according to Thiroux, 1980) should be an accompanying factor. Good and right should also exist equally for all: that is, justice should be seen to be done, not only exist as a principle. When, because of limited resources, justice cannot be administered with total fairness, some will always get the bigger share of the cake. The question of priorities therefore comes into play: will it be the cancer patient, the child, or the hip operations performed? It may not be a question of doing good so much as how harm can be avoided, particularly for those who cannot shout or who have no strong advocates, like elderly people or those who are mentally handicapped and ill. Indeed, would these people benefit from advocates? Truthfulness has a strange habit of turning up in unexpected situations, and it may not be a question of advocacy, but of justice. That leads to rights: people have a right to expect and get care, but not at any price. People should not be used as means to ends. Private health care may

be a good thing in itself, but only if it is not used as a means to overlooking the more stark inequalities.

If 'caring is the human mode of being' (Roach, 1987), then caring is what matters most of all. Nurses have always seen caring as their particular hallmark. This caring, characterised by listening and respecting the other and working from within a committed relationship, will enhance both the patient/client *and* the nurse. This is indeed an *ideal*, but after all only ideals attract the highest human values.

References

Binnie, A. (1984). *A Systematic Approach to Nursing Care*. Open University Press, Milton Keynes.

Byrne, D.J., Napier, A. and Cuschieri, A. (1988). How informed is signed consent? *Institute of Medical Ethics Bulletin*, 37, 3.

Campbell, A.V. (1984). *Moral Dilemmas in Medicine* (3rd ed.). Churchill Livingstone, Edinburgh. (page 91ff)

Carlisle, D. (1991). Protecting patients. *Nursing Times*, 87(8), 52–53.

Chapman, C.M. (1980). The rights and responsibilities of nurses and patients. *Journal of Advanced Nursing*, 5, 127–134.

Department of Health. (1991). *Local Research Ethics Committees*. Available from DoH Store, Health Publications Unit, No.2 Site, Manchester Road, Heywood OL10 2PZ.

Faulder, C. (1985). *Whose Body Is It?* Virago Press, London.

Fletcher, J. (1967). *Moral Responsibility: Situation Ethics at Work*. SCM Press, London.

Frankl, V. (1962). *Man's Search for Meaning*. Pocket Books, New York. (page 101)

Gillon, R. (1986). *Philosophical Medical Ethics*. John Wiley and Sons, Chichester.

Inglesby, E. (1988). Moral matters. *Nursing Times*, 84(19), 49.

Jameton, A. (1984). *Nursing Practice: The Ethical Issues*. Prentice-Hall International, New Jersey.

Jung, C.G. (1964). *Man and His Symbols*. Picador, London. (page 49)

Keirsey, D. and Bates, M. (1984). *Please Understand Me*. Prometheus Nemesis Book Co., Del Mar, California. (page 22)

Niebuhr, H.R. (1963). *The Responsible Self*. Harper and Row, New York.

Roach, M.S. (1987). *The Human Act of Caring*. Canadian Hospital Association, Ottawa.

Thiroux, J. (1980). *Ethics; Theory and Practice*. Glencoe Publishing Co., Encino, California.

Tschudin, V. (1992). *Ethics in Nursing: The Caring Relationship* (2nd ed.). Butterworth-Heinemann, Oxford.

United Kingdom Central Council for Nursing, Midwifery and Health Visiting. (1985). *Advertising*. UKCC, London.

UKCC. (1986). *Administration of Medicines*. UKCC, London.

UKCC. (1987). *Confidentiality*. UKCC, London.

UKCC. (1989). *Exercising Accountability*. UKCC, London.

UKCC. (1992). *Code of Professional Conduct* (3rd ed.). UKCC, London.

UKCC. (1992). *The Scope of Professional Practice*. UKCC, London.

Walsh, P. (1985). Speaking up for the patient. *Nursing Times*, 81(18), 24–26.

Webb, C. (1987). Speaking up for advocacy. *Nursing Times*, 83(34), 33–35.

Suggestions for further reading

Benjamin, M. and Curtis, J. (1986). *Ethics in Nursing* (2nd ed.). Oxford University Press, New York.

Fuchs, V.R. (1983). *Who Shall Live?* Basic Books, New York.

Jennett, B. (1986). *High Technology Medicine*. Oxford University Press, Oxford.

Rachels, J. (1986). *The End of Life : Euthanasia and Morality*. Oxford University Press, Oxford.

Rowson, R.H. (1990). *An Introduction to Ethics for Nurses*. Scutari, Harrow.

Seedhouse, D. (1988). *Ethics, the Heart of Health Care*. John Wiley and Sons, Chichester.

Thompson, I.E., Melia, K.M. and Boyd, K.M. (1983). *Nursing Ethics*. Churchill Livingstone, Edinburgh.

Wells, R.J. (1989). Ethics, informed consent and confidentiality. In *Nursing the Patient with Cancer*, Tschudin, V. (ed.). Prentice Hall, Hemel Hempstead.

14

DEVELOPING THE 'PERSON' OF THE PROFESSIONAL CARER

Paul Barber

This chapter is for those who give care and as such is a source of support for the reader. It offers ways of developing further insight into, and understanding of, how we may care for ourselves and others.

The author leads the reader from an analysis of what happens in the real world of caring to an exploration of ways of developing personal insights and understanding of how we may facilitate care for ourselves and for others. Throughout the chapter value is placed on the *person*, whether the giver or receiver of health care.

The themes of personal and professional growth and development feature throughout the work.

The chapter includes reference to and discussion of:

- Ways nurses function, survive and protect themselves from stress

- Factors which may influence care and the nurse-patient relationship

- Processes of understanding and change as they affect the way care is perceived and given

- Ways of 'seeing' and understanding reality. Reference is made to transactional analysis, qualities of care and adaptation which may lead

to changes and growth within the individual

- Ways of 'being', of being receptive, open to each other and self-aware

- The inter-relationship between thinking, feeling and sensing. This is followed by detailed consideration of styles of facilitation and intervention and their place in health care

The author leaves the reader with a profound message – to know and understand ourselves is the way to the understanding and care of others.

Personal development cannot be separated from professional development; each rests upon the other. Show me how well you share of yourself, understand your own interpersonal processes and are able to communicate this to others, and I'll know how good or bad your nursing care is.

The insights of this chapter have been hard won. As a student nurse I felt devalued and vulnerable, a small cog in the hospital machine. I did not feel listened to by senior colleagues, my questions remained unanswered and my concern with professional 'survival' seemed to displace any aspirations I had towards personal **growth**. Eventually I 'learnt the ropes' and started to develop the area that gave me the greatest satisfaction, namely, my ability to express myself through 'care'. Strangely enough, though care was said to be at the root of nursing, I saw little demonstrated. As a nurse amongst other nurses I felt uncared for. As a staff nurse I voiced my views with more confidence; I also met much resistance. As a charge nurse the fight was really on and I became aware of the enormous influence brought to bear by the institution on those who dare to suggest change. My resilience owed less to my skills than to my stubbornness. Eventually I read more, met other dissatisfied carers, and in sharing, started to develop my own conceptual framework. I try to share a little of this in what follows.

Much of my own growth appears like a letting-go of my defences – rather than the gaining of new skills – as if by unclogging my perceptions I started to appreciate others and care for myself with more honesty. As an educator and therapist I have let go of a lot more. In recent years I have reflected on my earlier journey as a student nurse and begun to value how much my clients and students have taught me. This work is theirs as much as it is mine.

Surviving (the nurse as an untherapeutic agent)

Historically, nursing has rarely been viewed as being a maturing or sensitising influence, in fact, often the reverse (Altschul, 1972; Ashworth, 1980).

Entrants to the profession are observed to commence full of questions, enthusiastic and committed to the ethic of care, but by the time of registration the brighter and more inquisitive amongst their number tend to have left under a cloud of frustration, and those who stayed have done so at a cost, such as a loss of humour, person sensitivity and self-worth (Olsen and Whittaker, 1961). This is sad, for much potential for personal development exists within nursing. All the ingredients are there; nurses face those natural crises of life that further character development, they have responsibility for the care of other individuals, and are required to develop personal and relationship skills within their work. They also have a team available to support and counsel them. This is the potential; it is not the fact, for most nurses are encouraged by their work climate to act contrary to the ideal and divorce themselves from their clients' crises, fear to accept and use their responsibility, are undeveloped in areas of personal skill, have blunted sensitivities, suffer constant interpersonal stress and are unsupported by colleagues.

Nursing makes incessant demands upon an individual's reserves of counselling and relationship skill, both of which are largely ignored in **traditional** patterns of basic training (Lamond, 1974).

Nurses work in areas where disease, death, personal loss and the anxieties which arise from these are commonplace; but they are ill prepared to shape 'therapeutically', or to learn interpersonally from, such life crises. Consequently, nurses are more likely to block off their person sensitivity, displace their attention from themselves onto tasks at hand and turn a blind eye to the lessons and wisdom available to them.

Displacement and **denial** are natural defences when individuals are thrown into insecure situations without the necessary skills – and relationship skills were, until comparatively recently, glaringly absent from most training curricula.

In unsafe environments 'survival skills' appear to be more necessary than growth-inducing ones. In nursing, survival mechanisms have all too often triumphed over other features of learning. When you feel insecure and vulnerable you are apt to grip too tightly onto practicalities, focus upon the details of your role and place an inordinate degree of effort in maintaining your professional **status** and personal distance. Everything is viewed as needing a firm outline. There is no time for abstract conceptual reflection. Security is perceived as emanating from tangibles, well-designated roles and maintenance of 'what is' rather than speculation upon 'what might be'. Concerns with 'structure', 'status', and the use of 'power' then come to overshadow relationships.

Undercurrents of **crisis management** and the drawing-up of protective boundaries around nurses frustrate their learning. Anything new is viewed as a threat. In order to learn, individuals must first let go of their prejudices, risk a little uncertainty and appreciate that some discomfort is required as a natural process of 'releasing the old' to 'let in the new'. Discomforts such as these may be equated with 'growing pains', those feelings of unfamiliarity when you leave the tried and tested parts of your life behind a little before the new role you attempt to play becomes you.

'Growing pains' may take us by surprise, producing those fresh awarenesses and confusions that accompany times of transition; when we go for an interview, start a new job or attempt something risky. Simply, they are states of emotional energy we may draw upon to achieve a little extra sensitivity. They are common to the newly qualified staff nurse who first takes charge of a ward.

Too many people view their emotions as 'symptoms' rather than 'energies'. Emotions threaten intellectual clarity; thinking becomes less clear as feelings draw attention to bodily sensations. As most of us have been taught to think – but not to feel – we may see feelings as getting in the way.

Social life is dependent upon a taught reality maintained via right thinking and cultural values.

Professions likewise emphasise an intellectual 'taught reality' which is dependent upon clear thinking. This is no mean thing. Education of the intellect is essential, but, we must retain perspective; intellectual cognition is but a feature – not the essence – of an individual. There are other realities open to us associated with feeling, our physical senses, and that ever hard to define perceptive organ we term **intuition**. Nurses need to value all these differing orientations to reality if they are fully to appreciate the situation and sensibilities of their clients.

'Patients' are people who are thrust into strange surroundings while undergoing a crisis of living; intellectual clarity does not come easily to them. An appreciation of emotional and intuitive functioning must be at the fore of care assessment, caring interventions and evaluation.

During times of crisis when unruly emotional energies pervade us, we see ourselves as powerless; depression may ensue as our energies reach a low ebb and we become subject to recriminative and self-deprecative thinking. At our most stressed we may regress to childlike states where we are pre-occupied with our intuitions and a world of fantasy, and if brought before psychiatrists may – even at this time – be labelled 'psychotic' and in need of care.

To recognise these states in clients is but half the story. Nurses need to be in touch with their own *thinking*, *sensing*, *feeling* and *intuitive* processes and have some understanding of how these may be therapeutically shaped to solicit health. This is what holistic models of nursing request of the nurse (Rogers, 1970).

Nurses *must* work towards evolving a sensitivity to the above processes within themselves if they are to develop empathy. The word 'must' is emphasised, for without movement into these areas the nursing profession can never progress. Time after time enquiries have been produced, reports implemented and re-organisations acted upon within our care institutions, but apart from a little tarting up of instrumental activity and the managerial or educational structure, little has really changed. You don't create lasting change from merely placing an old ingredient into a new box. Nursing has been subject to re-appraisal and many oddly shaped new wrappings, but its core has been little touched.

The *nursing process* promises to change all this, not so much in its watered down form of producing ever more records and making the nurse into a ward clerk, but in its more creative mode where the 'process' becomes a socially alert, interpersonal one.

When nurses come to appreciate the full implication of their role as social interactors, perhaps then 'process' changes will be enacted within the profession so that nursing education will be centred and 'growth-orientated', and personnel development will supersede the imposition of systems of control in nursing management. If we fail to 'care for care givers' or to counsel and develop **experientially** the 'humanity' of our new entrants to the profession, where will they find a 'role model' of caring from which to learn?

Nursing can be a caring experience for client and carer alike and solicit personal development in each. This is no pipe dream; we have the necessary knowledge base (Barber, 1990), the skills have been developed (Barber and Dietrich, 1985), and the care climate is ripe for change (UKCC, 1986), but first, let us contemplate the costs to the profession if these features remain unimplemented and we go on as before.

Harming (the nurse as a persecutor)

Self-worth and personal competence take quite a battering in professional preparation. Before an individual can 'professionally belong' they must survive numerous 'rites of passage' – the least of which may be formal examinations – before they become accepted by their colleagues. Dealing with sudden death and handling oneself during crises, counselling relatives, and balancing the conflicting demands of client and institution all relate to this. Proving oneself personally and building emotional competence is all part of the hidden agenda, but you are usually left to your own devices to achieve this.

Facilitating the care of others is a taxing science and an exhausting art. Professions which are empowered to cater for, monitor and/or control the casualties of society take a great deal of stress onto themselves (Edelwich and Brodsky, 1980). Acting as professional parents on society's behalf, nurses receive all the conflict associated with parenting and parenthood. They may be over-invested with responsibility by society and those who employ them, be expected to demonstrate unrealistic levels of expertise even when poorly resourced, and akin to all parents be apportioned undue blame when those they care for deteriorate. In the same way that we distanced ourselves from our parents to acquire adulthood, so our clients may need to reject us to achieve a better sense of their own independence. In this sense the care relationship is often experienced as intrusive and intimate for nurse and client alike, and too close for comfort.

The price of holding an authoritative position and the personal cost of this in terms of intrapersonal dis-ease is nowhere more intense nor better attested than within nursing (Menzies, 1960; Barber, 1991). Indeed, nursing provides us with a lesson as to how the best of intentions may, due to relational stress, end in harm.

Glancing through the nursing journals, one meets glaring examples of insensitive social practice. As I write this account I pause to pick an old *Nursing Times* from a pile near my desk. Inside I find two examples. In an article entitled 'Facing up to disfigurement', Pamela Holmes (1986) describes the case of a girl in her twenties who needed surgery for two brain tumours. 'Her face was badly disfigured and it didn't help that her hair had been shaved off. Anxious about seeing her mother for the first time since this traumatic surgery, the girl approached the ward sister to ask if there was anything that could be done to improve her looks. The sister, who was standing in a group of student nurses, suggested she "put a bucket on her head".' Later in the same article, a client describes her experience of returning to the ward after facial surgery. 'When I was brought back from theatre', she says, 'I didn't have a dressing over my face and all the patients came over to my bed to have a look at what the surgeons had done. It was the most humiliating and degrading thing to have happened.'

Further, in the same journal, another author relates the following. 'Some time ago I interviewed a psychiatric nurse who, in a deliberate and measured tone said: "We are looking after people here who are off their rockers, barmy"' (Vousden, 1986).

From my own clinical experience the above accounts ring true. In the mid 1960s, while training for the nursing of mentally handicapped people, I encountered both mental and physical cruelty; it was commonplace to see nurses teasing residents or forcing food quickly down the throats of severely disabled clients so as to have time later to relax and watch the TV. The care of residents was often jokingly referred to as 'farming', and the individuals so 'cared for' as 'animals'.

In mental nurse training this was little improved. The staff were very cohesive and powerful and 'care' often masqueraded as rigid regimes of control where staff interests could be presented at the expense of the client group. Staff boundaries were heavily defended and the trappings of nursing status were made much of. For example, keys were dangled from nurses' belts; white coats were worn with pride; badges of office were worn on lapels and ***authoritative*** professional interventions were the norm.

In general nursing I have found similar non-therapeutic attitudes and behaviours. On the medical wards all patients were forced to sleep, wake, and wash at the same time; visiting was restricted; nursing routines were performed – often without purpose – and the patients' feelings and opinions were ridden over roughshod. Before surgery the anxieties of pre-operative patients were ignored and clarifying information routinely withheld. Patients who asked for clarification or argued their case were unpopular, everything seemed to be structured to induce a ***learnt helplessness***

(Seligman, 1975). Both medical and surgical wards perpetuated the unforgivable sin of encouraging their clients to die alone; isolated in side rooms far away from others.

There are many reasons we may cite to excuse these actions. Indeed, some may have been performed with the very best of intentions. But the fact remains, they are insensitive, unhealthy, and run counter to therapeutic care and practice.

With the above in view, and mindful of an earlier concept which stated that stressed people cannot transmit care, reflect upon the following passage which describes the plight of a client whose request to delay a pain-killing injection so that he might better engage with his relative who had travelled some 200 miles to visit brought him in contact with the hard edge of professional politics. This passage also serves to remind us of how rigid we may become and how insulating professional defences can be:

'On what I thought to be my third post-operative day – but was in fact my fifth as I had been unconscious for two days post-operatively – I was approached just before visiting time by the ward sister who told me she was going to give me a pain-killing injection prior to getting me up and sitting me in a chair. As Anna was travelling up from Surrey to visit me, and as the injection cited made me sleepy, I enquired if this could be delayed so that I might remain alert during visiting. This suggestion was not favourably received: I was lectured on how important it was to get up. I agreed, but enquired whether two hours would make such a difference, and repeated my rationale. This did not go down well; I was told I must do as she asked. For whose benefit was this injection being given, I asked. The tempo now increased; we both had the bit between our teeth. I said, with respect, as a client I had a right to be heard; it was important to my own well-being for me to fully contact my kin – they were my lifeline. She objected. Surely, I argued, in these days of nursing process and client-centred care my request was a reasonable enough one to make. She stormed off. My visitors came and went. With their departure I had my injection, was helped out of bed and sat in a chair. While attending to me the sister said nothing. I did not feel forgiven for querying her instructions. A few hours later I heard laughter, the junior nurses and sister were playing, flicking water at one another. When she realised I was watching the sister stopped. I seemed to represent a problem for her, and suspected I had been "hit by a projection". A little after this a doctor was called, and following much flirtive glancing the sister came out to tell me I was being transferred out from intensive care. I asked the sister if this meant I was out of danger. She made no answer, but returned to the office where the doctor remained. More flirtive glances ensued. I checked myself, surely I was not becoming paranoid; I had earlier been told I would be here for at least a week more. A change of environment felt quite daunting; especially separation from that meaningful contact forged with the night staff. Within the hour porters came to collect me. When a nurse came over to carry the intravenous drips I asked her to relay to the sister and doctor the message that I did not respect their professional cowardice; she looked embarrassed and I doubt if this was relayed.

My move from intensive care felt ill-prepared and emotive. On the positive side, I was aware that I had the resemblance of an emotion forming within me; a potential for anger; confirmation of my ability to experience emotions again'

(Barber, 1991)

Understanding (the personal cost of nursing care)

In the late 1950s Isabel Menzies Lyth, while conducting a study into low levels of nursing morale, identified ways in which nurses have traditionally structured the social fabric of their clinical environment so as to avoid facing up to, confronting, and dealing with intrapersonal and social stress. More recent application of her work (Barber, 1991) suggests her findings have meaning today for those who work in organisational settings and engage in practitioner-client relationships.

Menzies' study, concerned with the 'Nursing Service of a General Hospital', described the stress that nurses met in the following terms:

'The direct impact on the nurse of physical illness is intensified by her task of meeting and dealing with psychological stress in other people including her own colleagues. It is by no means easy to tolerate such stress even if one is not under similar stress oneself. Quite short conversations with patients or relatives showed that their conscious concept of illness and treatment is a rich intermixture of objective knowledge, logical deduction, and fantasy . . .

'Patients and relatives have very complicated feelings towards the hospital, which are expressed particularly and most directly to nurses, and often puzzle and distress them. Patients and relatives show appreciation, gratitude, affection, respect; a touching relief that the hospital copes; helpfulness and concern for nurses in their difficult task. But patients often resent their dependence; accept grudgingly the discipline imposed by treatment and hospital routine; envy nurses their health and skills; are demanding, possessive and jealous . . .

'Relatives may also be demanding and critical, the more so because they resent the feeling that hospitalisation implies inadequacies in themselves. They envy nurses their skill and jealously resent the nurse's intimate contact with "their" patient . . .

'The hospital, particularly the nurses, must allow the projection into them of such feelings as depression and anxiety, fear of the patient and his illness, disgust at the illness and the necessary nursing tasks. Patients and relatives treat the staff in such a way as to ensure that the nurses experience these feelings instead of, or partly instead of themselves . . .

'Thus, to the nurses' own deep and intense anxieties are psychically added those of the other people concerned'

(Menzies, 1960)

I make no apology for quoting the above study at length; too few nurses have examined this work or availed themselves of its message. Indeed, many nurses have forgotten to reflect, preferring to act out their stresses through 'doing', rather than confronting and resolving them. Little has changed since Menzies' study. We have modern units, models of nursing at the fore of current practice, but the same old stresses remain, for we have not yet acquired the research awareness and interpersonal skills to deal with the legacy of stress we have inherited via our caring tradition.

Tradition is the more powerful because it is covert and beyond obvious question; what you cannot see you cannot fight.

Traditional power is prescriptive; it allocates power to historically significant agents (such as the hospital institution). This is in direct contrast to the negotiated authority of 'research'.

In such climates questioning is a rarity and 'change' unacceptable. Unanalysed customs are enshrined where tradition is adhered to rigidly, and ward staff subgroups develop a tribal character. Functionally, traditions provide a sense of permanence and orientate us to an interactive framework, but when oversubscribed they rob us of creative interpretation and interactive space. The values and **collusions** that emanate from traditional practice – nursing's hidden curriculum – are outlined in Menzies' work.

In the same study, Menzies ascribed the following techniques as ploys to alleviate face-to-face anxiety; they were seen as systems of collusive agreements – often unconscious – via which interactive anxieties were dissipated.

(1) Splitting up the nurse–patient relationship
(2) **Depersonalisation**, **categorisation** and denial of the significance of the individual
(3) Detachment and denial of feelings
(4) The attempt to eliminate decisions by **ritual task performance**
(5) Reducing the weight of responsibility in decision-making by checks and counter-checks
(6) Collusive social redistribution of responsibility and irresponsibility
(7) Purposeful obscurity in the formal distribution of responsibility
(8) The reduction of the impact of responsibility by delegation to superiors
(9) *Idealisation* and underestimation of personal development possibilities
(10) Avoidance of change

It is to be hoped that the above are relics of nursing practice rather than characteristics of its present.

We must redress those defences isolated by Menzies' study if nurses and nursing are to progress – for these are symptoms of a failure to evolve, to face up to the realities of care and to acquire the necessary relationship skills; they are what we must progress from in order to grow as a profession (Barber and Norman, 1987).

Lest you are in danger of too readily believing that Project 2000 and 'the modern nurse' have eradicated the above social dynamics from care, I submit below an extended breakdown of Menzies' categories along with specific examples of the same, gleaned whilst a participant observer/patient within a surgical ward.

Splitting up of the nurse–patient relationship

Here tasks are seen to demand more attention than individuals; patients are treated all the same, personal distinctions are reduced, clinical duties pre-scribed and listed. Little opportunity is afforded for development of one-to-one relationships; nurse–client relationships are strongly discouraged and professional distance strongly reinforced.

Example: I noted – while a patient in hospital – that nurses were constantly on the look-out for physical jobs to do. This behaviour was strongly reinforced; for example, when a senior member of staff en-countered juniors talking to clients, jobs were quickly found for them to do in areas distant from the individual they had engaged in conversation.

Depersonalisation, categorisation and denial of individual significance

Patients are referred to by their medical condition rather than names. Uniformity of response and client management, attitude and performance is encouraged; individuality and creativity are dis-couraged.

Example: My own experience testifies to this; I was rarely referred to by my name, but rather identified by my diet, condition, or yet again by my con-sultant surgeon – 'Dr X's thorax'!

Detachment and denial of feelings

Staff are expected to exert strong controls over their feelings; shows of emotion are discouraged and involvement is feared. Staff are disciplined rather than counselled and told what to do rather than listened to or really heard. Clients' feelings are gen-erally ignored and systems of control predominate over systems of care.

Example: Every nurse within the ward appeared to have two forms of presentation or communication style. To colleagues their tone of voice was feel-ingless and businesslike, and to patients jollying, rather patronising in a playful way, and chiding. When a patient died, no time was set aside for appraisal or mourning. In consequence nurses plunged themselves into ward tasks with increased energy and were seemingly even more desperate to keep themselves busy.

Decisions reduced and avoided via an adherence to ritual and routine

The anxiety of free choice is replaced with instru-mental activity and nursing procedures; decisions are shelved until new policies are formed. Ques-tioning is discouraged and new ways resisted.

Example: To take night sedation at any other than the usual time or to request pain-killers outside of the medicine round produced pronounced ten-sion. Relatively simple requests from patients, such as to delay night sedation or to sleep through breakfast after a sleepless night, were referred by junior staff to seniors, such was the fear of em-ploying one's own initiative.

Responsibility diluted by checks and counter-checks

Individual action is actively discouraged; every-thing has a tendency to be obsessively recorded. Trust of others – and their skills – is a rarity, fear of failure a constant motivator.

Example: Even aspirin, a common enough drug in the home, was given out in a manner one would expect of a deadly poison. My temperature, pulse and respiration, which I could easily take for my-self as a trained nurse, just had to be done for me. Strangely enough, what appeared on my observa-tion chart, the record of my pulse and temperature, was given much more credence than those symp-toms I was able to report as an experienced prac-titioner. Blood pressures recorded by juniors were nearly always checked routinely by senior staff, and observations by patients generally given little weight.

Collusive redistribution of responsibility and irresponsibility

Authoritative parts of oneself are displaced onto seniors and irresponsible parts onto juniors; conse-quentially seniors are seen as parents and juniors as 'childlike'. Personal power is denied and pro-fessional autonomy and personal initiative are largely left unused.

Example: It was commonplace to hear juniors being chastised for supposed errors openly in front of their patients. Likewise deviations from routine – for whatever reason – brought quick rebuke. Everything was seemingly directed at keeping the status quo.

Responsibility avoided by generalisation and role obscurity

Roles are unspecified, responsibilities blurred and boundaries largely undefined. Ample space is provided for excuses to be found, conflicts ignored and personal responsibilities disowned.

Example: Alongside the need to record things obsessively and to keep the routine operative was another, conflicting thread; here, practitioners would refer everything back to the next level of seniority. This seemed to be in part good sense, to avoid being told off for using initiative, but also appeared to have the flavour of getting back at seniors and acting out passive anger at the system. Seniors in like manner tended to select those individuals who were less compliant or whom they appeared to dislike for the more tedious jobs. Open disagreements and dislikes were thus avoided, kept under wraps, and punitive power play enacted with the professional veneer well and truly intact.

Delegation to superiors of professional and personal choice

Disclaimed responsibilities are forced upwards to seniors. Staff perform well below their level of competence and skills, and responsibility is shirked.

Example: Largely due to the aforementioned dynamics, seniors were forever overloaded with petty decisions. This in turn re-affirmed what appeared to be a personal need in themselves; to be seen as a 'work hero', a person who gives their all and never shirks decisions, an all-giving, all-powerful, indispensable being. Seniors here appeared dangerously close to burn-out.

Idealisation of self and underestimation of the potential to develop

Homage is paid to the belief that 'nurses are born rather than made' and selection of the 'right' people is emphasised over training and professional and/or personal development. Maturity and responsibility are allocated to rank rather than to individual merit.

Example: Personal and professional status within the clinical setting seemed to revolve around rank and rank ordering. This gave immense power to those who knew the routine, the system, and other power holders of the hospital. By venerating those who had remained longest in the hospital or one of its specialist areas, routine was safeguarded and change all too successfully resisted.

Avoidance of change

The full consent of everyone is sought before change can take place so progress is as fast as the slowest team member involved. Problem confrontation is avoided; change is avoided for fear of the necessity to restructure existing social defences.

Example: Understandably, in the light of all the above restrictions, change all but failed to permeate the clinical setting. Upon the wall of the nursing office was a chart of various nursing models, individualised Kardex reporting of patients occurred, but I was never interviewed by a nurse in my two month stay nor was a care plan produced. Things just went on as they always had done.

Looking at the above social defences, observed in the 1950s and confirmed more recently by my own experiences, I ask myself: do things ever change? When I speak to professional trainees who have reaped the benefit of many years of 'sociology', 'experiential learning' and 'communication studies', they nearly always believe the above to be historical to professional practice. With more thorough reflection and application to their own areas of work, this view changes. Indeed, in line with my own observations (Barber 1991), they generally report that the above defences are alive and flourishing within their own place of work.

Reflection

Reading the 'Rules and Orders for the Government of the Royal Hospitals of Bridewell and Bethlem', published 1778, I note the duties of the Matron as: 'to take care the rooms are in every respect in decent order'; 'to let in the women prisoners at all hours of the night should they be brought: and to keep due decorum among them'; 'to take upon her the charge of and be answerable for all the women prisoners'; 'to attend women prisoners when they are burning their straw and cleaning their wards'; 'to take care when the doctor prescribes any medicines'; 'to see that the women's prison be washed once a week and fumigated with tar'.

Though this is a historical document over 200 years old, there is something familiar to me. Then, just as now, routines stand in the way of communication and personal care, and individuals are lost within institutional systems which are supposed to care for them, but which in fact do more by way of managing and controlling them.

Changing (learning to grow)

'Change' is an interpersonal process, a natural consequence of growth and a requisite of education and personal development. At the last analysis we have no choice but to make 'change' our friend. Nothing is for ever, nothing is permanent, all is in flux. Accepting this fact is the hardest part of change; all too often we have been taught to believe in permanence. We rarely contemplate our own death – that ultimate change awaiting us – or comprehend 'our reality' as a momentary grasping at ever-flowing experience. Everything around us and within us is dynamic.

Our pretence to maintain a sense of permanence is understandable; it offers a palliative security. Change implies threat, the letting go of the old known ways. Change is hard work. Successful living requires you to ride upon the crest of the wave of change. To do other than this is to diminish your contact with the world, to retreat into fantasy, to segment yourself, hide from the here-and-now and deny much of your potential; it is also unhealthy.

Health is a state of mind, the ability to make contact with and experience such positive emotions as joy, love, and a sense of fulfilment while having the confidence to take risks and live life creatively (Wilson, 1975). Intellectual and physical functions are secondary yardsticks of health to these. Health is an emotionally energised state, and nurses – who concern themselves with the facilitation of health in others – must appreciate both their own and their clients' emotional experience.

Two possible responses to change are illustrated in Fig. 14.1. These responses are suggested to be either positive and supportive of healthy outcome, or negative and unhealthy.

Carl Jung suggested there were four major ways of relating to the world: thinking, feeling, sensing and intuition (Jung, 1957).

'Thinking' and 'feeling' are concerned with the way you judge and/or value things. Do you see life from a rational objective standpoint, or are you more inclined towards an inner worldview informed by subjective experience and emotion?

'Sensation' and 'intuition', by contrast, are ways of perceiving and gathering information from your environment. Here, you may look out upon the world primarily through your five senses or through intuitive knowing informed by inner certainty.

All these references are important. The science of care is informed by thinking and sensation, the art or expression of care by intuition and feeling.

By self-observation and paying attention to how we use the above dimensions, we may discover a little about how we adapt to change and process the environment.

The art of working through, enjoying and gaining from change is dependent upon our acceptance of it. Acceptance starts the whole process off. Personally, I have found it useful to 'check out' myself when meeting change. To do this I stop, reflect, and explore my 'thoughts', 'senses', 'feelings' and 'intuitions'. I can do this for such diverse issues as a change of job, a quandary of care, the meaning of a recently experienced dream, a life crisis, an essay topic, or indeed, to explore options open to me. I also employ this technique to enable students within my workshops and clients with whom I am working therapeutically to appreciate where they are *now*. For example, if I consider my own immediate reality while writing this tract, the following awarenesses arise:

Thoughts: I'm thinking where best to take this chapter, whether to introduce styles of intervention or continue with the theme of adaptation to change.

Sensations: I'm aware of being warmed by the open fire to my left, cool down my right side, and of my attention being drawn to the flakes of snow falling gently outside the window.

Feelings: I'm feeling low in emotional energy, satisfied with today's work on this chapter, but tired and emotionally flat.

Intuitions: I'm tired and in need of a rest, I will be unable to proceed with clarity unless I take time out of writing for a while.

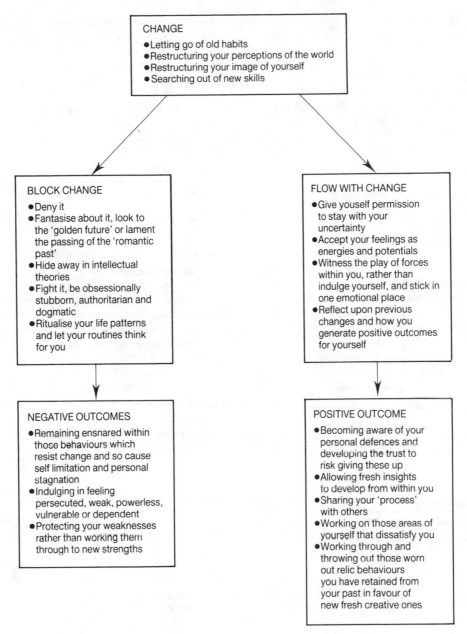

CHANGE
- Letting go of old habits
- Restructuring your perceptions of the world
- Restructuring your image of yourself
- Searching out of new skills

BLOCK CHANGE
- Deny it
- Fantasise about it, look to the 'golden future' or lament the passing of the 'romantic past'
- Hide away in intellectual theories
- Fight it, be obsessionally stubborn, authoritarian and dogmatic
- Ritualise your life patterns and let your routines think for you

FLOW WITH CHANGE
- Give youself permission to stay with your uncertainty
- Accept your feelings as energies and potentials
- Witness the play of forces within you, rather than indulge yourself, and stick in one emotional place
- Reflect upon previous changes and how you generate positive outcomes for yourself

NEGATIVE OUTCOMES
- Remaining ensnared within those behaviours which resist change and so cause self limitation and personal stagnation
- Indulging in feeling persecuted, weak, powerless, vulnerable or dependent
- Protecting your weaknesses rather than working them through to new strengths

POSITIVE OUTCOME
- Becoming aware of your personal defences and developing the trust to risk giving these up
- Allowing fresh insights to develop from within you
- Sharing your 'process' with others
- Working on those areas of yourself that dissatisfy you
- Working through and throwing out those worn out relic behaviours you have retained from your past in favour of new fresh creative ones

Fig. 14.1 *The demands of change on the individual*

Thoughts: I'll be more able to continue this work tomorrow, I will try to stop thinking about work until the morning.

Sensations: I'm aware of a sensation of relief at deciding to stop and am aware of my attention drifting away from writing.

Feelings: I'm feeling glad to turn away from my work, and am aware of a feeling of excited anticipation in recommencing afresh tomorrow morning.

Intuitions: I'm freer than I suppose, but in fantasy I make myself feel trapped in order to work harder and quicker; that is, I threaten myself into hard work.

My solution seems to stem from my self-awareness; in knowing where I am now and my present state of need, I can relinquish my work until morning. This process is detailed in Fig. 14.2 so you may sample it yourself.

Reflection

How do you rate yourself in the manner you evaluate and/or constitute your own worldview; are you primarily a thinker or feeler? Indicate this on the continuum below:

Thinking————————————**Feeling**

In which main way do you gather information; via your five senses or intuition? Indicate this on the continuum below:

Sensing————————————**Intuition**

How different are you in various settings – at home or work? Or when you lead a team or yet again are a member of it? That is to say, does your rank or status affect how you behave?

It might be interesting for you to examine your nursing notes. What do you portray of yourself in your records; your thoughts or feelings, sensory awarenesses or intuitions? Personally, I have been surprised by the high ratio of intuitive data I find in professional records which are taken as statements of fact.

Seeing (a transactional view of nursing)

Possibly you are starting to ponder just where this discussion is leading. We have identified the lack of relevant preparation in nursing education, the blocks which occur to frustrate personal development, and untherapeutic practices. Change has been addressed – along with those behaviours that enable growth-promoting outcomes – and an awareness exercise has been suggested. But so what?

I have attempted to write this chapter in much

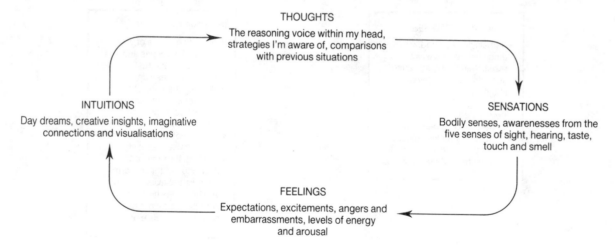

PROCESS

I am aware of thinking . . . . .
I am aware of sensing . . . . .
I am aware of feeling . . . . .
I am aware of imagining . . . . .

Fig. 14.2 *Awareness check sheet*

the same way as I approach the care of clients. I have introduced my biases and beliefs, provided evidence so that you might understand something of their origin, and shared my own process while directing attention upon 'the present'. What impressions are you left with?

Sometimes we must move slowly if we are to learn. A major fault of the nursing profession is that it spent too much time trying to define 'essences' but failed to appreciate 'existence' and its everyday reality. Many of its theorists would have been better employed exploring how nurses may make better contact with the clinical world in which they work.

Awareness is itself a potent agent of change. Nurses have rarely sought intimate contact with their world – rather distancing themselves from it – with the consequence that little has changed.

Nurses have denied their clients' internal states, paid homage to intellect, but divorced themselves from intuition, feelings and the evidence of their senses. They have forgotten to be 'aware' and 'research-minded'. Nurses have let managerial rituals do much of their thinking for them; likewise the impulse to keep busy in hands and feet has replaced much reflection. Qualitative supervision is a rarity, and there is little counselling or support (Moscato, 1976).

I am attempting to address all this by emphasising personal awareness, individual perception, and self-analysis of moment-to-moment function. The more self-aware nurses become (I suggest), the less blind they will be to what they do professionally, and how they manage their care role.

Transactional analysis (***TA***), a theory of human development and relating, may help here. Eric Berne (1967), the originator of transactional analysis, suggests that as infants grow they become aware of two images of themselves. Firstly, they are aware of their own emotions and physical

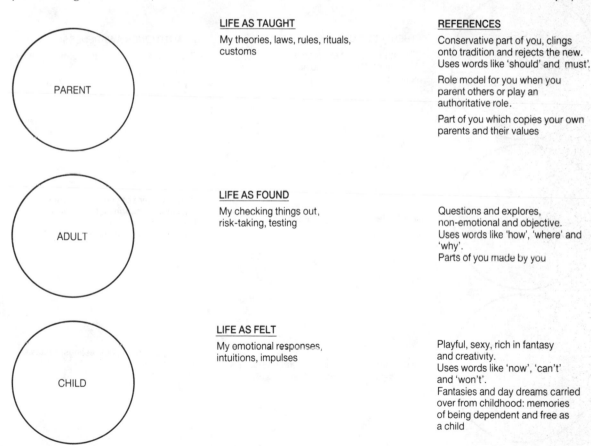

LIFE AS TAUGHT

My theories, laws, rules, rituals, customs

REFERENCES

Conservative part of you, clings onto tradition and rejects the new. Uses words like 'should' and must'.

Role model for you when you parent others or play an authoritative role.

Part of you which copies your own parents and their values

PARENT

LIFE AS FOUND

My checking things out, risk-taking, testing

Questions and explores, non-emotional and objective. Uses words like 'how', 'where' and 'why'. Parts of you made by you

ADULT

LIFE AS FELT

My emotional responses, intuitions, impulses

Playful, sexy, rich in fantasy and creativity. Uses words like 'now', 'can't' and 'won't'. Fantasies and day dreams carried over from childhood: memories of being dependent and free as a child

CHILD

Fig. 14.3 *A transaction model of ego function*

needs; secondly, they are aware of the expectations of their parents. Their own feelings provide an impression of themselves from the driver's seat, and the social viewpoint of their parents gives them a mirror with which to assess themselves.

Parents provide their children with a model of social behaviour. Consequently the infant, in loving, respecting and imitating his parents, internalises a social perception of the world. His orientation to his parents' world causes the development of an inner '**parent** ego' of his own, while his experience of his own emotional energies, his playful fantasies and creativity forms the bounds of his own '**child** ego'. Last to evolve, and very much linked with the growth of mobility, independence and questioning, is his '**adult** ego', his view of the world as he found it and checked it out to be.

This model is illustrated in Fig. 14.3. Three orientations to the world are evident. The 'parent ego' serves to relate us to the social world and '*life as taught*'; that is, our cultural beliefs and values. Under this is placed the 'adult ego', an exploratory and assessment mechanism that relates to everyday reality and '*life as found to be*'. Below is the 'child ego' which orientates us to our vulnerable, childlike qualities – along with the creativity and energies of '*life as felt*'.

Taking this model into the realms of the nursing profession and the roles carers play, further insights are available. Nursing has an abundance of rules, theories and rituals; it is overtly concerned with the structuring of the care experience and the formation of care strategies. Simply, training and practice encourage the nurse to perceive herself primarily as a 'parent' figure. A similar process occurs in the preparation of physicians, but unlike

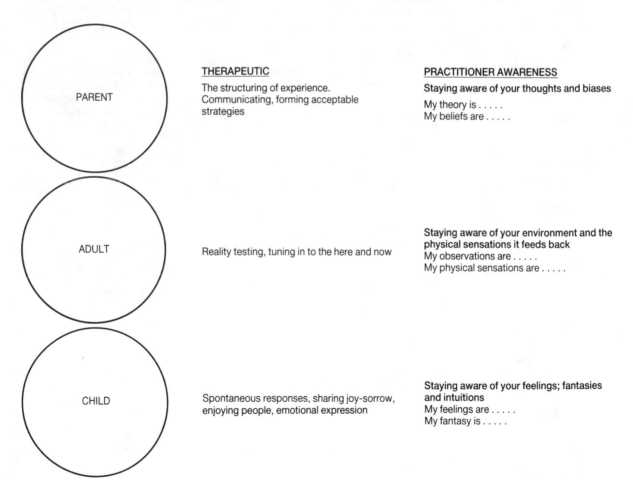

THERAPEUTIC

The structuring of experience. Communicating, forming acceptable strategies

Reality testing, tuning in to the here and now

Spontaneous responses, sharing joy-sorrow, enjoying people, emotional expression

PRACTITIONER AWARENESS

Staying aware of your thoughts and biases

My theory is . . . . .
My beliefs are . . . . .

Staying aware of your environment and the physical sensations it feeds back
My observations are . . . . .
My physical sensations are . . . . .

Staying aware of your feelings; fantasies and intuitions
My feelings are . . . . .
My fantasy is . . . . .

Fig. 14.4 *Transactional qualities of care*

nurses, they are taught to exercise more autonomy and to validate the reality of their experiences; their 'adult' function is more developed through 'research-mindedness'.

If we combine those experiential insights from the self-awareness exercise — Fig. 14.2 — with transactional analysis and the nursing role, we observe that awareness of theories and beliefs puts us in touch with our socially construed 'parent'; awareness of our observations and physical sensations relates to functional reality and our 'adult', while recognition of our feelings and fantasies places us in touch with the energies available within our 'child' (Fig. 14.4).

The above egos are valuable to us and relevant to nursing, but the strengths of each ego (i.e. the social awareness and intellectual structuring of the 'parent', the reality orientation and testing of the 'adult', and creative energies of the 'child') are rarely facilitated — with conscious intent — in nurse education or in clinical practice.

It is a sad fact that most educational and clinical relationships are predominantly 'parent to child' ones (Moscato, 1976). That is to say, professionals tend to adopt the roles of authoritative and critical parents, the 'know bests' who seek to control and impose their will upon others. Interactively, the resulting pecking order is often that represented in Fig. 14.5.

The issuing of authoritative demands, the withholding of information, and the absence of sharing, counselling and research-minded dis-cussion leads to rigid role performance which encourages seniors to relate to juniors as childlike and naive entities, and juniors to **idealise** and **project** 'parent-like' images and personal responsibilities upon the seniors. This corresponds with Menzies' (1960) findings in her study:

> 'Each nurse tends to split off aspects of herself from her conscious personality and to project them into other nurses. Her irresponsible impulses, which she feels she cannot control, are attributed to her juniors. Her painfully severe attitude to these impulses and burdensome sense of responsibility are attributed to her seniors. Consequently, she identifies juniors with her irresponsible self and treats them with the severity that self is felt to deserve. Similarly, she identifies seniors with her own harsh disciplinary attitude to her irresponsible self and expects harsh discipline. There is psychic truth in the assertion that juniors are irresponsible and seniors harsh disciplinarians. These are the roles assigned to them. There is also objective truth, since people act objectively on the psychic roles assigned to them'

Interactions returning to seniors thus reinforce the original transferences and counter-transferences (Fig. 14.6). In this situation, reality orientation is poor, personal awareness and self-awareness are lost and although feelings and stresses are experienced, they are denied and ignored. Burn-out and disillusionment follow naturally in such climates.

A healthier and far more therapeutic culture evolves when 'adult to adult' interactions are the pre-

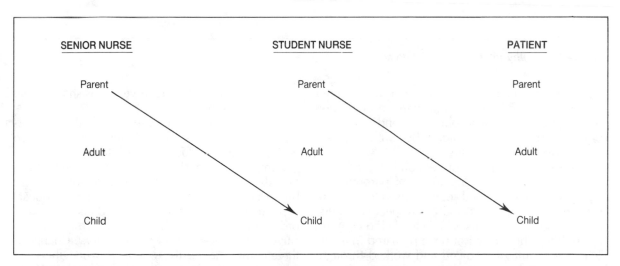

Fig. 14.5 *Authoritative interactions*

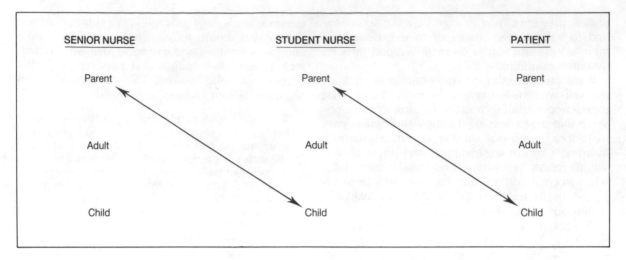

Fig. 14.6 *Responding to authoritative interactions*

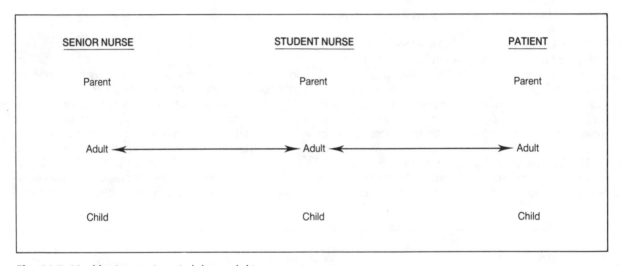

Fig. 14.7 *Healthy interactions (adult to adult)*

vailing norm (see Fig. 14.7). Material stored in our 'parent' and 'child' egos is primarily archaic and serves to orientate us to our social and emotional pasts (Harris, 1973). The adult, by contrast, orientates us to everyday reality.

Too often the nursing profession has bred in its practitioners an overstrong degree of 'parenthood', along with such parental social fears as losing control, losing self-respect and the respect of others. As a consequence, nurses have tended to conform too rigidly. They have not been prepared in a way where fears may be voiced and worked through; their preparation is nearer one of 'papering over the cracks'; their superficial veneer is shallow and prone to fracture.

Nurses are taught primarily to hide their vulnerabilities from others – and themselves – but in so doing they also reduce their sensitivity.

Bump the skin and it gives, stretches and returns quickly to normal in a fluid and flexible fashion; bump a blister and – no matter how hard it appears superficially – it cracks, weeps and takes an extraordinarily long time to heal. Nurses cover the sensitive bits of themselves with blisters. Change is threatening and costly to nurses when their defences are so brittle. Change must address the individual – rather than the system in which individuals operate – and specifically, it must be felt, checked out, and evaluated experientially.

Behaviour to facilitate your 'adult' function and ability to adapt is suggested in Fig. 14.8. Try out these behaviour cues in your nursing role. Goals I have found it especially useful to work towards are 'Giving myself permission to stay with my uncertainties', and 'Allowing myself to make mistakes'. The path of your enquiry is just as sacred as mine, and your own findings are much more relevant for you.

Being (living and caring in the 'now')

Let us leave both 'nursing' and the 'care role' for a while and examine a little further the concept of 'existence'. The need to focus upon 'existences' –

rather than 'essences' – was touched on earlier. When we seek out the essence of a thing we must of necessity confine, measure and define it. In doing this there is a tendency for us to fit the object under examination into a frame of reference already known to us; 'not seeing the wood for the trees' is an example of the danger in this type of thinking. Our contact with 'direct experience' is reduced by this means; for example, if I go for a walk at dusk and see in the distance an object I cannot identify, my imaginative perception runs riot. I squint to perceive the object more clearly, and tilt my head to one side to listen for any tell-tale noises to help recognition. I sense myself becoming aroused by expectancy and surprise within me. I approach the object tentatively for fear of a heaven-only-knows-what encounter. I am also truly alive.

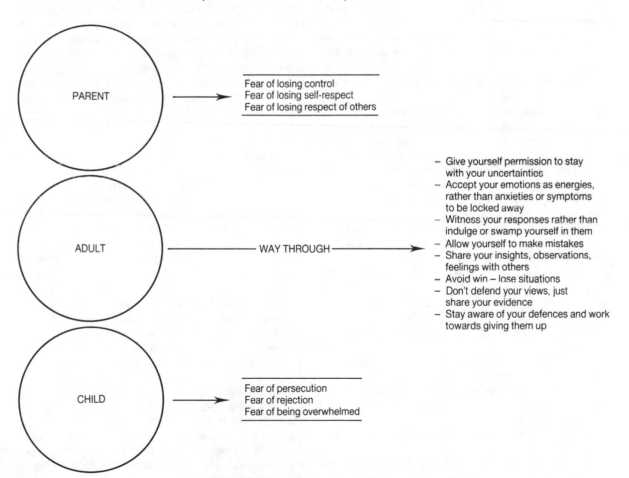

Fig. 14.8 *A transactional view of personal adaptation*

If, as I draw nearer, I identify the object as an old tree root – suddenly my enquiring stops. 'It's only an old tree root', I repeat to myself as I walk on. Could I recognise it again or have I learnt anything from it? Sadly, no. By defining what I believe it to be – the 'essence' of it – I cease to be moved.

Sometimes the same thing happens with interpersonal perception. In married life, for example, partners define and label each other with such judgements as 'they don't care', 'things will never improve', 'they'll always be the same' – and they stop looking, listening, being imaginatively aware of or emotionally moved by the other. A similar process can also happen in nursing care. Definition of the 'patient' as dependent and needing, or of 'nurses' as independent and caring, can cause stereotypical perceptions that hinder the transmission of care (Stockwell, 1972). The humanity within each individual may then be lost.

Concentration upon 'definition' may increase our knowledge but at the cost of our understanding.

To broaden our perceptions and widen our appreciation we must view things in the raw, stay open and receptive and withhold those definitive judgements that get in the way of listening to and hearing others. We need to capture some of our earlier childlike enthusiasm and interest in the world and to be fully committed to our own existence and the existences of others. As an individual's self-awareness grows, so too does his sense of 'existence'.

Anything that clogs up or blocks off our perceptive machinery interferes with our ability to contact our 'existence' directly.

Self-actualisers – individuals who maintain peak performance (Maslow, 1967) – demonstrate an ability to:

– perceive reality efficiently, and to tolerate uncertainty
– accept themselves and others for what they are
– be spontaneous in thought and behaviour
– be problem-centred rather than self-centred
– have a good sense of humour
– be highly creative
– be resistant to enculturation, although not purposely unconventional
– demonstrate concern for the welfare of mankind
– deeply appreciate the basic experiences of life
– establish deep satisfying interpersonal relations

with a few, rather than many, people
– look at life from an objective viewpoint.

The above characteristics suggest that acceptance, spontaneity, joy and a sense of wonder are vital to growth, and provide a springboard for discovery of what to aim towards for maximum health.

We earlier identified four perceptive functions: thinking, sensing, feeling, and intuition. Figure 14.9 isolates what are suggested to be 'growth-inducing' and 'non-growth-inducing' aspects of these functions. The shaded parts of the 'thinking function' suggested to be antagonistic to healthy and aware performance are: fears of losing control (earlier related to TA); irrationality; being judgemental and critical, of shallow intent and displaying empty niceness.

Growth-promoting orientations of 'thinking' – which are portrayed as unshaded – are order and clarity; the acceptance of responsibility and nurturing; the planning of strategies; values of right and wrong; social alertness and an awareness of relevant theory and knowledge.

Not only the quality of 'thought' but its distinction from other functions is desirable. If the boundaries of our 'thinking', 'sensing' and 'feeling/intuition' overlap, confusion and disorientation result.

The consequences of perceptual confusion and blurring are portrayed diagrammatically in Fig. 14.10. When 'thinking' overlaps with 'sensing', prejudice (i.e. unexplored and unvalidated social bias) occurs. When 'sensing' overlaps with feelings and intuitions we become deluded, for untested feelings of the world can develop; unclear boundaries between 'thinking' and 'feeling/intuition' may flood our intellect with irrational fears. Lastly, profound overshadowing of all three functions is seen to relate to **psychotic** states when theories, sensory impressions and those meanings and values we attach to the world become jumbled and distorted. The more jumbled we become, the more unaware and unconscious we are of our own processes; this is denoted by increasing shade within the diagram. The more shadow you have within your personality, the less aware you are of yourself and the less able you become to make positive gains from your experiences. Growth lies in the *working through and resolution of your shadow*, and nursing involves the **facilitation** of this process in others.

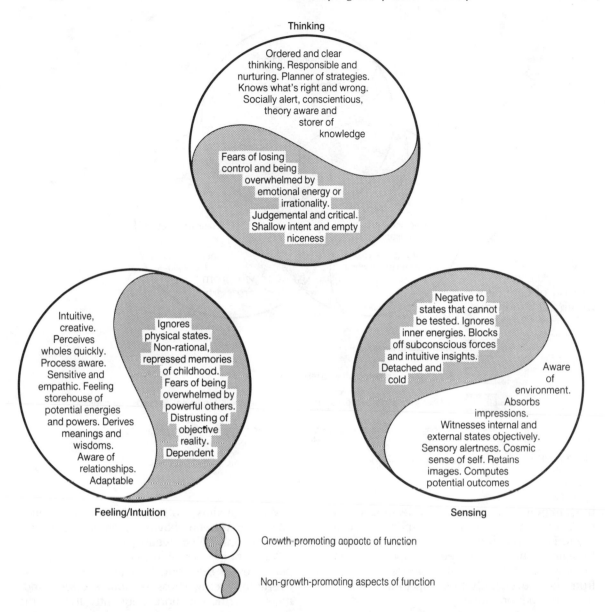

Thinking

Ordered and clear thinking. Responsible and nurturing. Planner of strategies. Knows what's right and wrong. Socially alert, conscientious, theory aware and storer of knowledge

Fears of losing control and being overwhelmed by emotional energy or irrationality. Judgemental and critical. Shallow intent and empty niceness

Intuitive, creative. Perceives wholes quickly. Process aware. Sensitive and empathic. Feeling storehouse of potential energies and powers. Derives meanings and wisdoms. Aware of relationships. Adaptable

Ignores physical states. Non-rational, repressed memories of childhood. Fears of being overwhelmed by powerful others. Distrusting of objective reality. Dependent

Feeling/Intuition

Negative to states that cannot be tested. Ignores inner energies. Blocks off subconscious forces and intuitive insights. Detached and cold

Aware of environment. Absorbs impressions. Witnesses internal and external states objectively. Sensory alertness. Cosmic sense of self. Retains images. Computes potential outcomes

Sensing

Growth-promoting aspects of function

Non-growth-promoting aspects of function

Fig. 14.9 *Growth-promoting and non-growth-promoting qualities of thinking, sensing, feeling and intuitive functions*

Facilitating (enabling health to grow)

The less shadow you carry with you the more potential you have to share. Simplistically, personal growth might be represented as a movement from darkness into light (see Fig. 14.11). 'Health' is balance, growth is 'Super-health'.

If we relate the findings of Menzies and our earlier discussion of nursing to our model, some interesting features develop (see Fig. 14.12). Here nurses are portrayed as being very 'head' motivated, intellectually stuck in issues of being right or fearing being wrong. Their orientation to reality is also seen as seriously impaired, for there is a

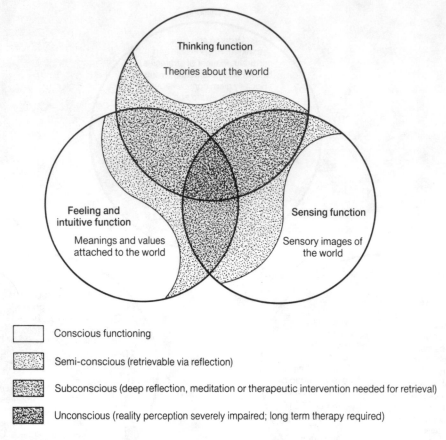

Conscious functioning

Semi-conscious (retrievable via reflection)

Subconscious (deep reflection, meditation or therapeutic intervention needed for retrieval)

Unconscious (reality perception severely impaired; long term therapy required)

Fig. 14.10 *Model of dysfunction: consequences of perceptual confusion and blurring*

blocking-off of intuitive insights leading to a denial of feelings and a negative response to change. There is not much fun in such nursing, nor room for enjoyment. Because feelings and intuitive functions are denied expression, the energies arising from these eventually build up to threaten objective work performance.

Nurses judiciously exercise control of themselves and their environment, demonstrating a brusque businesslike exterior in their performance of all those 'tasks-at-hand'. The maintenance of this facade is an expensive process, especially in terms of 'burn-out' and personal cost (Edelwich and Brodsky, 1980). To deny your emotionality leads to fear of the emotionality of others, for their anxiety in turn stimulates your own. Defensive ploys of displacing emotional energy onto work, the 'work hero' syndrome, are then commonly found.

When anxiety-motivated behaviours predominate over other behaviours, emotional burn-out and physical collapse easily ensue.

Many nurses are able to describe first-hand experiences of burn-out; they are used to working overtime, facing stress without support, and to meeting criticism more frequently than nurture. Because of this, they end up denying their own psychological and physical needs. Such circumstances light the fuse of burn-out. Sickness rates are often high. It is no wonder that declarations of sickness are preferable to other expressions of discontent or exhaustion when the workplace is geared to the care of others, when systems of instrumental activity over-ride person perception, and discipline takes the place of counselling – and when no one either listens to your feelings or sees the real you behind your role.

Attention was drawn earlier to the way senior

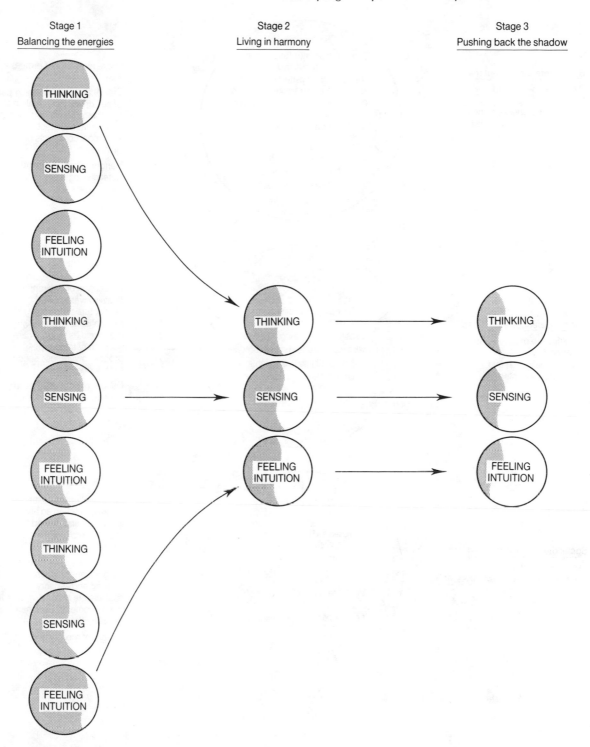

Fig. 14.11 *Model of adaptation and personal growth: stages of therapeutic change*

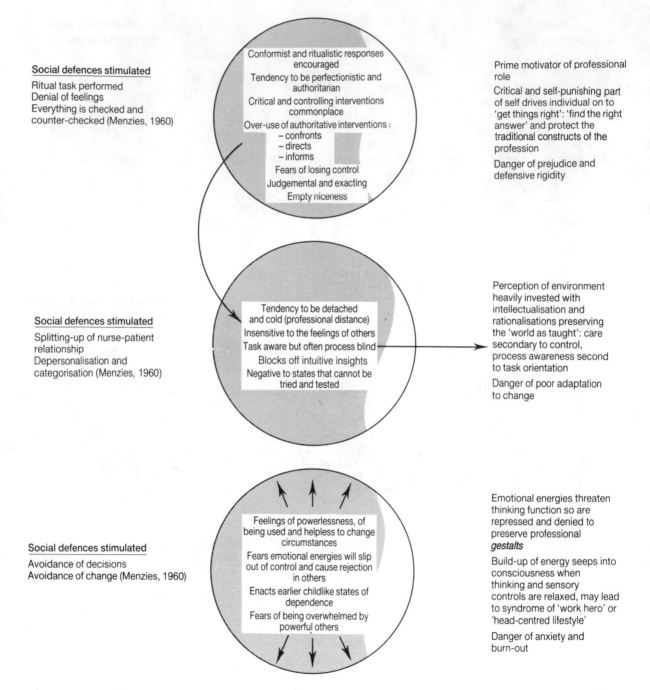

Social defences stimulated

Ritual task performed
Denial of feelings
Everything is checked and
counter-checked (Menzies, 1960)

Conformist and ritualistic responses
encouraged
Tendency to be perfectionistic and
authoritarian
Critical and controlling interventions
commonplace
Over-use of authoritative interventions :
  – confronts
  – directs
  – informs
Fears of losing control
Judgemental and exacting
Empty niceness

Prime motivator of professional
role

Critical and self-punishing part
of self drives individual on to
'get things right': 'find the right
answer' and protect the
traditional constructs of the
profession

Danger of prejudice and
defensive rigidity

Social defences stimulated

Splitting-up of nurse-patient
relationship
Depersonalisation and
categorisation (Menzies, 1960)

Tendency to be detached
and cold (professional distance)
Insensitive to the feelings of others
Task aware but often process blind
Blocks off intuitive insights
Negative to states that cannot be
tried and tested

Perception of environment
heavily invested with
intellectualisation and
rationalisations preserving
the 'world as taught': care
secondary to control,
process awareness second
to task orientation

Danger of poor adaptation
to change

Social defences stimulated

Avoidance of decisions
Avoidance of change (Menzies, 1960)

Feelings of powerlessness, of
being used and helpless to change
circumstances
Fears emotional energies will slip
out of control and cause rejection
in others
Enacts earlier childlike states of
dependence
Fears of being overwhelmed by
powerful others

Emotional energies threaten
thinking function so are
repressed and denied to
preserve professional
gestalts

Build-up of energy seeps into
consciousness when thinking and sensory
controls are relaxed, may lead
to syndrome of 'work hero' or
'head-centred lifestyle'

Danger of anxiety and
burn-out

Fig. 14.12 *Personal costs of the traditional nursing role*

nurses adopt an 'authoritative' role. Authoritative perceptions of oneself and others further the critical 'parent' role previously discussed. Authoritative interventions differ in type and kind from those *facilitative* interventions that further personal growth. A drastic re-orientation is required if the nursing profession is to be kinder to its practitioners and clients. The philosophy of facilitation provides this.

The philosophy of facilitation has been detailed by Carl Rogers in his many texts (see, for example: Rogers, 1967 and Rogers, 1983). Rogers makes the following points about the role of the facilitator.

(1) A *facilitator has much to do with setting the initial mood or climate of a group's experience.* If his own basic philosophy is one of trust in the group and in the individuals who compose the group, then this point of view will be communicated in many subtle ways.

(2) A *facilitator helps to elicit and clarify the purposes of the individuals as well as the more general purposes of the group.* If he is not fearful of accepting contradictory purposes and conflicting aims, if he is able to permit the individuals a sense of freedom in stating what they would like to do, then he is helping to create a climate for learning. There is no need for him to try to manufacture one unified purpose in the group if such a unified purpose is not there. He can permit a diversity of purposes, both contradictory and complementary, to exist in relationship to each other.

(3) A *facilitator regards himself as a flexible resource.* He does not downgrade himself as a resource. He makes himself available as a counsellor, lecturer, and advisor, a person with experience in the field. He wishes to be used by individuals and by the group in the ways which seem most meaningful to them – in so far as he can be comfortable in operating in the ways they wish.

(4) *In responding to expressions, a facilitator accepts both the intellectual content and emotional attitudes, endeavouring to give each aspect the approximate degree of emphasis which it has for the individual or the group.* In so far as he can be genuine in doing so, he accepts rationalisations and intellectualising, as well as deep and real personal feelings.

(5) *He takes the initiative in sharing himself with the group – his feelings as well as his thoughts – in ways which do not demand or impose but represent simply a personal sharing which students may take or leave.* Thus, he is free to express his own feelings in giving feedback to students, in his reaction to them as individuals, and in sharing his own satisfactions or disappointments. In such expressions it is his 'owned' attitudes which are shared, not judgements or evaluations of others.

(6) *In his function as a facilitator of learning, he endeavours to recognise and accept his own limitations.* He realises that he can only grant freedom to the extent that he is comfortable in giving such freedom. He can only be understanding to the extent that he actually desires to enter the inner world of another. He can only share himself to the extent that he is reasonably comfortable in taking that risk.

Facilitation puts 'people' firmly back into the care process. 'Systems' are secondary here to individual response. The above suggestions are readily applicable to those models of care collectively termed the 'nursing process'; indeed, they give the interactive foundation we need to prevent their freshness being swamped by the restraints of traditional practice.

Rogers' work on facilitation suggests a philosophy which enables the provision of a care climate in which education and care-giving may be maximised. But we need to know specifically what skills are necessary to inculcate the above.

Rogers suggests that the characteristics of caring relationships are related to how well individual carers work through their own interpersonal and personal baggage, the doubts they have regarding care – for example:

'Can I be caring in some way which will be perceived by the other person as trustworthy, as dependable, or consistent in some deep sense?'

'Can I be expressive enough as a person for what I am to be communicated unambiguously?'

'Can I let myself experience positive attitudes toward this other person – attitudes of warmth, caring, liking, interest or respect?'

'Can I be strong enough as a person to be separate from the other?'

'Am I secure enough within myself to permit him his separateness?'

'Can I let myself enter fully into the world of his feelings and personal meanings and see these as he does?'

'Can I accept each facet of his personality that a client presents to me?'

'Can I act with sufficient sensitivity in the relationship, so that my behaviour will not be perceived as a threat?'

'Can I free him from the threat of external evaluation?'

'Can I meet this other individual as a person who is in the process of *becoming*, or will I be bound by his past and my past?'

Further analysis of what we may do in the therapeutic relationship comes from the work of John Heron (1990). Heron describes two main orientations – or, as he calls them, *styles* – of intervention; the 'facilitative' and the 'authoritative'. Under the heading of *Authoritative Interventions*, he places those occasions when individuals speak from the power they invest within themselves and their role; *prescriptive, informative* and *confronting* modes of approach are cited here.

Conversely, under the heading of *Facilitative Interventions*, Heron stipulates those times when an individual attempts to attune to another and function in a person-centred fashion to enable that other to explore and take responsibility for himself. Under this category, Heron places *cathartic, catalytic* and *supportive* interventions. A fuller explanation of these terms is given in Table 14.1.

Six category intervention analysis, as Heron calls this system, is a valuable tool for assessing professional intentions and performance. It has opened my eyes to those options I have at my disposal in education and clinical practice alike.

Most nursing models state the importance of a healthy nurse–client relationship but fail to give a reference for these skills. Now you have one. *Authoritative interventions* frame the contextual and task boundaries of nursing care; *facilitative interventions* shape the interpersonal exchange process; both dimensions are also therapeutic and help you clarify clinical intent.

'Task' orientation contains a high frequency of *prescriptive, informative* and *confronting* interventions that 'tell people what to do'. Facilitative interventions are rather at the heart of the psychotherapies; they are essential components of nondirective counselling.

Both authoritative and facilitative interventions are necessary in holistic care.

Table 14.1. *Heron's six category intervention analysis*

Authoritative			Facilitative		
1.	Prescriptive	*Give advice, be judgemental/ critical/evaluative* A prescriptive intervention is one that explicitly seeks to direct the behaviour of the client, especially behaviour that is outside or beyond the practitioner–client interaction	4.	Cathartic	*Release tensions in, encourage laughter/crying* A cathartic intervention seeks to enable the client to experience painful emotion
2.	Informative	*Be didactic, instruct/inform, interpret* An informative intervention seeks to impart new knowledge and information to the client	5.	Catalytic	*Be reflective, encourage self-directed problem-solving, elicit information from* A catalytic intervention seeks to enable the client to learn and develop by self-direction and self-discovery within the context of the practitioner–client situation, but also beyond it
3.	Confronting	*Be challenging, give direct feedback* A confronting intervention directly challenges the restrictive attitude/ belief/behaviour of the client	6.	Supportive	*Be approving, confirming, validating* A supportive intervention affirms the worth and value of the client

Hildegard Peplau, a notable nursing theorist (see Chapter 12), has made the following statement:

'Nursing is a service for people that enhances healing and health by methods that are humanistic and primarily non-invasive'

(Peplau, 1987)

In context of this statement, it would seem more appropriate for today's nurses to err more in the direction of facilitative interventions than of authoritative ones.

Reflecting (the nature of nursing care)

The foremost duty of anyone who wishes to be an effective care-giver is to work on the self; we are each our own most important therapeutic tool.

Enriched, self-aware people make good nurses; emotionally impoverished, unaware people do not.

It would appear that in the past nursing has sought to produce impoverished, unaware practitioners to benefit its traditionally rigid system (see Fig. 14.9). This is now changing; there is promise of person-centred care in the implementation of nursing models, awareness training via experiential encounter in nurse education, and a political awareness in the use of advocacy as a care skill — notably in the nursing of mentally handicapped people.

With the nursing process established in general nursing, the psychosocial perspectives of psychiatric nurses have become increasingly relevant to general care. Nurses of the future could reasonably be expected to synthesise the empathic relating, political and educational awareness that nurses from the discipline of mental handicap employ; the interactive skills and **psychotherapeutic** insights used by mental nurses; and the physiological awarenesses and cognition that general nurses incorporate in their work.

All of the above must be incorporated into our therapeutic arsenal if we desire to fulfil the ideal of 'holistic care'. Sociological insights flow from mental handicap, psychological insights from mental illness, and physiological ones from general care.

As man is a physiological organism who correlates his world in psychological terms and defines reality in social ones, all dimensions must be combined.

Nursing is suggested in this chapter to be an *interpersonal process that relates scientifically derived insights to clients in empathic humane ways, while educating these clients to ways of thinking, feeling and relating that maximise their ability to grow in a self-directed and therapeutic way.* Nurses need cognitive skills to learn and understand these processes involved in health; they need empathy and an interest in the human condition; they need insight into their own unique composition, together with an ability to develop personal and interpersonal relationship skills so that they may share these insights with others. That body of theory and research findings derived from care is the *science* of nursing, while the expressive, empathic and relating aspects of nursing constitute its *art*. Therapy is both an art and a science.

Expressing (dynamics of care)

The nursing profession needs to *develop* its therapeutic arts. It has nursing models, a bank of theory extending back some 50 years but, from examination so far, it appears that nurses have developed more instrumental skills than expressive ones.

One is reminded of the 'Nursing Procedure Books' produced by many health authorities, emphasising instrumental vision across a host of 'care' activities, respectful of which tray or trolley arrangement to use and supportive of the philosophy that care can be reduced to the memorising of appropriate rituals safeguarding 'the right way' of doing things. All tend to be devoid of expressions of care or interpersonal nurse–client exchange; procedure books are one of the profession's horror stories.

Possibly this may sound radical to some. If so, it is not inappropriate, especially if it exposes the professional sterility we incur from the use of a pseudo-scientific and reductionist vision. Nursing has produced many more sheep than goats. Sheep make poor carers and are a far from potent symbol of assertion or advocacy.

Intuitively, I feel that when I am ill and low in energy I will want — and need — those who care for me to be assertive, to defend my rights and be strong enough to accept my pains, frustrations and angers, so that these may be expressed and released by me as they arise. I don't want to feel I must be on my behaviour, scared to vent those emotions that naturally percolate from disease states; simply, I want to be able to give myself permission to be real and to express my suffering in realistic terms. Expression is therapeutic; when energies are summoned, they demand release. ***Repression***, by contrast, has been linked to much somatic disturbance (Cox, 1983). Cathartic skills, that is the ability to enable a client to release his emotions, are crucial though oft forgotten caring skills.

In Fig. 14.13, we return to the work of Heron and stipulate cathartic interventions. These take therapeutic courage to initiate, sensitivity of timing and practice to use expertly. Cathartic interventions also require a fair degree of personal maturity in the practitioner. This is a part of that future therapeutic territory nurses need to make their own. Cathartic interventions are not rarified specialist psychiatric techniques, but tools all nurses require; anxiety is common to all hospital admission (Franklin, 1984).

In November 1984 the UKCC published a *Code of Professional Conduct* (UKCC, 1984 and 1992). Here, 14 recommendations were added to the Nurses' Charter (see page 336). Recommendations 4, 8 and 11 call for assertion and advocacy, qualities that require personal awareness and skills in confrontation.

Interpersonal awareness is likewise supported by recommendations 2, 7 and 13.

Recommendation 13 is especially intriguing; our earlier citation of the cost of professional care upon carers is supported. Maybe the suggestions in this chapter are not as radical as I supposed them to be after all. As for our late discussion of cathartic skills, what better way to address the stress of colleagues (Holmes, 1986) or the physical, psychological and social frustrations of clients (UKCC, 1986) than to facilitate their release so that they may be recognised, evaluated and therapeutically redressed?

Creating a workable synthesis

My dream is of a nursing profession where those we care for enter at times when life crises cause them to be patients, and as such may depend upon us and regress – if need be – and receive the nurturing they require; of a nursing profession that will encourage these individuals to share in their care as co-therapists in a regime that is primarily client-centred until, at a time preceding discharge, the recipients of our service truly become clients and care is client-directed in character.

Giving permission:
  'It's OK if you cry with me'

Removing physical blocks:
  'Try taking deep breaths'/'Say that and make a movement at the same time'

Picking up physical movements:
  'Exaggerate that arm movement ... that facial expression ... etc'

Noting mismatches between verbal and non-verbal behaviour:
  'You say you're upset and you're smiling'

Inviting earliest memory of an event or feeling:
  'Who did you first say that to?'

Repetition:
  Inviting repetition of a word or phrase — 'Say that again louder'

Catching the thought:
  Noting eye movements, facial expressions and inviting the verbal communication of thought. 'What are you thinking now?'

Role play:
  (a) 'What would you say if she was here now?'
  (b) 'Act as though you were her ... What is she saying?'

Monodrama:
  (a) Invite the client to play two or more conflicting roles
  (b) Invite the client to address his feelings: 'If you could talk to your anger, what would you say to it?'

Exploring fantasy:
  'What might happen if you allowed yourself to do that?'

Focusing:
  Inviting the client to identify an emotion bodily.
  'Where is your anxiety? .... point to it .... can you intensify it?'

Addressing hidden agendas:
  'Who do you want to say that to?'
  'What would you really like to say?'

Touch:
  Gently touching a client's hand or shoulder
  Massaging tense muscle groups

Fig. 14.13 *Examples of cathartic interventions*

But I'm discontent, I wish to make my dream reality. I am aware I am taking a risk in this chapter by sharing myself with an audience I have already identified as unsympathetic, namely my own profession.

Taking risks arouses energy. Pulling off these

risks in positive and creative ways breeds confidence. Failing, and indeed I might fail, provides one more experience to learn from and is nothing to fear. If I try my best there is nothing more in my power to be done; believing in this relieves me of much unnecessary stress.

You too can do no more than your best. It is important as a care-giver to define clearly your boundaries – how much can you reasonably give? Do you know when to say no? It is imperative that you care for yourself. It is not selfish to safeguard your own resources but logical and necessary. Unless you learn to 'care' for yourself – and experience such care – how will you be able to care for others?

Finally in this chapter I would like to share my own care orientation. My client group is comprised mainly of clinical nurses, educators and managers; some come from the field of social work and a few are individuals who seek therapy. Whether I function as an educationalist or as a therapist, the same rules apply. I *attune* myself to my positive perceptive functions (Fig. 14.9), stay cognisant of the role interactions available (Fig. 14.4), am mindful of Rogers' philosophy of facilitation, note my intentions and those interactions open to me (Table 14.1) and share with my clients the insights that arise from our interaction and the rationale of my work. To evaluate my performance I employ the experiential exercise (Fig. 14.2) described on page 354.

My intention is primarily an educational one and seeks to solicit growth of insight and self-directed problem-solving within clients. I view myself as a resource. As I view nursing as an interactive process, the approach outlined appears suitable for clients suffering physical, psychological or social ill health.

As a general nurse I would seek – where possible – to educate my client to self-care, share the reasoning behind the specialist medical procedures and investigations performed and use the disease state as a learning experience whereby clients gain new insights into their disease process and develop physiological care skills or preventive measures to forestall their condition recurring and aggravating their lifestyle.

As a mental nurse I would seek to intervene in my client's life crisis, educate him – where possible – about his emotions and behaviours, relay insights that enable him to understand those personal and interpersonal dynamics that trigger malfunction, and help him to identify his support agencies.

As a nurse for mentally handicapped people I would concentrate upon educating my client towards independent social functioning, and facilitating experiments of living where he may advance his capacity to enjoy, grow and maintain healthy modes of performance in keeping with his individual desires and abilities.

In all of the above areas my attention is focused upon the here-and-now reactions that occur between us. I stand on my senses and those patterns perceived from the interactive environment, but am ever mindful of my own intellectual and intuitive resources.

Care is a feeling state besides a string of growth-promoting strategies. Fig. 14.14 attempts to correlate a few of those features I have related to my work.

As a facilitator I witness myself and the environment via my senses, intellectually share my knowledge and social orientation, and allow my feeling and intuitions to suggest creative and empathic responses while using those authoritative or facilitative interventions relevant to immediate care. All is dependent upon how well I can contact – and remain with – the unbreaking wave of my client's experience; if I fail to tune in and 'stay with' him, my therapeutic potential is weakened.

In this chapter I have endeavoured to share my own facilitative style. I hope it has stimulated your own creative and imaginative processes, helping you to reflect upon, and synthesise, your own unique vision.

Nursing is at a crossroads. It can go through the motions of being a profession, or it can develop its therapeutic potential. If the latter road is chosen, nurses must refine their skills to the level of a therapy. Nurses are interactive agents. Whether they are concerned with physical or psychological health, their role is essentially that of a facilitator who supports, nurtures and educates others to independence. Their uniqueness lies in the therapeutic manner in which they use themselves and their interpersonal skills. All else is determined by the orientation of their discipline.

General nurses have specialist knowledge of physical disorder. Psychiatric nurses have specialist knowledge of psychological disorder. But, in the last analysis, they both need person sensitivity, an understanding of the dynamics of a caring relationship, counselling skills, and suf-

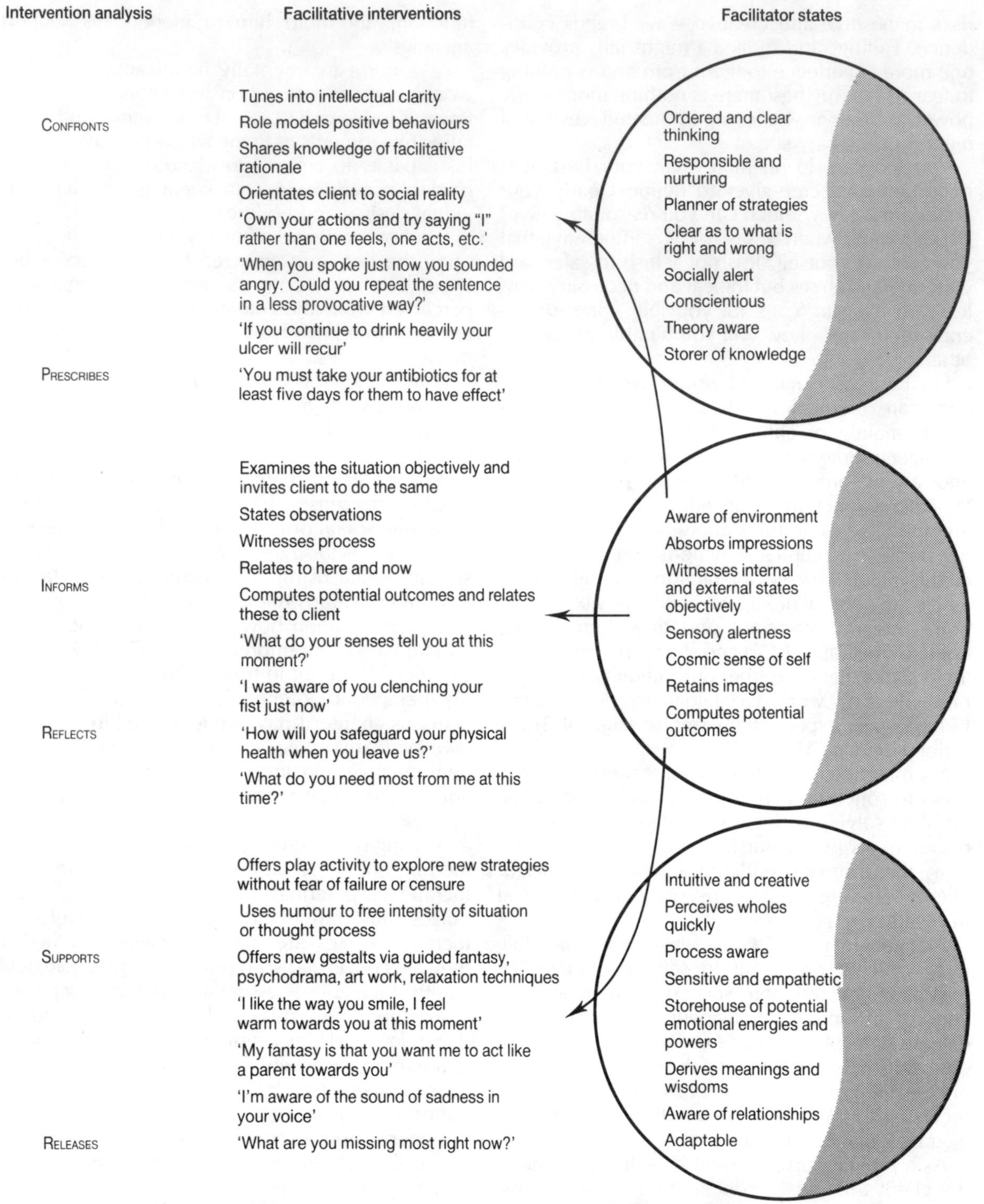

Intervention analysis	Facilitative interventions	Facilitator states

CONFRONTS

Tunes into intellectual clarity

Role models positive behaviours

Shares knowledge of facilitative rationale

Orientates client to social reality

'Own your actions and try saying "I" rather than one feels, one acts, etc.'

'When you spoke just now you sounded angry. Could you repeat the sentence in a less provocative way?'

'If you continue to drink heavily your ulcer will recur'

PRESCRIBES

'You must take your antibiotics for at least five days for them to have effect'

Ordered and clear thinking

Responsible and nurturing

Planner of strategies

Clear as to what is right and wrong

Socially alert

Conscientious

Theory aware

Storer of knowledge

Examines the situation objectively and invites client to do the same

States observations

Witnesses process

Relates to here and now

INFORMS

Computes potential outcomes and relates these to client

'What do your senses tell you at this moment?'

'I was aware of you clenching your fist just now'

REFLECTS

'How will you safeguard your physical health when you leave us?'

'What do you need most from me at this time?'

Aware of environment

Absorbs impressions

Witnesses internal and external states objectively

Sensory alertness

Cosmic sense of self

Retains images

Computes potential outcomes

Offers play activity to explore new strategies without fear of failure or censure

Uses humour to free intensity of situation or thought process

SUPPORTS

Offers new gestalts via guided fantasy, psychodrama, art work, relaxation techniques

'I like the way you smile, I feel warm towards you at this moment'

'My fantasy is that you want me to act like a parent towards you'

'I'm aware of the sound of sadness in your voice'

RELEASES

'What are you missing most right now?'

Intuitive and creative

Perceives wholes quickly

Process aware

Sensitive and empathetic

Storehouse of potential emotional energies and powers

Derives meanings and wisdoms

Aware of relationships

Adaptable

Fig. 14.14 *Relationship of facilitation to functions and personal awareness*

ficient maturity and self-awareness to share of themselves, working therapeutically through, and with, the life crises of others. As agents of intervention in the crises of others, nurses must have worked through their own emotional and professional baggage.

Well, this is the theory; are you up to acting as a therapeutic agent, facing yourself and contacting the reality of a truly caring relationship? The future of the profession is dependent upon you and the quality of your care.

Glossary

Adult: Ego state of transactional analysis concerned with testing reality and computing outcomes. Correlates with 'life as found to be' (see Berne, 1967)

Authoritative: A style of responding characterised by *prescriptive, confronting* and *informative* interventions (See Heron, 1990, and *six category intervention analysis*)

Categorisation: Act of labelling people and events so as to confine them to a classification, rather than appreciate them for what they are

Child: Ego state of transactional analysis concerned with feelings and expression, and addressing 'life as felt' (see Berne, 1967)

Collusion: A conspiracy by some individuals – often people in controlling roles – to preserve their power covertly: i.e. the 'professional collusion' of a nurse and doctor to withhold information from a client, often justified on the grounds of confidentiality

Crisis management: Management that addresses change primarily in response to a crisis, rather than reflecting upon and planning for progress and the unexpected

Denial: The pushing from consciousness of unwanted awareness

Depersonalisation: Loss of a sense of oneself, along with feelings of non-being

Displacement: A subconscious defence mechanism where an individual receives feeling from one situation and expresses it in another where it does not belong: for example, you are reprimanded by your boss but express your frustrations upon your colleagues

Experiential: An approach – often linked with teaching – where the authority of individual experience is emphasised in the acquisition of knowledge. Emphasises the affective (feeling) rather than cognitive (intellectual) aspects of function

Facilitation: The art of enabling others to explore and resolve their own problems rather than

doing this for them and inducing independence (see *facilitative, six category intervention analysis* for examples of facilitative interventions)

Facilitative: A style of responding characterised by *cathartic, catalytic* and *supportive* interventions (see Heron, 1990, and *six category intervention analysis*)

Gestalt: The perceptive pattern held by an individual as a product of his mental, emotional and environmental state at any one moment. Alludes to perception as being active and interpretive rather than a passive reception of external events

Growth: An individual's movement towards greater awareness, positive self-regard, enhanced personal and interpersonal skills and sensitivity

Idealisation: Investing idealistic values in an object or person (for example, the projecting of 'parent-like' qualities on a teacher by a student who may then feel unrealistically safe and cared for)

Intuition: Those internal awarenesses and insights seemingly unconnected with external reality, but often appearing to have wisdoms of their own. May be linked with fantasy and creativity

Learnt helplessness: A chronic form of dependence induced by authoritative methods of care which demotivate clients to care for themselves

Parent: Ego state of transactional analysis concerned with the social world and 'life as taught' (see Berne, 1967)

Projection: Placing our own feelings on another and responding to these feelings as if they originated and belonged there. A subconscious mental defence mechanism

Psychosis: A disordered mental reaction where there is loss of contact with conventional reality and withdrawal from usual social intercourse. A condition necessitating much psychiatric time and effort to address

Psychotherapy: The helping of another by a practitioner trained to a specific counselling mode

Repression: The exile of unpleasant memories and material from consciousness, linked to mental defence mechanisms and cited to explain some of the content of the 'unconscious mind'

Ritual task performance: The reduction of behaviour to a right procedure. May be used defensively to limit personal involvement and disturbing feedback (see Menzies, 1960)

Six category intervention analysis: A model of intervention classification after Heron (1990) who distinguishes between *authoritative* and *facilitative* styles of responding

Social defences: Ways in which social systems are evolved to defend participants from disturbing features of their role – for example, the carer from the distress of the client (see Menzies, 1960)

Status: The respect and value the society invests in a role – for example, the bestowing of professional status on certain workers

Tradition: That body of common practice which supports historically derived meanings and behaviours

Transactional analysis: A model of ego structure and development suggested by Berne, 1967, where personality is classified as consisting of *parent, adult and child* egos, the interplay of which produce characteristic behaviours and may be used to analyse interactions

References

Altschul, A. (1972). *Patient–Nurse Interaction*. Churchill Livingstone, Edinburgh.

Ashworth, P. (1980). *Care to Communicate*. RCN, London.

Barber, P. (1990). *The Facilitation of Personal and Professional Growth through Experiential Groupwork and Therapeutic Community Practice*. Unpublished PhD thesis, University of Surrey.

Barber, P. (1991). Caring; a therapeutic relationship. In *Nursing: A Knowledge Base for Practice*, Perry, A. and Jolley, M. (eds.). Edward Arnold, Sevenoaks.

Barber, P. and Dietrich, G. (1985). The skills of the nurse, caring for people with mental handicap. In *Making Interventions. A Learning Package for Nurses*, Barber, P. and Dietrich, G. (eds.). ENB, London and Sheffield.

Barber, P. and Norman, I. (1987). An eclectic model of staff development. In *Using Nursing Models: Mental Handicap – Facilitating Holistic Care*, Barber, P. (ed.). Hodder and Stoughton, Sevenoaks.

Berne, E. (1967). *Games People Play*. Penguin Books, Harmondsworth.

Cox, T. (1983). *Stress and Health*. Macmillan Press, Basingstoke.

Edelwich, J. and Brodsky, A. (1980). *Burnout: Stages of Disillusionment in the Helping Professions*. Human Sciences Press, London.

Franklin, B. (1984). *Patient Anxiety on Admission to Hospital*. RCN, London.

Harris, T. (1973). *I'm OK, You're OK*. Pan Books, London.

Heron, J. (1990). *Helping the Client: A Creative Practical Guide*. Sage Publications, London.

Holmes, P. (1986). Facing up to disfigurement. *Nursing Times*, 82(34), 16–18.

Jung, C. (1957). *The Undiscovered Self*. Mentor Books, London.

Lamond, N. (1974). *Becoming a Nurse: A Registered Nurse's View of General Student Education*. RCN, London.

Maslow, A. (1967). Cognition of being in peak experience. *Journal of Genetic Psychology*, 94, 43–66.

Menzies, I. (1960). *The Functioning of Social Systems as a Defence Against Anxiety*. Tavistock Pamphlet No. 3, London.

Moscato, B. (1976). The traditional nurse–physician relationship: a perpetuation of social stereotyping. In *Current Perspectives in Psychiatric Nursing*, Kneisl, C. and Wilson, H. (eds.). Mosby, St Louis.

Olsen, V. and Whittaker, E. (1961). *The Silent Dialogue*. Jossey-Bass, San Francisco.

Peplau, H. (1987). Tomorrow's world. *Nursing Times*, 83(1), 29–32.

Rogers, C. (1967). *On Becoming a Person*. Constable, London.

Rogers, C. (1983). *Freedom to Learn for the Eighties*. Merrill, Columbus, Ohio.

Rogers, M. (1970). *The Theory Basis of Nursing*. F.A. Davies, Philadelphia.

Seligman, M. (1975). *Learned Helplessness*. Freeman, Oxford.

Stockwell, F. (1972). *The Unpopular Patient*. RCN, London.

United Kingdom Central Council for Nursing, Midwifery

and Health Visiting. (1984). *Code of Professional Conduct* (2nd ed.). UKCC, London.

UKCC. (1986). *Project 2000. A New Preparation for Practice*. UKCC, London.

UKCC. (1992). *Code of Professional Conduct* (3rd ed.). UKCC, London.

Vousden, M. (1986). Talking to patients. *Nursing Times*, 82(34), 32–35.

Wilson, M. (1975). *Health is for People*. Darton, Longman and Todd, London.

15

CARE OF THE PERSON IN PAIN

Beatrice Sofaer

Physiology Section by John Foord

This chapter serves as a reminder to readers of the implications and effects of pain. The chapter emphasises the uniqueness of the experience of pain for each individual and offers the reader ways in which nurses may assess, support and care for those in pain.

The chapter refers to:

- Differences between acute, chronic non-malignant and chronic malignant pain

- Some personal accounts of experiences of pain

- Physiological aspects of pain

- Psychological and emotional factors as they affect nurses and patients including reference to pain tolerance and pain threshold

- Pain assessment tools which may be used by nurses with patients

- Treatments for and management of acute pain and chronic pain which are followed by references to particular patient groups, for example:
  – children
  – women
  – those with learning difficulties
  – the elderly

This short chapter is dedicated to the memory of a friend, Professor Terry Davidson, former Head of the Department of Anaesthetics, Hadassah Hebrew University Hospital, Jerusalem. He was a unique, *humane* being and was much respected and loved by patients, nurses and medical colleagues alike. He was instrumental in encouraging me to pursue a career in education, particularly in relation to pain management with patients.

To have experienced his warm friendship and wisdom was to have had a rich experience in life.

To have witnessed his courage and determination in the face of his own suffering and pain was a humbling experience.

A frustrating challenge

In recent years much has been written to help us manage pain with patients. So much has been written in fact that it would be quite impossible even to summarise it all in one chapter. This chapter is intended therefore to serve as a reminder of some of the principles involved and to encourage and stimulate further interest among readers. Furthermore, it would not be possible to cover all aspects of pain therapies and relevant research in one chapter. The primary intention is to relate the content to the other chapters in the book so that readers will feel able to integrate and apply some of the principles when nursing people in pain. In addition, the reference list will enable other aspects of the topic to be explored according to the various interests and curiosity of each reader.

One cannot make definitive statements about pain management because pain is a subjective phenomenon and it is impossible to feel what another person feels. It is possible, though, for us to try out one or more available treatments or therapies, sometimes with success. Collaboration with medical or other health professionals is important in facing the difficult and often frustrating challenge of combatting pain. Treatment is often only partially helpful. It is a frustrating challenge because there remains a great deficit in education about pain both for the nursing and medical professions. There is a considerable body of knowledge which has been built up over the past decade but, even allowing for this, pain is managed poorly for the most part, one reason being its frequent omission as a subject in medical and nursing curricula. This omission is being gradually remedied. The most difficult principle for health carers to comprehend seems to be the idea that pain is a very *subjective* phenomenon.

This means that even though it is essential to have a knowledge of factors contributing to pain and its expression, each person's experience has to be viewed and treated in an individual way. Getting this message across, and the resulting consequences for treatment, constitutes a major problem. Fagerhaugh and Strauss (1977) have noted also the complexity of pain management and the effect of ward routines on pain expression and control which has been defined as an important possible area for research (Weisenberg, 1977).

Differences in pain entities

Although medical doctors do the prescribing, we as nurses cope with the overall 'behaviour' of our clients/patients as sensitively as possible. Sometimes we have to do this in the light of little knowledge about their cultural backgrounds, experiences and personalities, all of which may affect responses to pain. Sometimes people in pain behave in a way which is contrary to the way they would like to be seen to behave – because the pain they are experiencing is too much for them. It is wise to keep an open and accepting mind when trying to help people in pain and to avoid developing prejudices and stereotyped beliefs. There is a wide variation within and between people in experience and expression of pain, be it acute pain, chronic non-malignant or chronic malignant pain. These different pain experiences are known as *pain entities*.

(1) *Acute pain* is that which is of a sudden onset and foreseeable end – for example, renal colic, post-operative pain and pain associated with trauma.
(2) *Chronic non-malignant pain* is that which lasts beyond the 'expected' time of healing and which may or may not be associated with ongoing pathology, for example rheumatic pain and chronic back pain.
(3) *Chronic pain occurring towards the end of a person's life* is usually associated with malignancy.

One can experience any of these pain entities at any stage in one's life, from infancy to late adulthood. The stage of life, of course, in itself is an 'experience' which may affect the way that pain is expressed and tolerated.

Neurophysiology of pain

Pain systems

There appear to be two different pain systems that convey pain information from injured skin and/or body tissues to the brain. Both pain systems synapse with neurones in the dorsal horn of the spinal cord in the *substantia gelatinosa* (from its gelatinous texture; Fig. 15.1).

The majority of the ascending neurone pathways in both pain systems are contralateral; that is, they cross over to the opposite side of the brain.

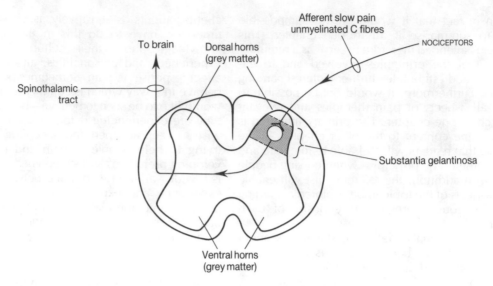

Fig. 15.1 *Transverse section through spinal cord showing some of the structures involved in pain transmission*

(a) **Fast pain system**: pain that is sharp, well-localised (e.g. pinprick or knife cut) and of short duration. This system is usually activated by noxious mechanical stimuli, and is thought to be a more recent evolutionary development. Morphine and other opiates have little or no effect on the fast pain system.

(b) **Slow pain system**: pain of a burning, aching type, poorly localised and frequently associated with tissue destruction. This system is usually activated by severe thermomechanical and algogenic (Greek *algos* pain + *-genes* born) chemical stimuli. It is present in the more primitive vertebrates that have little or no cerebral cortex, and so is thought to be an older pain system (Thompson, 1985). Morphine and other opiates have a very powerful blocking action on the slow pain system.

The origin of pain

The point at which a stimulus (e.g. mechanical, thermal, chemical, etc.) achieves a sufficient magnitude to begin to elicit the awareness of pain is known as the *pain threshold*. Although various factors may elevate (e.g. distraction, ethanol, shock, etc.) or lower (e.g. inflammation, injury, etc.) the pain threshold, it is usually fairly similar for most individuals; skin pressure threshold is about 2 kg, and skin temperature threshold range is about 43 to 47°C (Emslie-Smith *et al.*, 1989). Tissue damage

directly or indirectly releases chemical substances (*algogens*) that activate specialised receptors which detect tissue damage (*nociceptors*). Nociceptor stimulation produces the sensation of pain, thus the terms pain and nociception are often used synonymously (Mackenna and Callander, 1990). However, Stephen Barasi argues that the term nociceptor rather than pain receptor is preferred (Barasi, 1991).

There are two types of nociceptor. Their key properties are:

(a) The **high threshold mechanoceptors (HTM)** only respond to intense mechanical stimulation. HTM afferent axons (nerve fibres that conduct sensory nerve impulses to the spinal cord) belong to the myelinated A delta or Group III fibres (see later and Fig. 15.2).

(b) The **polymodal nociceptors (PMN)** respond to various noxious stimuli, including;
(1) noxious mechanical stimulation
(2) noxious heat stimulation, temperatures of above 43°C (approximately)
(3) stimulation by chemical irritants.
PMN afferent axons belong to slow conducting unmyelinated C or Group IV fibres (see later and Fig. 15.2).

Substances possessing algogenic properties include:

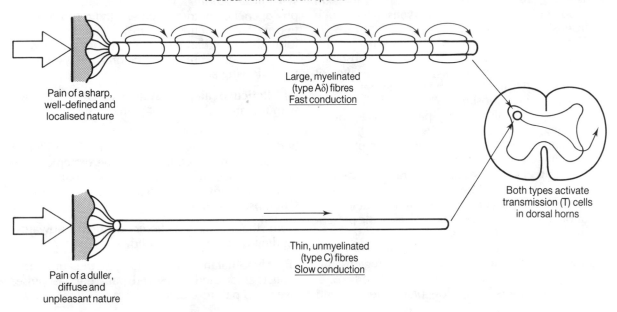

Afferent nociceptor fibres

Two types of nerve fibres transmit pain impulses from periphery to dorsal horn at different speeds

Pain of a sharp, well-defined and localised nature

Large, myelinated (type Aδ) fibres
Fast conduction

Both types activate transmission (T) cells in dorsal horns

Pain of a duller, diffuse and unpleasant nature

Thin, unmyelinated (type C) fibres
Slow conduction

Fig. 15.2 *Peripheral nervous system pain pathways*

(a) **Pain-producing substance (PPS)**: a *polypeptide* (a long chain of amino acids linked together by peptide bonds) with pharmacological properties resembling those of bradykinin. PPS is believed to be the result of the action of various *proteolytic* (protein-splitting) enzymes released during tissue damage on a plasma protein component or components.

(b) **5-hydroxytryptamine (5HT or serotonin)**: released from damaged platelets during injury.

(c) **Acetylcholine**: even in high dilution will immediately give rise to pain.

(d) **Prostaglandin E$_2$**: produced in inflamed tissue, does not directly induce pain but can potentiate the algogenic effects of 5HT and bradykinin. Non-steroidal anti-inflammatory agents (e.g. acetylsalicylic acid, indomethacin) block prostaglandin synthesis by inhibiting the enzyme *prostaglandin synthetase*, so producing an indirect analgesic effect.

Pain pathways to the brain

(a) **The fast pain system**: the peripheral nerve fibres of this pain system are relatively small, myelinated A delta or Group III fibres (Fig. 15.2). The conduction velocity is about 5 to 30 metres per second. Their nociceptors service only skin and mucous membranes (Thompson, 1985). The fast pain impulses are conducted from the substantia gelatinosa by the neospinothalamic pathway to the reticular formation terminating in two thalamic nuclei. This pathway is also known as the *oligosynaptic ascending system* (OAS). It travels in close association with the primary somatic sensory system that mediates touch and pressure senses, and so is phylogenetically (in developmental terms) the more recent pain-conducting system.

The two thalamic nuclei are the ventrobasal complex (the same structure that relays primary somatic senses of touch and pressure) and the posterior nucleus. Both of these nuclei relay fibres to the sensory cortex where precise information about the location and nature of the painful stimulus is presented.

(b) **The slow pain system**: the peripheral nerve fibres of this pain system are tiny, unmyelinated C or Group IV fibres (Fig. 15.2). The conduction velocity is about 0.5 to 2 metres per second. Thus, slow pain messages from the foot can take up to 2 seconds to reach the brain.

The C fibre nociceptors service all of the skin and body tissue except brain nervous tissue which is insensitive to pain.

The afferent unmyelinated C fibres synapse with the T (transmission) cell fibres in the substantia gelatinosa. The terminal axons of these afferent unmyelinated C fibres, when activated, release the neurotransmitter *substance P* which activates the T cells, so transmitting slow pain messages up to the brain.

Substance P is a peptide (a short chain of amino acids, linked together by peptide bonds) discovered in 1931 in a dried extract of acetone powder of a neural tissue extract. The 'P' stands for powder but has come to mean pain, at least in relation to the C fibres. In addition to being present in unmyelinated C fibres as a neurotransmitter, substance P is also found in the spinal cord pain pathways and in a number of brain regions, including the basal ganglia and cerebral cortex.

The T cell fibres of the slow pain system ascend to the brain stem as the paleospinothalamic pathway. This pathway is also known as the *multisynaptic ascending system* (MAS; Fig. 15.3). It is phylogenetically (developmentally) a more primitive pain-conducting system and follows a more tortuous route than the OAS fast pain pathway.

At the brain stem, the MAS forms relays through the following structures:

(a) **Reticular alerting system (RAS)**: concerned with the arousal aspect of pain.

(b) **Periaqueductal grey (PAG)**: a region of cell bodies surrounding the brain stem and midbrain aqueduct. The PAG appears to be extremely important in the sensation and control of pain; it may be critically involved in learned fear and anxiety (Thompson, 1985).

From the PAG, the fibres continue upwards, sending branches to the following:

(a) **Hypothalamus**: accounting for the autonomic aspects associated with severe pain, e.g. fast pulse, sweating, pallor, etc.

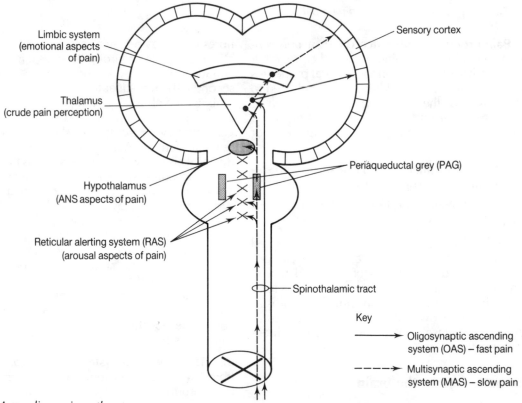

Fig. 15.3 *Ascending pain pathways*

(b) **Intralaminar nuclei** (a portion of thalamus): the thalamus appears to be the site of crude pain perception.

(c) **Limbic system** (portions such as the amygdala): the limbic system appears to contribute to the emotional aspects of pain, e.g. qualities which Melzack describes as wretched, terrifying and vicious (Melzack, 1990).

The ascending MAS fibres finally terminate in the sensory cerebral cortex.

The organisation and role of these higher slow pain system regions is uncertain. However, Melzack (1990) argues that such a slow transmitting, multi-synaptic system is well suited for producing the diffuse, subjective unpleasant experience of pain that will persist for some time after the injury has occurred. He further suggests the possibility that such emotional and motivational aspects of pain would help ensure that a wounded animal, having survived the cause of injury, would feel so miserable as to remain inactive long enough to heal.

Brain opiates and the pain control mechanism

In 1967, Avram Goldstein, at Stanford University, proposed the idea of cerebral endogenous opiate-like chemicals. Solomon Snyder and Candice Pert (Johns Hopkins University), in 1974, demonstrated that radio-active naloxone (a potent, specific morphine-antagonist) binds specifically to neurone receptors in several brain regions, especially throughout the slow pain system. In the same year, the opiate receptor was discovered. Opiate receptors exist in the brains of all higher vertebrates. They are present in the substantia gelatinosa, reticular formation, PAG, hypothalamus, thalamus, basal ganglia and many of the limbic structures; certain of these regions (e.g. cingulate gyrus, hippocampus, amygdala and mammillary body) appear to be particularly involved in the experience of pleasure, pain and emotion. In short, opiate receptors are distributed throughout the slow pain and pleasure systems of the body (Thompson, 1985).

In 1975, John Hughes and Hans Kosterlitz, from Aberdeen University, isolated a substance having the same actions as morphine and named it *enkephalin* ('in the head'). Enkephalin exists in two penta-peptide forms known as *met-enkephalin* and *leu-enkephalin*. A penta-peptide is a peptide which consists of a chain of five amino acids linked together by a peptide bond. The first four amino acids in both enkephalins are identical, only the terminal amino acid is different. In met-enkephalin, it is a sulphur-containing amino acid called *methionine* (met = methionine). In leu-enkephalin, it is an amino acid called *leucine* (leu = leucine).

Subsequently, other brain opioids have been discovered. The whole group are termed either *endorphins* (*endo*genous m*orphine*) or *brain opioids*.

(a) Enkephalins are present in nerve terminals of a number of brain regions, particularly in the slow pain system. At present they are believed to act as opioid neurotransmitters (Thompson, 1985).

(b) Beta-endorphin is much a larger molecule than the enkephalins. It is found almost entirely in the pituitary gland and is derived from a larger precursor pituitary molecule, 'big ACTH', from which ACTH, beta-endorphin and other hormones are made. At present, beta-endorphin is considered to be a pituitary gland hormone having opioid properties (i.e. actions similar to morphine).

(c) Other brain opioids have been discovered, e.g. Goldstein at Stanford has isolated *dynorphin*, a substance that is said to be more than 200 times more potent than morphine. The chemical structure and synthesis of dynorphin is still being determined.

Function of brain opioids

The exact function of brain opioids remains uncertain but the most obvious possibility is the release of these substances by the pituitary and certain neurones in response to stress, so minimising pain and enhancing adaptive behaviour; e.g. minor injury received during athletic or some other vigorous activity, but not noticed at the time.

Enkephalin-containing neurones are found in close association with the lower (spinal) levels of the slow pain system. These spinal cord enkephalin interneurones appear to act synaptically by inhibiting the neurotransmitter release of substance P by the incoming unmyelinated C fibre impulses, so preventing T cell activation (Fig. 15.4). Therefore, any nerve fibre that activates these spinal cord enkephalin interneurones will control (or *gate*) the amount of slow pain received from injured tissues to be conducted to the brain via the MAS slow pain pathway (Fig. 15.4).

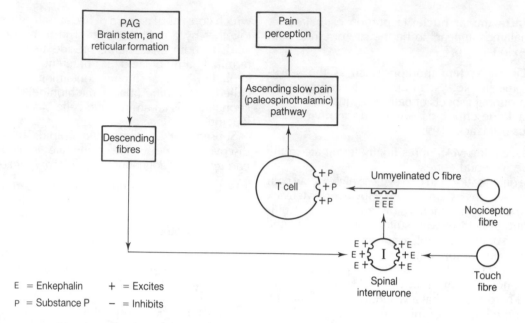

E = Enkephalin   + = Excites
P = Substance P   − = Inhibits

Fig. 15.4 *A possible physiological model for the gate theory*

Enkephalin-releasing spinal interneurones (neurones that interconnect with other neurones in the brain and spinal cord) appear to be influenced by impulses from the following nerve fibres:

(a) Large diameter afferent (LDA) sensory fibres which excite the interneurones, causing enkephalin release which inhibits substance P release from activated unmyelinated C fibres, so preventing T cell activation and thus closing the pain gate (Fig. 15.5). This gate model goes some way towards explaining the following analgesic phenomena:

(1) Why stimulating LDA activity by rubbing the skin in a painful area can sometimes help lessen the pain;
(2) The effectiveness of transcutaneous electrical nerve stimulation (TENS) in pain control by the selective stimulation of LDA activity;
(3) Some of the analgesic effect induced by acupuncture which could also be due to the stimulation of LDA activity.

However, activated afferent nociceptor unmyelinated C fibres activate the substantia gelatinosa T cell by releasing substance P and by directly inhibiting interneurone enkephalin release, so opening the pain gate (Fig. 15.6).

Therefore T cell activation will depend on the algebraic summation of the opposing impulse traffic of the LDA fibres versus the nociceptor C afferents. The final outcome (i.e. the pain gate being open or closed) depends on the afferent fibre system with the greatest impulse traffic in that situation. For example:

(1) When the nociceptor unmyelinated C afferent impulse traffic is greater than the LDA fibre traffic, T cell activation will occur and open the pain gate (Fig. 15.6).
(2) When the LDA fibre traffic is greater than the nociceptor unmyelinated C afferent impulse traffic, T cell activation does not occur and the pain gate is closed (Fig. 15.5).

(b) Descending pathway fibres originating from the sensory cortex, PAG and brain stem reticular formation terminate in the dorsal horn of the spinal cord where they excite enkephalin interneurones and so close the pain gate (Fig. 15.7).

These pathways contain opioid peptides (e.g. enkephalins, endorphins and dynorphin) which appear to act as neurotransmitters or neuromodulators. Their existence goes some way towards explaining how the brain can influence the severity of pain perception.

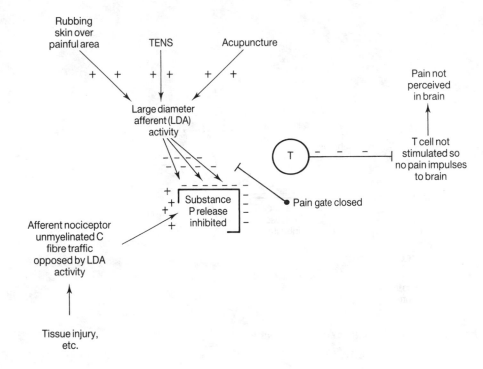

Fig. 15.5 *Pain gate closed by large diameter afferent (LDA) stimulation*

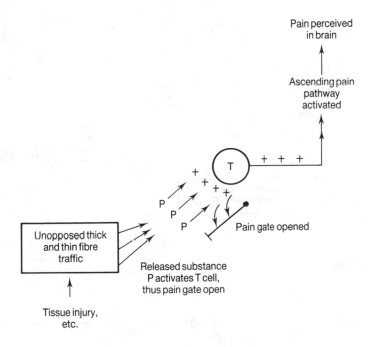

Fig. 15.6 *Tissue injury opening pain gate*

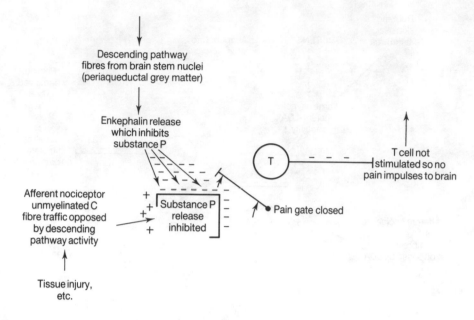

Fig. 15.7 *Pain gate closed by higher centre influences*

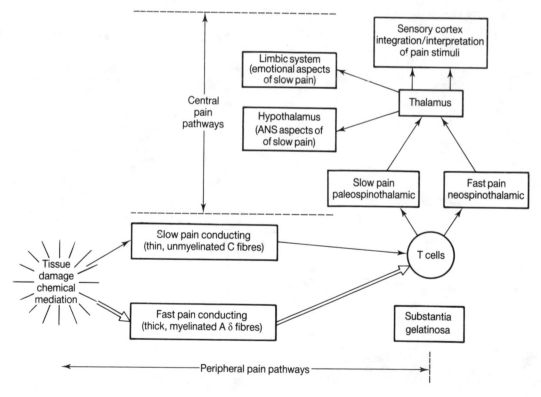

Fig. 15.8 *Summary of pain pathways*

Summary of key points (Fig. 15.8)

Two different pain systems exist in the human body:

(a) **Fast pain system** – conducts pain that is sharp, well-localised and of short duration. Activated by noxious mechanical stimulation which stimulates the HTM nociceptors. Myelinated A delta (Group III) afferent fibres then rapidly conduct the fast pain impulses from tissues to the substantia gelatinosa.

The OAS part of the spinothalamic pathway rapidly conducts the fast pain impulses to the sensory cortex via the thalamus.

(b) **Slow pain system** – conducts pain of a burning, aching type and is poorly localised. Activated by noxious thermomechanical and irritant chemicals producing tissue damage, this releases algogens, such as PPS, which stimulate the PMN nociceptors.

Unmyelinated C delta afferent fibres then conduct the slow pain impulses from injured tissues to the substantia gelatinosa, where substance P is released which activates the spinothalamic pathway T cells.

The MAS part of the spinothalamic pathway conducts the slow pain impulses to the sensory cortex via a number of subcortical structures, including RAS, PAG, hypothalamus, thalamus and limbic system. Involvement with some of these structures is responsible for the wide range of biological and psychological aspects of slow pain, e.g. RAS (arousal), hypothalamus (autonomic nervous system) and limbic system (emotional).

Brain opioids are a range of natural peptides and polypeptides which have slow pain analgesic properties. Spinal cord enkephalin inhibits substance P release, so closing the pain gate. Activated LDA fibres and the descending fibres originating from PAG and brain stem reticular formation close the pain gate by releasing spinal cord enkephalin.

This pain gate model helps explain some of the analgesic effects produced by rubbing a painful injured body area, TENS and some aspects of acupuncture.

Pain and pathology

Chapter 6 of this book discusses pathology. In the context of pain management it is important to note that the absence of pathology does not mean absence of pain (we may not have sufficiently sensitive methods for detecting the pathology). Presence of pathology does not mean presence of pain either. Presence or absence of pain may or may not result in expression of pain by a person. This may be confusing for health professionals, but it is a useful thought to keep in mind when caring for a patient. Being a patient may not be a pleasant experience, as the next section demonstrates.

On being a person in pain

Pain is unpleasant. People who are in pain and who are left to suffer pain sometimes become out of control and are forced into an unhappy situation of becoming impolite. Then they may be labelled as 'difficult' or 'uncooperative'. The following comments are true accounts from patients who 'were left to suffer' by staff. They are offered as food for thought.

Post-operative experience

'The day after my operation I asked the nurses to give me a narcotic to help me sleep. They said they could only give it for the immediate twelve hours post-operatively and would not call the doctor. I just wished the dear Lord would have taken me that night.'

(The patient was a medical doctor himself.)

Three years later

'When I went back to the surgeon and explained that I was having pain around the area of the scar three months after my operation he just didn't believe me; now three years later my family don't believe me. Sometimes I just lie on the bed and cry. My life has changed. The relationships with my family and friends have altered. I try to get on with my life. If only this damn pain would go away.'

(The patient was a 37 year old married house-wife unable to work because of chronic pain.)

Towards the end of life

'This pain is terrible. The doctors tell me I have another three months to live. I can't go on like this. Every day I feel worse. I am losing my self-respect and self-esteem. I want to be able to shave myself and walk to the toilet alone. It's living with the uncertainty that is so awful. I have made my will. I have bequeathed my body to medical science. I have discussed my dying with my wife. So what now? We hang on waiting. Every day is just waiting and waiting and living with this uncertainty. Or should I say dying with this uncertainty.'

(The patient was a man of 62 with carcinoma of the pancreas. He died two weeks later.)

The reader may wish to contrast the statements above with those following:

Post-operatively

'The nurses used a pain assessment chart. They explained that for each patient pain is an individual experience and so, to ensure that I didn't experience unnecessary pain after the operation, they came to my bedside frequently and asked how I was for the first few days after the surgery. The result was, of course, that we were able to avoid unnecessary pain. It was a great help to me to know that they cared, for almost certainly I would have felt uncomfortable having to ask for pain-killers as happened to my aunt when she had the same operation a few years ago.'

(This patient was a 30 year old lady who had had a foot operation.)

The above quotation demonstrates good collaboration between patient and nurses in assessing and controlling the patient's pain.

Six years after the onset

'Even though I know I will never be rid of the pain completely it is helpful to know that I am not being brushed under the carpet by you (the doctor). Sometimes it helps to meet other patients who suffer chronic back pain and we go together (my husband and I) to the back pain meetings. What is needed is more information for the public and for the caring professions. People tend to shy away from patients in pain. I know I have to get on with my life and I cry from time to time and sometimes I bang my fists against the wall. I have to give way to my feelings sometimes. It is helpful to me to know that I can keep in touch with the pain clinic and not feel abandoned. I know that I am *believed*. I am very grateful for that. It gives me some courage.'

(The patient was a 52 year old lady.)

At the end of my life

'I know I am going to die. It is not nice to die. But that is the way it is. The uncertainty is what is so awful. Just being able to talk about it in an honest and straightforward way is helping me to cope.'

(The patient was a 62 year old man with carcinoma.)

Communication skills

As well as knowledge about various pain-relieving treatments, communication skills are central to the issue of relieving pain – be it acute or chronic. Understanding something of the psychological factors in relation to pain may also be important, bearing in mind that each patient is unique and each experience different. Speculation may often contribute to day-to-day management of pain. Be that as it may, the following may be of some help when we think about the problems involved for it is thought that psychological and cultural factors may play a part in pain expression and behaviour.

Acute pain and chronic pain

Acute and chronic pain are different entities and need to be viewed in different ways. *All* pain should be believed. Nurses and all health carers should be aware that management is different for different pain entities. As Sternbach (1974) noted, chronic pain is usually destructive. That is to say, it destroys – physically, socially and psychologically. Acute pain, on the other hand, may be seen as both a warning and an indication of actual tissue damage, thus promoting survival. When acute pain is not relieved, as may be the case when post-operative pain is not assessed with individual patients, feelings of resentment against staff and fear of future hospitalisation may occur. In recalling her experience in hospital, one patient said, 'I couldn't go through taking that pain again. It was terrible. I just would not go in again if I knew the same thing was going to happen to me' (Sofaer, 1992). Sometimes patients feel out of control when their pain is unrelieved and later may feel they have to apologise to staff for aggressive behaviour. No patient should be put in this situation. Dignity and self-respect are important and nurses should strive to maintain these for people entrusted to their care. It is no good saying to a patient, 'You are not due for your pain-killers yet' or, 'Try to hang on a little longer'. Pain is pain and *can* be relieved, especially when it is acute. Relieving chronic pain is a different matter. Nurses should be aware that social, financial and physical changes will probably have taken place in a person's life with the advent of chronic pain, accompanied by erosion of confidence and the will to live. Different therapies and combinations of therapies may have to be attempted.

The feelings of nurses

It goes without saying that sometimes when a patient's pain is unrelieved, nurses feel helpless and distressed. There may be a tendency to avoid the patient. This may lead to unhappiness for the nurse. Indicating to a patient that she is willing to listen to, and be with, the patient is a positive way for her both to help a patient with pain and to feel less helpless. This is particularly applicable when a person is near the end of his life and expresses a need to share his thoughts. One nurse who worked in a hospice said, 'You have to be alert to the important cues from a patient, sometimes these are non-verbal but you *know* the patient wants you to stay with him. . . . He's really saying, "Nurse, do not walk away from my pain".'

Emotional aspects of pain

Undesirable feelings of anguish commonly accompany painful experiences. These may be expressed verbally in a variety of disagreeable ways which demonstrate one or more of the common concomitants of pain, such as fear, anxiety or depression. Interactions between emotional distress and pain are complex. Emotional distress may not only be a component of pain but may be manifested as a consequence of pain or a cause of pain. Acute pain provoked by tissue damage often initiates fear and anxiety. It may be that the greater the fear, the greater the sensitivity to the perceived injury. Usually there is depression associated with chronic pain. Chronic pain has very serious repercussions for the quality of life when there is little hope for relief. The longer a person suffers pain the more depressed he may become due to the disabling lifestyle which may be forced upon him.

Some people are blasé in the face of severe pain while others become angry and resentful to family, friends and health carers. There is a wide variation in coping mechanisms, and each person requires individual assessment of his psychological and social difficulties. Therapeutic interventions for patients who suffer chronic pain must reflect consideration of both physical and psychological aspects of their experience.

Because it is widely recognised that the central nervous system plays a large part in the pain experience, the psychological aspects of pain are being given increasing attention. This means that psychological interventions may often be used in conjunction with physical therapies to help pain sufferers. Many of the strategies used are concerned with how a person perceives and copes with pain and his interpretation of it rather than the elimination of the pain.

Some psychological factors and strategies

In order to help people in pain, it is useful to have an understanding of the psychological factors associated with pain. This applies whether or not a person is at home or in hospital. In terms of the application of useful psychological strategies for patients, it is widely assumed that preparing patients for a possible medical or dental procedure is beneficial. It is not known exactly which 'ingredients' of information-giving are important. However, it is thought that realistic information which is accepted and understood is helpful in allowing a patient to build psychological defences, particularly prior to surgery. An early study by Janis (1958) described the process of mental rehearsal as an important factor in helping a patient to avoid resentment, fear and disappointment. Other researchers have doubted Janis's point about fear and anxiety. Cohen and Lazarus (1973) have suggested that *denial* may be more useful as a coping strategy. Personality may be an important consideration, therefore, when deciding what information ought to be offered to help people to cope. De Long (1970) suggested that copers (people who try to deal with stress) and non-specific defenders (those who use both coping and avoiding strategies) seem able to accept more detailed information than avoiders (those people who avoid stress). The difficulty we face as nurses in the clinical setting is trying to define and distinguish between these groups of people. Ideally, it would be helpful to know what a person's personality was like before the onset of a painful experience so that his behaviour could be understood more easily by the carers.

It is important that we deal with pain from both physical and psychological standpoints, and that we do not regard pain as a symptom of illness only. Several research projects have explored the relationship between personality and **pain tolerance** and **pain threshold**. On the whole, pain thresholds have been shown to be lower for introverted people in comparison to extraverted people, but extraverts were shown to report pain more freely. Bond and Pearson (1969) showed that extravert patients were given analgesics more often than introverts. Petrie (1967) identified three kinds of person (the reducer, the augmenter and the moderate) who are different from each other in the way they experience pain. The reducer tends to decrease what he perceives, while the augmenter increases what he perceives. The moderate neither reduces nor augments. Dealing with individual behaviour and the acceptance of that behaviour without prejudice is important if pain is to be relieved. As a rule *acceptance* of what a person says about his pain is fundamental to management. However, in situations where a patient finds it difficult to express the need for relief, one has to be careful to ensure that suffering is avoided. It is important for the nurse to observe individual coping styles and to accept the wide variation without criticism. It could be helpful for nurses to record how a person sees himself normally and how his attitude changes in illness. If nothing else, the knowledge that staff are interested may be helpful in reducing anxiety – particularly if fear is related to the possibility of pain. There is a case for nursing research to help the profession in this area by investigating ways in which patients might be assessed psychologically on admission to hospital.

Giving information

Suggestions have been made that nurses may help to relieve anxiety by giving information and by teaching patients coping strategies (Johnson *et al.*, 1970). The idea behind using these interventions is that, by knowing what to expect, anxiety will be reduced and so possibly will pain. However, it is important to know what is *usual* for an individual; if a person is normally very anxious or very resistant to anxiety, explaining and giving information may prove to be of little help. The nurse must be prepared for a wide variation in individual responses to possible painful events. Pain is a warning to the body and it may also act as a threat to the personality. Anxiety may manifest itself as uncooperative behaviour, and the nurse should be prepared to respond in an understanding way in such situations. As mentioned above, depression is usually present and, in chronic pain, may manifest itself. Coping with chronic pain is bad enough. Coping with despair makes life and living more difficult. It is not unknown for a patient with chronic pain to attempt to end his own life.

Dealing with the possible psychological problems associated with pain is a challenging task. Developing a relationship with a patient and trying to learn about his normal coping abilities can be invaluable. Discussing feelings with a patient may give us clues as to how he copes.

Avoid labelling

Patients should not be labelled and value judgements should not be made about their behaviour. 'Being good' or 'being cooperative' is irrelevant. What is important to a patient is that he is believed and accepted as an individual. 'Pain is what a patient says it is and exists when he says it does' (McCaffery, 1983). Disapproval should not be shown towards patients because this could interfere with pain assessment. That patients undergoing the same or similar operations will experience the same amount of pain is a myth. For further discussion on the uniqueness of the individual the reader is referred to Sofaer (1992). The amount of tissue damage is not an indicator of the intensity and length of time a patient will experience pain. Signs of suffering may well be suppressed even though a patient is experiencing pain. Patients may or may not show objective signs of pain such as elevated blood pressure. Knowing that patients may adapt to pain both behaviourally and physiologically is important. Tiredness may also affect expression of pain.

Cultural factors relating to pain

An individual's liability to tolerate pain may be affected by his upbringing. There is no correct way for people to react to pain. Weisenberg (1977) has suggested that an important influence on pain expression is the family which transmits cultural norms to children. The meaning attached to pain within a particular group may be important in considering appropriate therapy. For some people, a particular or potentially painful event may be accepted as 'painful' whereas for others it may be seen as tolerable.

Pain assessment

There is a growing awareness of the usefulness of pain assessment. It provides a means whereby nurses can document the site of pain with a patient or a relative, and subsequent changes can be noted. There are no strict rules regarding times of assessment of pain. In general, the time interval of occurrence of pain and its assessment will not be the same for each patient in acute pain but will vary according to the time of administration of pain-relieving strategies, be they analgesics, local anaesthetic blocks or other less invasive procedures. In the case of pain associated with cancer, a body chart may be used to show the distribution of the pain by a patient. The London Hospital Pain Chart (Fig. 15.9) used with patients suffering protracted pain has proved helpful in this respect.

Work in the area of assessing pain in the nursing profession was pioneered by Jennifer Raiman in the 1970s at the London Hospital. There is an urgent need for practising nurses to learn more about application of these tools with patients, both at home and in clinical settings. Before rushing into pain assessment, it is essential that the nurse familiarises herself with information about the patient. A basic prerequisite is the acceptance of the individual nature of pain and the acceptance of individual differences in expression of pain. Pain is a subjective experience, so assessing it in the clinical area presents complex problems. If there is not agreement between a patient's account of a painful experience and the expectations of doctors and nurses in relation to that pain, then the caring professions may try to explain the patient's experience as 'being in the mind' without realising that all pain is real and needs to be managed with patients. Although assessing pain through verbal reports by patients may present problems, very often this is all we have to rely upon. Rating scales are sometimes used to assess changes in intensity and duration of pain. As far as post-operative pain is concerned, pain assessment charts may be useful. Their use should be explained to a patient prior to surgery so that unnecessary pain may be avoided. Close cooperation is called for between medical and nursing colleagues so that pain relief is administered according to the needs of an individual rather than according to a four-hourly regime – see the post-operative pain charts in Figs. 15.10 and 15.11 (Sofaer, 1992).

Logistic problems faced by nurses

Behavioural changes may, of course, take place in any painful situation. People in acute pain react in all sorts of ways. We see acute pain post-operatively, in accident and emergency settings and in intensive care units. The treatment of acute pain is discussed below. It is important to administer relief and maintain control of the pain. A major problem faced by nurses is the difficulty in assessing and treating pain in the shocked patient with multiple injuries, and then persuading medical colleagues that patients *do* require pain relief. Further problems may occur when a patient is in acute pain and (as in the case of accident and emergency departments) may have to wait to see a doctor. It would be helpful then for nurses to employ non-invasive methods of pain relief – such as distraction techniques – so that patients may be helped to focus on a stimulus other than discomfort and pain.

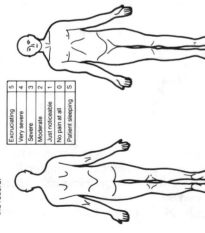

This chart records where a patient's pain is and how bad it is, by the nurse asking the patient at regular intervals. If analgesics are being given regularly, make an observation with each dose and another *half-way between* each dose. If analgesics are given only 'as required', observe 2-hourly. When the observations are stable and the patient is comfortable, any regular time interval between observations may be chosen.

TO USE THIS CHART ask the patient to mark all his or her pains on the body diagram below. Label each site of pain with a letter (i.e., A, B, C, etc.).

Then at each observation time ask the patient to assess:

1. The pain in each separate site since the last observation. Use the scale above the body diagram, and enter the number or letter in the appropriate column.

2. The pain overall since the last observation. Use the same scale and enter in column marked **OVERALL**.

Next, record what has been done to relieve pain:

3. Note any analgesic given since the last observation stating name, dose, route, and time given.

4. Tick any other nursing care or action taken to ease pain.

Finally, note any comment on pain from patient or nurse (use the back of the chart as well, if necessary) and initial the record.

Excruciating	5
Very severe	4
Severe	3
Moderate	2
Just noticeable	1
No pain at all	0
Patient sleeping	S

DATE _____

SHEET NUMBER _____

PATIENT IDENTIFICATION LABEL

TIME	PAIN RATING										ANALGESIC GIVEN (Name, dose, route, time)	MEASURES TO RELIEVE PAIN							COMMENTS FROM PATIENTS AND/OR STAFF	Initials
	BY SITES								OVER ALL			Lifting	Turning	Massage	Distracting activities	Position change*	Additional aids*	Other	Specify where starred	
	A	B	C	D	E	F	G	H												

Fig. 15.9 *The London Hospital pain observation chart (Reproduced by kind permission of Jennifer Raiman)*

PAIN ASSESSMENT CHART

Ward 28

Sheet No. 1

Patient's Name: Mrs MacDonald

Hospital Number: 00 7413

Put a tick in the column which best describes the pain since the last recording

Date	Time	No pain or sleeping	Slight pain	Moderate pain	Severe pain	Pain bad as it could be	Signature of nurse	Site	Comment and/or nursing action	Analgesic given Name	Dose	Route	Time
13.6.92	11.00		✓				P.Smith	abdomen	analgesic given with antiemetic	Diamorphine 5mg		I.M.	11.00
	12.10			✓			P.Smith	abdomen	Discussed with Sr. analgesic given	Diamorphine 5mg		I.M.	12.15
	13.30	✓					P.Smith	—					
	14.30	✓					P.Smith	—					
	15.30			✓			S/N McCallum	abdomen	Analgesic and Antiemetic given	Omnopon	15mg	I.M.	15.35
	16.30	✓					S/N McCallum	—	appears more settled				
	18.00	✓					S/N McCallum	—					
	20.00	✓		✓			S/N Ford	abdomen	washed and turned mi. pain following analgesic given	Omnopon	15mg	I.M.	20.10
	22.00	✓					S/N Ford	—	Turned and settled down.				
	24.00	✓					S/N T.Burns	—					
14.6.92	01.45		✓				S/N T.Burns	abdomen	Analgesic given.	Omnopon	15mg	I.M.	01.45

Fig. 15.10 A pain assessment chart showing how one patient's pain was assessed and effectively relieved following surgery

PAIN ASSESSMENT CHART
Ward 8.

Sheet No. 1

Patient's Name: Mrs Fraser
Hospital Number: 274306

Put a tick in the column which best describes the pain since the last recording

Date	Time	No pain or sleeping	Slight pain	Moderate pain	Severe pain	Pain bad as it could be	Signature of nurse	Site	Comment and/or nursing action	Analgesic given Name	Dose	Route	Time
23.8.92	16.45				✓		P.Jones	abdomen	Requested Dr. to increase dose (refused)	Diamorphine 2.5mg		I/M	17.10
	17.40			✓			P.Jones	abdomen					
	19.10		✓				P.Jones	abdomen					
	20.20	✓					P.Jones						
	21.15			✓			P.Jones	abdomen	Requested Dr. to increase dose (refused)	Diamorphine 2.5mg		I/M	21.20
	22.00			✓			J.Gort	abdomen					
	23.20			✓			J.Gort	abdomen	Analgesia	Diamorphine 2.5mg		I/M	23.25
24.8.92	24.00	✓					J.Gort						
	02.00		✓				M.Fishman	abdomen					
	03.30	✓					M.Fishman						
	04.00				✓		M.Fishman	abdomen	Analgesic given	Diamorphine 2.5mg		I/M	09.00
	07.30	✓					M.Fishman						
	06.00	✓					M.Fishman						

Fig. 15.11 A pain assessment chart showing how the relief of moderate pain was delayed

Treatment of acute pain

Generally speaking, methods of pain relief which 'physically enter' the body (such as analgesics and/or nerve blocks) are often used to counter acute pain. There are therapies, however, which may be helpful to a patient and which lie within the province of nurses. These are known as non-invasive. The nurse may or may not wish to explain to patients methods such as distraction, guided imagery or relaxation. The quality of the relationship between nurse and patient will influence the patient's willingness to try out different techniques. Another non-invasive method of pain relief is Transcutaneous Electrical Nerve Stimulation (TENS) discussed on page 393. Many nurses are learning how useful TENS can be to patients in achieving both acute and chronic pain relief.

In the Accident and Emergency Department or for acute pain management, entonox (a 50/50 mixture of nitrous oxide and oxygen from one cylinder) may be used advantageously. It is rapidly effective and can be self-administered.

An anticipatory approach is useful in treating acute pain. With the use of analgesics it should be noted that undertreatment may cause 'clock watching' by a patient, giving rise to psychological problems. A fear of addiction (be it on the part of staff or of patients) arising from the treatment of acute pain is unfounded. Pain should be relieved *immediately* and, in order to maintain the patient's comfort, analgesics should be given before severe pain returns. The only effective method of control for severe pain is the use of narcotics. Observation of individual responses to analgesia is important and the nurse should be aware that possible adjustments of dose and timing may need to be discussed with both the individual patient and the medical colleagues who prescribe medication. Nurses should be alert to the danger of changing to a less potent analgesic too soon. When a narcotic is used, a narcotic antagonist such as naloxone should be available should narcotic-induced respiratory depression develop. (It should be noted that naloxone is relatively short-acting and it may have to be repeated more than once.) For less severe pain, analgesics such as the non-steroidal anti-inflammatory (NSAID) drugs may be prescribed. Whereas narcotic analgesics act on the central nervous system, non-steroidal anti-inflammatory drugs act peripherally at the site of pain. McCaffery (1983) has summarised the nurse's power and responsibility in relation to administration of medication for pain relief. According to her summary, the nurse is generally expected to:

(1) determine whether or not the analgesic is to be given and, if so, when;
(2) choose the appropriate analgesic when one or more is ordered;
(3) evaluate the effectiveness of the analgesic at frequent, regular intervals following each administration;
(4) be aware of, and alert to, the possibility of side effects from the analgesic;
(5) report promptly and accurately to the doctor when change is needed;
(6) advise the patient about his use of analgesics, both those on prescription and those available over the chemist's counter.

The literature on analgesics is extensive and the reader is advised to consult Sofaer (1992) for an introduction to the subject. For a more thorough insight McCaffery (1983) is very useful. For an in-depth understanding of post-operative pain treatment, you should consult Hoskins and Welchew (1985), *Post-operative Pain: Understanding Its Nature and How to Treat It.*

Table 15.1. *Strategies for controlling acute pain*

- Rest and comfort
- Analgesics
- Local anaesthetic nerve blocks
- Distraction
- Imagery
- Relaxation
- Acupuncture
- Transcutaneous electrical nerve stimulation (TENS)

Table 15.1 gives a list that may be useful when considering options and strategies for controlling acute pain. Apart from the use of analgesics which are prescribed by medical colleagues and the use of nerve blocks which are carried out in certain circumstances, usually post-operatively, by anaesthetists, the other strategies mentioned in this list are within the province of the nurse.

Rest and comfort

People in pain feel tired. Ward routine may involve waking patients in hospital at an hour when most sensible people – especially those who are unwell – would prefer to sleep. It is high time that nursing practice followed the lines of common sense and afforded *extra* rest and sleep to people who have suffered, are suffering, or are likely to suffer pain. All other therapies should be used in conjunction with rest and sleep. A useful way to ensure this would be to supply all post-operative patients with wax earplugs to cut out background noise from the hospital environment and an eye shield to cut out the light. At the very least, patients could be advised to provide these for themselves as part of their efforts towards self-care and self-protection from the busy setting they will find themselves in.

Distraction

Distraction refers to the situation when a person focuses on a stimulus other than pain. It may be a useful strategy to try – especially when there is a good relationship between the nurse and patient. Some people have their own way of distracting themselves. Do be careful though: just because a person is distracting himself, it does not mean he is not suffering.

Distraction may help to increase tolerance for pain. Sometimes one can plan a distraction with a patient. It can be useful during a short procedure or while waiting for another kind of therapy to take effect. It is frequently used during childbirth. Talking, concentrating on a particular object whilst massaging a part of the body slowly and rhythmically can be a useful short term strategy to distract a person from pain. Using imagination, either by looking at pictures or photographs or by thinking about music, can be a powerful distraction especially if one encourages the use of the senses. One patient used a picture of a snow scene on the wall of a clinic and with encouragement from the nurse, she managed to distract herself for about 20 minutes while analgesics were beginning to work. She imagined what she would hear, what she would see around her and what she would feel were she in the snow. While she was using her imagination she forgot about the pain although it was still there.

Distraction usually depends on external stimuli while imagery depends on the mind. The patient referred to above was using imagery in conjunction with and as part of distraction.

Imagery

The use of imagination can be very powerful. It may be taught to a patient for self-use or may be guided by the nurse. Sometimes it may be preceded by a relaxation technique. Relaxation is discussed in the next section. One young patient was able to use imagery to distract herself from pain during a painful dressing. She closed her eyes and imagined she was in a place where she liked to be. With the guidance of the nurse she was able to smell whatever she imagined (in this case it was the scent of lilacs). In addition, she imagined warm sunshine on her skin and she 'heard' children playing in a garden close by. By the time all this had taken place, the painful dressing was completed. To demonstrate the usefulness of this technique to a group of 15 nurses, they were taken blindfolded one spring evening into a garden where there was a heavy scent of flowers. They were asked to imagine they could smell various scents ranging from fish and chips to coffee and fresh baked bread. Thirteen members of the group said they succeeded. When the blindfolds were removed they all smelt the flowers! When asked to identify spices (again blindfolded) only three of the 15 correctly identified spices that, when seen in powder form, they all recognised. They were quite surprised to find that it was possible to imagine sounds and scents. Believing in their own ability and sharing the experiences gave them confidence to try out the techniques with patients.

Relaxation

Relaxation results from freedom from mental and physical tension. Relaxation may be achieved by various means; sometimes people use yoga or meditation. Progressive exercises provide another way to relax. Muscle relaxation training may be useful in helping a person to get off to sleep. Progressive tension of muscles followed by relaxation of muscles in the different parts of the body (in sequence from toes to head) can be taught to a patient pre-operatively for use post-operatively, for example. A technique suggested by McCaffery is as follows:

(1) Breathe deeply and clench your fists

(2) Breathe out and go limp as a rag doll
(3) Start yawning.

Repeat these instructions as often as necessary. Step one should always be followed by step two and step three can be repeated alone at intervals (McCaffery, 1983).

Transcutaneous electrical nerve stimulation (TENS)

TENS is a non-invasive method of pain relief. Its exact mode of action is not known but it is thought that TENS activates peripheral nerve endings in much the same way as does vibration. This therapy was developed by Wall and Sweet (1967) and essentially it can be used to treat pain which is localised and of somatic or neurogenic origin. Sports injuries, pain associated with fractured ribs and post-operative pain are examples of situations where it may be used in the treatment of acute pain, and it may also be useful in the treatment of peripheral nerve injuries and chronic back pain. As shown in Fig. 15.12 the TENS system consists of a stimulator contained in a box about the size of a pack of cigarettes and a battery-powered electronic pulse generator. Two or four (or more) electrodes are connected by lead wires to the stimulator. The electrodes are secured to the skin of the patient and a mild electric current is applied to the skin via the electrodes.

The current can be adjusted by the patient who can control the intensity and quality of stimulation. Sterile electrodes are available for use in post-operative pain. Most stimulators can be used continuously for 24 hours or the electrodes can be detached until stimulation is required (see Figs. 15.12 and 15.13).

The nature of chronic pain

So far, comments related to pain entities and pain assessment have been of a general nature and intended to provide a framework for specialist care. It is especially important that nurses caring for patients with chronic illness and pain appreciate the nature of the depression which often accompanies chronic pain. The following poem from a patient gives us some insight into the isolation experienced through the burden of chronic pain.

'What does it feel like? Pain and more pain.
Darkness and silence and pain. Constant pain.

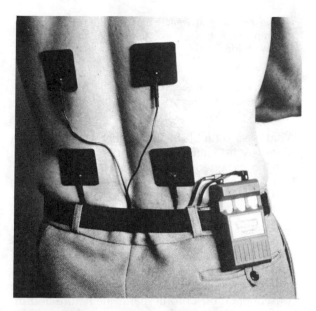

Fig. 15.12 *Placement of electrodes and lead wires attached to TENS*

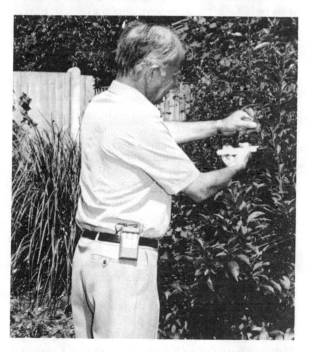

Fig. 15.13 *Patient is able to tend his garden while experiencing relief of pain from the TENS unit*

And no one can reach me . . . no one has the
sympathy, the wisdom, the courage, to find their
way inside

My wilderness of pain.

To find the right words.
Or maybe you, for *you've* helped *me* speak.'
                          (David. Jerusalem, May 1985)

What is so difficult for us to deal with in helping
patients who suffer from chronic pain is the fact
that the experience is different for each person.
That means that for each occasion we listen to the
problems, we are dealing with a new situation for
us. Listening to the difficulties of patients who attend pain clinics, one is often struck by how much
there is to learn and how little one knows. Although one can say in general terms that patients
are likely to experience depression, social, economic and sexual problems in relation to, or as a
consequence of, chronic pain, the nature and intensity of those problems, like the pain itself, is
subjective and will vary from patient to patient.
The first step in developing skills to help a patient
is to believe him. The next step is to allow him to
talk about how he feels about his pain experience.
The skills developed in learning about counselling
are an important part of helping patients in pain.
Living with pain is a burden, both physically and
emotionally. Nurses could be very helpful, too,
in initiating group discussions with patients and
helping them to help each other by talking through
problems and difficulties.

There are many situations and/or diseases which
cause chronic pain in varying degrees from severe
and disabling pain to pain of a milder and less
disabling nature. Wall and Melzack (1984), in
grouping aspects of diseases in which pain may
predominate, have differentiated between soft
tissue and peripheral damage such as found in
osteoarthritis and myofascial (muscle) pain, deep
and visceral pain as found in abdominal and
gynaecological pain, pain associated with nerve
and nerve root damage such as in amputation pain,
pain caused by carcinoma which may involve both
bone and soft tissue, and pain caused by disease
damaging the central nervous system such as that
which may occur as a result of lesions of the spinal
cord.

Pain clinics

People who suffer chronic pain are most often re-

ferred to pain clinics. For most people this is the
end of the road. Most are relieved to find a sympathetic doctor and/or nurse who believes that
they are in pain. One patient stated 'Nobody believed my pain . . . but you do. I feel a bit better
already.'

By the time people have reached a pain clinic,
they will have developed beliefs about their pain.
It has been suggested (Williams and Keefe, 1991)
that taking the opportunity to assess these beliefs
may be valuable in enabling health professionals
to identify treatments which will be acceptable to
the patient.

Treatment of chronic pain

Reference has already been made to the burden
borne by a person suffering from chronic pain.
Sometimes people find themselves being referred
to doctor after doctor in the search for relief and
often search out unconventional treatments. Table
15.2 gives the reader an idea of some of the techniques available to help people suffering from
chronic pain.

In the case of pain associated with non-
malignant conditions, it is advisable when medication is prescribed to use a drug that does not
have an abuse potential. Sometimes psychotropic
medicines, especially antidepressants and phenothiazines, may be useful in relieving chronic pain;
for example, amitriptyline may reduce the severity
and frequence of migraine.

TENS may be used to treat many types of chronic
pain. Some people using TENS may achieve good
relief whereas others experience none.

Acupuncture is a system of medicine developed
by the ancient Chinese. Some acupuncturists use
traditional Chinese acupuncture, needling the skin
at certain points by rotating or stimulating fine
needles. Other acupuncturists use trigger points
which are sensitive regions in the muscle or connective tissue. *Acupressure* is where pressure is
applied to a trigger point. McCaffery (1983) discusses possible areas for acupressure.

Hypnosis induces an altered state of reality in
a trusting relationship. It can be used to modify
perception of pain. Special training and supervision are required in order to use hypnosis. Self-
hypnosis is a very useful tool for the patient in pain
to have at his disposal.

Therapies which may be used by nurses in the
treatment of chronic pain are the same as those in

Table 15.2. *Techniques available to help alleviate chronic pain*

Comfort	Rest and sleep
Medicines	Analgesics
	Psychotropics
	Anticonvulsants
	Tranquillisers
Central modulation	Explanation
	Relaxation
	Imagery
	Hypnosis
	Distraction
	Family therapy
Peripheral and central modulation	Heat, cold
	Vibrotherapy
	Massage
	TENS
	Acupuncture
	Acupressure

Nerve and tracts interruption	Pharmacological
	   – local anaesthetic
	   – chemical nerve
	     blocks

	Surgical – *cordotomy*

	Heat
	   – *radiofrequency*
	     thermocoagulation
	     of nerve roots

	Cold – cryotherapy
Other	Physiotherapy Mud baths Hydrotherapy

the treatment of acute pain. Their use is different, however. The nurse may be instrumental in teaching strategies to patients for use at home according to their own needs. Learning to cope with pain is a problem for people and the nurse may wish to recommend literature for patients to read, such as Lipton (1984).

Counselling skills may be very helpful to a nurse when trying to help a person suffering chronic pain. Identifying areas of a person's life which may have been eroded as a result of chronic pain and discussion of realistic goals for the future are important in striving for hope in future living. For a deeper understanding of the difficulties faced by people who suffer chronic pain, the reader is referred to Finer and Milander, 1985. For further guidelines on the role of the nurse the reader is referred to Boore et al., 1987.

Pain associated with cancer

Pain may or may not be associated with cancer. Where there is pain and life expectancy is short, patients should be given analgesia in sufficient strength, quantity and frequency to control pain (Twycross and Lack, 1983). The possibility of addiction to narcotics is unimportant. The syringe driver is a vital piece of equipment.

When the syringe driver is in use, the injection should be given through a separate intravenous cannula and not through the 'Y' connection into an existing infusion tube. The reason for this is that if the cannula becomes blocked, the narcotic could pass back up the infusion tube and subsequently enter the circulation too rapidly should the blockage in the cannula suddenly clear.

The basis of managing pain associated with cancer is again to individualise the treatment. The idea of a simple 'analgesic ladder' is advocated by several medical colleagues. Generally speaking, this first involves the selection of a drug from the group known as mild analgesics. When this is not effective a moderate analgesic is substituted, and when this is not effective opioid analgesics are used. This is advisable rather than trying an alternative drug from the same level. For a thorough overview of treatment of cancer pain, the reader is referred to Twycross and Lack (1983). As with other pain entities, analgesics may be used in conjunction with other appropriate therapies.

Chapter 27 deals with the last days of life. There is little to add and yet much to be said. Whatever the care provided, it will be related to the place of care. If it takes place at home then the environment will be homely. If it takes place in hospital, the environment will be clinical. Even with the best will in the world and the most caring doctors and nurses, a hospital is a hospital. The sights and sounds are hardly conducive to peace. The hospice movement has worked to change this and has provided a model of caring where individual needs can be met. There can be no doubt that usually a person who is nearing the end of his life is, to quote a medical colleague, 'in bad shape and knows it'. The best and most useful thing we can do as nurses is to practise openness, honesty and caring. That is to say, to communicate in a way that conveys our respect for a fellow human being. Nurses feel very uncomfortable when they are put in a situation of withholding information about impending death from relatives or fellow health professionals because of lack of communication skills. A nurse recently mentioned that when she approached the doctor on her ward and discussed the fears and worries of a particular patient and the difficulties of staff in dealing with evasive answers, he was willing to listen and they were able to agree on an approach which involved truth and honesty both with the patient and relatives. The patient was then 'free' to discuss the pain of dying with his relatives and the staff. It was not a happy situation, but it was an honest one and for the most part free of tension. Trust between members of staff and between staff and patient is an important part of pain relief. For further information on this important aspect of nursing, the reader is referred to Latham (1991).

Special groups with special needs

Some specific points need to be made in relation to groups of people who have special needs when it comes to relieving their pain, in particular the elderly and the very young. Both these groups may experience difficulties when expressing needs and present difficulties to nurses in relation to assessment of pain. In addition, people who have mental illness or learning difficulties suffer pain too and their needs present special problems for carers.

Pain relief with elderly people

It has been pointed out (Harkins, 1987) that an age-related loss of sensitivity to painful stimuli has not been well documented in either laboratory or clinical studies. The implications for management of pain mean, therefore, that we must be cautious not to underestimate the need for pain control in elderly people. Harkins also suggested that 80% of older individuals have *at least one* condition which is likely to be associated with pain. Melding (1991) pointed out the deficiency of studies to do with pain and elderly people.

The problems of psychological and sensory changes which may accompany ageing have to be taken into account when assessing pain with an elderly person. It is difficult to assess the level of pain of a patient with communication difficulties especially if he is demented or disoriented. When medication is provided it may also prove difficult to assess its efficacy. There is the possibility of misinterpretation of signs. One nurse, commenting on the problem, stated that the attitudes of staff and lack of knowledge about the process of ageing often result in a 'quasi-military style and approach' to pain relief in caring for elderly people. The solutions to difficulties experienced by patients and staff are not easy. It may be possible, through *careful* observation and by monitoring usual behaviour, to detect changes which may lead one to suspect a patient is suffering pain. Increased agitation or aggression may be indicators. Helping an elderly person through clear and unhurried explanation is important. Involvement of family and friends (as well as other health care professionals) in assessing pain can sometimes help us to respond to individual needs. It is important therefore to try and find the level of communication of an elderly person and to use speech and language that is acceptable.

In trying to highlight some problems in caring for elderly people in pain, Sofaer and Ziv (1987) suggested that, where concentration seemed to be impaired, removal of distracting visual and auditory stimulation during communication could help. Only one person communicating at any one time with a confused person is important. The use of repetition of speech and touch may help a person to focus attention. Avoidance of harassment may be accomplished through asking about needs in a simple way. One student drew up a plan and applied it in caring for an elderly confused person (see Fig. 15.14).

It is a genuine cause for concern that a patient might be suffering. For this reason communication skills need to be developed and practised by nurses in order to relieve pain. You have to communicate

---

(1) Approach the patient in an open and friendly way

(2) Identify yourself... 'I am Rachel and I will be looking after you today'

(3) Use of clear, softly modulated speech

(4) Turn off the radio or TV during nursing care

(5) Use short sentences ... 'Are you cold?' 'Here are your tablets'

(6) In asking questions, wait for a response before asking another. Use repetition and the same tone if not understood

(7) Avoid double questions

(8) Use touch

(From Sofaer and Ziv, 1987)

Fig. 15.14 *Plan to be applied in caring for an elderly, confused person*

in order to assess pain and you have to assess pain in order to relieve it.

Walker *et al.* (1990) have shown that personal coping strategies are important for elderly patients in the community in order for them to control chronic pain.

The pain of children

Obviously there is a wide difference in life experiences between the very young and the very elderly patient. Nevertheless there may be some similarities which affect pain expression in these two groups. A child is in the process of acquiring a vocabulary, while an elderly person may be losing vocabulary due to deterioration of the senses (Eland, 1985). As Melzack (1987) says, 'it hurts to watch a child suffer'. He further mentions that treatment of pain in children has been dominated by the myth that children do not feel pain as intensely as adults. McGrath and Unruh (1987) have presented evidence that infants feel pain from birth. They suggest that there are three important areas where health carers have responsibilities to ensure pain control:

(1) Anaesthesia for operative procedures
(2) Post-operative pain and other medical conditions
(3) Relief of pain caused by injury and disease.

Their clinical guidelines include suggestions to select appropriate analgesics to match the level of expected pain, to control pain with regular rather than 'prn' schedules, and to avoid injections by substituting sublingual, rectal, intravenous or oral medications. They stress the importance of providing a supportive and interesting environment as a way of utilising distraction through play. Their recommendations for the management of post-operative pain to be part of the standard care plan applies across the board to children and adults alike. The reader is advised most strongly to consult McGrath and Unruh since there has, until recently, been a dearth of material published on pain control for children.

People with learning difficulties

This group of people may suffer unnecessarily due to lack of knowledge and information of the health care professionals. Some patients may show, for example, self-injurious behaviour. There may be a tendency for nurses to think that these patients do not feel pain to the same extent as 'normal people'. The breaking of such behavioural patterns is extremely difficult and requires motivation and experience on the part of the nurse. It could be that an individual starts this behaviour because of boredom with life and the stimulus of hurting oneself is under the person's control and relieves the boredom. This then could become a learned behaviour.

When people with learning difficulties have a specific illness or disease, picking up pain cues from them may be difficult. Close observation of changes in behaviour and communication with relatives or others who know the person well is very important if pain is to be identified and controlled. When such a patient is admitted to hospital, nurses are often scared because of their lack of experience in dealing with people who have learning difficulties. In such situations it should be possible to have someone stay in hospital with the patient who understands and can communicate with them and sometimes on their behalf.

Doctors specialising in pain therapy sometimes reveal how 'lost' they feel when faced with a patient with learning difficulties who is possibly in pain. How can the pain they are experiencing be assessed? One doctor described a situation where he was called to see a patient who had an abdominal tumour. The patient was blind and deaf and had learning difficulties. In any situation where such a patient may be suffering pain, it is absolutely essential to have a resource person to translate 'cues'. Skill is required to observe the behavioural changes in such patients. Also, as Fischbacher (1991) notes, some such individuals have a 'surprising tolerance to pain' and because communication with them can prove difficult, it is important to carry out a physical examination.

Women and pain

Crook (1985) has suggested that there is no consistent evidence to suggest that gender is a factor in the individual's pain tolerance or pain threshold. There are, however, certain conditions which affect either males or females. As Chapter 17 relates specially to the care of women, some discussion will be devoted to pain which is 'special' to the female gender.

Pain of a gynaecological nature may be acute or chronic. Acute pain may be due to such conditions as abortion, tubal pregnancy, acute pelvic inflammatory disease and torsion of an ovarian cyst. Chronic pain may be due to recurrent cyclical pain such as dysmenorrhoea, or pain associated with endometriosis, chronic pelvic inflammatory disease, displacement of the uterus, or pain due to a malignancy in the pelvic cavity (see also Chapter 17).

When pelvic pain lasts for several months and is not cured by medical or other methods, laparoscopy may be carried out followed by surgery if necessary. The role of the nurse is wide and varied in the treatment of gynaecological pain. She will often be called upon to offer information and/or counselling. When a patient expresses the need to discuss matters of a private nature with a nurse, it is important that privacy is respected and such discussions are not overheard by other patients. The guidelines for pain relief are the same as for other patients suffering acute or chronic pain.

The pain of labour

Childbirth is uncomfortable and severe labour pain may produce serious long term emotional consequences (Bonica, 1984). This could be a problem for future pregnancies and affect the relationship between a mother and her child and/or her partner. For an excellent guide to the use of analgesia and anaesthesia in childbirth, the reader is referred to Liu and Fairweather (1991).

Professional development

Learning about pain relief is a major task for the nurse. It requires an attitude of mind that allows patients to have control over their own pain and to maintain self-respect. It also means that patients must be encouraged to feel that *they do not have to suffer*. In terms of responsibility the nurse can choose how she moulds the situation. She can make an active effort; for example, she can choose to assess pain at times other than traditional drug rounds. She can involve other colleagues in discussions on how best to individualise pain relief for patients. She can request and seek out more information on different methods of pain relief according to her specialty. She can read books and articles on developments in pain research and therapy. She can encourage attendance at workshops and seminars to help herself and colleagues to manage pain better.

The power to make pain relief happen with patients belongs to the nurse. Professional development involves taking on responsibility to communicate better with medical colleagues and working together so that patients will not suffer unnecessarily. Pain relief is part of our ethical commitment to caring. Edwards (1984) has identified two areas where ethical values are important. First, there is the duty *not* to inflict pain unnecessarily during the course of investigations and, second, there is the duty to relieve pain as much as possible by whatever means possible. Sometimes pain relief gets forgotten; in the effort to treat an illness it may not be seen as a priority. In treating infection, for example, it is important to relieve the pain as well. In planning care for ill people, good communication is paramount to relief of pain. In this respect, nurses bridge the gap between patient and doctor and are often in a position (because of their increasing exposure to interdisciplinary contacts) to influence communication (Sofaer, 1983).

Making links

Nurses' experiences in communication skills are useful and important for making links with colleagues. Sometimes occupational therapist colleagues may be consulted regarding social and environmental situations. In the community setting, and where nurses are caring for people suffering chronic pain, it is important for the nurse to be knowledgeable about different pain-relieving strategies and to have the courage to use them. Because direct communication is possible with other health care professionals, particularly where a patient is receiving analgesia, pain assessment in the form of home recording charts can be helpful. These may be used to assess the necessity of increasing, decreasing or changing prescriptions. As always, pain assessment should be done *with* and not on a patient or client. At home the family may wish to be involved in helping to assess and relieve pain. Often relatives and friends are very worried about pain and feel guilty if they are not involved in care. In the community the nurse sees the person at home and gleans some understanding of his social setting and home environment. This may help the nurse to assess the support systems in the family and to feel her way in helping the patient and his family to cope with pain. The kinds of things that affect the lives of patients at home are to do with the physical environment and the contact and interaction people have with family members and society. Pain affects the quality of life for the sufferer and this is reflected in their social setting. Assessment of the social situation may, therefore, be an integral part of 'pain' assessment.

Hospital and community nurses should explore together the 'pain problems' and coping difficulties of their patients and clients so as to gain a deeper understanding of coping strategies and individual circumstances and of the complementary roles of nurses to each other and other health carers.

'The pain of nursing'

There is so much to be said about pain. This chapter really only touches the tip of the iceberg. Pain can take acute and chronic forms. It is often part of life and sometimes part of death. We cannot avoid it, but we can help to relieve it. Nurses have that opportunity yet people still suffer pain unnecessarily. There is a growing momentum within the medical profession to make advances in the field of pain research and therapy. 'Nurses *must* get in on the act' (Wall, 1988). The way forward is to increase knowledge and communication skills so that our patients will not suffer unnecessarily. The reader is advised to consult the recommended literature. It will take time and there is much to learn. It may be that the more you learn the less you know, but then you will have to consider whether it is better to know that you don't know, or not to know that you don't know. It is your own insight that will take you forward and help you to help others. There will be difficulties and risks to take: good luck.

Glossary

Acupressure: Pressure exerted on certain points on the body. Usually pressure is applied to traditional acupuncture points using the thumb or the index finger

Acupuncture: A system of medicine developed by the ancient Chinese where fine needles pierce the skin at certain points on the body. The needles are rotated or stimulated

Cordotomy: A neurosurgical procedure carried out on the spinal cord to cut pain pathways

Pain threshold: The least stimulus intensity at which a person perceives pain

Pain tolerance: The greatest stimulus intensity causing pain that a person is prepared to tolerate

Psychotropics: A group of drugs which include antidepressants and phenothiazines which may sometimes relieve chronic pain

Radiofrequency thermocoagulation of nerve roots: Destruction of nerve roots by heat using a special electrode under X-ray conditions

Vibrotherapy: Electric or battery-operated vibrators of varying shapes and sizes are available and may be used by patients to provide pain relief

References

Barasi, S. (1991). The physiology of pain. *Surgical Nurse*, October, 14–20.

Bond, M.R. and Pearson, I.B. (1969). Psychological aspects of pain in women with advanced cancer of the cervix. *Journal of Psychosomatic Research*, 13, 13–19.

Bonica, J.F. (1984). Labour pain. In *Textbook of Pain*, Wall, P.D. and Melzack, R. (eds.). Churchill Livingstone, Edinburgh.

Boore, J.R.P., Champion, R. and Ferguson, M.C. (1987). *Nursing the Physically Ill Adult* (Chapter 9). Churchill Livingstone, Edinburgh.

Cohen, F. and Lazarus, R.S. (1973). Active coping processes, coping dispositions and recovery from surgery. *Psychosomatic Medicine*, 35, 375–379.

Crook, J. (1985). Women in pain. In *Perspectives on Pain*, Copp, L.A. (ed.). Churchill Livingstone, Edinburgh.

De Long, R.D. (1970). *Individual Differences in Patterns of Anxiety Arousal, Stress Relevant Information and Recovery from Surgery*. PhD thesis, University of California.

Edwards, R.B. (1984). Pain and the ethics of pain management. *Social Science and Medicine*, 18, 515–523.

Eland, J.M. (1985). The role of the nurse in children's pain: psychosocial factors. In *Perspectives on Pain*, Copp, L.A. (ed.). Churchill Livingstone, Edinburgh.

Emslie-Smith, D., Paterson, C.R., Scratcherd, T. and Read, N.W. (1989). *Textbook of Physiology* (11th ed.). Churchill Livingstone, Edinburgh.

Fagerhaugh, S.Y. and Strauss, A. (1977). *Politics of Pain Management*. Addison Wesley, New York.

Finer, B. and Milander, B. (1985). Living in chronic pain. In *Persistent Pain, Vol. 5*, Lipton, S. (ed.). Grune and Stratton, New York.

Fischbacher, E. (1991). The assessment and delivery of health care. In *Caring for People with Mental Handicaps*, Fraser, W.I., MacGillivroy, R.C. and Green, A.M. (eds.). Butterworth Heinemann, Oxford.

Harkins, S.W. (1987). Pain in the elderly. *Pain Supplement 4*. Elsevier, Amsterdam.

Hoskins, J. and Welchew, E. (1985). *Post-operative Pain: Understanding Its Nature and How to Treat It*. Faber and Faber, London.

Janis, I.L. (1958). *Psychological Stress*. John Wiley and Sons, New York.

Johnson, J.E., Dabbs, J.M. and Leventhal, H. (1970). Psychological factors in the welfare of surgical patients. *Nursing Research*, 19(1), 18–20.

Latham, J. (1991). *Pain Control*. The Lisa Sainsbury Foundation Series. Austen Cornish, London.

Lipton, S. (1984). *Conquering Pain*. Martin Dunitz, London.

Liu, D.T.Y. and Fairweather, D.V.I. (1991). *Labour Ward Manual* (2nd ed.). Butterworth Heinemann, Oxford.

Mackenna, B.R. and Callander, R. (1990). *Illustrated Physiology* (5th ed.). Churchill Livingstone, Edinburgh.

McCaffery, M. (1983). *Nursing the Patient in Pain*. Harper and Row, London.

McGrath, P.J. and Unruh, A.M. (1987). *Pain in Children and Adolescents*. Elsevier, Amsterdam.

Melding, P.S. (1991). Is there such a thing as geriatric pain? *Pain*, 46, 119–121.

Melzack, R. (1987). Foreword in *Pain in Children and Adolescents*, McGrath, P.J. and Unruh, A.M. (eds.). Elsevier, Amsterdam.

Melzack, R. (1990). The tragedy of needless pain. *Scientific American*, 262(2), 19–25.

Petrie, A. (1967). *Individuality in Pain and Suffering*. University of Chicago Press, Chicago.

Sofaer, B. (1983). Pain relief: the importance of communication. *Nursing Times*, 79(49), 32–35.

Sofaer, B. (1992). *Pain: A Handbook for Nurses* (2nd ed.). Chapman and Hall, London.

Sofaer, B. and Ziv, L. (1987). Problems of pain in the elderly. In *Proceedings of the Ninth Third Open Conference of the Workgroup of European Nurse Researchers*, Kirjayhtyma Oy, Helsinki.

Sternbach, R.A. (1974). *Pain Patients: Traits and Treatments*. Academic Press, New York.

Thompson, R.F. (1985). *The Brain: An Introduction to Neuroscience*. W.H. Freeman and Company, New York.

Twycross, R.G. and Lack, S.A. (1983). *Symptom Control in Far Advanced Cancer: Pain Relief*. Pitman, London.

Walker, J.M., Akinsanya, J.A., Davis, B.D. and Mercer, D. (1990). The nursing management of elderly patients with pain in the community; study and recommendations. *Journal of Advanced Nursing*, 15, 1154–1161.

Wall, P.D. (1988). Chronic pain: more than one answer? Lecture to Leeds Polytechnic students and staff.

Wall, P.D. and Melzack, R. (1984). *Textbook of Pain*. Churchill Livingstone, Edinburgh.

Wall, P.D. and Sweet, W.H. (1967). Temporary abolition of pain in man. *Science*, 155, 108–109.

Weisenberg, M. (1977). Pain and pain control. *Psychological Bulletin*, 84(5), 1005–1044.

Williams, D.A. and Keefe, F.J. (1991). Pain beliefs and the use of cognitive-behavioural coping strategies. *Pain*, 46, 185–190.

Suggestions for further reading

It is strongly recommended that readers explore further some of the titles cited in the reference list. Another useful text is:

Melzack, R. and Wall, P.D. (1988). *The Challenge of Pain*. Penguin Books, Harmondsworth.
Also:

Bourbonnais, F. (1981). Pain assessment: development of a tool for the nurse and patient. *Journal of Advanced Nursing*, 6(4), 277–282.
and
Raiman, J. (1986). Monitoring pain at home. *Journal of District Nursing*, 4(11), 4–6. This paper explores the use of a patient-maintained diary in the management

of pain experienced by a terminally ill patient nursed at home.

For the nurse who is particularly interested in the treatment of pain in children, the following will be useful:

Eland, J. (1988). Persistence in paediatric pain research: one nurse researcher's efforts. In *Recent Advances in Nursing: Excellence in Nursing*, Johnson, J. (ed.). Churchill Livingstone, Edinburgh.

Mills, N. (1990). Pain behaviour in infants and toddlers. *Nursing Times*, 86(23), 54.

Price, S. (1990). Pain: its experience, assessment and management in children. *Nursing Times*, 86(9), 42–45.

Useful texts on physiology are:

Green, J.H. (1989). *An Introduction to Human Physiology* (4th ed.). Oxford University Press, Oxford.

Hinchliff, S. and Montague, S. (eds.) (1988). *Physiology for Nursing Practice*. Baillière Tindall, London.

16

CARE OF THE PERSON WITH AN INFECTION

Kate Ward

The aim of this chapter is to provide the reader with an understanding of the transmission, prevention and control of infection, as well as discussing the individual needs of a person with an infection.

The chapter includes the following topics:

- Body defences
- Transmission of organisms
- Reaction of the body to infection
- Needs of the person with an infection
- Controlling the spread of infection

- Investigation and control of an outbreak of infection
- Hospital acquired infection (HAI)
- Surveillance and audit
- Education and training

'The chief indictment of hospital work at this period is not that it did no good, but that it positively did harm . . . The common cause of death was infectious disease; any patient faced the risk of contracting a mortal infection'
(McKeown and Brown, 1955).

Progress has obviously been made since the 18th century, to which the above relates, but for a significant number of people who acquire infections in hospital, perhaps progress has not been great enough. Infection is associated with pain and distress, and, at times, with mortality. As the patient who suffers from infection is not confined to just one specialty or one section of society, it is necessary for all those involved in the care of the sick and the healthy both to understand and also

to practise methods by which infection can be prevented or controlled.

The work of Lister and his followers, the advent of antibiotics and the increase in knowledge of infectious agents and their mode of spread could give rise to the assumption that infections no longer pose the problem they used to. Unfortunately, with the difficulties caused by antibiotic-resistant organisms, new conditions such as AIDS and a reluctance to reject practices which can only be described as 'ritualistic', infection remains a considerable threat to health. The care of the person with an infection is still an important part of the health carer's role.

Nurses need to understand how infection is spread to promote prevention and control. For individual patients, nurses must anticipate the problems that may arise due to infection in order to prescribe appropriate nursing care, and must appreciate and participate in the important activity of health education to increase public safety and well-being.

Body defences

In order to prevent and control infection, the nurse must begin by understanding the way in which the human body protects itself against the entry of micro-organisms. Disease and trauma very often affect these defences; for example, an abdominal wound breaches the protective function of the skin, making the patient more susceptible to infection. If the nurse appreciates this fact, preventive measures can be included in nursing care plans and the risk of wound infection reduced. The first part of this chapter outlines some of the body defences.

The skin

The skin is one of the main protective organs of the body. It not only protects the deeper and more delicate organs but also acts as a substantial barrier against the invasion of micro-organisms. Fatty acids which are secreted in sebum help to inactivate micro-organisms that are not normally resident on the skin.

Any break in the skin, for example a wound or a puncture from a needle, may result in micro-organisms gaining entry to the body.

The eye

The continuous flow of tears from the lachrymal and other glands is responsible for keeping the conjunctiva moist and healthy. These secretions contain *lysozyme* (an enzyme with antibacterial properties) and other antimicrobial substances. However, their main action is to wash away foreign particles and they are aided in this function by the lids which pass over the surface of the eye every few seconds when blinking.

The conjunctiva may become infected by organisms in a number of ways: via the circulation (as is the case with the measles virus), by mechanical means (by organisms on the fingers or carried by flies), and during birth (by gonococci, for example).

The mouth

Saliva contains antimicrobial substances, lysozyme and **secretory antibodies**. It also removes micro-organisms mechanically by its flushing action. Should these functions be disturbed, the normal balance of oral micro-organisms could be upset. In certain circumstances, such as when a patient becomes dehydrated, the flow of saliva is reduced. This allows the number of bacteria to increase significantly, resulting in the patient having a foul mouth. Gum infections may occur when the resistance of the mucosa is lowered due to a vitamin C deficiency.

Certain areas of the teeth are readily colonised by bacteria. When dietary sugar is used by the bacteria contained in plaque, the resulting acid decalcifies the tooth, eventually resulting in dental caries.

The respiratory tract

The lower respiratory tract is lined with mucous membrane covered with ciliated columnar epithelium. Foreign particles which enter the tract are wafted back up to the throat by ciliary action. Particles entering the upper respiratory tract are moved down to the throat in a similar way and swallowed. The alveoli are lined with macrophages which **phagocytose** micro-organisms (see also Chapter 5).

Damage or disturbance of mucociliary function may occur for a number of reasons including viral infections, chronic bronchitis, cigarette smoking and the use of indwelling tracheal tubes.

The gastro-intestinal tract

The mucus protecting the epithelial cells throughout the tract appears to act as a mechanical barrier and contains secretory antibodies which protect the individual against infection. Many bacteria prefer slightly alkaline conditions and certain intestinal micro-organisms (for example, salmonella) are more likely to cause infection when either the host's production of acid is reduced, or if the organism is protected by food particles.

Enzymes and bile may also inhibit the growth of **pathogenic** organisms. While the normal bacterial flora are in a balanced state, colonisation by other pathogenic bacteria tends to be resisted. However, the balance can be upset by, for example, broad spectrum antibiotics which may allow an over-growth of antibiotic-resistant micro-organisms.

Babies who are breast-fed are more able to resist colonisation by pathogenic bacteria because of the metabolic activity of lactobacilli. As the predominant bacteria in the large intestine, lactobacilli produce acid and other factors that inhibit growth of other micro-organisms. Lactobacilli are lacking in bottle-fed babies, making them susceptible to infections caused by organisms such as pathogenic strains of *Escherichia coli*.

The urogenital tract

The female urethra is approximately 5 cm long — much shorter than the male urethra (approximately 20 cm long). This lack of length enables micro-organisms to enter the female bladder more readily and cause infection.

Normally, urine flushes the urinary tract every hour or two. This frequency of voiding reduces the chances of micro-organisms gaining access and becoming established. Urine itself provides an excellent growth medium for bacteria if it is not too acid. If there is any disturbance in the flow of urine, or if a residue of urine is retained in the bladder following incomplete emptying, the entire urinary tract will be susceptible to infection.

There is some evidence that the bladder wall has some intrinsic antibacterial activity but this mechanism is not fully understood.

The vagina is protected from colonisation by many micro-organisms from puberty until the menopause. During this reproductive period the vaginal epithelium contains glycogen due to the action of circulating oestrogens. A lactobacillus (*Doderlein's bacillus*) which colonises the vagina metabolises glycogen to produce lactic acid which gives the vagina a pH of about 5.0. This pH together with other products of metabolism inhibits the growth of all but a select group of non-pathogenic bacteria.

Transmission of organisms

Just as the understanding of body defences enables a nurse to prevent and control infection, so a knowledge of the ways organisms are transmitted will help in both the planning and implementation of care for a patient with an infection. If the way in which the infection is spread is appreciated, measures can be taken to block the spread of the

infective agent and reduce the risk of cross-infection. Examples of this could be the wearing of masks for certain infections transmitted by droplets, or the wearing of gloves to prevent contact spread of diseases like salmonella.

The degree to which bacteria are shed, their virulence and the number required to cause infection are all factors that influence the ease with which such micro-organisms are transmitted (Table 16.1).

Table 16.1. *The major routes of transmission of infection*

(1)	**From human to human:**	– Respiratory and salivary spread
		– Faecal-oral spread
		– Venereal spread
		– Bloodborne spread
(2)	**From *vectors* to humans (zoonoses):**	– Insects (for example: *Malaria* – mosquitoes; *Typhus* – fleas, ticks, mites)
		– Animals (for example: *Brucellosis* – cattle; *Rabies* – dogs; *Salmonellosis* – cattle, poultry)
		– Insect/Animal (for example: *Plague* – rats via fleas; *Yellow fever* – monkeys via mosquitoes)

Respiratory and salivary spread

Infection transmitted by the respiratory tract depends on micro-organisms being contained in airborne particles (aerosols). Coughing, sneezing or even talking will expel droplets from the respiratory tract and transmit most forms of virus infection (for example, influenza, poliomyelitis) and such bacterial diseases as diphtheria, meningococcal meningitis and pneumonia. It is estimated that as many as 20,000 droplets are produced in a sneeze and that during the common cold, for instance, many of these will contain virus particles. A number of viruses, such as the mumps virus and the cytomegalovirus, can infect the salivary glands and may be transmitted on hands or objects contaminated by saliva. Saliva is exchanged during kissing and infections can be transmitted in this way among all age groups. Spitting, which ejects both saliva and secretions from the lower respiratory tract, may transmit organisms — particularly those such as the tubercle bacillus which are resistant to drying.

Staphylococcus aureus may be shed from the nose and perineal area in small amounts but occasionally a person is found to shed large amounts of this organism. These 'dispersers' are responsible for heavy environmental contamination and are a particular hazard should they work in an operating theatre.

Faecal-oral spread

Faeces may contain micro-organisms that cause intestinal infections. Faecal contamination of the environment, which can result from diarrhoea, may transmit such organisms. Organisms which are resistant to drying can remain infectious for long periods outside the body. An example of this is the tetanus spore which is shed in large numbers in the faeces of domestic animals and may cause infection following a cut or abrasion sustained in the garden.

Contamination of food or water used for drinking can effectively transmit micro-organisms from faeces to mouth.

Spread via urine

Although urine may transmit infection in similar ways to faeces, transmission of micro-organisms shed from the urogenital tract generally depends on mucosal contact with susceptible individuals.

Venereal spread

Although semen is an unusual vehicle for the transmission of micro-organisms, it may contain, for example, cytomegalovirus and HIV (Human Immunodeficiency Virus), both of which can be transmitted during sexual intercourse.

Spread via human breast milk

Human breast milk may contain HIV, the mumps virus or cytomegalovirus. It is difficult to ascertain at present how effective a vehicle of transmission breast milk is, but HIV has been shown to have been transmitted by this route (Peckham, 1988).

Bloodborne spread

Transmission of infection through blood may occur as a result of inoculation wounds, trauma, transfusions of blood or blood products, and from bites of bloodsucking insects such as mosquitoes, fleas and ticks.

The reaction of the body to infection

There are a number of ways in which the body overcomes invading micro-organisms and these will now be discussed in general. Greater detail can be obtained from immunology and microbiology textbooks.

Cells and antibodies

Both cells and antibodies have a part to play in developing immunity to infection. Lymphocytes are small cells with large nuclei. There are two types of lymphocytes; *B lymphocytes* and *T lymphocytes*. The B lymphocytes become plasma cells which produce antibodies. T lymphocytes, associated with the thymus gland, produce soluble substances which activate *macrophages*. Macrophages are large motile cells which phagocytose and destroy micro-organisms. Polymorphonuclear cells, also motile, have a similar role to macrophages in phagocytosis and destruction of micro-organisms and are the main constituent of the pus produced in many infections.

Antibodies produced by plasma cells are carried in the blood to the infected area. These antibodies normally appear at the time of recovery from the infection and frequently persist for long periods after recovery. They are not only responsible for aiding recovery but may also give protection against further infection. Apart from clinical and subclinical infectious illnesses providing protection against further infection from a number of diseases, it is also possible to acquire artificial immunity (*active immunity*). Certain preparations (*vaccines*) are used to induce an artificial immune response. There are three main types of vaccine: those containing *attenuated micro-organisms*; those containing *killed micro-organisms*, and those containing the *products of micro-organisms* (altered *toxins* called toxoids). Passive immunity, in which the antibodies required come from another person or animal, may be acquired naturally or artificially. Natural passive immunity is usually acquired by the newborn child at the time of birth when maternal antibodies traverse the placenta. The baby also receives secretory *IgA* antibodies via colostrum during breast feeding. These antibodies persist for approximately six months during which time the baby is afforded partial protection in its encounters with many infectious agents. The infectious agent is able to multiply only to a limited extent, but it is sufficient to stimulate the baby's own immune response and whilst preventing significant disease, this mechanism allows the baby to acquire active immunity. Immunoglobulins provide artificial passive immunity against such diseases as hepatitis B.

An important non-immunological resistance factor is **interferon** which is formed in response to infection by nearly all viruses.

Inflammatory response

The inflammatory response is also involved in the fight against infection and involves three important post-defence systems: tissue fluid, the lymphatic system and phagocytic cells.

Inflammation focuses all the circulating antimicrobial factors (such as polymorphonuclear cells, macrophages and antibodies) on the site of infection and is essential for the proper functioning of the immune defences. The local signs of inflammation are:

(1) *Redness and warmth* due to vasodilation;
(2) *Swelling* due to vasodilation plus cell and fluid exudate;
(3) *Pain* due partly to pressure on sensory nerve endings by exuded fluid, especially if the space in which it can expand is limited, and partly to the release of substances which stimulate these nerves – for example, **histamine, serotonin, kinins** and prostaglandins. Prostaglandins may act by lowering the threshold of response to other pain-producing substances;
(4) *Loss of function* which results from the foregoing factors.

Chronic inflammation occurs when an infection is persistent. Episodes of tissue damage alternate with repair, resulting in the formation of granu-

lation tissue (consisting of capillaries, histiocytes and lymphocytes) and then fibrous tissue. The resulting granuloma is an attempt to wall off the infected area.

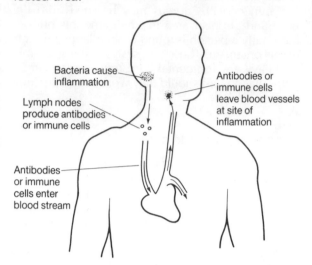

Fig. 16.1 *Diagram showing immune response to an infection*

Pyrexia

Pyrexia is a rise in body temperature and is one of the most frequent and familiar responses to infection – whether the infection is largely restricted to the body surfaces (for example, the common cold or influenza) or is obviously generalised (for example, measles, typhoid, malaria). The temperature rise results from an increase in metabolic rate stimulated by the response to the micro-organism. This, together with reduced food intake, results in high excretion of nitrogen in the urine. There is rapid wasting of body fat and muscle if the fever is prolonged.

The common mediator of the febrile response in infectious disease is known as **endogenous pyrogen**. This is present in inflammatory exudates and in the plasma during fever. Endogenous pyrogen acts on the temperature regulating centre in the anterior hypothalamus, resetting the body thermostat. The **cell-mediated immune response** in the infected host is also a cause of pyrexia, as demonstrated in tuberculosis and brucellosis.

The normal body temperature is 36.6°C, having a **diurnal** range from 36.3–37.2°C and being highest in the evening. There is very little variation of temperature in a healthy person. The temperature is decreased in conditions which produce dehydration, severe haemorrhage, and marked toxaemia, as well as in conditions of shock and collapse. An increase in temperature may be caused not only by infection but also by metabolic disorders and disturbances of the heat regulating centre.

Several studies have addressed factors which affect the accuracy of temperature recordings (Blainey, 1974; Eoff and Joyce, 1981; Boylan and Brown, 1985). These factors include the appropriateness of the site and the length of time the thermometer remains in situ. In the study of 50 children by Eoff and Joyce, the accuracy of the temperature recording from the rectal site was compared with that from the axillary site. The results showed a mean difference of 0.49°C for the total group tested. They concluded that as the axillary site is safer physically and less distressing psychologically it should be recommended as the site of choice. Although the aim of taking a temperature is to have as accurate a reading as possible, Mitchell (1973) indicates that the recorded temperature is only an estimate of the body temperature at any given time.

Pyrexia is defined clinically as the body temperature persistently exceeding 37.5°C when recorded either orally or rectally. Diseases may be characterised by either rapid or gradual onsets of pyrexia.

A rapid onset is characterised by a quick rise in temperature, reaching the highest point within hours of the onset of the illness. It is frequently preceded by an attack of shivering. It is at this point that febrile convulsions can occur in children.

A gradual onset is when the temperature rises a little each day taking several days or a week to reach its maximum point.

There are also different types of pyrexia and in some circumstances, an emerging pattern can be of great value in aiding diagnosis. For example, relapsing fever (a systemic spirochaetal disease) is characterised by periods of fever lasting 2–9 days alternating with afebrile periods of 2–4 days. The number of relapses varies from one to ten or more and each pyrexial period terminates by crisis. Malaria may begin with an indefinable malaise followed by a shaking chill and rapidly rising temperature, usually accompanied by headache and nausea and ending with profuse sweating. After an interval free of fever, the cycle of chills,

fever and sweating is repeated, either daily, every other day or every third day.

The sudden decline of the pyrexia to normal temperature, accompanied by a drop in the pulse and respiration rate, is known as *crisis* (Fig. 16.2). Crisis occurs in cases of untreated lobar pneumonia. A gradual decline in the temperature from a very high temperature to a normal recording, usually over a period of days, is called *lysis* (Fig. 16.3) and occurs, for example, in cases of untreated scarlet fever.

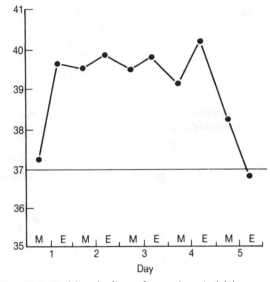

Fig. 16.2 *Sudden decline of pyrexia – 'crisis'*

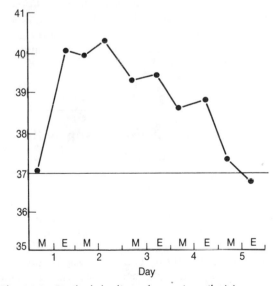

Fig. 16.3 *Gradual decline of pyrexia – 'lysis'*

Rigor

A severe attack of shivering known as a *rigor* may occur at the onset of an infection which is characterised by a rapid rise in temperature (for example, pneumonia), as well as during the course of infective diseases and conditions. There are three distinct phases to a rigor: the first or cold stage is characterised by uncontrollable shivering, cold skin and tachycardia. Despite the fact that the patient feels outwardly cold, the temperature is in fact rising rapidly during this phase. During the second or hot stage, the temperature may continue to rise and the patient is hot and restless, frequently complaining of thirst and a headache. In the third phase, profuse sweating occurs with a fall in temperature and an improvement in the pulse rate and volume.

The needs of a patient experiencing a rigor change rapidly, necessitating constant observation, re-assessment and updating of the care plan. Each stage will require very different care. For example, warmth in the form of extra blankets and hot drinks should be provided for the patient during the cold stage, whereas during the hot stage, blankets should be removed and heat loss facilitated by fan therapy and tepid sponging, through convection and conduction. The application of cold compresses or ice packs will help alleviate the associated headache. Extra fluids should be encouraged during the sweating phase.

Throughout all three phases, recording of temperature, pulse and respiration rate provide information on the course of the rigor and the patient's general condition. Reassurance and support of the patient during what can be a very distressing and frightening experience is vital.

The needs of the person with infection

Physical, psychological and, in some instances, social needs are experienced by people with infections or infectious diseases. The infective process produces a number of symptoms, principally pain and pyrexia, which cause physical distress. Psychological and social needs vary widely but the following two examples demonstrate the types of problem requiring consideration when planning appropriate care.

Example 1: Scabies

Except for the rare crusted or Norwegian scabies, this disease is transmitted only by close skin-to-skin contact (Robinson, 1986). It is understandable, therefore, that in the past scabies ran rife in homes and institutions where overcrowding was a problem. For this reason scabies was, and in some people's minds still is, associated with cramped, dirty conditions and therefore considered a 'dirty disease'. When scabies is discovered either in the community or in hospitals there is often, particularly among the elderly population, shame in having such a disease. Nurses and other carers may show a reluctance to be in contact with infected patients although the treatment is rapid and safe and the risk minimal, if the correct precautions are taken. Should an outbreak occur within a nursing home or day hospital for elderly patients, the stigma associated with scabies may be such that patients refuse to stay in, or attend, such establishments.

It is important when dealing with a case or outbreak of scabies to ensure that psychological and sociological factors are considered, and that steps are initiated to overcome problems that may arise in these areas, as well as carrying out the treatment of the disease and its symptoms.

Example 2: Human Immunodeficiency Virus (HIV)

Human immunodeficiency virus (HIV) belongs to a family of viruses called *retroviruses*. Retroviruses contain in their core an enzyme called *reverse transcriptase* which converts the viral ribonucleic acid (RNA) into a deoxyribonucleic acid (DNA) copy in the infected host cell (Christie, 1987). HIV infects the host target cells, T_4 lymphocytes, by binding to a receptor, CD_4, found on the surface of the cell. T_4 lymphocytes are of vital importance in inducing and controlling the immune response to infection (Bowen *et al.*, 1985). HIV has been found in neurons and glial cells of the brain and many of the central nervous system manifestations of HIV infection, for example AIDS dementia complex (ADC), are attributed to the direct destruction of these cells by the virus (Grimes, 1991; Lambert, 1991).

In the early stages of HIV infection, the cellular immune deficiency is of a minor character but as the T_4 cells become depleted the risk of serious infection, e.g. *Pneumocystis carinii* pneumonia, and certain neoplasms such as Kaposi's sarcoma, increases. The range of disease manifestations resulting from HIV infection is wide and complex. For detailed information about the virus and the associated complications, further reading is necessary (e.g. Grimes, 1991; Lambert, 1991; Pratt, 1991).

Just as the physical manifestations of HIV are complex so are the psychological reactions and an understanding of these is critical to caring for a person with the infection. The various reactions can be divided into three main areas: reaction to learning that one is HIV positive; reaction to becoming symptomatic; and reaction to dying.

Anxiety is the predominant reaction when a person submits themselves for a HIV test, and whilst awaiting the result. There is worry and fear about the long term implications of a positive result. Once the HIV positive status is known there are a number of psychological responses that may be experienced: denial, anger, depression and thoughts of suicide, feelings of guilt and self-blame, and fear of rejection.

As the person with HIV becomes symptomatic some of these initial reactions may become more intense, particularly as in addition they may experience job loss, impoverishment and social isolation. The fear of giving HIV to others (particularly sexual partners) presents additional stress. The diagnosis of HIV often initiates an intensified need for physical contact and emotional intimacy. Healthy but frightened partners, concerned family and friends may unwittingly withdraw, reinforcing the person's sense of being alone.

As the disease progresses the person with HIV may become pre-occupied with finding ways of maintaining or improving their health. This can include alternative therapies and special diets. In the later stages pain relief and preparing for death may be the dominant feature. During this period there is a great reliance on others including partners, friends, family, volunteers and health care workers to provide basic needs and comforts.

The nursing care of people with HIV infection needs to be holistic and flexible to meet their complex physical and psychological needs. Health care workers must be aware of how their own actions and attitudes can increase the feeling of isolation and rejection that may be felt. The Department of Health and professional bodies including the UKCC have provided advice on the prevention of infection (DoH, 1990), testing, treatment and care of AIDS sufferers (UKCC, 1987) and confidentiality (UKCC, 1984).

Consideration of these two examples makes it clear that the physical and non-physical needs of the patient with an infection must be assessed in accordance with the type and severity of the infection. The needs of a patient with a urinary tract infection obviously differ widely from the needs of a patient suffering from septicaemia. Account must also be taken of the modes of transmission and the measures required to prevent spread.

Whilst it is usually a medical responsibility to diagnose and treat the underlying cause, it is a nursing responsibility to assess and meet the patient's needs resulting from symptoms of infection. To illustrate this the care plan shown in Figs. 16.4–16.6, using an adaptation of Roper's activities of daily living (Roper *et al.*, 1990), raises a number of problems and potential problems which may be experienced by a patient who is pyrexial and in pain and outlines the general principles of care. Rationales have been added to explain why specific nursing actions have been prescribed.

> Mrs Rose Thorn aged 63 years was admitted to a surgical ward with abdominal pain. Following diagnosis of appendicitis an appendicectomy was performed. Mrs Thorn's recovery was uneventful until the third day when the wound became red and inflamed and she was discovered to be pyrexial.

Fig. 16.4 *Profile: Mrs Rose Thorn*

All care plans must be dated and signed, and in order to assess whether expected outcomes are achieved, nursing interventions must be evaluated. When the expected outcome has not been achieved, re-assessment of the problem with the patient and formulation of new interventions will be necessary.

Caring for the person with an infection

Specific needs and problems arising from the characteristics of certain diseases must also be considered when planning nursing care; for ex-

Activity of living		
1. **Communication**	(a)	Anxious and distressed due to excessive sweating and feeling 'hot'
	(b)	Discomfort and generalised pain around wound area
2. **Eating and drinking**	(a)	Mouth clean but dry – Mrs. Thorn is able to carry out her own oral toilet
	(b)	Lips free from cracks
3. **Personal cleansing and hygiene**	(a)	Excessive sweating – needs help with personal hygiene. Unable to wash without assistance
	(b)	Red, inflamed wound
4. **Mobilising**	(a)	On continued bedrest – able to move freely within the bed. Has not needed assistance to turn
	(b)	*Waterlow score* = 10 (Waterlow, 1985)
	(c)	Pressure areas intact and free from redness
5. **Sleeping**	(a)	Finds it difficult to sleep – due to sweating and generally feeling unwell
	(b)	Discomfort from the effects of the wound infection, causing restlessness

Fig. 16.5 *Assessment: Mrs Thorn*

ample, rashes, vomiting, diarrhoea and constipation.

Two examples are given to illustrate this point.

Problems due to skin rashes

Both rubella (German measles) and chickenpox (varicella) are characterised by rashes that can cause pruritus (itching). The rash caused by rubella is *macular* (i.e. a collection of flat spots differing in colour from the surrounding skin). The rash associated with chickenpox begins as red *papules* which become *vesicular* within a few hours, purulent within 48 hours, and dry up forming scabs after three to four days. A papule is a small lump raised above the surface of the skin and a vesicle is a small blister.

The itching can be alleviated by applications of soothing lotions, for example calamine, or creams.

Failure to prevent scratching may result in the patient acquiring secondary bacterial infection of the skin lesions, sometimes resulting in scarring.

Problems due to vomiting, diarrhoea and constipation

In a similar manner to rashes, vomiting, diarrhoea and constipation are specific characteristics of certain infectious diseases – particularly those of the gastro-intestinal tract. The severity and frequency of diarrhoea and vomiting are often part of the clinical picture of the disease (see Table 16.2).

Table 16.2. *Infectious diseases of the gastro-intestinal tract: characteristics*

1. **Bacillary dysentery**
   Typically a sudden onset of abdominal pain, followed by diarrhoea which decreases rapidly after one to four days. Vomiting is uncommon

2. **Staphylococcal food poisoning**
   Usually associated with salivation, nausea, vomiting and abdominal pain with a rapid incubation period of one to six hours. Diarrhoea occasionally occurs

3. **Salmonella food poisoning**
   Symptoms usually include diarrhoea, vomiting and fever starting after an incubation period of 12 to 24 hours (may be up to 36 hours)

4. **Typhoid fever**
   Typhoid is not typically a diarrhoeal disease and is much more often associated with constipation

Careful observation and recording of the frequency, severity and appearance of bowel actions and vomiting episodes may provide valuable information for the diagnosis of gastro-intestinal infections.

Nursing care plans must address not only the patient's physical needs, such as dehydration, exhaustion, skin cleansing and protection, but also psychological issues. A patient nursed in the middle of a ward may find it very embarrassing to have to ask frequently for a bedpan or help to get to the lavatory. Sounds and odour can cause further embarrassment. For these reasons the patient may prefer to be nursed in a single room even if the condition is not infective. If at all possible, such a room should have its own toilet and washing facilities.

Fig. 16.6 *Care plan for Mrs Thorn*

Activity	Nursing Action	Rationale	Expected Outcome
Communication Communication has become difficult for Mrs Thorn because she is so uncomfortable 1. Problem of sweating due to pyrexia causing discomfort and distress	(a) Advise patient to wear cotton night clothes	Cotton absorbs sweat more effectively than synthetic fibres and feels cooler to the skin	Patient will state that sweating has been reduced to a tolerable level
	(b) Reduce bed clothing to one sheet and counterpane. Avoid use of polythene drawer sheet	The temperature should be reduced gradually to avoid the patient becoming chilled. Plastic will increase sweating	Being comfortable will enable her to begin communicating effectively
	(c) Ensure that patient is in a well ventilated and draught free situation on the ward	To aid the loss of heat by convection but prevent chilling and any subsequent shivering	
	(d) Provide a bed cradle to allow air to circulate freely around the body	To promote loss of body heat by convection	
	(e) Wash/bathe patient 8 hourly when awake, more frequently if requested. Change clothing and bed linen when moist or at patient's request	To keep skin cool and the patient free from the effects of sweating, thereby enhancing comfort and well-being	
	(f) Provide constant reassurance and an explanation for all procedures	To relieve anxiety and distress	
	(g) Fan therapy as prescribed if body temperature is raised above 38.3°C. Set angle of fan to move through 180° just above skin surface	By reducing pyrexia the patient feels more comfortable, associated headaches can be relieved and sleep induced. By cooling air above the body, heat is lost by convection and shivering, which would increase pyrexia, avoided	
	(h) If fan therapy proves ineffective, tepid sponging as prescribed. Use tepid water (21°C) applied with disposable flannels. Place cooled flannels in groins, axillae, on forehead. Renew as they become warm. Making long, sweeping, strokes, wipe over surface of the skin using one cool flannel per stroke	Fan therapy and tepid sponging are normally prescribed by medical staff as a rapid reduction in the body temperature can, in rare circumstances, result in collapse. Heat is lost from the body by the evaporation of moisture left on the surface of the skin	

Activity	Nursing Action	Rationale	Expected Outcome
2. Potential problem of increased pain levels due to wound infection	(a) Provide bed cradle	By removing the weight of the bed clothes from the wound site, pain, which may be enhanced by pressure, will be relieved	Patient will state that pain has been reduced to acceptable levels
	(b) Monitor and record level, character and distribution of pain and give prescribed analgesia as appropriate	Pain differs in its character (e.g. throbbing, stabbing, 'pressure') and its distribution according to the site of infection. Every patient reacts differently to pain and by careful observation, the differing needs can be identified and appropriate care prescribed in order to reduce emotional distress (Latham, 1986; Creasia and Parker, 1991)	
Eating and Drinking 1. Potential problem of dry and cracked lips and the formation of *sordes* in a dirty mouth due to dehydration resulting from loss of fluid through sweating	(a) Offer citrus fruit drinks 4 hourly when awake	Citrus fruit drinks stimulate the flow of saliva which will help to keep the mouth clean and moist	A moist, clean mouth
	(b) Offer mouth washes after meals and more frequently if desired	The mechanical action of the mouth washes cleans and refreshes the mouth, particularly for patients who are vomiting or unable to take normal diet and fluids (Shepherd *et al.*, 1987)	
	(c) Provide toothbrush and toothpaste or denture cleansing agent after meals or more frequently if desired	To remove debris and freshen the mouth	
	(d) If lips become dry and cracked apply vaseline after meals or more frequently if necessary	The use of strong solutions of glycerine should be avoided as they absorb moisture from the mucosa causing drying by the osmotic action (Gooch, 1985)	
2. Potential problem of dehydration due to loss of fluid through sweating	(a) Encourage patient to drink hourly amounts of diluted citrus fluids which should be kept refrigerated or have ice added	The amount, nature and frequency of the fluid intake should be discussed with the patient to ensure cooperation. Cool fluids are more refreshing and acceptable to the patient	Hydration maintained

Activity	Nursing Action	Rationale	Expected Outcome
	(b) Record fluid intake and urine output and observe for signs of dehydration (dry mouth and tongue, sunken eyes, loss of skin elasticity and reduced urine output)	The loss of fluid from sweating is difficult to quantify and it is therefore necessary to observe and report signs of dehydration in order that any further action required can be taken	
Personal Cleansing and Hygiene 1. Potential problem of hair becoming greasy due to excessive sweating through pyrexia	Wash hair at least weekly and more frequently if necessary. Apply dry shampoo and brush well if patient is unable to cope with disturbance of hair washing	To remove grease and dirt from hair. Dry shampoo removes grease effectively with the minimum of disturbance	Clean, tangle-free hair
2. Potential problem of hair becoming tangled and knotted due to continued bed rest	(a) Brush and comb hair carefully morning and evening or more frequently if necessary	To remove knots and tangles	
	(b) Loosely plait or tie long hair back from face	By loosely confining the hair away from the face and neck, long hair is less likely to become tangled and knotted	
3. Potential problem of eyes feeling dry and sore	Bathe eyes as necessary with 0.9% normal saline	To soothe and moisten eyes	Moist, clean eyes
4. Problem of inflamed wound following surgery	(a) Dress wound each day with dry dressing using an aseptic technique. Observe for leakage and wound breakdown. Send swab to microbiology if leakage occurs	Daily redressing is necessary for aseptic observation of the wound. Microbiological culturing of the swab may result in a change to more appropriate antibiotic therapy	Healed wound
	(b) Give antibiotic therapy as prescribed		
Mobilising 1. Potential problem of pressure sore development due to continued bed rest	(a) Re-assess and record Waterlow Score every 48 hours until bed rest discontinued	Re-assessing factors such as mental state and mobility will allow appropriate nursing care to be prescribed. Various risk assessment scales may be used (Barratt, 1990) to identify patients at risk of developing pressure sores	Unblemished skin over pressure areas

Activity	Nursing Action	Rationale	Expected Outcome
	(b) Encourage patient to change position at least every two hours. If necessary offer help to re-position every 2–4 hours	Regular and frequent changes of patient's position will relieve pressure and is often all that is required to prevent pressure sores developing (Torrance, 1981)	
	(c) Observe pressure areas (e.g. sacrum, heels) at times of washing/ bathing, or at least four times daily	The reporting and recording on a regular basis of skin condition and any changes will ensure that appropriate nursing care is prescribed	
	(d) Keep skin clean and dry paying particular attention to skin creases. Do not use talcum powder	Sweat will accumulate in axillae, groins and under the breasts. Talcum powder will tend to form lumps in these areas and increase soreness	
Sleeping 1. Actual problem of disturbed sleep pattern and inadequate rest due to pyrexia	(a) Ask patient whether a wash/blanket bath prior to settling down in the evening is required	These measures will help to induce sleep by reducing some of the effects of the pyrexia (e.g. thirst, sweating)	Maximum sleep and rest
	(b) Offer a drink (e.g. Ovaltine, cocoa) late evening according to patient's preference		
	(c) Check with the patient whether any particular measures normally help her to sleep (e.g. positioning, night light)		
	(d) Night sedation as prescribed (if necessary)		

Controlling the spread of infection

To control the spread of infection it is necessary, at times, to isolate the source of the infection. This source can be either the whole patient or the site of infection – for example, the wound. The aim is to confine the organism and block its route of spread. Crow (1989) describes this as isolating the disease not the patient.

Isolation procedure

The nature and severity of the infection, the method of transmission and the susceptibility of other patients and carers influence both the necessity for and the selection of the most appropriate type of isolation procedure.

The way in which isolation precautions have been assigned to various communicable diseases has changed over the years (Jackson and Lynch, 1985). It was in 1963 that Shooter, O'Grady and Williams described a simplified guide to the management of patients with such diseases. Each communicable disease was assigned to one of three degrees of isolation:

(1) Barrier nursing in the open ward;
(2) Barrier nursing in a ward cubicle;
(3) Isolation in an infectious disease hospital or unit.

Some advice was given on basic precautions required when dealing with, for example, linen and crockery. Gradually this system of categorisation became more sophisticated and the Center for Disease Control in Atlanta, USA (1970), published the first edition of *Isolation Techniques for Use in Hospitals* which described seven categories of isolation. Similar categories were recommended by Bagshawe, Blowers and Lidwell (Table 16.3) in a series of articles published in 1978. The simplification of these systems, whilst making compliance easier, does in fact lead to major disadvantages for patients.

In placing all infections with similar modes of transmission into one isolation category, there is little flexibility for individualised patient care and over-isolation may result. By 1980 it was considered in America that this approach to isolation was out of date due to:

- the increased use of intensive care units and associated invasive procedures;
- the emergence of antibiotic-resistant organisms;
- the inappropriate assignment of isolation precautions;
- non-compliance with isolation policies;
- the presence in many hospitals of infection control nurses and other staff members with specific knowledge and commitment to managing isolation precautions more effectively (Haley et al., 1985).

Between 1981 and 1983 the Center for Disease Control re-evaluated the strategy for isolation precautions and guidelines were produced (Garner and Simmons, 1983) offering two fundamental approaches to applying isolation precautions.

One was the category system (Table 16.4), modified on the basis of current clinical information, and the other was called disease-specific precautions. This second approach is a system for assigning a specific set of isolation precautions for

Table 16.3. *Early isolation category system for classifying infectious diseases (Source: Bagshawe, Blowers and Lidwell, 1978)*

CATEGORY OF ISOLATION AND BASIC PRECAUTIONS	EXAMPLES OF DISEASE OR INFECTING AGENT
High security Separate purpose-built unit ***Negative pressure isolators***	Marburg disease Lassa fever
Strict Single room Gowning lobby Own toilet/bedpan Sterilisation unit Gown and plastic apron Gloves and mask	Pulmonary anthrax Staphylococcal pneumonia
Standard Single room (preferably with gowning lobby and wash basin) Negative pressure ventilation Own toilet/access to bedpan Sterilisation unit Gowns or plastic apron Gloves	Herpes zoster Influenza
Stool-urine-needle Accommodation as for standard isolation Gowns or plastic aprons and gloves when in contact with patient or excreta or blood	Hepatitis B Shigella

each infectious disease (Table 16.5) and allows more flexibility in the type of precautions required for individual patients.

The requirement for flexibility is illustrated by considering two patients with the same communicable disease. One patient is 74 years old, confused and with restricted mobility, who has been admitted to a ward caring for elderly patients with diarrhoea, and finally diagnosed as having salmonellosis. Using the scoring system suggested by Bowell (1990), this patient's risk of spreading infection to others can be assessed using a scale of:

No risk   = 0
Medium risk   = 2
High risk   = 3

Table 16.4. *Isolation categories defined by Garner and Simmons 1983*

Isolation	No. diseases in category	Examples of diseases
Strict	11	Lassa fever
Respiratory	12	Haemophilus influenzae infections
Tuberculosis *(acid-fast bacilli)*	1	Pulmonary and laryngeal tuberculosis
Enteric	42	Salmonella
Contact	47	Staphylococcus aureus
Drainage/secretion	38	Purulent material, drainage or secretions
Blood/body fluid	16	Hepatitis B
Sub-total	167	
No. of isolation precautions necessary	108	
TOTAL	275	

(Source: Haley *et al.*, 1985)

Mr Jones

Diagnosis of salmonella =	3
Persistent diarrhoea =	3
Faecal incontinence =	3
Confusion =	3
TOTAL	12

The other patient is a young woman also diagnosed as having salmonella but whose diarrhoea is less severe. She has been admitted to a surgical ward because of abdominal pain.

Ms Flower

Diagnosis of salmonella =	3
Diarrhoea 3–4 daily =	2
Continent =	0
Mentally alert =	0
TOTAL	5

These examples demonstrate the difference in the risks that are presented to other patients and staff. In the past, using a category system, both patients would be nursed using the same precautions. This might lead to over-isolation for Ms Flower and insufficient precautions being taken for Mr Jones. By using disease-specific precautions, Mr Jones would be placed in a single room because of his incontinence, diarrhoea and confusion, and gloves and aprons would be worn by staff when in contact with faeces and contaminated surfaces. Mr Jones would require a high level of nursing input to care for his physical and psychological needs.

Ms Flower on the other hand would be accommodated in the main ward as she would be self-caring and unlikely to contaminate the environment. Gloves and aprons would not be necessary as staff would not be coming into direct contact with the infectious material, i.e. the faeces.

It is evident that by using some form of assessment coupled with a number of general principles, it is possible to provide an individualised care plan for anyone suffering from a communicable disease, whilst at the same time keeping other people safe from the risk of infection. However, for this approach to be successful there must be adequate information provided at all levels to ensure that decisions on the type of accommodation and precautions required are made on a sound clinical basis and are not dependent on guesswork and rituals.

Isolation techniques

Whatever system of isolation precautions is used, there are a number of principles which help to achieve the aim of confining the organism and blocking its route of spread. If these principles are applied when planning the care of a person with a communicable disease, it is possible to develop safe and sensible isolation techniques whilst at the same time reducing the psychological effects to a minimum.

Accommodation

The requirement for a single room can be determined by simple selection criteria (Crow, 1989). A single room is necessary when the patient has an airborne disease or when the patient cannot confine and contain his body fluids.

The room should contain a sink for handwashing as well as toilet/bathing facilities. Patients with airborne infections such as chickenpox should be nursed in single rooms equipped with negative

Table 16.5. Disease-specific precautions – isolation techniques

Disease	Incubation period	Infective material	Mode of spread	Period of infectivity	Single room	Apron	Gloves	Mask	Management of contacts	Comments
Brucellosis	1–3 weeks, occasionally 6–7 months	Exudate	Inoculation	Duration of illness	No	No	When handling exudate	No	None	None
Chickenpox	11–21 days	Respiratory and lesion secretions	Airborne and contact	7 days after the appearance of the last vesicle	Yes	Yes	Yes	Yes if non-immune	Protect non-immune staff and patients, etc.	Gamma-globulin available for susceptible patients, e.g. immune-suppressed
Diphtheria	2–7 days	Respiratory secretions	Airborne and contact	From onset until 3 negative swabs obtained	Yes	Yes	Yes	Yes if non-immune	Swabbing of all contacts and prophylaxis	
Gas gangrene	2–7 days	Not transmitted from man to man	None	None	No	No	No	No	None	
HIV	Variable	Blood, serum-derived body fluids, e.g. semen + vaginal fluids	Inoculation	Duration of infection	No	No	When in contact with blood and body fluids	No	None	Detailed information available in national and local policies for specific procedures
Salmonella	12–72 hours	Faeces	Faecal/oral	Duration of illness	Occasion-ally	When in contact with faeces	When in contact with faeces	No	Stools from affected contacts	Food handlers dealt with by Environmental Health Officers

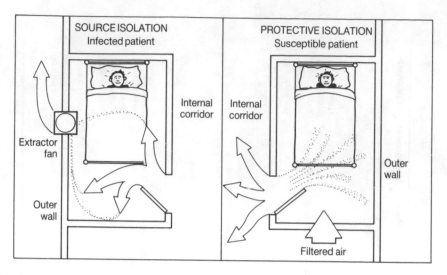

Fig. 16.7 *Airflow patterns of negative and positive pressures*

pressure ventilation (Josephson and Gombert, 1988) (Fig. 16.7). This type of ventilation will prevent contaminated air from entering corridors outside the room.

To help reduce the feeling of isolation, rooms used for this purpose should preferably have a good outlook and be provided with glass partitions between the room and the rest of the ward.

The use for isolation purposes of single rooms attached to general wards is now quite widespread although there are still other facilities available offering different degrees of protection. These include:

- general hospital isolation or infectious diseases wards;
- infectious diseases hospitals/units;
- high security isolation units.

Protective clothing

The decision as to which articles of protective clothing are required for individual cases is, as previously mentioned, entirely dependent on the way the particular infection is spread, the type of care being given and the patient. For example, when entering a room to talk to a patient with salmonella there is no need to put on gloves and apron but if the same patient requires help with using the toilet, then such items would be worn to prevent risk of cross-contamination. Whilst assessing the need for protection it is necessary to consider the various items of protective clothing available.

Gowns/plastic aprons

Transfer of organisms from the clothing of staff is possible but not a major problem (Ayliffe *et al.*, 1982). However, the wearing of protective gowns or aprons is an accepted part of isolation or barrier nursing techniques, particularly when handling infectious material.

A plastic apron affords better protection than a cotton gown for several reasons. Disposable plastic aprons are cheap, impermeable to bacteria and water (Lidwell *et al.*, 1974; Ransjo, 1979) and easy to put on. It is uncommon for the shoulder area of the uniform to become contaminated (Babb *et al.*, 1983) and the area of maximum contamination is the front of the uniform at bed height (Ayton *et al.*, 1984). They can be re-used provided one apron is allocated for use with one particular patient and it is dry and the ties intact. It has been shown that an apron can be re-used on a number of occasions without a significant rise in microbial load (Babb *et al.*, 1983) due to the 'plateau effect' which occurs on environmental surfaces. Freshly deposited micro-organisms replace those dying off due to lack of moisture and nutrients. It must be emphasised that if plastic aprons are used more than once for the same patient, it is essential that the wearer can distinguish the inside from the outside of the apron. This can be done by some form of marking. If the apron is visibly soiled it must be disposed of and it is advisable to have a set period for re-use, e.g. one per shift.

Masks

Masks are now generally considered to contribute little to patient or staff safety. The situations where a mask may be of value have been reduced significantly over the last few years. Nurses or staff with colds do not need to wear masks to protect patients – they should not be on duty! The Subcommittee of the Joint Tuberculosis Committee of the British Thoracic Society reiterated in 1990 that the wearing of gowns and masks by staff was unnecessary when caring for people with tuberculosis, even smear-positive pulmonary tuberculosis (i.e. when there are sufficient tubercle bacilli in the sputum to be seen on direct examination). Patients with measles, chickenpox or shingles, for example, should only be cared for by staff who are immune to these diseases and who will, therefore, not need to wear a mask. Recently further evidence has confirmed earlier work (Orr, 1981; Laslett and Sabin, 1989) that during quiet breathing, few if any nasal bacteria are expelled into the air, despite heavy colonisation of the nose. Mitchell and Hunt (1991) concluded that the routine wearing of masks by all staff working in a modern operating room with positive pressure ventilation is a costly and unnecessary ritual.

These examples illustrate the growing evidence that rarely does a face mask need to be worn as protection for either staff or patient. In fact, there are greater hazards associated with the mishandling of masks, e.g. handling the mask, possibly to remove it, followed by touching the patient without washing the hands first. On the rare occasions when a mask is necessary, it must be the same type as used in theatres, i.e. an efficient filter type.

Gloves

Hands play a major role in the spread of infection by contact. Handwashing (Watson, 1978) and glove-wearing therefore have a particularly important part to play in the prevention of spread by this route. Gloves prolong the effect of hand disinfection as well as reducing cross-contamination of the hands from infected sites and equipment (Lowbury et al., 1981).

It is generally accepted that a fitted latex glove should be used in these situations. They are comfortable, do not slip off during procedures such as bedmaking, and are unlikely to split. Unless the procedures are aseptic there is no need to wear a sterile glove. The gloves should be disposed of after use and all staff must be aware that wearing a pair of gloves is not a substitute for handwashing (Linden, 1991)

Caps and overshoes

Neither caps nor overshoes serve a useful purpose in the care of a person with an infection or infectious disease. Closefitting caps which cover all of the hair are used in areas where there is a risk of infection from *Staphylococcus aureus* which is found in the hair or from the shedding of hair itself, for example in catering departments (HMSO, 1970), theatres and sterile service units. However, there is no need to protect the staff's hair from the patient. The use of caps is therefore unjustified as part of the isolation technique.

The wearing of plastic overshoes as a method of controlling infection is considered to be both ritualistic and unacceptable (Carter, 1990). Any organisms on the floor will remain there harmlessly unless they are introduced to a susceptible host via hands or equipment. Overshoes themselves can act as a source of cross-contamination (Bentham, 1979) during the donning and removal process. Carter observed a large proportion of staff did not wash their hands after putting on and taking off the overshoes.

Handwashing

The most effective method of preventing the spread of infection is still the act of handwashing and hand disinfection (Daschner, 1985). There is a great variation in both quality and frequency of handwashing practices (Sedgwick, 1984). Despite understanding the importance of handwashing, the number of times that staff report they have washed their hands is often well above the frequency actually observed (Broughall et al., 1984; Williams and Buckles, 1988). Taylor (1978) demonstrated with the use of dye the areas of the hand most frequently not washed (Fig. 16.8). A number of people have used Feldman's criteria for handwashing evaluation (cited in Taylor, 1978; Gidley, 1987) (Fig. 16.9) to assess handwashing techniques. In Taylor's study the mean score was 14 for registered

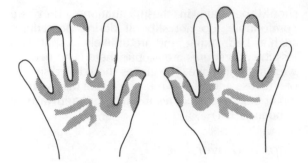

Fig. 16.8 *Areas commonly missed during hand washing*

nurses, 12 for enrolled nurses and learners and 10 for auxilliaries out of a maximum score of 20.

There are three types of handwashing (Phillips, 1989): social, using soap and water; antiseptic, using an antiseptic detergent solution or an alcohol hand rub; and surgical, which usually requires washing for a total time of three minutes using an antiseptic detergent. Following contact with known or suspected contaminated surfaces and materials, staff should use an antiseptic detergent solution or alcohol hand rub.

Research has shown there is no doubt that infrequent washing and poor technique continue to cause infection to spread via hands. Patients may also be instrumental in spreading infection this way. A study by Pritchard and Hathaway (1988) showed that of 20 male patients, 60% did not wash their hands after using the toilet. Only half of the ambulant patients and none of the non-ambulant patients did so. In three of the four non-ambulant patients, the nurse did not offer to assist with handwashing nor did the patients request help. This research highlights the need for nurses to ensure that both patients and visitors are reminded of the importance of handwashing. Information leaflets should be available explaining why isolation is required and what precautions are needed with particular emphasis on handwashing.

Equipment

Over recent years there has been increasing awareness of the need to decontaminate or dispose of equipment which has been in contact with blood, serum or other body fluids, and equipment used on or by patients in isolation (DHSS, 1987a). The Health and Safety at Work Act (HMSO, 1974)

Scores

Used soap
2 Visible lather
0 No contact with soap

Used continuously running water
2 Did
0 Did not

Positioned hands to avoid contaminating arms
2 Held hands down so that water drained from fingertips into sink
1 Held hands parallel with arms so that water drained from hands into sink
0 Held hands so that water drained onto arm

Avoided splashing clothing or floor
2 No splashing
1 Minimal splashing
0 Vigorous splashing

Rubbed hands together vigorously
2 Vigorous rubbing
1 Minimal rubbing
0 No rubbing

Used friction on all surfaces
2 Dorsal, ventral, interdigital
1 One or two of the above
0 Did not use friction

Rinsed hands thoroughly
2 All surfaces: dorsal, ventral, interdigital
1 One or two of the above
0 Did not rinse

Held hands down to rinse
2 Did
0 Did not

Dried hands thoroughly
2 Dried all surfaces
1 Dried one or two surfaces
0 Did not dry

Turned tap off with paper towel
2 Did
0 Did not

Fig. 16.9 *Feldman's criteria for handwashing evaluation (cited in Taylor, 1978; Gidley, 1987)*

states: 'Manufacturers are required to ensure that their employees are not put at risk, for example, by handling items that may be contaminated as a result of their use in health care or in a laboratory'. The National Health Service has a similar duty of care towards its employees and all staff have a responsibility to ensure that neither patients nor staff are put at risk from inadequately cleaned and decontaminated equipment.

Disposable or autoclavable equipment should

be used whenever possible and the amount of equipment taken into the isolation room kept to a minimum. Certain pieces of equipment, e.g. sphygmomanometers and stethoscopes, should be used exclusively by the patient and kept in the room until the discontinuation of isolation precautions. They should then be decontaminated appropriately. The methods of disinfection should be detailed in a policy agreed by the Control of Infection Team (Collins and Josse, 1990). Advice should include the method of decontamination to be used (e.g. chemical, low temperature steam, autoclaving), the frequency and any particular requirements, e.g. dilution factors and protective clothing to be worn.

Waste disposal

HIV infection has raised the public's concern with regard to the disposal of clinical waste, in particular the disposal of contaminated sharps (BMA, 1991). Even though clinical waste, excluding contaminated sharps, does not necessarily present a greater infection risk than many other items which are handled with less concern (Collins and Josse, 1990), recent legislation has led to the introduction of even more stringent regulations covering the disposal of clinical waste (HMSO, 1990a).

It has previously been recommended that waste from patients with some types of infection should be double-bagged (Bagshawe et al., 1978). However, this technique is now considered unnecessary and it is recommended (Health and Safety Commission, 1982) that such waste should be placed in yellow coloured plastic bags which are of a minimum gauge of either 800 if low density or 400 if high density. These bags of waste must be disposed of by incineration. Used sharps must be disposed of in a approved pattern sharps box (DHSS, 1976/1978) for final disposal by incineration.

Infected linen should be enclosed in totally water-soluble bags, or bags with a soluble strip, at the bedside to prevent the dispersal or transference of organisms. The bag is designed so that it remains intact until placed unopened in a washing machine, where part or all of the bag will dissolve to release the contents. As wet linen may partially dissolve the strip or bag during storage, it is advisable to place it in another ordinary plastic bag. Information on colour coding of linen bags and the various aspects of storage, transportation and washing of linen, including infected linen, are contained in Department of Health guidelines (DHSS, 1987b).

Psychological care

The overall response of the patient to isolation is one of stress (Denton, 1986). Children and elderly people will need particular support. It should be remembered that elderly patients may become confused, particularly if they suffer from some form of sensory deprivation, e.g. impaired sight or deafness. Communication may also be difficult if there are language barriers. Every effort must be made to compensate for these deficiencies by providing, for example, a telephone, television, reading matter, a radio. Frequently newspaper, library and sweet trolleys pass by an isolation room without thought being given to the fact that the isolated patient is probably in greater need of such services. Staff not directly involved in the care of patients with communicable infections, such as domestic staff, are often frightened of the perceived risk of infection to themselves and their families. An explanation as to the precautions that need to be taken will often be sufficient to overcome their fears and encourage them to enter the room and provide a normal service to the patient.

Visitors should not normally be restricted. They must receive an explanation, accompanied by written information, as to the precautions they must take and some supervision might be necessary during the first visit. Mothers visiting children with infections should not handle other babies and children on the ward. Visitors who are not immune to certain infectious diseases, e.g. chickenpox, must be made aware of the risk of infection and discouraged from visiting, particularly if they are pregnant.

The routine use of disposable crockery and cutlery for infectious patients in the past increased the patient's feeling of being 'dirty' and isolated. The use of such items is unnecessary as there are few instances where a dishwashing facility with a final rinse temperature of 80°C is not available either at ward level or in the main kitchen. Special precautions do not need to be taken for either the delivery of meals or the return of used crockery or cutlery (Maki et al., 1979).

Investigation and control of an outbreak of infection

The control methods required to prevent the spread of infection from one person to others have been discussed above, but there are obviously situations where a number of people have already been affected and it is necessary to take immediate action to investigate and control an outbreak of infection. Such outbreaks are not confined to hospitals and, therefore, the principles involved apply as much in the community as they do in the hospital situation.

Those involved in controlling and investigating an outbreak of infection often include microbiologists, infection control nurses, consultants in communicable disease control, infectious disease specialists, epidemiologists and environmental health officers.

Recommendations detailing action to be taken should an outbreak of infection occur are available from a number of sources. Gailbraith (1984) considered that several main activities are required to investigate and control an acute episode of infection, some of which are undertaken simultaneously. These main activities may include those detailed in Table 16.6.

Some diseases are notifiable by law to the proper officer of the local authority (see Table 16.7). Although this is often the Consultant in Communicable Disease there is no statutory requirement for it to be so (HMSO, 1984). There are some differences in the diseases that require notification between England and Wales, Scotland and Northern Ireland.

The proper officer has a surveillance duty in that he/she must notify the Chief Medical Officer and district health authority of any serious outbreak of any disease, including food poisoning.

The Department of Health and the Welsh Office have set up the Communicable Diseases Surveillance Centre in Colindale, London, to help coordinate the investigation and control of communicable diseases in England and Wales, and their expert advice is often sought by local teams involved in an outbreak of infection.

Hospital acquired infection

A hospital, or *nosocomial*, infection is an infection acquired by patients or members of staff whilst staying or working in a hospital. This type of infec-

Table 16.6. *Activities required to investigate and control an acute episode of infection*

1. **Preliminary inquiry**
   (a) Establish that the problem exists
   (b) Confirm the diagnosis
   (c) Formulate a preliminary hypothesis for the cause of the episode
   (d) Undertake immediate control measures if necessary

2. **Identification of infected persons**

3. **Collection of data**
   Including names, ages, sex, occupation, recent whereabouts, date of onset of illness, clinical description of disease

4. **Analysis of data**

5. **Control**
   Which may include isolation of infected patients, closure of ward or wards, restriction of staff movements between wards, surveillance of contacts, examination of all staff and patients for carriage, bacteriological specimens, survey of procedures and practice, equipment and buildings, etc.

Table 16.7. *Notifiable diseases: the list for England and Wales*

Acute encephalitis	Ophthalmia neonatorum
Acute poliomyelitis	Paratyphoid
Anthrax	Plague
Cholera	Rabies
Diphtheria	Relapsing fever
Dysentery (amoebic and	Rubella
bacillary)	Scarlet fever
Food poisoning	Smallpox
Leprosy	Tetanus
Leptospirosis	Tuberculosis
Malaria	Typhoid fever
Measles	Typhus
Meningitis	Viral haemorrhagic fever
Meningococcal	Viral hepatitis
septicaemia	Whooping cough
(without meningitis)	Yellow fever
Mumps	

AIDS is a disease for which provision is now made in the 1988 Regulations, but it is not notifiable

tion may be associated with sepsis or other forms of infective illness which becomes apparent whilst the patient is in hospital or following discharge. Hospital acquired infection (HAI) can either be a result of cross-infection, when the infection is acquired from **exogenous** sources outside the patient's body (for example, staff, visitors, other patients, equipment and the environment), or as a result of self-infection when it is termed **endogenous** (Fig. 16.10).

A number of infections are obviously acquired in hospital but there are situations where difficulties arise in deciding whether the infection has been acquired in hospital or prior to admission.

Pathogenic micro-organisms associated with HAI may be transmitted directly or indirectly from a number of sources, including infected wounds, the nose or faeces of carers, contaminated food or fluids (Ayliffe, 1983). Transmission may also occur from a reservoir, where organisms survive outside the body – for example, on static equipment, furniture or floors. Mobile objects such as dust particles, blankets and toys can act as vehicles, carrying pathogenic organisms to a patient (Fig. 16.11).

Hands are the most important mode of spread of infection and the environment (e.g. surfaces, fixtures and fittings) probably the least. Many of the sources and routes of infection, however, cannot be considered as separate entities. Hands (contact) and air (aerosols, skin scales), for example, may be the linking factors between many infective sources.

Certain pathogenic organisms are particularly associated with HAI and it is of interest to note that the strains of bacteria have changed within this century. Streptococcal infections which predominated in the 1930s were replaced during the 1940s by staphylococcal infections.

In recent years, *Pseudomonas aeruginosa, Klebsiella* spp. and other **Gram-negative** bacilli have become increasingly important causes of infection (Selwyn *et al.,* 1964). 'Opportunistic' organisms, such as *Pseudomonas aeruginosa,* rarely cause infection in environments other than those found in a hospital. These particular organisms are often resistant to many antibiotics and are able to flourish under conditions in which most pathogenic organisms cannot multiply. Patients who are particularly susceptible, as a result of receiving immunosuppressive drugs or because of certain diseases, are affected by a number of normally

ENDOGENOUS INFECTION

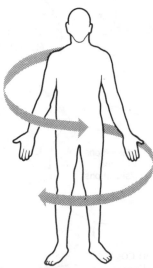

Micro-organisms originate from
the patient's own body

EXOGENOUS INFECTION

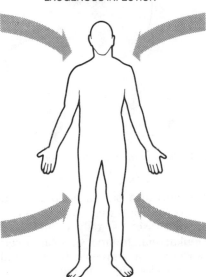

Micro-organisms originate from
other people or inanimate objects

Fig. 16.10 *Endogenous and exogenous infection*

non-pathogenic fungi and viruses which cause severe and sometimes fatal infections. Arthropod parasites (such as scabies and lice) can also be transmitted in hospital.

Patients' resistance, both general and local, to

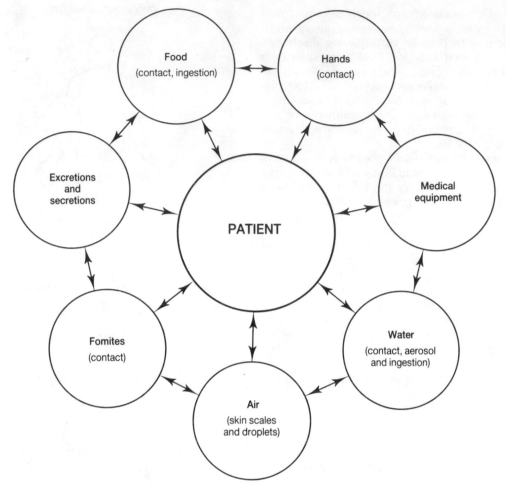

Fig. 16.11 Risks of infection to patients

infection must also be considered. A number of factors adversely affecting patients' general resistance include diseases such as uncontrolled diabetes, leukaemia, trauma such as severe burns, and poor nutrition. Impaired blood supply to the tissues, e.g. following prolonged pressure and the presence of necrotic tissue or blood clot in which bacteria can survive and multiply without interference from the body's natural defences, reduce the patient's local resistance. Susceptibility to local sepsis is increased by foreign bodies including sutures and prostheses. Invasive procedures, for example insertion of intravenous devices, surgical operations and instrumentation such as catheterisation (Selwyn, 1991) allow access of bacteria to tissues which are normally protected against con-

tamination (Fig. 16.12). The meninges, endocardium and urinary tract have a very low resistance to bacterial invasion and are particularly susceptible to infection from 'opportunist' organisms.

Infection hazards vary from ward to ward and from department to department. Intensive care units and neonatal units must be considered high risk areas due to the high number of invasive procedures performed, the amount of antibiotics used, and the use of equipment such as suction units and life-support systems. Patients undergoing surgery are at particular risk during operations when susceptible tissues are exposed, often for several hours. For this reason, operating theatres with their relatively high number of human and inanimate sources of infection must also be considered as

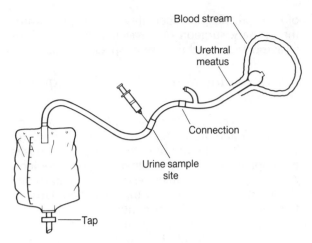

Fig. 16.12 *Entry points for bacteria: indwelling urinary catheter*

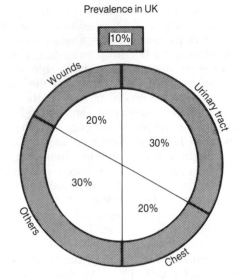

Fig. 16.13 *Prevalence of hospital acquired infection (HAI)*

high risk areas. Infectious disease units are obviously areas where there is an increased risk of infection but because staff are specially trained and procedures and policies are strictly adhered to, the actual risk is usually minimal.

Correctly performed medical and surgical procedures and careful use of antibiotics and other chemotherapy reduce the risk of HAI, but the unavoidable use of immunosuppressive drugs and steroids, as well as advances in surgical and medical techniques, place a significant number of patients at risk.

Much infection can be prevented and consequent morbidity and mortality rates reduced. However, the incidence of endemic infections in many hospitals has not decreased over the years.

Health care workers (nurses, doctors, laboratory, portering, laundry, CSSD and domestic staff) are all exposed from time to time to special hazards or infection due to the nature of their work. The Health and Safety at Work Act 1974 and more recently the Control of Substances Hazardous to Health Regulations (COSHH) (HMSO, 1988) require action on the part of both the employer and employee to reduce such risks to a minimum.

Prevalence of hospital acquired infection

Results of the 1980 prevalence survey (Meers et al., 1981) showed that 9.2% of patients studied were suffering from hospital acquired infections. An approximate breakdown of this overall figure is shown in Fig. 16.13. Similar rates have been

demonstrated in other surveys. Certain factors including the type of patient, the length of hospital stay and the type of operation or treatment influence the frequency and severity of the infection. From different studies, there seems to have been little change in the rate of HAI in the UK over recent years and it would appear that we are failing in our efforts to control infection in hospitals. This is probably partly due to the fact that surgical and medical techniques and treatments (heart transplants, total hip replacements, etc.) have advanced dramatically and that there is an increased population of susceptible patients, e.g. those who are elderly or immunosuppressed. However, there still remains evidence that erratic and unstandardised methods of asepsis and hygiene contribute to the continuing high proportion of patients who become infected during their stay in hospital. It is necessary for all staff caring directly or indirectly for patients to be aware of the importance of controlling HAI and to have an understanding of the principles used in the prevention of cross-infection.

Costs of hospital acquired infection

As with any infection, the patient with a hospital acquired infection suffers both physically and psychologically and there may be financial implications. A patient who is admitted into hospital for routine surgery is justified in believing that he will be in for a set number of days and after a period of convalescence will be returning to work. If, however, this patient acquires a wound infection, his stay in hospital becomes extended; it can be weeks or even months before he is able to return to full employment. The effect on the family's finances can be extremely serious, particularly if the patient is self-employed, and extended sick leave may even put his job in jeopardy. The implications of an HAI can, therefore, be far-reaching for the patient and it is not surprising that in the United States such infections feature frequently in cases of litigation. Indeed, such cases are starting to be heard in the UK (Cooke, 1989).

HAI also has implications for the health service. Bed occupancy is prolonged, which inevitably affects waiting lists and increases the cost of the patient's admission. A report by the Hospital Infection Working Group (DHSS, 1988b) includes information on the cost to the NHS in England and Wales of HAI. The report estimates that some 950,000 bed days are lost each year on average – a monetary cost of £111 million.

Studies in the United States have differed in their findings with regard to the length of extra stay in hospital for infected patients. Haley et al. (1981) reported that in three hospitals studied, the extra stay due to HAI varied from 3.1 to 4.5 days. However, Rubenstein et al. (1982), using another method for assessment, gave a more detailed analysis and produced the figures shown in Table 16.8.

Table 16.8. *General surgical and orthopaedic patients. Extra stay in hospital due to acquired infection (Compiled from Rubenstein et al., 1982)*

INFECTION	EXTRA DAYS
Urinary infection	5.1
Wound infection	12.9
Post-operative fever of unknown origin	8.0
Multiple infection	13.0

Freeman and McGowan (1981) included the following patient characteristics as being potentially important in the study of HAI: age, primary diagnosis, admission, vital signs, previous infections and health care prior to admission. The hospital characteristics that they considered to be potentially important included date of admission, the type of hospital, hospital speciality and hospital ward, the primary surgeon or physician, the use of invasive devices and the use of special units.

Individual incidence of hospital acquired infection

It is perhaps difficult to realise just how devastating a hospital acquired infection can be, particularly when, in the majority of cases, the patient makes a complete recovery from their original problem. An example of HAI which results both in morbidity and mortality is the urinary tract infection. Urinary tract infections (UTI) continue to be the most common of the hospital acquired infections.

The Public Health Laboratory Service prevalence survey in 1980 found that, of the 9.2% of patients who contracted HAIs, UTIs accounted for 30.3%, and of the 8.6% patients who were catheterised, 21.2% were shown to have a urinary tract infection, compared with 2.9% in the non-catheterised group (Meers et al., 1981).

A study funded by the Department of Health as a result of these findings looked in detail at 294 newly catheterised patients, each one for a period of 14 days. It monitored the patient and the drainage system and studied factors which might influence the patient's likelihood of acquiring bacteriuria (Crow, 1986).

The results showed, among other things, that the daily rate of catheterisation was 11 per 1000 of the initial patient population and that 44% of patients who had been catheterised for more than 48 hours developed *bacteriuria*. Bacteriuria has been defined as the 'presence of bacteria in bladder urine' (Medical Research Council, 1979). Contamination can occur with organisms from the anterior urethra or insertion of the catheter. The organisms involved might be, for example, coagulase negative staphylococci (*Staphylococcus epidermidis*), which is found on the skin, or faecal flora such as *E. coli*. Bacteriuria may develop into a UTI. It is commonly believed that a urinary tract infection is a benign, easily treated condition and for many patients this is quite true. However, due to organisms spreading from the infected urinary tract into the blood, a much more serious complication occurs – septicaemia. Septicaemia affects between 1–3% of patients with a catheter associated UTI (Clifford, 1982) and has an associated mortality in many hospitals of approximately 30% (Stamm, 1978). It is estimated that two in every 1000 patients catheterised in the UK die as a result of hospital acquired urinary tract infections (Meers and Stronge, 1980).

Despite improvements in catheter drainage systems and increased staff awareness regarding the need to look after them correctly (Schaffner, 1984), there continues to be a real need for staff education on all aspects of catheter care (Glenister, 1990a).

A great deal of research has been done on procedures associated with catheter care, including bag emptying (Glenister, 1987), disconnection of closed urine drainage systems (Platt *et al.*, 1983), meatal cleansing (Burke *et al.*, 1981) and bladder washouts (Stickler *et al.*, 1987).

The development of standards of practice for the catheterisation of patients and care of the drainage system must be based on scientific evidence and ways of measuring the effectiveness of these standards investigated.

Large outbreaks of hospital acquired infections

In 1984 at the Stanley Royd Hospital, Wakefield, an outbreak of salmonella food poisoning affected over half the inpatients (in 1984 there were 830 patients in the hospital) resulting in 19 deaths (DHSS, 1986a). In 1985 at the Stafford District General Hospital there was an outbreak of legionnaires' disease. A hundred and one outpatients were considered to be affected by the outbreak and in total, 28 patients died (22 definite cases and six possible cases) (DHSS, 1986b). The resulting investigations into both these outbreaks highlighted shortcomings in procedures, policies and standards in various areas. The recommendations made by the Committee of Inquiry into the Stanley Royd outbreak in particular has had wide repercussions for all NHS hospitals. From October 1986, NHS premises where food is prepared, cooked and stored (including ward kitchens) are no longer covered by Crown Immunity and therefore those responsible for these areas have become liable for offences against the various Food Hygiene Acts and can be prosecuted.

A particular strain of methicillin-resistant *Staphylococcus aureus* has been responsible for outbreaks of infection in many parts of the world (Marples *et al.*, 1987). The organism, the epidemic methicillin-resistant *Staphylococcus aureus* (EMRSA), is characterised by the ease with which

it spreads (Phillips, 1991). It is spread mainly via hands, although airborne dispersal on skin scales can occur. The most serious effects of EMRSA outbreaks have been seen among patients in surgical intensive care units, neonatal units, dermatology wards and burns units. Although there is no evidence that EMRSA is more virulent than any other *S. aureus*, a study from Hong Kong (French *et al.*, 1990) established that it is no less virulent than more sensitive strains. Outbreaks have not always been associated with significant clinical infection but immunocompromised, debilitated patients or those with open wounds are at particular risk from infection and deaths do occur (Phillips, 1991).

There is general agreement that the costs of controlling strains of EMRSA are less than the cost of ignoring them, particularly when the costs of potential legal action are included. Guidelines on the control of EMRSA are available from several sources, including a report from the combined Hospital Infection Society and British Society for Antimicrobial Chemotherapy (1990). Advice is given on the care of a known infected patient or carrier from the time of admission through to discharge, including isolation requirements, treatment, decontamination of colonised staff and microbiological procedures.

Prevention of communicable disease and infection

The cost in morbidity, mortality and money of HAI has led to the development of a structured system of control. In 1941 a recommendation was made by the British Medical Research Council that a full-time officer be appointed to supervise the control of surgical sepsis (Medical Research Council, 1941). A further MRC report advised, in 1944, that every hospital should have a multidisciplinary Infection Control Committee, but there was really no progress made before 1959, when the advice was reiterated by the Standing Medical Advisory Committee during a pandemic outbreak of staphylococcal infection. In the same year the first appointment was made for a full-time nurse to work with a medical microbiologist to investigate and control an outbreak of staphylococcal infections. The hospital was the Torbay Hospital in Devon and the medical microbiologist Dr Brendan Moore of Exeter, whose idea led to the development of the role of the infection control nurse (ICN) (Gardner *et al.*, 1962). The ICN and the infection control doctor work together to form the nucleus of the Infection Control Team. A survey in 1986 showed that the majority of infection control doctors were consultant microbiologists (Howard et al., 1988).

A joint Department of Health and Public Health Laboratory Services working party was set up in 1985 to consider the revision of departmental guidance on the control of infection in hospitals. In 1986 the Secretary of State for Social Services set up a Committee of Inquiry into the future development of the Public Health Function. The two resulting reports, Public Health in England (DHSS, 1988a) and Hospital Infection Control (DHSS, 1988b), have confirmed and extended the structure for the control of infection both in hospitals and the community. The Public Health in England Report recommended that a medical practitioner be appointed to have executive responsibility for necessary action on communicable disease and infection control, and be responsible for linking the vital work undertaken by microbiologists and control of infection teams within hospitals with cases of infection outside. The appointed doctor is known as the Consultant in Communicable Disease Control (CCDC) based in the health authority's Department of Public Health Medicine.

Over recent years the National Health Service and its employees have become increasingly responsible in law for ensuring the safety of both patients and staff (HMSO, 1987). The NHS and Community Care Act (HMSO, 1990d) has now removed Crown Immunity generally from health service bodies. One of the consequences is that the NHS becomes liable under existing legislation governing the disposal of clinical waste as well as the new requirements of the 1990 Environmental Protection Act. The removal of Crown Immunity affects all staff and there is a much greater awareness, at all levels, for the need to adhere to the regulations, particularly those already mentioned and others recently introduced, for example, the Food Safety Act (HMSO, 1990c) and the Food Hygiene (Amendment) Regulations (HMSO, 1990b).

Surveillance and audit

Surveillance and audit have become increasingly important as a means of monitoring standards of practice within the health service. The importance of target-setting and audit in relation to infection

control is recognised, as is the need to reduce as far as possible the incidence of hospital acquired infection. It has been suggested that targets should be set on the basis of what can be achieved through good practice, and that medical and clinical audit will allow continuing development of both target-setting and monitoring.

A number of quality assurance tools can be used to monitor various infection control procedures, for example, Monitor (Goldstone et al., 1984), National Association of Theatre Nurses Quality Assurance Tool (NATN, 1987) and the King's Fund Organisational Audit (1990). An audit tool specifically for monitoring adherence to infection control policies and procedures, particularly in the environment, has been developed by the author (Ward, 1991). The scoring mechanism enables it to be used as a performance indicator for inclusion in quality programmes.

Despite a great deal of work, both nationally (Glenister, 1990b) and internationally (Haley, 1988), there remain differences of opinion in this country as to the most effective way of carrying out surveillance of infection.

Any surveillance programme must include patients who have been discharged. Whereas the majority of hospital acquired infections – particularly wound infections – were in the past identified in hospital, there is an increasing chance that with shorter inpatient stays, these will not now be discovered until after discharge.

Education and training

To reduce the levels of infection, both in hospitals and the community, it is necessary for the principles of good practice not only to be known but also to be implemented. Studies have shown that, despite knowledge of appropriate practices, staff do not always incorporate such knowledge into their work (Linden, 1991). Larson (1988) identifies three major obstacles to behavioural change: lack of skills and knowledge; lack of systems and supplies; or lack of motivation. However, Larson, and Williams and Buckles (1988), showed that increasing knowledge did not necessarily bring about increased behavioural compliance with infection control procedures. It appeared that lack of motivation rather than lack of knowledge was the most important cause of low compliance.

Strategies to overcome lack of skills and knowledge include not only teaching programmes for health care workers but for also the general public.

All health care workers should become health educators by providing information and guidance on matters which will encourage the general public to become responsible for their own health, and by doing so preventing, and even in some cases eradicating, infections and infectious diseases.

Nurses are in a unique position, by virtue of their frequent and sustained contact with patients, to carry out this role in all health care settings (see also Chapter 3).

Perhaps the most vigorous infection-related health education campaign ever seen in this country has been in association with AIDS. Leaflets, posters and the mass media have been used in a concerted effort to heighten the public's awareness of facts about and methods of preventing AIDS. It is hoped that by altering high risk behaviour patterns such as sexual promiscuity, unsafe sex and intravenous drug abuse, the spread of this virus will be curtailed.

However, in this programme, as in others, it is proving difficult to sustain a lasting change in behaviour and attitudes and more research is required to provide answers to the very difficult problem of motivating such changes.

Conclusions

As stated at the beginning of this chapter, the aim has been to provide the reader with an understanding of certain aspects concerning infection – its transmission, prevention, containment and, most importantly, the related patient needs and nursing responsibilities. The subject is far-reaching and it has only been possible to discuss these aspects in relatively general terms. However, it is hoped that the chapter has proved successful in illustrating that the needs of the patient with infection are complex, in both physical and psychological terms. In order to ensure the well-being of the affected patient and the safety of other patients and staff, a sound knowledge of the principles involved is necessary, together with an awareness that only by applying such principles diligently will effective standards of care be achieved.

Glossary

Acid-fast bacilli: The mycobacterium group of organisms, e.g. mycobacterium tuberculosis, are not readily seen by *Gram-stain* method. They are examined by an acid-fast or Ziehl-Nielsen stain, hence the term 'acid-fast bacilli' (AFB), or Ziehl-Nielsen (ZN) positive when one of the mycobacteria are seen

Active immunity: Induced by using inactivated or attenuated live organisms or their products. Live attenuated vaccines include those for poliomyelitis (OPV), measles and rubella, and BCG vaccine. Bacterial and viral vaccines such as whooping cough, typhoid and inactivated poliomyelitis (IPV) vaccines contain inactivated organisms

Cell-mediated immune response: Specific immunity which does not depend upon antibody or complement but is instead due to an interplay between macrophages and T lymphocytes

Diurnal: Having a daily cycle

Endogenous: Originating or produced within the organism or one of its parts

Endogenous pyrogen: A substance contained and released by neutrophils which is partly responsible for the development of fever during acute inflammation. It is a lipoprotein probably released during phagocytosis which acts on the thermoregulatory centres of the brain

Exogenous: Originating or produced outside the organism

Gram-staining: Staining methods are employed to make use of the fact that different chemical substances within the body of the bacteria are stained different colours by different stains. Gram's method uses a mixture of violet dye and iodine to stain the magnesium ribonucleate, found in some bacteria, a deep purple. This purple stain cannot be readily washed out by alcohol. Bacteria stained in this way are known as *Gram-positive*. When other bacteria without magnesium ribonucleate are stained in the same way, the purple dye can easily be washed out by alcohol. These microbes are called *Gram-negative*

Histamine: A compound found in all cells produced by the breakdown of *histidine* (a basic amino acid). Histamine release may lead to itching

IgA: The most important antibody class in external secretions – intestinal, bronchial and nasal secretions, saliva, tears, colostrum and milk. Their function is to provide local immunity against infectious agents in the gut and respiratory tract by combining with and neutralising them before they can gain entry into the body.

IgA is the main antibody in milk and breast milk and provides protection for the sucking infant against enteric organisms

Interferon: An antiviral protein produced by T cells and often present in serum during virus infection. Interferon production can be stimulated by inactivated and living virus, by viral nucleic acid, and also by artificially synthesised double-stranded RNA. Macrophages may also produce interferon

Kinins: Biologically active polypeptides which are produced by the action of enzymes known as *kallikreins* on a kinin-precursor called *kininogen*. The best known kinin is *bradykinin* which produces extravascular smooth muscle contraction, vasodilation, increased permeability, pain and possible margination and emigration of leucocytes

Negative pressure isolators: A PVC tent in which the pressure can be regulated. For source isolation the pressure is kept below atmospheric pressure. This negative pressure is just visible in the slight concavity of the tent (Bowell, 1986)

Pathogenic: Disease-producing. A term applied to bacteria, for example

Phagocytose/phagocytosis: A process by which the attacks by bacteria upon the living body are repelled and the bacteria destroyed through the activity of the white blood cells, principally polymorphonuclear leucocytes

Secretory antibodies: In the humoral antibody response, protein molecules known as antibodies (*immunoglobulins*) are produced in the circulation. There are five subgroups of immunoglobulins, of which IgA is one. IgA has a special structure ('the secretory piece') which allows it to be secreted and is especially prominent in the gastro-intestinal tract and in the salivary glands

Serotonin: A substance released from platelets on damage to the blood vessels. It acts as a potent vasoconstrictor and, in the central nervous system, acts as a neurotransmitter

Sordes: Crusts consisting of food, microorganisms and epithelial cells that accumulate on teeth and lips during febrile illness or when a patient takes nothing by mouth

Vector: A carrier, especially one that transmits disease. A biological vector is usually an insect in which the infecting organism completes part of its life cycle. A mechanical vector transmits the infecting organisms from one host to another but is not essential to the life cycle of the parasite

Waterlow Score: A scoring system used to assess the degree of risk of a patient developing a pressure sore. It is combined with advice on preventive measures required to minimise the risk

References

Ayliffe, G.A.J. (1983). Epidemiology. In *Seminar. Control of Hospital-Acquired Infections*. Noble, W.C. (ed.). Update Publications, London.

Ayliffe, G.A.J., Collins, B.J. and Taylor, L.J. (1982). *Hospital-Acquired Infection: Principles and Prevention* (1st ed.). John Wright, Bristol.

Ayton, M., Babb, J.R. and Mackintosh, C. (1984). *Report of an Infection Control Nurses' Association Working Party on Ward Protective Clothing. Section A1–11. Gowns and Aprons*. ICNA, privately published.

Babb, J.R., Davies, J.G. and Ayliffe, G.A.J. (1983). Contamination of protective clothing and nurses' uniforms in an isolation ward. *Journal of Hospital Infection*, 4, 149–157.

Bagshawe, K.D., Blowers, R. and Lidwell, O.M. (1978). Isolating patients in hospital to control infection. Part IV – Nursing procedures. *British Medical Journal*, 2, 808–811.

Barratt, E. (1990). Pressure sores in intensive care. *Intensive Therapy and Clinical Monitoring*, September/October, 158–164.

Bentham, A.J. (1979). An investigation into a cross-infection problem in a cardio-thoracic unit. *Proceedings of the Tenth Annual Symposium of the Infection Control Nurses Association*. ICNA, privately published.

Blainey, C.G. (1974). Site selection in taking body temperature. *American Journal of Nursing*, 74(10), 1859–1861.

Bowell, B. (1986). Nursing the isolated patient: Lassa fever. *Journal of Infection Control Nursing, Nursing Times*, 33, 72–81.

Bowell, B. (1990). Assessing infection risks. *Nursing*, 4(12), 19–23.

Bowen, D.L., Lane, H.C. and Fauci, A.S. (1985). Immunopathogenesis of the Acquired Immunodeficiency Syndrome. *Annals of Internal Medicine*, 103, 710–714.

Boylan, A. and Brown, P. (1985). Temperature. *Nursing Times*, 81(16), 36–40.

British Medical Association. (1991). *Hazardous Waste and Human Health*. Oxford University Press, Oxford.

Broughall, J.M., Marshman, C., Jackson, B. and Bird, P. (1984). An automatic monitoring system for measuring handwashing frequencies in hospital wards. *Journal of Hospital Infection*, 5, 447–453.

Burke, J.P., Garibaldi, R.A., Britt, M.R., Jacobson J.A., Conti, M. and Alling, D.W. (1981). Prevention of catheter associated urinary tract infections. *American Journal of Medicine*, 70, 655–658.

Carter, R. (1990). Ritual and risk. *Nursing Times*, 86(13), 63–64.

Center for Disease Control. (1970). *Isolation Techniques for Use in Hospitals*. DHEW Publication No. HSM 71–8043. US GPO, Washington DC.

Christie, A.B. (1987). *Infectious Diseases* (4th ed.). Churchill Livingstone, London.

Clifford, C. (1982). Bacteriuria – a possible consequence of urinary tract infection. *Proceedings of the Conference organised by the Nursing Practice Research Unit at Northwick Park Hospital*, London.

Collins, B. and Josse, E. (1990). The patient's environment. In *Infection Control: Guidelines for Nursing Care*, Worsley, M., Ward, K.A., Parker, L. et al., (eds.). ICNA, privately published.

Cooke, E.M. (1989). Hospital infection control and medico-legal problems. *Journal of the Medical Defence Union*, Winter, 62–65.

Creasia, J.L. and Parker, B. (1991). *Conceptual Foundations of Professional Nursing Practice*. Mosby, St Louis.

Crow, R.A. (1986). *Study of Patients with an Indwelling Urethral Catheter and Related Nursing Practice*. University of Surrey, Nursing Practice Research Unit.

Crow, R.A. (1989). *Asepsis, the Right Touch*. Everett Companies, Louisiana, USA.

Daschner, F.D. (1985). Useful and useless hygiene techniques in intensive care units. *Intensive Care Medicine*, 11, 280–283.

Denton, P.F. (1986). Psychological and physiological effects of isolation. *Nursing*, 3, 88–91.

Department of Health. (1990). *Expert Advisory Group on AIDS. Guidance for Clinical Health Care Workers. Protection against Infection with HIV and Hepatitis Viruses*. HMSO, London.

DoH. (1991). *The Health of the Nation. A Consultative Document for Health in England*. HMSO, London.

Department of Health and Social Security. (1976/78). *Specification for Containers for the Disposal of Used Needles and Sharp Instruments – Specification No. TSS/S330, 015 11/76 and 74/78*. HMSO, London.

DHSS. (1986a). *The Report of the Committee of Inquiry into an Outbreak of Food Poisoning at Stanley Royd Hospital, 1986*. HMSO, London.

DHSS. (1986b). *First Report of the Committee of Inquiry into the Outbreak of Legionnaires' Disease in Stafford in April 1985*. HMSO, London.

DHSS. (1987a). *Decontamination of Health Care Equipment Prior to Inspection, Service, Repair or Disposal*. HN(87)22. HMSO, London.

DHSS. (1987b). *Hospital Arrangements for Used and Infected Linen*. HMSO, London.

DHSS. (1988a). *Public Health in England. Report of the Committee of Inquiry into the Future Development of the Public Health Function*. HMSO, London.

DHSS/PHLS Hospital Infection Working Group (1988b). *Hospital Infection Control: Guidance on the Control of Infection in Hospitals*. HMSO, London.

Eoff, M.J. and Joyce, B. (1981). Temperature measurements in children. *American Journal of Nursing*, 81(5), 1010–1011.

Freeman, J. and McGowan, J.E. Jr. (1981). Differential risks of nosocomial infection. *American Journal of Medicine*, 70, 915.

French, G.L., Chene, A.F.B., Lung, J.M.L., Mo, P. and Donnan, S. (1990). Hong Kong strains of methicillin-resistant and methicillin-sensitive Staphylococcus aureus have similar virulence. *Journal of Hospital Infection*, 15, 117–125.

Gailbraith, N.S. (1984). Investigation and control of an acute episode of disease. *Medicine International*, 2, 1–7.

Gardner, A.M.N., Stamp, M., Bowgen, J.A. and Moore, B. (1962). The Infection Control Sister: A new member of the control of infection team in general hospitals. *Lancet*, 2, 710–711.

Garner, J.S. and Simmons, B.P. (1983). Guideline for isolation precautions in hospitals. *Infection Control*, 4, 245–325.

Gidley, C. (1987). Now wash your hands. *Nursing Times*, 83 (29), 41–42.

Glenister, H. (1987). The passage of infection. *Journal of Infection Control Nursing, Nursing Times*, 83(22), 68–73.

Glenister, H. (1990a). The catheterised patient. In *Infection Control: Guidelines for Nursing Care*, Worsley, M., Ward, K.A., Parker, L., et al. (eds.). ICNA, privately published.

Glenister, H. (1990b). Investigating infection acquired in hospitals. *Nursing Times*, 86(49), 46–48.

Goldstone, L.A., Ball, J.A. and Collier, M.M. (1984). *Monitor: An Index of the Quality of Nursing Care*. Newcastle upon Tyne Polytechnic Products LTP.

Gooch, J. (1985). Mouth care. *Professional Nurse*, 1(3), 77–78.

Grimes, D. (1991). *Infectious Diseases*. Mosby, St Louis.

Haley, R.W. (1988). The legacy of SENIC: Strategies for reducing infection rates. *Proceedings of the Second International Conference on Infection Control, organised by the Infection Control Nurses' Association of Great Britain*. CMA Medical Data Ltd., Cambridge.

Haley, R.W., Garner, J.S. and Simmons, B.P. (1985). A new approach to the isolation of hospitalised patients with infectious diseases; alternative systems. *Journal of Hospital Infection*, 6, 128–139.

Haley, R.W., Schaberg, D.R., von Allmen, S.D. and McGowan, J.E. Jr. (1981). Extra charges and prolongation of stay attributable to nosocomial infections: a prospective interhospital comparison. *American Journal of Medicine*, 70, 51–58.

Health and Safety Commission. (1982). *The Safe Disposal of Clinical Waste*. HN(82)22. HMSO, London.

HMSO. (1970). *Food Hygiene Regulations*. HMSO, London.

HMSO. (1974). *Health and Safety at Work Act*. (HS (R) 6). HMSO, London.

HMSO, (1984). *Public Health (Control of Diseases) Act*. HMSO, London.

HMSO. (1987). *NHS Amendment*. HMSO, London.

HMSO. (1988). *Control of Substances Hazardous to Health Regulations (COSHH)*. HMSO, London.

HMSO. (1990a). *Environmental Protection Act*. HMSO, London.

HMSO. (1990b). *Food Hygiene (Amendment) Regulations*. HMSO, London.

HMSO. (1990c). *Food Safety Act*. HMSO, London.

HMSO. (1990d). *NHS and Community Care Act*. HMSO London.

Hospital Infection Society and British Society of Antimicrobial Chemotherapy. (1990). Revised guidelines for the control of epidemic methicillin-resistant Staphylococcus aureus. *Journal of Hospital Infection*, 16, 351–377.

Howard, A.J., Selkon, J.B., Gillett, P., Sanderson, P.J., Selwyn, S., Shanson, D.C. and Taylor, L.J. (1988). Infection control organisation in hospitals in England and Wales, 1986. *Journal of Hospital Infection*, 11, 183–191.

Jackson, M.M. and Lynch, P. (1985). Isolation practices: a historical perspective. *American Journal of Infection Control*, 13, 21–31.

Josephson, A. and Gombert, M. (1988). Airborne transmission of nosocomial varicella from localised zoster. *Journal of Infectious Diseases*, 158(1), 238–242.

King's Fund Centre. (1990). *Organisational Audit (Accreditation UK)* (2nd ed.). King's Fund Centre, London.

Lambert, H.P. (1991). *Infections of the Central Nervous System*. Edward Arnold, London.

Larson, E. (1988). Psychology of change in infection control. *Proceedings of the Second International Conference on Infection Control, organised by the Infection Control Nurses' Association of Great Britain*. CMA Medical Data Ltd., Cambridge.

Laslett, L.J. and Sabin, A. (1989). Wearing of caps and masks not necessary during cardiac catheterisation. *Catheterisation and Cardiovascular Diagnosis*, 17, 158–160.

Latham, J. (1986). Assessment, observation and measurement of pain. *Professional Nurse*, 1(4), 107–110.

Lidwell, O.M., Towers, A.G., Ballard, J. and Gladstone, B. (1974). Transfer of micro-organisms between nurses and patients in a clean air environment. *Journal of Applied Bacteriology*, 37, 649–656.

Linden, B. (1991). Protection in practice. *Journal of Infection Control, Nursing Times*, 87(11), 59–63.

Lowbury, E.J.L., Ayliffe, G.A.J., Geddes, A.M. and Williams, J.D. (1981). *Control of Hospital Infection: A Practical Handbook* (2nd ed.). Chapman and Hall, London.

Maki, M.G., Alvarado, C.J., Hassemer, C.A. and Zilz, M.A. (1979). Relation of the inanimate environment to endemic nosocomial infection. *New England Journal of Medicine*, 307, 1562–1566.

Marples, R.R., Richardson, J.F. and Roberts, J.I.S. (1987). Methicillin-resistant Staphylococcus aureus. *Proceedings of Infection Control Nurses' Association Conference*. Blackpool, 1986. CMA Medical Data Ltd., Cambridge.

McKeown, T. and Brown, R.G. (1955). Medical evidence related to English population changes in the eighteenth century. *Population Studies*, 9(6), 125.

Medical Research Council. (1941). *The Prevention of 'Hospital Infection' of Wounds*. MRC War Memorandum No. 6. HMSO, London.

Medical Research Council. (1944). *The Control of Cross Infection in Hospitals*. MRC War Memorandum No. 11. HMSO, London.

Medical Research Council Bacteriuria Committee. (1979). Recommended terminology of urinary tract infection. *British Medical Journal*, 2, 717–719.

Meers, P.O., Ayliffe, G.A.J., Emmerson, A.M., Leigh, D.A., Mayon-White, R.T., Mackintosh, C.A. and Stronge, J.L. (1981). Report on the National Survey of Infection in Hospitals, 1980. *Journal of Hospital Infection*, 2(Supplement), 1–51.

Meers, P.O. and Stronge, J.L. (1980). Hospitals should do the sick no harm. Urinary tract infection. *Nursing Times*, 76(30)Supplement.

Mitchell, N.J. and Hunt, S. (1991). Surgical face masks in modern operating rooms – a costly and unnecessary ritual. *Journal of Hospital Infection*, 18, 239–242.

Mitchell, P. (1973). *Concepts: Back to Nursing*. McGraw-Hill, New York.

National Association of Theatre Nurses. (1987). *Quality*

Assurance Tool (2nd ed.). BUPA Printing Division, Kent.

Orr, N.W.M. (1981). Is a mask necessary in the operating theatre? *Annals of the Royal College of Surgeons of England*, 63, 380–392.

Peckham, C.S. (1988). Mother-to-child transmission of HIV infection. The European Collaborative Study. *Lancet*, ii, 1039–1043.

Phillips, C. (1989). Hand hygiene. *Journal of Infection Control Nursing, Nursing Times*, 85(37), 76–79.

Phillips, I. (1991). Epidemic potential and pathogenicity in outbreaks of infection with EMRSA and EMREC. *Journal of Hospital Infection*, 18(Supplement), 197–201.

Platt, R., Polk, B.F., Murdock, B. and Rosner, B. (1983). Reduction of mortality association with nosocomial urinary tract infection. *New England Journal of Medicine*, 307, 637–642.

Pratt, R.J. (1991). *AIDS: A Strategy for Nursing Care* (3rd ed.). Edward Arnold, London.

Pritchard, V. and Hathaway, C. (1988). Patient handwashing practice. *Journal of Infection Control Nursing, Nursing Times*, 84(36), 68–72.

Ransjo, U. (1979). Attempts to control clothes-borne infection in a burns unit. 3. An open-roofed plastic isolator or plastic aprons to prevent contact transfer of bacteria. *Journal of Hygiene*, 82,385.

Robinson, R. (1986). Scratching the surface. *Nursing Times*, 34,71–72.

Roper, N., Logan, W.W. and Tierney, A.J. (1990). *The Elements of Nursing* (3rd ed.). Churchill Livingstone, Edinburgh.

Rubenstein, E., Green, M., Molan, M., Amit, P., Bernstein, L. and Rubenstein, A. (1982). The effects of nosocomial infections on the length and costs of hospital stay. *Journal of Antimicrobial Chemotherapy*, 9(Supplement), 93.

Schaffner, W. (1984). Priorities in infection control: the impact of new technology. *Journal of Hospital Infection*, 5,1–19.

Sedgwick, J. (1984). Handwashing in hospital wards. *Nursing Times*, 80(20), 64–67.

Selwyn, S. (1991). Hospital infection: the first 2500 years. *Journal of Hospital Infection*, 18(Supplement A), 6–64.

Selwyn, S., McCabe, A.F. and Gould, J.C. (1964). Hospital infection in perspective – the importance of Gram-negative bacilli. *Scottish Medical Journal*, 9,409–417.

Shepherd, G., Page, C. and Sammon, P. (1987). Oral hygiene – the mouth trap. *Nursing Times*, 83(19), 24–27.

Shooter, R.A., O'Grady, F.W. and Williams, R.E.O. (1963). Isolation of patients in hospital. *British Medical Journal*, 2, 924–925.

Stamm, W.E. (1978). Infections related to medical devices. *Annals of Internal Medicine*, 89,764–769.

Standing Medical Advisory Committee/Ministry of Health. (1959). *Staphylococcal Infections in Hospitals*. HMSO, London.

Stickler, D.J., Clayton, C.L. and Chawla, J.A. (1987). The resistance of urinary tract pathogens to chlorhexidine bladder washouts. *Journal of Hospital Infection*, 10,28–39.

Subcommittee of the Joint Tuberculosis Committee of the British Thoracic Society. (1990). Control and prevention of tuberculosis in Britain: an updated code of practice. *British Medical Journal*, 300, 995–998.

Taylor, L.J. (1978). An evaluation of handwashing techniques. *Nursing Times*, 74(3), 108–110.

Torrance, C. (1981). Pressure sores 2: predisposing factors. The at risk patient. *Nursing Times*, 77(7), 5–8.

United Kingdom Central Council for Nursing, Midwifery and Health Visiting. (1984). *Confidentiality. An Elaboration of Clause 9 of the Second Edition of the UKCC's Code of Professional Conduct for the Nurse, Midwife and Health Visitor*. UKCC, London.

UKCC. (1987). *AIDS – Testing, Treatment and Care*. UKCC, London.

Ward, K.A. (1991). Infection Control Audit. Paper given at the Infection Control Nurses' Association Conference, Edinburgh, September 1991. To be published.

Waterlow, J. (1985). A risk assessment card. *Nursing Times*, 27(49), 51–55.

Watson, K. (1978). Medical microbiology. *Nursing Mirror*, 146(5), 32–33.

Williams, E. and Buckles, A. (1988). A lack of motivation. *Journal of Infection Control Nursing, Nursing Times*, 84(22), 60–64.

Suggestions for further reading

Ayliffe, G.A.J., Collins, B.J. and Taylor, L.J. (1990). *Hospital Acquired Infection: Principles and Prevention* (2nd ed.). John Wright, Bristol.

British Medical Association. (1989). *Infection Control*. Edward Arnold, London.

Christie, A.B. (1987). *Infectious Diseases Vols. 1 & 2* (4th ed.). Churchill Livingstone, London.

David, J.A. (1986). *Wound Management: A Compre-hensive Guide to Dressing and Healing*. Martin Dunitz, London.

Grimes, D. (1991). *Infectious Diseases*. Mosby, St Louis.

Hare, R. and Cooke, E.M. (1991). *Bacteriology and Immunity for Nurses* (7th ed.). Churchill Livingstone, Edinburgh.

Lambert, H.P. (1991). *Infections of the Central Nervous System*. Edward Arnold, London.

Lowbury, E.J.L., Ayliffe, G.A.!., Geddes, A.M. and Williams, J.D. (eds.) (1981). *Control of Hospital Infection: A Practical Handbook* (2nd ed.). Chapman and Hall, London.

Maurer, I.M. (1978). *Hospital Hygiene*. Edward Arnold, London.

Mims, C.A. (1982). *The Pathogenesis of Infectious Diseases* (2nd ed.). Academic Press, New York.

Pratt, R.J. (1991). *AIDS: A Strategy for Nursing Care* (3rd ed.). Edward Arnold, London.

Westaby, S. (1985). *Wound Care*. Heinemann Books, London.

Worsley, M., Ward, K.A., Parker, L., Ayliffe, G.A.J. and Sedgwick, J.A. (eds.). (1990). *Infection Control: Guidelines for Nursing Care*. ICNA, privately published.

Acknowledgement

The author and publishers would like to thank ICI for their kind permission to reproduce Figures 16.7, 16.8 and 16.10 to 16.13 taken from: Ayliffe, G.A.J. and Taylor, L.J. *Infection Control: A Slide Library for Infection Control Nurses*. Produced by ICI (Imperial Chemicals Industries).

17

WOMEN'S HEALTH CARE

Dinah Gould

The aim of this chapter is to introduce and discuss the care of women in health and when health fails. The focus is on the promotion and awareness of health.

The chapter includes the following:

- Exploding myths concerned with women's position in society and with their health

- Women's bodies and women's lives:
  —The menstrual cycle
  —Menstrual problems
  —Ectopic pregnancy
  —Miscarriage
  —The menopause

- Promoting health: women's needs and health-related choices:
  —Contraception
  —Abortion
  —Infertility
  —Sexually transmitted diseases
  —Cervical screening
  —Breast screening
  —Hormone replacement therapy
  —Female incontinence

The position of women in society is changing. Because history has been dominated by men it was once argued that this must be the product of women's biological destiny (English and Ehrenreich, 1973). There is plenty of evidence to suggest that in the past women's health has been sapped by repeated childbearing and the burden of caring for the rest of the family (Shorter, 1984). However, modern feminist writers argue that, except in their obvious anatomical differences, women are not fundamentally different from men in terms of physical strength or intellectual capacity. Oakley (1985), a sociologist, and Webb (1985), a nurse, have both undertaken considerable research in this sphere, pointing out that much of what is commonly accepted as 'natural' feminine behaviour is

actually learned from early childhood. Girls in the past, and to some extent today, were expected to play with dolls not trains, to cry when they were hurt, and to develop interests like sewing and cooking rather than scientific or technological hobbies. 'Typical female behaviour' is thus the product of sexual stereotyping, and the myth that women should maintain exclusively domestic interests has only been slowly eroded.

Educational opportunities for girls are still narrow compared to those for boys, especially in social classes IV and V. Sharpe (1984) describes how attitudes concerning the education of girls (with emphasis on home-centred skills and relatively superficial treatment of technological and scientific subjects, including maths) have persisted. At the turn of the century, when compulsory education was introduced, girls were expected to learn how to look after husband, home and children. Sharpe's work illustrates the grave difficulties faced by working women who have young families. There is undoubtedly a shortage of good childcare facilities at reasonable cost. The ideas of Bowlby (1947), promulgated in the 1950s, suggested that small children remain entirely dependent on the presence of their mothers unless they are to be psychologically damaged. Such attitudes have done little to improve childcare facilities, even though more recent evidence tends not to support Bowlby's views (Rutter, 1987).

Many women feel guilty when they divide their attention between domestic ties and paid employment, even if they have had good educational opportunities and expect to find fulfilment in an interesting career. The classic work of Rappaport and Rappaport (1975) points out that even in privileged families where both partners work in highly paid jobs, it is still generally the woman rather than the man who faces the greatest demands made by domestic and childcare arrangements.

From these studies it emerges that whatever her social class, educational status or employment, it is most often the woman who has to cope with the demands of running a home and organising the care of children, especially when they become ill.

These studies are relevant to nurses because the health care of women, whether taking place in hospital or the community, cannot be separated from the everyday pressures facing the female client. This chapter is about the care of women, and its focus will be on promoting health and awareness of health, not just on the treatment needed when a visit to the doctor or hospital admission is necessary.

Women are the greatest consumers of health care in the UK, therefore health education provided for a woman is likely to reach the rest of her family, especially since it is usually the female partner who, for example, chooses food and decides how it should be prepared.

The nurse's role

Nurses working in a variety of different settings are well placed to help and advise women: health visitors, practice nurses, occupational health nurses, school nurses, midwives, nurses involved in family planning, and district nurses who may visit the home, officially to provide care for an elderly relative. Many women need specialist gynaecological advice at some stage in their lives, but even so, they may not be admitted to hospital. Today a great deal of treatment takes place in the outpatient clinic or on a day-care basis. Even if hospital admission is necessary, the length of stay is generally quite short. The pressure of work on gynaecology wards is often very high, leaving little time to get to know individual patients and their information needs (Gould, 1982). Much could be done to provide information during the time spent waiting in the outpatient department. Research has shown that women may be dissatisfied with the after-care received following routine gynaecological surgery, especially in terms of the information provided about recovery and return to normal activities (Webb, 1983). From the results of Webb's study, it emerged that women are often concerned about coping when they return home, and do not always have all the practical help they require. Clearly it is vital for nurses involved with female patients to recognise that women coming into hospital often worry as much about the domestic situation as their own health. Webb's study has yet to be replicated but more recent work (Oakley, 1985; Oakley et al., 1990) suggests that women who receive good emotional and social support during pregnancy are likelier to have fewer problems during labour and healthier babies, emphasising the value of care in the community.

Exploding the myths

As we enter the 1990s a number of myths persist concerning the nature of family life in the UK, the role played by women at home and at work, women's health and the difficult decisions which must sometimes be faced by women and their families concerning health care, childbearing and childrearing.

Family structure

Many people carry a pleasing image of 'typical' family life — working father, housewife mother and two children, with grandparents and other significant people in the locality providing support. However, only 5% of families are believed to accord with this ideal (Graham, 1984). Most women in the UK (about 60%) are in paid employment, mainly service employment such as cleaning, catering, nursing, teaching or technical work; at work as well as at home the role of a woman is to look after other people. This type of work is generally not well paid, though often forming an important contribution to family income. It is usually the woman who sacrifices her job when the first child is born, remaining at home until the youngest goes to school. Most then work part-time to fit in with the demands of the family. Job-sharing has become an option in recent years, but it is still not possible for many women because in practical terms it can prove difficult to organise. Those in gainful employment end up working extremely hard as they take on a dual role as employee and family carer. Men provide help in the home, but evidence suggests that they are unlikely to relieve their partners of childcare and housework even when unemployed (Graham, 1990).

Today one marriage in three will end in divorce and if there are children, they usually live with their mother, resulting in a situation which does not accord with the ideal model presented at the opening of this section. Other family units differ in that care is provided for elderly relatives. Much informal care within the community is given by women, who may be single or married, confirming that women are the greatest consumers of the health care services because they receive health care not only for themselves, but on behalf of their dependents (Graham, 1990; Arber, 1990).

Traditionally, the British family was an extended one (see Bott, 1968) but today small family units tend to have become widely separated in geographical terms through need to work where employment (the man's in most cases) is available. Although close relatives may keep in frequent contact through visits and telephone calls this does not provide the same type of support as in the past when female relatives living nearby could give practical help and emotional support in times of financial hardship, illness and, particularly, when children were small. Today the woman at home with young children is at risk of depression, especially if she lacks a close relationship with her partner or became motherless herself when young (Brown and Harris, 1978). A classic study by Paykel and Weisman (1974) reported that going out to work is important to women not only for financial reward, but because feelings of self-esteem and self-worth are promoted, reducing the likelihood of depression. It is unfortunate, therefore, that in the UK, childcare facilities for working

women are generally in short supply and expensive. The problems which young women at home with small children face are well known to health visitors, especially those who work in deprived areas where physical isolation may become acute through housing (tower blocks with broken lifts, lack of play areas, etc.), fear of going out alone in violent neighbourhoods, and lack of transport. Although most families have access to a car, priority is usually given to the man travelling to work. Shopping with small children, especially when using public transport, can be stressful for all concerned. At the other end of the scale is the elderly woman, physically frail but often providing care for her partner, or newly widowed and becoming accustomed to living alone after a lifetime of partnership and joint decisions (Arber, 1990).

Other myths that need exploding concern the victims of violence and rape. Orr (1984) has provided evidence to show that violence towards women is not related to social class, age or stage in family life. She points out that many episodes are never reported to the police through shame or fear of stigma, and that even when reported, help from the health and welfare services does not seem to be provided readily in most cases. Health visitors and others working with women in the community can only recognise difficulties and help to find solutions if they reject the stereotype of the battered woman held by the general public; such women are not 'to blame' for their plight, and it is not helpful to provide advice along the lines of what we would do if in the same situation. Many women in this position still genuinely care for their partners and are bound to them by other ties such as children or financial dependence. The first step in providing help is to listen non-judgementally, and to encourage an exchange of feelings between both partners, in an attempt to save the marriage or relationship if this is desired.

Rape, the ultimate form of violence against women, is defined as entry of the penis beyond the labia majora without the woman's consent (HMSO, 1976). It is considered a serious crime with a maximum life imprisonment, although most people are aware from media coverage that sentences are often much more lenient. The 1976 Act recognises two categories of rape:

(1) Statutory rape when the girl cannot consent because she is below the legal age (16 years in the UK);

(2) Forcible rape, when the woman is made to have sexual intercourse against her will or when her assailant is reckless as to her consent. This situation is now considered possible within marriage.

Legal wrangles, which always take place in a Crown Court before a jury, centre around whether the victim is able to provide evidence that she withheld consent (Moore, 1985). The assailant may persuade the court that at the time he believed that consent was given.

The related but more loosely defined crime of sexual assault (indecent assault) involves forced penetration of mouth by penis, vagina or anus by an object, touching breasts, buttocks or genitals or forcing the woman to touch the male genitalia.

The incidence of sexual crimes is difficult to establish, though figures are provided annually by HMSO, because many women do not report them for fear of the media and because police reception of victims is often as stressful as the incident itself, though in recent years services have been vastly improved in many localities. Several special reception centres have been established where women can receive attention from female officers, and a positive attempt has been made to make surroundings more pleasant and the experience of examination less intimidating (Di Nitto, 1986).

Sadly, women who have been raped are sometimes considered to have 'deserved' what has happened, and rape is popularly supposed to occur mainly to the young who behave provocatively and carelessly. In fact, many rapists are known to the victims and assaults (which are by no means restricted to young women) have frequently occurred in the middle of the day, within earshot of other people, in well-lit urban areas (Foley, 1979; Moore, 1985).

Women's bodies and women's lives

Throughout the 19th century it was widely believed that women's lives were dominated by the functioning of their reproductive systems (English and Ehrenreich, 1973). Removal of the uterus (*hysterectomy*) was considered not only physically hazardous but also likely to result in psychiatric illness, as it was thought that all females were emotionally attached to their uteri and would mourn the loss of childbearing capacity and menstruation. The work of authors like Webb (1983) and Gath

(1980) have shown that this is not true, although women benefit from careful emotional preparation and value the provision of information before they undergo gynaecological procedures. However, the menstrual cycle plays a central part in the lives of most women. Its commencement (*menarche*) marks reproductive maturity and menstruation is frequently associated with a certain amount of discomfort and inconvenience. The **menopause** is regarded as an unwelcome milestone in the ageing process by some women, although welcomed by others who are experiencing menstrual discomfort, and is marked by physical and emotional changes. Women usually keep a record of when they expect to menstruate for convenience and are particularly likely to do so when attempting to plan or avoid pregnancy. This section will discuss some of the problems women face when coping with menstruation and menstrual problems, opening with a description of physiological control.

The menstrual cycle

The structure of the female reproductive tract is shown in Chapter 5. Unlike the male, who produces sperm from puberty until the end of his life, females are fertile from the age of the menarche until the menopause, which usually occurs in the late 40s or early 50s. Eggs are released cyclically, and in a typical adult female the average length of the menstrual cycle is about 28 days.

Many women have considerably shorter or longer cycles, and this may lead to difficulties

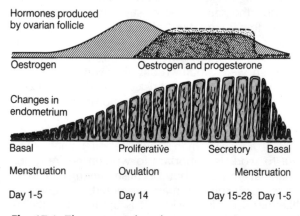

Fig. 17.1 The menstrual cycle

when trying to plan or prevent pregnancy. Variation in length and irregularities are particularly common when menstruation first starts and as the menopause approaches.

Physiology of the normal menstrual cycle

The first day of the cycle is regarded by convention as the first day of menstruation (Fig. 17.1). Usually bleeding lasts about five days. The length and amount of bleeding considered 'normal' by individuals is subject to considerable variation. Menstrual problems, including unpredictability and variability, worry so many women that all nurses need to understand how the menstrual cycle operates in order to provide reassurance and advice in terms their patients can understand.

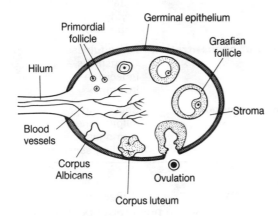

Fig. 17.2 *Section through an ovary showing development of the Graafian follicle*

Eggs (ova) ripen under the influence of oestrogen. Figure 17.2 shows a section cut through an ovary. Embedded in the connective tissue of this small organ are large numbers of ova waiting to develop. All the eggs a female will ever have are already present in her ovaries by the seventh week of her gestation. Many of them degenerate without maturing. Physiologists are still not sure why one or occasionally two ova are selected to mature during a particular cycle.

The egg develops during the first half of the cycle, its cells divide and then begin to release further oestrogen into the bloodstream. The egg is surrounded by a capsule called the *Graafian follicle*, which gradually moves towards the surface of the ovary where it can be detected with the **laparoscope**. Fluid secreted by the dividing cells collects inside the Graafian follicle. As the pressure builds up the egg is suddenly forced out of the follicle, through the wall of the ovary and into the abdominal cavity.

In a typical 28-day cycle, ovulation will occur on day 14, often accompanied by a transient pain called *Mittelschmerz*. Throughout this first proliferative phase of the cycle, oestrogen primes the uterine lining to prepare for possible pregnancy. After ovulation, the empty follicle (now known as the *corpus luteum*) persists on the surface of the ovary and releases progesterone. The **endometrium** becomes thicker and develops extra blood vessels and stores of glycogen. This secretory phase of the cycle lasts from ovulation until menstruation. If conception does not occur the corpus luteum shrivels up and the supply of female sex hormones abruptly ceases. The thickened lining of the uterus degenerates because the blood vessels that have developed suddenly constrict, cutting off the blood supply to the surface cells. For an interval lasting four or five days, the remains of these cells, mucus and blood drain away through the vagina as menstrual loss, which averages about 70 ml.

Hormone control of the menstrual cycle by the pituitary gland

Secretion of oestrogen and progesterone is controlled by two hormones released from the anterior pituitary. In the first half of the cycle follicular stimulating hormone (FSH) stimulates the follicle to develop and release oestrogen. Stimulation for the production of FSH itself comes from the hypothalamus which delivers a substance called *Releasing Factor* to the pituitary. Half way through the cycle a surge of Releasing Factor stimulates the pituitary to release the second hormone, luteinising hormone (LH). LH stimulates ovulation.

Although the mechanisms controlling release of FSH and LH are not completely understood, regulation seems to be mainly by negative feedback (see Chapter 5). Production of FSH is increased by Releasing Factor and diminished when levels of circulating oestrogens reach a critical threshold level (see Fig. 17.3). Similarly, progesterone from the corpus luteum inhibits LH release.

When ovulation occurs, core temperature rises slightly (up to 1°C) due to release of progesterone. The egg remains viable for about 36 hours, so it must be fertilised at this time if pregnancy is to

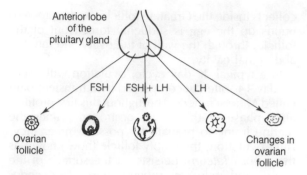

Fig. 17.3 *Control of secretion of ovarian hormones*

Table 17.1. *Principal features of the premenstrual syndrome*

Fluid retention	Weight gain
	Painful, heavy breasts
	Abdominal distension
	Feeling bloated
Pain	Headache
	Backache
	Muscle stiffness
	Fatigue
Autonomic reactions	Dizziness/faintness
	Nausea
	Vomiting
	Sweating
	Hot flushes
Mood changes	Tension
	Irritability
	Crying
	Depression
Loss of concentration	Forgetfulness
	Clumsiness
	Indecision
	Insomnia
Miscellaneous	Chest pain
	Palpitations
	Numbness
	Tingling sensations

occur. The time before ovulation and following it, once the egg is no longer viable, is theoretically a 'safe period' when unprotected intercourse cannot result in pregnancy. However, people wishing to use a 'natural' method of contraception should be warned that the safe period can never be regarded as absolutely safe, because the length of the cycle may vary. The rise in temperature is so slight that many women are unable to detect it accurately.

Menstrual problems

Most women probably experience a certain amount of discomfort with their periods from time to time. Early cycles, which are often *anovulatory* (not resulting in release of an egg), are usually painless. Later the girl may complain of a range of physical or emotional reactions before menstruation.

Premenstrual syndrome (PMS)

The cyclical appearance of a cluster of symptoms in the second half of the menstrual cycle was first described by the American gynaecologist Frankle in the 1940s, but much subsequent research has been undertaken in the UK by a GP, Katrina Dalton (1971). She documented the individual experiences of large numbers of women in her practice, revealing that prior to menstruation many women complained of minor physical and emotional upsets (see Table 17.1), while for others problems could be severe. Statistics collected over the years suggest that criminal offences committed by women often occur just before menstruation and at least one charge of murder has been altered to manslaughter on these grounds (Lancet, 1981).

For many years gynaecologists paid little atten- tion to PMS, but recently there has been an up- surge of interest and numerous books and articles have been written on the subject, many with the layperson in mind (Beard, 1984). Its cause remains elusive, although a number of theories exist. Various hormone deficiencies or excesses have been suggested, especially of the sex hormones and those responsible for fluid balance. A team of researchers working at a London teaching hospital have suggested that PMS may be caused or made worse by vitamin B deficiency, and believe that supplementing the diet with vitamin B_6 tablets ap- pears to have beneficial effects. Women can be encouraged to help themselves by purchasing their own tablets and working out the regime that seems most helpful. Vitamin tablets are cheap and pre- scriptions unnecessary. Treatment using another vegetable extract called *gamma linoleic acid* (oil of evening primrose) also seems promising.

Women who seek medical advice may be given diuretics to reduce fluid retention and possibly mild tranquillisers, but much depends on the cultivation of a positive attitude and recognition that PMS does not indicate weakness. Crying may help to reduce tension. Discussion with a partner and other family members may increase awareness of PMS and help to create understanding. Some women find benefit from joining a self-help group, reporting that ventilation of feelings with others in the same situation is helpful, though this does not necessarily have to occur when PMS is actually being experienced and may be more fruitful when it is not. To avoid 'blaming' PMS for every emotional upset or pain, some women keep PMS diaries to document when symptoms are most likely to occur (see Table 17.2). There is evidence that self-help measures, such as deliberate attempts to relax, discuss the issues with partner and family, take vitamin supplements and generally adopt a healthy lifestyle, can improve the quality of life for those with PMS (Kirpatrick *et al.*, 1990).

Dysmenorrhoea

Dysmenorrhoea is defined as pain experienced during menstruation. There are two types: *primary dysmenorrhoea*, diagnosed in the absence of demonstrable pelvic pathology, and *secondary dysmenorrhoea* when the woman is found to have some pelvic disorder or the pain can be attributed to an IUCD (intra-uterine contraceptive device).

For many years victims of primary dysmenorrhoea, like those of PMS, were unlikely to receive a great deal of sympathy from doctors, particularly as they are usually young women who otherwise enjoy good health and the pain can be guaranteed to go away when menstruation ceases, with no lasting ill effects. This was unfortunate for, as teachers, school nurses and those involved in the care of young women are all too well aware, period pains can be severe enough to disrupt work, educational and social activities. Its distribution is quite distinct from pain due to secondary dysmenorrhoea (see Fig. 17.4). A more enlightened attitude is now emerging, as it has been established that primary dysmenorrhoea is due to excess *prostaglandin F2*. Prostaglandins are locally produced hormones, meaning that they act rapidly on or near the same tissues responsible for secretion, rather than being transported relatively long distances from the gland of origin to target tissues, as is the case in classic hormonal control. Many prostaglandins have been identified and all have the general effect of increasing the contractility of

Table 17.2. *Sample PMS diary*

| Name .... | **Month** .... |

Record how you feel each day according to the five point scale below under the column headed 'Problems'. In the column headed 'Symptoms noted' describe how you feel. Circle each day you menstruate.

1. No symptoms
2. Some symptoms beginning/just noticeable
3. Moderate symptoms, but under control
4. Symptoms not really under control, but bearable/ coping is possible
5. Symptoms not controlled at all/not coping at all

Day of cycle	Problems	Symptoms noted
1		
2		
3		
4		
5		
6		
7		
8		
9		
10		
11		
12		
13		
14		
15		
16		
17		
18		
19		
20		
21		
22		
23		
24		
25		
26		
27		
28		

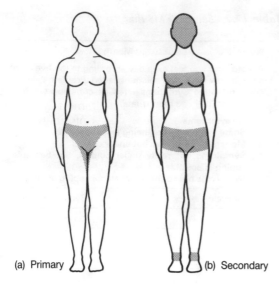

Fig. 17.4 *Distribution of pain in primary and secondary dysmenorrhoea*

smooth muscle. Prostaglandin F2 is secreted by the endometrium, inducing the *myometrium* (muscular layer of the uterus) to contract, resulting in cramping pain. Contractions also result in local ischaemia to the muscle, adding to pain. Prostaglandin F2, released in large quantities, gains access to the systemic circulation, resulting in nausea, vomiting, elevated temperature, diarrhoea and faintness.

The reason for elevated prostaglandin levels is assumed to be related to some mechanism associated with establishing menstrual flow, especially as pain is worse when a period commences or when it is particularly heavy. Aspirin breaks down prostaglandins and is therefore an effective analgesic in the treatment of primary dysmenorrhoea. For those who suffer extreme pain, more powerful anti-inflammatory drugs such as mefenamic acid (Ponstan) can be prescribed. These are most effective if tablet taking can begin before a period is anticipated.

Secondary dysmenorrhoea is not usually experienced until the woman reaches her mid-twenties and is usually described as a dragging rather than a cramping pain. As it results from pelvic abnormality, the advice of a doctor is necessary before effective treatment aimed at removing the cause can begin. The nurse responsible for menstrual assessment therefore needs to be aware of the different ways in which primary and secondary dysmenorrhoea are likely to present.

Heavy menstrual bleeding

Some women experience heavy menstrual loss, known in medical terminology as *menorrhagia*. This is sometimes, but not necessarily, associated with pain.

A number of different gynaecological conditions can result in the distressing symptom of menorrhagia. Among the most common are **fibroids** (leiomyomata), benign tumours of the myometrium which may occur singly or in large numbers. Fibroids may be so large that the doctor and sometimes even the woman herself can feel them on palpation, or they may be small and numerous. Small fibroids may be asymptomatic. Women can be reassured that fibroids never become malignant. Bleeding becomes excessive because fibroids increase the surface area of the uterus, as shown in Fig. 17.5, which also demonstrates possible locations at which they develop and the different types.

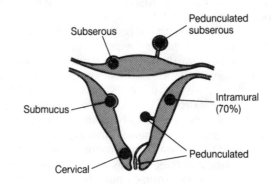

Fig. 17.5 *Uterine fibroids*

Endometriosis is a rather less common but very distressing cause of menorrhagia, usually associated with pain. Endometrial tissue develops ectopically (i.e. outside the uterine cavity) on the surface of the uterus or other pelvic structures and sometimes at sites distant to the pelvic cavity. Wherever it is positioned, ectopic endometrium responds to cyclical changes induced by the ovarian hormones, so that at each menstruation it bleeds. The blood, unable to escape, tends to form cysts, so-called *chocolate cysts* named after the altered appearance of the trapped blood. These cause pain. Endometriosis also tends to occur in women who are childless, but whether this is the cause or result of childlessness remains to be established. The cause of the condition itself is also open to debate. Cells destined to become endometrium may reach the wrong destination during embryonic development, but this does not explain why some women develop patches of endometrium in surgical scars. A second theory holds that reverse menstrual flow, escaping via the fimbriated openings of the uterine tubes into the pelvic cavity, can result in lesions, but the manner in which tissue gains access to organs outside the pelvis, as it very occasionally does, is not suggested.

A third condition likely to result in menorrhagia is *dysfunctional uterine bleeding*, a rather vaguely defined condition in which hormonal imbalance, occurring particularly during the second half of the cycle, results in over-stimulation of the endometrium to result in excessive bleeding.

The treatment of menorrhagia depends on diagnosis and the woman's wishes. For some, heavy periods become tolerable once they can be reassured that there is no likelihood of malignant disease, but for others bleeding interferes with work, family and social activities to such an extent that medical intervention seems their only recourse. Most women moved to seek the help of their GP will have a pelvic and vaginal examination. A very careful menstrual history will be taken. Fibroids may be palpated. A woman who complains that her periods have gradually become increasingly painful and heavy, with discomfort developing insidiously throughout the second half of the cycle is describing the classic signs and symptoms of endometriosis, especially if she is childless. A blood test will be performed to detect iron deficiency anaemia which will need treatment with iron supplements orally or a blood transfusion in hospital if very severe. Practice nurses are well placed to provide advice about diet and emotional support. Many of the women interviewed by Gould (1985a) described poignantly the distress and embarrassment caused by their heavy periods.

The investigation most commonly performed to find the cause of menorrhagia entails hospital admission to undergo *dilation and curettage* (D and C). This is a diagnostic procedure in which the **cervix** is gradually opened with an instrument to allow biopsy of endometrial fragments for examination in the laboratory. The woman is admitted to hospital the evening before surgery, or on the same

morning if day surgery is planned, and receives a light general anaesthetic following routine preoperative preparation. She can go home the next morning or later that evening providing she has recovered from the anaesthetic, has someone to collect her and her home circumstances will enable her to rest. D and C is a common procedure and Table 17.3 outlines the information the woman will need at every stage from admission to planning discharge.

Remember that although this minor operation is a routine hospital event it will seem anything but routine to the person undergoing it. She will experience a range of feelings which among others could include: anxiety, fear, embarrassment, and relief that something is at last being done about her problem periods. Core care plans for individuals undergoing the same physical procedure have obvious advantages in a gynaecology ward where patient turnover can be very rapid, but they will only contribute to care of high quality if the woman is able to discuss her needs, including requirements for specific information. In this situation, several women may be admitted to a ward on the same day, apparently to undergo the same operation although their symptoms and the likely cause of their bleeding may well differ. Myths concerning female disorders still abound and nurses can do much to promote clear understanding of approaches to diagnosis, emphasising that D and C is not intended as a cure.

Hysterectomy

Under anaesthesia the woman is relaxed, permitting a thorough pelvic examination. Other findings will be reported later when staff in the histology department have been able to examine tissue fragments under the microscope. The woman will be invited to return to the hospital outpatient department 5–6 weeks later to discuss the results and treatment options available to her. This can be a very stressful experience. Nurses in the ward can prepare the woman by reminding her to write down any questions she may wish to ask the doctor in advance. She may also benefit from the support of her partner or a close friend or relative while she is waiting to see the doctor.

Treatment of menorrhagia depends on the cause of heavy bleeding and what is acceptable to the woman. A single large fibroid can be removed and the uterus left (*myomectomy*), but women whose

Table 17.3. *Information needs of a woman who is to undergo dilation and curettage*

1. The date and time of her hospital appointment and where she is to go

2. What is likely to happen when she sees the gynaecologist:
    a) She will be asked about her previous medical, obstetric and menstrual history (the length of her cycle and the character of her periods, i.e. whether they are heavy, whether she experiences symptoms of the premenstrual syndrome or has pain)
    b) Her method of contraception, if any
    c) She will be examined by the gynaecologist, but a nurse will be present throughout to provide emotional and if necessary physical help (i.e. getting on and off couch)
    d) Gynaecological examination will probably include examination of the breasts and genital area, with a bimanual pelvic examination to assess the size and position of the uterus. Fibroids and polyps can be detected by this examination. A cervical smear may be taken

3. What D and C involves: she will be given a light general anaesthetic, allowing a more thorough pelvic examination to take place while she is relaxed and asleep. The cervix will gently be dilated by an instrument (dilator) then a second instrument (curette) will be used to obtain some material from the uterine lining to be sent to the laboratory for examination

4. Why this examination is necessary: D and C can help detect fibroids and polyps, and provides information about hormonal response of the endometrium during the second stage of the menstrual cycle which may be helpful in diagnosing the cause of some types of heavy menstrual bleeding or infertility. It may also be used to detect malignant change. It is evident that women with a diverse range of conditions are subjected to this same diagnostic procedure and this may be puzzling to women admitted to hospital apparently with very different health problems. It should be emphasised that D and C is a diagnostic procedure and not a form of treatment, although for some women with heavy periods it may effect temporary relief

5. The date of her hospital admission, where she should go and what she will need to bring with her. Some hospitals have a policy of day surgery for this operation, but the woman will only be able

to go home if she is sufficiently well and recovered from the anaesthetic and can be taken home by a responsible friend or relative. She should not be in the house alone that night – she needs to know this in advance so that contingency plans can be made.

6. Details of routine pre- and post-operative care. She should be warned that she will be bleeding slightly when she wakes up, and that when she first gets out of bed the bleeding may appear to become a little heavier: blood pools in the vagina when lying supine and drains through gravity when upright

7. Before leaving hospital she should know:
    a) That slight bleeding is to be expected for a few days, but medical advice should be sought promptly if it becomes copious, offensive or persists for more than a few days
    b) Sanitary towels rather than tampons should be used because the cervix has been dilated and it is sensible to reduce any chance of introducing infection
    c) She may return to work as soon as she feels ready. For some women this may be up to a week afterwards
    d) Her next period may arrive unexpectedly early or late
    e) The time and date of her next outpatient appointment

families are complete may prefer to undergo hysterectomy (see Fig. 17.6). For a woman who has yet to experience the menopause, total abdominal hysterectomy is likely to be performed. The body of the uterus and cervix are removed, but the ovaries are left unless there is evidence of disease. This is very important for the premenopausal woman because unpleasant symptoms such as hot flushes can quickly follow removal of the ovaries due to oestrogen withdrawal.

It is important for the nurse to know the type of operation that her patient is to have so that she can provide relevant information. As Fig. 17.6 shows, subtotal hysterectomy leaves the cervix intact, therefore any woman undergoing this procedure will still need cervical screening. Malignant cells often develop at this site and for this reason subtotal hysterectomy is seldom performed today.

Wertheim's hysterectomy is a radical procedure performed when there is evidence of advanced malignancy of the genital tract. As well as the

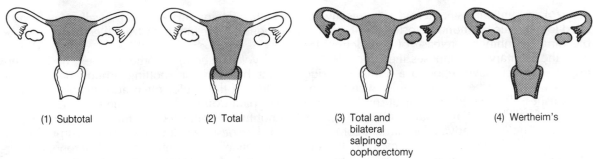

(1) Subtotal (2) Total (3) Total and bilateral salpingo oophorectomy (4) Wertheim's

Fig. 17.6 *Types of hysterectomy*

uterus, the ovaries, uterine tubes and surrounding lymph ducts are all removed, and often only one third of the vagina remains. Clearly women must be told about this, because as well as no longer menstruating or being able to have children, their sexual activity will be restricted.

Giving information to a woman undergoing hysterectomy

Hysterectomy is a routine operation, performed annually on large numbers of women, but for the individual it represents a completely new and threatening situation. Women must be warned about what to expect when they come into hospital, and nurses need to find out what knowledge each patient has about the operation, as misconceptions are quite common.

A second important aspect of care is to ensure that the patient and her family appreciate that when she returns home it may be some time before she feels completely well. Gould (1982) found that the length of time before recovery could be considered complete was a highly individual phenomenon, varying considerably between one person and another.

Gould's research indicated that women who have chosen to have a hysterectomy do not tend to become depressed. However, tiredness, tearfulness and boredom may be problems, especially during the early days at home when usual routine is disrupted. These possible effects must be discussed before discharge, and opportunity should be provided for both partners to express any anxieties about their sexual activity. Gould's work does not suggest that deterioration is likely; in fact, if discomfort and the need for contraception are removed, sex may become more enjoyable. However, women for whom sexual relationships have

not been entirely satisfactory may be disappointed if they anticipate that the operation will solve all their problems.

Histology report findings should be discussed when they become available; the woman may secretly fear that a malignant growth has been found, and she may worry needlessly because she is afraid to ask.

Alternatives to surgery

From time to time the number of hysterectomies performed in the UK and USA have been used as evidence that too many operations are being performed, sometimes needlessly, especially when, as in the case of dysfunctional uterine bleeding, no organic lesions are found. Some authorities argue that before surgery is offered an attempt should be made to quantify the amount of blood lost each month. This is rarely practical as it involves saving and weighing sanitary protection, an inconvenience which few women, already weary with the ill effects of menorrhagia, would choose to undergo. Most doctors assume, probably correctly, that if the woman considers her menstrual bleeding problematic *then for her it is a cause for distress* and the subjective nature of her judgement becomes irrelevant. Nevertheless, some women do not wish to have surgery and for these drug therapy may be an alternative. Antifibrinolytic agents (e.g. aminocaproic acid) taken in tablet form during menstruation may help prevent excessive bleeding by inducing coagulation. Oestrogen and progesterone given as the combined pill (see page 458) can relieve dysfunctional uterine bleeding very effectively by correcting hormonal imbalance, but this is not usually regarded as suitable for an older woman approaching the menopause. Another drug sometimes prescribed is danazol, a synthetic sex steroid, chemically related to the male hormone testosterone. It reduces bleeding by inhibiting release of gonadotrophins from the pituitary and opposes the effects of oestrogen. Women have reported a number of side effects which can be unacceptable: weight gain, hot flushes, loss of libido, hirsutism (excessive growth of hair, including facial hair) and increased appetite. Another disadvantage of danazol is that bleeding tends to recur once therapy stops. In view of the effects of this drug and its tendency to control symptoms rather than cure, it is not surprising that many women prefer to undergo hysterectomy.

Intermenstrual bleeding

Intermenstrual bleeding (*metropathica haemor-rhagica*) is bleeding in between menstrual periods. There are a number of causes, some minor where bleeding is really only an inconvenience, others of a more serious nature. For this reason any woman who experiences unexpected bleeding should be encouraged to seek medical advice. A few of the conditions a nurse is most likely to encounter are discussed here.

Polyps These are benign growths which develop on the cervix, sometimes growing large enough to protrude down into the vagina. Their epithelial covering is friable and delicate, so trauma (e.g. from sexual intercourse) can make them bleed. Polyps never undergo malignant change, but can be inconvenient and distressing. The woman will require examination under anaesthesia and the polyps can be excised surgically at the same time.

'Breakthrough' bleeding from the pill Combined oral contraceptives (see page 458) operate by the oestrogen and progesterone they contain acting on the pituitary gland to prevent ovulation. Modern low dose pills contain very small amounts of oestrogen and women who take them may sometimes experience slight 'breakthrough' bleeding or 'spotting'. This often resolves after the first few cycles but if recurrent can be a cause of dissatisfaction with this method of contraception. Women should always be given the opportunity to discuss their feelings about contraception when visiting the family planning clinic because dissatisfaction can result in low motivation to take pills and inevitable unplanned pregnancy. The progesterone-only pill, which contains no oestrogen at all, may also be responsible for intermenstrual bleeding.

Midcycle bleeding Some women notice very slight bleeding or spotting around day 14, the middle of the cycle, often accompanied by transient pain (Mittelschmerz). The cause of bleeding is not fully established but may be due to temporarily low oestrogen levels before the corpus luteum commences the secretion of progesterone, the hormone which, together with oestrogen, is responsible for the continuing development of the endometrium throughout the second part of the menstrual cycle. Pain may be caused by the irritant effect of fluid surrounding the ovum gaining access to the pelvic cavity. Women can be reassured that midcycle pain and a show of blood are normal. They may be valuable markers of the fertile period to women and their partners trying to avoid or achieve pregnancy.

Malignancy Carcinoma of the cervix is the eighth most common cause of cancer among women in the UK (Gould, 1990), and receives wide publicity as it is a preventable disease with well-established risk factors and a method of screening known to be effective, providing women present themselves for investigation. Table 17.7 on page 467, where cervical cancer and the earlier premalignant changes of cervical intra-epithelial neoplasia (CIN) are detailed, shows that the disease is managed medically according to the stage that it has reached. Sadly, many women are reluctant to be screened and the first change of which they become aware is bleeding, commonly occurring after intercourse. Although the disease is often advancing by this time, treatment is available and much can still be done to improve future health prospects.

Carcinoma of the body of the uterus traditionally affects older women, but in recent years the age of those affected appears to be reduced, possibly because incidence is in some cases linked to high oestrogen levels which may result from prolonged use of the combined pill or hormone replacement therapy (page 469). It is a malignancy which progresses much more slowly than cervical cancer and as the endometrium is affected, the very thick wall of the myometrium may help reduce local spread. Again, bleeding may be the first indication that something is amiss, especially for the woman who experienced her last menstrual period some time ago. Nurses whose work brings them into contact with the general public outside and in hospital can promote awareness by advising that all post-menstrual bleeding should be investigated promptly. Older women may need a great deal of encouragement to go to a doctor, dreading pelvic examination and the possibility of further investigation (dilation and curettage). Even if malignant change is detected, the prognosis for cancer of the body of the uterus is good.

Missing periods

The technical term for absence of menstruation is *amenorrhoea*. There are two types: *primary amenorrhoea* when the girl or woman has never had a period, and *secondary amenorrhoea* when established menstruation has ceased. The most common reason for secondary amenorrhoea is an entirely normal physiological event – pregnancy. In this section, several causes of amenorrhoea are discussed, some related to pregnancy, others not.

Delayed menarche

Most girls experience their first menstrual period between the ages of 11 and 14, though the menarche can occur as early as nine years of age or as late as 17 and still be regarded as normal. Most girls value being like their friends, however, and begin to worry if they are the only one in the crowd who has not yet had a period. Discussion with a school nurse can be helpful; she can point out that most people are a variant on what is normal and that as the menarche is generally experienced once a girl has reached a critical weight threshold (dependent on her height and body build), those who are small for their age frequently have their first period relatively late. She may weigh the girl and make some enquiries about diet and appetite. Anorexia nervosa, which is not uncommon in this age group, is known to delay the menarche or cause periods to stop until the weight lost has been regained. If the girl is still worried or has reached the age of 16 or so, then a visit to the GP or a gynaecologist may be reassuring.

When she sees the doctor the girl can expect to be examined. As this will be her first experience of a pelvic examination, very careful preparation and explanation will be required. The doctor will inspect the breasts to determine whether they have begun to develop as they should and look for signs that the other secondary sexual characteristics (e.g. pubic and axillary hair) are becoming apparent. In the case of a young girl, a rectal rather than a vaginal examination is usually performed to provide information about the internal pelvic structures. Genuine pathological delay of the menarche is rare, but this type of examination will give a fair idea of any problems if they exist. If there is no evidence of development of the breasts and no body hair or an unusual distribution, then a chromosomal or hormonal problem is indicated, with treatment depending on its cause. If development is proceeding as expected, the girl could have an imperforate hymen blocking the escape of menstrual blood. Treatment consists of hospital admission (a day or two) and a minor surgical procedure to allow the blood to escape. Old, altered blood provides a very good medium for infection so the girl must be advised of the need for scrupulous hygiene.

Vaginal atresia is a rare condition in which the vagina, which begins as a rod of tissue canalising into a hollow organ during embryonic development, remains as a solid wall of tissue. This must be removed and a pack inserted to ensure that **adhesions** do not form. Often this condition is accompanied by other abnormalities of reproductive function such as a small or poorly developed uterus. These are often possible to correct by surgery but may have implications for future fertility.

Secondary amenorrhoea

Infrequent, irregular periods may be no more than an inconvenience to women until they try to plan pregnancy. Nurses who work in family planning clinics can do much to help by providing advice about the menstrual cycle in terms the woman and her partner can readily understand and by pointing out that although text books always describe the typical 28-day cycle with ovulation and therefore fertility occurring around day 14, the reality for many women is quite different. Where periods come far apart, it is helpful to know that it is the first half of the cycle which is open to wide variations in length. Ovulation is always followed 13–14 days later by menstruation (unless pregnancy supervenes), so intercourse should occur frequently around this time. The nurse can also take the woman's menstrual history from which it may be possible to determine whether or not she is ovulating. Anovulatory cycles (those in which no egg is released) occur from time to time in most women. Indications of failure to ovulate include painless, relatively trouble-free periods with no breast soreness or other symptoms of PMS. These findings may be confirmed by measuring levels of the sex hormones in the blood at critical stages in the cycle or in the urine, as oestrogen and progesterone, like a great many other hormones, are broken down in the liver and excreted mainly via the kidneys. As the endometrium responds to circulating levels of oestrogen and progesterone, medical investigations for amenorrhoea or infertility may involve D and C to obtain endometrial fragments for histological examination.

Failure to ovulate may be the result of systemic disease such as thyroid dysfunction or may involve the reproductive organs and their hormones. Young women who have taken oral contraceptives for some time may discover that it takes a while for menstruation to become re-established. This problem is less common than frequently supposed and is amenable to treatment if necessary. For women trying to become pregnant clomiphene, given at a critical time in the cycle, will stimulate ovulation and is associated with a high degree of success. For those women who fail to respond, carefully monitored treatment with Pergonal (chemically identical to **human chorionic gonadotrophin**) may be successful. The whole topic of infertility and the meaning of childlessness is discussed on page 463.

Disorders of early pregnancy

A missed period may be the woman's first indication that she has become pregnant, although those who have conceived before may recognise very early breast soreness, even before the period was due. In some circumstances, however, pregnancy may not be normal and it is at this very early stage that the woman may need urgent gynaecological intervention. Etopic pregnancy, threatened and inevitable miscarriage (abortion) are discussed below.

Ectopic pregnancy

Ectopic pregnancy occurs when the fertilised egg embeds at some location other than the wall of the uterus. The most usual site is in the uterine tube at a point called the *ampulla*, which is slightly more

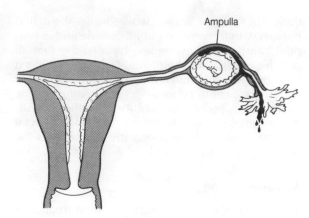

Fig. 17.7 *Ectopic pregnancy*

dilated than the rest of the tube (Fig. 17.7). Occasionally implantation may take place outside the tube, in the abdominal cavity.

Ectopic pregnancy is potentially a life-threatening condition, and it is becoming more common. As the egg divides and the embryo grows bigger it erodes surrounding tissues, including blood vessels, leading to bleeding, severe pain and circulatory shock. Macafee (1984) quotes figures to show that between 1973 and 1975, 21 women in England and Wales died of ruptured ectopic pregnancy, and that one ectopic pregnancy can be expected for about every 175 live births. One of the biggest dangers is that the patient may not realise she is pregnant because pain often begins before she has had time to miss a period.

The typical scenario is of a woman who is complaining of acute pelvic pain brought to the Accident and Emergency Department. Vaginal bleeding may occur, but it will not resemble a normal period. To save time, preparation for theatre is minimal. A laparoscopy (examination under anaesthetic in which a fine fibre-optic instrument is used to examine the pelvic and reproductive structures) will confirm the presence of ectopic pregnancy. All or part of the affected uterine tube will be removed (*salpingectomy*). Depending on the amount of damage, the doctor may attempt to repair the affected tube. After this operation most patients are ready to go home within a few days, but time should be spent with the patient and her partner so they can discuss their feelings; sometimes couples feel that ectopic pregnancy is somehow their 'fault'.

Often an alternative method of contraception

must be found, as ectopic pregnancy is particularly likely to occur in women who use an IUCD because the passage of the egg may be interrupted. There is also some risk that pregnancies unsuccessfully prevented by post-coital contraception (the 'morning-after' pill) will also be ectopic. There is a somewhat higher risk of developing pelvic inflammatory disease (PID) when an IUCD has been inserted, and since this may interfere with fertility, women with only one remaining uterine tube should be discouraged from using an IUCD.

Miscarriage

Miscarriage is the layperson's term for accidental **abortion**. To many people the word abortion implies only therapeutic abortion, and this should be remembered in discussions with patients.

There are several ways of classifying spontaneous (non-therapeutic) abortion (Fig. 17.8) (see Lewis and Chamberlain, 1990). If there is pain but only slight vaginal bleeding (spotting) and the uterine cervix is not dilated, the pregnancy may still be saved. The care of a woman and her partner in this situation is illustrated in Figs. 17.9 and 17.10.

> Elizabeth Cohen is 25 years old, and has been married for two years. She was 11 weeks pregnant when she was admitted to the Accident and Emergency Department with lower abdominal and back pain (slight) and vaginal bleeding. The pregnancy had been planned. Elizabeth was very distressed. Neither she nor her husband Jacob has been in hospital before, and they know of no one else who has had a miscarriage. An ultrasound examination performed before Elizabeth arrives in the ward indicates that the pregnancy is still viable.

Fig. 17.9 *Assessment/history: Elizabeth Cohen*

Types of spontaneous abortion

Inevitable abortion means that the pregnancy cannot be saved. Bleeding is heavier and bright red, accompanied by pelvic and back pain due to uterine contractions. The **cervical os** is dilated. If all the products of conception are lost, abortion is said to be complete (see Fig. 17.11).

Because the risk of infection following incomplete abortion is high, it is the policy in most hospitals to perform an *evacuation of retained products of conception* (ERPC). Under a general anaesthetic, the woman's uterine lining is gently scraped with a curette passed up through the dilated cervix and the remaining products of conception removed. If this is not done and the woman

Threatened abortion ⟶ Inevitable abortion

Normal pregnancy

Complete or incomplete abortion

Death of fetus *in utero* and non-expulsion = missed abortion

Habitual abortion if this happens more than twice for two consecutive pregnancies

Fig. 17.8 *Types of abortion*

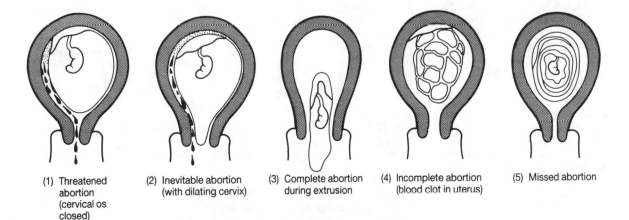

(1) Threatened abortion (cervical os closed)

(2) Inevitable abortion (with dilating cervix)

(3) Complete abortion during extrusion

(4) Incomplete abortion (blood clot in uterus)

(5) Missed abortion

Fig. 17.11 *Types of spontaneous abortion*

Fig. 17.10 Care plan for Elizabeth Cohen

	Elizabeth Cohen: threatened abortion	
Activity of Living Assessment	Problems	Goals
Maintaining a safe environment *Vital signs.* Pulse 90 beats/min. BP 110/80. Vaginal loss: slight, bright red. Elizabeth complains of backache and abdominal cramps, but says that neither is severe. Ultrasound examination performed at 12.30 am has shown that the pregnancy is viable	1P – hypovolaemic shock if there is excessive bleeding from the placental site and abortion becomes inevitable 2P – increased backache and abdominal pain if abortion becomes inevitable 3P – the need for evacuation of retained products in theatre if abortion becomes inevitable 4P – the need for blood transfusion if bleeding becomes severe	Recognise the signs of shock and haemorrhage. Inform medical staff promptly. Ensure that all documentation is correct should Elizabeth require emergency preparation for theatre Ensure that the results of Elizabeth's blood tests are recorded in her case notes in case the need for emergency blood transfusion arises
Communicating Elizabeth looks pale, tired and frightened. She says that she and her husband are anxious. She is tearful because she has overheard the nurse saying she has 'a threatened abortion'. Her husband is very angry about this	**20.02.1992 1.30 pm** A – Elizabeth and her husband are worried because she is bleeding and has come into hospital. They are still afraid that she could lose the baby. Both are angry about the conversation they have overheard	Elizabeth and her husband will feel less anxious. They will understand the meaning of the term 'abortion'. Both will understand the treatment Elizabeth will receive, and why
Breathing Respiratory rate – 22/minute. Deep, not irregular. Not cyanosed	**20.02.1992 1.30 pm** 1P – respiratory arrest following haemorrhage from placental site and hypovolaemic shock 2P – respiratory obstruction due to vomiting (says she feels nauseated)	(1) Elizabeth will not experience respiratory problems due to shock (2) Elizabeth will not experience respiratory problems due to obstruction of the airways
Eating and drinking Elizabeth says she feels nauseated. Says this is her usual reaction to fear/anxiety. Time of last meal: breakfast at 8.30. Time of last drink: coffee at 11.30	**20.02.1992 1.30 pm** 1P – vomiting 2P – mouth sore and feels dry from anorexia 3A – nausea	(1) Elizabeth will not vomit (2) Elizabeth's mouth will feel moist and comfortable. She will not feel thirsty (3) Elizabeth will no longer feel nauseated
Eliminating Elizabeth last emptied her bladder at 12.30 p.m. after ultrasound was performed. She has not opened her bowels since yesterday	**20.02.1992 1.30 pm** 1P – Elizabeth may find it difficult to pass urine while she is confined to bed 2P – Elizabeth may become constipated while confined to bed. She will be unable to take aperients, as this may stimulate the uterus to contract	(1) Elizabeth will pass urine without difficulty (2) She will not become constipated

Care plan – Roper's model (Roper *et. al.*, 1985). *P = Potential* problem. *A = Actual* problem

Nursing Intervention	Evaluation	Signature
Monitor vital signs four-hourly Inform medical staff of any change in condition Identify Elizabeth with a wristband, and check with her that all details are correct	**20.02.1992 4.30 pm** Elizabeth's condition is stable. Her pain has diminished. The need for surgery is unlikely Reassessment of this care is needed. Reassess 21.02.1992	*C. Dale*
Elizabeth and her husband will be given explanations about the term 'abortion' in medical parlance. They will understand the reason for Elizabeth's treatment and be given the results of the ultrasound examination	**20.02.1992 5.30 pm** Elizabeth and her husband feel reassured and understand what is happening to them **24.02.1992 2.30 pm** Elizabeth and her husband are satisfied with their care	*C. Dale* *L. Strong*
(1) Observe respiratory rate four hourly Observe depth and volume, skin colour of extremities (2) Observe vaginal loss (see **maintaining a safe environment**) (3) Reduce nausea and the likelihood of vomiting (see **eating and drinking**)	**20.02.1992 5.30 pm** Elizabeth's respiratory rate is 20/minute, deep and regular. She is not cyanosed	*C. Dale*
(1) Now that ultrasound examination has shown that the pregnancy is viable, Elizabeth will not need to go to theatre. She may eat and drink normally (2) Elizabeth will receive mouthwashes and have the opportunity to clean her teeth (3) Elizabeth will be reassured and nursed in a quiet part of the ward so she will feel less anxious	**20.02.1992 5.30 pm** Elizabeth is drinking freely and no longer feels nauseated	*C. Dale*
(1) Elizabeth will drink at least two litres of fluid daily and be offered bedpans frequently. She will be given privacy to use them. Her urinary output will be monitored daily (2) Elizabeth will eat a diet from the hospital menu containing foods rich in fibre. She may get up to the WC once daily	**20.02.1992 5.30 pm** Elizabeth's urinary output is monitored. She has passed 300 ml. of urine **21.02.1992 8.00 pm** Elizabeth is passing adequate amounts of urine. She has opened her bowels once (1,500 ml/24 hrs)	*C. Dale* *C. Dale*

Activity of Living Assessment	Problems	Goals
Personal cleansing and dressing Elizabeth's standard of hygiene is good. She is wearing a hospital gown provided in A and E	**20.02.1992 1.30 pm** 1A – Elizabeth feels exposed and uncomfortable in the hospital gown, especially as she is bleeding vaginally 2A – unfamiliar clothes add to her discomfort and anxiety	Elizabeth's husband will bring her own nightclothes from home as soon as possible
Controlling body temperature Temperature 37.5°C on admission. Elizabeth says she is cold, and her skin feels cold	**20.02.1992 1.30 pm** 1A – Elizabeth complains of cold and feels cold to the touch 2A – Elizabeth is wearing only a hospital gown 3P – Elizabeth could develop pyrexia due to sepsis	Elizabeth will no longer complain of the cold Elizabeth's temperature will remain within normal limits
Mobilising Elizabeth says she felt uncomfortable on the hospital trolley in A and E, but she can move freely	**20.02.1992 1.30 pm** 1P – Elizabeth will be confined to bed 2A – bedrest may result in soreness and backache 3P – bedrest may result in deep venous thrombosis (DVT)	(1) Elizabeth will not complain of discomfort (2) She will not develop soreness or backache (3) She will not develop DVT
Working and playing Elizabeth's normal activities are disrupted by sudden hospital admission	**20.02.1992 3.30 pm** 1P – Elizabeth will become bored by enforced bedrest. She will worry about how her husband is managing at home	Elizabeth will be able to find some activities that will amuse and distract her while confined to bed. Her husband will tell her about events at home
Expressing sexuality Elizabeth is tearful. She says this was a wanted pregnancy (her first)	**20.02.1992 3.00 pm** 1P – threatened loss of pregnancy may have a damaging effect on Elizabeth's body image and self esteem. She may worry that she will be unable to carry future pregnancies to term. Her husband may have similar worries	Elizabeth and her husband will feel able to voice their fears to one another, to the hospital staff and show their emotions
Sleeping and resting Elizabeth says she normally sleeps well, about eight hours (11 pm–7 am) per night. Since she has been pregnant she has occasionally had to get up to pass urine. She is not yet resting in the day	**20.02.1992 3.30 pm** 1P – Elizabeth's usual sleeping habits may be disrupted by ward activities, anxiety and urinary frequency	Elizabeth will sleep eight hours a night, undisturbed

Nursing Intervention	Evaluation	Signature
Elizabeth is reassured that she will not need to get out of bed in the gown, and that her own belongings will be provided as soon as possible	**20.02.1992 5.30 pm** Elizabeth is wearing her own nightclothes and feels more comfortable	C. Dale
Monitor temperature four-hourly Provide Elizabeth with extra bedclothes Elizabeth's husband will bring her own nightclothes from home Instruct Elizabeth to take good hygienic measures to prevent ascending vaginal infection. Provide her with sterile sanitary towels	**20.02.1992 5.30 pm** Elizabeth no longer feels cold. Her temperature is now 36.8°C **24.02.1992 2.30 pm** Elizabeth's temperature remains within normal limits. She has no evidence of sepsis	C. Dale L. Strong
Elizabeth will be positioned comfortably in bed She will be encouraged to change her position frequently She will be taught leg exercises to prevent DVT Her pressure areas will be examined for signs of inflammation	**20.02.1992 2.30 pm** Elizabeth is comfortable in bed **20.02.1992 8.30 pm** Elizabeth is comfortable, and moving in bed **24.02.1992 2.30 pm** Elizabeth has not developed inflammation over her pressure areas and has no DVT	C. Dale L. Strong
Elizabeth is occupied by books from the hospital library and by sewing brought by her husband. She is kept informed of events at home	**24.02.1992 2.30 pm** Elizabeth spends part of each day reading and sewing. She is happy about the way her husband is coping at home	L. Strong
Provide clear explanations of all that is happening. Reassure Elizabeth and her husband that the pregnancy is still viable. Explain that threatened miscarriage is an extremely common event in early pregnancy and that many pregnancies continue undisturbed	**24.02.1992 2.30 pm** Elizabeth and her husband feel happier about the situation which they have discussed with their nurse. Elizabeth has been visited by a previous patient whose pregnancy continued satisfactorily despite an early episode of vaginal bleeding	L. Strong
Elizabeth will be given a bed in a quiet part of the ward She will be given the opportunity to empty her bladder before settling for the night Her nursing care will be organised so that she is undisturbed between 11 pm and 7 am	**21.02.1992 8.00 pm** Elizabeth says she has slept quite well. She has not been disturbed between 11 pm and 7 am	C. Dale

subsequently complains of fever, malaise and an offensive vaginal discharge, then she has a septic abortion. This condition has been associated with criminal 'back street' abortions but can nevertheless occur following spontaneous, incomplete abortions.

Aetiology of abortion

Quite a high percentage of pregnancies end spontaneously in abortion. Estimates vary and the precise number is probably impossible to calculate accurately because some abortions occur so soon after conception that the woman is unaware that she was ever pregnant, noticing only that her period was later and rather heavier than usual. The IUCD, which works by preventing implantation of the fertilised egg, blurs the dividing line between contraception and abortion.

Most spontaneous abortions take place between the sixth and twelfth week of pregnancy, because the corpus luteum left behind after the egg is released from the ovary is ceasing to produce progesterone. Progesterone secretion is necessary for the continuance of pregnancy and also comes from the placenta, but at this early stage the placenta may not be sufficiently developed to secrete all the progesterone necessary to maintain pregnancy. Alternatively, abortion may occur because of maternal ill health, especially pyrexia. There may be some uterine abnormality such as *bicornuate uterus* (Fig. 17.12), which interferes with the growing fetus, but more often the woman has an incompetent cervix, which dilates as the pregnancy advances. The woman can be admitted at 14 weeks gestation and a **Shirodkar suture** used to draw the lips of the cervix together (Fig. 17.13). It must be removed towards the end of pregnancy so that labour can begin.

Habitual abortion

The term habitual abortion is used when a woman has had three or more successive spontaneous abortions. About 20% of these patients have an incompetent cervix. In other cases a malformed uterus may prevent the baby developing properly. Incompetent cervix was once considered a risk of therapeutic abortion, especially if performed several times. However, modern pregnancy tests allow pregnancy to be detected as early as the day a menstrual period was expected and, if performed

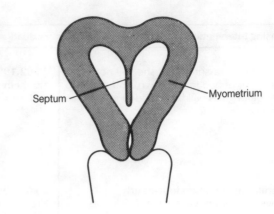

Fig. 17.12 *Bicornuate uterus*

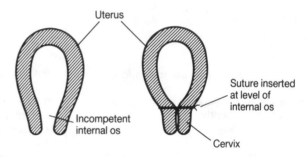

Fig. 17.13 *Shirodkar suture*

early, abortion need not dilate the cervix as a very fine plastic catheter may be used, so damage and loss of future pregnancies may no longer be feared.

Emotional reactions to spontaneous abortions

Nurses need to be sensitive to the feelings of women who are admitted to hospital with spontaneous abortion, particularly since the patient will be unwilling to confide in anyone who seems unsympathetic, and may therefore prefer not to divulge all the details of her past gynaecological history. Although many spontaneous abortions are due to fetal abnormality investigations do not usually proceed until several have occurred in succession, often leaving the woman wondering about what has gone wrong. Being told by well-meaning people that miscarriage was 'probably for the best' is poor comfort.

Spontaneous abortion has not evoked a great deal of interest among nurse researchers. Oakley (1984), a sociologist who has a particular interest in women's health, conducted a study among women who had experienced spontaneous abortion. Although her study could be criticised for the method used to obtain the sample (requesting information from volunteers, so that women with unresolved problems may have been particularly willing to respond), Oakley found disturbing evidence to suggest that women experience grief and feelings of loss after miscarriage, which health care professionals, including nurses, do little to allay.

Missed abortion

Missed abortion happens when pregnancy has started but the fetus has died and not been expelled. The normal signs of pregnancy gradually regress and concern will arise when the uterus ceases to enlarge. If this happens early in pregnancy, a small haemorrhage may take place with blood collecting between the placenta and the uterine wall. The blood clot is called a *carnous mole*. If pregnancy is more advanced the fetus shrivels up, becoming mummified. Dark brown vaginal loss indicates that all is not well. The products of conception must be removed, either by dilating the cervix and aspirating the uterine contents or by inducing uterine contractions with prostaglandins, because the retained products of conception could result in sepsis. The idea of the baby dying but remaining inside the uterus may seem very unpleasant to the woman, who will need a great deal of support whichever method is used.

The menopause: problems associated with the cessation of menstruation

Like puberty, the menopause is a normal physiological event, although it has come to be associated with numerous myths and half-truths (Gould, 1985b). Possibly the menopause is seen in Western society in a negative light because it is proof that the woman is growing older and ageing itself is regarded in a negative way in our culture.

Numerous problems – both physical and emotional – have been attributed to the menopause, including headaches, vertigo, depression, loss of interest in sex and, of course, the notorious hot flushes. Several researchers have set out to time the onset of these discomforts, and in order to do so they have defined the term menopause precisely. The *menopause* is defined as the last menstrual period, while the *climacteric* is the time leading up to and around the last period. Critical examination of most studies reveals that many symptoms are actually experienced during the climacteric, and they tend to be perceived as most troublesome by women who are already unhappy.

The majority of these studies have been undertaken by doctors (e.g. Nolan, 1986), but they are of interest to nurses who meet women in this age group wherever they work, whether in hospital or the community. Problems such as menorrhagia or stress incontinence often bring middle-aged women to the gynaecology clinic or ward, but many others may not seek help or realise that anything can be done to help. Nurses need a sound understanding of the normal physiological changes expected at the menopause to enable them to give clients appropriate advice and support.

Physiological changes at the menopause

At the menopause the ovaries stop releasing oestrogen. This causes changes to occur in the vagina. The layer of cells lining the vaginal walls becomes thinner, lubrication decreases and the pH changes, reducing the population of bacteria called lactobacilli normally colonising the vagina throughout reproductive life. Foreign micro-organisms, like the yeast infection *Candida*, can invade and set up inflammatory changes associated with a vaginal discharge. This condition is sometimes called senile vaginitis, although it often affects younger women. Treatment with fungicidal creams and pessaries will alleviate this condition. Sometimes the woman's quality of life at this time can be greatly improved by relieving these minor but troubling symptoms, combined with sympathy and the opportunity to discuss anxieties, but for others the menopause can result in genuine depression. Some women perceive themselves as less attractive and possibly less valuable once their children have grown older and more independent. Loss of interest in sex can have a psychological component if the woman holds a deep-rooted belief that sex without the possibility of conception is without purpose. Such feelings may not be rational, for they may be entertained by women who have been practising contraception effectively for years and who have not seriously considered the possibility of having another child.

Nobody can make these dissatisfactions go away but women can be helped, through counselling, to perceive the natural events occurring in their bodies in a more positive light, and to develop a lifestyle that is as healthy as possible. Weight gain, tiredness and boredom are not inevitable with the onset of middle age, and with more time available as children become independent, there is the opportunity to develop new interests, to take more exercise and to experiment with healthy eating. Without the need for contraception and freed from the discomforts and inconvenience accompanying menstruation, sex may become more enjoyable.

Some women do benefit from specialised help and they may be referred to a gynaecologist who has a particular interest in menopausal problems. Often the first step is to obtain a blood sample to ensure that the woman is actually menopausal. When the ovaries cease to produce oestrogen, negative feedback to the pituitary gland is interrupted and the resulting higher levels of FSH and LH are detectable in the blood.

Among the more far-reaching effects of oestrogen withdrawal is the possibility of developing osteoporosis, which increases risk of bone fractures with age. This effect may be reduced by hormone replacement therapy (HRT) discussed on page 469.

Promoting health: women's needs and health-related choices

In the previous section we discussed the influence of reproduction and reproductive function on women's general health, emphasising that although menstruation and the cyclical changes accompanying it do not govern female health and happiness in the 1990s, they may still contribute towards it. In this section we focus on some of the considerations women may give to the type of care they choose: whether to undergo screening procedures or not, which type of contraception to choose and the setting in which to receive care. Some women, for example, would approach their own GP to receive contraceptive advice, others prefer a family planning clinic, while a third group cope entirely without medical or nursing intervention when controlling fertility. Note that some of these 'health-related' choices are as much to do with social as health needs: the woman and her partner who decide to plan or avoid pregnancy, to undergo treatment for fertility or have a therapeutic abortion are making decisions which will affect their physical and emotional status now and in the future. It is equally important to remember that many women may be admitted to hospital for part of their care, perhaps to undergo an operation or investigation, but this forms only a brief interlude in treatment for a condition or situation, such as infertility, which may be ongoing and have existed for a long time. This section opens with a discussion of contraception, as it is a need common to many women throughout their reproductive lives.

Contraception

Women have always tried to control their fertility. Before understanding of reproductive physiology was complete, these attempts had little rationale and many were unsuccessful. Even today our knowledge of some of the effects of the contraceptive pill and intra-uterine contraceptive device (IUCD) remains incomplete, despite the large numbers of women who use them.

Although the great majority of people who live in the UK probably do use some method of controlling their fertility, all nurses who play a role in women's health should remember that there are exceptions, and that people belonging to some religious and cultural groups do not wish to use artificial methods of birth control. David Lodge (1983) describes, in a humorous but compassionate account, the trials of a young Catholic couple who already have three children, but feel that their religious teaching precludes the use of any form of contraception other than the 'safe period'. Methods of contraception fall into four main groups:

(1) Natural methods (including abstinence)
(2) Barrier methods

(3) Hormonal methods
(4) Sterilisation

Natural methods of contraception

Natural methods of contraception demand a sound understanding of the normal menstrual cycle and its variations (see page 438) by the nurse or lay teacher who provides instruction and by the people who adopt this method.

A team of researchers in Australia have developed another natural method of contraception based on observable cyclical changes in the character of mucus secreted by the cervix (Billings and Westland, 1980). Throughout most of the cycle cervical secretion is scanty, but around ovulation the mucus becomes slippery and forms long strands. This change in consistency helps penetration by sperm. Women can be taught to observe these changes and to record them on a chart to help interpretation; however, this method of birth control requires considerable self-discipline and mutual understanding between partners. Spermicides cannot be used on fertile days because they interfere with the interpretation of cervical mucus. It must be emphasised that motivation plays a major role in the use of natural methods. They are suitable only for dedicated couples who have a close and lasting relationship.

Barrier methods of contraception

Perhaps the oldest barrier method, also constituting a natural method, is coitus interruptus (withdrawal), when ejaculation is not allowed to take place in the vagina. Coitus interruptus has been heavily criticised because sperm can be released before ejaculation has occurred. Coitus interruptus requires some skill, and is said to be associated with a certain amount of psychological distress in one or both partners. However, Potts and Diggory (1983), who have written extensively on the relative merits of different forms of contraception, point out that since coitus interruptus requires no purchases and no intervention from any health professional, it is not possible to make accurate estimations of the number of people who use it, nor of their success.

Sex is a private activity and many people prefer not to discuss it either with health professionals or anyone else. Their privacy must be respected.

Some people may neither want nor expect 100% effective contraception. Despite the message portrayed by the media, a large number of people who enjoy healthy sex lives are neither young nor single but in a stable relationship of long standing, and the arrival of a baby, although not strictly planned, may not be a disaster.

This situation is different for those who, for economic or other reasons, definitely do not want to risk pregnancy. Nevertheless, the condom or sheath, a barrier method (Fig. 17.14), is still one of the most popular methods of contraception because it is cheap and easily obtainable. It requires no medical intervention and gives some protection against sexually transmitted disease. If it is used correctly with a chemical spermicide, it is estimated to be highly effective. Those seeking advice about reliability can be reassured that reputable companies test their products exhaustively.

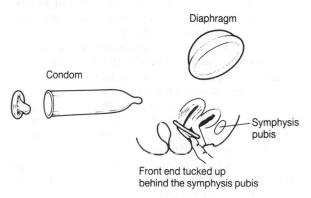

Fig. 17.14 Barrier methods of contraception

The other barrier method in common use is the diaphragm or cap. Several different types are available, but in order to achieve 98–99% safety each must be used with a chemical spermicide. The cap has distinct advantages over the sheath. It can be placed in position over the cervix before intercourse takes place and if properly positioned, it should not be felt by either partner. The chief disadvantage of the cap is that it must be fitted initially by a doctor or nurse, and the woman must be taught how to use it. This demands some skill. The woman must be able to locate and recognise her cervix, and feel confident that the cap is properly in place, otherwise there is a real risk of pregnancy. Some women do not like touching their genitalia.

However, this method is non-invasive, for it

does not involve taking any drugs other than topically applied spermicide, and it does not disturb metabolism in any known way.

The cap gained favour in the 1950s but following the advent of the pill its popularity waned. Nowadays, with the accent on healthy lifestyles and the dangers of repeated drug usage made well-known, many people are showing renewed interest in the cap. Some women are beginning to combine barrier methods with the safe period, using caps or condoms only at times of the month when conception is likely (Renn, 1986).

Oral contraceptives

The role of the pituitary gland and ovaries in the production of hormones was not fully understood until the beginning of this century. It was soon appreciated that if ovulation could be inhibited, conception would be avoided. This did not become a practical possibility until long after the discovery of oestrogen in 1933, for oestrogen and progesterone were not synthesised by biochemists for another decade. Clinical trials of oral contraceptives began in 1956 in Puerto Rico, spurred on by the endeavours of politicians, economists and health professionals to contain the world's rapidly growing population. Much work needed to be done, however, before the female cycle could be properly controlled with doses of oestrogen and progesterone sufficient to prevent conception and bleeding, but low enough to avoid the side effects associated with steroid hormones.

The combined oral contraceptive pill is highly efficient. Providing that it is taken correctly, the failure rate is 1 in 10,000 (usually associated with user error rather than the method). The way in which the combined pill prevents ovulation is shown in Table 17.4.

Failure is a considerable problem for women who have not been taught how to take oral contra-

Table 17.4. *Effects of the combined oral contraceptive pill in preventing conception*

1. Inhibits ovulation (action of oestrogen)
2. Thickens cervical mucus, making it impenetrable by sperm (action of progesterone)
3. Makes the endometrium unreceptive to ova (both hormones)
4. Disrupts transport of sperm along the uterine tubes (both hormones)

ceptives correctly or what to do if they forget to take a pill. Nurses often have to give or reinforce this information.

In recent years there has been growing disenchantment with the combined pill, because of the increasing number of associated side effects. Nurses need to be aware of the problems patients may experience, and the information about the pill made available to the public. Some of this material is heavily biased either in favour of or against the pill (Grant, 1985) so it is difficult for both nurse and client to evaluate the current state of knowledge. A recent review of the literature evaluating possible links between pill-taking and breast, endometrial and ovarian cancers concludes that at present our knowledge is still too incomplete to provide definitive advice for clients (Knowlden, 1990). According to this author, it seems prudent to discourage the use of oral contraceptives merely to regulate menstruation, as has occasionally happened in the past. Pauses in pill-taking could be a sensible precaution when a woman is not sexually active. Some doctors recommend a change of use to another form of contraception after four years or so, but there is no research evidence to suggest whether this is beneficial or how long a break in pill-taking should be. The views of women concerned about pill-taking should be taken into careful consideration, as the anxious individual who suddenly abandons pill-taking without contraceptive advice may soon become pregnant: amenorrhoea following the pill is said to occur frequently and to be a problem among those who wish to conceive, but statistical evidence appears to be lacking.

One possible alternative to the combined pill is the progesterone-only pill, which has to be taken every day at the same time. Ovulation is inhibited in about 40% of cycles. Contraception is achieved mainly because progesterone causes the cervical mucus to become thick, preventing penetration by sperm. The progesterone-only pill has been described as a 'barrier form of contraception taken orally'. Progesterone alone is slightly less effective in preventing pregnancy than if taken with oestrogen, and some women complain of symptoms which mimic those of early pregnancy. Although these may disappear with continued use, menstruation may be erratic, or breakthrough bleeding may occur throughout the cycle. Many of the side effects attributed to the combined pill have not been identified among women taking progesterone, but it is only fair to point out to women requesting this method that less research has so far been conducted (see Guillebaud, 1984) with the progesterone-only pill.

Intra-uterine contraceptive devices (IUCD)

The remaining method of contraception to be described, the IUCD, cannot easily be fitted into any of the categories discussed so far, since it operates by making the endometrium hostile to implantation of a fertilised egg. Interference with endocrine function is not thought to occur, although the number of white blood cells in the uterine lining is known to increase and locally acting prostaglandins may speed up the passage of the egg through the uterine tube, causing it to arrive in the uterus at too early a stage of development for implantation to occur.

Different types of IUCD are available (see Fig. 17.15), but all must be fitted by a doctor, and the threads which will be used to remove the coil when it is changed must be checked from time to time by the user, to ensure that the IUCD remains in the correct position.

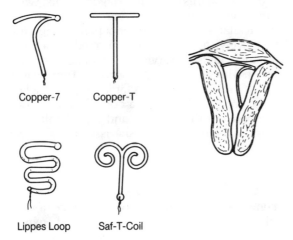

Copper-7   Copper-T

Lippes Loop   Saf-T-Coil

Fig. 17.15 *Types of intra-uterine device*

The IUCD is a safe though not infallible method of contraception, ideal for someone who feels she may forget to take pills or who is unhappy with oral contraceptives. It is effective as soon as it is fitted, and except for checking the position of the threads after each menstrual period and the occasional visit to the clinic to ensure that all is well,

its use involves no other action on the woman's part. Devices incorporating copper or progestogens need to be changed annually. Others can remain *in situ* for years as long as there are no problems.

In the past few years attention has focused on the coil as a possible cause of pelvic pain and heavy periods. At first, these reports tended to be dismissed by doctors and nurses but Potts and Diggory (1983) suggest that the IUCD may cause or aggravate these problems and therefore every opportunity should be given to allow the woman to express her feelings, especially since the IUCD may have been chosen in the absence of any other method perceived as suitable.

Sterilisation

Sterilisation is the ultimate form of contraception. Although both tubal ligation in the female and vasectomy in the male can sometimes be successfully reversed, this depends very much on the individual case and the method of sterilisation originally used by the surgeon. Therefore people requesting sterilisation should be advised to regard it as permanent. This decision should not be taken lightly either by the client, his or her partner, the surgeon who will perform the sterilisation, or the nurse who provides information and counselling. Even so, the number of people in the UK who have been sterilised is rising and very few psychological problems have been reported – provided that sterilisation has been the choice of the individual and not performed after therapeutic abortion.

In the female, the uterine tubes are tied, severed or occluded by slipping a ring round the tube (Fig. 17.16) resulting in immediate sterilisation. A general anaesthetic and an overnight stay in hospital may be necessary, although an increasing number of operations are now performed on a day care basis. This latter situation is possible because a fine fibre-optic instrument called a laparoscope is inserted through a small incision in the abdominal wall and used to visualise the pelvic contents. The laparoscope can also be used in diagnosing the cause of pelvic pain, which may be due to inflammation of the uterine tubes (*salpingitis*) or ectopic pregnancy.

Vasectomy (Fig. 17.17) involves cutting the vasa deferentia so that sperm are prevented from travelling down the urethra. Instead, they are absorbed. Sterilisation is not immediate, and at least three

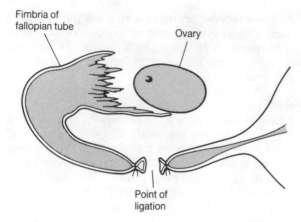

Fig. 17.16 *Female sterilisation*

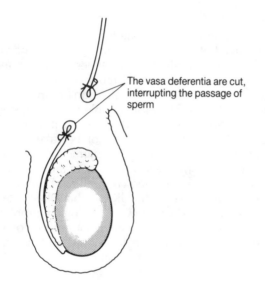

Fig. 17.17 *Male sterilisation (vasectomy)*

negative sperm counts must be obtained before unprotected intercourse can be considered safe.

Family planning: the role of the nurse

Nurses have accepted family planning as an official part of their role since the 1950s, but provision of this service did not become an essential part of the NHS until 1974 – although the demand for safe and effective contraception has been (and still is) increasing. Prevention of unplanned pregnancy is part of normal, everyday life, not a cure for an illness. It seems, therefore, more a nursing responsibility than a medical one, particularly since nursing education is more orientated toward health and the exploration of personal feelings than that of doctors. At the present time, nurses do not prescribe oral contraceptives but those who have received an appropriate training can perform many other procedures (such as fitting vaginal diaphragms) as an extended part of their role. Every woman is an individual and the options available to each will differ. Adequate discussion and time spent exploring feelings can help to avoid an inappropriate decision and much unhappiness. Providing the correct atmosphere and encouraging people to discuss the range of options available to them takes more skill than writing a prescription.

Therapeutic abortion

The decision to end an unplanned or otherwise problematic pregnancy is one of the ethical and moral dilemmas faced by women, with or without the support of partner or family. Today it is possible to detect pregnancy as early as the day on which a period was due, because technology has made available reliable pregnancy testing kits which can detect the first early increase of the hormone human chorionic gonadotrophin (HCG) in the bloodstream at this very early stage. Results, which depend on carefully following instructions, become available within an hour of performing a test. Alternatively, tests can be performed by a GP, a pregnancy advisory service or in some cases by a chemist who advertises the service. The decision made as a result of the test is far less easily reached, and the woman may need a considerable amount of support from her family and from health care professionals, especially if she is young and feels unable to confide in parents.

The Abortion Act

Greenwood and Young (1976), who trace how the original 1967 Abortion Act was passed, explain that it was considered necessary to legalise and make safe the illegal therapeutic abortions which were suspected to take place.

Termination of pregnancy has been performed since time immemorial, often without official approval of the government, medical profession or religious bodies. It could be argued that abortion has always been available to those able and willing to pay, whether for safer private operations or the more questionable services of the 'back street' abortionist. The number of illegal operations actually performed could never be determined, although it is generally considered that women whose pregnancies had been illegally aborted by unskilled hands were at risk of infection (septic abortion) and haemorrhage. Performed in this way, abortion could be fatal.

It was believed that when the Abortion Act (Table 17.5) was passed, the need for illegal operations would disappear, and that the need for legal abortion would not be great. In fact the number of operations taking place every year has increased since 1967, and by no means all of them are performed on young or single women.

Table 17.5. *Conditions of the 1967 Abortion Act*

(1) Allowing pregnancy to continue would involve greater risk to the woman than if pregnancy was terminated
(2) Allowing pregnancy to continue would result in greater risk of physical or emotional damage to the woman than if it was terminated
(3) Allowing pregnancy to continue might risk physical or mental health of existing children
(4) There is a substantial risk that the pregnancy, if not terminated, might result in the birth of a seriously mentally or physically handicapped child

Amendments to the Act were made in 1991 in response to growing concern about late abortions, as it is now possible to keep alive a fetus born at 25–26 weeks gestation, whereas the old Act permitted termination up to 28 weeks. Abortions are now legal up to 24 weeks. In other ways the Act has changed very little.

Therapeutic abortion must be carried out in an NHS hospital or approved premises. About 120,000 take place annually but since 1977 the number of abortions performed under the NHS has declined, with an accompanying increase in the number performed in private clinics, often on a day care basis (OPCS, 1983). The availability of the service under the NHS and the willingness of doctors to make referrals and to perform abortions may be the underlying reasons for this trend. Webb (1985b) describes the unsympathetic attitudes which nurses working on gynaecology wards tend to adopt, and Neustatter and Newson (1986) report how women faced with the prospect of 'shopping around' to find a sympathetic consultant may prefer to pay for private care.

Moral dilemmas

The morality of destroying potential human life by terminating pregnancy has troubled many people for centuries, not least nurses and doctors who may feel that their work is concerned with enhancing the quality of human life, not destroying it. No nurse is compelled to assist in an abortion procedure against her conscience, but she has a duty to participate in treatment needed to save the life of or prevent injury (mental or physical) to a woman who is undergoing abortion. Webb's research study clearly indicated that while many nurses working on gynaecology wards believed that women undergoing abortion needed special understanding, they were unable to give it and, even more worryingly, seemed unable to recognise their failing. Clearly it would be in the best interests of all concerned if nurses involved in caring for women who undergo therapeutic abortion should have chosen to do so, and been given the opportunity to explore their own feelings. Psychological care before and after the procedure is of the upmost importance.

Numerous researchers have set out to document the feelings of women who have had therapeutic abortions. Their conclusions almost certainly reflect the bias of the people who have conducted them, at least to some extent. Few people manage to remain impartial about this emotionally, politically and spiritually charged issue. Undoubtedly many women experience relief when the possibility of an unwanted baby is removed, but relief will not necessarily diminish the grief that they may continue to feel for months or years after the event. Although technically abortion is available in the UK to all those who legally require it, the decision whether or not to terminate a pregnancy cannot be undertaken lightly.

Methods of therapeutic abortion

One of the benefits of legal abortion has been the development of new and increasingly safe methods of terminating pregnancy, providing it is detected early and the operation takes place in the first *trimester*. In private clinics and to a lesser extent in the NHS, early abortions are performed after a local anaesthetic has been injected into the cervix. A fine suction catheter is introduced into the uterine cavity and suction is applied by means of a low power suction pump. After ten weeks

Table 17.6. *Methods used to terminate pregnancy in the first and second trimesters*

1. Suction termination of pregnancy (STOP) up to 13 weeks gestation
2. Dilation and curettage
3. Extra-amniotic instillation of prostaglandin (into the uterus via Foley catheter)
4. Intra-amniotic instillation of prostaglandin (into the amniotic space via a needle inserted through the abdominal wall)
5. Medically induced with prostaglandin-stimulating drugs which induce powerful uterine contractions. RU486 (Mifepristone)

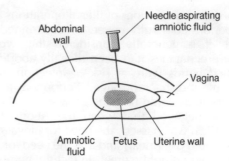

Fig. 17.18 *Amniocentesis*

gestation some dilation of the cervix is necessary so that a slightly wider catheter (12 mm) can be used to aspirate the uterine contents. Methods employed to terminate pregnancy are summarised in Table 17.6.

Late abortions

The number of late therapeutic abortions performed is small compared to first trimester ones, and the patient and her partner require a great deal of psychological support. Often the patient is very young, and has been slow to recognise the symptoms of pregnancy or too frightened to tell anybody. In other cases the abortion may be

performed because fetal abnormality has been detected. *Amniocentesis*, the procedure used to detect abnormality, cannot be attempted until the sixteenth week of gestation. It involves the removal of a small quantity of the fluid surrounding the fetus, through a fine needle inserted into the uterus via the abdominal wall, for laboratory examination (Fig. 17.18). Cells shed from the fetus can be grown in the laboratory and tested for genetic abnormalities and the presence of unusual proteins which accompany some congenital defects. A protein called *alpha-fetoprotein* is associated with spina bifida, for example. Several weeks must pass before the cells have multiplied sufficiently to be examined, therefore pregnancy will be even further advanced before results are available.

A newer technique, chorionic villus biopsy or

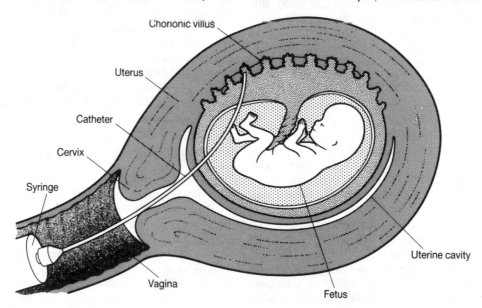

Fig. 17.19 *Chorionic villus biopsy*

sampling (Fig. 17.19), is increasingly being used to detect chromosomal abnormalities, as it can be performed between the eighth and twelfth week of gestation and yields results within 24 hours. Pieces of chorionic villus are obtained for examination. These are derived from the fetus so contain the same genetic make-up and do not have to be grown in culture. Chorionic villus sampling is clearly better than amniocentesis in this respect, but is known to increase risks of miscarriage and may possibly be associated with limb abnormalities according to recent research (Firth *et al.*, 1991). Such tests should not be considered routine until more extensively evaluated.

In the next section we consider further issues concerning rights to decide whether to become a parent.

Infertility

Infertility is defined as difficulty in conceiving a child – perhaps a kinder term would be *subfertility*. The condition can either be primary or secondary. In *primary infertility* the couple have never been able to conceive a child. *Secondary infertility* is said to exist when pregnancy has previously occurred, followed by apparent inability to conceive again. Estimates suggest that about one couple in every six have this problem (Stanway, 1980).

Traditionally, most women expected to marry and have children, to the extent that those who did not were sometimes considered unusual (Dominion, 1956). Views are now slowly changing. As career opportunities improve, some women now choose to remain childless or deliberately postpone childbearing until their late twenties or thirties. Delay may be sufficient to bring problems because fertility is at its peak in the early twenties. Even when an older woman manages to conceive, the pregnancy is more likely to end in miscarriage, possibly because of developmental problems with ageing oocytes, the cells from which ova are derived (Narot *et al.*, 1991).

Considerable unhappiness may be generated by the inability to conceive once a couple decide they would like to start a family. Disappointment is just as keen amongst those who experience secondary infertility, particularly when a couple remarry after divorce. Even though one or both partners may have had children during the previous marriage they may wish to have another baby together. Inability to conceive can put strain on any marriage, and may itself sometimes provide impetus for divorce.

Incidence and causes of infertility

In approximately one third of the couples unable to conceive, the problem lies with the woman. Approximately another third are problems connected with the male partner and among the remainder there will probably be difficulties concerning both. Investigations may begin with the male partner because these are more easily undertaken.

When a couple first seek help for infertility, the doctor will take a thorough medical history before any tests are done. This is because some problems are solved relatively easily. Stanway (1982), in his book designed to help the layperson, explains how some couples, despite their intelligence and apparent sophistication, may have very limited knowledge of reproductive function. Sometimes failure to conceive occurs because the menstrual cycle is unusually long or short, and therefore intercourse is not planned to occur at the optimal time of ovulation. Despite the picture portrayed in the media, interest in sex varies between individuals, and some people go through life happily with their partner, having intercourse only once or twice a month. In other cases the couple may be poorly informed about the mechanisms of sexual intercourse itself. Cases where the female urethra has been enlarged due to penetration are not unknown. Naturally this situation is profoundly embarrassing to the people concerned. Couples are usually seen together by the doctor and often the nurse will be asked afterwards to clarify his explanations. Sometimes information given to the nurse provides a clue to the problem.

Inflammatory conditions involving the pelvic organs can lead to scarring and the delicate fimbriae of the uterine tubes can become blocked, creating a barrier between the sperm and egg. Adhesions following pelvic surgery can have the same effect. Damage can also follow sexually transmitted infections, especially salpingitis caused by *Neisseria gonorrhoeae*, the bacteria causing gonorrhoea, and *Chlamydia trachomatis*.

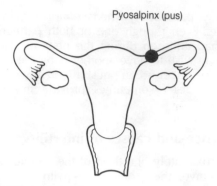

Fig. 17.20 *A pyosalpinx*

Gonorrhoea is an extremely common sexually transmitted infection. Contact tracing of affected partners is of great importance because women often do not realise they have been infected. The bacteria can damage the epithelium of the uterine tubes. Pus may build up, leading to the formation of an abscess, *pyosalpinx* (Fig. 17.20). The patient feels unwell, runs a temperature and is usually admitted to hospital with acute abdominal pain. Diagnosis is by laparoscopy. Antibiotics are needed to destroy the infection, and the patient is usually kept in bed until the inflammation subsides, since rest helps to reduce the inflammatory response and lessens damage. In other cases the woman may not be admitted to hospital, but chronic inflammation may permanently damage the uterine tubes. Damage can be avoided providing the infection is diagnosed and treated effectively soon after onset. A single large dose of penicillin taken orally is effective although there is now some evidence of micro-organisms becoming resistant to penicillin. In this instance, other antibiotics such as atetracycline are used. Health education is important both immediately and in the long term. Sexual intercourse is inadvisable until repeated tests have shown infection to be destroyed.

The risk of developing a sexually transmitted infection increases with the number of partners, and advice may need to be given about the use of condoms as a barrier against infection.

Diagnosis and treatment of infertility

Diagnostic tests can be performed to determine whether the uterine tubes are patent. In the X-ray department, a radio-opaque dye is injected into the vagina and its passage up the genital tract can be visualised on an X-ray screen. If the tubes are patent, dye will spill into the abdominal cavity. This examination is usually performed in the outpatient department. The dye causes the uterine tubes to go into spasm, resulting in considerable pain. It is best for the patient to be collected by a relative or friend and she will need to rest before she feels ready to travel home.

Because this test is unpleasant and invasive, doctors usually prefer to perform a sperm count on the male partner before the woman is investigated. Mobility of the sperm is noted together with the number of dead and damaged cells contained in the ejaculate. Some malformed sperm will always be present, but large numbers of dead, inactive or sluggishly moving sperm suggest subfertility.

Occasionally sperm are inactivated by the secretions of the female genital tract. This is detected by performing a post-coital test. The couple are asked to have intercourse in the morning. The woman attends the clinic as soon as possible afterwards (within three hours) so that some of the secretions withdrawn from the cervix can be examined to detect activity of the sperm.

Other causes of infertility may concern the female endocrine system. Hormone imbalances may interfere with menstruation or prevent ovulation. Anovulatory cycles can be detected by keeping careful records of daily temperature, since the rise in temperature before ovulation will not occur. The nurse can teach the woman how to use temperature charts and thereby involve her in her own care.

Blood tests to measure the levels of female hormones will supplement this information, and treatment with fertility drugs may result in pregnancy.

Benign tumours of the pituitary gland may interfere with hormone production. This is not the most common cause of infertility, but one that nurses must know about since it can be detected readily by skull X-ray.

The oral contraceptive pill has sometimes been implicated in fertility problems. Several months may pass before the cycles return to normal and ovulation occurs, but few women actually need treatment to recommence normal cycles after they have taken the pill.

The nursing response

Nursing patients troubled by fertility problems demands considerable sensitivity combined with interpersonal and educative skills. Some people attend the clinic for months, even years, and occasionally no physical reasons for their difficulty can be found. They benefit from seeing the same nurse, who is sympathetic to their concerns and who can help them to take a realistic view of their chances of achieving pregnancy. A number of myths concerning fertility and fertility treatments are held by the public and the nurse should help dispel these. It is widely believed, for example, that stress reduces the chances of conception, but there is no evidence of this; indeed, women under great stress trying to avoid pregnancy may still conceive. There is also an idea that if a couple can adopt a baby they cease to be so concerned about their own fertility and later tend to conceive. Although occasional reports of this phenomenon exist, it does not often happen. As research progresses and more becomes known about the causes of infertility, it is gradually losing its mystique.

Sexually transmitted disease

As some sexually transmitted diseases can result in reduced fertility, we have already spent some time discussing the nature and damaging consequences of infections such as gonorrhoea and chlamydia. A number of other sexually transmitted diseases exist which, though they do not interfere with fertility in the same way, result in unpleasant symptoms which may significantly reduce quality of life and have, in some cases, other long-lasting side effects.

An infection familiar to a great many women is that caused by yeasts, particularly *Candida* ('thrush') already discussed in relation to the menopause (see Fig. 17.21). There is no doubt that yeasts can be spread from one partner to the other during intercourse, but also some evidence that non-sexual spread can occur via fomites (objects which transfer infection) such as the contraceptive vaginal sponge (see Rashid *et al.*, 1990). Again it is women rather than men who usually develop symptoms. For women this takes the form of an irritant, thick white discharge, though less typically a thin, scalding fluid discharge may result. The social and economic consequences of *Candida* should not be underestimated as the itching and

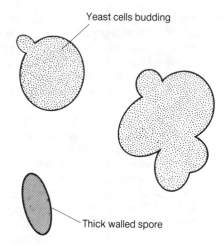

Fig. 17.21 *Candida albicans*

discomfort may be sufficient to disrupt work as well as sleep and social activities. Some women appear to be prone to recurrent attacks of *Candida*, but the underlying reason has never been found. Oral contraceptives and being a diabetic are often blamed, but a review of the literature (Rashid *et al.*, 1990) failed to find any real evidence in support of this. Poor hygiene, though often implicated, does not appear to be a significant causative factor either and there is no real evidence that underclothing operates as a reservoir of infection despite harbouring spores. Cotton underwear is certainly more cool and comfortable for sufferers, but disinfectant soaks and boiling do not appear to help. Long term victims of *Candida* need sympathetic understanding and encouragement to persevere with treatment, which can be depressing as it involves the use of fungicidal creams and pessaries which to many women are messy and unaesthetic.

A second infection to which women fall victim, but which seldom causes symptoms in men though they may carry it, is the flagellate protozoan *Trichomonas vaginalis*. Women complain of a most offensive discharge which may be treated with metronidazole. Again treatment is unpopular as the course must be completed and infection resolved before intercourse is recommended. Metronidazole should not be taken in combination with alcohol and this should be impressed on the woman, as fits have been reported.

Genital herpes causes repeated attacks of painful blisters and there is thought to be a possible association between the virus responsible and increased risk of developing cervical carcinoma. As in the case of many virus infections, cure is not possible, although use of topical agents, such as acyclovir, applied as soon as blisters appear may help reduce the severity of an attack. Herpes is infectious only when virus particles are shed from the surface of moist lesions, so women can be reassured that between attacks they are unlikely to infect their partner. Other self-help measures include promotion of a healthy lifestyle as attacks tend to occur when the individual is generally 'run down' and the immune system is compromised.

Like the herpes virus, the papilloma virus responsible for genital warts is also associated with increasing risks of developing cervical carcinoma. Warts are transmissible, but as they have a long incubation period (several months) it is not always possible to determine when or how infection occurred. They may be removed chemically by topical application of agents such as podophyllin or trichloroacetic acid, but motivation is required as treatment can take weeks and may be painful. Warts developing on the cervix itself may not be visible and the woman may not suspect that she is infected.

Women who have a history of genital herpes or warts are currently recommended to have cervical smears performed annually (see page 467).

Treating sexually transmitted diseases

Women who have developed a sexually transmitted infection require treatment promptly to avoid damaging side effects and also for their own peace of mind, but the setting in which treatment is available is open to choice. Some women prefer to visit their own GP, others may ask for advice at a family planning clinic or may be referred to a gynaecologist. However, the most efficient and comprehensive service is offered by a department of genito-urinary medicine (special clinic) where nurses and doctors receive training to cope with the emotional and social as well as the physical needs of people who have developed a sexually transmitted infection. Diagnosis can usually be made at the first visit and treatment can begin immediately. The entire service is confidential and clinics are organised with the needs of busy, otherwise healthy working people in mind, often open until late in the evening so there is no embarrassment about taking time off work. There is evidence that the great majority of people who attend such a clinic are highly satisfied with its services and are particularly grateful for confidentiality (Munday, 1990).

Carcinoma of the cervix and cervical screening

There has been great concern in recent years about the apparent increase in carcinoma of the cervix, especially in very young women. Some people have blamed this on increasing promiscuity and widespread use of oral contraceptives. Evidence (Lewis and Chamberlain, 1990) suggests that an infective agent may be at least partly to blame, for the risk of developing the disease appears to be related to having sexual intercourse with a large number of different partners and having the first experience of intercourse at an early age. Carcinoma of the cervix is exceptionally rare among women who are celibate (for example, nuns) and among those practising the Jewish faith, where males are circumcised. It has been suggested that some infective agent, probably a virus, may be transferred from male to female during intercourse. Large epidemiological studies (see Knowlden, 1990) have variously implicated the pill as a predisposing factor, or ruled it out, and the research evidence is mixed.

All these factors are important for health professionals who need to be aware of the information acquired by anxious women from the media, but a sense of proportion must be kept. Not every woman who has taken the pill or had multiple sexual partners will be at risk, nor will every woman succumb from exposure to a particular chemical or infective agent; much will depend upon the state of her immune system at that particular time. It would certainly be wrong to label every patient with carcinoma of the cervix as promiscuous.

Cervical screening

One of the reasons for the apparent increase in the number of women diagnosed as having carcinoma of the cervix is advance in technology, making early detection possible. In Scandinavia and the Netherlands, rigorous screening of the population has led to very successful early treatment. In Britain the picture is not so bright, because the women who take advantage of the service tend to be middle class, while those shown to be at greatest risk, belonging to social classes IV and V, tend not to respond to health education campaigns.

As part of their role as health educators, nurses need to encourage women to come forward for screening at regular intervals. They should also be able to reassure women that the test is quick and painless, with results becoming available within a few weeks. The equipment used to perform the Papanicolaou cervical smear test is shown in Fig. 17.22. A Cuscoe's speculum is used to separate the walls of the vagina, thus making the cervix visible, and a wooden spatula is used to scrape cells gently from the cervix and transfer them to a microscope slide. Prepared slides are then stored in a special fixative solution until they can be examined by a hospital laboratory technician. Some doctors do not tell patients routinely about test results unless they are abnormal, but this can cause needless worry unless women are warned in advance. It is also important to impress upon women that early premalignant changes (see Table 17.7) may revert to normal without further intervention, although careful monitoring of the situation is considered good medical practice.

Microscope specimens can easily become damaged, making repeat tests necessary, or abnormality may be due to a minor infection such as *Candida* which is easily treated. Whatever the reason for a repeat test, the nurse contacting the

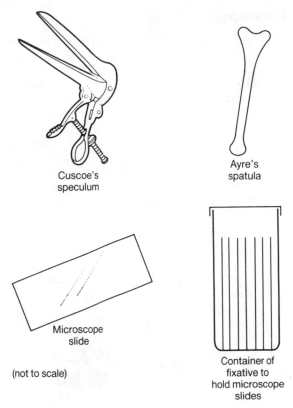

Cuscoe's speculum

Ayre's spatula

Microscope slide

(not to scale)

Container of fixative to hold microscope slides

Fig. 17.22 *Equipment needed for a Papanicolaou smear test*

woman should explain why it is necessary so as to avoid causing undue anxiety.

Table 17.7. *The cervical intra-epithelial neoplasia (CIN) staging system and the clinical staging for cervical carcinoma CIN system (premalignant)*

Stage	Histological change	Treatment	
CIN I	Mild dysplasia (reversible)	Laser	
CIN II	Moderate dysplasia	Laser	Completely curable
CIN III	Severe dysplasia grading into overt early malignancy, not yet invasive	Laser/cone biopsy	

Stage	Clinical staging malignant	Treatment	Five year survival value
0	Malignancy not yet invasive	Cone biopsy	Curable
1	Limited to cervix		81%
2	Spread to upper third of vagina/lower part of uterus	Wertheim's hysterectomy	60%
3	Involvement of parametrium	Radiotherapy	30%
4	Infiltration of bladder/rectum/distant metastases	Sometimes with palliative surgery	8%

Colposcopy

Early malignant lesions of the cervix can be investigated by colposcopy. A **colposcope** is used to visualise and magnify the cervix, and areas of abnormal cells can be removed by laser treatment or cryotherapy (destruction of the cells by intense cold). Careful assessment of patients is necessary before treatment, because though outpatient treatment is possible, those who are unduly nervous may feel happier having a general anaesthetic, especially if any lesions are present on the vulva. If the lesions have begun to invade the cervix, admission to hospital is necessary because removal will involve a cone biopsy (Fig. 17.23). More extensive growths will require radical surgery, followed by chemotherapy or radiotherapy.

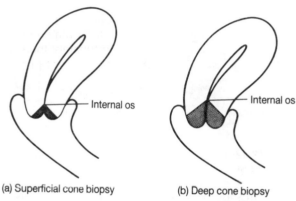

(a) Superficial cone biopsy   (b) Deep cone biopsy

Fig. 17.23 *Cone biopsy*

Breast screening

Cancer of the breast is the most common malignancy affecting women in Western society, and one of the most common causes of death (Gould, 1990; Gillies, 1988). One woman in 14 can be expected to develop carcinoma of the breast in Britain today, and many of them will ultimately die of their disease. However, the vast majority of lumps do not turn out to be malignant. Health educationalists are keen for women to report abnormalities as soon as they have detected them. Early diagnosis is the key to effective treatment and those women who, on examination, turn out not to have cancer at all could be spared much worry.

The aetiology of breast cancer remains obscure, although it has been linked with a Western diet high in saturated fat, and the practice among women in developed societies to delay their first pregnancy and to discontinue breastfeeding early – if indeed they ever try to breastfeed at all. The use of the oral contraceptive pill certainly appears to decrease benign breast disease, but the same cannot be said of cancer itself, since malignancy of the breast appears to depend on oestrogens for growth. Evidence that the pill actually promotes breast cancer is confused at the present time, but the incidence is higher in obese women and it is known that adipose tissue produces one of the hormones belonging to the oestrogen family.

Views about breast screening are changing. Stanway, writing for the general public in 1982, argued that breast screening was really not worth the high cost that would be involved, given that many women never develop the disease anyway, and that the necessary monthly examinations may well cause a lot of worry and 'false alarms' among women whose attempts at self-examination are inexpert. More recently, cancer specialists in the USA and Scandinavia have reported that national screening programmes and early detection can help to reduce mortality associated with breast cancer, and that women should be encouraged to attend for regular examination. In the UK women under 50 may not receive mammography routinely.

Treatment for breast cancer has long had a bad press, because it traditionally took the form of a mutilating radical mastectomy, which involved removing not only all breast tissue but the underlying muscle and lymph ducts as well. Apparently, this did not always prevent spread and later recurrence of the disease – probably because once an appreciable number of cells had lodged in the axillary lymph nodes, smaller clumps had probably managed to travel even further.

The new approach, which involves removing a minimum amount of tissue followed by carefully controlled doses of radiotherapy, is not only less disfiguring but seems a good deal more effective in halting spread of the disease for an appreciable number of years. Recent evidence suggests that if surgery is performed before day 3 of the menstrual cycle or after day 12 when there is either low secretion of oestrogen or when oestrogen and progesterone are secreted together, prognosis is considerably improved (Badwe *et al.*, 1991). Although these findings are tentative, some surgeons are changing their practice.

Whatever approach to treatment is selected, the emphasis today is on improving the quality of life of the individual woman. Although more breast cancers are identified in young women today, the majority still occur in the older age groups when all tissues, including malignant ones, grow slowly. Such women may live for many years, ultimately dying of an unrelated disease.

In view of these findings it seems sensible to encourage women to get to know the appearance of their breasts and their texture, so that abnormalities can be detected and reported early. Self-examination is best performed after menstruation when the glandular tissue is least active, and does not feel lumpy. Lesions can best be detected if the woman feels each breast systematically in turn using the pads of the fingers, which are the most sensitive, and working in a circular motion until all the tissue has been palpated (Fig. 17.24). Suspicious lumps can be examined in more detail by X-ray mammography and xeroradiography, which are non-invasive and painless techniques.

Nurses working both in hospital and the community can do much to help their patients, by teaching them how to examine their own breasts and by pointing out that although still a serious and by no means uncommon disease, breast cancer need not inspire the fear with which it was once associated.

Hormone replacement therapy

The decision of whether or not to take hormone replacement therapy (HRT) faces women as they approach the end of their reproductive years. It is of advantage in the short term because it may help reduce uncomfortable menopausal symptoms such as hot flushes and in the longer term may reduce the effects of osteoporosis. Unfortunately there is a certain amount of evidence to suggest that HRT may be associated with increased risk of de-

---

The breasts are best examined after menstruation when they are least likely to be affected by hormonal fluctuations

(1) Start the examination in the bath or shower, as the hands glide most easily over the skin when it is wet. Use the undersides of the fingers – they are the most sensitive. Move them gently over every part of the breast, checking for any hard lumps or irregularities. Use the right hand for the left breast

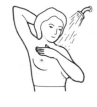

(2) Much information can be gained just by looking. Inspect your breasts with your arms by your sides. Next raise your arms above your head and look for any changes in the contour of each breast, especially swellings, nipple changes or dimpling (when the skin takes the appearance of orange peel). Breasts are rarely symmetrical or the same size

a
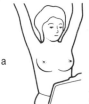
b
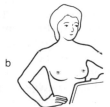

(3) Lying down with a pillow beneath the shoulder, explore each breast with the tips of the fingers in a circular motion. It is important to develop a system so that no part of the breast escapes examination. Finally, squeeze the nipple gently between index finger and thumb – discharge is abnormal except during lactation

a
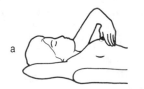
b
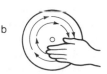
c
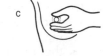

Remember that most lumps turn out to be non-malignant

Fig. 17.24 *How to examine your breasts*

veloping endometrial cancer (Knowlden, 1990) and as with issues such as contraception and abortion, nurses need to be aware of the options open to their patients and their possible side effects so that each woman can make an informed choice about the treatment she agrees to have. HRT may clear up troublesome symptoms, but it is not an elixir of youth and anyone allowed to believe otherwise is likely to be disappointed. Women who choose this option can be reassured that side effects are reduced by using natural hormones, not synthetic ones as in oral contraceptives, and that by taking tablets three weeks in every four they reduce the amount of hormones actually taken. Withdrawal bleeding occurs during each weekly break in pill-taking, but is not true menstruation though sufficient to require sanitary protection. Pregnancy is not possible.

Female urinary incontinence

Urinary incontinence is a problem that often presents in middle life, especially among women who have had several children and difficult deliveries, because damage can occur to the supporting muscles of the pelvic floor. Figure 17.25 shows how these muscles support the pelvic organs like a hammock. The strength of the pelvic muscles is naturally reduced because they are perforated by the urethra and anus. In females, the vagina further weakens the pelvic supports. Straining the abdominal muscles by coughing or becoming overweight brings added problems. As the pelvic supports weaken, the uterus sags down into the vagina, and incontinence occurs because the wall of the uterus bulges against the bladder (*cystocele*). The close anatomical relationship between the uterus, vagina and bladder is shown in Fig. 17.26. The bladder may not be able to empty properly, so infection develops. Running, laughing or coughing causes urine to be passed involuntarily. This is called stress incontinence. Added to this there may be backache and an uncomfortable sensation that 'something inside' is displaced downwards. Sometimes the prolapsing uterus pushes against the rectum (*rectocele*) causing pain and discomfort on defaecation.

Unless medical advice is sought, symptoms are likely to become worse. Going out can become a

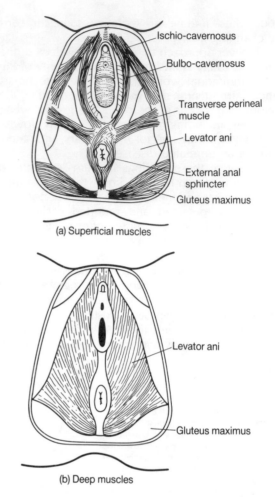

(a) Superficial muscles

(b) Deep muscles

Fig. 17.25 *Muscles of the pelvic floor*

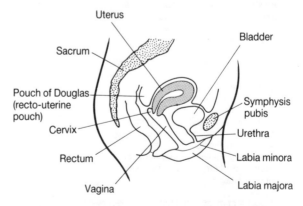

Fig. 17.26 *Section through the pelvis showing the female reproductive organs*

nightmare, with fears of soiling clothes and furnishings. Some women resort to sanitary protection. Prevention should begin during antenatal care, when women are taught pelvic floor exercises, and they should be encouraged to continue these after childbirth. Women should be taught how to lift heavy objects correctly, and if their jobs entail heavy manual work the occupational health nurse can provide advice.

Investigating urinary incontinence

When a woman complains of urinary incontinence the precise cause must be established so that effective treatment can be provided. The nurse's role is to support her patient during a series of uncomfortable and often embarrassing investigations. As well as taking a general medical and obstetric history, the doctor will perform vaginal and rectal examinations to find out if the uterus is descending. Other causes of incontinence do exist, so examinations may also take place in the Department of Urodynamics to determine the capacity of the bladder before there is desire to empty it, and whether filling and emptying take place normally. This is likely to be most distressing for the patient, since she may be required to pass urine in front of several other people, in an unnatural or uncomfortable position, for example in front of an X-ray screen. She will need the nurse to explain exactly what will happen before the day of the investigation and to comfort her afterwards.

Conclusions

This chapter has focused on the care of women in hospital and the community. It is important that nurses who work in the hospital setting do not forget that ill health or health problems begin in the community, and that it is to the community that a woman will return, perhaps to other worries, when her hospital treatment is over. Many health problems today are avoidable, and nurses can do much to provide information about health-related issues wherever they encounter female patients or clients. Those who work on gynaecology wards have a special responsibility to ensure that women know what to expect during longer term recovery at home, and are prepared for any difficulties they may meet.

We have shown that, today, women's wellbeing does not revolve entirely around such issues as menstruation, but the cyclical, hormone-dependent changes associated with reproductive functioning have wide implications not only for health, but for social and family life.

Glossary

Abortion: Expulsion of the products of conception from the uterus before the 28th week of pregnancy. It may be performed therapeutically or occur spontaneously

Adhesions: Scar tissue that results from inflammation, either as a result of infection or surgical intervention, and which may cause dysfunction as the damaged tissues stick together

Cervical os: Opening in the cervix permitting direct communication between the vagina and uterine cavity

Cervix: Narrow, lower part of the uterus projecting down into the vagina

Colposcope: Low power binocular microscope used to examine the cervix

Endometrium: Lining of the uterus, shed every month during menstruation

Fibroids: Benign fibrous tumours of the uterine wall (more correctly called *fibromyoma*)

Human chorionic gonadotrophin (HCG): Hormone released from the placenta during pregnancy. Detection in the urine forms the basis of modern pregnancy tests

Laparoscope: Telescopic fibre-optic instrument used to view the contents of the pelvic cavity

Menopause: The last menstrual period. A series of physiological changes in middle age results in the cessation of menstrual periods

Pyosalpinx: Collection of pus in the uterine tube, forming an abcess

Shirodkar suture: A suture drawn around the cervix like a purse string in order to prevent miscarriage due to incompetent cervix

Trimester: First, second or third three months of pregnancy

References

Arber, S. (1990). Revealing women's health; re-analysing the General Household Survey. In *Women's Health Counts*, Roberts, H. (ed.). Routledge, London.

Badwe, R.A., Gregory, W.M. and Chandry, M.A. (1991). Timing of surgery during the menstrual cycle and survival of pre-menopausal women with operable breast cancer. *Lancet*, 337, 1261–1262.

Beard, M. (1984). *Understanding Pre-menstrual Tension*. Pan Books, London.

Billings, A. and Westland, A. (1980). *Natural Family Planning*. Allen Lane, London.

Bott, E. (1968). *Kinship and Network*. Tavistock Publications, London.

Bowlby, J. (1947). *Childcare and the Growth of Love*. Penguin Books, Harmondsworth.

Brown, G.W. and Harris, T. (1978). *The Social Origins of Depression*. Tavistock Publications, London.

Dalton, K. (1971). *The Menstrual Cycle* (2nd ed.). Pantheon, New York.

Di Nitto, D. (1986). After rape: who should examine rape survivors? *American Journal of Nursing*, 86(5), 538–540.

Dominion, J. (1956). *Marital Breakdown*. Penguin Books, Harmondsworth.

English, D. and Ehrenreich, B. (1973). *Complaints and Disorders*. The Feminist Press, New York.

Firth, H.V., Boyd, P.A. and Chamberlain, P. (1991). Severe limb abnormalities after chorionic villus sampling at 56–66 days gestation. *Lancet*, 337, 762–763.

Foley, T.S. (1979). Counselling the victim of rape. In *Principles and Practice of Psychiatric Nursing*, Stuart, G.W. and Sundeen, S.J. (eds.). Mosby, St Louis.

Gath, D.M. (1980). Psychiatric aspects of hysterectomy. In *The Social Consequences of Psychiatric Illness*, Robins, L. (ed.). Brunner-Mazel, New York.

Gillies, C. (1988). The epidemiology of human cancer. In *Oncology for Nurses and Health Care Professionals* (2nd ed.), Tiffany, R. (ed.). Harper and Row, London.

Gould, D.J. (1982). Recovery from hysterectomy. *Nursing Times*, 78(42), 1769–1771.

Gould, D.J. (1985a). Understanding emotional need. *Nursing Mirror*, 160(1), Research Forum, 2–5.

Gould, D.J. (1985b). The myth of the menopause. *Nursing Mirror*, 160(23), 25–27.

Gould, D. (1990). *Nursing Care of Women*. Prentice Hall, London.

Graham, H. (1984). *Women, Health and the Family*. Wheatsheaf Books, Brighton.

Graham, H. (1990). Behaving well: women's behaviour in context. In *Women's Health Counts*, Roberts, H. (ed.). Routledge, London.

Grant, E. (1985). *The Bitter Pill*. Corgi Books, London.

Greenwood, V. and Young, J. (1976). *Abortion on Demand*. Pluto Press, London.

Guillebaud, J. (1984). *The Pill*. Oxford University Press, Oxford.

HMSO. (1976). *Sexual Offences (Amendment) Act*. HMSO, London.

Kirpatrick, M.K., Brewer, J.A. and Stocks, B. (1990). Efficacy of self-care measures for perimenstrual syndrome (PMS). *Journal of Advanced Nursing*, 15, 281–285.

Knowlden, H.A. (1990). The pill and cancer: a review of the literature. A case of swings and roundabouts? *Journal of Advanced Nursing*, 15, 1016–1020.

Lancet. (1981). Editorial: Premenstrual syndrome: a disease of the mind? *Lancet*, 2, 1238–1240.

Lewis, T.L.T. and Chamberlain, G.V.P. (1990). *Gynaecology by Ten Teachers* (15th ed.). Edward Arnold, London.

Lodge, D. (1983). *The British Museum is Falling Down*. Penguin Books, Harmondsworth.

Macafee, J.C.A. (1984). Ectopic pregnancy. In *Contemporary Gynaecology*, Chamberlain, G. (ed.). Butterworths, London.

Moore, J. (1985). Rape and the double victim. *Nursing Times*, 81(19), 24–25.

Munday, P.E. (1990). Genitourinary medicine services: consumers' views. *Genitourinary Medicine*, 66, 108–111.

Narot, D., Bergh, P.A. and Williams, M.A. (1991). Poor oocyte quality rather than implantation failure as a cause of age-related decline in female fertility. *Lancet*, 337, 1375–1377.

Neustatter, A. and Newson, G. (1986). *Mixed Feelings: The Experience of Abortion*. Pluto Press, London.

Nolan, J. (1986). Developmental concerns and the health of mid-life women. *Nursing Clinics of North America*, 21(1), 155–165.

Oakley, A. (1984). *Miscarriage*. Fontana, London.

Oakley, A. (1985). Social support in pregnancy: the 'soft way' to increase birthweight? *Social Science and Medicine*, 21(11), 1259–1268.

Oakley, A., Rajan, L. and Grant, A. (1990). *Social Support and Pregnancy Outcome*. Report from the Thomas Coram Research Unit, University of London.

Office of Population Censuses and Surveys. (1983). *Abortion Monitor*. HMSO, London.

Orr, J. (1984). Violence against women. *Nursing Times*, 80(17), 34–36.

Paykel, E. and Weisman, M. (1974). *The Depressed Woman: A Study of Social Relationships*. University of Chicago Press, Chicago.

Potts, M. and Diggory, P. (1983). *Textbook of Contraceptive Practice*. Cambridge University Press, Cambridge.

Rappaport, D. and Rappaport, S. (1975). *Dual Career Families*. Penguin Books, Harmondsworth.

Rashid, S., Collins, M. and Kennedy, R.J. (1990). A

study of candidosis: the role of fomites. *Genitourinary Medicine*, 66, 137–142.

Renn, M. (1986). If the cap fits. *Nursing Times*, 82(4), 22–27.

Roper, N., Logan W.W. and Tierney, A.J. (1985). *The Elements of Nursing* (2nd ed.). Churchill Livingstone, Edinburgh.

Rutter, M. (1987). *Maternal Deprivation Reassessed* (2nd ed.). Penguin, Harmondsworth.

Sharpe, S. (1984). *Double Identity: The Lives of Working Mothers*. Penguin Books, Harmondsworth.

Shorter, E. (1984). *A History of Women's Bodies*. Pelican Books, Harmondsworth.

Stanway, A. (1980). *Why Us? Infertility*. Granada, London.

Stanway, A. (1982). *Alternative Medicine*. Penguin Books, Harmondsworth.

Webb, C. (1983). Hysterectomy – dispelling the myths. *Nursing Times* Occasional Papers. Paper 1, 79(47), 52–54. Paper 2, 79(47), 44–46.

Webb, C. (1985a). *Sexuality, Nursing and Health*. John Wiley and Sons, Chichester.

Webb, C. (1985b). Barriers to sympathy. *Nursing Mirror*, 160(1), Research Forum 5–7.

Suggestions for further reading

Broadley, F. (1986). Cervical cancer. *Nursing Times*, 82(24), 29–30.

Department of Health and Social Security. (1987). *Breast Cancer Screening*. (The Forrest Report). HMSO, London.

Gould, D. (1989). *Care of Women: A Gynaecological Perspective*. Prentice Hall, Hemel Hempstead.

Hull, M.G.R. (1985). Population study of the causes, treatment and outcome of infertility. *British Medical Journal*, 2, 1693–1697.

Oliver, G. (1989). Gynaecological tumours. In *Nursing the Patient with Cancer*, Tschudin, V. (ed.) Prentice Hall, Hemel Hempstead.

Thomson, L. (1989). Breast cancer. In *Nursing the Patient with Cancer*, Tschudin, V. (ed.) Prentice Hall, Hemel Hempstead.

Westrom, L. (1981). Incidence, trends and risks of ectopic pregnancy in a population of women. *British Medical Journal*, 1, 15–18.

Yule, R. (1984). Cervical cancer – screening and prevention. *Nursing Mirror*, 159(13), 37–39.

Webb, C. (1986). *Using Nursing Models: Women's Health*. Hodder and Stoughton, Sevenoaks.

Books to be recommended to women and their partners

Health Education Authority. (1991). *Thrush: A Self Help Guide*. HEA, London.

Last, P. and Rushton, A. (1990). *Women's Health Questions Answered*. Thorsons, London.

Mosse, J. and Heaton, J. (1990). *The Fertility and Contraception Book*. Faber and Faber, London.

Useful addresses

Endometriosis Society
65 Holmedene Avenue, London SE24. Tel. 081-737 4764

Hysterectomy Support Group
C/o Anne Webb, 11 Henryson Road, Brockley, London SE4 1HL. Tel. 081-690 5987

Miscarriage Association
18 Stoneybrook Close, West Bretun, Wakefield, West Yorkshire, WF4 4TP. Tel. 0924 885515

National Association for the Childless
318 Summer Lane, Birmingham, B19 3RL. Tel. 021-359 4887

National Osteoporosis Society
P.O. Box 10, Barton Meade House, Radstock, Avon BA3 3JB

Women's Health Concern
P.O. Box 1629, London SW19 3LP.

Womens' Reproductive Rights Information Centre
52/54 Featherstone Street, London EC1

The address and phone number of your local **Rape Crisis Centre** should be given in the area telephone directory

18

MATERNITY CARE

Anne Thompson

The aim of this chapter is to provide the reader with 'building blocks' for the study and care of women undergoing the experience of childbearing. From pre-conception through pregnancy and delivery, the emphasis is on childbirth as a normal life event in which the mother is helped to take an active part.

The chapter includes the following topics:

- Childbearing – social aspects
- The maternity care experience
- The setting for childbearing
- The changing face of maternity care
- Alternatives in care – choice
- The carers – team midwifery
- Preparation for childbearing
- The childbearing woman
- Pregnancy
- Antenatal care
- Lifestyle in pregnancy
- Preparation for labour and parenthood

- Mothers with special needs in pregnancy
- Labour and delivery
- Care in labour
- Delivery
- Emergency delivery
- Postnatal care
- The baby
- Infant feeding
- Babies born too soon, too small, unwell
- When pregnancy fails

Some 700,000 babies are born in England and Wales each year. Yet each birth is a unique event. Few other moments have quite so much power to alter the pattern of people's lives.

Childbearing: the social aspects

The arrival of a new baby – especially if it is the first one – changes the web of relationships in which its mother and father have lived until then. Whatever the situation a baby is born into, the long processes of childbearing and childrearing are likely to have considerable impact on the physical, emotional and social life of the mother. Whether she is married or single her lifestyle is inevitably going to be altered, often from well before the birth.

The enormous development of the maternity services in this century reflects society's awareness of the special provisions which have to be made to ensure that mothers and babies get the best possible start in their life together. It may be a truism to reflect that each new baby is an assurance of the continuity of human life. Nonetheless, each new generation has a deep symbolic and cultural meaning for its own family and for society. Any future depends on them. The seeds of that future are nurtured by the special protection which family and state offer the pregnant woman and her newborn child, however minimal that protection may sometimes be.

With this in mind the student will understand why the knowledge of the behavioural sciences outlined elsewhere in this book is as relevant to the provision of good maternity care as is a grasp of the physiological changes brought about by pregnancy. The psychological, sociological and interpersonal aspects of care are implicit throughout this chapter as it describes the processes involved in childbearing. Some insight into human interaction in terms of role theory, communication and self-perception will help the student understand patterns of behaviour she might otherwise overlook as unimportant. Too easily, maternal mood swings and anxiety are explained away with 'that's what pregnancy does to them', when often what women are trying to express is closely linked to a new awareness of their changing, and sometimes frightening, responsibilities (Macintyre, 1984).

The maternity care course

This chapter is designed to provide a basis for students undertaking the statutory experience in maternity care and care of the newborn. It could well serve as an introduction to their new careers for pre-registration (direct entry) students as well. A chapter in a general text such as this can only attempt to provide the essential elements of a many-faceted subject. It will be successful in so far that the student uses these 'building blocks' as points of departure for her own study and reflection. The references and suggestions for further reading at the end of the chapter should help further exploration of the subject.

The chapter itself will continue with a description of the setting for childbearing and the types of care available for the pregnant mother. The anatomy and physiology relevant to childbearing will appear throughout the text related to the processes of pregnancy, labour, delivery and the **puerperium**. The care appropriate to each stage is described, with special stress on childbearing as a normal life event in which the mother is helped to take the most active part possible.

Experience in maternity care and care of the newborn

This part of the student's training is intended to offer some experience of the needs of childbearing women and their babies. The course aims to develop the perception of childbirth as a natural and normal event, while providing some understanding of those occasions when something goes wrong.

Courses vary widely in length and content, and each college of nursing and midwifery will have its own objectives for this part of training. During the weeks spent on the maternity unit, students will normally gain experience of the whole range of care provided by the local maternity services, from the booking clinic at the beginning of pregnancy to the return home of a mother and her baby after delivery. Where possible, time is spent with the community midwife and there may be a visit to a Special Care Baby Unit too.

Students sometimes take a little time to adjust to the rhythm and special requirements of a service where people are not sick. Most find, however, that the presence of the babies makes a fine topic of conversation in the early days when they are gaining confidence. Students soon develop the listening and observation skills which are so important in a unit where young parents are learning to care for their babies. The art of encouraging mothers to become independent and skilful in the care of their babies is learned from the permanent members of the maternity unit staff, and students often discover that mothers will ask them questions that they will not 'bother' other members of staff with.

The setting for childbearing

Even a short time spent in a maternity unit will familiarise the student with the wide variety of family patterns into which babies are born.

Family structures

With a national trend towards young marriages, a steady increase in single parent families and a one in three divorce rate (Ermisch, 1990), the complexity of family structures also increases. Second or third marriages are common and these may have children from either or both previous marriages in addition to the new baby. The first baby of a new marriage is often the occasion of considerable tension and anxiety, however much it is desired, and there may well be a long gap between a woman's 'first' and 'second' family. A gap of 24 years was recently claimed by an improbably young-looking mother of forty. Learning to mother a small baby again after so many years, to 'make space' for it in well-established lives, can be difficult when childbearing has been deferred for whatever reason.

Sensitivity is needed to recognise the needs of the very young as well as the much older mothers. Both are likely to suffer from lack of confidence which neither will want to admit. Well-timed, tactful support can stop lack of confidence degenerating into depression.

Fathers and partners

Fathers' and partners' presence and support at all stages of pregnancy and childbirth is so common now that it is easy to forget that not all take spontaneously to the role that is thrust upon them by modern maternity practice. Cultural or ethnic tradition may make it either difficult or inappropriate for them to share the experience of delivery. It is important to recognise and respect this, while ensuring alternative support for the mother.

Where fathers or partners do wish to take part, it is important that they are positively welcomed, whether in antenatal clinic, parentcraft classes or the delivery suite. They too need to learn what to expect, as well as what is expected of them. Couples who share the preparation of their baby's arrival in this way frequently find their relationship strengthened. Where the father has been well prepared and is able actively to care for his partner during labour, he stops being a helpless onlooker

and has, instead, his own sense of achievement, a real share in their great event (Jackson, 1984).

Siblings

Brothers and sisters of the new baby find their established world badly jolted, and as a result often show their anxiety by aggressive behaviour or reverting to babyhood practices. A stay in hospital for their mother only adds separation to their miseries.

The new baby's arrival needs to be discussed and planned for well ahead of the event with the other children. Meeting the baby for the first time can be magical or awful – much depends on the age of the sibling as well as the preparation – and it can be one of the most fascinating moments a student may observe.

Ethnic groups

Nursing in almost any of Britain's big cities will bring the student in contact with people of widely differing racial, cultural, ethnic and religious backgrounds. Because of the deep social significance of the birth of a baby, the maternity staff in any area need to familiarise themselves with the beliefs and customs which prevail among the population they serve.

Women from ethnic minority groups may well receive poorer than average care simply because of problems of communication and lack of knowledge on the part of the staff. A number of studies have highlighted these problems and the *Asian mother and baby campaign* is one example of a project designed to improve women's experience of pregnancy and childbirth by educating the staff about special needs and providing link workers to improve communications (Ahmed and Watt, 1986).

The changing face of maternity care

Forty years ago, more than half of all deliveries in this country still took place at home. When birth happened in hospital the father was rarely present and the midwife conducted the labour and delivery unless there was some complication.

The picture is very different now. Some 99% of all deliveries take place in hospital, where electronic monitoring and medical surveillance are the norm in most cases. Fathers, or other companions, are normally welcome partners in the care of the woman in labour and they may remain present even throughout forceps deliveries and caesarean sections. The midwife is still the senior member of staff present at some 78% of deliveries (Robinson, Golden and Bradley, 1983), but she works in very close liaison with the specialist obstetric team.

These facts mark a dual shift in the traditional pattern of care. The first is towards much closer monitoring of every stage of pregnancy, labour and delivery, with consequently more frequent medical intervention. The second shift is towards the 'humanisation' of maternity care, particularly in the delivery suite, with a conscious effort being made to offer the parents more choice in the care they receive.

The father's presence at delivery was a turning point in the style of care offered in childbirth. Since then the work of obstetricians such as Frederick Leboyer and Michel Odent has provided an impetus towards the creation of a less clinical, more empathetic environment for birth. In the mid 1970s, midwives all over the country dreamed up schemes for transforming delivery suites which looked like operating theatres into something a little more homelike.

For many women labour is their first experience of hospital and may be closely associated with ideas of pain and death, absorbed from family life and the media. The introduction of familiar furnishings – comfortable chairs, pictures, plants and even carpets – may have seemed irrelevant and superficial to some, but it represented a serious concern to create a less threatening atmosphere for birth. Now, in the 1990s most British hospitals claim to encourage mothers to prepare their own birth plans and express their preferences for care, so giving them a sense of having some control over events.

Pressure groups and feminism

Various organisations such as the National Childbirth Trust (NCT), the Association for the Improvement of Maternity Services (AIMS) and the Association of Radical Midwives (ARM) have articulated the growing need of women to regain some personal control over decisions about where and how they give birth. Although the move towards more readily available home confinement has not resulted in a great increase of babies born outside hospital, it has played an important part in

making hospital staff examine the type and quality of the care they provide in an effort to provide alternative choices which combine the maximum safety and satisfaction (Tew, 1990).

Alternatives in care

In theory at least a woman has the choice of where she would prefer to be delivered. In practice this freedom is often severely curtailed by considerations of safety and the effective constraints of health authority policies.

The alternatives available may vary between health authorities, but they normally include the following possibilities for childbirth.

Hospital. Consultant unit 'Full-stay'

This used to mean between 7–10 days. In a time of health service cutbacks, the stay is often shortened to three days or less. Although many mothers appreciate returning home as soon as possible, in areas of urban deprivation it may be advisable to encourage a longer stay for mothers with poor socio-economic backgrounds.

Hospital.'Early transfer'

Mothers return home with their babies to the care of the community midwives one or two days after delivery. Those with other young children at home usually prefer this choice. The transfer is arranged during pregnancy with the community midwife, who will visit the home to make sure that arrangements will be suitable for a very new baby and a newly delivered mother.

'DOMINO' scheme

This stands literally for DOmiciliary Midwifery IN and Out.

The mother books with her community midwife for her antenatal care and delivery in hospital. She returns home six hours or so after delivery and the community midwife continues her care. This system seems to combine the advantages of home and hospital care in a satisfying manner, but provision for it is patchy throughout the country, mainly because DOMINO deliveries are very demanding on an already stretched community midwifery service. Where it does exist it has often been found an acceptable alternative for mothers for whom home birth is not a viable option.

General practitioner units

Although many GP units have disappeared in the last decade, those which still exist are usually much appreciated by their local community. Many are now no longer isolated little units but are located close to the delivery suite of a district general hospital, where care can rapidly be transferred from the primary health care team to the obstetric specialist team if an emergency occurs.

Home confinement

Not more than about 1% of women have their babies at home now (OPCS, 1990). Few general practitioners, even those who are on the official Obstetric List, wish to accept responsibility for these confinements. Although a midwife can, and sometimes has to, deliver a woman unaided it is obviously preferable for her to do so with medical back-up. Parents who request a home birth should have the advantages and disadvantages clearly explained to them and constructive alternatives offered if their choice seems unwise.

In every case a woman's choice of place of confinement needs careful consideration to see if it is suitable in view of factors such as her medical and obstetric history, her age and social circumstances.

The carers

Modern maternity care requires a team approach in order to provide the best possible service. Some of the main participants in that team are shown in Fig. 18.1

The midwife

The World Health Organisation definition of a midwife is given in Fig. 18.2. In Britain midwives were first required to be licensed to practise in 1902 when the Midwives Act was passed. Although practice varies widely within the European Community, the minimum range of skills a mid-

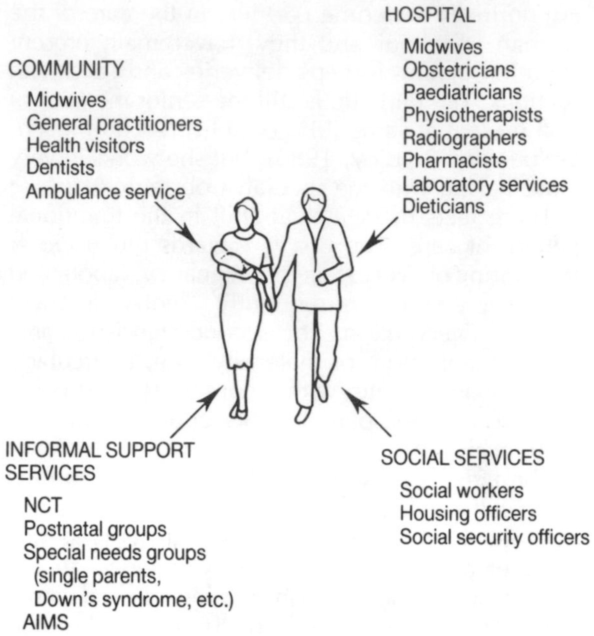

COMMUNITY

Midwives
General practitioners
Health visitors
Dentists
Ambulance service

HOSPITAL

Midwives
Obstetricians
Paediatricians
Physiotherapists
Radiographers
Pharmacists
Laboratory services
Dieticians

INFORMAL SUPPORT SERVICES

NCT
Postnatal groups
Special needs groups
 (single parents,
 Down's syndrome, etc.)
AIMS

SOCIAL SERVICES

Social workers
Housing officers
Social security officers

Fig. 18.1 *Obstetric services*

wife should be permitted to practise was published in the Midwifery Directives in 1980 (Fig. 18.3).

The English word *midwife* comes from the Saxon meaning *with woman* – a succinct account of the nature of the midwife's role.

Professor Kloostermans, a Dutch obstetrician and vigorous defender of midwifery practice, is quoted as saying, 'Throughout the world, there exists a group of women who feel mightily drawn to giving care to women in childbirth. At the same time maternal and independent, responsive to the mother's needs, yet accepting full responsibility as her attendant, such women are natural midwives. Without the presence and acceptance of the midwife, obstetrics becomes aggressive, technological and inhumane' (Oakley and Houd, 1990; page 2).

In the UK, the legal framework permits the midwife to work with a considerable degree of professional autonomy. How individual midwives interpret this in practice depends not just on their personal preference but also on the constraints imposed by local health authorities and by other members of the maternity services team, midwives as well as obstetricians. The small but steady growth of Midwifery Practice Units around the country is witness to midwives' willingness to

The Definition of a Midwife

The definition of a midwife adopted by the International Confederation of Midwives and International Federation of Gynaecologists and Obstetricians in 1972 and 1973 respectively, following amendment of the definition formulated by the World Health Organisation, was amended in 1990 by the ICM to read as follows:

A midwife is a person who, having been regularly admitted to a midwifery education programme, duly recognised in the country in which it is located, has successfully completed the prescribed course of studies in midwifery and has acquired the requisite qualifications to be registered and/or legally licensed to practise midwifery.

She must be able to give the necessary supervision, care and advice to women during pregnancy, labour and the post-partum period, to conduct deliveries on her own responsibility and to care for the newborn and the infant. This care includes preventative measures, the detection of abnormal conditions in mother and child, the procurement of medical assistance and the execution of emergency measures in the absence of medical help. She has an important task in health counselling and health education, not only for the women, but also within the family and the community. The work should involve antenatal education and preparation for parenthood and extends to certain areas of gynaecology, family planning and child care. She may practise in hospitals, clinics, health units, domiciliary conditions or in any other service

Fig. 18.2 *The definition of a midwife (ICM 1990)*

assume full professional responsibility for their decisions. In such units, obstetricians are used in a truly 'consultant' role, since midwives will refer women to them should problems arise. In many more traditional units, midwives are using research evidence about intervention in labour and women's wishes with regard to childbirth to establish a similar pattern of care, one which encourages the woman to have confidence in her own ability to give birth. Students may find very wide variations in the degree of independence with which midwives choose to or are able to practise.

Pregnancy and childbearing

There has been increasing evidence in recent years of the important part parental health prior to conception plays in the outcome of pregnancy. As a

The Activities of a Midwife

The activities of a midwife are defined in the European Community Directive 80/155/EEC Article 4 as follows:

Member states shall ensure that midwives are at least entitled to take up and pursue the following activities:

1. to provide sound family planning information and advice
2. to diagnose pregnancies and monitor normal pregnancies; to carry out examinations necessary for the monitoring of the development of normal pregnancies
3. to prescribe or advise on the examinations necessary for earliest possible diagnosis of pregnancies at risk
4. to provide a programme of parenthood preparation and a complete preparation for childbirth including advice on hygiene and nutrition
5. to care for and assist the mother during labour and to monitor the condition of the fetus *in utero* by the appropriate clinical and technical means
6. to conduct spontaneous deliveries including where required an episiotomy and in urgent cases a breech delivery
7. to recognise the warning signs of abnormality in the mother or infant which necessitate referral to a doctor and to assist the latter where appropriate; to take the necessary emergency measures in the doctor's absence, in particular the manual removal of the placenta, possibly followed by manual examination of the uterus
8. to examine and care for the newborn infant; to take all initiatives which are necessary in case of need and to carry out where necessary immediate resuscitation
9. to care for and monitor the progress of the mother in the postnatal period and to give all necessary advice to the mother on infant care to enable her to ensure the optimum progress of the newborn infant
10. to carry out the treatment prescribed by a doctor
11. to maintain all necessary records

Fig. 18.3 *The activities of a midwife*

result there has been an effort to encourage people who are thinking of starting a family to evaluate their own state of health.

Preconceptual care

As yet there is little provision for preconceptual care within the NHS. Nonetheless, individual GPs and midwives, as well as private sector groups such as Foresight, now offer counselling, basic screening and advice to would-be parents.

A careful history elicits information about lifestyle, eating habits and contraceptive practice. Enquiring about smoking, drinking and medication (especially drug abuse), allergies and chronic infection provides the basis for discussion and advice designed to help the parents choose the adjustments they will need to make to provide the most favourable circumstances for a pregnancy.

The childbearing woman

In order to understand the processes involved in conception, pregnancy and birth, some knowledge of the relevant structures and their function is essential. This knowledge provides an important part of the information on which a pattern of care at each stage of pregnancy can be based.

Details of the non-pregnant female genital tract will be found in Chapter 17, together with an account of the menstrual cycle, the starting point for understanding the processes of reproduction. It will probably be helpful to read the section in Chapter 17 before continuing with the description of pregnancy which follows. Throughout her maternity care course, the student will find constant reference to a sound midwifery textbook invaluable (e.g. Bennett and Brown, 1989).

The beginning of pregnancy

The process of *ovulation, fertilisation* and *implantation* is shown schematically in Fig. 18.4.

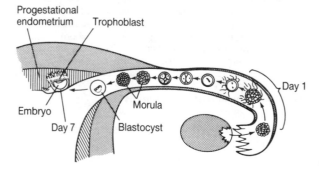

Fig. 18.4 *Fertilisation and implantation of the ovum*

Fertilisation

When the ripe Graafian follicle ruptures on the surface of the ovary on about the 14th day of the menstrual cycle, the ovum is ejected into the wide-open end of the uterine (Fallopian) tube, the *am-pulla*. The ovum is propelled along the tube by the rhythmic contraction of the muscle walls and the movement of *cilia* in the fluid which acts as a transport medium.

Fertilisation normally takes place up to 36 hours after ovulation. If it does not occur the ovum degenerates and the menstrual cycle continues uninterrupted. Of the millions of spermatozoa that are ejaculated into the vagina at intercourse, only a relatively small number will reach the ampulla, where fertilisation usually takes place. The use of the electron microscope has permitted observation of the moment of conception. Only one of the spermatozoa struggling to penetrate the outer wall of the ovum succeeds, helped by the release of **acrosomal** enzymes. This penetration seems immediately to inhibit the entry of further spermatozoa.

The fertilised ovum is known as a **zygote**. Humans normally have 46 **chromosomes**, the structures that carry genetic information determining the particular characteristics of a person. The chromosomes are grouped in pairs. At fertilisation one chromosome of each of the 23 pairs remains in the ovum as a result of a special form of cell division known as **meiosis** (see Chapter 6). These combine with the 23 chromosomes carried in the cell nucleus of the spermatozoon to form the zygote, which now carries a total of 46 chromosomes necessary for the new human being. The future baby's sex is determined by the father at conception, as the sperm cell contributes one of its two possible sex chromosomes, X for female or Y for male, to the X chromosome present in the ovum.

Zygote development and implantation

Rapid cell division takes place as the zygote travels down the uterine tube. By the 4th-5th day, a small ball of cells called a **morula** exists. This develops a cavity containing an inner cell mass, the future **embryo**, and an outer wall of **trophoblast**, the future placenta and membranes. This tiny structure, now called the **blastocyst**, reaches the rich bed of the endometrium. This stage is known as implantation (Fig. 18.4). The blastocyst then throws out small shoots, known as *primary chorionic villi*, to draw essential nutrients from the maternal tissues surrounding it. This 'seed-bed' endometrium is now known as the **decidua** throughout pregnancy.

The diagnosis of pregnancy

A woman usually first suspects she is pregnant when she fails to menstruate at the normal time. Her suspicions can be confirmed by the use of one of the many pregnancy tests which are available. This can be done through her GP, or she may prefer to buy a kit herself at the chemist. An early morning specimen of urine is tested against a sensitive reagent to show the presence or absence of *human chorionic gonadotrophin* (HCG), a pregnancy-specific hormone produced by the trophoblast.

Amenorrhoea is not an infallible sign of pregnancy. Other signs which may indicate that a woman is pregnant are listed in Table 18.1.

Table 18.1. *Probable signs of pregnancy*

- Breast tenderness, tingling and enlargement, the appearance of **colostrum** in later weeks
- Frequency of micturition
- Recurrent nausea and vomiting
- Skin changes, including darkening of the areolar tissue around the nipples and the development of the 'dark line of pregnancy' on the lower abdomen
- In later weeks abdominal enlargement and fetal movements will be observable

Few doctors now use internal vaginal examinations to confirm pregnancy, since surer and more acceptable means are available. As well as the HCG immunoglobulin test already mentioned, these include:

(1) **Ultrasound** – a technique using high frequency sound waves to create a visual image of internal body structures. It can be used, if necessary, to identify the presence of one or more gestational sacs in the uterus from as early as four weeks after conception. Ultrasound plays a large part now in the management of pregnancy, especially when things go wrong, and students will often have the opportunity to see the **fetus** on the scanning screen.
(2) *Fetal heart sounds* can be heard by *Doppler* sonography from about 10 weeks, and through the trumpet-shaped Pinard's stethoscope from about 24 weeks.
(3) *Palpation*. In later weeks the midwife or doctor can palpate fetal parts and fetal movements, both definite signs of pregnancy.

The date of delivery

Once she is sure of being pregnant the next question the woman wants answered is, 'When is my baby due?'. If she has a regular menstrual cycle, the quickest and most common way of finding out is to do the calculation shown in Fig. 18.5. Mothers should be reminded, however, that babies often ignore their 'expected date' and can arrive safely a week or two either side of the day they are due.

NB. This calculation is only reliable for women with a regular menstrual cycle

(1) Find out the first day of the woman's last period
(2) Add seven days to that
(3) Then add nine calendar months

This will give her expected date of delivery (EDD)
For example (1) 17th May 1992 (2) 24th May 1992
(3) 24th February 1993

Fig. 18.5 *Calculating the expected delivery date (EDD)*

When the menstrual cycle is irregular, calculation is unreliable and ultrasound measurement is invaluable for estimating the period of **gestation** to within 4–5 days. This is done by comparing various measurements of fetal growth, particularly the **biparietal diameter**, with standard growth charts.

The changes caused by pregnancy

The changes brought about in a woman by the presence of a developing fetus affect the whole person. All her body systems, her mind and her emotions are involved. The changes are 'masterminded' by the endocrine system and are designed to enable the body to adapt to its new tasks of sustaining the fetus, labour, delivery and, eventually, lactation.

The endocrine system

This system is considered first, since it regulates the other changes which occur. No attempt will be made here to describe the complex and sensitive feedback mechanisms by which the different hormones interact and become effective at different stages (see Chapter 5). The activity of the most important is described below.

(1) *Human chorionic gonadotrophin* (HCG), already mentioned, is produced by the trophoblast and maintains the **corpus luteum** in the ovary until the placenta is functioning effectively.

(2) *Progesterone* is produced by the corpus luteum and increases greatly once the placenta takes over at about 10–12 weeks. Progesterone maintains the decidua, relaxes smooth muscle and connective tissue throughout the body and causes breast changes, including the development of glandular and duct tissue.

(3) *Oestrogens* have similar origins to progesterone, although the fetus also plays some part in the metabolism of *oestriol*. Oestrogens cause tissue growth in the breasts and the uterus. Fluid retention and the inhibition of lactation during pregnancy result from the high levels of oestrogens.

(4) *Human placental lactogen* (HPL) is produced from the placenta and promotes tissue growth and fat metabolism.

(5) *Relaxin* from the placenta mainly relaxes connective tissue.

(6) *Prolactin* from the anterior pituitary is present but inhibited in pregnancy. Once oestrogen levels fall at delivery, it becomes active and stimulates lactation.

(7) The activity of *pituitary*, *adrenal* and *thyroid glands* is also altered in pregnancy.

Largely as a result of these extensive hormonal changes, other systems are affected as described below.

Blood and circulatory system

There is a 30–40% increase in blood volume during pregnancy, with a consequent rise in cardiac output. The main component of the blood volume increase is plasma. This means that although there is an absolute rise in total haemoglobin content, the mean haemoglobin concentration falls in the second trimester of pregnancy, an effect known as *haemodilution*. Although recent studies (Montgomery, 1990) have questioned the routine use of iron supplements in pregnancy, it is generally recognised that once a woman's haemoglobin falls below 10.5 g/dl, fetal demands make extra iron necessary.

The increased circulating blood volume is accommodated by peripheral vasodilation caused by progesterone. As a result the blood pressure usually drops slightly in the second trimester. The uterus and breasts receive an important increase in blood flow necessary to support tissue growth.

Other changes in the blood during pregnancy include a raised *erythrocyte sedimentation rate*, (ESR), an increase in leucocytes and in fibrinogen levels. Many of the changes increase the blood's ability to coagulate. This is obviously intended to prevent bleeding, but also results in a tendency to form thrombi, especially when other predisposing factors such as obesity, immobility or varicosities are present.

Urinary tract

The kidneys have a higher *glomerular filtration rate* (GFR) as a result of the raised blood flow. Sugar appears in the urine of some women because the renal threshold is lowered. Although this is not normally significant, the blood sugar levels must be investigated if it happens more than once since diabetes can become evident for the first time in pregnancy.

Progesterone causes the smooth muscle wall of the ureters to kink and dilate. This provides an opportunity for *urinary stasis* to occur, with a resultant risk of ascending infection.

Mechanical as well as hormonal influences bring about changes in pregnancy and the growing uterus can irritate the bladder in early pregnancy causing frequency of micturition. The same thing can happen at the end of pregnancy when the engaging head descends into the pelvis, causing pressure.

Digestive tract

The relaxing effects of progesterone result in reduced peristalsis and slower stomach emptying. The cardiac sphincter is lax and gastric reflux together with pressure on the diaphragm from the fetus in late pregnancy can cause heartburn. Constipation is a further consequence of sluggish alimentary tract activity.

Respiratory system

There is a 20% increase in oxygen consumption to supply fetal needs. The diaphragm rises in late pregnancy and some ribcage flaring may occur. Dyspnoea is sometimes a problem at the end of pregnancy.

Skeletal system

The softening action of progesterone and relaxin on cartilaginous tissue results in a small degree of destabilisation of certain joints, especially of the pelvis. With the mechanical effect of the growing fetus causing some lordosis in late pregnancy, the mother may experience considerable discomfort and less mobility.

Skin changes

An increase in melanocyte activity results in darkening of certain areas, as previously mentioned. An increased peripheral blood flow results in more active sebaceous and sweat glands. Stretch marks, or **striae gravidarum**, may appear on the abdomen, or even the breasts as they increase in size. New striae are pinkish in colour. They become faded and silvery in subsequent pregnancies.

Metabolic changes

The most obvious of these changes is the weight gain. Its components are shown in Fig. 18.6. The average gain is about 12 kg throughout the whole pregnancy, although the major part of this gain, some 10 kg, takes place in the second half of the nine months.

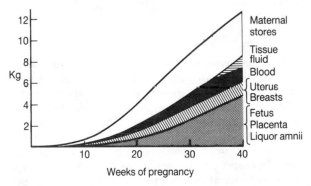

Fig. 18.6 *The components of weight gain in normal pregnancy*

Fat and carbohydrate metabolism are altered and about 4 kg is laid down as fat 'reserves', to provide for lactation later.

The alteration of her body image brought about by pregnancy can be a source of distress or a source of pride for the mother-to-be, and a sensitive carer will be aware of this, providing her with the opportunity to discuss it if she wishes.

The mind and emotions

It is not surprising that a woman undergoing the changes described in this section should react to them emotionally. 'Mood swings' are a recognised feature of pregnancy and the puerperium and are probably attributable as much to the huge increase in hormone levels as to the mother's perception of and natural anxieties about pregnancy and childbirth. Elation and tears follow swiftly upon each other in this situation and the midwife has to be alert to the mother's moods, perhaps especially when they are unexpressed. She may need to help male partners develop their awareness of the origins of seemingly 'irrational' alterations in order to be able to provide much needed support.

Changes in the reproductive system: the uterus

This small, hollow, muscular organ, normally buried deep in the pelvic cavity between the bladder and the pouch of Douglas, undergoes drastic change in size, weight, shape and position during pregnancy (see Table 18.2).

The body, isthmus and cervix of the uterus are shown in Fig. 18.7. There are three layers of endometrium (decidua), myometrium and perimetrium. The myometrium undergoes the most changes with its complex structure of muscle fibres increasing in size and number by at least tenfold.

Table 18.2. *Changes in the uterus*

	Pre-pregnant	Term
Weight	60g	1000 g
Size	7.5cm long 5.0cm wide 2.5cm deep	30cm long 25cm wide 20cm deep
Shape	Small pear — Globular — Ovoid	
Position	Pelvic cavity	Abdominal cavity

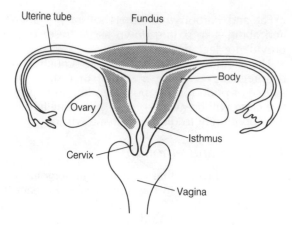

Fig. 18.7 *The uterus*

The upper two thirds of the uterus, the body, meets the cervix at an area called the isthmus. This small (7 mm) region expands to 7.5 cm at term and, together with the cervix as it becomes effaced, forms the lower segment of the uterus, a thin-walled structure.

The cervix remains largely unaltered in pregnancy. The cervical canal is closed at either end by an internal and external os and is filled with a thick, jelly-like mucus *operculum* or plug. This appears at the onset of labour as the slightly blood-stained 'show', when the cervix begins to dilate.

The blood supply to the uterus is from the ovarian and uterine arteries, through greatly enlarged and distended blood vessels supplying the chorio-decidual space, where the placenta is attached.

The growth of the uterus is used as a clinical measure of fetal well-being. It can be palpated and measured abdominally and Fig. 18.8 shows the average fundal size in relation to the weeks of gestation. Wide variations from normal are possible.

The vagina

The vagina softens and becomes more extensible as a result of increased blood supply and hormone levels. A whitish, non-offensive discharge (leucorrhoea) is normal in pregnancy and should be explained to the mothers. Alteration in vaginal pH means that vaginal thrush (*moniliasis*) is common in pregnancy.

The ovaries

Normal ovarian function is suspended during preg-

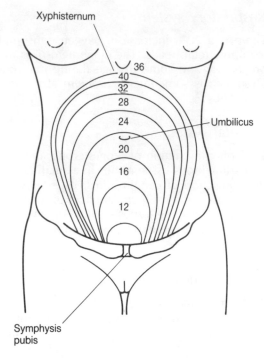

Fig. 18.8 *Fundal heights in relation to weeks of gestation*

nancy. In the first weeks the corpus luteum produces oestrogen and progesterone until the placenta is sufficiently developed to take over this task.

Supports

The reproductive organs are supported by a powerful system of muscles and ligaments which form the pelvic floor and perineal body. The stress of childbirth can weaken them (Fig. 18.9).

Breast changes

The breasts will be described in detail when lactation is discussed (page 506). Changes occur very early in pregnancy as hormonal activity promotes glandular growth. After the initial 'tingling' sensation breasts begin to grow in size from the 6th week onwards. This growth is enormously variable between women. The areola and nipple darken and become prominent, with Montgomery's tubercles evident on the areola. These small structures produce sebum to prevent the nipple drying out. Some women with fine skin have a prominent

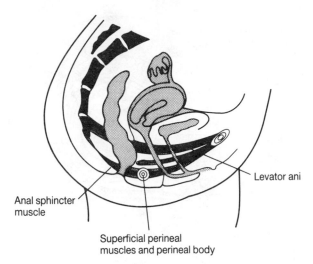

Anal sphincter
muscle

Levator ani

Superficial perineal
muscles and perineal body

Fig. 18.9 *The muscles of the pelvic floor, sagittal section*

web of bluish veins visible. Colostrum is secreted from about the 16th week of pregnancy.

The minor disorders of pregnancy

What the doctors call 'minor disorders' may actually be major discomforts for the mother. They have the advantage of being self-limiting, since they disappear once pregnancy is over, if not before. On the whole there are no 'cures', only palliative measures such as support tights for varicose veins; small, frequent meals for nausea; increased fibre for constipation; and extra pillows in bed for heartburn. The most common problems arise as a result of the hormonal and pressure changes discussed in this section and have already been mentioned in relation to the affected systems.

The development of the fetus and placenta

The fetus grows from the inner cell mass described earlier. The growth is supported by a parallel growth of the trophoblast, which later becomes the placenta. New techniques of photography and fetoscopy have allowed us to follow this marvellous evolution from a cluster of cells to a full-term baby and there are some superbly illustrated texts and films now available which show this growth in detail. The illustrations in Fig. 18.10 show the fetus at various stages of development. Technological advances in Special Care Baby Units mean

that some babies of 23–24 weeks gestation are now able to survive despite very immature body systems.

The placenta

The placenta and membranes with the umbilical cord provide the fetus' life-support system. From the 12th week of pregnancy its tasks are:

(1) To produce hormones to support the fetus (see above)
(2) To provide a means of nutrition, excretion and respiration
(3) To protect the fetus from infection and from the effects of drugs.

The placenta is not always efficient at all of these tasks, and babies are sometimes born small or deformed because of placental failure.

The placenta and umbilical cord are inspected carefully at delivery. Their appearance is described in the account of the third stage of labour (page 497).

The amniotic fluid or liquor provides a cushion for the fetus, who is mobile and active in about 1000 ml of fluid in the amniotic sac at term. The two membranes, the *chorion* and *amnion*, enclose and protect the fetus and placenta and are active in hormone production.

Antenatal care

At the beginning of this century there was virtually no provision for antenatal care. A woman just booked a doctor (if she was well off) or a midwife (if she wasn't) to attend her once she went into labour. People gradually realised that the outcome of pregnancy could be improved by care during pregnancy and by the 1920s the concept of antenatal care was accepted. The relative effects of socio-economic factors and obstetric care on the steadily declining perinatal mortality rates are difficult to distinguish, but Fig 18.11 shows the extent of that decline, an improvement which has transformed the experience of childbirth for thousands of women who no longer have to face a high risk to themselves or their babies.

More recently schemes such as the Cowgate project in Newcastle (Davies and Evans, 1990) have demonstrated beyond doubt that, properly used, appropriate antenatal intervention can and

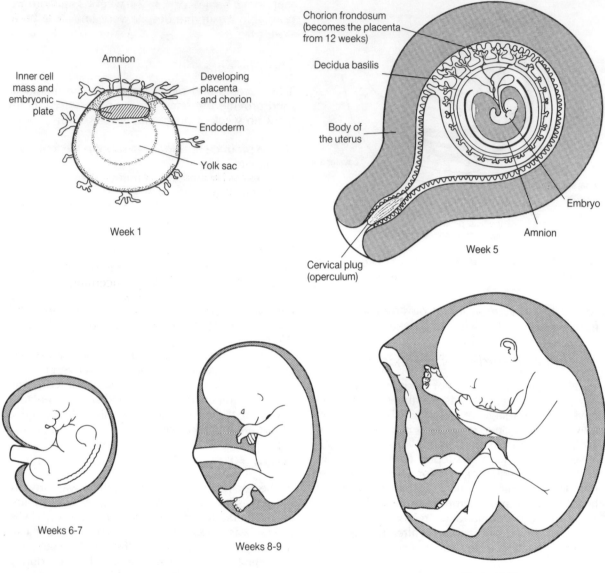

Week 1

Week 5

Weeks 6-7

Weeks 8-9

Weeks 15-22

Fig. 18.10 *The development of the fetus*

does reduce perinatal mortality and morbidity. What has been questioned is the value of patterns of care which have become ritualised. Media focus on rushed and crowded clinics is making maternity services search for alternative solutions which combine fewer visits with continued high levels of safety (Field, 1990).

To meet the frequently expressed need for greater continuity of care, a wide variety of innov-

ative schemes, usually taking some form of 'team midwifery' (Flint and Poulengeris, 1987), have been developed in the UK. Comparisons are difficult to make precisely because of the many different local interpretations of the 'team' concept – only time and careful evaluation will show how effective such initiatives are in providing the personalised care which women need during pregnancy and childbirth.

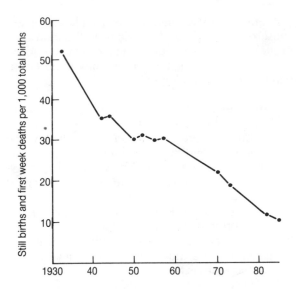

Fig. 18.11 *Perinatal mortality 1931–1985 (figures supplied by OPCS)*

The aims of antenatal care

Mothers, midwives and doctors are all likely to have a slightly differing version of what they hope to achieve by antenatal care. Most, however, would accept the list given in Table 18.3 as a basis for good care.

Table 18.3. *The aims of antenatal care*

- A safe pregnancy and delivery resulting in a healthy mother and baby
- The identification and management of any deviation from normal
- Preparation for labour and parenthood
- Prevention of the onset of avoidable complications
- An emotionally satisfying experience
- *You might like to add to this list*

Planning and implementing care

Achieving these aims is a matter of teamwork between the mother, the midwife and the doctor. A major component of the teamwork is communication. The style of communication, and the attitudes transmitted by the people communicating, contribute to making or breaking the relationship

of trust on which satisfactory care depends. For this reason the initial welcome to the hospital clinic where the mother comes for the first time to book is enormously important (Methven, 1982). The challenge for the midwife is somehow to enable the mother in her care to 'feel special' even when she is being seen in a clinic of 80–90 other pregnant women.

Booking

The cornerstone of good antenatal care is a carefully taken history of the pregnant woman. This is one of the most worthwhile moments in midwifery practice, for in a private one-to-one interview the midwife has the chance not only of acquiring the essential information which will guide the subsequent care but of initiating a relationship with the mother which will encourage her to express her own hopes and fears concerning her pregnancy and delivery.

Each midwifery unit has its own system of notes, and many are becoming computerised. The essential elements of a booking interview should include details of a woman's *social background* (for example, her occupation and her accommodation), her *marital status*, her history of *smoking*, *drinking* and *drug usage*, her *previous obstetric history*, and the history of her *present pregnancy*. In addition, she should be asked about her *relevant medical and surgical history*, and her *family medical and reproductive history*. Her wishes and expectations about delivery and her plans for feeding the baby should also be discussed fully. Increasingly this is done by getting the mother to complete a birth plan.

This history will form the personal database on which judgement about future courses of action will be made. It should provide enough information to alert the obstetric team to potential hazards ahead (for example, a family history of hereditary disease or a maternal history of recurrent abortion).

Table 18.4 lists the investigations which are commonly undertaken in early pregnancy. The haemoglobin and antibody tests are repeated in the third trimester to make sure no problems are arising. Ultrasound screening may be repeated to confirm a satisfactory fetal growth rate or to verify the position of the placenta.

Table 18.4. *Routine pregnancy investigations*

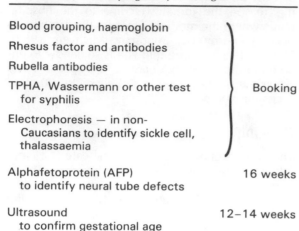

Blood grouping, haemoglobin	
Rhesus factor and antibodies	
Rubella antibodies	
TPHA, Wassermann or other test for syphilis	Booking
Electrophoresis — in non-Caucasians to identify sickle cell, thalassaemia	
Alphafetoprotein (AFP) to identify neural tube defects	16 weeks
Ultrasound to confirm gestational age	12–14 weeks

Table 18.5. *Frequency of antenatal visits*

- At booking
- × 1 per month for first 6 months of pregnancy
- × 1 per fortnight for 7th and 8th months of pregnancy
- × 1 per week until delivery

Patterns of care

Patterns of care should be worked out according to individual need and the responsibility is often shared between the woman's GP and the hospital consultant obstetric unit. The classical frequency of antenatal visits is shown in Table 18.5, although this may vary with different regions. Where consultant services have been centralised, getting to hospital clinics can be an expensive and tedious experience for a woman (particularly if she has other small children) and some areas are experimenting with peripheral consultant clinics.

Communication between the GP and the hospital clinic is assured by the use of the Co-operation Card carried by the woman. This carries all the essential details about the woman and should be filled in at each visit during pregnancy, so that information is complete and up to date. In many centres women are now carrying their own notes. This not only gives them a certain sense of control but dramatically reduces the frustration which occurs when notes cannot be found by the Medical Records Department.

A number of women, either by choice or because of an associated problem, will attend only the hospital throughout pregnancy. Whether the visit occurs in hospital or community it must contain the following elements:

(1) An assessment of the woman's general well-being and emotional state
(2) Blood pressure estimation — to identify the onset of hypertensive problems
(3) Maternal weight should be recorded — to see whether the changes are within accepted norms
(4) Urine should be tested for the presence of glucose, protein, ketones or blood
(5) A physical examination should be given — a general one at booking, an abdominal one at subsequent visits.

Abdominal examination

This is done in pregnancy for the following reasons:

(1) To estimate the growth of the fetus
(2) To affirm that growth is compatible with the period of gestation
(3) To identify the lie, presentation, position and attitude of the fetus
(4) To identify **engagement** of the presenting part
(5) In order to hear the fetal heart.

A midwife has to learn to 'see with her hands' and becomes skilled in interpreting what she feels (see Table 18.6). She can teach student nurses to discover how the baby is lying. When carrying out the examination she can involve the mother by encouraging her to feel her baby's head or back. As always with physical examinations, it is important that the mother has an empty bladder and

Table 18.6. *Abdominal examination: what it includes*

Looking	Observation, to see the size and shape of the abdomen and any scars or stretch marks. The baby can sometimes be seen moving
Feeling	Palpating in order to identify the factors listed above
Listening	Auscultation, to hear the rate and rhythm of the fetal heart

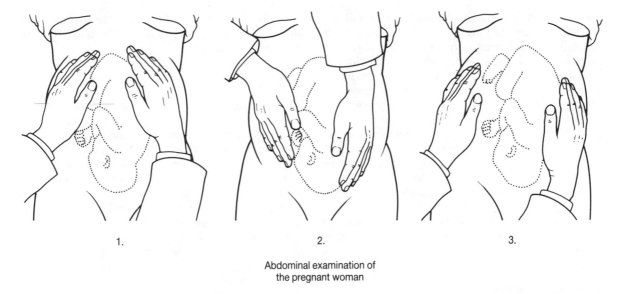

1.   2.   3.

Abdominal examination of
the pregnant woman

Fig. 18.12 *Abdominal examination of the pregnant woman*

that she is lying comfortably with her head and shoulders supported.

The use of the midwife's hands is shown in Fig. 18.12. She explains what she finds to the woman and makes a record in the notes.

Maternity benefits

A number of facilities are offered to the pregnant woman. Although most are offered through the Department of Social Security, the woman should be informed of what is available when she books at the clinic. Explanatory leaflets are available in clinics and Social Security offices. The regulations governing statutory maternity benefits change so frequently that midwives have to ensure that they obtain up to date information from the local Social Security office.

Communication

It cannot be overstressed how important effective communication is to satisfactory and satisfying care in the entire childbearing year, from conception to the postnatal visit. Rushed, crowded clinics, often with inadequate assurance of privacy, are a major handicap and make the staff's task especially difficult. In addition the special needs of those who have a limited ability to understand what is said or done to them must be provided for. In many areas language is a common barrier, but low social status,

poor education or handicap such as deaf mutism can all mean that the essentials are not transmitted to the mothers. Student nurses, less involved in the responsibilities of management of a clinic, may be able to take time to be attentive to these more needy mothers.

Lifestyle in pregnancy

Motivation towards a healthier lifestyle is usually high in pregnancy, since most women are very keen to do all they can to assure the well-being of their babies and many realise the extent to which their own habits can affect the child they are carrying. From the earliest days the midwife has an opportunity to help women understand what they can do to help ensure their own and their baby's health.

Areas which may need discussion include sleep, rest, physical exercise, sexual intercourse and personal hygiene. Nutrition, smoking, drinking and drugs deserve special consideration.

Nutrition

Maternal tissue growth and fetal development make special demands on the mother's metabolism. Dietary habits vary so widely across cultural and socio-economic groups that it is valueless to generalise about what constitutes a suitable diet. Each mother needs specific advice in the light of her own preferences and habits. This is best offered by a dietician, who will sometimes be present in the antenatal clinic. Where this is not possible the midwife should be able to discuss the altered needs of pregnancy and suggest practical ways in which the woman might increase her protein, iron, calcium, vitamin and fibre intakes, which are economically realistic and acceptable to her.

Vegetarians, and more especially vegans, pose special problems in terms of providing for fetal demands, and expert advice can be particularly useful here in order to ensure adequate protein intake and protect the mother and the fetus against the effects of anaemia.

Harmful social practices

Education for childbearing involves making people aware of the damaging effects which some social practices can have on the developing fetus. It is important not to be alarmist or dogmatic about this. The Health Education Authority produces attractively presented literature which states the case against smoking, alcohol and drugs in pregnancy and this can be reinforced by providing the occasion for discussion of these issues in private. Anything which requires people to alter their lifestyle has to be carefully thought through, and the midwife needs to be prepared to listen rather than to lecture. She must be aware of the research findings on which the arguments against these practices are based, their effects on the fetus and the newborn, and be ready to offer practical suggestions to help the mother who wants to change her habits.

Smoking

Fetal oxygenation is reduced with the inhalation of tobacco smoke. Smoking is shown to affect the fetus adversely and is one of the topics best considered before embarking on a pregnancy. Smoking increases the risk of spontaneous abortion and reduces fetal growth by about 200g on average. Although many mothers see no disadvantage in the latter, long term effects have been shown in the children of chronic smokers. Where smoking is associated with other factors calculated to undermine health, such as inappropriate nutri-

tion, poor housing conditions and recurrent respiratory infection, the effects on the fetus may be serious (Black, 1985).

Drinking

Research studies vary widely in their reporting of the known effects of drinking on the fetus. It seems beyond doubt that 'binge' drinking in early pregnancy or persistent heavy drinking can do extensive fetal damage. Fetal alcohol syndrome has been described as a result. Mothers need to be alerted to this danger in a world where alcohol consumption, together with female alcohol addiction, is rising steeply (Plant, 1986). Accurate figures are difficult to obtain, but Rossett, Weiner and Lee (1983) found between one and three babies per 1000 in the USA were severely affected by maternal alcohol intake.

Drugs

Drug taking falls into two categories: *medication* and drug abuse.

Most women are now well aware of the risks of medically unsupervised self-medication in pregnancy and are very willing to avoid all but the most medically essential drugs.

Drug abuse is a more serious matter, however. The problems of drug dependency are increasing rapidly. In 1985 there were thought to be some 20,000 users of heroin and similar substances in London alone (Kroll, 1986). There are no simple, short answers to a problem which is symptomatic of profound social disorder. The maternity units of most inner city areas are now familiar with the distressing picture offered by drug-dependent parents and their affected babies.

The effects of drug dependency may be compounded by co-existing problems such as herpes simplex II, HIV and hepatitis.

When genital herpes is active, the baby is delivered by elective caesarean section. HIV seropositive women may prefer to avoid becoming pregnant at all because the full extent of the long term consequences for the babies remains unknown as yet (Pinching, 1987), although the transmission rate from mother to baby at birth is thought to be in the region of 13% (European Collaborative Study, 1991).

Known or suspected drug-dependent mothers need specialist support through pregnancy and close liaison between the maternity services and the social services is essential if the baby is going home to a precarious environment.

Preparation for labour and parenthood

All maternity units and most community services offer a programme of parentcraft education. As with so many services, it is often the already reasonably well provided for who use it and continual efforts have to be made to devise schemes that will appeal to a wider audience. There are already some successful initiatives, especially for very young single mothers. These may find it daunting to join a group of mothers in their mid-twenties to thirties with a well established pattern of family life but respond well to groups of their peers (Evans and Parker, 1985).

The aims and content of parentcraft classes

Parentcraft classes are primarily a confidence-building exercise. Their major objectives fall into three broad categories: the acquisition of *psychological support* (from peers and from professionals); of *information* (what to expect in pregnancy and labour, the basis for choice, and birth plans); and of *skills* (in relaxation and baby care).

Many series of classes include an 'early bird' class soon after booking to prepare women for the early months of pregnancy and the growth of the fetus, as well as the choice of layette.

In the third trimester the remaining classes (which are often weekly) deal with topics such as *infant feeding, labour* (often over several sessions), *pain relief*, the *delivery* itself, then care *after* delivery and baby care.

Relaxation in preparation for childbirth usually forms part of each class.

There is commonly a parents' evening for couples, where the father's role is explored, and a tour of the maternity unit so that there is at least some familiarity with the place where the great event is to take place.

It is helpful if various members of staff can share responsibility for the parentcraft session so that parents become familiar with them. Sessions need to be as varied as possible, allowing opportunity for discussion and sharing of experiences and anxieties. Up to date films or videos and well produced pamphlets reinforce teaching and stimulate discussion, but nothing replaces an informed, enthusiastic midwife to answer the many questions which parents-to-be ask.

NHS classes are complemented in many areas by those offered by the National Childbirth Trust and run in members' homes.

Whatever the format selected for parentcraft education, it is geared as much to creating an atmosphere of trust between midwives and parents as to transmitting information. While it is important that women reach their confinements clear about what is happening to them, it is just as important that they have developed a sense of confidence in their attendants which will allow them, the clients, to participate as fully as they wish in the preparation for and birth of their child.

Women with special needs in pregnancy

A certain number of women will have their pregnancies complicated by associated medical conditions. These include women with pre-eclampsia, diabetes, cardiac and renal conditions, epilepsy, **sickle cell anaemia**, the physically or mentally handicapped as well as the very young and much older mother. Unfortunately, space does not allow consideration here of their special needs and the student is referred to larger midwifery texts. Since the maternity care course is intended to offer an experience of normal pregnancy, only one exception to that norm will be discussed here — because of the frequency of its occurrence.

Pregnancy induced hypertension (PIH), pre-eclampsia

PIH occurs in the second half of pregnancy and is characterised by the presence of two of its three cardinal signs, hypertension (>140/90 or 15 mmHg above the baseline diastolic), oedema and proteinuria. Its origins are still unknown but, if neglected, its outcome can be drastic for both mother and baby. Pregnant women may develop the disease to the point of fitting with eclampsia and the fetus may be so nutritionally deprived as a result of the placental damage caused by this condition that it may be born very small (intra-uterine growth retardation, IUGR, resulting in a light-for-dates baby) or succumb to lack of oxygen during birth.

More consistent antenatal care has been successful in reducing the risk of severe PIH developing by picking up the early warning signs. This explains the universal attention to blood pressure, urinalysis and weight gain in antenatal clinics.

Rest may prevent the condition worsening, but its management is hotly debated. Once PIH is detected, close monitoring of fetal growth and well-being is undertaken and fetal movement charts, serial ultrasound and **cardiotocograph (CTG)** tracings may be used. If proteinuria sets in, the pregnancy is usually brought to an end by early induction of labour. This is for two reasons. At this stage the fetus is no longer being adequately nourished by the placenta and the worsening maternal condition will only be improved once delivery is achieved.

Labour and delivery

At the end of nine months, pregnancy ends with the onset of labour, the process by which the fetus and placenta with its membranes are expelled from the uterus. In a short maternity care course the student will only be able to follow a very small number of labours. The following description of the processes of labour should help her understand the needs and care of the mother and baby.

Labour falls naturally into three stages, although the onset of the first and second stages are not always very distinct.

The first stage lasts from the onset of regular painful contractions, which cause cervical dilation, to full dilation of the cervix. This is usually between 10–12 hours.

The second stage continues from full cervical dilation to the birth of the baby – about an hour.

The third stage lasts from the birth of the baby until the expulsion of the placenta and membranes – about 7–10 minutes.

The times given are for primiparae. Women who have already had a baby usually have rather more rapid labours, usually about 8–10 hours. If no **oxytocic** injection is given in the third stage, this will take about 20–30 minutes.

The onset of labour

It is not yet known what causes the onset of labour, but a woman may think it has started if any of the following occur:

(1) A blood-streaked mucoid 'plug', the *operculum*, is lost from the vagina (a 'show')
(2) Low backache develops
(3) Painful uterine contractions start and become stronger and more frequent
(4) The membranes rupture, allowing amniotic fluid to escape ('waters breaking').

Women are warned about these signs during pregnancy. If their waters break they are advised to come into hospital without delay because of the risk of infection or cord accident. Otherwise they are usually advised to come in once contractions are well established – not leaving it too late for those who have already had a baby and are likely to be quicker this time.

Labours vary as much as mothers do. Short easy ones and long tedious ones can both fall into the 'normal' parameters established by the classic definition of 'spontaneous vaginal delivery by the vertex of a normal, live fetus within 24 hours of the onset of labour'. They will need a very different approach, however.

Before continuing further with patterns of care a brief account of the different stages of labour is given.

The physical process

There are three major factors to consider when thinking about what happens in labour. They have traditionally, and usefully, been described as *the powers* (the uterine muscle and the mother's effort), *the passenger* (the fetus), and *the passages* (the bony pelvis and genital tract). The *powers* enable the *passenger* to negotiate the *passages* as described below.

First stage

The strong muscles of the myometrium contract and retract with a rhythmic flow from the fundus to the cervix. This gradually pushes the fetus further down the birth canal (descent) and increases fetal flexion. By the end of the first stage of labour, contractions usually come every 2–2½ minutes and last about 50–60 seconds. They are much more powerful than at the onset of labour. The cervix, often effaced before labour starts, dilates to form one continuous canal with the vagina when full dilation is reached. The membranes, if not ruptured artificially, often break with the first contractions of the second stage. The various stages are shown in Fig. 18.13.

Second stage

The passenger descends further as the contractions of the fundus become expulsive and the mother starts active pushing. Rotation of the head brings the smallest diameters into the pelvic outlet and the vertex appears at the vulva. Continued effort allows the head to glide over the perineum and be born. It is swiftly followed by the shoulders, which have turned in the pelvis to fit under the pubic arch, and the body is born.

Third stage

The great expulsive contractions of the end of the second stage greatly reduce the available space inside the uterus, and the placenta is forced off the uterine wall as the myometrium, emptied of its passenger, contracts right down. The membranes peel away from the decidua and slide down the birth canal, helped by the weight of the placenta. Labour is complete once the placenta and membranes are delivered, although a traditional 'fourth' stage includes inspection for possible tears, inspection of the placenta and membranes for completeness, and making the mother and baby comfortable for the first hour or so after birth.

Care in labour

The care described will use a hospital setting, since some 99% of all deliveries occur there and that will be where the student nurse gains her first experience of childbirth.

Assessment

In the time between being warned that a mother is coming in and her arrival in the delivery suite, a midwife has an opportunity to look at the notes.

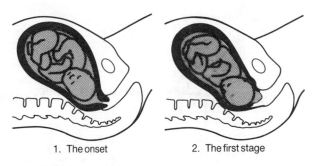

1. The onset   2. The first stage

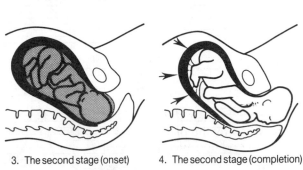

3. The second stage (onset)   4. The second stage (completion)

Fig. 18.13 *The process of labour: (1) The onset; (2) The first stage; (3) The second stage (onset); (4) The second stage (completion) (reproduced by kind permission of the Health Education Authority)*

This will give her some idea of the mother's background as well as vital information about this and previous pregnancies which could affect her management of labour. A birth plan makes the mother's expectations clear. With this information to hand the midwife welcomes the mother and her partner and makes an initial assessment of the situation. The mother is likely to be tense and anxious on her arrival in the delivery suite, even when well prepared, and a warm, open and friendly manner goes a long way towards relaxing her.

Some essential information is obtained, such as the time of the onset of contractions and whether the membranes have ruptured. During the conversation the midwife notes the effect that the contractions have on the mother. After the mother has passed urine, which is tested for signs of problems such as pre-eclampsia or dehydration, she is gently examined abdominally, just as she was in the antenatal clinic, and the fetal heart is auscultated. A CTG tracing is often done at this stage as it shows how the fetus is responding to contractions (Fig. 18.14).

A vaginal examination may complete the assess-

Normal trace — Ultrasound

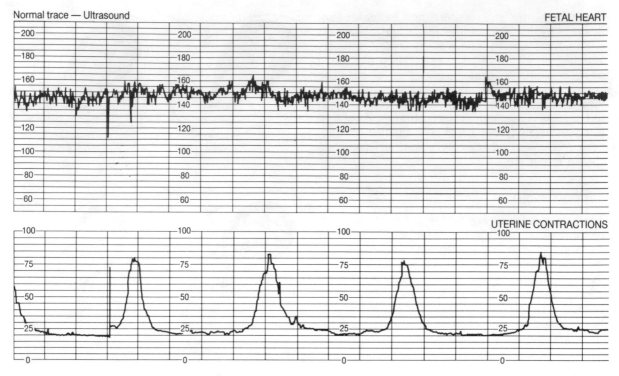

Fig. 18.14 Cardiotocograph tracing (CTG)

ment, in order to confirm the presentation and determine the dilation of the cervix. All findings are carefully recorded on the **partogram** in the notes, and the mother has their significance explained to her.

Planning

At this stage, if labour is neither too rapid nor too advanced, there is sufficient information for the midwife and mother to discuss the strategy for the management of labour. Major points to consider should include: *mobility* and the preferred position for delivery, *pain relief, nutrition* and *hydration, general comfort* (including bladder care), the *prevention of infection, fetal monitoring,* and the assessment of *progress.*

Mobility will depend on factors such as the choice of analgesia, the need for continuous monitoring, and the mother's preferences. To be free to wander around with her companion shortens the tedious hours of early labour and facilitates the descent of the fetus.

Pain relief is far too large a subject to be covered fully here. The level of pain experienced in labour varies widely and is affected by some of the many factors shown in Fig. 18.15. Antenatal education should have helped the mother form her ideas about her preferences for pain relief. The range of available methods can seem bewildering. Table 18.7 gives a list of possible techniques, the first three of which are in widespread use.

Pethidine is still the most commonly used analgesic in labour. A narcotic drug, given by intramuscular injections of doses from 50 mg-150 mg, it

Table 18.7. *Methods of pain relief in labour*

Pethidine

Entonox (NO_2 + O_2)

Epidural

TNS (transcutaneous nerve stimulation)

Psychoprophylaxis

Hypnosis

Acupuncture

Yoga

White sound

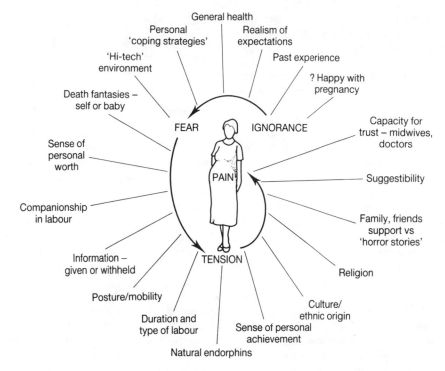

Fig. 18.15 *Factors influencing pain perception in labour*

is reasonably effective but fairly short acting as it starts wearing off after about two hours. The baby's respiratory centres may be affected, leaving him drowsy and floppy after birth, although an efficient antagonist, Narcan, is available. Some mothers experience nausea with pethidine and an anti-emetic is often given with it.

Entonox is the name of the apparatus which is used to deliver a self-administered mixture of nitrous oxide (NO_2) 50%, and oxygen (O_2) 50%. Breathed from the onset of the contractions, the gas can be quite effective in pain relief, especially for shorter labours. The gas is breathed off rapidly and has little or no effect on the baby.

Epidural analgesia has become widespread in recent years and is usually very effective. *Marcain* (*bupivacaine*) or a similar drug is injected via a fine catheter into the epidural space by a senior anaesthetist. The dose is 'topped up' by midwives when necessary. The legs become floppy and heavy and there is a tendency towards a sudden drop in blood pressure (*supine hypotensive syndrome*). If this occurs the mother must be turned on her side. The long, fine plastic catheter is removed after delivery.

Nutrition and hydration. Stomach emptying is notoriously inefficient in labour. As a result, and because the need for a general anaesthetic could arise in an emergency, most obstetric units avoid solid food once labour has started. Women are usually given sips of water only, with some form of antacid to reduce the effects of inhaled vomit, should this occur. Ketoacidosis is a real risk if dehydration occurs, with adverse effects on the fetus and the mother, but is unlikely where labour is not allowed to go on for too long and intravenous fluids are used.

General comfort (*including bladder care*). Labour can become messy and miserable if attention is not paid to small details such as adequate pillows, fresh linen, a damp flannel. A bath can be a great help and morale booster during the first stage. If the membranes are ruptured frequent changes of sanitary pad are necessary.

A full bladder is painful and inhibits contractions. It can be dangerous in the third stage as it may prevent the uterus from contracting efficiently, giving rise to bleeding. It is important to ensure that the bladder is emptied at regular and reasonably frequent intervals – not less than two-hourly, even if in late labour or with an epidural this means using a catheter.

Prevention of infection. Invasive techniques such as vaginal examination, epidural analgesia, application of fetal scalp electrode (FSE), or operative delivery present opportunities for infection and care must be taken to reduce this risk by keeping interventions to the strict minimum and scrupulously maintaining asepsis.

Fetal monitoring. The response of the fetus to the stress of labour may be monitored by simple auscultation with Pinard's stethoscope, Doppler effect equipment such as a sonic aid or CTG (mentioned above). Part of planning care is to determine whether monitoring should be continuous or intermittent, though some units require continuous monitoring as a matter of policy. The reassurance offered by the CTG tracing is invaluable where there is any question of the fetus being compromised but the machine has a terribly mesmerising effect and too easily becomes the focus of attention. The appearance of **meconium** in the liquor at any stage is a sign of fetal distress and needs investigation and action.

Assessment of progress. Because labour is a dynamic process it is important to evaluate progress regularly. Maternal and fetal well-being are constantly observed, with maternal blood pressure recorded at frequent intervals in the first and second stage. The mother's pulse and temperature are monitored on a regular basis, and an abdominal assessment of the length, strength and frequency of the contractions is made half-hourly. The clinical assessment is completed by a vaginal examination, at about four-hourly intervals, which will yield information about the state of the cervix and the descent of the head. When all this information is plotted on a partogram, it is possible to identify delay in the normal sequence of labour and plan action accordingly.

Implementation

The assessment and action plan described above establish the intervention which will be chosen by the midwife to ensure that labour continues as smoothly as possible.

Evaluation

Many midwives find it valuable to visit the mothers they have delivered a couple of days after the birth to discover how they feel about the experience.

Delivery

As the time for delivery draws near, levels of concentration in the labour room rise. The transition phase, between the end of the first stage and the onset of the second, is especially trying for the mother and she may need a lot of extra encouragement to get through it. Talking should be limited to the midwife's instructions guiding the mother through the birth of her baby. The partner, too, will help with encouragement and physical support.

Positions in labour

Although most births still take place in a well-supported semi-recumbent position, there is a growing use of alternatives, such as squatting and all fours, since they are known to increase the size of the pelvic outlet and uterine activity increases with an upright posture. Mothers and midwives need to have prepared for these well before delivery if they are to be successful. Birthing chairs also help the mother maintain a more favourable position for delivery, though she has less freedom of movement than in other positions. Water births have received a lot of publicity recently but there is insufficient research evidence as yet to establish their value. There is growing use of water as an alternative means of pain relief during the earlier part of labour, even where delivery is planned for 'dry land'.

The second stage

Once it is clear that the second stage has begun, and the mother feels the urge to push, she is helped to coordinate her breathing and muscular effort. The fetal heart is monitored, by CTG or with a Pinard's stethoscope, between each contraction. Although some deceleration of the heart rate is common with second stage contractions, there should be a swift return to normal each time.

The advancing head has to negotiate the sharp pelvic curve before appearing at the vulva. The perineal muscles stretch and thin, moving backwards to permit the head to be born. Occasionally the outlet has to be enlarged by a single incision into the perineum, an **episiotomy**, if the fetus shows signs of distress or the perineum is especially rigid.

The mother needs to be kept aware of her progress and some like to be able to see for themselves with a mirror. The last expulsive efforts as the head distends the vulva can be very frightening – she feels she is tearing apart and needs lots of reassurance to continue. The midwife meanwhile simply waits, watching the response of the perineum to the advancing head while keeping the anus covered with a soft pad, her hand lightly poised to control the head should the mother make a sudden expulsive effort. The surrounding area is protected with sterile towels and is maintained as clean as possible.

As *crowning* occurs, the widest part of the advancing head distending the vulva, the mother is encouraged to let the uterus do the rest of the work as she breathes rapidly in and out, allowing the fetal head to glide millimetre by millimetre over the perineum. As the face appears any excess mucus can be wiped away and the midwife feels round the neck for the umbilical cord. She may have to clamp and cut this before delivering the baby's trunk, or it may be sufficiently loose to slide over the shoulders as they are born. With the next contraction the shoulders rotate into the anteroposterior diameter of the pelvis and the anterior one is delivered first under the pubic arch. The baby's body curves upwards over its mother's abdomen as the rest of the body is born and warm dry towels protect the wet, slippery body from the cold. The mother can hold her baby securely while the next stage is completed – she is often so enthralled by the sight of her baby that she hardly notices as the placenta is delivered.

The third stage

It is common practice to give an oxytocic preparation, syntocinon or syntometrine, as the anterior shoulder is born. This causes a strong uterine contraction which separates the placenta from the uterine wall and prevents excessive bleeding. The midwife attempts to deliver the placenta with the first contraction after the baby's birth. Holding the uterus back with one hand behind the symphysis pubis she applies steady countertraction on the cord and the placenta and membranes are usually delivered within about five minutes. Some mothers prefer not to have the injection and wait for the slower, unaided natural processes of placental separation and descent to take place, in which case no attempt at cord traction is made.

Once the placenta and membranes are delivered the midwife checks that the uterus is firmly contracted and that there is no excess blood loss before examining them for completeness and measuring the blood loss, which is usually about 150–200 ml. Before leaving the mother to do this she will gently and rapidly inspect the vulva and vagina for tears. Damage to the area, whether it is a tear or an episiotomy, needs to be repaired as soon as possible, both for the mother's comfort and to improve chances of healing (Sleep, 1984).

Appearance of the placenta

At delivery, the placenta is about 20 cm wide and 2.5 cm thick in the middle. The maternal surface which has been adherent to the uterine decidua is dark red, fleshy and divided up into large lobes and smaller *cotyledons*, groupings of the chorionic tissue described above (page 485). These small cotyledons may get torn and left behind at delivery, so the midwife must examine the placenta carefully.

The fetal surface is covered by the other fetal membrane, the *amnion*. It is greyish and shiny and carries thick blood vessels to and from the umbilical cord – a twisted structure about 50 cm long carrying two arteries and one vein.

The membranes usually form a neat sac with a hole in it, if they are not ragged. Membrane fragments left in the uterus are as dangerous as cotyledons, giving rise to infection and haemorrhage if left unnoticed. This explains the importance of the examination of the placenta and membranes straight after delivery.

Immediate care after delivery – 'the fourth stage'

The first hour after delivery is unique for the baby and its parents and they need time together in peace, to begin to get used to each other. The baby is usually alert and responsive and if put to the breast will probably delight its parents by sucking strongly – the best start for a mother who plans to breastfeed.

The midwife will complete her delivery by

checking the mother's temperature, pulse and blood pressure. She will make sure the *lochia* (the discharges from the genital tract after delivery) are not abnormally heavy, for postpartum haemorrhage remains a possibility. The baby is usually weighed, measured, securely labelled and wrapped in clean linen at this stage. The couple can then be safely left with a cup of tea and a bell to call the midwife if they need her. She is free to check the placenta, clear and clean her trolley and complete the essential records of the delivery which include:

(1) The case notes, partogram and co-op card
(2) The birth register
(3) The Notification of Birth for the District Medical Officer.

Other documents will be required according to local policy.

Eventually the mother can turn her attention from the new baby and will feel, and look, a new woman after a 'wash and brush up' A clean nightdress, freshly brushed teeth and hair and an empty bladder work wonders for her comfort.

The midwife makes a final check to make sure the uterus is well contracted before transferring her to a postnatal ward with her baby. It is useful at this stage to remind her partner of visiting times and possibly how long she is likely to stay in hospital.

When things go wrong

A too-slow labour may exhaust both mother and baby. The fetus may become distressed or lie awkwardly in the pelvis. These and other causes require intervention by acceleration with oxytocic drugs or by operative delivery, forceps, vacuum extraction or lower segment caesarean section (LSCS). These labours not only need extra surveillance but the mothers, who may feel 'failures' because unable to have a normal delivery, will need a great deal of support and explanation before, during and after the event.

Emergency delivery

Emergency delivery can occur anywhere, anytime, in a crowded shop or on an open moor. Few situations call for such rapid improvisation and cool thinking. Emergency delivery happens rarely, but

when it does a nurse is expected to cope. The mother needs immediate help. Your ability to supply that help effectively will be a permanent source of pleasure and pride for her and you long after it is safely over.

A few straightforward principles sensibly applied should ensure a happy outcome (see Fig. 18.16).

- Stay with the mother – stay calm! Assess the situation rapidly

- Send for help – emergency obstetric unit. If alone – cope

- Co-opt bystanders (if any) to provide
  - warm cover for mother (coats, rugs)
  - clean wraps for delivery and baby
  - physical support and comfort
  - privacy

If no bystanders, do what you can, including wash hands

- <u>Let nature take its course: no interference</u>
Breathe with her as head emerges – no pushing
Keep delivery area clean
Talk her through it – she's probably terrified
One hand poised over the baby's head – no rapid expulsion
If the cord is round the neck – slip it up and over

- Deliver the baby into clean, dry wraps on mother's abdomen
Clear mucus from nose and mouth
Stimulate breathing if delayed
Discard wet wraps, replace with dry covers

- Leave the cord alone – don't cut or clamp it

- Do not attempt to deliver the placenta – just make sure the mother is not bleeding. If she loses more than two cupfuls of blood put the baby to her breast. The uterus will contract and the bleeding should stop

- If the placenta drops out, wrap it in a plastic bag

- Tell the mother how marvellous she is – keep her warm, but <u>no</u> hot sweet tea till after the obstetric team arrives

---

Fig. 18.16 *Principles for dealing with an emergency delivery*

Postnatal care

A new phase begins with the transfer of the mother and baby from the delivery suite to the postnatal ward. The long waiting, the careful preparation, the apprehension are all over. The dream has become reality and lies curled in its mother's arms or in the cot beside her. Labour, the great mental and physical hurdle, is safely over and the mother's relationships with her attendants are subtly altered. The time for close dependence is past and now she has to learn how to assume with confidence the new range of responsibilities and skills required by the arrival of her baby.

Patterns of care

The care of mother and baby should be carried out as one process. They are separated here only for the purposes of description.

The duration of stay in hospital varies from a few hours to more than a week according to the mother's needs and local policy. Her care in the first ten postnatal days is carried out by a midwife. This may be extended to 28 days if necessary. The community midwifery service is responsible for the mothers and babies once they are at home.

Wherever the newly delivered mother and her baby are looked after, the care follows a similar pattern. Its main objectives can be described as shown in Table 18.8.

Changes in the puerperlum

As with the antenatal period, good care is based on a knowledge of the physiological changes which

Table 18.8. *Postnatal care: the main objectives*

- Provision of adequate rest and nutrition to promote rapid recovery from labour
- Establishment of a satisfactory feeding pattern
- Education of the mother in essential baby care skills
- Development of mother/baby relationship
- Avoidance of infection, early identification of problems (for example, anaemia, breast engorgement)

occur. The early postnatal period is the beginning of the puerperium, the time when the genital organs return to their non-pregnant state. It usually lasts about six weeks. Unless a woman is fully breast-feeding, ovulation often occurs by the end of the six weeks, and the menstrual cycle resumes.

Involution is the name given to the reduction in size of the reproductive organs which happens in the days after delivery. Tissue atrophy and autolysis occur as hormone levels fall.

The uterus

The uterus weighs 1000 g at the end of labour and can be felt well contracted below the umbilicus. By the end of the first week it is scarcely palpable above the symphysis pubis and by six weeks it has returned to its non-pregnant size and weight, 60 g. This great change occurs because the uterus continues to contract and retract, reducing the blood supply to the decidua. This, together with transudate from the healing placental site, is passed from the genital tract as *lochia*. The lochia change in colour and quantity over the postnatal period, from a moderate fresh red blood loss immediately after delivery, through the brown or pinkish discharge of the fourth or fifth days, to the colourless discharge of the second week.

Other organs

The uterine tubes, the vagina and the vulva almost regain their original shape, size and position. The perineal muscles, even if damaged during delivery, can be helped back to normal tone by regular exercise.

Body systems

The body systems which underwent the changes described at the beginning of this chapter return to normal very quickly with the withdrawal of the high levels of placental hormones. The urinary tract may have been damaged at delivery and the mother can experience difficulty with micturition in the first couple of days. This is made worse by a naturally occurring diuresis as oestrogen levels fall and the circulating fluid volume finds its pre-pregnant level.

The digestive tract remains sluggish for a few days and, together with a painful perineum, may make constipation a problem. An increase in dietary fibre and fluids may be sufficient to overcome this, though many women need the initial help of suppositories on the third or fourth day.

Emotions

Sudden changes in hormone levels, sheer weariness, pain, the 'reality shock' of her new baby, filling breasts and broken sleep may all conspire to shake a woman's normal equilibrium and tears come easily on about the fourth day, often for no obvious reason. A kind, matter-of-fact approach, comfort, and some privacy are normally all that is needed to tide her over until she feels able to cope again.

The breasts

Breast changes associated with lactation are dealt with later in the section on infant feeding, but it is worth noting here that the whole issue of lactation can be a source of great anxiety and women need support and encouragement through the early experimental days of breastfeeding. Women who do not breastfeed may still experience considerable discomfort as their breasts fill about the third day after delivery and they will need advice about well-supporting brassières and analgesia until they settle.

Care in the puerperium

Given basic good health and sound emotional support, most women recover very quickly from the fatigue of late pregnancy and stress of labour. The midwife's care, at home or in hospital, is designed to ensure that the mother makes the necessary adjustments to her new role as smoothly as possible while her body returns to its non-pregnant state. A number of observations are made each day to make sure this is happening (see Table 18.9).

Hygiene, nutrition, rest and exercise, together with instruction in baby care, are the foundations of effective postnatal care.

Hygiene

The stretched and bruised birth canal provides an ideal site for infection, so personal hygiene is particularly important. Frequent baths, or showers with use of the bidet, and careful drying help keep the perineal area clean and promote healing if it

Table 18.9. *Care in the puerperium: observations*

General condition	Sleep, rest, mood, appetite, micturition and bowel activity
Breast and nipple state	Any soreness, flushing, tension
Uterine involution	Height of fundus
Lochia	Amount, colour
Perineal healing	Haemorrhoids
Legs	Oedema, tenderness, varicosities

Temperature and pulse are recorded twice daily for the first three days, once daily thereafter

has been damaged. Sanitary pads need frequent changing and tactful reminders about the importance of handwashing in the prevention of cross-infection may be in order.

Nutrition

Nutrition is particularly important if the mother is breastfeeding, though all women will need a high protein diet after the energy expended in labour. The quality of the food is important for the healing of tissues and for milk production. A third-day haemoglobin check will identify any anaemia, which can be corrected by oral iron supplements. A high fibre diet will help early constipation and the old wives' tales warning new mothers not to eat fruit can be ignored – as long as it is not eaten to excess.

Rest and exercise

Rest and exercise have to be nicely balanced. Rest is hard to achieve in the average postnatal ward and staff need to be alert to signs of strain or the results of being over-visited. Physiotherapists are rare now on postnatal wards, but simple exercise sheets and a few words of encouragement and explanation from staff as they carry out the daily care will help those mothers who are keen to get back into shape again as soon as they can. Pelvic floor exercises are simple, not too strenuous, and can be practised anywhere, at any time, to restore muscle tone as soon as possible.

Baby care instruction includes daily care and

feeding preparation and is dealt with in the next section.

Care of particular mothers may include giving an injection of Anti-D antibodies or rubella vaccination.

Anti-D antibodies

Mothers with a Rhesus negative blood group carrying a Rhesus positive baby are at risk of forming antibodies which could destroy the red blood cells of any subsequent Rhesus positive baby. An injection of Anti-D immunoglobulin is given to Rhesus negative mothers soon after delivery to neutralise the effect of any fetal D antigen which may have entered the mother's circulation during delivery.

Rubella vaccine

The rubella virus can cross the placenta and cause serious fetal abnormalities if the disease is contracted in pregnancy. Schoolgirls are offered protection and currently about 86% accept. Mothers who are found to be non-immune to the virus during their pregnancy are offered the injection after delivery. They are advised not to become pregnant for at least three months after the injection because of the risk of fetal damage.

Problems

Three of the more serious problems of the puerperium are:

(1) *Infection* – this can be localised in the breasts, the urinary tract or uterus, or it can be systemic. Infection requires early identification and treatment. In the uterus it may be due to retained products of conception which require evacuation under general anaesthetic
(2) *Postpartum haemorrhage* (PPH) has similar causes and needs urgent action
(3) *Clot formation* is a post-delivery hazard, especially where there has been an operative delivery. Early mobilisation has reduced this risk considerably.

Discharge

Midwives have a statutory obligation to care for a woman and her baby for ten days after delivery. This duty may be extended to 28 days if it seems appropriate. Responsibility is then transferred to the health visitor, who has a statutory duty towards all children under five.

Before discharging a mother, the midwife (in addition to her usual observations) will discuss the mother's arrangements for family planning and if she wishes it, will advise her about alternatives suitable for use in the puerperium. Women vary greatly in their approach to resuming sexual intercourse after delivery and individuals may want or need to discuss this. Once perineal healing is complete intercourse can take place, but some women may prefer to wait longer and need to be encouraged to talk about this with their partners.

The address of the Child Health Clinic and a reminder about immunisation programmes available for the baby are left, together with a phone number to use in case of an emergency.

The mother is asked to visit her GP, for a postnatal check up, six weeks after delivery. He will make sure her body has returned to normal and that she is coping happily with her new responsibilities. He may take a cervical smear and, if she wishes, fit an intra-uterine contraceptive device (IUCD) at this visit.

New mothers can feel terribly isolated and lonely. Local support groups have grown up in many areas and provide the companionship which might otherwise be lacking. Many midwives keep a list of such local groups to offer their newly delivered mothers.

The baby

Birth brings about dramatic changes in the baby's environment. Noise, space, light, touch are all qualitatively different from the life of the womb. The 'life-support' system of umbilical cord and placenta is literally cut off and immediate, radical adjustments have to be made if the baby is to make the transition safely into the outside world. Happily the vast majority adjust swiftly and successfully. The midwife and (where trouble is anticipated) the paediatrician are there to help when there is any delay in making these adjustments.

First needs

The baby's immediate needs include:

(1) *A clear airway*: before his lungs expand with his first gasp he may need mucus removed from his nasopharynx with a soft catheter before he can breathe comfortably
(2) *Warmth*: there is a 17°C drop in temperature between the inside of the uterus and the average delivery suite. A newborn baby is wet, has a poorly developed heat-regulating centre, a large skin surface to body mass ratio, and loses heat very fast unless he is dried and wrapped immediately. Snug against his mother's abdomen, covered with warm dry towels he will maintain his temperature. Any baby who needs help to start breathing needs special care taken to keep him warm during resuscitation measures
(3) *Security/love*: although recent studies have questioned the theoretical bases for the bonding process described by Klaus and Kennell (1976), humanity and common sense would seem to indicate that usually the best place for a baby to come to terms with its new environment is in its mother's arms as soon as possible. One of the most marvellous moments in midwifery happens when the fuss of delivery is over and one sees the baby gazing wide-eyed at its equally wide-eyed parents.

Immediate care: the Apgar score

The baby's condition at birth determines any special care he may need straight away. This is usually assessed by use of the Apgar score. Midwives evaluate the baby's condition at one minute and five minutes after delivery – by which time most babies are pink and vigorous, scoring 10/10. The score, which uses five criteria, is shown in Table 18.10.

Cord clamping and division

The cord may be clamped before or after it stops pulsating. If it is left to stop beating the baby will receive a few extra ml of blood from the placenta. Initially the cord is usually clamped and cut between two steel artery forceps. Later, when the baby is being weighed and identified a plastic clamp is fixed firmly a couple of centimetres from

Table 18.10. *Apgar scoring system*

Sign	0	1	2
Heart rate	Absent	Slow — below 100	Over 100
Respiratory effort	Absent	Weak cry Gasping	Good cry
Muscle tone	Limp	Some flexion	Well flexed Active
Reflex irritability	No response	Some response Grimace	Good response Cry, cough
Colour	Blue/pale	Body pink Extremities blue	Pink

the abdominal wall. This remains in place for 36 hours until there is no risk of haemorrhage from the cord stump and is then removed with special clamp cutters. The cord stump should be checked regularly in the first hours after delivery to ensure there is no blood loss.

Once the mother is comfortable after delivery the midwife will complete the first examination in front of her where she can watch and learn about her baby.

Observations

The baby is weighed. Normal, **term** babies weigh about 3200–3500 g. Two people usually check the delivery weight to safeguard against errors.

In many units the baby's temperature is taken and recorded at this stage.

Identification

There are various systems in use for identifying new babies. The most common seems to be a double plastic bracelet for wrist and ankle, though babies are adept at slipping out of them. These bracelets may be paired with one on the mother's wrist, with the same name and identification number. She should be invited to check these for accuracy with the midwife before they are fixed on the baby. Cot labels are used, with extra details of delivery and the baby's weight. Such precautions may seem excessive but mix-ups occur periodically, with enormous distress to all concerned, so it pays to check that babies are clearly identified at all times.

Examination

A systematic but swift examination is made at this stage. Its purpose is to identify any external abnormalities so that action can be taken as soon as possible. It also reassures the vast majority of parents whose babies are found to be flawless. A first impression of the baby's well-being has been obtained from the Apgar score. This is now amplified by checking visually and by palpation (see Table 18.11).

Table 18.11. *Physical examination of the newborn*

Weight and temperature	Recorded
The head	Sutures, fontanelles, both eyes and the baby's mouth — this to exclude defects in the palate or even, occasionally, teeth.
The neck, trunk and arms	A special check is made on the number and formation of digits and palmar creases
The abdomen and genitalia	For any obvious abnormalities
The lower limbs and feet	Again, attention is paid to the number and formation of toes and correct position of the feet. Inward curving talipes equino varus may be positional and temporary or, occasionally, need orthopaedic correction
The back and spinal column	To exclude occult spina bifida
The anus	Patency is ascertained
Measurement	The head circumference (35cm) and length (50cm) are checked and recorded
Urine and meconium	A note is made if these are observed in the delivery suite

Vitamin K (konakion)

Because babies metabolise inadequate amounts of vitamin K at birth, an injection of synthetic vitamin K is commonly given to protect them from haemorrhagic disease.

Screening tests

The initial examination may be complemented by a number of subsequent tests to detect problems in the new baby. The two most common are for *congenital dislocation of the hip* and a hereditary condition called *phenylketonuria*.

(1) *Congenital dislocation of the hip* can be identified by the midwife or paediatrician as they use Barlow's or Ortolani's test to examine the baby. If the head of the femur is found to be displaced, initial management may include the use of double nappies or a splint to maintain the thighs abducted. The orthopaedic surgeons usually assume responsibility for care of these babies.

(2) *Phenylketonuria* is an inborn protein metabolism defect which affects one in about 10,000 babies. Milk feeding results in dangerously high levels of the amino acid *phenylalanine* in the blood. Although the condition is entirely treatable by suitable diet, severe brain damage occurs if it remains undetected. Screening by use of a heel-prick blood sample for the Guthrie or Scriver test is therefore offered for all new babies on the sixth or seventh day of life, after a couple of days or more of milk feeding.

Understandably, the mother will be concerned about everything that is done to her baby and a clear, straightforward explanation of why these and other tests are offered will reduce her anxiety and should precede any intervention undertaken by the staff.

Teaching baby care

As soon as the mother feels well enough she should be encouraged to take on the care of her baby. The midwife will, however, check the baby each day to make sure all is well. By her own attitude she can teach the inexperienced mother how to talk to her baby and play with him as he is cared for, even though at first she may not recognise the baby's response. Recent research has extended our knowledge of a newborn's perceptual skills and mothers are often excited to discover for themselves how much their babies are aware of.

Keeping the baby clean, comfortable, well fed and loved responds to his basic needs, as does the initial care described above. The principles established at delivery continue, with special attention to the need for hygiene and the prevention of infection where there are several babies and many attendants. Individual equipment and care by the mother reduce infection.

Hygiene

Daily care is directed at keeping the baby's fine skin clean and in good condition. Bathing policies vary at different units, but mothers need to be taught how to handle their babies when bathing them. Very few babies ever seem to get dropped but mothers as well as student nurses seem to think they will let the baby slip.

Bathing is not necessary every day. A thorough daily toilet is adequate, checking and cleaning the face and body creases, especially the napkin area, which may need protection with vaseline from sticky meconium in the first day or two.

Water should be used to wash the buttocks at each napkin change.

The eyes are left untouched unless they are moist, when a soft wool swab in boiled water (that has cooled) or saline will often be sufficient. The nostrils and ears should not be probed either.

The cord stump

Mothers often dislike having to care for the cord and are relieved when the stump falls off after about 5–7 days. The stump is kept clean and dry with a spirit swab each time the napkin is changed. A bacteriostatic powder is used once a day in some units. Any moistness or offensive smell must be reported and investigated immediately. Further research is needed to determine the most affective type of cord care (Salariya and Kowbus, 1988).

Midwife's observations

During the daily care the midwife is attentive to changes in the baby's condition, his temperature, colour, muscle tone and skin condition. She looks in his mouth to make sure there are no signs of *candida* (thrush, monilia) and makes sure the eyes show no signs of infection. Nail beds and dry, flaking creases are other possible sites of infection.

The baby's stools

The midwife will teach the mother about the changes she can expect in her baby's stools. The dark green sticky mass of meconium gives way to a lighter, still sticky, rather greeny-brown stool at about 24–36 hours and is followed by the bright, thin, mustard grainy stool of breast feeding or the darker yellow, more substantial stool of artificial feeding. Stool patterns in breast-fed babies can vary enormously and mothers need to be reassured that this is quite normal.

Weight

After an initial weight loss most babies regain their birthweight by the end of the first week of life. In most units they are weighed every three or four days.

Sleep

After a time of post-delivery alertness babies often sleep for long periods for the first day or so. After that the pattern may be very erratic for three or four days until they establish their own rhythm – which rarely seems to coincide with their parents' sleep patterns.

Crying

Crying can be a source of great stress and anxiety, though mothers learn quickly the different sounds of hunger, discomfort, pain or simple boredom.

Baby care: some problems

During the days after delivery a number of common problems can arise. They rarely become serious if spotted and treated early and it is important to explain this to the mothers.

Caput succedaneum and cephalhaematoma

These are both the direct result of labour on the soft, unfused bones of the baby's skull (Fig. 18.17). *Caput succedaneum* is a simple oedematous swelling on the baby's scalp. It is present at birth but disappears within 24 hours. *Cephalhaematoma* appears later, usually as a result of a difficult labour. Bleeding below the periosteum of the soft skull bones causes a raised swelling. Though it may sometimes be bilateral it does not cross the

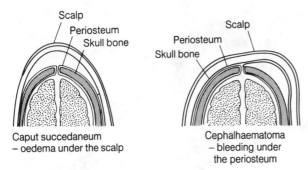

Scalp
Periosteum
Skull bone

Scalp
Periosteum
Skull bone

Caput succedaneum
– oedema under the scalp

Cephalhaematoma
– bleeding under
the periosteum

Fig. 18.17 *Caput succedaneum and cephalhaematoma*

suture lines, as it is contained by the periosteum. It may take a few weeks to subside.

Jaundice

Babies are born with an excess of red blood cells and a fairly immature enzyme system. This combination means that bilirubin from the superfluous red blood cells is not cleared quickly from the system. It appears as a yellow tinge to the skin and conjunctiva. Phototherapy treatment breaks down the toxic fat-soluble bilirubin into water-soluble bilirubin which can be excreted by the gut and kidneys. This avoids the risk of brain damage resulting from *kernicterus* (yellow staining of the basal brain cells). While under the light, the babies have their eyes covered for protection. They need extra fluids and may well develop runny stools. Physiological jaundice reaches a peak on about the fifth day and has faded by the end of the first week.

Other, more serious forms of jaundice result from Rhesus incompatibility, infection or bile duct obstruction.

Sticky eyes

Sticky eyes are a common response to the dust of open wards. A purulent discharge signifies the serious condition of *ophthalmia neonatorum*, which is usually the result of infection from the vagina by organisms such as the gonococcus or chlamydia. This needs urgent, vigorous treatment to avoid permanent damage to the baby's eyes.

Infant feeding

The choice of feeding method is usually made well before birth and, not surprisingly, family influences have been found to be more persuasive than professional ones in the choice between artificial and breastfeeding (Thomson, 1989). A number of mothers will switch to artificial feeding after a few days, unsure of their ability to breastfeed successfully and sometimes discouraged by the difficulties of the early days, especially where there is insufficient support available.

Whichever way a mother chooses to feed her baby, she needs to feel happy about her choice and confident that she can cope with its demands. It is important not to overstep the mark between encouragement of breastfeeding and propaganda which could make non-breastfeeding mothers feel second rate.

Whichever way a baby is fed, a number of basic principles well grasped will make it a good experience for the baby. Most people enjoy their food and babies, on the whole, are no exception. Few of us would appreciate being shaken awake and presented with a meal when we are not hungry but sleepy. Hospitals have recognised this, after years of rigid four-hourly feeding routines, and now most babies except the very small and ill are fed when they are awake and hungry. This is usually at more frequent intervals in breastfed babies.

A baby should be dry and comfortable for his feed and held close to his mother's body where he feels secure. In the first 24 hours he may vomit some mucus and even refuse feeds, but once the stomach has been cleared of mucus he normally accepts and retains feeds happily. Each baby has his rhythm for feeding and the greedier 'gulping' ones will need more frequent breaks in feeding to rest and bring up wind they have swallowed.

Breastfeeding

Cleanliness, convenience, relative cheapness, the transmission of antibodies and important trace elements, and the most appropriate nutritional balance for babies are among the many advantages claimed for breastfeeding. On the negative side some women find it repugnant, inconvenient, too tying, and dislike not knowing how much the baby gets at each feed. Some fathers dislike the idea as well.

Only the essentials of breastfeeding can be described here and the student is recommended to any of the many good texts available to deepen her knowledge. A warm, unhurried and encouraging approach is as important as knowledge of physiology in successful establishment of lactation in first-time mothers. The influence of emotional well-being on the mother's ability to feed her baby is well documented. Tension, pain or anxiety — from whatever source — effectively inhibit the milk flow or 'let down reflex'. It follows that time spent making the mother more at ease is likely to be rewarded by her pleasure and boosted confidence in her improved ability to feed her baby.

The structures and process of lactation

The breasts enlarge in pregnancy and milk-producing glandular tissue is laid down. The structure of the breast is shown in Fig. 18.18. A series of ducts leads back from the nipple and its surrounding areolar tissue into the lobes and lobules where, under the influence of prolactin from the anterior pituitary gland, clusters of grape-like alveoli are squeezed by the web-like myoepithelial cells which surround them. These contract under the influence of oxytocin, secreted by the hypothalamus and released from the posterior pituitary, but stimulated by the act of suckling.

Since milk production is a supply-and-demand circuit, it is important that the demand be started as soon as possible after delivery and repeated frequently to maintain the stimulus. The neuro-hormonal reflex arc is shown in Fig. 18.19.

Practical considerations

Once progesterone and oestrogen levels drop after delivery, prolactin levels rise and colostrum, the high protein yellowish clear fluid secreted during pregnancy, is replaced by milk on about the second or third day. Painful **engorgement** of the breasts associated with the onset of lactation can be considerably reduced by early and frequent suckling. The full, tense breasts of the fourth and fifth days need the support of a well-cut brassière and the comfort of a warm bath, perhaps even a mild analgesic. Careful positioning of the baby from the first feed will help reduce the incidence of sore nipples and improve the milk flow (Fisher, 1987). The baby needs to be well supported with his chest close to his mother's, his face reaching up to the nipple so that his chin is firmly under the areolar tissue while he is sucking. This will not be possible if he is swaddled in layers of blanket with his arms across his chest.

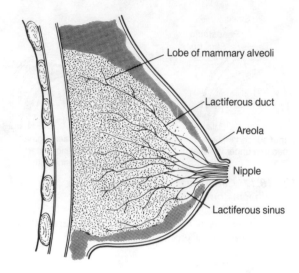

Fig. 18.18 *The structure of the breast — cross-section*

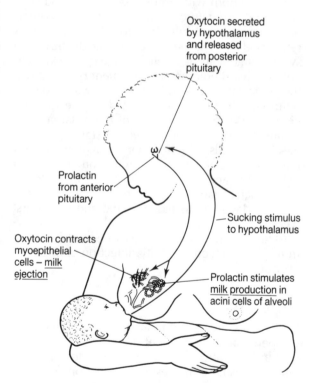

Fig. 18.19 *The neurohormonal arc of lactation*

Babies seem to learn very quickly, but the first few feeds are necessarily experimental. For some babies and their mothers the whole thing goes marvellously well from the beginning. The vast majority need more time and lots of patience before the art of breastfeeding is mastered to their mutual satisfaction.

One of the most rewarding sights of postnatal care is that of a mother contentedly nursing her baby just a couple of days after the whole thing had seemed so messy, painful and complicated that she nearly gave up.

Artificial feeding

Whether or not a mother plans to use artificial milk to feed her baby, she should know how to make up a feed and how to store feeding utensils safely at home. She may always need to use a bottle in an emergency – or she may simply wish to offer a drink of water. Ward staff need to make sure that all mothers have a chance to learn about preparing feeds before they go home. This is especially important now that most hospitals use pre-packed milk in bottles, for mothers have no opportunity to watch the mixing of feeds unless teaching sessions are provided.

The midwife can advise on the choice of feed from the many modified cows' milk formulae available. All of them are now near to human milk in composition although, obviously, they cannot offer the living components such as the high levels of antibodies (see Table 18.12).

Table 18.12. Constituents of milk

	Colostrum	Human milk	Cows' milk
Protein	8.0%	1.5%	3.5%
Carbohydrate	3.5%	7.0%	4.5%
Fat	2.5%	3.5%	3.5%
Minerals	0.4%	0.2%	0.75%
Water	85.6%	87.8%	87.75%

Preparation of bottle feeds

Every packet of milk has detailed instructions for feed preparation printed on it, but it should not be assumed that all mothers can read or understand them. In today's hospitals, for example, many mothers may come from non-English-speaking countries. A clearly demonstrated routine will permit her to learn by observation and, eventually, practice.

Cleanliness and correct proportions are the two

Table 18.13. A step-by-step procedure for preparing feeds

- Boil kettle, allow to cool
- Clean working surface, wash hands, collect sterile bottle, teat, cap and cover, powder measure
- Fill bottle with required amount of cooled boiled water (for example, 120ml)
- Add requisite number of scoops of powder (for example, four scoops levelled off but not packed down)
- Cap the bottle well and shake
- Test for temperature with a drop on your wrist before feeding

most important principles to be underlined in teaching feed preparation. A step-by-step procedure is outlined in Table 18.13.

Feeds can be made in a jug for a period of not more than 24 hours if they can be stored in a refrigerator. They are best kept in the feeding bottles filled with the required amount. These just need warming back to body temperature before feeding the baby.

After feeding or preparing feeds, all equipment must be carefully washed and rinsed. Teats should be turned inside-out under a running tap to make sure no curds are left.

Clean equipment is stored in a plastic container containing a proprietary hypochlorite solution such as Milton which must be renewed each day. Only glass or plastic utensils should be kept in the tank, since metals are corroded by hypochlorites.

In a real emergency feeding bottles and teats can be boiled, but this can prove inconvenient as a long term measure.

Feeding

Babies fed by bottle need to be held as closely as breastfed babies have to be. Many fathers enjoy the opportunity to share feeding their babies. Mothers should be shown how to hold the bottle so that the teat is always full of milk, to avoid the baby swallowing air.

After any feed a baby should be winded and then tucked down on his front or on his side to sleep, to avoid the risk of asphyxiation from inhaled milk if he vomits or regurgitates.

For the first day or so after delivery babies need only small quantities of feed, but by the end of the first week they will need about 150 ml per kilo of baby weight per day.

Born too soon, born too small, born unwell

Special Care Baby Units (SCBU) exist in most major maternity units and many also have neonatal intensive care units (NICU) for babies who need ventilation.

Many simply small babies who used to be cared for in SCBU are now nursed next to their mothers in the postnatal wards. This overcomes the major disadvantage of the SCBU, separation of mother and baby. It brings its own problems of ensuring adequate rest for an anxious mother, warmth and safety from infection for a specially vulnerable new baby, and proper supervision if the ward is busy. 'Transitional care wards' seem to provide a helpful answer in many units, where special care staff retain responsibility for, or at least close liaison with, the ward.

In the SCBU itself there is limited accommodation for parents, who may have long journeys from home. Staff try to involve them as much as possible in the care of their babies, although the sight of a 650 g tiny baby of 26 weeks gestation being ventilated is daunting to most nurses, and terrifying to the baby's parents.

The maternity care course student may be able to visit the unit and will probably stop, fascinated, not just by the tinies in the nursery but by the display of 'before and after' pictures which is often posted at the entrance. How such miniscule babies ever grow into tearaway toddlers may seem a mystery, but it is consoling evidence to many parents waiting anxiously for their own newborn to find the strength to breathe on his own.

Mothers in the postnatal wards who have babies in the SCBU are conspicuous by the lack of a cot beside them. When they are not beside the incubator in the SCBU they are usually grateful for a chance to talk to a sympathetic student about their frail new baby who carries such a weight of hope and fear.

When pregnancy fails

Sadly, pregnancy does not always result in the birth of a live healthy baby. Spontaneous abortion (miscarriage), fetal abnormality leading to a choice of voluntary termination of pregnancy (VTOP), stillbirth or severe neonatal abnormality can all ruin the dreams of a couple who embark on pregnancy.

Each of these conditions means grief and loss and possibly death. Midwifery unit staff are trained to help couples living through the devastation brought by these situations. It is unlikely that maternity care course students will have much direct contact with such bereaved parents. Nonetheless, it is common enough to have a woman at booking clinic admit to one or more such events in her life. They should *not* be noted for their clinical relevance and then glossed over, for surprisingly often one finds that this is the first time the woman has had the chance to talk her grief through with a professional. It is important to take time to listen, not least because her attitudes to the new pregnancy may be strongly coloured by the bad experience.

Where fetal abnormality (for example spina bifida or congenital heart disease) has occurred, and where there is a history of hereditary disease (such as Duchenne muscular dystrophy), professional genetic counselling services are available – usually at a regional centre, where there are facilities for full investigation and special tests such as prenatal echocardiography.

Conclusions

The maternity care course is short, and very different from any other experience the student meets in training. Nonetheless, it is often the course that students remember most vividly, partly because many of them can identify easily with the young mothers they care for. The students should finish the course confident that they understand better the needs and hopes of the mothers, have some appreciation of the problems facing young parents and the processes of childbearing and can offer simple, straightforward, advice to women who may approach them for help in the future.

Students should also be aware of the changing state of midwifery, where efforts are increasing to make partnership in care a more genuine reality and client choice a factor which shapes service provision. A critical view of the social and political determinants which provide the setting for maternity care should enable students to react with greater insight and sensitivity to the situations of pregnant women and their families.

Glossary

Acrosome: Head of spermatozoon

Amenorrhoea: Absence of menstruation

Biparietal diameter: The distance between the salient points on the parietal bones of the skull – about 9.5 cm in a term baby

Blastocyst: The hollow ball of cells formed by the *conceptus* (see below) during the pre-embryonic stage of development

Cardiotocograph (CTG): An electronic monitoring device displaying fetal heart and uterine muscle activity

Chromosome: Thread-like strands of cell nucleus carrying genetic material

Colostrum: A fluid material precursor of milk found in the breasts in pregnancy and for the first couple of days after delivery

Conceptus: The complete products of conception

Corpus luteum: Remnants of the ruptured Graafian follicle

Decidua: The lining of the uterus during pregnancy

Embryo: The developing conceptus from 21 days till the eighth week of pregnancy

Engagement (of the presenting part): Said to occur when the widest presenting diameters have passed through the pelvic brim

Engorgement: Painful swelling and tension in the breasts due to overfilling of veins and lymphatics

Epidural: The name given to a form of local analgesia administered into the epidural space of the spinal column

Episiotomy: A surgical incision of the perineum which enlarges the vulval opening

Fertilisation: The fusion of sperm and ovum to form the zygote

Fetus: The developing embryo after the eighth week of pregnancy until delivery

Gestation: Pregnancy

Implantation: Embedding of the blastocyst in the decidua

Meconium: The contents of the fetal intestinal tract, the first stool

Meiosis: A form of cell division peculiar to reproductive cells (gametes) resulting in a reduction in the number of chromosomes present (see also Chapter 6)

Morula: The clump of cells formed by the developing zygote

Ovulation: Release of the ovum from the ruptured Graafian follicle

Oxytocin: A drug which causes the uterus to contract

Partogram: A chart displaying the progress of labour

Puerperium: The period of time after delivery during which the genital tract returns to its non-pregnant state

Sickle cell anaemia (disease or trait): An inherited blood condition of people of mainly negroid origin, which may result in severe anaemia

Striae gravidarum: Stretch marks under the skin caused by pregnancy

Term: Used to described the maturity of a baby born within two weeks either side of its expected date of delivery

Trophoblast: The outer layer of cells of the developing conceptus

Ultrasound: The use of high frequency sound waves to transmit an image of tissue surfaces onto a screen

Zygote: The fertilised ovum

References

Ahmed, G. and Watt, S. (1986). Understanding Asian women in pregnancy and confinement. *Midwives Chronicle*, 99, 98–101.

Black, T. (1985). Smoking in pregnancy revisited. *Midwifery*, 1, 135–145.

Davies, J. and Evans, F. (1990). Care in the community. In *Midwifery: Excellence in Nursing, The Research Route*, Faulkner, A. and Murphy-Black, T. (eds.). Scutari, London.

Ermisch, J. (1990). *Fewer Babies, Longer Lives*. Joseph Rowntree Foundation, York.

European Collaborative Study. (1991). Children born to

women with HIV-1 infection; natural history and risk of transmission. *Lancet*, 337, 253–260.

Evans, G. and Parker, P. (1985). Preparing teenagers for pregnancy. *Midwives Chronicle*, 98, 239–240.

Field, P.A. (1990). Effectiveness and efficacy of antenatal care. *Midwifery*, 6, 215–223.

Fisher, C. (1987). Breast feeding. *Journal of Maternal and Child Health*, 6, 52–57.

Flint, C. and Poulengeris, P. (1987). *The Know Your Midwife Report*. Published by the authors and available from 49 Peckarmans Wood, London SE26 6RZ.

Jackson, B. (1984). *Fatherhood*. Allen and Unwin, London.

Klaus, M.H. and Kennell, J.H. (1976). *Maternal-Infant Bonding: the Impact of Early Separation or Loss on Family Development*. Mosby, St Louis.

Kroll, D. (1986). Heroin addiction in pregnancy. *Midwives Chronicle*, 99, 153–157.

Macintyre, S. (1984). Consumer reaction to present day antenatal services. In *Pregnancy Care for the 80s*, Zander, L. and Chamberlain, G. (eds.). RSM and Macmillan Press, London.

Methven, R. (1982). The antenatal booking interview: recording an obstetric history or relating to a mother-to-be? *Proceedings of Research and the Midwife Conference*, 63–76, available through the Royal College of Midwives, London.

Montgomery, E. (1990). Iron levels in pregnancy – physiology or pathology? Assessing the need for supplements. *Midwifery*, 6, 205–214.

Oakley, A. (1989). Who cares for women? Science versus love in midwifery today. *Midwives Chronicle*, 102, 214–220.

Oakley, A. and Houd, S. (eds.). (1990). *Helpers in Childbirth: Midwifery Today*. Hemisphere Publishing Corporation, New York.

Office of Population Censuses and Surveys. (1990). *Birth Statistics: Review of the Registrar General on Births and Patterns of Family Building in England and Wales, 1988*. OPCS, London.

Pinching, A.J. (1987). HIV, AIDS and pregnancy. *Journal of Maternal and Child Health*, 12, 146–150.

Plant, M.L. (1986). Drinking in pregnancy and fetal harm: results from a Scottish prospective study. *Midwifery*, 2, 81–85.

Robinson, S., Golden, J. and Bradley, S. (1983). *A Study of the Role and Responsibility of the Midwife*. NERU, Chelsea College, London.

Rossett, H.L., Weiner, L. and Lee, A. (1983). Patterns of alcohol consumption and fetal development. *Journal of the Americal College of Obstetrics and Gynecology*, 61(5), 539–546.

Salariya, A.M. and Kowbus, N.M. (1988). Variable umbilical cord care. *Midwifery*, 4, 73–79.

Sleep, J. (1984). Episiotomy in normal delivery – management of the perineum. *Nursing Times*, 80(48), 51–54.

Tew, M. (1990). *Safer Childbirth? A Critical History of Maternity Care*. Chapman and Hall, London.

Thomson, A.M. (1989). Why don't women breastfeed? In *Midwives, Research and Childbirth, Vol. 1*. Robinson, S. and Thomson, A.M. (eds.). Chapman and Hall, London.

Further reading

Alexander, J., Levy, V. and Roch, S. (1990). *Midwifery Practice Series – Antenatal, Intrapartum and Postnatal Care* (3 vols.). Macmillan, London.

Bennett, V.R. and Brown, L.K. (1989). *Myles Textbook for Midwives*. Churchill Livingstone, Edinburgh.

Bryan, E.M. (1983). *The Nature and Nurture of Twins*. Baillière Tindall, Eastbourne.

Cartwright, A. (1979). *The Dignity of Labour*. Tavistock Publications, London.

Chamberlain, G. (1984). *Pregnant Women at Work*. RSM and Macmillan Press, London.

Enkin, M., Keirse, M. and Chalmers, I. (1989). *A Guide to Effective Care in Pregnancy and Childbirth*. Oxford University Press, Oxford.

Garcia, J., Kilpatrick, R. and Richards, M. (1990). *The Politics of Maternity Care. Services for Childbearing Women in Twentieth Century Britain*. Clarendon Press, Oxford.

Green, J.M. (1990). Prenatal screening and diagnosis; some psychological and social issues. *British Journal of Obstetrics and Gynaecology*, 97(12), 1074–1076.

Inch, S. (1988). *Birthrights*. Hutchinson, London.

Leboyer, F. (1976). *Birth without Violence*, Wildwood House Ltd., London.

Nilsson, L. (1984). *A Child is Born*. Faber, London.

Oakley, A. (1979). *Becoming a Mother*. Martin Robertson, London.

Odent, M. (1985). *Entering the World – the Demedicalisation of Childbirth*. Penguin Books, Harmondsworth.

Panos Institute. (1990). *Triple Jeopardy: Women and AIDS*. Panos Publications, London.

Royal College of Midwives. (1991). *Successful Breastfeeding* (2nd ed.). Churchill Livingstone, Edinburgh.

Royal College of Midwives. (1991). *Towards a Healthy Nation* (2nd ed.). RCM, London.

Towler, J. and Bramall, J. (1986). *Midwives in History and Society*. Croom Helm, London.

World Health Organisation. (1986). *Birth in Europe*. Public Health in Europe 26. WHO, Copenhagen.

Useful addresses

National Childbirth Trust
Alexandra House, Oldham Terrace, Acton, London W3 6NH.

La Leche League
(Breastfeeding help and information)
BM 3424, London WC1V 6XX.

Health Education Authority
(Health promotion)
78 New Oxford Street, London WC1A 1AY.

Stillbirth and Neonatal Death Society (SANDS)
28 Portland Place, London W1N 4DE.

Twins and Multiple Births Association (TAMBA)
59 Sunnyside, Worksop, Nottinghamshire, S81 7LN.

Gingerbread
(Support for single parents)
35 Wellington Street, London WC2E 7BN.

CRY-SIS
(Support for mothers with crying/sleepless babies)
BM Cry-sis, London WC1 3XX.

MIDIRS
(Midwives Information and Resource Service)
Institute of Child Health, Royal Hospital for Sick Children, St Michaels Hill, Bristol, BS2 8BJ.

The Royal College of Midwives
15 Mansfield Street, London W1M 0BE.

19

THE CARE OF CHILDREN

Sally Glen and Janice Colson

This chapter focuses on issues central to child health which is interpreted as a positive state of well-being in the child. It sets out to explore the changing nature both of health problems in children and their families, and of health care.

The chapter differs from others in that it is divided into three distinct sections:

(1) The family
(2) Child development
(3) Nursing processes in health promotion.

Each section is presented complete with its own references section and expanded glossary. Suggestions for further reading, however, are listed at the end of the complete chapter.

Throughout the chapter, the child is referred to in the female gender, unless this is clearly inappropriate.

The discussion of child health is complicated by the fact that we have little factual information about children's health, only about their ill health and death. Secondly, the health problems of today's children are both complex and quite unlike those that prevailed in the past.

For children and adults, the causes of many modern illnesses lie in the complex relationships between the environment and health. The determinants of child health care are not predominantly biological but are related to the child's social and economic environment (Black Report, 1980).

Environmentally induced stress is greater today as the family is being redefined; as the physical environment, the work environment, socio-economic conditions and political and cultural factors undergo rapid change. Changes in lifestyle undoubtedly affect child health and are manifest in symptoms of family, social and behavioural distress — such as child abuse, sexual abuse, accidents, and childhood suicide.

Environmental effects on the health of children are demonstrated by the disproportionate toll of organic diseases on children in social classes IV and V. For example, the Black Report suggested that a child born to unskilled manual parents is *still* more than twice as likely to die before her first birthday than is the child of professional parents. Class inequalities are especially marked in the first year of life. Throughout childhood, accidents and respiratory diseases are still significant causes of death and disability within these two social groups.

Class differences in children's health are related to parental income, poor housing, lack of warmth, overcrowding, hazardous domestic appliances, poor hygiene, and the absence of a rapid means of communication with the outside world. Many of the most critical problems that face children and their families result from events and circumstances largely beyond their control. Economic factors including unemployment and low wages, government housing policies and social policies, have a powerful impact on children's health.

There is a potential relationship between adult disease and disability and childhood illness – and between the needs of families and the health of their children. Childhood illness deriving from dilapidated housing, overcrowding, inadequate nutrition, or hazards within the environment may well reflect parental needs. For example, needs for employment in order to afford to house and feed a family adequately; for help to overcome alcoholism; for day care to get some relief from the frustration of spending all day, every day in a two-roomed highrise flat with four underclothed, underfed, crying, pre-school children; for an adequate bus service in order to get to jobs, services and day care.

A central theme of this chapter is therefore the inter-relationship between the needs of families and the health of their children, and between the child and her socio-economic milieu. Consequently the chapter reflects a social model of health.

Central to the medical approach (epitomised in the term 'paediatric nursing') has been the idea that child health means freedom from ascertainable clinical disease, an approach governed by the identification of ill health. The social model of health represents a different emphasis, interpreting health as a positive state of well-being.

A child 'health' policy based on such a concept would be founded on creating good homes, balanced towns, and the evolution of stimulating but not abrasive or self-destructive social relationships. Child health has implications for policy outside the health system. There are professions other than medicine and nursing, and organisations and services other than the NHS, which play an important part in contributing to child health.

Although we cannot deny the importance of dealing with the complex illnesses that continue to plague children – leukaemia, genetic and congenital problems, and occasional life-threatening infections – our ability to treat and prevent them will not serve to make the majority of children function more effectively. Social problems and the management of everyday environmental stresses now have a direct bearing on whether children grow up healthy or unhealthy.

This chapter therefore attempts to approach the problems of contemporary child health from a broader perspective. Without this broader view, our understanding of the specifics, and subsequently our decisions about how best to improve matters, become distorted or irrelevant. The chapter not only reflects the changing nature of health problems experienced by children and families but also the changing nature of health care.

It is important to remember that caring for the health of children encompasses not only the care provided by nurses and doctors, hospitals and health centres, but also that provided by friends and relatives, social services and charities. Indeed, with the development of active consumerism, there has been a shift in the balance of power away from the professional. However, individual parents' right to participate in their own child's treatment is not widely advocated.

There is no attempt to address the less common health problems, experienced by a small percentage of children and families. Instead you are asked to reflect on the all-important question – do the services nurses and other health professionals provide really make a difference in terms of improving people's health?

Reference

DHSS. (1980). *Inequalities in Health*. Report of a research working group (The Black Report). HMSO, London.

SECTION 1: THE FAMILY

This section includes the following topics:

- What has the family to do with child health?

- What is family centred nursing care?

- Social change and the family

- Family structure and child health

- Influential factors in family life

- Political participation and the nursing advocate

- Cultural differences between families

- Families experiencing disturbed relationships

- Child protection

- Child abuse
  - its aetiology
  - prevention
  - management and nursing intervention
  - Failure to thrive families

- The role of the health visitor in working with families under stress

The family is the focus of a great deal of surveillance within the health and social services, which underlines its importance in relation to child health.

What has the family to do with child health?

The family will influence the physical, social and psychological well-being of the developing child in the following ways.

(1) The child's relationships with other family members, and the social and economic circumstances of the family of which she is a part, can exert a powerful influence on her experience of health and disease. That experience may in turn affect family life.

(2) The family is widely seen as a source of nursing care. This function has become more pertinent with the government's increasing emphasis on community care. However, given that women still bear primary responsibility for children, it is they who have to adjust their lives to meet these obligations. Children's illness, for example, is not a legitimate or customary reason for men taking time off work in Britain.

(3) A source of information about health and disease. Adult members decide when to seek professional help in caring for the health of children.

(4) The family is a site for the nurture and socialisation of children.

The family will be a recurring theme throughout this chapter.

What is family centred nursing care?

One of the fundamental goals of nursing children is to provide *family centred nursing care* (Forfar, 1989; While, 1991). This is in part based on the premise that, since the family is a system, no one individual can be effectively cared for if that care does not consider the other members who both *affect* and *are affected* by the member seeking nursing care.

Nurses who care for children must acknowledge this relationship because it is the family which is largely responsible for the child and most significantly enhances or hinders that child's development.

Family centred nursing of children implies *either* caring for the child directly, or assisting a family member to care for the child who is developmentally healthy – as well as the child who may deviate from the norms.

Family centred nursing of children *always* implies consideration of *all* family members in planning and providing care for children, whether in the home, the community, or in hospital.

Social change and child nursing practice

Social change influences the family and therefore child nursing practice (Forfar, 1989). There are deeply held beliefs in our society about what is normal and abnormal in family life, both in terms of the composition of families, and in terms of the roles and relationships within them. There are also strong assumptions about an idealised past when families were more stable and more caring than they are today.

One of the major problems we encounter in studying the family is that myths have been created which are simply not true. An excellent example is the myth of the extended family of the past giving way to the nuclear family of the present, with an associated loss of sense of community. In fact, the nuclear family (that is, a group comprising parents and children alone) has been in existence for a very long time.

Such beliefs draw on prevailing assumptions about the correct form of family life of which we need to rid ourselves. Stereotypes about the nuclear family, the extended family, the role of the mother, the role of the housewife, need to be demystified and destroyed.

The family is not a static entity. Over centuries, in the UK as elsewhere, there have been changes in the types of families people live in and in the

relationships between individual family members. Indeed, mention of the word 'family' conjures up an extraordinary range of meanings and associations. Some of these developments have implications for health and disease and are illustrated in Fig. 19.1.

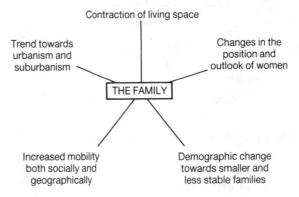

Fig. 19.1 *Social change and the family*

Social change and the family

These social changes raise many questions for the nurse caring for children and their families.

– When a child is seriously ill or dying why do we expect the mother to devote herself to the child and are highly critical of anything less?

– Paediatric community nursing services and paediatric day care facilities undoubtedly have great advantages such as mitigating the associated adverse effects of separation; however, can we expect the isolated mobile nuclear family and the one parent family to bear the strain of caring for a sick child at home?

Family structure and child nursing practice

More recently statistics have seemed to challenge the primacy of the nuclear family. Yet extended, nuclear, and single parent families are generalisations. Such labels offer the nurse little guidance for interaction. Even families that may seem to fit the nuclear patterns are often found to have created social support systems among neighbours and friends that are strongly reminiscent of the extended family; and the term 'single parent' is almost meaningless.

More specific classifications are illustrated in Fig. 19.2.

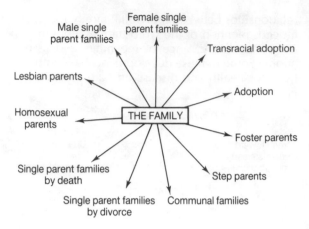

Fig. 19.2 *Diversity of family structure*

One parent families

A great deal of concern has been focused on the circumstances of parents and children in one parent families, for they may well face greater hazards to their health than other types of family.

People in one parent families tend to have lower incomes and this may adversely affect health. The physical and emotional pressures of caring for children alone may also take their toll on the health of the parent. Nevertheless it is not inevitable that life in a one parent family will pose a greater threat to health than life in any other sort of family. Some lone parents feel that their situation is considerably improved, especially if they previously had insecure or unhappy marriages.

It is wrong to assume that all one parent families, or for that matter all two parent families, form homogeneous groups. Although the majority of lone parents are women, almost a quarter are men. The marital status of lone mothers varies. Almost half are divorced and a further quarter separated, and there are as many single mothers as widowed mothers. The actual experience of divorce, separation, single parenthood and bereavement may differ significantly, but these elements of **diversity** are associated with important differences in income levels and poverty.

Homosexual and lesbian parents

Normality versus abnormality is not the topic of this discussion. Rather, it is the recognition that children are being raised by homosexual and les-

bian parents and therefore the nurse will inevitably be working with such family units.

In society, women who raise children on their own or without men challenge the normal idea of the family. In addition to this, the lesbian mother has to cope with her rejection of being a 'traditional woman' and ultimately, a 'real mother'. The greatest concern most researchers have about sexual preference of the parents is its influence on the children. However, the obvious fact is that many men and women who develop homosexual preferences grew up in heterosexual homes.

Many lesbian and male homosexual relationships have permanence, faithfulness and a shared life. However, if a lesbian mother leaves her family, her lesbianism may be used as evidence against her in a court case for custody of her children. There are also problems for male homosexuals who want children since adoption agencies give preference to heterosexual parents, and courts are more likely to grant custody to the mother than to the homosexual father.

Family structure and the nurse

The nurse must be aware of her feelings and beliefs about these various family forms and how they might influence her nursing practice. However, when one is confronted with so many different family lifestyles and child-rearing practices it may be difficult to remain objective. To examine one's values does not mean one agrees with the choices other people have made regarding lifestyles. It does mean that one attempts to understand the grid through which one views another's lifestyle.

In assessing families, it is important to view them from the perspective of their strengths. No family should automatically be considered weak or fragmented simply because it does not fit the traditional nuclear mode. Indeed traditional roles (that is, roles clearly defined on the basis of sex and family position) are not functional in most families today. Clearly defined roles do not allow for individual uniqueness or particular family needs, both of which are major concerns in modern families.

Consequently we have identified for the first time the inherently value-laden character of professional work with children and families. This theme will inevitably recur throughout the chapter. Professional intervention in families' lives is based on assumptions as to what constitutes happiness, health, adjustment and maturity. Such assumptions cannot be proven and there is considerable danger that the nurse's assumptions about what is best for the child and family will be different from the clients'. Thus the question of the character of the care offered is crucial, otherwise the vulnerability of the child and her family may well be abused (see also Chapter 13).

Influential factors in family life

The family environment refers to anything external to the family unit. It includes other people, the material world, and non-material factors such as social systems, institutions, political structures and value systems – to name but a few. The family and the environment are constantly in a state of mutual interaction in which both are simultaneously shaping and being shaped. Each individual family has arrived at its present condition through a process of development and interaction with the environment through time. In addition, the family as a social institution has been shaped by a long historical process of interaction with other social institutions down through the ages.

When assessing families it is useful to view the family as it functions within its environment in terms of its internal interaction. **Influential factors** are outlined in Fig. 19.3.

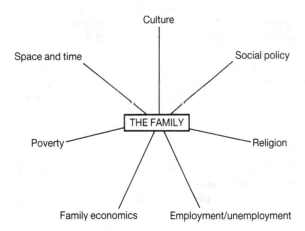

Fig. 19.3 *Influential factors in family living*

Space

A consideration of family space might be included in the nursing assessment, plan and intervention. Table 19.1 lists a number of questions that may be relevant at this stage.

Table 19.1, *Consideration of family space: questions for the nursing assessment*

How much space, in terms of rooms, does each family member have?

Is this enough?

Does it present problems?

How happy are you with where you are living?

Do you get on with your neighbours?

Accidents in childhood and overcrowding are undoubtedly linked. Townsend (1979) found that 41% of one parent families and 29% of households headed by a partly skilled or unskilled worker lived in overcrowded conditions compared to 5% of households headed by a professional or managerial worker.

There are many specific dangers to children in poor housing, from faulty electrical wiring and unsafe window catches to badly lit stairs and non-safety glass in doors. All these hazards cost money to put right, which is beyond the reach of families on low incomes. Simple safety equipment (such as a saucepan guard for the cooker or a stair-gate) may be too costly; similarly, cheap but relatively hazardous forms of heating (such as paraffin stoves) may be all a family can afford.

Poor circumstances outside the home may also be important (Child Accident Prevention Trust, 1989). Townsend (1979) found that 44% of children aged between one and four years, living in families with a partly skilled or unskilled parent, had no safe place to play near their home. This was in contrast to 25% of children in the same age group with professional or managerial parents. He also found that 43% of children aged between one and ten in one parent families had no safe place to play.

Time

It can be argued that areas of potential problems affecting families in modern society, such as effects of urbanisation, excessive time devoted to watching television, and possibly commuting, are basically problems of time rather than problems of interpersonal competence and that time-structuring holds the solution to these problems.

There are a number of important time-related assessments that the nurse might make in her work with some family units. For example, she can ask the following questions:

(1) Are there periods during the day for quiet or private communion between partners, parent and child, or for individual solitude?
(2) How much freedom is accorded to individual family members to schedule their own personal activities?

Family communication

The family provides the primary orientation to and training for communication and since communication is critical to family functioning, it might be necessary to include an assessment of communication patterns in the provision of nursing care.

Families experiencing interactional problems often exhibit communication patterns that are negative in content, confusing, contradictory or restricted. The members may share comments that are mainly of a complaining or devaluing nature. They may confuse each other by giving incongruent messages on verbal and non-verbal levels: a mother may give her child a verbal command whilst her behaviour implies that the child need not obey. The communication may be contradictory, leading to anxiety and uncertainty on the part of the person to whom it is directed. For example, children may be instructed not to resort to the use of falsehoods, whereas they observe the parents doing precisely this.

Families can differ tremendously in the ways they communicate non-verbally. For some, the physical expression of affection is frequent, spontaneous and unlimited with regard to age or family position. In these families, for example, it may be a commonly accepted practice for the father to embrace his teenage son. Families may also vary in the ways in which they express feelings symbolically through behaviour such as gift giving or locking of doors.

When the nurse interacts with families and observes their communication patterns, she may tend to assess and understand these behaviours in the light of her own particular cultural and familial orientation. Thus, it may be easy for her to misunderstand or misinterpret what is happening in a situation unless she is sensitive not only to the content but also to the meanings that are attached to the communication by the participants.

Another problem in communication is often experienced by immigrant families or by English families with regional or cultural speech patterns that differ from those of the community with which they interact.

A need may be indicated in these situations for the nurse to enact the advocate role to ensure that families and agencies or systems are communicating in such a way that family needs are recognised and met and that family rights and responsibilities are respected.

Family economics

Money is the most frequent reason for quarrelling between partners, and economic instability is a major cause of marital failure. Another aspect of the problem, which has become increasingly pertinent, is that many families are in such financial distress that their major concern is bare subsistence.

Nurses have often been reluctant to involve themselves in the financial situations of the families with whom they work. With increasing acceptance of holistic ideas of health care, nurses must begin to view their role as one of involvement with the total family in all major aspects of its life. The nurse must be aware of the interaction of family economics with other factors critical to family health and welfare. Many health visitors can confirm that a frequent problem identified by the families they visit is one of financial distress. The distress is not limited to lower income families, but is also experienced by middle class families. It is important, therefore, that nurses use their knowledge about available resources and agencies in order to refer the family appropriately for help.

Poverty

The hazards to children and the pressure on parents that poverty can create are more easily grasped if the circumstances of an actual child's life are described. Consider for example the case study given in Fig. 19.4.

Parents do clearly carry some responsibility for their children's health, but in conditions such as these the task may be particularly difficult. Furthermore, health promotion directed at the individual or the family has less chance of success if the socioeconomic environment remains outside the control of the individuals involved.

When subsistence is a problem, health is not a

The family, comprising two parents and four children under five, lived in grossly overcrowded conditions in a tenement flat, which appeared to consist of a large kitchen (i.e. six feet or more wide) and one other room. The child who was the subject of the study shared a bed with two of her younger siblings in one room while the other three members of the family slept in the kitchen. There was no bathroom or hot water supply, and the only lavatory was outside and shared by other households. The family did not have such basic items of equipment as a refrigerator, washing machine or spin dryer, nor did they have access either to a telephone or car. There was, however, a black and white television set.

Fig. 19.4 *Case study from Osborn, Butler and Morris, 1984*

primary family goal. If the family is struggling to pay the rent and provide food, clothing and other basic necessities, the parents may not be vitally interested in keeping the children's immunisations up to date – especially when this involves long waits, possibly paternalistic and condescending attitudes displayed by health care providers, and the problems and expense related to transport that a clinic visit often entails.

Nurses need to be aware constantly that their values may be different from those of the low income families with whom they work. This awareness will help to avoid the labelling and blaming that often results when the nurse evaluates the family's behaviour in the light of her own value system.

Advocacy

Another facet of family centred care with low income families is *advocacy*. The nurse who assumes the advocate role represents the family's interests as it seeks to cope with the health and social security systems. In this role the nurse perceives herself as primarily accountable to the family.

Similarly, intervention by the health visitor advocate is often vital to the effective functioning of the low income family. Faced with a bewildering display of social services bureaucracy, the family may be at a loss.

Political participation and the nurse advocate

In a larger sense the nurse may act as advocate for low income families by her **participation in the political process**. The much greater poverty experienced by women in one parent families stems from a variety of factors. The continuing wage differentials between men and women are especially important, making it difficult for single women to get reasonably paid work. These problems are compounded by the lack of jobs with suitable hours and the scarcity of child care provision, which may well force women back onto State benefits.

Women from ethnic minorities are over-represented among one parent families so that racial discrimination in jobs and housing will make their situation particularly difficult.

Both individually and collectively, nurses may give active support to legislation that ameliorates social and economic factors such as those affecting low income families.

Work

Employers have only recently begun to notice the effect of the family on workers' effectiveness and to appreciate how the work situation affects the total family.

Although work and family situations may sometimes be mutually supportive, at other times they may conflict. The demands of the workplace may create severe strains on family relationships. In most traditional nuclear families, the father spends more time at work than with the family. In fact, if a man desires to reduce his interaction with the family, he may use work as an excuse to withdraw.

Shift work can produce a variety of problems for the family, depending on the particular shift that is worked. Working the night shift can increase friction between partners. Alternating work on afternoon and night shifts may lead to inability to establish regular eating and sleeping patterns. Night work leads to a decreased social life but increases time available for housework and child care.

The demands of the job often present problems for families. Transfers, promotions and work-related travel may all subject the family to stress. Transfers mean that children must leave neighbourhood and school friends and establish new social ties. This often involves a temporary loss of status for the child.

Extensive work-related travel leads to changes in family roles and functions. Fathers may experience guilt and travel fatigue. An important effect is that the father misses out on experiencing significant family events.

When mothers work, child care becomes a problem. Although in an ideal situation both parents are equally involved in child care, in reality the mother is usually the main caretaker.

Pre-school provision – nurseries and play groups

There has been a focus of attention on pre-school provision in the last two decades. This concern is, in part, related to a continuing concern for a fair start for children whatever their circumstances.

Government policy

Families in the UK are constrained by government policies – legalities surrounding compulsory education, marriage, divorce and child custody.

Compulsory education has a marked effect on family life, since from approximately the age of five the child spends a considerable portion of the day in school and receives a large measure of socialisation there. As a result the child is exposed to authority figures, information and values beyond those provided by parents and family.

The law regarding divorce regulates the manner in which families become legally disconnected and controls subsequent management of their inter-related finances and the care of dependent children.

As the nurse considers individual families, she must assess the influence of factors such as these in more specific detail. However, it should be appreciated that families are not merely passive in their relation to government decisions. Changes in collective family behaviour and values have led to alterations in laws. An example of this is the change in divorce and child custody laws, reflecting the value placed on more equitable privileges and responsibility for both partners in the divorce.

Religion and spiritual needs

The impact of religion on family life in general, and on behaviour related to health and sickness in particular, is obvious. Often religious preferences are intermeshed with the cultural background of families, making them an even more salient aspect of the lifestyle. Among the family patterns affected by religion are relationships between its members, family power configurations, responsibilities of parents and children, diet, use of leisure time and finances, attitudes toward family planning and divorce, beliefs regarding health and illness, and the use of health care facilities.

A number of religions affect families' attitudes to health care through precepts determining which (if any) medical or health-related procedures are appropriate for their followers. This has often led to conflict between families and health care providers, especially when certain interventions have been refused on behalf of dependent children.

In assessing the religious aspects of an individual family the nurse must be careful to maintain an open and non-judgemental attitude. Often the family may value adherence to their religious convictions much more highly than a conflicting health goal that is valued by a nurse. It is also important to avoid the pitfall of religious stereotyping of families and failing to assess with accuracy the extent to which each individual family adheres to the tenets of their religious preference and the extent to which they have made alternative decisions.

Culture

As the nurse attempts to individualise care based on cultural understanding, it may be helpful for her to focus on a few areas in which cultural differences are important.

Family constellation and power structure

In some cultural groups the paternal uncles or some other non-paternal relative may hold power. For example, the nurse may find that some parents from the Far East or Middle East are reluctant to make decisions. If the nurse does not know whom to approach for health care decisions she may feel that the family are being evasive or uncooperative.

Sex roles

The sex roles ascribed to males and females by the culture present another area of health concern. The division of labour within the family and variation in training and discipline of male and female children are a few of the areas affected by what are considered proper roles for males and females. The nurse must be aware of these differences as she plans family centred child care.

Diet

The nurse must be aware that much of what she has learned, and much of what is published, about nutrition is culturally biased towards the food preferences of white middle-class individuals. Nutritional counselling must begin with the identification of the typical diet and food consumption patterns of the family. The use of culturally appropriate literature or consultation with a dietician (or both) may be necessary (DoH, 1989a and 1989b).

Cultural differences in beliefs and behaviour

Not only are illness-states culturally defined, but also who will be consulted and which kinds of treatment are appropriate are culturally determined. Health professionals are beginning to realise that traditional, culturally relevant practitioners (such as shamans, witch doctors and medicine men) are often sought in preference to doctors and nurses. In the past the typical reaction has been to discourage and ridicule the use of the traditional practitioner. As more is learnt about the relationship between belief and healing, progressive health professionals are learning to work cooperatively with traditional practitioners for the benefit of the child and her family.

The nurse should include in her assessment the identification of health practices and practitioners that the family believes to be appropriate for care. She should be sensitive to the religious basis for family beliefs related to health. When family values have been explored the nurse is able to add an important dimension to her care-planning by incorporating the family's cultural health beliefs.

However, while it is helpful for the nurse to have a basic understanding of the culture of a given family, this should not blind her to what actually characterises that family in a cultural sense. Assumptions or biased expectations must not replace accurate assessment of each individual child and family.

Families experiencing disturbed relationships

So far in this chapter the emphasis has been on interactional patterns. This section continues the theme, placing the emphasis on disturbed relationships.

Common disturbances in the relationship between children and parents include:

(1) Inflexibility in the style of parenting
(2) Inappropriate expectations of parents
(3) Parent–child mismatch
(4) Parental misconceptions regarding the child.

Inflexibility in parenting styles

The nurse may see parenting practices that are functional for one child but quite dysfunctional for another. One basis for these differences lies in the children's temperaments or their fundamental, individual approaches to life.

Inappropriate expectations

Sometimes parents relate to their children in a manner that reflects inappropriate expectations for the child in relation to her age or capabilities.

Often they lack the knowledge necessary for anticipating what their child can be expected to do or comprehend. During periods of stress, even informed parents sometimes relate inappropriately to their child.

Parent–child mismatch

One particular child may not fit her parents, but she could be loved and nurtured by another set of parents for the very qualities that set off stressful interactions within her biological family.

Parental misconception

Disturbed parent–child interactions may be related to the parents' misconceptions about the child. A child affects her parents by the way she responds to them, and by the way they, the parents, perceive her, the child.

The parents' perception may be related not objectively to the child's looks or behaviour but to a projected attribution. 'She looks like your sister, whom I don't like' or 'She looks just like me at that age' are examples of common parental reactions.

Child protection

Child protection generally replaces the term child abuse. It implies a positive approach to children who may be in need and prevention of abuse rather than action after the event. However, in some instances the term abuse may still be applied; for example, with sexual abuse. Historically, the abuse of children was an invisible problem. According to Kempe and Kempe (1978), maltreatment of children has survived into the late 20th century, virtually unchallenged because two beliefs remained strong:

(1) Children were seen as their parents' property and it was taken for granted that parents had the right to treat their children as they saw fit (Freeman, 1989).

(2) Children were seen as their parents' responsibility and for many centuries harsh treatment was justified by the belief that severe physical punishment was necessary to maintain discipline, transmit educational decisions and expel evil spirits.

Today, children of all ages, whatever their family and cultural background, remain vulnerable for a variety of reasons. However, in recent years changes in the outlook and sensibilities of our society have caused an increased awareness of the need to address the issue of child protection constructively. Under the aegis of child protection, three major initiatives have occurred.

Firstly, the Social Service departments, who have the primary responsibility for the protection of children, are encouraging the development of multi-agency training in child protection at four levels. This requires the cooperation of health professionals, the police and probation officers with Social Services.

Secondly, the opening of the telephone helpline **Childline** and its attendant publicity has created an increased awareness of all forms of abuse and the need for victims to have a safe and confidential helpline.

Thirdly, in October 1991 the Children Act (HMSO, 1989) was introduced. This Act replaces almost all of the previous items of legislation relating to children and provides a single coherent framework for the welfare of children. Whilst the implications of the Act extend far beyond the protection of children from physical injury and sexual abuse, it would seem appropriate to make brief mention of some of the key points here.

The Children Act

The Children Act passed in 1989 was introduced in October 1991. It is the most comprehensive piece of legislation Parliament has ever enacted about children. Previously the law relating to the care of children, their upbringing and protection was rather fragmented and inconsistent. The aim of the Act is to facilitate improvements through radical changes to the law, producing a consistent single statement. It simplifies the law, making it explicit and flexible to the advantage of the child. Three key issues from the Act are highlighted below.

Children's rights

The rights of children have been discussed widely in recent years. Although much of this discussion has related to the wider political status of children it also has implications for child protection. The Children Act increases the status of children, stating 'the child's welfare is paramount' and that the child must always come first when a decision is made about him or her. In addition, the child must be consulted and his or her wishes taken into account when decisions are being made.

In adhering to this legislation it is important to remember the child's age and stage of development and to be aware of the inappropriate perception of children as mini-adults able to decide their future.

Parents' rights become parents' responsibilities

The aim of this change in terminology is to acknowledge that parents have a duty and obligation to care for their children rather than 'rights' over them. The Act presumes that childrearing is best carried out by the parents within the family home, with the State giving support when necessary, rather than intervention. This implies that all services relating to child care will need to provide more support for the family.

The Act stresses the need for partnership in care with the parents. This is a concept which has been incorporated into the philosophy of children's nursing for some considerable time.

Children in need

A child is defined as being in need if:

- he or she is unlikely to achieve and maintain or to have the opportunity of achieving or maintaining a reasonable standard of health or development without provision by the local authorities;
- his or her health and development are likely to be significantly impaired without the provision of such services;
- he or she is disabled.

The Children Act is not solely concerned with children in need of protection. It brings together for the first time the public and private law relating to children. Briefly, public law concerns those areas where society intervenes in the actions of individuals (such as care proceedings). Private law addresses the behaviour of individuals towards each other; for example, with whom the child should live following divorce of parents.

In summary, the Children Act is concerned with the rights of all children in every circumstance.

When is a child in need of protection?

The following categories are now identified on the *Child Protection Register*:

- Physical injury or the likelihood of physical injury;
- Emotional abuse or the likelihood of emotional abuse;
- Neglect;
- Sexual abuse.

A child may fall into one or more of these categories at any one time and therefore be in need of protection.

Aetiology of physical injury, emotional abuse and neglect

Three elements are commonly present in families where children may be in need of protection. These are abuse of the parent(s) themselves as children; perception by the parent(s) that the child is different; and occurrence of a family crisis that alters living conditions.

Injury to the parent(s) themselves as children

The potential for non-accidental injury to children often results from the parents themselves having been victims of non-accidental physical injury as children. Such parents are likely to be isolated individuals who cannot trust or relate to other people beneficially. The parents have a poor self-image, are impatient, and often in conflict with each other about many things. Their family systems perpetuate a discipline that makes use of physical punishment. The spouse of the offending parent may be so passive that he or she does not intervene to spare the child from injury.

Perception by the parent(s) that the child is different

These parents have unrealistic expectations of their children: the child who is abused may be perceived as different by one or both parents. Often the child will have been unwanted, and parents may have experienced stress at the birth. The child may have special problems such as retardation, prematurity, or a congenital defect that triggers the abusive pattern in the parents. A difference between the child's temperament and that of the abusive parent often exists, making the child seem unacceptable or undesirable to this parent. Sometimes the precipitating factor is simply a developmental task that the child is attempting to master under unrealistic parental demand.

Occurrence of a family crisis that alters living conditions

The family often endures a crisis or a series of crises, such as drastic changes in its living conditions or financial situation.

The aetiology of incest and other forms of sexual abuse

A discussion of incest or other forms of sexual abuse of children is likely to evoke strong feelings of revulsion or disbelief among readers. These are the same feelings that have caused professionals to shy away from the problems and to underestimate the extent of their severity.

Sexual abuse

Sexual abuse is defined as the involvement of dependent, developmentally immature children and adolescents in sexual activities that they do not fully comprehend, and to which they are unable to give informed consent. It includes *paedophilia* (an adult's preference for or addiction to sexual relations with children), rape and incest.

Incest

This is usually hidden for years and only comes to public attention during a dramatic change in the family situation, such as adolescent rebellion or delinquent acts, pregnancy, venereal disease, psychiatric illness, or something as trivial as a sudden family quarrel.

Father-daughter incest accounts for approximately three quarters of incest cases. It is usually non-violent, but most fathers incestuously involved with their daughters are introverted personalities who tend to be socially isolated and family orientated. In the silent agreement among husband, wife and daughter, each plays a role unless a crisis occurs; one of these crises is public discovery.

The treatment of incest, however, is likely to be successful and to result in three desired goals:

- Stopping the practice;
- Providing individual and later group treatment for the victim and her parents;
- Helping to heal the victim's wounds by permitting growth as a whole person, including the ability to enjoy normal sexuality.

Identifying infants and children who may be in need of protection

Diagnosing physical injury or neglect

The injured or neglected child's behaviour depends on many factors including age; developmental level; the specific pattern of relationships in the family; what injuries have been received; and whether injury has been a continuing situation or a single event. Abused children may be irritable or apathetic.

The index of suspicion for the nurse should be triggered by certain factors in the history and signs and symptoms (see Table 19.2).

Table 19.2. *Warning signs: physical injury*

History indications	Physical signs and symptoms
Unexplained trauma. Evasive or contradictory accounts of how trauma occurred	Evidence of general neglect
	Failure to thrive
Pattern injuries caused by belt loops or electric cords and burns, or hand imprints	Poor skin hygiene
	Irritability
	Delayed motor, social, language and cognitive development
Reluctance to give information	Bruises
Delay in seeking medical care	Abrasions
	Burns
Previous history of similar episodes or multiple visits to various hospitals	Soft tissue swelling
	Human bites
Multiple poison ingestions or 'accidents'	Eye damage
Inappropriate reaction to severity of child's injury	Lesions or injuries in various stages of healing
Abusive verbal exchanges between child and parent	Fracture or dislocation of extremities
	Unexplained genital or severe abdominal injuries
	Coma
	Convulsions
	Symptoms of drug withdrawal or intoxication

Diagnosing sexual abuse

In order for sexual abuse to be identified, the child must be carefully examined for evidence of oral, anal or genital penetration. Tests are carried out to determine the presence of semen or venereal disease. It is important that the nurse explains what is to be done clearly, thoroughly and in language the child can understand. A girl may feel uncomfortable with a male doctor or nurse and may be unwilling to be examined by him. The child is likely to be upset and frightened by physical contact, especially in the genital area. The role of the nurse and the doctor should be explained to the child as well as the procedures to be performed. Uncertainty provokes anxiety and simple explanations reduce a significant source of stress for the child.

Protection of potential/actual victims

Protection from all forms of injury/abuse is extremely important. Health visitors and nurses working in the community, nurses working in obstetric units, accident and emergency departments and children's wards are in strategic positions to identify those children who, potentially, are in need of protection.

Antenatal observations

The nurse should assess the parents' attitude towards the pregnancy. Is the pregnancy wanted or not? Are the parents depressed? Is the pregnancy publicly acknowledged or denied?

Enquiries should be made about social support for the mother. Nursing care includes recognition of family situations or excessive stress such as job loss, inadequate income or housing. Several children to care for or children born very close together can cause strain on the mother's energy or relationship difficulties between the parents.

The role of the nurse is to work in a team with the obstetrician, health visitor, social worker or other appropriate team members to try and resolve as many problems as possible during the pregnancy and to offer counselling in relation to those situations that cannot be changed.

Post-natal observations

What are the parents' initial responses to the baby? Do they talk to their baby, recognise cues, establish eye contact, play with her? The nurse can help the mother to see likeable characteristics in her child and can point out the baby's capabilities. The nurse should observe parents' reactions to care giving: whether they recognise the baby's needs and the way they offer care.

Working with parents to protect the child

The health visitor or obstetric nurse may need to offer counselling related to childrearing practices beginning antenatally or in the newborn period.

The health visitor's role is very much that of a health educator. She visits 'high risk families' regularly (as determined by local health authority policy) and discusses with parents themes such as developmental expectations and child care skills, appropriate to the child's age. Parents may also need guidance to develop more appropriate ways of interacting with the child during stressful periods. The health visitor can discuss with parents the fact that temperaments do clash, but ways to cope with those aspects of their child's personality that conflict with their own can be learnt.

These duties frequently bring the health visitor into a long term relationship with the family; she becomes a friend and confidante as well as a health care professional. This position makes the health visitor a vulnerable practitioner, especially when a case of abuse is suspected. In such a situation practitioners should maintain a focus on the child as the primary client whose interests must transcend those of the parent when there is any conflict. School nurses and teachers may also find themselves in similar complex and sensitive situations with the child in need of protection and her family.

Management and nursing intervention

Child protection is a situation that involves the entire family. Health professionals must consider every member of the family because each individual member affects and is affected by every other member. The nurse can promote harmony among parents and children by praising positive interactions and parenting behaviours. She can help parents to identify the child's attributes and unique qualities. The nurse can make the infant available to parents, facilitating the bonds of attachment after delivery and in the post-natal period in the hospital.

Care of the child

The child needs to experience consistent behaviour towards her by nurses. Play is particularly important. The nurse should also encourage positive interactions between the child and parents and pleasant feelings from the child toward the parents while the child is being cared for in the hospital setting.

Care of the parent

The nurse can reinforce any positive parenting efforts by actively involving the parents in the planning of care. On the other hand, the nurse should avoid forcing participation when the parents are not ready for care giving. The nurse can praise the parents' concern for their child, and reinforce competent child care behaviour. As a team member the trained nurse provides mothering of the abusive parents to help fulfil unmet needs; she can also model healthy mothering behaviours for the parents.

The trained nurse and health visitor can teach realistic growth and development expectations and childrearing options to the parents, mostly through demonstration, role modelling, and discussions on management of the child's development, such as toilet training.

The trained nurse and health visitor may help the family members reduce crisis in the home by referring them to Social Services, housing departments or other appropriate agencies.

Discharge planning

When a child is admitted to hospital with a possible non-accidental injury an exchange of views is required between well-informed members of senior status from the various services who are involved with the problem. The case conference facilitates contact between the various disciplines.

The composition of a typical conference is illustrated in Fig. 19.5. It is essential that attention should be paid to the requirements of any experienced professional who has ethical considerations to express. It is at this stage that matters of confidentiality arise, particularly in relation to the disclosure of medical information about the parents or about family matters which have become known because of a previous involvement with the family.

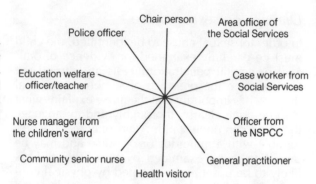

Fig. 19.5 Composition of a typical case conference

Usually a *key worker* is allocated the responsibility of carrying out the decision of the conference and the child's name may be placed on the *At Risk Register*. This is a register maintained by the local Social Services department. The key worker is then given the responsibility of working with the family and monitoring the child's well-being.

Families where a child fails to thrive

The failure of a child to thrive without organic cause is one evidence of family disorganisation and can occur in all socio-economic circumstances.

The family's first plea for help may be to seek advice from the health visitor, school nurse or GP for their child. Or they may be reported by a neighbour to the Social Services department or the NSPCC (National Society for the Prevention of Cruelty to Children).

The home environment of infants and children who fail to thrive may be so limited or threatening that they fail to grow and develop 'without organic reason'.

Aetiology

The child's **failure to thrive** may be due to a nutritional deficiency or organic disease; however, it may also be the result of a disturbance in the relationship between the mother and the child.

The precipitating factors underlying the disturbance are varied. The infant may be the result of an unwanted, unplanned or stressful pregnancy. The infant's birth may have been a difficult one, or by caesarean section; she may have been premature or she may have some birth-associated illness or congenital defect. The baby's appearance or temperament may be displeasing to the parents, or they may attribute some defect to her when none is apparent. The mother and child may have been separated after delivery. The parents may lack information about infant care and development, and expect responses from their child that conflict with the child's needs, development and abilities. For example, some young parents are disappointed to discover their baby does not 'love' them as they expected but demands a lot instead.

History taking

The manner of questioning and the types of questions asked may seem threatening to parents. The nurse must be tactful and support the parents adequately. A helpful attitude in which the nurse is concerned about the child and also about the parents' feelings is likely to elicit the most information. The nurse needs to know about the antenatal history and the perinatal events, the infant's feeding history, and the child's health history. The nurse will observe and ask questions about parent-child relationships and the child's developmental attainment at home.

Care of the child in hospital

The nurse manager or her deputy should limit the number of care-givers to a **primary nurse** each shift with an **associate nurse**(s) to relieve the primary nurse.

The basic care is the same as for any child of similar age, but more time may be needed, especially for feeding. Extra attention should be paid to holding the child, cuddling her and eliciting eye contact. Special attention to the skin is sometimes required because of alterations in the general nutritional state, bulky, acid stools or frequent vomiting.

During hospitalisation, nursing care includes ongoing monitoring of the child. The nurse will record the number, character, colour and consistency of the stools; she may test the stools for occult blood and for sugar. (If the infant is unable to absorb properly from the gut, sugar will be present in the stool.) The nurse should check the pH of the stool — if it is less than 5.5 this means that acid is present from metabolic breakdown products. The weight of the child is documented at the same time each day, under similar conditions. An accurate record of intake and output is made. The nurse will also work with the dietician in regard to planning the diet so that the child will have an optimum intake for 'catch-up growth' while at the same time overfeeding is avoided.

Nursing care of the child's mother/father

The child's mother and father should be welcomed and included in the child's care. However, parents should not be coerced into participating until they are ready. Sometimes it is necessary to plan care that requires parents to be absent — temporarily feeding and nurturing is done by the nurses and the weight gain is evaluated while the child has been separated from the parents.

The trained nurse 'mothers the mother' by providing emotional nurturing. This is often done most effectively through role-modelling demonstration and positive reinforcement of the parent's efforts by the infant's primary nurse.

In spite of all the nurse's guidance and tact, parents may feel threatened — particularly if the child improves during hospitalisation during which no treatment other than feeding, nurturing and stimulation has been provided. Parents need to have their insecurity alleviated and their self-esteem built up as they begin to succeed in caring for their child.

The nurse can listen to the mother and help her work through the negative feelings that have disrupted healthy interaction with the child. The nurse can also help the mother to allay her feelings of guilt about the diagnosis.

Documentation of observations during treatment

The primary nurse and associate nurses who care for the child must build upon each other's findings and those of others in the care team. In the case of an infant they should:

(1) Document the ways in which the child is held and fed, how eye contact is initiated by the mother/father, together with descriptions of and the facial expressions of the child and of the mother during interactions
(2) Note what the mother does with the child —

play, talk, hold, stroke – and the child's response

(3) Note how the care-giver refers to the baby and whether she talks about the baby at all. This is an indication to others of how the mother perceives the child

(4) Record the mother's responses to the baby's cues; for example, how does the mother respond when the baby looks at her, when she cries, when she reaches toward her, during motor activity?

(5) Note the responses of the infant to the mother's overtures, the baby's reaction to the mother's feeding rate and the way she is being held.

Prevention

In the broadest sense, nurses (as community members and providers of health care) can have an impact on the prevention of failure to thrive. Obstetric nurses can initiate antenatal classes; school nurses can initiate discussion with pupils – not only about physical effects, but also about the psychological and social effects that children may have on families.

Obstetric nurses can intervene with counselling to parents in situations of high-risk pregnancy, premature birth, caesarean sections and the birth of a handicapped child.

At home, health visitors can help parents to learn and interpret their child's cues and gain a sense of self-esteem from their interactions. Child health clinics held by health visitors provide excellent opportunities to model and teach positive parenting techniques.

The health visitor's role in working with families in stress

The health visitor is at a unique advantage in helping families in stress, in that she can be eclectic and select from other disciplines interventions that will be helpful to clients.

The health visitor is often the first professional helper with whom the family shares its stress and distress. Their request for help is often not explicit; it may be a report of some symptom to a health visitor that leads her to suspect stress. She must

therefore be observant of family interactions and alert in her history taking to those patterns that characterise the dysfunctional family. She can then either use her own skills to intervene or refer the family to agencies that can help them.

Role model

The health visitor acts as a role model, demonstrating how to relate to others in an autonomous and caring manner. She can teach people how to look at things, feel, touch and respond in ways that bring them pleasure instead of the pain of dysfunction.

Teacher and counsellor

The health visitor's function as teacher or counsellor requires that she intervene to help reverse the family's stress. She can provide information to help parents correct knowledge deficits or misconceptions about parenting options, or to develop mental expectations.

Her counselling efforts can reinforce the fact that each child is unique. Parents should be assured that temperaments do clash, but ways to cope with those aspects of their child's personality that conflict with their own can be learned. Parents may also need guidance to develop realistic ways of interacting with their child during periods of stress.

Health visitors, obstetric nurses and children's ward nurses can lend themselves to families as parent surrogates for a time. When a nurse intervenes to assist a mother or father with parenting tasks, she nurtures them in the present and also may be caring for parts of their personalities that suffered deprivation and unresolved hurts during their own childhood. Specifically, the nurse's interventions are aimed at giving parents permission to enjoy their children and instruction in how to relate to them. Together, nurse and parents can plan how to initiate actions whereby parents can satisfy their own needs in order that they, in turn, can give to their children. These experiences can stimulate parents to take charge of their own life and decide how they will behave.

Working as a team member

The health visitor and the ward nurse can increase their effectiveness by participating in an interdisciplinary team. The team offers the advantage of balancing the multiple problems of the stressed family with the energies and skill of experts from several disciplines. The team approach offers each individual professional the emotional reinforcement needed to withstand the stresses that typify this family unit. The nurse's specific role within the team and interaction with the family depend on several factors, including the team's composition and her particular expertise.

Self-care/family care

An emphasis on patient self-care (i.e. family self-care) is found in the writings of Orem (1989) whose nursing model has particular relevance to child and family care. Orem places 'self-care' at the centre of her definition of what she describes as 'the art of nursing'. She distinguishes three types of nursing system which define the respective roles of nurse and child/family:

(1) *The wholly compensatory system*
   This system is required when the child and family's capacities for self-care are temporarily or permanently destroyed. The nurse therefore cares for the child directly.
(2) *The partly compensatory system*
   This system is used when the child and family's capacities are restricted to a greater or lesser degree. The nurse therefore assists a family member to care for the child.
(3) *The supportive-educative system*
   This system is used when the child and family need only guidance, support or teaching to enable them to care. The nurse is a health educator and hence an enabler.

Conclusions

This section has demonstrated throughout its content the critical role of the family in the adaptation, integration and development of the child. The theme that the family is society's primary source for the provision of the growing child's biological, psychological and sociological needs has been explored. Two important questions have been considered.

(1) *What has the family to do with child health?*

There is an inter-relationship between the individual child's experience of health and disease and the family's social and economic circumstances. This relationship underlines a premise central to issues and debates related to child health – that is the acknowledgement that health does not exist in a social or political void. Child health is determined by the socio-economic milieu and not purely by health care provision.

(2) *What is family centred care?*

The concept of family centred care is pivotal to the care of children. It reflects, within this specialty of nursing, a shift of emphasis towards caring for children within the context of their families.

When planning and implementing child care we must acknowledge that it is the family that is largely responsible for the child and to which that child must ultimately be accountable. This implies caring for the child directly or assisting a family member to care for the child.

Social change and the nursing of children

The chapter has continued with an examination of some of the social changes which have influenced the 'family unit' and hence child nursing practice. Stereotypes and myths about the nuclear family, the extended family, one parent families, homosexual and lesbian families have been explored. All these family units have been portrayed from the perspective of their strengths; furthermore it has been stressed that 'families' are highly individualistic in terms of structure and lifestyles and therefore should not be stereotyped.

Families experiencing disturbed relationships

Finally, disturbed family relationships and the implications for child health have been discussed. All families have phases when they function well and other periods when they function poorly. However, families that function poorly on a long term basis place their children in physical, emotional, social and intellectual jeopardy. Particular attention has been paid to two specific problems – children in need of protection and failure to thrive.

At its best, family life fulfils a human need which

is not fully met by any other arrangements or institutions. Despite its limitations the family remains the most powerful influence in the lives of most of us.

Glossary

Advocacy: The definition in most general dictionaries is that advocacy is 'the act of defending or pleading the case of another' (Kohnke, 1982). This definition does not apply to most of the situations that the practising nurse encounters. The role of the nurse advocate is to inform the client and family and then to support them in whatever decision they make. The most important personal attribute for the advocate to possess is open-mindedness. Open-mindedness allows the advocate to listen to, and hear what the client/family are saying. The nurse advocate must also have an understanding of her own attitudes, values and beliefs. Such personal knowledge allows the advocate to hear and understand the attitudes, values and beliefs of others without identifying with them. The advocate allows others to have different values and beliefs. Open-mindedness is extremely important, for the advocate must be able to present information as objectively as possible and to allow clients/families to make their own decisions, even when those decisions differ from the advocate's personal judgement

Associate nurse: When the primary nurse is off duty she delegates responsibility to an associate nurse, who works according to the plan worked out by the primary nurse. Except in an emergency situation the plan of care is not altered without consultation with the primary nurse (see *primary nursing* below)

Childline: A voluntary initiative launched in 1986, this telephone helpline has been taking hundreds of calls daily and logging many more attempted calls. Victims of abuse can be assured of confidentiality and remain anonymous if they wish

Child Protection Register: Registers of children who have or are believed to have been abused have existed since the 1960s under a succession of different titles. Child Protection Registers are the most recent. These consist of lists in each area administered by either Social Services or the NSPCC; they are strictly confidential. Only named professionals from the agencies concerned may have access

Diversity of family structure: Such diversity includes female single parent families, transracial adoption, foster parents, step-parents, communal families, single parent families by divorce, single parent families by death, homosexual parents, lesbian parents and male single parent families

Failure to thrive: May be due to a nutritional deficiency or organic disease, or may be the result of a disturbance in the relationship between the parent and the child

Family centred nursing care: One of the fundamental goals of nursing children. Based on the premise that, since the family is a system, no one individual can be effectively cared for if that care does not consider the other members who both affect and are affected by the member seeking nursing

Influential factors in family living: The family and the environment are constantly in a state of mutual interaction in which both are simultaneously shaping and being shaped. Influential factors include culture, social policy, religion, employment or the lack of it, family economics, poverty, space and time

Political participation: The nurse who assumes the advocate role represents the family's interests as it seeks to cope with the health and social security systems. In this role the nurse perceives herself as primarily accountable to the family; in a larger sense she may act as advocate for low income families by participation in the political process

Primary nursing: A system of work organisation first described by Manthey et al. (1970), who were concerned by the fragmentation of patient care and by the diffuse, collective responsibility for care in hospital nursing. They suggested that these two factors prevented nurses from providing professional care to individual clients. Consequently an organisational pattern enabling each nurse to take continuous responsibility for the total nursing care of between three and six patients was developed.

A primary nurse is responsible and accountable for the care of her own group of patients.

The primary nurse works with her patients and plans their nursing care. She also plays a major role in the implementation of care. The primary nurse liaises with doctors and paramedical staff and will be the main contact for child/family education. She works with the child/family planning and preparing for discharge

Social changes which affect the family: Involve factors such as the trend towards urbanism and suburbanism, increased mobility (both socially and geographically), demographic change towards smaller and less stable families, changes in the position and outlook of women

References

Child Accident Prevention Trust. (1989). *Basic Principles of Child Accident Prevention*. CAPT, London.

Department of Health. (1989a). *Present Day Practice in Infant Feeding*. HMSO, London.

DoH. (1989b). *The Diets of British School Children*. HMSO, London.

Forfar, J. (ed.). (1989). *Child Health in a Changing Society*. British Paediatric Society/Harper and Row, London.

Freeman, M. (1989). Principles and processes of the law in child protection. In *Child Abuse and Neglect: Facing the Challenge*, Stainton Rogers, W., Hevey, D. and Ash, E. (eds.). Open University/Batsford, London.

Kempe, R.S. and Kempe, C.H. (1978). *Child Abuse*. Fontana/Open Books Original, London.

Kohnke, M.F. (1982). *Advocacy, Risk and Reality*. Mosby, St Louis.

Manthey, M., Ciske, K., Robertson, P. and Harris, R. (1970). Primary nurse: a return to the concept of 'my nurse' and 'my patient'. *Nursing Forum*, 9(1), 65–83.

Orem, D. (1989). *Nursing: Concepts of Practice* (3rd ed.). McGraw Hill, New York.

Osborn, A.F., Butler, N.B. and Morris, A. (1984). *The Social Life of Britain's Five Year Olds: A Report of the Child Health and Development Study*. Routledge and Kegan Paul, London.

Townsend, P. (1979). *Poverty in the United Kingdom*. Penguin Books, Harmondsworth.

While, A. (1991). *Caring for Children: Towards a Partnership with Families*. Edward Arnold, London.

SECTION 2: CHILD DEVELOPMENT

This section includes the following topics:

- What do we mean by 'child'?
  - social determinants
  - personal determinants
- Inter-relationship between society and the individual child's development
- Principles of development
  - quantitative and qualitative development
  - transactional models of development
  - genetic factors
  - the developing child as part of a system
- Concepts central to child development
- Play
  - some theories
  - its contribution to child development
  - social characteristics of play
  - content of play
  - helping parents to promote play

The whole of childhood includes a continuous process of growth and development. Any nurse caring for children should have some understanding of this process and its implications.

Why study growth and development?

Studying child development enables the nurse to know what to expect of children at any given age. Such knowledge is necessary for the nurse to develop and deliver a plan of care that is age-appropriate and relevant to the needs of the child (Herbert, 1990).

Understanding human developmental processes also helps us to see the reason why some conditions or illnesses are more prominent in certain age groups.

Nurses working with children require developmental knowledge to teach parents accurately, so that they can contribute positively to their children's optimal growth and development (Laishley, 1987).

The foremost question to be considered by the nurse is:

'How does the problem which brings the child into my care (health state, physical trait, temperament, parental disharmony, social condition) affect this child's ability to function physically; to learn and think; and to perceive and accept herself in a way that allows her to relate socially to others? Furthermore, how does this factor affect the family's ability to support their child in these tasks?'

This approach maintains the focus on the *whole* child, in the context of her family.

The developmental psychologist

The task of the developmental psychologist is, in effect, a two-fold one: to identify and describe age-related changes in behaviour, and to provide an explanation for the phenomena identified.

Age can never be regarded as an explanatory concept. Age itself does not cause behavioural change. For example, four-year-old children generally have larger vocabularies and are capable of producing more complex utterances than two-year-olds, but the explanation for this does not lie in the fact that the former are two years older than the latter. Chronological age is simply a convenient way of measuring the time in which experiential, maturational and physiological processes occur (see Table 19.3).

Definitions of a child

There is considerable leeway in what we mean by the term 'child'. The variations involve an inter-relationship between biological, social and personal determinants (see Table 19.4).

Commenting on data from various other cultures, Goodman (1967) noted that, 'people rarely dichotomize between childhood and adults as we do and even fewer conceive of a murky transitional phase of adolescence . . . The Western concept of the child as a creature of emotions, physically fragile and easily damaged is almost without parallel'.

Table 19.3. *Birth to adulthood: the principal biological, social and personal transitions of an average childhood and adolescence (optional transitions are shown in square brackets)*

Age/years	Women	Both sexes	Men
0.5		Registration of birth	
3		[Playgroup]	
5		Compulsory schooling begins	
10		Can be held responsible for a crime	
		Physical changes of puberty may begin	
12	Menarche (39% of girls menstruating)*		
16		Age of heterosexual consent	Puberty complete (only 0.6%
		Minimum school-leaving age	of boys have testicles still
		Minimum age of marriage (requires parental consent)	undescended) *
		[Parenthood may commence]	
		[Full-time employment may commence]	
17		Eligible for armed services	
18		Able to vote	
		Can marry without parental consent	
		Eligible for council house tenancy/ mortgage	
21			Age of homosexual consent

* Percentages relating to menstruating and testicular development taken from National Child Development Study, 1958

Table 19.4. *Definitions of a child: biological, social and personal determinants*

Biological determinants	Social determinants	Personal determinants
– Do babies become children at about a year with the acquisition of certain skills?	– Is someone a child until he leaves school at 16 years, or even later?	– Is it important to state categorically an age when someone is no longer a child, or should we look for signs of personal qualities (such as 'responsibility' or 'good sense') supposed to be adult attributes?
– Does childhood end at puberty, around 11 or 12 years?		

We cannot give childhood a culturally universal fixed beginning and end. We use the term to cover an enormous range of development.

The inter-relationship between society and the individual child's development

---

Various factors affect the individual child's development and one way of summarising these is illustrated in Fig. 19.6.

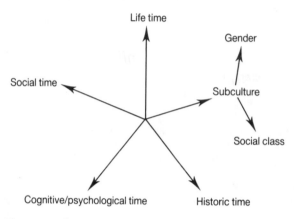

Fig. 19.6 *The inter-relationship between society and the individual child's development*

Life time

Chronological age is only loosely related to the major changes that occur in the body as a result of biological maturation. For example, the state insists that all five year olds start school – the same chronological age but not necessarily the same mental age.

Social time

Societies use the changes that occur as a result of biological maturation or increasing chronological age to delineate particular periods of development. Therefore the boundary between commonly defined stages of infancy, childhood and adolescence are fixed by the conventions of society. Whilst the onset of adolescence may be loosely related to puberty, its termination may occur by the achievement of legal maturity at eighteen, by marriage, or by entering into the labour force.

Historic time

Concepts of children and childhood alter. Children and childhood are not necessarily the same from century to century, nor even from decade to decade.

It is not merely a case today of earlier physical and mental maturity nor merely the effects of an earlier onset of menstruation, but the ways we view the state of childhood. In Western technological societies children are generally encouraged to explore the environment, to ask questions, to try things out. A child may be more in touch with the here-and-now than are her parents. Schools are sometimes forced to recognise this – for example computers in primary schools are often better understood by the nine year olds using them than by most of their parents.

Part of the so-called 'generation gap' is produced by successive generations being formed by different constellations of influences – political, economic and social events and institutions.

Population trends

The population structure in a society at a particular time may have a considerable influence on the course of development. In industrialised societies, there are always at least three age categories: an adult producer, dependent young people, and dependent old people.

Over the last 50 years there has been a decline in the numbers of children under five, despite a massive increase in infant survival rate. There has also been a vast increase in the percentage of the population who are aged 65 years and older, as a result of a declining death rate. This has considerable implications for the lives of young children in terms of their opportunities to form relationships, and the role of the **peer group**.

Cognitive and psychological time

Piaget (1969) identified the sensorimotor, preconceptual, concrete operational and formal operational stages in the development of thought processes. The infant according to Piaget is profoundly egocentric. The child is not capable of making any distinction between herself and what is not herself; she cannot draw the boundary which later (most of the time) is so obvious and so firm.

Kohlberg (1969) has developed a theory of moral development which is based on a Piagetian approach. Kohlberg suggests that before the age of six or seven, a child is not able to put herself in the position of another child. However by the age of about seven, during Piaget's period of concrete operations, she is able to do mental experiments which enable her to achieve an idea of how others might feel in similar situations.

Donaldson (1978) criticised some of the experimentation involved in Piaget's theory of cognitive development. Donaldson's own theories suggest that if one wants to see children at their most competent, one should not look at how they attempt tasks or questions set by psychologists, but at how they attempt tasks which they have set themselves in an environment which is meaningful and supportive to them. If Donaldson's views are correct, it seems likely that by observing children going about their ordinary lives we see examples of intellectual competence – such as logical reasoning or taking another's point of view – before the age of seven.

In the area of sex-role development, the two-year old child knows she is called a girl, but tends to use words as proper names. It is not until she has achieved a notion of classes and categories that she can begin to see herself as a member of the group of children called girls and then begin to identify with that group. Classifying or sorting of objects or people according to size, shape, colour, peer group, family and race develops gradually. A two-way classification is all that most children can cope with at the age of three to five years – the more complex classifications occur later during infant and junior school. Similarly the young child understands time only in relation to her own activities.

Social developmental stages cannot occur until the child has passed through a cognitive stage in which she is able to grasp general principles to guide her behaviour in situations in which she is not immediately involved.

A theme which runs throughout this chapter is the interaction of two important influences on a child's health – biological state and social milieu.

Biological transitions are shared by all children, whatever their cultural group or location. However, the meaning attached to these biological changes varies greatly. For example, the onset of menstruation may be openly discussed, a private mystery, or a source of embarrassment.

Transitions that are determined by society tend to have very little correspondence with the biological state of the child or adolescent. This is underlined by the fact that sexual maturity usually occurs several years before sexual relationships are permitted by law in the UK. Compulsory entry into school and the right to vote occur on a particular day, regardless of the physical, emotional or cognitive state of the child or adolescent.

In relation to the social milieu, economic circumstances are also an important influence on child health. Indeed, economic influences on child health are far-reaching. Health will be affected by both the social class into which the child is born and the prevailing social policies.

Subculture and the family

Each **subculture** has a pattern of experience which affects the pace of development. Boys or girls can be considered as belonging to different subcultures in society for which there are distinctive expectations about age-appropriate behaviour (Nicholson, 1977; Sharpe, 1976). These expectations are affected in their turn by the other groups to which a particular boy or girl belongs.

The pattern of language that a child develops in her family is often characteristic of the subculture to which the family belongs and will serve as a signal of subcultural membership to others. Therefore when a child begins **school**, which is a socialising influence, her style of language may well determine a set of expectations and attitudes that are associated with her group (Bernstein, 1964).

Biological time

Each child follows her own course of biological maturation and change. No two children are completely alike.

Discussion of biological time, social time, historic time, subculture, and cognitive and psychological time indicates that what happens to an individual child at a particular age can only be understood in terms of the particular processes affecting her at a certain time. In the absence of a knowledge of these processes, a child's age tells us relatively little about her psychological state.

Principles of development

The ways in which the whole child changes over time are both quantitative and qualitative in nature.

Quantitative changes

Growth comprises quantitative changes involving an increase in size of the whole child, or in the size and number of any of the child's parts. The change is measurable, usually in *centimetres* (height), *kilograms* (weight) or by an *increase in numbers present* (for example increased vocabulary, increased number of relationships with others, increased number of physical skills that can be performed). Such changes are easily observed or studied.

Qualitative changes

These refer to the 'leaps' (increased skill or capacity) in function that result from mastering a series of smaller steps. The qualitative component, called development, is more complex and less easily measured or studied.

Timing of quantitative and qualitative changes

To some extent this is controlled by a maturational process that involves the child's biological ability and environmental opportunity. For example, at approximately ten to 16 months, the child relinquishes the palmar grasp in favour of the more manipulative pincer grasp that will allow better investigation of the immediate environment. This does not happen, however, until the biological structures, increased muscle cells and nerve cell specialisation necessary to perform this action have developed.

Transactional model of development

During the course of development the child and the environment affect each other. Development is a continuous process of 'transactions' between the child and her environment, and the only way to understand that fully is to watch it as it happens. The transactional model of development is illustrated in Fig. 19.8.

The Alis are a Bengali family living in the East End of London. Mr Ali owns a local restaurant. Mrs Ali remains at home. There are four children — Shagna aged eleven and her siblings aged nine, seven and five.

Shagna has dark brown hair and sparkling brown eyes; she is wearing a dress with large buttons down the front. She later tells you she can button her dress all by herself. Her legs are in braces and her arms appear stiff. Shagna's mother is a thin, pleasant, but tired-looking woman. She says Shagna needs some assistance with bathing, dressing and feeding and she uses special utensils for eating. Although Shagna has a chronological age of eleven years, her physical abilities are approximately those of a four year old, while her intelligence has been evaluated at the twelve year old level. Emotionally and socially she appears to be at the level of a seven or eight year old child.

Shagna was diagnosed as having cerebral palsy when she was five months old. She has been followed by the Community Team for People with a Learning Disability. You are visiting Shagna in her home, with the health visitor member of the team.

Consider the following issues:

(1) What factors do you think might explain the variation in Shagna's developmental levels (physical, cognitive, emotional and social)?
(2) How might Shagna's disability influence her developing concept of her body-image and her self-concept?
(3) What effect might Shagna's disability have on her mother, her father, and her siblings?

Fig. 19.7 Profile: Shagna Ali

The profile of a child with cerebral palsy (Fig. 19.7) is given to encourage you to consider the ways in which a child transacts with the immediate environment, and how both become altered in the process.

The role of genes in development

It may appear from Fig. 19.6 that there is no role left for genes to play in development. However, this is as untrue as the belief that the environment interacts directly with the genes. We know that there are some features of the **genotype** that almost certainly affect development. Although the chromosomal abnormality explains *why* a child with

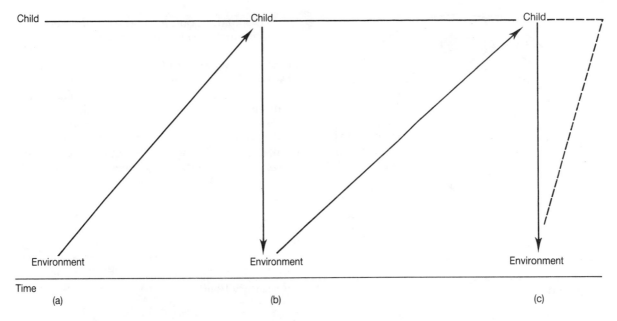

We can summarise the argument as follows:

- Development at point (b) is the result of the interactions between the environment and the child
- The environment at point (b) is partly a result of the child
- The child at point (b) is the result of interaction between the environment and the child at point (a), and so on

Fig. 19.8 *Transactional model of development (adapted from Sameroff and Chandler, 1975)*

Down's syndrome is retarded, it does not tell us *how*. In order to understand the abnormal development we need to know how the genetic factors affect development via the child and her environment. With our present state of knowledge, we are unable to provide an environment for Down's syndrome children which can be engineered to produce normal outcomes, but this has not been proved to be out of the question. Indeed recent advances in the education of handicapped children are showing more and more how optimal environments can produce faster and more normal development.

For normal development to occur, there has to be an appropriate and continuous interaction between the child and the environment. Children who start life with a normal genetic endowment following a normal pregnancy and delivery are able to develop normally given an appropriate environment. But children who start life with abnormal behaviour – whether for genetic or prenatal reasons – do not always stay abnormal. The result of the developmental process depends on the ex-

tent to which the environment can adjust to the child in order to produce a normal outcome. In the same way, children who start life normal can become abnormal if the environment in which they develop does not provide the right 'transactions' and if it is insensitive to the child's own influence.

The child as part of a system

At first the child relates mainly to her primary carer, then to the family, then to peers and teachers at school, and finally to members of the wider community (Herbert, 1991). This inter-relationship is illustrated in Fig. 19.9.

The child affects the mother (aunt, teacher or friend) as much as she herself is influenced by them. Early books on child development described a one-way process; now we are more confident in asserting that the process is two-way.

Trevarthen (1982) has argued that human infants are social beings at birth, ready to interact with others of their own kind. Therefore cognitive de-

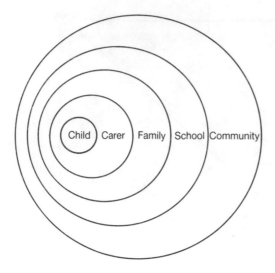

Fig. 19.9 *The developing child as part of a system*

velopment may result from the interaction between the innately social human infant and other humans who have already developed the relevant form of understanding. Infants seem to seek to share their 'knowledge' with their care-givers who usually treat the infants as if they do indeed comprehend more than they appear to. In this way, cognitive development takes root.

Concepts central to development

The following concepts are central to child development.

(1) The child is always part of a system. At birth this system is one of child–mother (or mother substitute). As the child's social interactions widen the system becomes child–family, then child–school and later child–community. The child affects the other members of this system as much as she is influenced by them. This perspective represents a shift in theories relating to child development. Early texts on child development described a one-way process; most now assert that the process is two-way.

(2) Heredity and transactions with the environment shape the child into a unique human being.

(3) Self-actualisation (achievement of potential) is the ultimate goal of human development.

In the early weeks of life it looks as if anything is possible cognitively, for the normal healthy infant has considerable cognitive potential. Infants have both the sensory equipment and the cognitive organisation to enable them to attend to all those aspects of the human environment which are relevant to their existence. As the months pass, selective exposure to certain experiences will mean that not all the possibilities will be actualised. Development is thus the sum of both loss and gain. An adult's construction of reality is the actualisation of one spectrum of possibilities and, by its existence, renders impossible the emergence of others.

Derived from these concepts are some commonalities of development, referred to as *principles of growth and development* (see Table 19.5).

(1) *Development is complex*
Human development is a continuous, irreversible and complex process that is lifelong. Inherent in this developmental process is ageing, which is most rapid during the fetal stage and is also lifelong.

(2) *Development has direction*
Human development follows a sequence: from *simple* to *complex* (for example, the child's ability

Table 19.5. *Principles of growth and development*

1. Development is complex

2. Development has direction
   - from simple to complex
   - from general to specific
   - from head to toe (cephalo-caudal)
   - from inner to outer (proximo-distal)

3. Development is predictable

4. Children develop uniquely

5. Children develop through conflict and adaptation

6. Development involves challenge

7. Development requires practice and energy investment

to make basic 'cooing' sounds before she learns to refine those sounds into speech); from *general* to *specific* (for example, the infant's acquisition of palmar grasp before she learns the finer control of pincer grasp); from *head* to *toe* (cephalo-caudally) – an infant gains neck and head control before she can control the movements of her trunk and limbs; from *inner* to *outer* (proximo-distally) – similar to the cephalo-caudal principle, in that the child learns control of the near structures before that of the structures further away from her centre. She is able to coordinate her arms to reach for an object before she has learned the hand and finger coordination necessary to grasp it.

(3) *Development is predictable*

The orderly sequence of development is invariable and although the precise age for the sequential steps to occur varies for each child, there is a general chronology that involves wide norm ranges to allow for these individual differences. For example, the age range for learning to walk is usually given as nine to 15 months, with the average age being 12 months.

A child will usually follow a consistent pattern with respect to either an early or late rate of development. Therefore, deviation from her own pattern may be more indicative of a problem than conforming to the norm.

However, the characteristics of growth and behaviour at each age, and the maturational changes that occur with increasing age are similar between children. The child cannot walk until she has mastered crawling, regardless of whether she follows an early or late pattern for achieving these characteristic behaviours or changes.

(4) *Children develop uniquely*

The sequence is the same for all children but the rate of development varies from child to child. It is essential for parents to understand this principle when they are tempted to compare one child to the detriment of another.

Every child has her own genetic potential for growth and development that cannot be exceeded but may be deterred or modified at any stage in the sequence. For example, although intellect is primarily set by genetic inheritance, a child's experiences will either stimulate or discourage her intellect. If she is malnourished, confined to her cot, offered few interactions with the people in her environment, she may not achieve intellec-

tually regardless of her genetic potential. Conversely, offered opportunities to experience the world from a number of positions (cot, floor, shoulder), fed on a nutritionally balanced diet, and provided with regular opportunities to interact (be spoken to, played with, cuddled) with the important people in her environment, the child is on her way to achieving her intellectual potential.

(5) *Children develop through conflict and adaptation*

Each stage in the developmental sequence has intervals of equilibrium and disequilibrium. Conflict arises out of the child's motivation to master her environment and her lack of the competence needed for that mastery. Equilibrium exists before the new environmental or maturational stimulus occurs that demands adaptation by the child, and after the child has developed the necessary competence to adapt to the stimulus. Disequilibrium exists in the interval between recognition of and desire to master (adapt to) the new stimulus until mastery is accomplished. Growing children repeatedly demonstrate their strength and competence to adapt and achieve if their environment gives them at least some support.

(6) *Development involves challenge*

Development comes about when a stable set of structures or organisational forms of mental activity are challenged by an external or internal event, or by change with which they cannot cope. This sets up disequilibrium. New structures are formed which are able to cope. Equilibrium is restored and a new developmental level is reached.

Social expectations for each developmental stage exist, and are called *developmental tasks*. The task of each stage is to overcome the problem or challenge that (because of her age) confronts a child. Delay or failure in task achievement makes further development more difficult. For example: Erikson (1963) defines the infant's emotional and social tasks as 'learning to trust'; Piaget (1969) defines the school-age child's intellectual task as learning to use symbols and the concepts they represent; a physical task of the toddler is learning to walk without aid.

(7) *Development requires practice and energy investment*

Although development is consistent and follows a pattern, this does not mean that it is steady across all areas.

Table 19.6. Development requires practice and energy investment

- During *infancy* the central focus of energy is on sensorimotor and physical growth

- The *toddler's* energy concentration is invested in her developing selfhood and body control

- The *pre-schooler's* investment is in language development

- Cognitive development and sociability require the bulk of the *school-age child's* energy

- The *teenager* exerts massive energy in development of her sexual and social identity and capacity for intimacy

Early achievement in one competency area may regress temporarily while some other aspect of that competency area or another is being stimulated, because a strong preoccupation exists to perfect the skill required for mastery of the newly confronted stimulus (see, for example, Table 19.6).

In summary, although human development is complex, it is continuous, it follows an orderly sequence and general chronological pattern, it involves task mastery, and it requires concentration of energy upon the task confronting the child at that particular time. Task achievement in one area of competence is not accomplished in isolation but interacts simultaneously with skills in other areas of competence to result in characteristic ways of behaving.

Play

Play is a difficult word to define. Numerous theories have been put forward to explain why and how children play.

Play as a preparation for adulthood

According to those who uphold this theory, the function of play is to enable the child to exercise skills necessary for adult life.

The value of this theory is that it recognises the functional value of play: practising and perfecting the skills needed in adult life.

Surplus energy theory

Those propagating this theory suggest that children play because excess energy accumulates, necessitating release through play. The exuberant activities of children are recognised to be a normal part of their development but play is not thought to accomplish any immediate goal.

Psychoanalytic theory

Theorists such as Freud and Erikson see play as a method used by children to relive certain powerful experiences and thus to come to terms with them. The use of play therapy to treat emotionally disturbed children is an outgrowth of the psychoanalytic view of play.

None of these theories is acceptable as a total explanation of play and none can be, for play means different things to different people at different times.

The contribution of play to child development

The varied theories of play suggest that play has something to do with every aspect of the developing child. A combination of these theories suggests that play contributes to the physical, intellectual, emotional and social development of children (see Table 19.7).

Developmental characteristics of play

The kind of play in which children engage is largely determined by their developmental stage. As a child grows and develops, her environment changes and so do her needs. From a developmental point of view, patterns of children's play can be categorised according to content and social character. In both there is an additive effect. Each builds on past accomplishments and some element of each is maintained throughout life.

Social character of play

The social character of play can be classified chronologically.

Table 19.7. *The contribution of play*

Active play encourages both gross and fine motor development	Physical development
Through active exploration of the environment and through passive play activities like watching television and reading	Cognitive development
Before a child is able to use words to describe what she sees, her experiences with space, sound, colour and relationships help her to form impressions about the environment. It is these early experiences and formation of multiple images that help her put words into use	Language development
Children can experiment in play and may then transfer learning to other situations	Stimulus for creativity
Children learn something of their abilities and how they compare with their peers	The development of self-insight
This is a life-long learning process. Children engage in fantasy play to explore feelings, lessen fears and work through conflicts. In games of pretending, imaginary playmates are safe recipients of aggressive impulses. Experiences that have frightened or excited a child may be re-enacted in play with imaginary participants. Through such play activities a child can express those intense feelings that may not be perceived as acceptable forms of behaviour in the real world	Expression of emotions
As play becomes more bound by rules so these become enforced more rigidly and group norms of right and wrong, fair and unfair are learned	Moral standards
Sex roles are rarely taught explicitly. Play provides many opportunities for covert instruction	Learning to play 'appropriate' sex roles

(1) Unoccupied behaviour

The child apparently is not playing but occupies herself with watching anything that happens to be of momentary interest.

(2) Onlooker

The child spends most of her time watching the other children play. She often talks to the children whom she is observing, asks questions or gives suggestions, but does not overtly enter into the play herself.

(3) Solitary independent play

The child plays alone and independently with toys that are different from those used by the children within speaking distance. She makes no effort to get close to other children.

(4) Parallel activity

The child plays independently but the activity she chooses naturally brings her among other children. She plays with toys that are like those the children around her are using, but she plays with the toys as she sees fit and does not try to influence or modify the activity of the children near her.

(5) Associative play

The child plays with other children. The conversation concerns their common activity; there is borrowing and lending of play material and mild attempts to control which children may or may not play in the group. All the members engage in similar if not identical activity. There is no division of labour, and no organisation of the activity of several individuals around any material goal or product. Instead of subordinating her individual interest to that of the group, each child plays as she wishes.

(6) Cooperative play

The child plays in a group that is organised for the purpose of making some material product, or of striving to attain some competitive goal, or of dramatising situations of adult life. There is a marked sense of belonging to the group or not belonging to it. The control of the group situation is in the hands of one or two of the members who direct the activity of the others. The goal as well as the method of attaining it necessitates a division of labour, the taking of different roles by the various group members, and the organisation of activity so that the efforts of one child are supplemented by those of another.

Content of play

Six categories of play have been identified. These are social–affective play; sense–pleasure play; skill play; dramatic play; formal play; and competitive play.

Each category of play builds on past accomplishments, and some element of each is maintained throughout life.

Social–affective play

Parents stimulate their infants and the infants' positive responses act as a reward to the parents so that a cyclical pattern of play develops.

Sense–pleasure play

This is stimulated by environmental variations in colour, movement, sound, taste and texture. The experience of sensing these variations is pleasurable, consequently the term sense-pleasure. For the infant, pleasurable experiences are expanded when she develops the manipulative and loco-motor ability to experiment with the sensations derived from play with water, sand and food. Activities of movement such as swinging, bouncing and rocking are examples of sense-pleasure play, as is the child's exploration of her own body.

Skill play

Skill play occurs when infants have developed the ability to reach out, grasp and manipulate. It consists of the repetitive practice of newly discovered abilities. For example, it is the challenge of a new video game rather than the sensation of playing it that motivates the child in skill play. The fascination that motivates skill play is the challenge of taking on a task which one is hardly capable of accomplishing. People of all ages are subject to this intrigue.

Dramatic play

In dramatic play a child tries out roles and identities drawn from her immediate home environment, and later from the world at large. The imitative quality of this play is obvious when a child mimics adults by talking into the telephone and dressing up in adult clothing. It is through imitation that a child identifies with the prominent people in her environment.

Dramatic play can take two forms – *reproductive dramatic play* or *productive dramatic play*. In reproductive dramatic play children attempt to re-create in their play a situation they have observed in real life or perhaps on the television or at the cinema. In productive dramatic play, by contrast, children create characters and themes that may be taken either from real life experiences or from their imagination.

Formal games

Formal play consists of simple, non-competitive games such as London Bridge. As children get older, their play becomes competitive (many sporting activities are competitive, for example).

Competitive games

In Western societies, as children grow older, they are encouraged to play competitive games. These range from board games to sports. Indeed adolescent boys who deviate from the norm of expressing intense interest in sport are often ridiculed. One might cynically argue that this meets the needs of a secular society whose principles are based on acquisition and profit and hence the need to produce a social character orientated to these principles.

The progression from social–affective play to formal games and from solitary play to cooperative play reflects the child's developing physical, intellectual and social skills. This process is obviously influenced by the child's social milieu. Economic necessity puts a severe constraint on play in some cultures. Lansdown (1984) reports that one group in Kenya have chores assigned to them by the age of three, thus time for play is restricted. Economic poverty also restricts the number and quality of toys available to many children but it does not follow that there is no play. Children are adept at using other materials such as mud, wood and stone.

Rich, imaginative play is less often observed in cultures where adults live narrow, restricted lives. It has also been suggested that different play experiences explain many of the differences in ability and attainment that are found between children of differing cultures. However, this a politically sensitive topic.

Helping parents to promote play

If the nurse has some knowledge of what constitutes normal, healthy play she can discuss with parents the importance of providing opportunities for play appropriate to the child's age. It should also be stressed that it is not necessary to buy expensive toys to promote children's development.

Working-class parents and parents from other cultures may regard play simply as a way in which children amuse and occupy themselves. Tizard *et al*. (1981) found that parents who take this view are often puzzled by, or even hostile to, the priority given by professionals to play.

Too many toys can be confusing and overstimulating to children. Excessive use of toys can frustrate a child's own resourcefulness to create play situations out of natural stimuli in the environment. Self-expression and the freedom to play according to their own needs is what is most beneficial to children.

Play: a summary

Numerous theories have been put forward to explain why and how children play. These include: children use play to practise the skills necessary for life; children play in order to release excess energy; in play children recapitulate the history of their race. Psychoanalysts see play as a means of reliving certain powerful experiences and thus coming to terms with them. This has formed the basis of play therapy. Play also advances physical, cognitive and language development and the learning of 'appropriate' sex roles. In addition to stimulating creativity, play facilitates the development of self-insight, moral standards and expression of emotions.

From a developmental point of view, patterns of children's play can be categorised according to content and social character. In both there is an additive effect. Each builds on past accomplish-

ments and some element of each is maintained throughout life. The social character of play includes unoccupied behaviour, onlooker play, solitary independent play, parallel activity, associative play and cooperative play. The content of play includes social–affective play, sense–pleasure play, skill play, dramatic play and formal games. The nurse's role as a health educator involves discussing with parents the importance of play.

Conclusions

In this section, the need has been stressed to maintain the focus on the whole child, including her family, whilst examining the different components of her development.

The question of why nurses who care for children require a knowledge of child development has been explored. At the most fundamental level, such knowledge is necessary for the nurse to develop and use a plan of care that is age-appropriate and relevant to the needs of the child. As the nurse becomes more skilled she can use such knowledge to teach parents so that they can contribute positively to their children's optimal growth and development.

Concepts related to development, which are often taken for granted, have been explored in this chapter. Age does not cause behavioural change, it is simply a convenient way of measuring the time in which experiential, maturational and physiological processes occur. What is meant by the word 'child' has been discussed – and the conclusions reached suggest that we cannot give childhood a culturally universal fixed beginning and end; rather that we use the term to cover an enormous range of development.

Througout this section the transactional model of development has been emphasised. The inter-relationship between society and the individual child's development has been discussed and it has been suggested that what happens to an individual child at a particular age can only be understood in terms of the particular processes affecting her at that time.

The transactional model of development is reflected in the idea that the developing child and the environment affect each other. Development is a continuous process of 'transactions' between the child and her environment. The child is therefore always part of a system. Thus the child affects the mother (aunt, teacher or friend) as much as she herself is influenced – it is a two-way process.

Concepts central to child development that have been discussed include: complexity; direction; predictability; uniqueness; development through conflict and adaptation; the importance of challenge; and the need for practice and the investment of energy.

Play is very much related to development. Through playing, children promote and advance development and their evolving capacity to participate in more complex interpersonal relationships.

A consideration of the different theories of play, the nature of play and its importance, has been given in this chapter.

Glossary

Genotype: Genes are hereditary factors, and the combination of genes that an individual plant or animal possesses is called its 'genotype'. Therefore an individual's genetic constitution is called his genotype. However, his actual appearance, which is the product of his genotype and the environment he has experienced, is called his 'phenotype' (see also Chapter 6)

Peer group as an agent of socialisation: The peer group or association of age-mates is produced, to a great extent, by the age-grading of the school. One of its functions may be to provide a particular child with a learning setting in which to exert influence. It may also enable the child to resist, through solidarity and support from friends, the socialising pressures of adults, such as teachers and parents. In changing societies, the peer group may enable the child to practise roles that she will act out in her future life, but which her parents have been unable to teach her

School as an agent of socialisation: The school introduces the child to the wider society where there are new patterns of authority and new possibilities for forming relationships. Even where there is no emphasis on competition at home, she will become aware that individuals are valued differently depending on what they can do. She will no longer be valued just for what she is as she progresses through the school; she will learn at some point that society has a pyramidal structure with a few places at the top, but with most people destined for a lower status

Subculture and the family as agents of socialisation: The family presents the infant with her first image of society in the context of its particular subcultural settings. The pattern of relationships that she meets serve as a first, powerful glimpse of the possible interactions between people.

It is almost certain that the child will learn a set of behaviours appropriate to her sex. From the moment of birth, boys and girls are usually treated differently by parents, brothers and sisters (Maccaby and Jacklin, 1975). Some researchers (for example, Newson and Newson, 1976) might argue, however, that boys and girls are not treated differently. Although much of our sex-role behaviour may be 'personally constricting', it is maintained and enhanced by institutions throughout our lives

References

Donaldson, M. (1978). *Children's Minds* (6th ed.). Fontana, London.

Erikson, W.W. (1963). *Childhood and Society*. Norton and Company, London

Goodman, M.E. (1967). *The Individual and Culture*. Homeward, Illinois.

Herbert, M. (1991). *Clinical Child Psychology: Social Learning, Development and Behaviour*. John Wiley, New York.

Kohlberg, L. (1969). *Stages in the Development of Moral Thought and Action*. Holt, Rinehart and Winston, New York.

Laishley, J. (1987). *Working with Young Children: Encouraging their Developmental Dealing with Problems*. Edward Arnold, London.

Lansdown, R. (1984). *Child Development Made Simple*. Heinemann, London.

Maccaby, E.E. and Jacklin, C.N. (1975). *The Psychology of Sex Difference*. Oxford University Press, Oxford.

Newson, J. and Newson, E. (1976). *Seven Years Old in the Home Environment*. Allen and Unwin, London.

Nicholson, J. (1977). *What Society Does to Girls*. Virago, London.

Piaget, J. and Inhelder, B. (1969). *The Psychology of the Child*. Basic Books, London.

Sameroff, A.J. and Chandler, M.J. (1975). Reproductive risk and the continuum of caretaking casualty. In *Review of Child Development Research 4*, Hurowitz, F.D. (ed.). University of Chicago Press, Chicago.

Sharpe, S. (1976). *Just Like a Girl: How Girls Learn to be Women*. Penguin Books, Harmondsworth.

Tizard, B., Mortimore, J. and Burchell, B. (1981). *Involving Parents In Nursing and Infant Schools*. Grant McIntyre, London.

Trevarthen, C. (1982). The primary motives for cooperative understanding. In *Social Cognition*, Butterworth, S. and Light, P. (eds.). Harvester Press, Brighton.

SECTION 3: NURSING PROCESSES IN HEALTH PROMOTION

This section includes the following topics:

- Promoting personal responsibility for health

- The nurse's teaching role
  - teaching parents
  - teaching children

- Communicating with children and parents

- children's cognitive and linguistic abilities
- the counselling role

- Health appraisal
  - taking a history
  - physical parameters

- Fluid and electrolyte balance
  - a key concept in child health

Promoting personal responsibility for health by children and their families may occur in a variety of settings including the well child clinic, the children's ward, the school, or any other setting where the nurse interacts with children and families.

Whatever the setting, the process by which the nurse motivates this responsibility for self-care is illustrated in Fig. 19.10.

Establishing rapport

The essentials for a cooperative relationship are trust, empathy, and genuineness, shared mutually by each person involved in the interaction. Each participant comes with her own values, needs and perceptions of what the relationship will accomplish.

Trust

Trust is most quickly established when the nurse responds in a consistent, non-judgemental manner that conveys acceptance of and alliance with the child and parent.

Empathy

Empathy is communicated to the child or parent

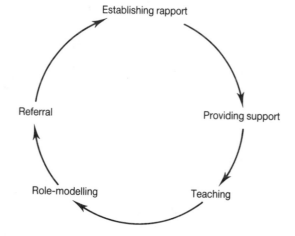

Fig. 19.10 *The process by which the nurse motivates responsibility for self-care*

when the nurse takes seriously the concerns expressed, whether they are expressed verbally or non-verbally. The nurse's questions, used to help her discover the child's and parent's perceptions of their needs, should demonstrate that she cares, that she considers them worthwhile, and that she wants to understand how they are feeling.

Genuineness

Being genuine is extremely important when dealing with children, as they are particularly alert to insincerity. The nurse should be honest with the child and the parent at all times and make no promises that cannot be carried out. If possible, the nurse should position herself at the child's physical level during any interaction and avoid artificial barriers (such as desks) between herself and her clients. A working relationship is seldom established immediately, and the child will frequently test the nurse to assure herself that the relationship with her is still stable. Often, the best approach to the child is through the medium of shared play. Parents respond more quickly when the nurse approaches parental needs first (even small ones such as making sure they are comfortable or that they have a cup of coffee).

When the nurse models the behaviours necessary for a good working relationship, her client (whether a child or adult) is given guidelines for her behaviour in the relationship. Once she becomes comfortable in this behaviour, cooperative interaction is possible.

Supportive nursing actions

The modern family often feels isolated from the wisdom of the older generation's extended family. Health professionals have recognised this fact and accepted greater responsibility for providing information and the support services that were formerly readily available within the family itself.

Unless parents have their own dependent needs met, we cannot expect that they will do well in meeting their child's developmental needs, encouraging her steadily to assume responsibility for her own health, hence giving reinforcement to their own credibility as parents.

Building parental self-esteem

Very simple actions by the nurse, if genuinely employed, will build parents' self-esteem. These actions can be carried out even during brief contacts with them. When the nurse addresses the parent (or child) by name, she communicates that she acknowledges him or her to be a recognisable, unique person rather than 'just another parent'. Casual statements by the nurse such as, 'Mrs Carpenter, you are feeding Donna properly. She is gaining just the amount in weight and height that she should be for her age', reassure the parent that positive changes are occurring in the child because of her care.

Equally supportive are comments that help the family see their child's positive responses to them – for example, 'Look how Adam follows you with his eyes? You are important to him. He looks for you', or 'Catherine talks about you frequently and pretends that she is you in her play on the children's ward'.

Not only do such statements support the parent's confidence in herself as a parent, they also stimulate positive feelings in the parent toward the child.

An approach that acknowledges the feelings, needs and well-being of the family (not just the child) is also supportive. A question such as 'How is the rest of the family reacting to David's temper tantrums?' or 'How are you managing your own need for rest while Patsy is ill?' communicates the nurse's understanding that the child's needs and behaviours affect all family members.

The nurse must support families within the context of their cultural beliefs, parenting practices, and selected lifestyle. She should also make use of every opportunity to convey confidence in the parents' ability to make health judgements and to trust their own feelings and their ability to act to promote the child's health. The feelings of success the nurse helps to engender in the child's parents in one situation encourage them to act successfully in others.

The nurse's teaching role

A large amount of nursing care in any setting is teaching. Because of the brevity of contact, the nurse should recognise that the whole time a parent is present is a precious teaching opportunity, and that each procedure or treatment carried out lends itself simultaneously to teaching.

Teaching may be formal in a planned situation such as parentcraft classes or school health education. More often, however, teaching is informal or incidental, occurring at any opportune moment and prompted by an immediately identified need.

The three most prominent forms of incidental learning are:

(1) Imitation of role models
(2) Task repetition
(3) Positive environmental feedback.

In any situation, *active* teaching is usually more

effective. Active teaching uses actions rather than words to convey the necessary information.

Role modelling is a technique that the nurse may use in order to teach actively. At any age, individuals learn more from the teacher's actions than from her words. This is especially true of adults who feel insecure in the parent role, since they tend to rely on imitation to learn skills. A second technique is the use of demonstration to clarify verbal instruction. A third is role playing, puppet play, games using role reversal, and psychodrama. These take more time but are extremely effective in increasing the learner's sensitivity to others' feelings or circumstances. A fourth technique is learner-participation in tasks, reinforced by visible or tangible rewards for effort as well as accomplishment. One learns best when one performs or practises under supervision those skills one must eventually manage on one's own. Rewards can be used to motivate repetition to master the task. As a general rule of thumb, the more educated the learner, the more likely she is to be able to learn through verbal or written instruction and logical explanation, with or without the use of active teaching techniques.

Teaching parents

Wellness behaviour is learnt. The overall concept of health, and the value it is given, indirectly influence health behaviour and the readiness with which it is learnt. The values parents hold towards health, the level of knowledge they have about health, and the extent to which they practise wellness behaviours greatly influence their child's development of healthy attitudes and behaviour. These facts indicate the relevance of teaching parents the principles of healthy living if the goal of developing self-initiated responsibility for health in their children is to be reached.

Several critical areas in which parents expect assistance have been identified (Hansen and Avadine, 1974). These are summarised in Table 19.8.

Underlying these many expectations brought to the health professional is the parents' desire to succeed in the care of their child and to receive encouragement from the professional that their parenting strategies can succeed.

Health-related topics are currently receiving a high priority in the media. The nurse should keep herself up-to-date in relation to this, since parents are likely to apply and question such information

Table 19.8. *Areas where parents require particular help and information*

- Child development and the parents' role in fostering positive development

- Childrearing issues and the rationale for approaches that the health professions recommend

- Child behaviour (including school, social and learning behaviour) and how to manage it

- The steps to take when caring for an ill child at home, and the rationale for this management

- Family issues and balancing the needs, care and problems of all family members

- How best to use and relate to members of the primary health care team and other community resources

- Identifying and managing problems and needs that parents themselves experience

- Family relationships related to issues such as personal and interpersonal crises, illness, divorce or separation, single parenting

and look to the nurse to answer their questions. The nurse should also consider the *political implications of health education*.

The trained nurse can employ a variety of techniques in assisting parents to gain knowledge and skills in parenting, such as applying teaching-learning theory. However, the teaching the nurse carries out as a role model (demonstrating to parents how to respond to their child through cuddling, talking, listening, touching and praise) is probably the most important knowledge she can impart.

Teaching children

If children are steadily to assume more responsibility for their own health as they grow, we need to teach them how to manage stress. They must learn ways to reduce stress in their environment, acquire effective coping skills, and develop an attitude that is orientated towards health rather than illness. Children need information about what to expect (what they will hear, feel, smell and see) during health care experiences. Similarly, if they are to initiate their own health care, they must learn how to approach health care providers and be assertive with them.

Table 19.9. *Typical age-related concepts of health, cognitive level, approach to teaching and expectations for self-care*

Age	Health concept	Cognitive level	Age-related teaching approach	Responsibility for self-initiated care
Infancy (0–1)	No concept, learns to assign value to needs on the basis of how well and how consistently they are met	Egocentric	Basic needs must be fully and consistently met	None — totally dependent on caretakers
Early childhood (1–4)	No concept; merely imitates behaviour of role models that are satisfying and/or earn reward	Egocentric; preconceptual; does not question own perceptions	Continue meeting basic needs but steadily demand that child master skills of daily living; model wellness behaviours; reward her imitations. Play with child to learn her perceptions since she cannot communicate them adequately	Some capacity to carry out tasks to promote own health if taught skills and allowed opportunity to take responsibility; likes to practise wellness behaviours
Middle childhood (5–8)	Recognises that health involves a series of health practices – (eat a balanced diet, brush teeth, stay clean, etc.)	Egocentric; concrete reality predominates	Encourage her to say what her health needs are, what caused any deficit, what she might do to resolve that need. Correct misperceptions. Use teaching techniques that provide her with tactile, visual, auditory and motor experiences	Can carry out many tasks to promote own health, seeks responsibility; practice is important. Can take independent action to identify many health needs and can identify some realistic solutions
Late childhood and pre-adolescence (9–13)	Concept of health as sense of physical well-being, for example 'feeling good', 'being fit'	Objective, systematic thought; questions and seeks validation and correction of own perceptions. Gradual increase in causal reasoning; still favours concrete reality	Share assessment and/or findings; this allows her to perceive changes in health status. Allow time for her to validate her perceptions of her needs and what actions should be taken, respect her views and opinions. Give simple rationale for health practices/procedures. Make invisible processes of health real with diagrams, models. Teach the skill/procedure then give the rationale in simple terms	Can plan for and take initiative to carry out most health needs if she has learned trust and autonomy. Can participate actively in managing her own health needs. Acute interest in health education. Can consider possible risks and benefits of health behaviours if allowed to participate in problem solving

Age	Health concept	Cognitive level	Age-related teaching approach	Responsibility for self-initiated care
Adolescence and young adulthood (14–21)	Concept of health as physical, emotional, social stability that is long term though superimposed brief illness may cause temporary instability. Evidenced by 'feeling good', being in control of self, being able to participate in desired activities	Realises realm of possible and hypothetical as well as the real. Develops theories. Craves details for egocentric purposes primarily	Important to have people whom she respects as role models to overcome peer group pressure. Honesty imperative to her cooperation. Present all details; relate them to her personally. Especially likes theoretical explanations and discussions. Allow discussion of the effects of health problems and health behaviours on her and her future. Let her determine the possible resolutions to her health needs and collaborate with her to determine management. Begin by presenting rationale for a skill procedure, then give details of performing it	Can assume full responsibility to identify her health needs, determine possible resolutions and carry them out. Can use concepts of wellness constructively in decision making

Acquisition of healthy behaviour by the child involves four processes:

(1) She must develop an awareness of health from role models.
(2) She must be exposed to developmentally appropriate information about wellness and health practices.
(3) If she is to learn responsibility, she must be included as an active participant (as early in life as possible) in making health choices so that she can master the problem-solving required to make healthy decisions about her life.
(4) She must be reinforced for her attempts and her successes in practising wellness behaviours.

Those teaching children health education must consider the child's thinking ability at various ages; the concept of health that is characteristic of her age; and the degree of independent action that she is realistically capable of for her stage in development. Table 19.9 describes these various characteristics for children at different age groups and their relevance in selecting an appropriate teaching approach.

Communicating with children and parents

Central to the process of communicating with children and parents is the nurse's understanding of herself and her awareness of the effect of her own communication. The way messages are formed (coded) and interpreted (decoded) is affected by how comfortable one feels in the presence of another. It is the nurse's goal to facilitate communication by creating an atmosphere of mutual acceptance.

Communications skills are some of the most important a nurse requires when nursing children in the context of family centred care. A nurse is able to accomplish very little unless parents and children feel accepted and comfortable in the relationship. For example, parents who feel that there is even the slightest possibility that they might be judged as incompetent are unlikely to reveal what they really feel about their children. Children are particularly sensitive and are unlikely to communicate with people who do not respect their worries and concerns.

Respect for each person as an individual is another central tenet of effective communication with parents and children. Communicating respect involves recognition that the views held by parents about bringing up children, health maintenance and children's roles may be opposite to those of the nurse. To respect parents as individuals is to recognise that longstanding family and cultural patterns are an integral part of their way of life and affect their view of parenting.

Children also need to be respected as individuals. It is easy to stereotype individual children by believing that because they are at a certain age they will behave in a prescribed manner. Each child has her own unique experiences that undoubtedly affect the way she talks and feels and how she interprets what is communicated to her. When the nurse is able to demonstrate her respect for the individuality of each family member, as well as for their needs, communication is likely to contribute to an effective parent-child-nurse relationship.

Integral to respect is the concept of acceptance of the whole person. To be accepting of a parent, a nurse must be able to appreciate that the child's temper tantrums produce intolerable frustration in the parent and may lead to physical punishment. The nurse does not have to agree with physical punishment to be accepting of the parent, but she should not make the parent feel less worthy. She should be able to accept the *need* that motivated the behaviour, rather than condemning the parent for the behaviour.

The nurse can show acceptance by encouraging expression of the feelings that led to the incident and thereby help a parent to identify alternative ways of responding to such stress.

Communicating with children involves a similar approach. The behaviour of the child does not have to be condoned even though her need is accepted.

Another tenet of effective communication with parents and children is *empathy*. Empathy means being able to perceive accurately how an experience *feels* for another person, from that person's

point of view. When dealing with children it means that one has to be able to see the world through the child's eyes to grasp what an experience means to her. Children express how they feel when they are quiet, when they talk, and especially when they play. To grasp how a child feels, attention must be given to *all* aspects of her behaviour, not just to her speech. Sensitivity to a child's non-verbal communication gives the nurse the most accurate sense of the child's true feelings, because children are often unable to talk about the way they feel.

When dealing with parents empathetically, a nurse does not offer advice or try to change the parent's way of thinking. Attempting to alter another person's thinking to fit in with one's own biases and beliefs is *evaluative* (not empathetic) behaviour.

The attitudes that the nurse holds about parents and children determine the quality of the relationship she can expect to develop. Her respect for the individual and acceptance of each family member in his or her own right are necessary before empathetic understanding can be communicated. It is the nurse's use of self and individuality that determines how the attitudes of respect, acceptance and empathy will be communicated. The parent-child-nurse relationship is shaped by the nurse's ability to use her own personal attributes in combination with her skills of communication.

Communicating with children

When communicating with a child it is important to recognise that each child is an individual who comes from a family. For example, a child who is encouraged to participate in decision-making in the home is likely to take an active role in decisions outside the home. A more dependent role is likely when the child comes from an adult-centred home in which children are expected to be submissive and are allowed little opportunity to contribute to family matters.

When communicating with children, always remember that they are people. Like everyone else they have ideas, and they need to feel important. It is essential that you take the time to listen to, and talk with, the child.

Children should be made to feel that their thoughts are significant enough to be heard and considered. It is particularly important that the child's view about health be heard and considered when health care is being planned. This is crucial if children are to participate in planning their own care. Research has suggested that children as young as five years old have ideas about health and can talk about health matters. The children in one study (Baker, 1980) defined health in a positive way as feeling good and being able to participate in desired activities.

If a nurse is to develop a relationship with a child in which she is trusted, she must be honest. Adults sometimes do not tell children the truth because they want to protect them. A fair approach to a child's question is an honest, straightforward answer. For example, if a child asks whether an injection will hurt the honest answer is 'yes', but one should also add the reassuring statement that it will be over quickly.

A nurse must be reliable in her relationship with a child so that an environment of trust is created in which the child feels secure. If promises are not kept the child may feel deceived. If it proves impossible to keep a promise this must be explained to the child.

Another area of potential deception is the offering of a choice when there is no choice. If small realistic choices are offered to a child this can give her a sense of importance and some control.

Setting limits is also important. A child without limits feels insecure. The 'testing' of adults by children should be recognised as a normal part of the process by which children receive feedback. Consistency and fairness in limit-setting provide security in child–nurse relationships and this will be beneficial to the child.

Communication by touch is a sensitive dimension. Treating children as objects to be indiscriminately patted, kissed and picked up without giving them a choice can communicate disrespect for them as persons. A child may be busy planning an important course of action when a nurse abruptly picks her up. When nurses meet their own needs of holding and cuddling with little regard for where the child was going or what she was about to do, touch has been used indiscriminately. A sensitive nurse will see the child as a person, observe what the child is doing and then use touch as a response to the needs of this individual and as a way to communicate affection.

Children also need privacy. Even at a young age a child's private thoughts should not be interrupted. The respect and confidence that children develop in their relationships with adults cannot be forced.

To communicate with children it is important to realise that emotions change rapidly. Hate can exist one moment and love the next. Respecting a child's emotions means allowing her to cry when she is hurt and to become angry when she is frustrated. This does not mean, however, that she should be allowed to be destructive or cause injury.

Children need time to get to know new people. An infant or a toddler may be frightened if approached and spoken to directly. When a child fears strangers it is more effective to speak first to the parent in the presence of the child and gradually to become acquainted with the child through the parent. It is important not to block the child's view of the parent so that she will not fear the parent has disappeared. A pre-school child might be approached through the medium of play, while a school-age child and adolescent need different approaches; they need to be spoken to directly, speaking secondly to the parent.

A child's height is obviously a disadvantage to any sense of power. Every attempt should be made to meet this person at eye level. This facilitates a greater sense of equality in the exchange from child to adult and from adult to child.

As children begin to understand and use words, it is important to have an understanding of the thought processes that affect the child's communication. It is important therefore to consider their cognitive and language abilities.

From two to seven years of age a child usually sees things from her own point of view (though this has been disputed by psychologists such as Donaldson, 1978, and Tizard and Hughes, 1984). It is difficult for her to understand why she cannot have a drink of water before an operation. She also makes causal errors by thinking that events that happen in proximity to each other are related. To give a child an injection immediately after she has been reprimanded for some unacceptable behaviour is both insensitive and destructive, because the child is likely to think that she received the injection *because* she misbehaved. Verbal explanations of the relationship between treatments and a child's state of health are not understood completely, but brief simple explanations should be given to increase her sense of well-being and security. It is important that acceptance and affection are communicated both verbally and non-verbally before, during, and after any painful event. Although a child does not understand the full implication of the words spoken to her, she understands (receptive language) more than is indicated by her speech (expressive language).

During the pre-operational stage children engage in pretending. A child's natural tendency to act out her feelings and experiences helps her to cope with the real world and can provide important information to others. Giving a child the opportunity to act out events which are about to happen to her may be more effective than verbal explanation.

At this stage children ask lots of 'why' questions. Armed only with their curiosity, logic and persistence, children tackle the task of making sense of a world they understand only imperfectly. Providing simple, concrete answers to 'why' questions helps the child to understand relationships and satisfies her curiosity. Answering the question is of greatest importance and should not be avoided.

Explanations that are given to children need to be expressed in concrete terms with reference to familiar happenings in their daily life. For example, time is understood when it is explained in relation to everyday events – after you wake up, have your breakfast and brush your teeth. Explanations such as 'There will be bright lights, the room will be cool, and they will take your picture with a large camera', gives the child concrete facts to think about and does not leave her prey to an imagination that is capable of perceiving an event as being far worse than it is in reality.

Between the ages of seven and 11 years, important advances are made that affect communication. The child's cognitive ability enables her to explore and consider many alternatives to a problem, but she is still bound to concrete thought. A school-age child must be given the opportunity to question and explore what is being said and what will happen to her. An increased understanding of her body and environment means that details must be painstakingly explained when describing an event that pertains to her body. It is especially important to encourage expression of fears when body integrity is threatened by invasive procedures.

The period between 11–15 years is when abstract thinking begins so that hypothetical situations can be created. The adolescent is no longer bound to concrete phenomena, and wishes to discuss values and ideals. She can hypothesise about how things should be done, especially when it involves her own future. She does not wish to be told what to do but will be much more cooperative if she is included in the decisions that are made regarding her.

Adolescents particularly need special respect for their thoughts and this should be communicated by avoiding prying into personal matters. They are also highly sensitive to non-verbal communication and need an environment of acceptance within which they feel free to express their view if they so desire (Neinstein, 1991).

Communicating with parents

Nurses must remember that parents too are individuals. Consequently the way parents view and feel about their parental role will differ with each individual. This accounts for phenomena that nurses may find troublesome; parents are individuals and therefore may disagree with each other.

The nurse must recognise that the way parents perceive their role will affect the communication process. Some parents may feel that they are expected to have certain feelings and respond in prescribed ways *because* they are parents. The nurse can dispel some of these erroneous ideas by acknowledging that their frustrations are normal reactions.

The nurse whose goal is to establish an atmosphere that encourages communication will be careful to avoid an attitude of 'talking to' but rather will use an approach that facilitates 'talking with' parents. To accomplish this, she will use the skills of silence, listening, and observation combined with her own personal characteristics of acceptance of others, respect for them, and empathy with them. A non-directive approach (using open-ended questions) usually creates an environment within which a parent feels accepted and is able to think through a problem and consider new ways of approaching it. The nurse's role, then, is to reflect the parents' thinking so that issues can be clarified more easily, and decision-making by the parents can be facilitated.

The goals parents set for themselves are more likely to be reached and to bring beneficial results to the family than are those the health visitor, school nurse or children's ward nurse sets for them.

Helping children to cope

Wherever teaching takes place, the nurse can use the same basic steps to help the child to develop problem-solving and coping abilities in health promotion. The only alteration required is in the approach taken, which must be adjusted to the child's age and cognitive capabilities. These steps are listed below.

(1) Ask the child what she thinks her problem or need is (she learns problem identification), and whether the problem is important to her (she learns to make health a priority). This information gives the nurse an understanding of the child's perception of her situation. This also indicates to the nurse how much information the child needs before she is likely to co-operate.

(2) The nurse then takes an additional history (preferably from the child and subsequently augmented by the parents) and carries out whatever assessment is indicated. Teaching occurs throughout this process as the nurse gives truthful explanations of what the child will see, hear, feel, smell, and taste during assessment procedures. An age-appropriate explanation is given for each procedure. Because young children acquaint themselves with the world through their physical senses, teaching should focus on this aspect of procedures. Young children may also require visual examples (for example, a pretend procedure done on a teddy) or sample sensation (for example, what a pinch of the skin feels like) so that they know what to expect. Older school-age children still need explanations about expected physical sensations, but they can usually understand from verbal explanations alone. Adolescents, although they want to know what physical sensations to expect, are likely to be much more interested in the rationale and consequences of each procedure.

(3) The child is presented with the findings revealed by the nursing assessment. This is a good opportunity to teach the names of body organs or to explain body processes (or both), as well as what it means when these are altered. How simple and concrete or complex and abstract this teaching must be will depend on the child's age and degree of understanding.

(4) The nurse interprets the findings to the child in terms of probable cause. For the young child who still perceives people as the cause of all events, the explanation should be prefaced by reassurance that the cause was *not* herself, her wishes, nor the wishes of others upon her. The child in late childhood or pre-adolescence has usually mastered causal relationships sufficiently well to grasp a simply presented scientific explanation. The adolescent or young adult will want a detailed scientific explanation. The provision of health information is critical at this time because this is when it has maximum relevance to the child personally.

(5) The nurse elicits the child's opinions of what she thinks ought to be done. One approach may be to ask the child to list the alternatives she can think of and why she thinks each would help (she learns problem-solving). This task should be the child's responsibility, with the nurse assisting only if the child cannot think of any alternatives on her own. Health education is then offered to correct any misconceptions to increase the child's knowledge of the situation so that she can identify more realistic alternatives, or to reinforce accurate perceptions of what will work and why.

(6) The child selects the alternatives she will carry out, alone or with assistance (she learns decision-making). Before she makes her selection, she should be informed if any of her alternatives are not acceptable because of local policy. The child's selection should be written down for her (and for those who will assist her to carry it out) and documented in the nurse's records. This becomes a contract between the child, the nurse, and the others involved, as to what must be done by each.

(7) The child is asked to identify the resources (personal or in the external environment) that she will need to use to carry out the alternatives. Health teaching that helps the child to become knowledgeable about personal, family or community resources available and how to use them is appropriate.

(8) The nurse asks the child what she will do if the same problem or need recurs (reinforcing child's ability to be responsible for her own health care).

When the child selects sound alternatives, this should be reinforced. Inappropriate decisions are

Early childhood   3 years – 5 years

(1) I will brush my teeth after breakfast and immediately before going to bed

(2) Before coughing or sneezing I will cover my mouth with
my hand or use a handkerchief

School-age child   6 years – 9 years

(1) I will try to remember to wash my hands after using the
toilet

(2) Whenever possible I will change my wet shoes and socks

Late childhood and early adolescence   10 years – 12 years

(1) I will try new foods or foods that have been cooked in a
way that is new to me

(2) I will consider the weather when I get dressed in the
morning

Adolescence   12 years and over

(1) I will listen to my parents' point of view in areas in which
we disagree and seriously evaluate their point

(2) I will bath or shower at least twice a week and wash my
hair at least once a week

Fig. 19.11 *Examples of realistic health behaviours at
given ages, as identified by Tackett (1981)*

not reinforced, and the nurse provides additional
information that will provide further clarification
of the problem and its cause, and to help the child
see the inappropriateness of the decision.

Tackett (1981) gives some examples of realistic
health behaviours which children have identified
at various ages (see Fig. 19.11).

This approach involves the child actively in identifying her health needs, finding viable solutions
and carrying them out. The nurse applies learning,
reinforcement and decision-making theories to
assist the child to become responsible for her own
wellness behaviours.

The counselling role

A counselling relationship, whether with a child
or her parents, is a two-way interaction involving
both verbal and non-verbal communication. Its
purposes are firstly, to come to a realistic definition
and/or resolution of a problem; secondly, to increase the client's awareness of herself and her
needs; and thirdly, to develop a broader under-

Table 19.10. *Potential areas of child/parent
development conflict*

Newborn and young infant	Feeding Crying Sleeping Bathing and dressing
Older infant	Feeding Weaning Separation Toilet needs Sleeping Crying Safety measures
Toddler	Self-feeding Decreasing appetite Toilet training Separation Tantrums Negativism Breath-holding Aggressive behaviour Discipline Childproofing
Pre-schooler	Speech Independence Sibling rivalry Sexual curiosity Bad dreams Phobias Discipline Safety rules
School-age	School adjustment Conduct disturbances Lying Cheating Stealing Bad language Aggressive behaviour School achievement Discipline
Adolescent	Independence (adolescent rebellion) Sexual activity Drug experimentation Peer group choices Delinquent behaviours Truancy Shoplifting Nutrition

standing of the situation which is causing conflict for the client.

Often counselling is the intervention required during developmental or situational crises. Table 19.10 describes common developmental conflicts in families for which the health visitor, school nurse or children's ward nurse is most often consulted. Table 19.11 describes some situational problems which may require counselling.

To be successful, the nurse counsellor must develop skills of astute observation, tactful questioning and objective listening. It is particularly important, too, that she is able to *allow* clients to choose their own alternatives and solutions.

The patient profile given in Fig. 19.12 relates to the problem of preparing a child for hospitalisation.

Health appraisal

The phrases *assessment* and *appraisal* of health are often used interchangeably; both can be defined as the act of evaluating the quality or status of health. Health appraisal gives the nurse the opportunity to collect information about the child's past and current health status and present problems, and to plan for action that may prevent future problems or identify conditions that may need follow-up assessment. The appraisal focuses primarily on the child but also explores family dynamics and cultural and environmental factors that may affect the child's development.

The main aim of a comprehensive assessment is to evaluate the child's physical, intellectual and emotional–social competencies.

Taking a history

There are three main aspects to history taking: interviewing the child herself, taking a child health history, and making a more general review of the wider systems (social and physical) in the context of which the child lives.

Interviewing

Interviewing the child or adolescent presents a challenge to the nurse because information must be gathered both from the child herself and from

Table 19.11. *Some situational problems requiring counselling (adapted from Browden, 1970)*

- Birth of a sibling
- Death in the family
- Adoption
- Divorce or separation
- Rape, incest, promiscuity
- Child with handicaps
- Entry into school and school readiness
- Preparation for hospitalisation

Claire Thomas, aged four years, is being admitted for adenoidectomy, myringotomy and insertion of grommets, planned for tomorrow morning. As you greet Claire and Mrs Thomas you notice Claire is smiling and she looks happy. Mrs Thomas, however, appears tense and is staring ahead. She glances at you when Claire says, 'Oh, we're not staying! I'm going to visit my grandma as soon as mummy has talked to the doctor.' Mrs Thomas whispers to you that she has been unable to prepare Claire for her surgery. 'She's too young to understand about it and honestly, Nurse, I just didn't know what to tell her.'

Consider the following points:

(1) Why is it important to prepare Claire for hospitalisation and surgery?
(2) Outline a plan for preparing Claire for admission. Include the information she should receive about hospital admission, pre-operative and post-operative care and the surgery itself.
(3) Would it be advisable for Mrs Thomas to stay with Claire during this hospital admission? If so, why?

Fig. 19.12 *Profile: Claire Thomas*

her caretakers. Equal value should be placed on the information received from the child and from the adult.

The interview is also a time to establish trust between the nurse, the child, and the parents. The nurse should try to arrange a relaxed accepting atmosphere. Privacy is very important. It is also very important to arrange for an interpreter if the child and family speak another language.

Communicating, by health care professionals, with a child and family requires active listening. The nurse must listen to what the child or parent says and tell them her perception of what has been said or implied. This allows the child or parent to verify the nurse's interpretation and provides the opportunity for clarification of any misinterpreted statement.

When asking questions, jargon and medical terminology should be avoided. Questions should be asked in a way that is non-threatening and non-judgemental. For example, instead of asking the child, 'Are you having any problems at school?', the nurse might ask, 'How do you like school?'. This approach does not judge or threaten the child by presupposing a problem or making her feel inferior.

How questions are asked is very important. The type of question may either facilitate the interview process or make it difficult: for example, the use of open as opposed to closed questions. Open questions allow the child or parent the opportunity to express views, opinions, thoughts and feelings. The closed question does just the opposite. 'How do you like school?' is an open question. A closed question would be, 'Do you like school?' which allows for only a *yes* or *no* answer.

Questions may also be direct or indirect. Direct questions are stated in a manner that generally requires a *yes* or *no* answer or specific information (such as 'How old are you?'). Indirect questions, or questions that do not seem to be questions, allow the child or parent to select or elaborate on information. 'It must be difficult coping with three children under five years old', is an indirect question that does not end with a question mark but obviously invites a response. Indirect questions express the interviewer's interest in what the child or parent has to say and allow the child or parent to give information in her own way.

A variety of these techniques and types of questions can be used in an interview, depending on the situation and the style of the interviewer. Certain kinds of information lend themselves to a particular technique. For example, direct questions may be used when collecting basic factual information, whereas open questions may be better when collecting information about family or social relationships.

Although each child is approached on the basis of her unique character, some general principles exist regarding the child's ability to contribute to the interview that are determined by her age and stage of development. Obviously, the infant and very young toddler will not have mastered language sufficiently to be interviewed verbally; however, they contribute a volume of information through their behaviour and other forms of non-verbal communication that the observant nurse can note and document.

The three or four year old has sufficient command of language to tell the nurse about her daily activities, so long as questions are put in terms she can understand. She may also be able to relate some characteristics of symptoms if they produce sensations she is currently experiencing (such as earache); however, memory for past sensations is vague at this age. The three or four year old child relates best to the nurse if the parents remain present throughout the interview.

School-age children can provide the majority of the current information about themselves and their family, school and daily life. Involving the school-age child conveys to her that the nurse thinks she is competent and responsible regarding her own health care. Parents can remain present during most of the interview; however, the school-age child should have some time alone with the nurse so that she can share things she feels unable to express in her parents' presence. The older school-age child is well able to report past events with accuracy, and will therefore be a significant informant about her own health history.

Generally, the adolescent can be independent in contributing necessary information. Once the interview is complete and a summary has been shared with the adolescent, she and the nurse together can discuss the problem and its management with the parent. A parent should remain nearby to provide any information about which the adolescent is unsure, or which she does not know. How much independence and responsibility the adolescent can assume for the prescribed care will depend on her maturity.

The interview incorporates not only verbal but also non-verbal communication. Body posture and facial expressions may influence the flow of the interview. How far apart the nurse and the child or parent are from each other also contributes to the effectiveness of communication. Most nurses select a distance of approximately two to three feet from the parent and child. It is difficult to establish a rapport or listen when the child and parent are sitting at some distance across the room.

A successful interview is based on:

(1) Appropriate verbal and non-verbal communication skills

Fig. 19.13 *Child health history: an outline*

The nurse will need to take a child health history outline which might include the following information.

Demographic information

(1) Name (nickname or preferred name)

(2) Address

(3) Date of birth

(4) Nationality

(5) Primary language spoken

(6) Name and address of GP

(7) Name and address of health visitor

(8) Name and address of play group/nursery

Reason for contact/admission

(1) State in child's or parents' own words the reason health care is presently being sought – problem or symptom
Onset – events coincident with onset, sudden or gradual, previous episodes, when they began

(2) Characteristics of chief complaint
  – *type or character* of complaint (for example pain: dull, sharp, aching, burning, radiating, itching, tickling)
  – *location* (if applicable): ask child to point to affected areas
  – *severity* (annoying, uncomfortable, incapacitating) and effect on normal daily activities (eating, sleeping, elimination, planning, mood)
  – *duration* (intermittent, persistent or continuous; interval between if intermittent)
  – *influencing factors* (precipitating, aggravating, relieving, ameliorating)
  – *present status* of complaint (getting worse, better, unchanged)

Past health history

Birth history

(1) Conditions of baby at birth
  Birth weight

(2) Any neonatal difficulties – feeding or sucking problems, cyanosis, jaundice, rashes

(3) Bottle fed? Breast fed?

Accidents

(1) Age at each accident

(2) Circumstances surrounding accident (cause, where occurred)

(3) Facts regarding accident
  – extent of injury
  – treatment received
  – complications or residual problems
  – child's reaction

(4) Any current problems associated with accident(s)

Illnesses

(1) Name of illness or infections
  – age when occurred
  – treatment received
  – complications or sequelae

(2) Names of childhood diseases
  – age when occurred
  – severity
  – treatment received
  – residual problems

Operations

(1) Date and age at each operation

(2) Why was surgery done?

(3) Outcome of surgery

(4) Child's reaction to each operation

(5) Any follow-up or complications?

Allergies

(1) Untoward responses to medications, food, animals, insect bites

(2) Type of reaction (hives, rash, swelling, rhinitis, nausea)

(3) Do symptoms occur seasonally?

(4) Do symptoms occur immediately or several hours after exposure?

Immunisation

(1) Type received

(2) Dates received

(3) Untoward reactions

Developmental history

(1) Motor development *milestones*

(2) Language development milestones

(3) Social development milestones

Current developmental status with regard to activities of daily living

(1) Eating and drinking
- How good is child's appetite?
- Bottle-fed? Breast-fed?
- If bottle-fed, what kind, how much?
- Amount in 24 hours? Number of feedings in 24 hours, length of each feed?
- If taking solids, what kind, portion size, how often?
- What kinds of food does she enjoy? Meats, vegetables, fruits,cereals, juices, eggs, milk?
- How often? What portion size? How does the child eat (spoon, fork, knife)? How does the child feed herself? Is she messy, neat? Does she use a cup?
- Food dislikes, food fads?

(2) Elimination
- What is the child's bowel pattern? Frequency, consistency?
- Discomfort?
- Is child toilet trained (at what age? accidents? day or night trained?)
- Any associated stresses with elimination habits? Enuresis?
- What word does the child use for potty/toilet?

(3) Sleep and rest
- When does the child go to bed? Does she sleep through the night? Nightmares? Night terrors?
- Difficulties with putting the child to bed?
- How many hours does child sleep in 24 hours?
- Naps (when, how long)? Difficulty falling asleep? Insomnia? Where does the child sleep? Does she have her own bed? How does the child wake (alert, fussy)? Does she need a teddy or other toy to comfort her in order to get to sleep?
- Any change in sleep patterns?

(4) Development
- How does child compare to siblings, peers?
- What can the child do now? (This should be age appropriate – for example, a 15 month-old walks, a three year old rides a tricycle)
- What kinds of games does the child like to play? How does she play with her peers?

(5) Personality
- Unusual behaviours (thumbsucking, nailbiting, masturbation)?
- How does the child describe herself?
- How do parents describe child's personality?
- What does the child do when she is angry, sad, afraid?
- How does child interact with teachers, classmates?

(6) Sexuality
- What does the child/adolescent know about secondary development, sexuality, menstruation, sexual exploration?
- Is the adolescent sexually active? Using birth control? Type, frequency of use, problems?
- Does the adolescent female know how to examine her breasts?

General review of systems

(1) General appearance	(6) Cardiorespiratory
(2) Condition of skin	(7) Gastro-intestinal
(3) Eyes	(8) Genito-urinary
(4) Ears	(9) Musculoskeletal
(5) Nose	(10) Neurological

Family profile

(1) Family members

(2) Familial and hereditary diseases

(2) The establishment of appropriate environmental conditions
(3) The use of a variety of direct and indirect interviewing techniques
(4) The establishment of a rapport with the parent and the child.

Child health history

The nurse will need to gather various items of information, as outlined in Fig. 19.13.

(1) *Demographic information*
Before beginning the interview the nurse intro-

duces herself, makes sure the child and parents are comfortable, explains the purpose of the interview, and then begins to collect basic demographic information. Much of this information may already be found in the child's notes and may only need verification as being correct.

(2) *Reason for contact*
The reason for contact is the specific reason for the child's admission to hospital. It is a brief statement recorded in the child's or the parent's own words. The reason for contact is often referred to as 'the chief complaint'.

(3) *Past health history*
Whenever asking questions it is helpful to explain the relevance of the questions and the importance of having this information. It should be explained to the parent that experiences during the child's early life may have significant effects on the child's physical, intellectual and emotional development.

The past health history includes a summary of any diseases, accidents, operations or hospitalisations the child has experienced before the present health history.

The type of immunisations the child has received as well as the dates of the initial series and last booster dosage (if appropriate) should be noted.

(4) *Developmental history*
Although parental memory may be hazy, such information may give insight into a current abnormality. Milestones are usually recorded in three categories: motor development, language development and social development.

Motor development milestones are: held head up, rolled front to back, and back to front, sat alone, crawled, pulled to stand, walked holding on and alone. For the older child, motor development history includes the age at which she rode a tricycle, hopped, skipped, ran, jumped and climbed stairs.

Language development milestones are: babbled, used first word, used two-word sentence, major method of communication (for example, sounds, words, actions), and the present vocabulary.

Social development milestones are: the child's or parent's description of the child's basic personality (usual mood, strong traits, difficult or weak traits); present and persisting fears; nervous behaviours; the way the child expresses feelings (ver-

bally, behaviourally, aggressively); how the child gets along with her parents, siblings, peers at school; type and quality of play, including who the child plays with; typical response to new situations.

A review of the child's current developmental status is also summarised with regard to skills relevant to daily living. The specific questions asked will depend on the child's age and development.

General review of systems

The general review of systems focuses attention on any deviation from health, thus allowing the nurse a more comprehensive picture of the child's health status and potential problems. The information received in this part of the history is invaluable even when it may appear unrelated to the present problem.

An outline of suggested areas for review of each body system is given in Fig 19.14. The nurse should use terms that are easily understood by the parent and child.

Family profile

One purpose of obtaining a 'family profile' is to identify possible stress factors that could affect the child and her family. A recent death or chronic illness of one of the family members may interfere with the normal function of the child and her normal developmental progress.

Physical assessment

When assessing a child physically it is important to provide a comfortable atmosphere and to be quick and efficient, creating as little anxiety as possible. To do this the nurse must determine what approach is developmentally appropriate for the child being assessed.

The nurse must take full advantage of opportunities as they arise. For example, she can observe the neurological, growth and developmental status of the child who is playing with toys in the room. The nurse may also listen to the child's speech and articulation when she talks to a parent or sibling in the room or when she answers questions during the history. It is also essential that the nurse explains each step and if possible makes a game of it. Children of any age exhibit modesty and this should be respected.

General	– Overall state of health?
	– Tiredness?
	– Recent unexplained weight loss or weight gain?
	– General ability to perform normal daily functions?
Skin	– Skin problems such as excessive dryness, pruritis, skin sensitivity?
	– Rashes?
	– Acne?
Eyes	– Known visual problems?
	– Wears glasses or contact lenses?
	– Eye infections?
Ears	– Hearing loss?
	– Ear infections?
	– Ear discharge?
Nose	– Nasal obstruction or difficulty with breathing?
Throat	– Mouth breathing?
	– Teething?
	– Hoarseness?
	– Difficulty swallowing?
Cardiorespiratory	– Trouble breathing, choking, turning blue?
	– Difficulty feeding?
	– Tires easily, difficulty running or playing?
	– Cough: wet or dry?
	– Wheezing?
Gastro-intestinal	– Bowel patterns, frequency?
	– Diarrhoea, constipation?
	– Bloody stools?
	– Vomiting?
Genito-urinary	– Enuresis?
	– Menstruation (when started, how often, amount, length of each menses, discomfort, problems)
Musculoskeletal	– Weakness?
	– Clumsiness, lack of coordination?
	– Abnormal gait?
Neurological	– Hearing problems?
	– Clumsiness, coordination problems?
	– Speech problems?
	– Unusual habits?
	– Smell?

Fig. 19.14 *Suggested checklist of questions to be asked in relation to a child's state of health on admission*

Measurements

Height and weight measurements reflect the child's overall growth.

Height

The method of assessing the child's height varies with age. The infant or young child is stretched out and her knees are extended. One way of measuring height is by the use of a sliding tool. The child's head is placed firmly at the head board while the movable end of the measuring stick is stretched until the child's heel touches the foot-board. The older child can stand against a standard balanced adult scale with a movable rod.

The height is recorded and plotted on a growth grid. Percentile charts with height, weight and head circumferences are usually used by health care professionals. The percentile charts use percentiles to show the distribution of height, weight and head circumference for a typical series of 100 children. For example, the 25th percentile indicates that 75 children are taller and 25 children shorter than the child being measured.

Generally a child on the 25th percentile will continue at about this percentile throughout her life. A child who suddenly has an increase to the

90th percentile or a drop to the 3rd percentile requires further investigation.

Heredity is a major factor influencing a child's height. Tall parents usually have taller children than shorter parents; however, abnormal shortness may also be due to chronic illness, heart disease, liver or kidney disease, allergies, malnutrition or growth hormone deficiencies.

Weight

Weight is also an important index of the child's growth and should be measured every time the child is seen at the clinic and whenever the child is sick. The same general considerations of growth and development that applied to height also apply to weight.

Infants are weighed without any clothing on a balanced infant scale. Older children can remain clothed without shoes and be weighed on an adult balanced scale. Depending on the child's age and the amount of privacy available, the child can undress down to her underwear.

Once a measurement has been taken, it is plotted on the growth chart. The weight generally follows the same percentile from one time to the next; any sudden decrease or increase should be evaluated. Percentile decrease may suggest malnutrition, acute illness, dehydration, emotional problems or chronic illness. Percentile increase may be related to overnutrition, oedema or endocrine disorders.

Some general rules exist regarding height and weight.

(1) Height and weight measurements provide important information, but a single measurement is of less importance than a series of measurements.
(2) The relationship between height and weight is significant. A child who falls at the 90th percentile for height and at the 3rd percentile for weight requires a more detailed assessment.

Head circumference

The brain achieves 75% of its adult size by three years of age. One half of total head growth occurs during the first year of life. Therefore the head circumference is usually measured every time the child attends the well child clinic. It is usually not taken after the child has reached her third birthday unless some abnormality exists.

A reliable reading of head circumference is obtained by using a paper tape measure around the broadest part of the head. The tape is placed over the occipital protuberance and the frontal bones. A newborn's head circumference is equal to or slightly larger than the chest circumference, a situation that continues until the child is about three years of age when the chest circumference becomes larger than the head size. Head circumference increases by four inches in the first year, and only two inches between the ages of one and seven.

The head circumference is plotted on a growth chart like the height and weight. As with the height and weight, serial measurement provide more information than a single measurement, and marked differences should be investigated.

Assessment of vital signs

The nurse should set out to reduce anxiety and gain cooperation when vital signs are being assessed. Older children and adolescents are treated in the same way as adults. Like adults they need adequate explanation of what is being done and need to be told the results. Younger school-age children may wish to participate – for example, they may help in taking their blood pressure by pressing the cuff down, holding the gauge or squeezing the bulb. Small children fear body mutilation with any intrusive procedure. The rectal temperature, for example, often arouses anxiety and stress. In young children it is usually advisable to check respirations and pulse first and temperature last. This order should produce greater accuracy, since rectal temperature-taking can produce sufficient anxiety and crying to alter the respiratory and pulse rate.

The normal oral temperature is between 35.5 and 37.5°C. Rectal temperatures are one degree higher and axillary temperatures are one degree lower than oral temperatures. When the temperature is recorded, the method for obtaining it must be noted.

The length of time allowed for accurate measurement of temperature depends in part on custom in various settings (Nichols and Rushkin, 1966; Nichols and Verkonick, 1967; Gooch, 1986; Closs, 1987). The advantage of electronic thermometers is that they require only seconds to

Table 19.12. Normal pulse and respiratory rates for specific ages

Age	Pulse (beats per minute)	Average pulse	Respirations
Newborn	70–170	120	30–40
2 years	80–130	110	25–32
4 years	80–120	100	23–30
6 years	75–115	100	21–26
8 years	70–110	90	20–26
10 years	70–110	90	20–26
12 years	70–110	85	18–22
14 years	65–105	85	18–22
16 years	60–100	85	16–20
18 years	50–90	80	12–24

register accurate temperatures, regardless of the route, and thus are especially helpful with young children.

Children often have elevated temperatures after vigorous playing or after eating. They may also have an increased temperature on very warm days. A pyrexia may also be produced by viral or bacterial infections, dehydration, tumours, poisoning or chronic infections. Hypothermia is seen in children who are shocked or chilled or it may be seen in infants with infections. If pyrexia exists, it should be evaluated and followed closely. Table 19.12 describes average pulse rates, respiratory rates and blood pressure readings at various ages.

General appearance

Observation of the child is important for the forming of an impression that can be verified or disproved later. The following are examples of some items used to develop a general appearance statement: physical appearance (ill or well), nutritional status, behaviour and degree of activity, facial expression, interactions with parents or nurse, consciousness level, speech or nature of cry, gait and coordination, and posture.

The general appearance statement focuses on the physical characteristics of the child's behaviour and should be a brief summary statement. An ex-ample of a general appearance statement is: 'Alert, smiling, well-developed, well-nourished toddler playing on her mother's lap and in no acute distress'.

Skin

The skin is assessed for colour, moisture, texture and turgor.

Colour

Normal skin colour varies from whitish pink to dark brown depending on race. Accurate skin assessment must take into consideration the variations in skin of each race. For example, children who are of oriental descent have a yellow skin tone that may appear to be jaundiced. Black children may often have bluish pigmentation around the gum lines or palate.

Erythema refers to an increased amount of oxygenated blood in the vasculature of the dermis. This condition is found in children who are pyrexial, have sunburn or localised infection, or who have been exposed to the cold (body parts exposed to the cold become a bright pink or red).

Cyanosis is a bluish tint of the skin due to a large amount of reduced haemoglobin in the capillaries. It is most obvious in the mucous membranes, conjunctivae of the lower eyelids and the nail beds. Children with congestive heart failure or congenital heart disorders are usually cyanotic. Cyanosis may also be evident in children with respiratory disturbances. *Acrocyanosis*, the bluish discoloration of the hands and feet which is often seen in newborn babies, is normal for the first few days of life; it is caused by an inadequate peripheral vasculature.

Skin that is *very pale* suggests a decrease in haemoglobin content, often secondary to anaemia or shock. In white-skinned people, pallor is noted by a loss of pink skin colouring; in black-skinned persons the skin becomes an ashen grey. Jaundice is seen as a yellow-green hue; this usually suggests an increased serum bilirubin level which occurs in children with liver or haemolytic blood disease. Jaundice is best discerned by blanching the skin and observing the blanched area for a subsequent yellow or yellow-green appearance. Examination of the skin for jaundice should be done in natural sunlight, as fluorescent light gives some normal skin tones a yellow colour. Areas in which jaundice is easily observed (particularly in dark-skinned races) are the sclera, the hard palate and the gums.

Moisture

Dry skin suggests a rising temperature, whereas a hot moist skin suggests a resolving fever.

Texture

Normal skin is smooth, soft and flexible. Skin that is rough and dry is seen in children who bathe very frequently or who are exposed to cold weather. It may also suggest an endocrine problem. Scaling present only between fingers and toes could be a sign of a fungal infection. Eczema often causes scaling of the cheeks and behind the ears, knees and elbows.

Turgor

One of the best indicators of nutrition and hydration is skin *turgor*. Normal skin turgor is elastic and taut. Turgor is evaluated by pinching the skin between thumb and forefinger, usually in the lower abdomen or calf, and noting the reaction of the pinched skin. If the skin returns promptly to the normal position it is assessed as elastic. Skin that does not promptly return may indicate a loss of turgor due to dehydration.

Oedema

Excess water that is stored in the skin is referred to as oedema and should be assessed to determine if it is pitting or non-pitting. The nurse's thumb is firmly pressed over the child's ankle protuberance for at least five seconds. After releasing the skin, any sign of indentation that lasts several seconds indicates pitting oedema. Oedema is seen in children who have allergies, kidney or heart anomalies, and malnutrition.

Lesions

Many skin lesions can be normal – for example, capillary haemangiomas (birthmarks), mongolian spots, freckles and *naevi* (moles). Other skin lesions such as cysts, port-wine stains or large hairy moles require further evaluation and possible referral. Lesions in the form of a skin rash are seen frequently in children of all ages. Heat-rash and nappy-rash are common in infants and young children. Another common condition is acne. This generally begins during adolescence (as a result of the increase in testosterone levels in both sexes) and can range from mild to severe.

Hair

Hair is examined for colour, length, distribution, cleanliness, amount and texture. Nutritional and endocrine disturbances may affect hair texture.

Pubic hair usually appears when the child is between eight and twelve years of age.

Axillary hair appears shortly after the onset of pubic hair. Adolescent males begin to develop facial hair approximately six months after the appearance of axillary hair. Hair that has appeared earlier than normal or excessive hair may be an indication of precocious puberty or could suggest an endocrine problem.

Nails

Characteristics such as smoothness, pitting, ridging and clubbing are carefully noted. Clubbing is sometimes a sign of chronic lack of oxygen often seen in children with congenital heart disease or chronic pulmonary disease. It can also be a normal familial trait. Adolescents and children who smoke heavily may have yellow nail tips.

Mouth

The nurse notes the lips for colour, oedema or lesions. The lips and the surrounding area are also inspected for pallor or cyanosis. Cherry-red lips are seen in children with acidosis or carbon monoxide poisoning. Unusual mouth odours should be noted as they can be clinically significant. Unusual odours are present in children with poor oral hygiene, dental caries, sinusitis, allergies, diabetic acidosis, malnutrition and diphtheria.

Children have two sets of teeth. The first teeth, milk or *deciduous* teeth begin eruption around six months of age. All 20 of the deciduous teeth have usually erupted by two and a half to three years of age. Permanent dentition begins at around six and progresses until all 32 permanent teeth have erupted. Delay in tooth eruption can be genetic or significant of underlying disease processes.

Salivary secretion is limited until three months of age when the salivary glands become more active. Absence of salivation may be caused by a pyrexia or dehydration. Excessive salivation is seen in children who are teething or who have caries or mouth infections. The amount, colour, consistency and odour of saliva are recorded if abnormal.

Gums should be inspected and palpated for colour and moisture. Inflammation, swelling, bleeding, tenderness and ulcerations should be noted. Inflammation and swelling are secondary to infection or poor oral hygiene. Inflamed, bleeding gums may be a result of decreased vitamin C intake or pyorrhoea. A black line along the margin of the gum may signify metal poisoning (such as lead poisoning).

The *buccal mucosa* (inner cheek region) is examined. The buccal mucosa is normally pink but black or brown areas may be seen in dark-skinned children. Koplik's spots (a group of grey-white spots) are seen on the buccal mucosa opposite the molars in the prodromal stage of measles. White patches on the oral mucosa, especially the tongue and hard palate, that cannot be scraped off indicate a yeast (monilial) infection called thrush caused by the fungus *Candida albicans*.

The normal tongue is pink and should fit in the mouth. A large protruding tongue is seen in chil-dren with Down's syndrome. The tongue becomes tender and red with severe anaemia.

Grey, irregular borders on the tongue can be considered normal or caused by allergies, fever or drug ingestion. Deep furrows on the tongue are seen in children with Down's syndrome. Scars could be the result of trauma or previous con-vulsions during which the tongue has been bitten. Gross tongue tremors when the tongue is stuck out are seen in children with cerebral palsy; fine tremors are seen with chorea or hypothyroidism.

The chest

The chest is examined for size, shape, symmetry and movement. The chest is round in the newborn but becomes more oval as the child grows. Normal respirations are generally abdominal in the infant and young child and become thoracic around seven years of age, although both are normal.

It is important to note the type, rate, rhythm and depth of respiration as well as the use of any accessory respiratory muscles.

Musculoskeletal system

The child is observed during her play activities, while walking about the room, and while per-forming tasks such as undressing. Symmetry of movement, position, general alignment, deform-ities, gait, extra digits and unusual posture are noted while the child is unaware that the nurse is observing her.

Fluid and electrolyte balance

Fluid and electrolyte balance is a key concept in child health. The reader is referred to basic texts of physiology for in-depth discussions of the be-haviour of fluids and electrolytes in the body (see also Chapter 5). Included here is a discussion of fluid and electrolyte balance as it applies to infants and children.

Assessing fluid and electrolyte balance in children

The nurse who cares for infants and children re-quires an understanding of the body's regulatory mechanisms to enhance her assessment skills and decision-making ability.

Body water compartments and internal distribution

Total body water at birth comprises 75–80% of body weight. During the immediate postnatal period there is a weight loss of approximately 19% of body weight. The infant's proportionate rapid weight gain during the first year of life is due primarily to an increase in adipose tissue. Since there is an inverse relationship between total body water and total body fat, the infant's weight gain is accompanied by a proportionate reduction in fluid volume. Therefore the internal distribution of fluids in an infant makes her vulnerable to high losses of fluid. In the child of around two years of age both the percentage of total body water and its internal distribution approximate that of an adult.

Extracellular fluid is easily lost and in the event of illness, trauma or stressful environmental conditions the infant is extremely vulnerable to fluid and electrolyte imbalances.

Regulation of fluid and electrolytes

Infants and young children are more vulnerable to rapid fluid and electrolyte imbalances than adults for various reasons; a major difference is their higher basal metabolic rate.

The increased metabolic rate of infants is due to their greater proportional surface area, growth needs and relatively large viscera and brain. The body surface area of an infant is proportionately two or three times greater than that of an adult. It is not until the child is two or three years of age that the relatively greater surface area is no longer present. An increased metabolic rate accounts for the rapid rate of water turnover. Finally, the homeostatic mechanisms of the body are less mature in infants and small children; thus when they become ill they are more vulnerable to imbalances.

Gains and losses

Gains and losses are more rapid during infancy and childhood, but in conditions of health this rapid turnover of water is of little consequence. It is when fluid and electrolyte losses are compounded by illness that infants and young children can quickly develop extracellular fluid volume deficit and suffer from electrolyte and acid-base balances. Furthermore an infant or child often cannot be persuaded to take fluids, whereas an adult will respond to explanation. Losses in a child on the other hand occur even more rapidly than in an adult. The losses that occur in such common occurrences as pyrexia, vomiting and diarrhoea quickly deplete the child's supply of energy, resulting in imbalance. The surface area through which losses occur (skin, lungs and gastro-intestinal tract) is proportionately greater in children than in adults. The kidneys, which regulate excretion, are less mature and ineffective therefore in conserving fluids and electrolytes to compensate for energy depletion and electrolyte imbalances.

The gastro-intestinal tract is particularly important in relation to fluid and electrolyte balance in children. In health there is a larger exchange of fluid in children as opposed to adults within the gastro-intestinal tract whereby water and sodium are reabsorbed and potassium is excreted. Any illness that affects intestinal absorption will therefore have a serious effect on the child's life because of the rapid and great losses that can occur through the gastro-intestinal tract.

The nurse's teaching role in the prevention of imbalances

One of the greatest responsibilities of the nurse is to teach parents how to prevent imbalances and how to detect early symptoms. A few basic principles regarding fluid intake and output should be discussed with the parents. These measures may prevent their child from developing more serious problems.

Over-dressing in relation to the environmental temperature causes increased sweating, resulting in both fluid and electrolyte losses. Parents should be advised to check the child's temperature early in illness and give the child extra fluids if she is pyrexial. Extra fluids should be offered to young children during hot weather and the number and saturation of nappies should be used as a guide to the need for additional fluids.

When vomiting or diarrhoea occurs parents should be advised to reduce solid and milk intake and give primarily clear fluids. However it is important that parents also understand how to increase the child's food intake gradually to avoid starvation.

Parents should be taught to identify early signs of imbalance so that treatment can be started. A child's eyes often lack lustre; she looks pale and is more irritable and demanding than usual in the early stages of imbalance. If a child's nappy proves to be dry at the usual times of changing, the parent should also check the mouth, tongue and lips for dryness. Often the nurse can help parents prevent the development of more serious problems if she takes the time to discuss these few early signs.

Assessment

A child's condition can change rapidly, and therefore assessments need to be made frequently and thoroughly. The nurse evaluates vital signs, body weight, skin colour and turgor, mucous membranes, fontanelles and eyes, intake and output and neurological status.

Vital signs

Evaluation of temperature is important because pyrexia increases the metabolic rate. A raised metabolic rate increases the amount of metabolic wastes, consequently extra fluids are required for excretion of wastes via the kidneys. Sweating results in the loss of body fluids and electrolytes and additional fluid loss accompanies a raised respiratory rate in association with pyrexia. However a subnormal body temperature may occur in the later stages of a volume deficit.

Pulse is evaluated for rate, quality and regularity. When extravascular fluid volume is reduced the pulse is rapid, weak and thready. Dehydration is associated with loss of potassium and results in *hypokalaemia*. Either a severe potassium deficit or excess causes a weak, irregular pulse.

Respirations are affected by fluid volume alterations, electrolyte imbalances and acid-base imbalances. Dehydration is often accompanied by metabolic acidosis; consequently there is an increased respiratory rate to compensate. However, an increased respiratory rate in metabolic acidosis is not always as obvious in a child as it is in an adult.

Blood pressure is an unreliable sign in infants and young children because of the elasticity of blood vessels; however it does add valuable information when evaluated along with other data.

Weight

Assessment of weight loss or gain is important. Weight loss can occur rapidly in children as a result of large fluid losses. Severity of **isotonic dehydration** is classified as mild, moderate or severe according to the weight that has been lost.

Weight gain during illness can be a sign of fluid retention resulting in pulmonary oedema or generalised oedema. If a dehydrated child gains weight suddenly the nurse should recheck the weight but also look for signs of fluid retention.

Skin assessment

The skin should be assessed for colour, temperature, turgor and moisture (see above, pages 563–564). The most common type of dehydration in children is isotonic dehydration and usually the skin is pale and dry and elasticity is decreased. The peripheral blood flow is also decreased; consequently the extremities become cool with poor capillary filling. The skin is a greyish colour, and if mottling occurs, it is an unfavourable sign.

The mouth and tongue are dry, tears and salivation are absent and an older child may be very thirsty.

Anterior fontanelle and eyes

The anterior cranial fontanelle and the eyes should also be assessed. If the fontanelles are still open they will be tense and bulging when there is a fluid excess and sunken or depressed when a child is dehydrated. Suture lines in the skull may become prominent in dehydration. The eyes are also sunken when a child is dehydrated.

Intake and output and urine specific gravity

A nurse's accurate assessment and recording of intake and output are vitally important when caring for children with fluid and electrolyte imbalances. The nurse should also check the specific gravity of the urine.

An infant's urine is usually dilute and so will show a low specific gravity. In the neonatal period this ranges from 1.001 to 1.020. A fluid excess in the body is reflected in a low specific gravity (1.010 or less) and a fluid deficit is reflected in a high specific gravity reading. After a period of fluid restriction specific gravity is often more than 1.025.

Oral fluid intake usually equals urinary output daily. Normal range for 24 hour urinary output varies with age as follows: in the neonate 50–300 ml; in the infant 350–550 ml; in the child 500–1000 ml; and in the adolescent 700–1400 ml. The nurse should be aware that if a child with a known fluid volume deficit excretes large amounts of urine, it is likely that the child has renal damage.

Common childhood conditions that result in a high volume of urine are pyrexia and infection. Due to the higher metabolic demand, there is increased waste production for the kidneys to excrete. Additional water is required to clear such wastes from the body.

Neurological and general behaviour

Behaviour changes are frequently reported by parents and are an important aspect of the nurse's assessment. A child with a fluid deficit may be lethargic or irritable, and an infant's cry may be high pitched and weak. Usually a degree of irritability is first noticed followed by lethargy. Extreme restlessness in a child may indicate a potassium deficit. Potassium deficits also cause abdominal distension, hypotonia and in severe cases flaccid paralysis. A calcium deficiency may result in a child's twitching, irritability and possibly eventual convulsions.

Conclusions

The theme running throughout this section has been that the nurse who works with children and their families must also work within the family's values and beliefs. An essential prerequisite is that the nurse should understand herself, her values and beliefs. Such self-knowledge can be the key to an effective relationship with children and their parents. Identifying what the nurse considers healthy and what she needs or requires to do to preserve her health is determined by her subjective reality. This also applies to children and their parents. What a child or her parents believe to be good or right for her influences whether or not she will engage in health-promoting activities. Conse-

quently the goals parents and children set for themselves are more likely to be reached and to bring beneficial results than are those that health visitors, school nurses, clinic nurses or children's ward nurses establish for children and parents.

Respect for the individuality of the child and each of her parents is a central tenet of child nursing. When working with parents, therefore, the nurse does not offer uncalled-for advice nor try to change the parents' way of thinking. Attempting to alter another person's thinking to fit in with one's own biases and beliefs is an evaluative gesture. When working with children it is important to remember that they are people who have ideas. The child's view about health should be heard and considered. Children also need to be helped to develop life skills (such as the management of stress in their environment) and to be assertive in their social interactions. These are prerequisites for health.

Health education is fundamental to the nursing of children and is concerned with facilitating personal responsibility for health. This will occur in the variety of settings in which nurses work with children – child health clinics, outpatients' departments, schools, children's wards, and within the home. However, the process by which the nurse facilitates responsibility for self-care is the same regardless of the setting. It includes establishing a rapport and providing support, teaching, counselling, and therapeutic referral.

Whenever teaching opportunities arise, the nurse takes the same basic steps to help the child to develop problem-solving and coping abilities in health promotion. The only alteration required is in the teaching approach taken which must be adjusted to the child's age and cognitive capabilities. This approach involves the child actively in the identification of her health needs, the finding of viable solutions, and the implementation of them. The nurse applies learning, reinforcement and decision-making theories to help the child become responsible for her own health behaviours.

Nursing assessment, as fundamental to the nursing process, has also been given a prominent place within this section. Again, nursing assessment demands active listening on the part of the nurse. The nurse actively listens to what the child or parent says, which helps to establish trust between the nurse, child and the parents.

Observation is an important component of nursing assessment. This requires the nurse to take full advantage of opportunities as they arise, for example observing the neurological growth and developmental status of the child while she is playing with toys.

When assessing vital signs the nurse may need to use special approaches that reduce anxiety and gain cooperation. Like adults, older children need adequate explanation of what is being done and should be informed about the results. Younger school-age children may wish to participate. Measuring the child's height and weight are important components of the assessment process because both are indicative of the child's growth. However, the nurse should bear in mind that a single measurement is less significant than a series of measurements.

Finally, this section discusses the significance of fluid and electrolyte balance in children because it is a key concept in child health. Infants and children are more vulnerable to rapid fluid and electrolyte imbalance than adults. As a health educator the nurse has a responsibility to teach parents how to prevent imbalances and how to detect problems at an early stage.

Glossary

Hypokalaemia: The term used to describe decreased serum potassium concentration. Normal serum potassium levels are 3.5–5.5 mmol/litre. The clinical manifestations of hypokalaemia may include muscle weakness, stiffness, paralysis, low blood pressure, cardiac arrhythmias, tachycardia or bradycardia, paralytic ileus, apathy, drowsiness, irritability and fatigue

Isotonic dehydration: Loss of water and salt in approximately balanced proportion. The observable fluid losses are not necessarily isotonic, but losses from other avenues make adjustments so that the sum of all losses (the net loss) is isotonic. Since there is no osmotic force present to cause a redistribution of water between the intracellular and extracellular compartments, the major loss is from extracellular fluid. This reduces the plasma volume and therefore the circulating blood volume – which affects skin, muscle and kidneys. Shock is a threat to life in isotonic dehydration and the child with this condition displays the symptoms characteristic of hypovolaemic shock. Plasma sodium levels remain within normal limits at between 135–145 mmol/litre

Milestones: Refer to *age-linked behaviours*. In a conducive environment the child will proceed through a series of developmental milestones (or stepping stones) and will not 'jump' from one stage to the next

Promoting personal responsibility for health: Health education is not solely or even primarily about bodily health and fitness. It is about enhancing the child's ability to make decisions governing her lifestyle and the child's developing insight into the repercussions these have for physical, mental and social development. The emphasis is on helping children to reach their own decisions, not on telling them what they should believe.

If children are to make decisions, then they should do so from a position of knowledge rather than ignorance. If children choose to smoke, for example, they have a right to do so but they should make such a choice knowing the consequences of their actions. In other words the nurse's role is to foster informed decision-making. The task is to help children clarify their values and make genuine autonomous choices rather than to impose approved values and coerce 'responsible' decision-making. However, it would be naive in the extreme to expect very young children to make certain kinds of decisions. The goal is to facilitate decision-making

References

Baker, P.A. (1980). Concepts of health, illness and hospitalisation. In *Five to Seven Year Old Children: Suggestions for Health and Education*. Unpublished MSc Dissertation, University of London.

Browden, J. (1970). Needs and techniques for counselling parents of young children. *Clinical Pediatrics*, October, 599.

Closs, J. (1987). Oral temperature measurement. *Nursing Times*, 83(1), 36–39.

Donaldson, M. (1978). *Children's Minds* (6th ed.). Fontana, London.

Gooch, J. (1986). Taking temperatures. *Professional Nurse*, 1(10), 273–274.

Hansen, M. and Aradine, C. (1974). The changing face

of primary pediatrics. *Pediatric Clinics of North America*, 21(1), 245–256.

Neinstein, L.S. (1991). *Adolescent Health Care: A Paediatric Guide* (2nd ed.). Urban and Schwarzenberg, Baltimore.

Nichols, G.A. and Rushkin, G. (1966). Oral, axillary and rectal temperatures: determinations and relationships. *Nursing Research*, 15, 307–310.

Nichols, G.A. and Verkonick, P.J. (1967). Placement time for oral thermometers, a nursing study replication. *Nursing Research*, 17, 159–161.

Tackett, J.J.M. (1981). Managing health. In *Nursing Concepts in Child Health*. W.B. Saunders, Philadelphia.

Tizard, B. and Hughes, M. (1984). *Young Children Learning*. Fontana, London.

CONCLUSIONS

It has been the intention in this chapter to present a broad perspective on caring for children; to provide a view of the complex inter-related issues concerned with health and illness. The approach has moved away from that reflected in many nursing textbooks about the care of children, which present highly structured, specially focused situations.

To augment this broader perspective, references and suggestions for further reading have been drawn from a wide array of health-related journals and books, to include information from those areas not 'traditionally' associated with courses related to child health; for example, politics and economics.

The issues raised should contribute to your efforts to work realistically and effectively with other health professionals towards improving the health of children and families. However, in order to collaborate, nurses and other health professionals need to acquire a common comprehensive understanding of those conditions and circumstances which affect health. The contents of this chapter are therefore intended to provide the foundation necessary to plan health care more realistically for selected individuals or groups of children and families.

By the end of this chapter you will probably have identified some questions which (if time permits) you may like to explore in more depth. For example:

(1) How do the health practices and lifestyles adopted by adults affect the health of their children?
(2) How do wealth or poverty, and being brought up in the country or the town, affect the health of children?
(3) Does screening for specific diseases and abnormalities benefit children's health?
(4) What is the effect on the health of children of such services as immunisation and health visitor surveillance?

In essence, this chapter is asking you to reflect on important questions, such as:

(1) What chances for life and health do various population groups have?
(2) Do the services provided by health professionals actually improve the health of those who receive them?

Suggestions for further reading

Motherhood

Dowrick, E. and Grundberg, S. (1980). *Why Children?* The Women's Press, London.

Hanscombe, G. and Forster, J. (1982). *Rocking the Cradle: Lesbian Mothers – A Challenge in Family Living.* Sheba Feminist Publishers, London.

McConville, B. (1987). *How to be A Mother: Is There Life After Birth for Women Today?* Century Hutchinson, London.

Oakley, A. (1981). *From Here to Maternity.* Penguin Books, Harmondsworth.

Rich, A. (1979). *Of Woman Born: Motherhood and Experience.* Virago Press, London.

Scarrs Dunn, J. (1987). *Mother Care/Other Care: The Child-care Dilemma for Women and Children.* Pelican, Harmondsworth.

Fatherhood

Barrett, R.L. and Robinson, B.E. (1986). Adolescent fathers: often forgotten parents. *Paediatric Nursing*, 12(4), 273–277.

Russell, G. (1983). *The Changing Role of the Father.* Open University Press, Milton Keynes.

Weinberg, T.S. (1985). Single fatherhood: how is it different? *Paediatric Nursing*, 11(3), 173–177.

Family relationships

Cohen, M. and Reid, T. (1981). *Ourselves and Our Children – A Book by Parents for Parents*. The Boston Women's Health Book Collective, Boston; Penguin Books, Harmondsworth.

The Open University Continuing Education Unit has developed a range of packs for parent groups which can be used within schools of nursing. They include:

Parents Talking: Family Relationships

Women and Young Children and are available from the Learning Materials Service Office, The Open University, PO Box 188, Walton Hall, Milton Keynes, MK7 6DH.

Nuclear families

Chester, R. (1985). The rise of the new conventional family. *New Society*, 72(167), 185–186.

One-parent families

Caring for Health. A report on health issues for one-parent families. From the National Council for One-Parent Families, 225 Kentish Town Road, London, BW5 2LA, or the Kings Fund Centre, 126 Albert Street, London, NW1 7NP.

Cashmore, E.E. (1985). *The World of One-Parent Families – Having To*. Unwin Publications, London.

McNeill Taylor, L. (1985). *Bringing up Children On Your Own*. Fontana, London.

Renvoize, J. (1985). *Going Solo: Single Mothers By Choice*. Routledge and Kegan Paul, London.

Siebert, K.D., Ganong, C.M., Hagemann, V. and Coleman, M. (1986). Nursing students' perception of a child: influences of information on family structure. *Journal of Advanced Nursing*, 11, 333–337.

Family and child care in a multicultural society

Beare, J. (1983). Parenthood in other cultures. *Nursing*, 2(10), 563–566.

Black, J. (1990). *Child Health in a Multicultural Society* (2nd ed.). British Medical Journal, London.

Henley, A. (1986). Nursing care in a multiracial society. *Senior Nurse*, 2(2), 18–20.

Stress and the family

Abuse in Families. Study Pack for O.U. Course P552. The Open University, Milton Keynes.

Burton, L. (1975). *The Family Life of Sick Children: A Study of Families Coping with Chronic Childhood Disease*. Routledge and Kegan Paul, London.

Dryden, W. (ed.). (1988). *Family Therapy in Britain*. Open University Press, Milton Keynes.

Harrisson, S. (1977). *Families in Stress*. Royal College of Nursing, London.

Jolly, J. (1981). *The Other Side of Paediatrics*. Macmillan Press, Basingstoke.

Stallard, P. (1992). Fresh thinking on family conflicts. *Professional Care of Mother and Child*, Part I, 1(3), 105–6; Part II, 2(1), 10–15.

Child protection

Camden, E. (1984). *If He Comes Back He's Mine: A Mother's Story of Child Abuse*. The Women's Press, Toronto.

Edward, K. (1987). Child abuse (incest). *Nursing Times*, 83(17), 47–50.

Elliott, M. (1985). *Preventing Child Sexual Assault: A Practical Guide to Talking with Children*. Bedford Square Press, London.

Kelly, S.J. (1985). Drawings: critical communications for sexually abused children. *Paediatric Nursing*, 11(6), 421.

Parton, N. (1985). *The Politics of Child Abuse*. Macmillan Press, Basingstoke.

Renvoize, J. (1982). *Incest: A Family Pattern*. Routledge and Kegan Paul, London.

Thiel Ryan, M. (1984). Identifying the sexually abused child. *Paediatric Nursing*, 10(6), 419.

Ward, E. (1984). *Father Daughter Rape*. The Womens Press, London.

For Children

Elliott, M. (1986). *The Willow Street Kids*. Piccola. Stories in the book are all true and are told by children to whom they have happened.

Film

Incest. Video, 26 minutes, colour. Thames Television. Afternoon Plus Service. A filmed report on young adults, both men and women, who were the victims of incest as children. The interviewees describe the effect this has had on their emotional development. Available from: Guild Sound and Vision Ltd., 6 Royce Road, Peterborough, PE1 S78.

Poverty and the family

Cornwell, J. (1985). *Hard Earned Lives: Accounts of Health and Illness from East London*. Tavistock Publications, London.

Harrison, P. (1985). *Inside the Inner City: Life Under The Cutting Edge*. Penguin Books, Harmondsworth.

Whitehead, M. (1987). *The Health Divide: Inequalities in Health in the 1980s*. Health Education Council, London.

Nursing process and nursing models

Cheetham, T. (1988). Model care in the surgical ward. *Senior Nurse*, 8(4), 10–12.

Friedman, M.M. (1981). *Family Nursing – Theory and Assessment*. Appleton Century Crofts, New York.

Reutter, L. (1984). Family health assessment – an integrated approach. *Journal of Advanced Nursing*, 9, 391–399.

Speer, J.J. and Sachs, B. (1985). Selecting the appropriate family assessment tool. *Pediatric Nursing*, 11(5), 349–355.

Stephenson, P. (1987). Models for action. *Nursing Times*, 83(29), 62–63.

While, A. (1986). Care planning: helping a handicapped child improve her walking. *Nursing Times*, 82(22), 52–55.

Communicating with children and parents

Gleeson, C. (1986). Ward management of nursing care: psychosocial needs. *Senior Nurse*, 3(4), 16–18.

Glen, S. (1983). Paediatric nursing: happy families. *Nursing Mirror*, 156(4), 24–6.

Streff, M.B. (1982). The counselling dimension of the nurse practitioner role. *Pediatric Nursing*, 8(1), 9.

Whaley, L.F. and Wong, D. (1985). Effective communication strategies for pediatric practice. *Pediatric Nursing*, 11(6), 429.

Health education – children and family

Anderson, J. (1986). Health skills – the power to choose. *Health Education Journal*, 45(1), 19.

Azarnoff, P. (1985). Preparing well children for possible hospitalisation. *Pediatric Nursing*, 11(1), 53–55.

Bradley, J. (1984). Do adolescents practice what they preach about health? *Pediatric Nursing*, 10(4), 285.

Denehy, J. (1984). What do school age children know about their bodies? *Pediatric Nursing*, 10(4), 296.

Elkind, D. (1984). Teenage thinking: implications for health care. *Pediatric Nursing*, 10(6), 383.

Glen, S. (1988). Altered body image in children. In *Altered Body Image: The Nurse's Role*, Salter, M. (ed.). John Wiley and Sons, Chichester.

Hellmann Kaufman, D. (1985). An interview guide for helping children make health care decisions. *Pediatric Nursing*, 11(5), 36.

Keenan, T. (1986). School based adolescent health care programme. *Pediatric Nursing*, 12(5), 365–369.

Maneady, D. (1986). Health concepts of pre-school children. *Pediatric Nursing*, 12(3), 195–197.

Mayall, B. and Grossmith, C. (1985). Using preventive child health services, *Health Visitor*, 58(11), 293.

Mayall, B. and Grossmith, C. (1985). Keeping children healthy. *Health Visitor*, 58(11), 317.

McLeavy, D. (1986). Helping children make decisions – the 'My Body' project. *Health Education Journal*, 45(1), 30.

Wood, S.P. (1983). School age children's perceptions of the causes of illness. *Pediatric Nursing*, 9(2), 101–108.

The role of the school nurse

Holliday, K., Carter, E. and Cardwell, E. (1985). The school nurse as a health educator. *Health Visitor*, 57(6), 182.

Nash, W., Thruston, M. and Baly, M. (1985). *Health at School: Caring for the Whole*. Heinemann, London.

Shannon, A. (1986). A process of change for school nursing. *Health Visitor*, 59(3), 91.

Wilde, C. (1986). Comprehensive school nurse. *Health Visitor*, 59(3), 92.

The role of the health visitor

Broomes, H.J. (1987). Health For All by the Year 2000: the role of the health visitor. *Health Visitor*, 60(1), 9.

Dean, C. (1985). Health Visitor/Paediatric Liaison Officer. *Health Visitor*, 58(8), 221.

Hall, D.M.B. (ed.). (1989). *Health for All Children. A Programme for Child Health Surveillance*. Oxford University Press, Oxford.

Robertson, C. (1988). *Health Visiting in Practice*. Churchill Livingstone, Edinburgh

Primary nursing

Hymovich, D.P. (1980). How children, mothers and nurses view primary and team nursing. *American Journal of Nursing*, 80, 2041–2045.

Physiology

Hinchliff, S.M. and Montague, S.E. (1988). *Physiology for Nursing Practice*. Baillière Tindall, London.

Genetic factors and development

Connor, J.M. and Ferguson-Smith, M.A. (1987). *Essential Medical Genetics*. Blackwell Scientific, Oxford.

Milunshy, A. (1980). *Know Your Genes*. Penguin Books, Harmondsworth.

Williams, J.K. (1986). Genetic counselling in pediatric nursing care. *Pediatric Nursing*, 12(4), 287–291.

General textbooks related to child development

Bee, H. (1989). *The Developing Child* (5th ed.). Harper and Row, New York.

Buckler, J. (1987). *The Adolescent Years*. Castlemead, Welwyn Garden City.

Cohen, D. (1987). *The Development of Play*. Routledge, London.

Department of Health. (1991). *The Children Act 1989: An Introductory Guide for the NHS*. Health Publications, Lancashire.

Department of Health and Social Welfare. (1991). *The Children Act 1989: Putting It into Practice*. Open University, Milton Keynes.

Mussen, P.H., Conger, J.J., Kagan, J. and Huston, A.C. (1990). *Child Development and Personality* (7th ed.). Harper and Row, New York.

20

MENTAL HEALTH NURSING

Meg Miller

In this chapter the reader will be introduced to knowledge and skills that need to be part of the nurse's repertoire if she is to give holistic care to patients in any setting.

Some of the factors that may contribute to the onset of mental illness are explored and illustrate the impact it can have on people's lives.

The history of psychiatry is briefly described to provide a background to the discussion regarding the development of services for people with mental health problems.

Profiles of a patient cared for in hospital and a client cared for in the community, with nursing care planned according to different nursing models, highlight the role of the nurse in this field.

The main themes developed are the following:

- Human relationships
- Self-awareness
- Interpersonal skills
- The concept of a mental health/ illness continuum
- The effect of mental health law on

the development of modern mental health services

- The role of the psychiatric nurse
- The value of nursing theory
- Care of a disturbed patient
- Ethical issues in psychiatry

Human relationships

Human relations theory derives from the **behavioural sciences** and from studies that have observed people interacting in all types of situations. Argyle (1988) has written extensively about the means by which humans communicate, especially non-verbally. Goffman (1967) informs us of the rituals human beings engage in during different encounters. For instance, he details the behaviours one person will adopt in order to save face and to save the face of other people in that encounter.

Animals and humans communicate constantly by non-verbal behaviour. Some human behaviour may derive from instincts by which many species survive. For example, pupil dilation is unconscious and therefore outside our control, but is a sign of attraction between two people. Blushing is perhaps more conscious, yet still outside our control. Other non-verbal communication will be intentional and voluntary, for example a mother shaking her head to reinforce the message to her baby that he must not touch an electric plug, or a footballer raising his arms in celebration of scoring a goal. Gestures and movements, facial expressions and eye contact, positions and postures all communicate a wealth of information between humans besides the verbal communication that often accompanies it.

Rules of encounter

Part of the process of **socialisation** into our culture is the learning of rules about social encounters. Sometimes we may not be aware of these rules unless they are broken, for example how much distance should be left between two strangers engaged in conversation or working on a transaction such as buying and selling. At times these rules are allowed to be broken. It would be considered the height of indecency if a shopkeeper were to stand up against a customer as closely as he might stand to a fellow traveller during the crowded tube journey home.

Just as there are a multitude of different ways in which we communicate non-verbally, so there are numerous rules of encounter which are learnt. These include the degree of eye contact to maintain, either when speaking or listening, where to look at a person when we are not looking directly into their eyes, the cues to pick up that it is our turn to talk or to listen, the degree of personal disclosure that is appropriate, what is acceptable to ask the other person and what is not. With each different type of relationship comes another set of rules: with strangers, friends, acquaintances, lovers, parents, children, teachers, therapists, policemen and other authority figures.

Consider the rules of encounter of the following:

— A relationship between two close female friends
— A relationship between a male manual worker and his exclusively male workmates
— A relationship between a bank manager and a customer
— A relationship between an adolescent schoolgirl and her mother
— A relationship between a 60 year old woman and her disabled mother
— A relationship between a father and his mother-in-law
— A relationship between a prisoner and a prison warden
— A relationship between a terminally ill person and a voluntary befriender

The chances are you will have thought about rules concerning touch and proximity, acceptability of certain topics of conversation, the extent to which one may express feelings honestly, deference to authority and use of language. While all relationships of this type can differ, there are nevertheless rules of encounter that we can identify.

Unfortunately, there is no handbook which outlines these rules, no highway code of relationships. We tend to learn them through trial and error as much as by learning the 'correct' way to behave according to the values of our parent(s) or parent figures. Relationships within the family are **dynamic**; in other words they are constantly changing. Husband and wife often become parents. Children progress through different stages of development and eventually leave home. They may become parents themselves, creating another generation. Some families break up and of these some are reconstituted, with children of different parents living as one family or having two quite distinct family lives. There is evidence that family stresses occur around transition points in the family life cycle, sometimes resulting in one or more members experiencing health problems (Carter and McGoldrick, 1989).

Relationships outside the family may be extremely varied as already indicated. We may be attracted to like-minded people, and to people who we see as leading very different lifestyles. Factors such as our class, culture and gender will inevitably affect the nature of our relationships, since they influence how we view others and how we believe they will view us.

Power relations

Individuals who come into contact with one another will experience themselves as more or less powerful depending on their position in society, their gender and their experience of the world through the process of socialisation (see Chapter 2). Anyone believing they are occupying a role that carries less power may experience oppression.

The professional helping relationship

Anyone who goes to a professional practitioner will be likely to experience themselves as less powerful than the professional person, particularly if the reason for requiring the service is that one is ill or debilitated.

Several authors refer to a crisis occurring within the professions. Ivan Illich (1977) is renowned for his attack on the professions, especially the medical profession, which he claims abuses the client through overstating its knowledge and expertise.

Heron (1990) recognises the need for professionals to redefine their relationship with the client, allowing the client greater autonomy in decision-making regarding his life, with the professional offering support and information from which the client may make informed decisions. While these principles may apply to any profession, it is the helping professions to which Heron was referring.

The following are expectations this author has of a relationship she enters into with a professional helper. The professional is a person of integrity, ensuring his knowledge is accurate and up-to-date. He is honest and prepared to acknowledge his limitations when my safety depends on this. He is able to listen to me without needing to assert his authority or infer that he knows me better than I know myself. He is committed to his work, i.e. to helping me, and is reliable and trustworthy. What I tell him will be treated with respect and kept confidential. He will show empathy, a regard for my vulnerability in confiding in him and an openness that allows me to know the real person, not just the professional. However, I do not want to feel that I need to help him, or that he has expectations of me, at least while I am in the position of seeking help for myself, other than that I am interested in using the help he offers.

As this is what I expect from another helper, it is what I aim to achieve as a nurse. Along with this goes an appreciation that I cannot know everything about the person who temporarily occupies the role of client, but that that person will be disclosing a lot of personal information, while I am not. I am in a powerful position therefore, notwithstanding

the client may perceive himself as a member of an oppressed group. The best I can do is to acknowledge this and guard against abusing that power.

This is not a list of professional rules, rather a set of professional values. As Heron emphasises, it is the striving to uphold these values in our work with clients that makes us worthy of clients' trust.

'Human skills are maculate skills, enriched by earthy granulation: they are more basic and worthwhile than any seemingly immaculate descriptions that may service them'

(Heron, 1990; page 14)

In other words, the very fallibility of humans when relating to one another is in itself a valuable quality, that cannot easily be conveyed in textbooks which outline the skills and qualities of effective helpers.

The concept of self-awareness

To some extent we all know ourselves. We are aware of what we do and of what happens to us. We develop a sense of self as we develop physically, intellectually and emotionally. The baby exploring his toes is learning that they are a part of him, that he can wiggle them, that they feel warm or cold, that he cannot see them when he has shoes on, and so on.

If getting to know ourselves is a developmental process, then we are unlikely ever to know ourselves completely. Kelly (1955) has considered how human beings construct a view of the world in order to be able to predict events. He claims that we construct a view of our 'self' through other people's view of us. As we grow and mature, the chances are that we will come to trust that people will react to us consistently; that some people will be similar to us in some ways and others very different; that certain behaviour will provoke certain reactions; that certain emotions will be reciprocated. We probably know what we like and dislike, what we are striving for and what we rate as achievements.

However, there are likely to be occasions when we do not fully know ourselves. We may be hurt by something somebody says and not really know why it has upset us so much. We may behave in a way that evokes certain reactions but deny any responsibility for these. We may find certain relationships problematic, for instance with the bank manager, with a friend who constantly depends on us for support, with men, with women, with our closest relatives. At these times it can be very useful to learn more about ourselves, to find reasons for our reactions and to recognise our behaviour patterns, so that we are free to change to be able to live our lives more positively.

Theories of the self

Sigmund Freud (1962) viewed the self as divided into three parts. As he saw it, the mind is made up of an **unconscious** part, comprising the id and the superego, and a conscious part, the ego. The id is the primitive part of our 'self', the instinctive uncensored drives and desires. The superego is the conscience, the moralising and critical part. The ego, the conscious, realistic, organising part of the 'self', constantly strives to maintain an equilibrium between the drives of the id and the superego. Freud believed that only through **psychoanalysis** could we gain access to the unconscious mind, by creating a unique relationship with a therapist, which, by constantly reminding us of our relationships in the past, enables us to come to understand our past and present behaviour.

In contrast, Carl Rogers (1951) believed that the self is made up of all the thoughts, feelings and values that a person has. He claimed that the individual experiences everything in relation to their self-concept. The closer our self-concept is to our self-ideal, the more fulfilled we are. Rogers' theory of client-centred helping depends on his belief that every person has an **innate** capacity to change and grow, to become a more fulfilled person, and that the therapist needs to be self-aware and willing to grow himself, with a belief in his fellow individual's capacity to change, in order to help.

Psychoanalysis and **psychotherapy** may seem drastic and expensive ways to develop ourselves as carers, yet a willingness to know ourselves more completely and an openness to change are desirable qualities, so that through our own personal growth we can create opportunities for clients to achieve fulfilment.

A less extreme and expensive way of affecting our capacity to change involves participation in a group in which we demonstrate a willingness to examine our behaviour and feelings, to hear from

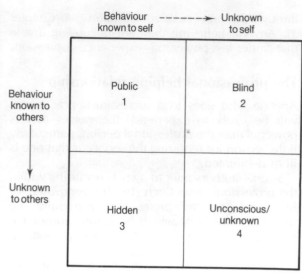

Fig. 20.1 *A Johari Window*

others how they experience us and to enact the role of that person into whom we wish to change.

A useful model for defining the terms of reference of such a group is named the *Johari Window* (Luft, 1970) (see Fig. 20.1) The model conceptualises four types of behaviour. Behaviour that is *public* is known both to oneself and others, while *unconscious* behaviour is known to neither. *Hidden* behaviour is that which is known to oneself but not to others, and *blind* behaviour is that which is known to others but not to oneself.

Through self-disclosure and feedback the group members aim to reduce the hidden, blind and unknown areas and enlarge the public areas (Fig. 20.2). Self-disclosure in this context comprises any

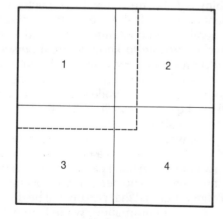

Fig. 20.2 *Developing self-awareness*

expression of feelings in the group, whether about oneself or others, while feedback is the direct verbal statements made to others about their behaviour (Smith, 1980).

Smith (1980) outlined a typological theory of change in individuals who are members of a ***sensitivity group***. The theory seeks to specify what happens when there is a mix of support and confrontation and when there is not. Smith proposes that confrontation alone leads to compliance on the part of the group member which is relatively short-lived, while support without confrontation can bring about changes in behaviour motivated only by the group member desiring to maintain rewarding relationships within the group. The most persistent form of learning or change is believed to take place if support and confrontation occur simultaneously. Smith terms this form of learning 'internalisation'. In other words, it is the individual's choice to change. Support refers to those behaviours that validate a person. Confrontation, in this sense, means giving feedback that challenges the person's perceptions of self.

Values clarification

One aspect that may be explored in the context of the group life of the student nurse is that of philosophy and values. Individuals can be asked to write down a statement of what they believe about humanity, discuss it, first with a partner and then in small groups. A joint philosophy for the group might then be formulated which embraces the students' common beliefs about people. This can be reviewed periodically as the students progress through their course, an exercise which in itself may indicate how change is taking place.

Another way of exploring values held by different members of the group is to ask students, before they have met any clients, to define nursing. During this exercise, there is likely to be some agreement and some dissent, depending on people's ideas of why they wish to become nurses. For example, if one person chose to be a nurse because she wants to help people by doing things for them that they cannot do themselves, this may conflict with another student's desire to help people to do more for themselves than they are able to at present. However, the same two people may be able to agree that nursing is about caring, which involves the nurse trying to understand how the patient is feeling.

A third exercise, which enables group members to learn to talk about themselves and to listen to each other, is one in which each student draws a symbolic picture of themselves as they think others see them on the front of a folded sheet of paper. On the inside of the sheet, they then draw how they see themselves. Having done this, they choose one other member of the group with whom they are prepared to share their pictures and the partners take it in turns to talk about them. The person describing their picture does not have to justify it or answer questions from their partner if they do not wish to. The partner's role is to listen and show respect for the pictures being shown them, only asking questions for clarification and not giving feedback unless it is asked for. These pictures are then kept by the individual and shared no further. However, the group can reconvene to discuss the exercise and feelings arising from it.

Discussing oneself in this way with others can be disturbing. Students may feel unprepared for the reaction to their beliefs and values from others in the group, and therefore feel exposed and become ***defensive***. For some, the exercises may act as a trigger, evoking feelings that have been aroused in the past which the ego has successfully ***repressed***. There may be ***group dynamics*** which inhibit people from being honest about themselves or with each other. For example, one member of the group may dominate and annoy other members by talking a lot, which at the same time allows them to keep quiet and avoid taking risks. If this situation develops unchecked, a mixture of dependence on the dominant member and resentment builds up, effectively halting the group in its endeavours to learn. Anger, which is commonly felt at this stage, may be directed at any member of the group who acts as leader or conductor, whose task it is then to point out how the group is behaving.

The setting of ground rules at the start of a group's life is helpful in enabling students to feel safe enough to do this kind of work. Bond (1986) suggests the following but emphasises the need for group members to decide their own.

(1) Confidentiality. Anything personal shared is kept confidential.

(2) Autonomy. Each person decides how much to disclose. Avoid probing or pressure. Ask 'Do you want to talk about this further?'

(3) No put-downs. Avoid judging or labelling, even as a joke.

(4) Reciprocity. Each person has the chance of equal time to be listened to.

(5) Each person speaks for themselves only, avoiding generalising. Tries to use 'I'.

(6) Avoid giving advice unless it is asked for.

(7) Tea breaks are breaks. Discussion ceases unless there is permission from the individual.

(8) Each person has the right to opt out.

(adapted from Bond, 1986)

Factors such as group size need to be addressed before such work is embarked upon. As colleges of nursing combine and form links with higher education, student intakes are increasing in size. Facilities for working in groups of 10–14 are essential for aspects of interpersonal skills training, as cited in Dickson *et al.* (1989) and Macleod Clark and Faulkner (1987).

The importance of self-awareness for nursing

This kind of learning can be invaluable for people who are working with clients in distress.

> 'The nurse who is aware of the complex nature of self is also likely to be aware of the complexities of the client, thus leading to care based on the whole person'
>
> (La Monica, 1979; page 469)

Peplau (1988) describes nursing as a therapeutic interpersonal relationship. Her theory incorporates the concept of nursing as 'a maturing force and an educative instrument', and the nursing process as a collaborative exercise between nurse and patient who, by coming to know and respect each other, together work at solving the problems faced by the patient.

Fundamental to the model is the belief that the nurse uses her unique personality as the tool she offers the patient to assist that individual to learn alternative ways of behaving. The patient is viewed as moving constantly along a continuum of dependence—independence with interdependence as a mature state.

Peplau defines the functions of the nurse as fivefold:

(1) Resource person
(2) Counsellor
(3) Surrogate or parent
(4) Leader
(5) Teacher

John Heron (1990) outlines how people in the helping role can select from six categories of intervention depending on the response they feel is the most effective. These categories are: prescriptive, informative, confronting, catalytic, cathartic and supportive. The first three categories he classifies as *authoritative*, the remainder as *facilitative* (see page 582).

Together with Smith's (1980) theory of using support and confrontation to effect change in people in a group setting, these two models of helping clearly rely on the helper having a sophisticated awareness of herself and the way in which she uses her 'self' for the patient's good. The Syllabus of Training for admission to Part 3 of the Professional Register, the Registered Mental Nurse (English and Welsh National Boards, 1982), specifies one of the skills to be acquired is 'the intentional and conscious use of self'. This might be interpreted as fulfilling two basic functions: supporting the patient until he finds the point on the dependence—independence continuum that is right for him (this may be further towards dependence if he is disabled or dying); and confronting the patient by offering herself as a real person with whom the patient may interact and therefore learn or relearn about himself and continue his growth towards interdependence.

The following examples illustrate how the nurse may work in this way.

Mrs Thompson, who is dying of cancer, is dependent on the nurse for her physical needs. In meeting these, the nurse acts in a supportive role. For her psychological and spiritual needs, Mrs Thompson requires the nurse to offer her 'self' with whom she can interact, and from whom she can expect honesty, integrity and respect, so that she may explore her feelings regarding her impending death and continue to grow in the sense of viewing her last days positively. The nurse may not be the person she chooses to use in this way, but by being self-aware the nurse can offer herself consciously for this purpose and understand if the offer is not taken up.

Peter is an 18 year old boy who has had his leg amputated. He has a great deal of dependence on others, at least initially, but all things being equal, he should be able to regain independence and also to mature through the experience, developing his capacity for interdependence, for example by helping others to be less frightened of disability. However, Peter suffers a prolonged **grief reaction** and becomes depressed, believing himself to be no longer the person he was and that therefore nobody will want to know him. Through his interaction with the nurse, Peter can learn that he is not simply someone who is no longer fit and ablebodied, but a person who is worth knowing even with only one leg.

The nurse herself will also mature through her interactions with patients if she allows herself to acknowledge the confrontation the patient faces her with; for example, her need to look after sick people, her prejudices, her reactions to pain, death, suicidal attempts or child abuse.

The dangers of the nurse not developing selfawareness are many. The nurse and patient may become mutually dependent and both stop growing towards interdependence. The nurse may herself adopt a patient role; for example, working out her own needs at the expense of the patient's. Support may be offered with no confrontation. This may mean the patient recovers from his immediate problem but does not grow from the experience. Confrontation with no support may make the patient withdraw, or regress, perhaps manipulating the nurse in order to get support, for example by refusing food or becoming incontinent.

The implications of this are that nurses require continuing support and confrontation themselves in the form of **supervision**. While staff support groups do occur in some mental health settings and areas such as intensive care units in general hospitals, there is still an enormous shortfall in support that the nurse requires. The availability of a staff **counsellor** is insufficient, as this suggests that the nurse requires therapy as opposed to supervision. While standards of care are expected to be improving against a background of diminishing resources, this will continue to promote tension.

Interpersonal skills

The term interpersonal skills is often used interchangeably with communication skills. In my opinion, communication skills are a category of interpersonal skills, which also comprise counselling skills, assertiveness, skills in managing oneself, skills in managing conflict and group facilitation skills. The latter involves use of all the others plus leadership skills. The first three of these skills will be discussed here. The others will be discussed later in the chapter or elsewhere in the book.

Communication skills

Macleod Clark *et al*. (1991) suggest that the purpose of communication skills is 'to ensure appropriate social contact and interaction'. They identify five objectives the nurse needs to achieve this:

(1) To give information
(2) To allow discussion and dialogue
(3) To allow expression of feelings
(4) To support and encourage
(5) To assess a situation

The skills required for this purpose include observation, listening skills, questioning skills, supporting and encouraging skills, use of non-verbal communication such as touch and silence, and being aware of one's limitations and how to refer the patient to a more experienced practitioner (Macleod Clark *et al*., 1991).

Counselling skills

Counselling skills are important if nurses are going to support patients in making decisions about their lives, solving problems and effecting changes in their usual patterns of coping.

Gerard Egan has developed a problem-solving model of counselling, the Skilled Helper Model (Egan, 1990). The model identifies three stages of the process: problem identification, goal development and action. Each stage needs a set of core skills, non-verbal and verbal. The non-verbal skills can be remembered using the acronym SOLER, which stands for **S**itting squarely, adopting an **O**pen posture, **L**eaning slightly forward, establishing **E**ye contact and **R**elaxing. While this may sound very prescriptive and rigid, Egan would assert that it is only by attending to one's body language in this detail that one can learn to attend adequately to the client.

Verbal skills of **active listening** include **para-**

phrasing, *reflecting*, *clarifying*, using **open questions**, *focusing* and **summarising**. In other words, the counsellor uses skills to help the client explore their problem without the counsellor adding anything of their own to this exploration. The skills convey the total attention that the counsellor is giving the client and a willingness on the part of the counsellor to understand the client's life as it is for them.

Many of these skills will be necessary for nurses in their everyday work with patients in any setting, regardless of their not being trained counsellors and the patients not asking for counselling. This is not to suggest that the nurse will be counselling as such, but that the understanding of the patient and his problems is an important part of the nurse's function. In hospital, nurses are the only practitioners who are in contact with the patients over the 24-hour period, so it is logical that they be equipped to respond to patients at those moments when their problems appear overwhelming, or they are grieving for their lost health, anxious about the future or feeling lonely. In the community, nurses are often in a position to offer support through listening and understanding the patient's situation and feelings.

Heron's model of six category intervention analysis (1990), first published in 1975 (referred to on page 580), is another framework for developing counselling skills. He identifies the interventions as:

AUTHORITATIVE　*Prescriptive*: giving advice, instructions
Informative: giving information, teaching
Confronting: challenging the client's existing self-perceptions
FACILITATIVE　*Catalytic*: enabling the client to explore a point further
Cathartic: encouraging the expression of feelings
Supportive: indicating the worth of the client

Burnard and Morrison (1991) have found that nurses on both the general and mental register find it easiest to use prescriptive and informative skills and hardest to use cathartic and confronting skills. This may be because of the rules of encounter referred to earlier. As expression of deep emotions and challenging people are not acceptable in everyday interaction, in Western culture in particular, so they may come harder as therapeutic skills. Yet the inappropriate use of questioning or a well-meaning 'Don't worry' when a patient is wanting to express strong feelings can greatly inhibit a person from coming to terms with their problems, and may cause the patient to withdraw from the nurse who has not understood him.

Assertiveness

Assertiveness is a skill nurses need to acquire in order to manage their own stress, respond appropriately to others' feelings and anxieties and to cope with situations of conflict.

To be assertive is to feel comfortable with oneself. The assertive person respects herself and is not afraid to ask for what she wants or to say how she feels. She also respects others in the same way and does not feel offended by others exercising their right to speak their minds. She accepts that she is not faultless and can make mistakes, but takes full responsibility for her own behaviour. She does not accept responsibility for others' behaviour and makes clear distinctions between helping others and feeling obliged to help even when she doesn't want to.

Alternative behaviours people use as coping mechanisms under stress are passivity, aggression and manipulation (Dickson, 1982). The passive person takes the blame for things, feeling guilty and anxious but not taking corrective action either. The passive woman may be nicknamed a 'doormat', being used and exploited because she will never complain, though inwardly she will be unhappy and may grouse about her lot to a friend whom she knows will not be able to change things either.

The aggressive person may hit out when upset or under stress, using abusive language and rejecting body language which she may afterwards regret. The aggressive person is often very competitive, needing to win all the time and prove her superiority. She will usually provoke an aggressive response; at least she will put others on the defensive, and people may get impatient with this way of getting what she wants and start resenting her.

The manipulative person is also aggressive but is too afraid of the reaction she will get to openly aggressive behaviour, so she disguises it. This indirectly aggressive style is perhaps the most difficult to conceptualise. Consider the following responses by four nurses to a request from a Senior Nurse to change their shift for the third time in one month. Which response matches with each of the four styles of interacting given above?

'Well, if you really cannot find anybody else to do it, I suppose I will.'

'I'm unwilling to alter my shift as it is the third time this month that I have done so, but I will ask the other nurses for you to see if anyone else would do it.'

'Oh no! Not again! Why is it always me you ask to change shifts? I have other interests besides nursing, you know.'

'Yes OK, I'll do it' (thinking 'I'm blowed if I'm going to let them shove me about like this'. Takes the day off sick.)

Hopefully, you will have identified the second response as the assertive one. Here, the nurse is using one of the assertion skills, workable compromise, which means 'being able to negotiate around a conflict of priorities' (Dickson, 1982; page 11). This and other skills can be learnt, so that the nurse can have a repertoire of skills from which to choose when the assertive response does not come naturally. Very few people are assertive all of the time in all their relationships. In some cases you may feel it is inappropriate to speak your mind however comfortable you might feel doing this in other situations. With the skills, you have the choice.

Skills acquisition

Throughout this section, skills have been identified but there has been little elaboration on each. This would be outside the remit of this chapter. However, it is also difficult, and inappropriate, to describe skills as if one could acquire them simply by reading about them and understanding what is meant by them. Skills need to be demonstrated and then practised by the learner under supervision from the teacher, and continually practised until they become a part of one's personality. Indeed, Burnard (1990) argues that there may be a 'factor X' in being interpersonally skilled, in other words that however hard someone practises the skills, they will only be successful in acquiring them if there is a certain factor present in their

personality. Whether this is true or not, skills of all kinds, including interpersonal skills, need practice.

The way in which interpersonal skills are introduced in the nursing curriculum will depend on the lecturer who plans this aspect of the course, and the time and resources allocated to it.

Microskills teaching is widely recognised as a suitable way of training students in communication (Hargie, 1986; Argyle, 1981; Trower et al., 1978). The advantages are that a complex skill can be broken down into manageable units, and the skills can be demonstrated without the student being overawed. Comparing communicating with the skills of driving a car may encourage students to accept that learning can be uncomfortable and to persevere with skills that they are unfamiliar with. Practically, it is difficult to do microskills teaching with large groups. There may be dangers with this method including students finding the environment unsafe to try new behaviours, and students may develop poor communication due to insufficient supervision. However, breaking a large group into small groups requires more time, teachers and classroom space.

Despite the problems, it is likely that at some point in your nursing course you will be asked to engage in *experiential learning*. This means that you will experience the feelings, thoughts and behaviours engendered by a simulation of a real situation, for example a game or through *role play* (Van Ments, 1983). These techniques are often found to be very useful by students, but are not always popular. This may be because students see themselves as being asked to do childish things in the classroom when they are used to taking considerable responsibility in their practical work on the wards or in the community. Sometimes students say role play is unrealistic, that it is not like the real situation. This is true. It is also true that the relationship with the patient, client, relative or other member of staff will not resemble the relationship between two students. One misconception around role play is that it is acting. It is not. It is using your *empathy* with people you have witnessed, or taking the part of yourself in a different context from that of the classroom, and exploring the experience for the learning you can derive from it. The object is not to entertain. You do not need to know a script. The fact of your using your empathy to imagine a role will bring with it its own script.

Experiential learning can be very powerful. Feelings are generated that students do not associate with classroom learning. Students have a right to skilled tuition and the recognition that learning in this way can be hard. Those who have assumed a role need help to **debrief** and **derole** before they move on to another learning situation.

My answer to critics of its use is this. Patients and their relatives are entitled to interpersonally skilled carers as much as to technically skilled ones. Skills need to be practised. If we do not practise and experiment in the relatively safe environment of the classroom, we inevitably practise on the patients. That is unethical.

The concept of a mental health/illness continuum

The concept of mental health is complex. The World Health Organisation definition of health in Chapter 3, which includes the notion of mental well-being, raises more questions than answers. Few could argue that they are always in a state of mental well-being, but does it follow that they are mentally ill?

An attempt at a definition of normality may throw more light on the issue. Atkinson *et al.* (1990) claim that certain traits are present in a normal person to a 'greater degree' than a person diagnosed as abnormal. These are traits such as a realistic perception of the world, awareness of self, self-control, an appreciation of one's own worth, an ability to give and receive affection in relationships, and volition to carry out daily living activities.

If we use these as criteria that, if absent, constitute mental illness, we may arrive at the conclusion that a person who does not demonstrate these traits needs help, but would we feel confident in saying they were mentally ill? After all, most of us would claim that our self-control or self-image is not too great on occasion. Even our perception of reality can be challenged if we are drunk or extremely tired, and we all know people whose rigid opinions lead us to perceive that their view of reality is very different from our own.

Perhaps it is a matter of degree or consistency, and of all people occupying varying points on a mental health/illness continuum. Certainly, the decision to pronounce someone mentally ill depends on contextual factors. It is all too easy to judge a person as mad when they are disturbing the peace, embarrassing us with their behaviour or being generally socially unacceptable.

Labelling theory

Scheff (1966) argues that people acquire labels from the social responses evoked by their behaviour. The term 'deviance', for example, he claims is attributed to a person by those whom the behaviour offends. The term 'mental illness' is expanding to encompass more and more forms of deviance that were previously regarded as criminal; for example, baby snatching, drunkenness and child abuse are seen to be due to psychological causes and therefore amenable to psychiatric treatment (Miles, 1987).

Psychiatrists might argue against this social construction of mental illness. They have exhaustive lists of criteria for every diagnostic category of mental disorder (World Health Organisation, 1975). Yet anomalies are rife. Labels of **schizophrenia** have often covered a wide range of incomprehensible behaviour. Research has shown that quite normal behaviour can be labelled as deviant by those who have a readiness to perceive someone as suffering from mental illness (Rosenhan, 1979).

Debate continues amongst sociologists, psychologists and philosophers with psychiatrists fiercely defending their concept of mental illness as a medical phenomenon. Meanwhile, consider the following statistics in the light of labelling theory:

(1) Black people are proportionately over-represented in those compulsorily detained in mental hospitals in the UK (Ineichen and Harrison, 1984; McGovern and Cope, 1987). A diagnosis of schizophrenia is significantly more commonly given to West Indians and West Africans compared to UK-born and other migrant groups (Carpenter and Brockington, 1980; Dean *et al.*, 1981). In a survey of detained patients in Birmingham in 1987, two thirds of West Indian patients were diagnosed as schizophrenic compared to one third of whites and Asians (McGovern and Cope, 1987).

A study at Springfield Hospital, South London, in 1984 revealed that in the case of 'uncooperative' patients, 87% of Afro-Caribbean patients as opposed to 36% of British patients were transferred to a locked ward (Bolton, 1984).

(2) One in five women takes tranquillisers and twice as many women as men receive treatment for affective disorders; of these, the ratio of working class to middle class women is 5:1 (Selig, 1988).

(3) A classic study in the 1950s showed that 78% of people diagnosed as suffering from mental illness were in social classes IV and V (Hollingshead and Redlich, 1958). Moreover, the kind of treatment a patient received varied with his social class, those in class V being most likely to receive custodial care alone, while those in classes I and II received the most expensive treatment. Subsequent studies have produced similar class differentials (Busfield, 1986; Selig, 1988).

The possible reasons for these differences in labelling and treatment practices are complex. Further reading is recommended and suggested at the end of the chapter. Suffice it to say here that there would appear to be sufficient evidence to support the claim by labelling theorists that:

> 'the psychiatric label, like other stigmatising labels, is most likely to be applied to those who are powerless to resist it'
>
> (Miles, 1987; page 191)

Stress and mental illness

Mental illness is commonly thought to be the outcome of a combination of predisposing and precipitating factors, the latter now being referred to as *stressors* (Schwabb and Schwabb, 1978).

Stress is a term used in common parlance to describe both the *stimulus* and the *response* of an individual when there is an imbalance between the environmental demands and the individual's capacity to meet them (Selye, 1974, Holmes and Rahe, 1967).

The contemporary model of stress is the *interactive* model which takes account of individuality and interaction with the environment. Lazarus and Folkman (1984) claim that the stress response arises from the individual comparing the demand, danger or threat imposed by the environment and their own ability to cope with it, and believing that they are unable to master the situation. Roth and Cohen (1986) considered the types of coping response adopted, categorising them into approach and avoidance strategies. Approach strategies would include direct action to solve a problem, while avoidance strategies would include denial of the existence of the problem.

There is now incontrovertible evidence that stress does affect health. Immune function is known to be depressed by life events such as bereavement (Schleifer *et al.*, 1982), marital disharmony and recent divorce (Kiecolt-Glaser *et al.*, 1987), and unemployment (Arnetz *et al.*, 1987). Cohen and Williamson (1991) propose three methods by which stress may influence people's illness behaviour. Firstly, stress may alter a person's biological susceptibility so that on exposure to pathogens, the person develops illness. Secondly, stress may initiate the activation of a latent pathogen so that the course of a disease is speeded up. Thirdly, stress may contribute to the maintenance of an ongoing pathogenic process, so that recovery is delayed. The authors suggest that a combination of physiological responses and health behaviours, e.g. poor diet, smoking, unsafe sex, drinking more alcohol and sleeping less, are responsible for the consequent health problems.

However, as the effects of stress on illness behaviour are not disease-specific, it is reasonable to assume they are often due to psychological processes influencing symptom-reporting and care-seeking rather than underlying pathology. Experiencing more physiological sensations due to the autonomic responses the stressor activates, the sufferer may label these as symptoms of disease rather than attribute them to the stress. Alternatively, the person may report symptoms and illness as ways of avoiding stressful situations, thereby influencing their seeking of medical care (Cohen and Williamson, 1991).

There is also considerable research showing that certain factors mediate the effects of stressful situations on a person's health. These include personality factors, beliefs regarding **locus of control**, the degree of social support a person enjoys, and self-esteem. It is not possible to expand on all these factors in this chapter, but the reader is referred to Chapter 9 and encouraged to follow up some of the suggestions for further reading given here.

Self-esteem

Self-esteem is the value we give ourselves. It is built up over years starting from the moment we are born, but it is constantly threatened when our self-image fails to live up to our ideal self.

The sort of things that promote our self-esteem are unconditional love from our parents or parent figures, safety and security while we are totally dependent, praise and acknowledgement of our achievements, commiseration with our disappointments, and celebration of our individuality and separate identity.

Threats to our self-esteem are, in the main, losses: loss of treasured objects and loved ones, loss of security, withdrawal of unconditional love, loss of face, loss of direction in our lives, loss of health and mobility. Bowlby (1980) claims that unresolved grief is often at the root of mental illness, which is not to say that any or even successive losses will predispose a person to mental illness, but that they have opted for avoidance coping strategies and the feelings of sadness, anger, despair and longing still reside unacknowledged in the person's psyche.

For many mentally ill people, self-esteem will be almost negligible. Some patients will have lost jobs, family, friends, independence and autonomy as a result of their illness. In addition, the stigma of being a patient in a psychiatric unit or hospital will further undermine any self-respect. One of the most rewarding aspects of psychiatric nursing is to help a person to restore their self-esteem.

Self-esteem is not only affected by personal life events. Social policy can also have negative effects on people's health, hence the importance of nurses being politically aware.

Unemployment and health

Unemployment is by no means a recent phenomenon. Any economy goes through recessions and recoveries with consequent effects on the availability of work, especially for skilled labour in industry. However, this inevitability makes unemployment a political issue which may be one reason for the dearth of research on this subject.

It is seen by some as a political device used to reduce inflation caused by wage demands and strikes, and has undoubtedly been exacerbated by the economic strategy of the 1980s. During periods of unemployment, there is less wage-bargaining, fewer hours lost through sickness, and less mobility between jobs – not, as might be argued, because of satisfaction and greater health of workers, but through fear of redundancy preventing the workforce from communicating their feelings and complaints (Fagin and Little, 1984).

It is important to consider the health of the employed as well as the unemployed in times of recession. Brenner (1979) published his findings of a study in *The Lancet* that showed mortality rates were directly proportional to unemployment rates, and that following economic recovery there continued to be significantly high mortality rates for two to three years. This study was criticised for its narrow approach in that other contributory factors such as nutrition and geographical inconsistencies were not taken into account. However, there does appear to be agreement that a rise in unemployment is directly associated with increased morbidity.

Unemployment and suicide

Many studies have found that there is a positive correlation between economic troughs and suicide and homicide (Fagin and Little, 1984), but others have found negative correlations and there is no conclusive evidence. A study conducted in Southampton by Shepherd and Barraclough (1980) showed that of a sample of 75 consecutive suicides, a high proportion had psychiatric histories, which raises the question of whether unemployment is a result of ill health or ill health a result of unemployment.

Nevertheless, there is evidence that unemployment is followed by changes in mental and physical health. While some people appear to respond favourably and become happier and more productive, the majority progress through recognisable stages similar to the grieving process.

(1) Initially there is a period in which the recently unemployed person experiences a 'holiday' feeling. Relationships within the family improve.

(2) This is followed by a period of anxiety and distress. Money is beginning to run short. There are times of frantic applications for jobs, interspersed with periods of lethargy. Relationships become strained, tempers frayed and social engagements virtually non-existent. Despite unemployment rates close to 50% within some towns, there is likely to

be self-imposed isolation of those out of work, suggesting that there still remains a stigma attached to being unemployed.

(3) Lastly, there is a phase of resignation and adjustment, usually after about one year of unemployment, when the person stops searching for jobs, lowers his expectations and resigns himself to a life of inactivity. Unlike the constructive resignation stage in the loss of a loved one, however, this phase is usually accompanied by loss of self-esteem, feelings of sadness, hopelessness, worthlessness, self-blame and a tendency towards isolation, suicidal thoughts, loss or gain in weight, violent outbursts, and abuse of alcohol and cigarettes. Spouses may also suffer from depression. Prescriptions for sleeping pills or tranquillisers are common as sleeping patterns are disturbed, and anxiety and irritability frequently result (Robertson, 1981).

Psychosomatic disorders are also reported, and may include psoriasis, backache, asthma, headaches and insomnia. Prolonged unemployment may also affect the children in the family, commonly in the form of behaviour problems, disturbances in sleeping and eating habits, and accident proneness (Robertson, 1981).

Fagin's study of 22 families showed that there was no common set of reactions and problems experienced by unemployed families. The breadwinner's attitude to his work and ability to use time constructively other than at work, financial status, relationships within the family, the spouse's employment status, the effect on family life of a member being ill, and prospects for future work all contribute to the physical and mental well-being of the families concerned (Fagin, 1981).

Recent studies have all confirmed that unemployment has negative effects on health, the link between suicide and *parasuicide* and unemployment being the most strongly established (Laurance, 1986). There is a need for more extensive research in this area, particularly to establish what alternatives may be found if society is to accept that full employment for all is no longer a realistic ideal. With advances in technology and a larger proportion of women joining the labour force, the establishment of such alternatives is essential for the continued health of our society.

Social factors in the onset of depression

While depression is a term loosely used by the general public, in psychiatric terms it is a diagnosis usually associated with distinct biological and psychological changes – for example, anorexia and weight loss, sleep disturbances, *psychomotor retardation*, loss of libido, low self-esteem, tearfulness and thoughts of suicide. Biochemical changes can occur in the brain.

The causal factors in depression are complex. Severe prolonged physical illness and pain, bereavement, or a pessimistic personality may all be factors. Even endogenous depression, so called because it is induced from within the person rather than due to external factors (reactive depression), is still thought to be related in some way to life events.

Brown and Harris (1978) carried out a study of women in Camberwell, South London, who were being treated for depression to elicit if there were common features underlying their illness. They discovered that there were four main factors which made women vulnerable to depression:

(1) Loss of mother before the age of 11;

(2) Three or four children under the age of 14 still living at home;

(3) Lack of employment outside the home if (1) and/or (2) apply;

(4) Lack of an intimate relationship and therefore nobody in whom to confide.

Low self-esteem was considered to be a common feature in all women who were vulnerable from all four factors. Factors such as the presence of young children meant that these women were less likely to be able to find employment outside the home, or to go to a GP when symptoms first appeared.

Brown and Harris also found that factors (1) and (2) correlated with the factor of low intimacy with partner and therefore nobody in whom to confide. Indeed, their conclusions focus more on hopelessness than on loss or lack of independence, and the fact that low self-esteem before a loss is crucial to the development of *generalised hopelessness*. They state that if perpetuated by vulnerability factors, low self-esteem 'can limit a woman's ability to develop an optimistic view about controlling the world to restore some sense of value'.

Finally, the study examined social class, and concluded that several factors may generate hopelessness in working class women that are not relevant in the case of middle class women. Firstly, poor housing was frequently a feature of the women they studied, and lack of response from authorities if they complained. Secondly, working class women were less likely to have contact with external agencies, for example, a solicitor, bank manager or insurance company, and seek their help with financial or housing problems. Thirdly, they had smaller networks of social contacts in whom they might confide if they had marriage problems. Problems were therefore of greater significance. For instance, poor housing, causing illness in a wage-earning member of a family, both rendered budgeting unmanageable and took longer to resolve.

Drug abuse – an example of avoidance coping

Since the 1970s there has been a rapid increase in opiate addiction according to figures issued by the Home Office. During 1991, the Home Office was notified of over 17,755 addicts, 65% of whom injected. Of that 17,755, 6923 were 'new' addicts that year compared to 5639 new addicts reported in 1989 (ISDD, 1991). Cocaine is also used by a broad section of the drug-using population. In the past three years, amphetamine misuse has increased along with use of lysergic acid diethylamide (LSD), the popularity of these hallucinogens growing with the trend for 'rave' parties (ISDD, 1991).

Despite the emphasis placed on opiate abuse by the media, use of minor tranquillisers such as Valium (diazepam), Librium (chlordiazepoxide) and Ativan (lorazepam) causes addiction problems to a far greater proportion of the population. Benzodiazepines are the most commonly prescribed drugs in Britain (ISDD, 1991), so there is no illicit manufacture of these drugs, but prescribed or stolen benzodiazepines, particularly temazepam, 'are widely misused by injection either as an alternative to heroin or as a drug of choice' (ISDD, 1991).

Excessive drinking of alcohol is also on the increase. Between 1970 and 1988 the consumption of alcohol per head increased by nearly 40% (HMSO, 1991). One in four men and one in 12 women are said to drink more than the recommended sensible number of units of alcohol per week. 750,000 people in the United Kingdom are seriously dependent on alcohol, and 40,000 deaths each year are alcohol-related (Royal College of Physicians, 1987). Prolonged alcoholism can cause hallucinations, epilepsy and dementia.

Figures show that young adults drink more than their elders. In the late teens and early twenties, consumption is 40–50% above the national average. A third of all children aged 13–16 years drink at least once a week. A survey conducted by the TV programme *Panorama* in 1987 found that 20% of all boys aged 15 years drink 20 or more units a week and there is evidence that girls are closing the gap (Holmes, 1990).

So far in this chapter the focus has been on factors that contribute to, and compromise, people's mental health as well as the skills nurses require to promote mental health in patients/clients they meet.

In each of the following scenarios, consider what has contributed to the person's mental state, drawing on your knowledge of sociology (Chapter 2) and psychology (Chapter 7) as well as human relations theory and your intuition.

Scenario 1

A woman who has been violently assaulted and raped is then subjected to a long interrogation by police and an intimidating courtroom examination. The accused is finally sentenced but only to 12 months imprisonment.

The woman is now afraid of the dark, of walking alone through streets and parks, of answering the door or telephone, and of social situations. She avoids any occasion where she might be expected to establish a relationship with a man, and especially an intimate one. She tends to blame herself for every mishap that occurs in her life.

Issues that you might have identified include: gender stereotyping, power and control, classical conditioning (generalisation of anxiety), defence mechanisms, lack of opportunity to express feelings and loss of self-esteem.

Scenario 2

A 17 year old boy has left home as a result of family conflict. Unable to find work without a fixed address, he ends up sleeping rough on the streets, starts taking drugs and is arrested by the police for stealing in order to pay for these. While on remand pending a court hearing, he attempts suicide.

Issues that you might have identified include: stages of psychological development, loss, stress and coping mechanisms, peer group pressure, family dynamics, loneliness and isolation, fear, lack of opportunity to explore feelings and consider alternative strategies, and social policy.

Scenario 3

An elderly widow lives in a flat in a high-rise council block. She has no friends, those she did have having died, and her only daughter doesn't visit. She is afraid to go out because the lifts frequently break down and the immediate environment is intimidating. She believes she has been mugged on numerous occasions, and that she is being poisoned by the people in the flat below by their gassing her through the floorboards.

A social worker visits her regularly but she is suspicious of him and often does not allow him access to her flat.

She can often be heard yelling for the police from her window, saying she is being murdered. She dials 999 for the police many times.

Issues you might have identified include: enforced isolation, demographic changes and lack of suitable housing and social facilities for the growing number of elderly people, age and sensory impairment, loss and grief, bystander apathy.

Treatment approaches and nursing care of people with mental illness in hospital and the community will now be addressed. A brief history of psychiatry serves to provide a background to the subsequent discussion.

The effect of mental health law on the development of modern mental health services

The history of psychiatry

Developments in psychiatry have been affected as much by legislation as by increase in knowledge and the views of physicians.

Mental health law has largely reflected the prevailing attitudes towards the mentally ill at the time of enactment. In 1890, for instance, the Lunacy Act legislated that those of unsound mind be isolated from the general public in large mental institutions by certification. Since so little was understood about the causes of mental illness, the emphasis was on protection of society from the mad. Lack of knowledge of mental illness also led to people of loose morals being incarcerated in these hospitals, which rendered them totally dependent on the institution within a number of years, thereby 'justifying' their original need to be there.

By the 1920s it was becoming apparent that some mental disorders had an **organic** base and could be treated, although the treatments were often bizarre (for example, insulin therapy in which the patient was rendered comatose for long periods of time, being roused for meals and toileting only). The Mental Treatment Act of 1930 reflected the growing realisation that not all mentally ill patients required compulsory detention. The term 'informal' as opposed to 'formal' was used for patients voluntarily accepting admission. The number of patients treated on a voluntary basis grew, and by the 1940s there was a movement spearheaded by Main (1968) towards the use of **sociotherapeutic** techniques such as group methods of treatment. The 1950s heralded a major change in the treatment of **psychotic** patients as the phenothiazine drugs were discovered to have a major tranquillising effect on disturbed patients. They could therefore be cared for in much more humane ways than previously, and were rendered more amenable to psychotherapy.

The Mental Health Act of 1959 (HMSO, 1959) laid emphasis on the development of community services. There followed a movement to unlock the doors of the mental hospitals to such an extent that there are few locked wards still in existence, despite the problems associated with treating patients who are disinclined to stay in hospital because they have no insight into their illness.

The 'open door' movement was so popular that plans were started in the 1960s to discharge patients back into the community, disband large mental hospitals and treat all psychiatric patients in their homes or in units attached to District General Hospitals. This was partly due to the description by Russell Barton (1976) and others of the effects of **institutionalisation**. Barton coined the term '**institutional neurosis**' which identified the common set of symptoms frequently observed in patients caused by lack of stimulation and motivation. Rehabilitation became the order of the day with all hospitals having **industrial** and occupational **therapy units**. The 1970s saw little progress in the move from hospital to community care of psychiatric patients. On the contrary, due to the reorganisation of the NHS in 1974 and the Report of the Committee on Senior Nursing Staff Structure (DHSS, 1966), little attention was paid to the mental health services.

In 1975, the government issued a White Paper, *Better Services for the Mentally Ill* (DHSS, 1975), in which were outlined plans for the development of psychiatric units within District General Hospitals. These were gradually to replace the large mental hospitals, and it was envisaged that community care would reduce the need for hospital care over time. Also outlined in this paper were plans for local Social Services to work with health authorities and the voluntary and private sectors to meet the needs of people of all ages suffering from mental illness, including those with long-term disabilities.

However, large mental hospitals remained full but under-resourced. Staff, too, suffered the effects of institutionalisation and there were a number of allegations of ill treatment on long-stay wards where nurses received little recognition or support for their work. The Report of the Working Group on Organisational and Management Problems in Mental Illness Hospitals (DHSS, 1980) found management to be sadly lacking in its organisation in these hospitals and education of qualified staff to be practically non-existent. Health authorities were therefore alerted once more to the need for transformation of mental health services.

In 1981, the DHSS published a handout, *Care in Action*, in which it was stated that certain ser-

vices were to be regarded as priority services by all health authorities. These were primary health care, and care of those who are elderly, mentally ill and mentally handicapped. Thus, while all other services were subjected to cuts in the early 1980s, these services were meant to expand and improve, continuing to carry out the master plan of reducing numbers of patients in hospital and building up community services.

The Mental Health Act of 1983 (HMSO, 1983) reflected the growing awareness of patients' rights: to information, to refuse treatments of a controversial nature, to have their drug treatment regularly reviewed. The new Act made explicit the need for doctors to consult with other professionals regarding detention and treatment of formal patients. There is also a section allowing nurses to detain a patient for up to six hours until a doctor can carry out an assessment. While under the 1959 Act the nurse was covered by common law for detaining against their will patients whom she deemed to require formal detention, the 1983 Act acknowledged the competence of the nurse to make such a judgement.

Conditions for detention – Mental Health Act 1983

Mental disorder is defined in the Act as a general category subdivided into 'mental illness, arrested or incomplete development of the mind, psychopathic disorder or disability of mind' (Section 1). Certain categories are then further defined (see Table 20.1).

Compulsory admissions

For a patient to be admitted against his will under the Act, certain conditions must apply.

(1) The patient must be suffering from mental disorder of a nature or to a degree which warrants detention in hospital;

(2) The patient does not agree to stay in hospital informally;

(3) The patient requires to be detained in the interests of his own health and safety or with a view to the protection of others.

Sections 2,3,4 and 5 allow for patients to be detained against their will. Section 2 lasts for up

Table 20.1. *Conditions for detention: the Mental Health Act 1983*

Severe mental impairment:	'A state of arrested or incomplete development of mind which includes severe impairment of intelligence and social functioning and is associated with abnormally aggressive or seriously irresponsible conduct on the part of the person concerned'
Mental impairment:	Defined in the same way as severe mental impairment except the phrase 'severe impairment' is replaced by 'significant impairment'
Psychopathic disorder:	'A persistent disorder or disability of mind (whether or not including significant impairment of intelligence) which results in abnormally aggressive or seriously irresponsible conduct on the part of the person concerned'
	Promiscuity or immoral behaviour by itself is not implied as falling within the categories of mental disorder, neither are sexual deviance or dependence on alcohol or drugs
	MIND (1983)

to 28 days and is specifically for observation and assessment of the patient as to his need for treatment and further detention.

Section 3 lasts for six months and is applied for if the patient requires treatment for prolonged periods and is unlikely to gain insight into his need for treatment despite its effect on his state of mind. This section may be repeated for six months and thereafter lasts for one year.

Sections 4 and 5(2) are 72-hour sections for emergency admission or detention of a patient already in hospital who decides he wants to leave and who is considered to be a danger to himself or others. Section 5(4) is the aforementioned section giving a registered mental nurse (RMN) or registered nurse for persons with a mental handicap (RNMH) the authority to invoke a 'holding power' in respect of a patient who wishes to leave the hospital when it appears to the nurse that the patient is suffering from mental disorder such that it is necessary for the patient's safety and the safety of others to restrain him from so doing, and it is impractical to secure the immediate attendance of a medical practitioner.

All but Section 5 require an independent application by an approved social worker or nearest relative besides the medical recommendation.

Section 136 may be used by the police to transfer a person from a public place to a place of safety if they consider him to be mentally ill.

Sections 37 and 41 are orders made by the court in respect of criminal offenders for whom treatment is deemed to be more appropriate than imprisonment on the evidence of two registered medical practitioners. Section 37, a hospital order, is used in the case of offences which would not have justified a substantial term of imprisonment, and patients may be discharged by the Responsible Medical Officer. On the other hand, patients on Section 41, a restriction order, are serious offenders and can only be discharged, or indeed allowed out of hospital at all, with the consent of the Home Secretary.

Patients' rights

Since authorities may make decisions that greatly affect a person's freedom, it is essential that the patient's rights are recognised and protected. Frequently, the patient is unable to assert himself in his own interests and relatives may either fear involvement or just not want to know. Advocacy is of paramount importance. The National Association for Mental Health (MIND) has long been watchdog for the rights of all psychiatric patients, and is responsible for many of the changes in the law in the patient's favour. Any patient who seeks representation regarding an appeal against formal detention or compulsory treatment may call on a member of MIND who will act on his behalf. If a patient wishes to appeal against his section, he must be given assistance in so doing. Nurses must allow him access to relevant information. The social worker who makes the application is obliged to inform the patient of his formal status, and ensure he is aware of his rights. A leaflet explaining his rights is also given to the patient, and it is often the nurse who is best placed to ensure that the patient understands the details.

Usually the patient must appeal within a set number of days if he wishes his case to be heard by a Mental Health Review Tribunal. This is a board consisting of an independent doctor, a solicitor and a lay person, who, having heard the case for the section by the Responsible Medical Officer and read his notes, will then hear the case of the patient, while other members of the multidisciplinary team may be called to give their opinion. The Tribunal will then make a decision in favour of either the responsible authority or the patient. An appeal may also be made to the hospital managers, who must then review the patient's situation within 72 hours. This appeal may be made by either the patient or his nearest relative.

The 1983 Mental Health Act saw the establishment of the Mental Health Act Commission. This body also acts as watchdog by making visits to hospitals, sometimes unannounced, interviewing detained patients and reading records. Detained patients must all be aware of their right to complain to the Mental Health Act Commission about their detention, treatment or general care if they are not satisfied that a complaint to the managers was promptly investigated.

The provision for aftercare for patients detained on Section 3 or 37 is also an addition in the 1983 act. Previously, care of the patient following discharge had not been covered by law, but in line with the plan to shift the emphasis on mental health care from the hospital to the community, rehabilitation both within and without the hospital is now addressed.

Services include: hostels, day centres, group homes, lunch clubs, training centres and social work support for ex-patients with problems of employment, accommodation or family relationships, all of which assist the client in the community, and cater for different needs of individual clients.

In practice, the provision of services for this group of people varies geographically, and resources in the community are not expanding as rapidly as they need to to cope with the exodus of patients from the mental institutions. Crucial to the successful rehabilitation of the patient in the community is the community psychiatric nurse (CPN). The CPN is generally attached to a GP practice and her functions are extremely diverse, ranging from organising clinics for administration of long-acting injections of phenothiazine drugs, to **family therapy** and **behaviour therapy**. CPNs also serve the vital function of educating the general public about the nature of mental illness, so that any stigma may be reduced and the ex-patient accepted as a neighbour.

CPNs are at the forefront in promoting mental health along with community mental handicap nurses. This is likely to be reflected in their title soon, since it is proposed that post-registration education of all community nurses take account of Project 2000 reforms, and that core skills of community nursing acquired in the pre-registration courses be supplemented by specific skills in post-registration modules leading to a qualification as a Community Health Care Nurse (UKCC, 1991).

The role of the psychiatric nurse

During the past two decades several nurse researchers have studied what psychiatric nurses actually do (Altschul, 1972; Towell, 1975; Cormack, 1976, 1983; Macilwaine, 1983; Powell, 1982).

These studies showed that although no theoretical basis existed for psychiatric nursing, the consumers, psychiatric patients, viewed the nurse as 'being positive and therapeutic' and that the skills of conveying respect, empathy and genuineness to patients gave nurses 'a unique opportunity to play a more specific, active and therapeutic part in patient care if they wish to do so' (Cormack, 1983; page 23).

Cormack's research highlighted the way the role of the nurse was developing in accordance with different philosophies on the causation and treatment of mental illness (see Table 20.2). More recent research has studied the effectiveness of nursing patients according to these different theoretical approaches. Reynolds and Cormack (1990) cite the following studies: hallucinating patients were relieved under the direction of nurses trained to use a counselling approach based on Peplau's Theory of Interpersonal Relations (Field, 1985); student nurses trained in the Rogerian client-centred approach were rated more highly on empathy scales by patients at the end of a series of interviews than at the start, suggesting a trusting relationship was developing (Reynolds, 1986); patients with major affective disorders were cared for by nurses using a cognitive/behavioural approach, which was found to be significantly more

Table 20.2. *Showing the emergence of nursing roles from popular viewpoints of **psychopathology***

Model of psychopathology	Emphasis and treatment		Role of the nurse	
ORGANIC	**Emphasis:**	Genetic factors Biochemical factors Physiological factors Neuropsychological factors	**Role:**	Doctor's assistant
	Treatment:	Physical treatments: ECT, drugs, psychosurgery	**Functions:**	Administration of medicines Provision of asylum Observation and reporting of behaviour Caring for patients before and after operations or ECT
PSYCHOTHERAPEUTIC	**Emphasis:**	Nature of the patient's interpersonal relationships especially the patient/ therapist relationship	**Role:**	Counsellor
	Treatment:	Talking to therapist, often about early life experiences Interpretations offered by therapist enable patient to gain insight into his behaviour	**Functions:**	Interactions and development of nurse/ patient relationships One-to-one planned nurse/ patient contact on purposeful basis Development of insight and self-help on part of patient
SOCIOTHERAPEUTIC	**Emphasis:**	Social functioning, adequacy and potential of patient	**Role:**	Creator of a wholesome ward atmosphere, and to influence routine and surroundings in the patients' interests
	Treatment:	Modification of the patient's ability to cope with everyday demands of living, and altering the immediate social milieu	**Functions:**	Involvement in group therapy Participation in networks of relationships between patients and staff
BEHAVIOURAL	**Emphasis:**	Helping the patient unlearn undesirable behaviour	**Role:**	Therapist role
	Treatment:	Direct treatment of symptoms by behavioural techniques, e.g. *desensitisation*, *exposure*, *flooding*.	**Functions:**	Application of behavioural techniques
		(*from* Clare, 1980)		(*from* Cormack, 1983)

effective than more traditional nursing approaches (Barker, 1988).

Leiba (1990) studied the training needs of nurses with respect to their ability to prevent, contain and manage violence. His findings include that training needs to be ongoing for all nurses from pre-registration students to qualified staff, and requires more resources than have been allocated to it to date. His study also suggests that staff support mechanisms need to be increased.

Two major studies involved work with the families of patients (Brooker, 1990; Watkins, 1988). A nurse researcher at Manchester University has reviewed the effectiveness of CPNs working with families of patients with schizophrenia (Brooker, 1990). The CPNs have been trained in the use of a **psychosocial** approach based on the theory that patients with a vulnerability to schizophrenia are more likely to develop symptoms when exposed to high levels of expressed emotion within the family. With encouragement from the CPNs, families are able to learn better ways of communicating.

Watkins (1988) has studied the effect of providing a night hospital for clients with organic brain disease, or **Alzheimer's disease**, on their carers. Approximately 5% of the population over 65 years old are affected by this disease, and more in older age groups (Medical Research Council, 1991). All mental functions are affected: memory, speech and mood, and eventually the person's physical condition deteriorates, so that total nursing care is required. This can be a great strain on carers, whose own mental health can be compromised by the stress of caring for such a dependent person (Llewelyn, 1989).

Compared to traditional respite care where a person is admitted to hospital for a period of 1–2 weeks to allow the carer to have a holiday, the night hospital provided 'the opportunity to relatives to have a night free, allowing them to rest or socialise undisturbed' (Watkins, 1988). Evaluation of the service has shown that carers have felt 'relief, pleasure and happiness' and clients have been found to become no more dependent. In fact, the nursing care delivered according to a modified form of Roper's Activities of Daily Living Model (Roper *et al.*, 1980) 'facilitated clients' independence in that they became no more dependent over a six month period of attendance than on initial admission' (Watkins, 1992).

Besides major nursing research studies being on the increase, initiatives have been taken such as the compilation of a manual of research-based psychiatric nursing procedures (Ritter, 1989), contributing to the development of a professional knowledge base.

Psychiatric nursing skills

In addition to the interpersonal skills outlined earlier in this chapter, the psychiatric nurse needs to develop other skills including those of assessment, relationship-building and group facilitation.

Assessment

Regardless of whether a person with mental health problems is admitted to hospital or cared for in the community, the nurse will be required to perform an assessment. This necessitates skills of observation, questioning and gathering information from a variety of sources. The kind of information sought depends to a certain extent on the model of nursing used. Examples are shown in Figs. 20.4 and 20.9.

Assessment will take many different forms. Initially the nurse will make an assessment from what she observes; for example, the person's state of dress may indicate whether he has been maintaining his personal hygiene or if he is disinhibited, flamboyant or meticulous. To some extent, his response to the nurse will indicate whether he is withdrawn, suspicious, confused or preoccupied, and whether or not his attitude to treatment is favourable.

A more comprehensive assessment may take as long as a week to complete, the nurse ascertaining through several interviews with the patient and with relatives, friends, social workers, teachers or employers (as well as through her own observations) exactly what the patient perceives as his problems, how this compares with others' views, how able he is to perform daily living activities, and so on. To obtain information from the patient about what he is experiencing, thinking and feeling, the nurse will need to build up a relationship of trust with him and this takes time.

Building relationships

Rogers (1967) asserted that this all-important aspect of helping rests on the helper developing qualities of respect, empathy and genuineness. If these are present, the relationship-building process is possible even if the patient is being detained involuntarily or being forcibly medicated. To illustrate this point these qualities are examined in more depth.

Respect. This quality comprises a willingness to be honest and an unconditional acceptance of the patient. It means the nurse not making assumptions, for example about what the patient wants to be called; or stereotyping, by assuming the patient's attitudes and behaviour will conform with her own, or with her ideas of mentally ill people. For example, if a nurse's jolly, lighthearted approach to a patient meets with a rejecting response, she is not respectful if she then tells the patient off for being rude, or teases him for being moody.

If a tall male patient is verbally aggressive, hostile and threatening, it is sometimes tempting for a petite female nurse to fob him off when he is demanding something which he cannot have – release from the ward, for example.

By approaching him with the words, 'I'm afraid you cannot leave the ward at present; you are not well, but as soon as you are well enough to go out we will go for a walk', the nurse demonstrates her respect for the patient by honouring him with the truth. Often, rather than becoming even more aggressive, the patient will accept this restriction, for a short while at least, and allow his attention to be directed towards some activity within the ward instead.

Empathy. Empathy is sometimes confused with sympathy, which is the process of identifying with someone else who has experienced the same phenomena. The patient who is describing his problems requires empathy: time, attention and a willingness to understand his situation. Empathising involves the nurse noticing the non-verbal communication accompanying the patient's words and responding by acknowledging both messages without adding any ideas of her own.

People who are mentally ill have often suffered rejection in the past from parents, partners or other helping agencies, and this can cause them to behave in such a way as to provoke further rejection, for example by answering a caring remark with abuse, or walking away from the friendly approach of the nurse. The nurse who remains friendly despite rebuffs and who makes herself available rather than forcing a relationship will do much to change this learned reaction.

Genuineness. Accepting the patient despite his hostility, and remaining friendly and empathetic despite the patient's behaviour, does not mean that the nurse has to deny herself the right to her own feelings. On the contrary, everybody is entitled to their emotions. A patient may make the nurse feel angry, upset, anxious, amused, indignant or happy. If allowed to know this, the patient learns how his behaviour affects others and thereby has the opportunity to change. If the nurse denies her feelings the patient can become confused and unable to predict how people will react to him. Showing emotion to patients is a skill that nurses need to learn. Spontaneous venting of feeling can be counterproductive as this may overwhelm the patient and cause him to become defensive, attacking or inappropriately affectionate. The response this provokes in the nurse may then bemuse the patient, who has received conflicting messages.

Group facilitation

A group can allow people a forum for expression of feelings, and receipt of support from others with similar problems whom they may perceive as more able to understand their feelings than their friends or family. Groups can also be effective in helping people to take responsibility for their own lives. The purpose of a group may be therapeutic or educational, or a combination of the two. Some groups specifically help people to change their ways of thinking, feeling and behaving. Others teach members skills or primarily provide support for people with a common problem (Corey, 1990).

Nurses facilitating a group may allow it to develop in its own way while ensuring that there is a balance of support and confrontation between members. Others may initiate an activity so that members can focus on something other than their relationships with each other, which can feel threatening and create resistance.

In the community, the nurse might choose to facilitate a group as a way of fulfilling her function as a promoter of mental health. For instance, she may run a group for people trying to give up smoking, people who want help with managing their stress, or people who have recently been bereaved.

Common uses of groups in wards include a regular community meeting for all staff and patients, a group for patients who are approaching discharge or have recently been discharged, and activity groups as part of occupational therapy. There may also be a staff group held on a regular basis in which staff members can express their feelings aroused by working on the ward, and work through differences and problems within the team that will otherwise mar the team's functioning.

An example of the nursing care of a patient in hospital – Jack

Jack is a 25 year old man who has been diagnosed as suffering from **paranoid** schizophrenia for the past five years (Fig. 20.3).

Jack's nursing care took place in a ward where a combination of Orem's model and Travelbee's model was used as the conceptual framework for nursing care. Orem's model (1985) is described in Chapter 12, so only Travelbee's model is outlined here.

Jack is the only son of a divorced couple. He used to live with his father, a 'hard and strict' man, who had been a soldier in the Polish army, and who is now retired at the age of 72 and lives in a rented bedsitter in London, showing little interest in Jack's whereabouts or developments.

Jack's mother also lives in London with his three sisters, aged 17, 19 and 21, but Jack has no contact with any of them.

He was admitted to the unit for rehabilitation having been referred from a large mental institution where he had been treated for five years for paranoid schizophrenia.

Fig. 20.3 *Case history: Jack*

Travelbee's interpersonal model of nursing

Travelbee (1971) sees a human being as 'a unique, irreplaceable individual' who 'is always in the process of becoming, evolving or changing' (page 26–7). Her approach to nursing emphasises the fact that both patient and nurse will be engaged in a human-to-human relationship.

Nursing, according to Travelbee, is:

'an interpersonal process whereby the professional nurse practitioner assists an individual, family or community to prevent or cope with the experience of illness and suffering, and, if necessary, to find meaning in these experiences'

(Travelbee, 1971; page 7)

Travelbee defines health by subjective and objective criteria, objective health being 'an absence of discernible disease, disability, or defect as measured by physical examination, laboratory tests, assessment by a spiritual director or psychological counsellor' (page 10) and subjective health status as being how the individual perceives his health.

By using a combination of Orem's and Travelbee's models, the nursing team on Jack's ward believed it had identified a framework that embodied its mental health nursing function: the rehabilitation of people who have been rendered incapable of self-care by their long term illness, and whose individual view of their state of health is confused by society's reaction to them. Orem's model provided a useful tool for assessment of self-care deficits. Travelbee underlines the dynamic interaction between nurse and patient, acknowledging that the patient's perception of his illness plays an integral part in the complex process of nursing. This is most important to remember when the patient sabotages his negotiated programme, as Jack tended to do.

When Jack was admitted to this unit for rehabilitation, an assessment was made of his self-care abilities using Orem's checklist of universal self-care requisites (see Fig. 20.4). Taking into account Jack's and the nurse's views, a care plan was formulated in Jack's first week on the ward (Fig. 20.5).

At this stage everything seemed to be straightforward. Jack appeared to have a certain degree of insight into his needs and self-care deficits which, together with the nurse, he formulated a plan to overcome.

Initially Jack was compliant with his programme though he did not mix with other patients. However, in some respects his behaviour deteriorated. His sleep pattern altered; he was going to bed late, having listened to music until 1.00 or 2.00am, and not getting up in the morning. He was becoming preoccupied with getting a girlfriend and was noticed to be masturbating quite frequently. An occupational therapy programme was organised for him in the day hospital but he rarely attended. His speech became quite bizarre except for regular statements of 'I want a girlfriend', 'I want to stay in bed', and 'I want to find a job'.

These formed Jack's perceptions of his problems and therefore it was necessary both for him and for the nurses to consider what it meant to him to remain a patient in hospital, in line with

SELF CARE REQUISITE	ASSESSMENT	HEALTH STATUS
(1) Sufficient intake of air, water and nutrition	Appetite good Enjoys cooking No difficulties in meeting these self-care needs	Subjective health status Understands he is ill and hears voices Describes himself as needing to sort himself out
(2) Satisfactory eliminative functions	No elimination difficulties	
(3) Activity balanced with rest	Erratic sleep pattern Takes sedation Unwilling to rise in the morning	Jack's view of his need for help
(4) Time spent alone balanced with time spent with others	Finds difficulty communicating with people, so spends a lot of time alone Preoccupied with finding a girlfriend and having sex Hobbies are solitary – listening to music and watching football on the television	'I want to live in a hostel. I want the social worker to find me a place and a job on a building site'
(5) Prevention of danger to self	No history of self-injury or crime Can become aggressive Smokes up to 30 cigarettes per day Misuses drugs and alcohol on occasion	Nurse's view Jack has distressing symptoms at times still
(6) Human functioning	Untidy in appearance but clean Usually normal speech pattern but has slight stutter and difficulty finding the correct words Expresses delusional beliefs, for example: – that radios and other people have power over his mind and so can control him – that he has occasional control over these and also cars and the TV – that he belongs to a previous life – that his face looks funny However he can respond rationally in conversation Mood appears flat though Jack says he is happy Orientation and memory are intact Attention span is poor	Poor view of himself – especially his sexuality Seems settled on the ward Signed .....(Jack Dee 12.7.92

Fig. 20.4 *Assessment sheet for Jack*

Long term aim	Objectives	Nursing intervention
That Jack be rehabilitated into a supportive hostel or similar environment	(1) That Jack be able to join in activities on the ward and learn about himself (2) That he look positively at his future and make constructive plans	Encourage Jack to join in ward activities e.g. ward meeting, games and conversations Assess for day hospital programme Observe for distressing symptoms e.g. his ideas concerning the radio Encourage him to talk about himself on a one-to-one basis and about his future

Fig. 20.5 *Care plan for Jack. Week one*

Problem	Aims and objectives	Nursing intervention
Patient's view of problem(s) 'I haven't got a girlfriend' 'Do I look all right?' **Nurse's view of problems** Jack is restless, tense and angry when dissatisfied. He lacks motivation, and is not following his day hospital programme. He has difficulty communicating in groups especially with women. He still displays symptoms of his illness.	**Long-term aim:** Unchanged **Objectives:** (1) That he complies with his day hospital programme (2) That he develops self-esteem	Ask Jack to get out of bed in the morning at ten minute intervals from 8.00 am so that he is up by 9.00 am Explain frequently why we ask him to do things, i.e. so that he will gain his independence Praise all special efforts or accomplishments and *reinforce* all acceptable behaviour Check he is following his day hospital programme and ask him about what he was doing each day Spend 30 minutes each day with Jack when not needing to get him to do something, so as to demonstrate his worthiness of attention and time, to increase his self-esteem

Signed .....*M. Hill*.......... Date *18.3.92*

Fig. 20.6 *Care plan for Jack. Week six*

Travelbee's belief as to the nature of nursing. However, one cannot approach the patient with such a question when he is stuck in a pattern of self-destructive behaviour and is only able to express his needs, thoughts and feelings in this way. Rather, the nurses needed to demonstrate through their relationship with Jack that they did believe he was able to change; that they did have faith in him as a human being capable of relearning to meet his own self-care needs; that he was worth the time, effort and attention put into his care despite his repeated sabotage of their attempts. Meanwhile, the care plan needed to be negotiated with Jack, and to reflect realistically his capabilities at that time (Fig. 20.6). This plan served to support and bring about a slow but gradual improvement in Jack's behaviour. Many other members of the multidisciplinary team worked in conjunction with the nurses to help Jack overcome his self-care deficits.

The speech therapist agreed to see Jack weekly to help him articulate his words better and express himself verbally more easily, so reducing his frustration and increasing his self-esteem.

The occupational therapists worked closely with the nurses to ensure that Jack's programme was carefully tailored to his needs.

Towards the end of Jack's stay in hospital, he started to attend a day centre outside the hospital, run by Social Services, to increase his indepen-

dence prior to his discharge. Although this was eventually achieved and Jack did obtain a place at the hostel, the overall period of rehabilitation was eight months, and there were many setbacks along the way. One of these was Jack's resorting to taking drugs and getting drunk on the ward when frustration, impatience or a sudden fear of 'recovery' overwhelmed him. Not only was this destructive towards himself but he would consume the alcohol on the ward, become drunk and aggressive (on one occasion he was physically violent) and upset the other patients, particularly those whose problems were alcohol-related.

At this point it became necessary to draw up a contract with Jack which would be binding, in that if it were not adhered to, a sanction of some kind would be applied, which would be considered by the multidisciplinary team and authorised by Jack's consultant psychiatrist (see Fig. 20.7). Though it was never stated, this was likely to have been discharge back into his father's care or to the previous institution, neither of which Jack relished.

This form of ultimate limit-setting is a necessary and caring way of helping a patient to control his own behaviour. The contract was not religiously adhered to by Jack (although he did not drink, use drugs or become violent again) but it was not meant to serve as a threat. What it did do was help Jack to develop some motivation to move on and, knowing exactly what was expected of him, to

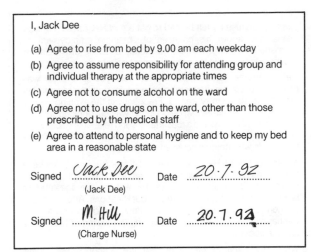

I, Jack Dee

(a) Agree to rise from bed by 9.00 am each weekday

(b) Agree to assume responsibility for attending group and individual therapy at the appropriate times

(c) Agree not to consume alcohol on the ward

(d) Agree not to use drugs on the ward, other than those prescribed by the medical staff

(e) Agree to attend to personal hygiene and to keep my bed area in a reasonable state

Signed   *Jack Dee*   Date   20·7·92
        (Jack Dee)

Signed   *M. Hill*   Date   20.7.92
        (Charge Nurse)

Fig. 20.7 *Jack's contract. Week twenty-two*

develop beyond the stage of testing limits. Freed from the inner struggle between that part of him still clinging to familiar, institutional dependent ways of coping and that part of him which was searching for independence and fulfilling relationships, he was able to move more steadily towards his long term goal.

It is doubtful whether the contract could have been used successfully earlier on in his stay in the unit, since the relationships he had formed with staff involved trust, knowledge of their care and concern and a greater self-respect, all of which were necessary for the contract to serve a useful function.

Jack's future in the hostel depends on all of these things. trust, development of relationships, and maintaining a reasonable level of self-esteem. It may not be a one-way ticket that he has bought out of hospital. There may be times when stressful life events force him to resort to his dependent, self-destructive behaviour. It is to be hoped, however, that a significant change has been achieved and relearning will be a less painful process. For him, perhaps, a stay in hospital of a few weeks will be comparable to a holiday – time out from the struggle to live up to society's standards.

An example of the nursing care of a client in the community – Harry

Harry's story is told in Fig. 20.9. The CPN assessing and supporting him chose Neuman's

model as the most appropriach to this particular individual.

In assessing Harry there were no major discrepancies between the CPN's perception of his situation and Harry's own. The problems (or what Neuman terms *stressors*) that were agreed upon can be itemised under the headings *intrapersonal*, *interpersonal* and *extrapersonal* problems (see Fig. 20.8).

Intrapersonal problems

(1) Depression
(2) Generalised, moderate anxiety
(3) Low self-esteem, and lack of self-confidence
(4) Low frustration threshold
(5) Excessive use of alcohol
(6) Guilt feelings and resentment towards father

Interpersonal problems

(1) Social isolation
(2) Difficulty in expressing emotions
(3) Anxiety in social situations

Extrapersonal problems

(1) Homelessness – unsatisfactory temporary hostel accommodation
(2) Unemployment
(3) Poverty

Fig. 20.8 *Stressors agreed upon by Harry and the CPN*

In marked contrast to the more serious kinds of mental disorder that CPNs have to deal with, Harry's mental state was not grossly abnormal. It was not necessary to refer him either to his GP for a prescription for psychotropic medication or to a psychiatrist for hospital admission. Although he complained of feeling depressed, his sleep and eating patterns were fairly normal and there was no retardation or other gross abnormality present in his cognition and behaviour. In other words, Harry was an unhappy man but he did not exhibit the symptomatology of severe clinical depression. He was coping with life but in a way that was harmful to him; he was stuck in a pattern of avoidance coping. Previously a successful person when things went his way, he lacked the resources to adapt effectively to change.

Viewed in terms of Neuman's model, Harry's lines of defence were penetrated by intrapersonal, interpersonal and extrapersonal stressors arising from the imbalance that existed between his personal system and the environment (Fig. 20.10).

Harry was a 28 ~~[redacted]~~ single man who was referred by his GP to the Community Psychiatric Nurse with a request for an assessment of his mental state. The GP suggested that Harry might benefit from CPN 'counselling and support'. The intervention that followed consisted of six one hour sessions held weekly in the health centre where the CPN was based.

The client was a short, stocky, rather overweight young man. He was clean, well-groomed and neatly dressed in casual clothes. He appeared uncomfortable and anxious initially but relaxed as the assessment interviews progressed. He was rational and articulate in his speech.

Harry complained that his life had taken a downward turn since he left the Army nine months before. Previously a contented, easy-going and confident man, he was now a worried and depressed man who had lost faith in himself. He had no job, no permanent accommodation, no family and no friends. This situation was causing him considerable anxiety: he worried constantly about his circumstances but felt powerless to change them. At times he experienced feelings of acute anxiety which were accompanied by distressing physical sensations such as a pounding heart, tremor and excessive sweating. He generally avoided social encounters because he felt he had nothing to offer other people and because he was ashamed of what he had become. While in contact with others he worried about the negative impression he felt he must be making on them, and afterwards he tended to re-enact the encounter in his mind and criticise himself for what he had or had not done.

Ruminations of this kind kept him awake at night, though he slept an average of eight hours. He was drinking more than he felt was good for him – up to eight pints of beer a day – whenever he had money. At times, while drunk, he felt an urge to smash property such as pub furniture and shop windows. He always managed to resist these urges but was afraid that one day he would 'snap' and cause a lot of damage. He did not understand why he got these feelings. At times he felt acutely depressed when he considered the mess he had made of his life and what the future held for him. On a couple of occasions he had briefly contemplated committing suicide by jumping in front of a bus or a tube train.

Harry had come to London one month previously from his native Newcastle. At the time of assessment he was staying in a hostel for homeless men which he said made him feel like 'a dosser'. He knew nobody in London and only undertook the journey because he felt he had to get out of Newcastle. He was pessimistic about his chances of obtaining employment or permanent housing. He had no money because of a delay in processing his claim for unemployment benefit.

Harry's mother died while he was very young and he was brought up by his father who worked in a shipyard until his retirement when Harry was 21. Frequently in the evenings Harry had to look after himself while his father was out drinking with his workmates. The two had a reasonably good relationship but were never emotionally close. Harry described his father as a man of few words who never discussed his feelings.

As an only child Harry felt lonely at times but was a sociable boy and he had many friends. He described a fairly normal childhood with the usual milestones. He was an average student leaving school without gaining any qualifications. After a variety of short-term jobs Harry joined the Army, and described this as the happiest period of his life, enjoying the feeling of belonging and the social life.

When Harry was 26 his father died after a short illness. Being stationed in Germany at the time, Harry was unable to visit his father before he died and has blamed himself for 'abandoning' him ever since. He returned to England and threw himself into his work in the Army. However, he had to take a series of fitness tests in order to qualify for progression in his chosen career. Knowing that he was overweight and drank too much, he undertook to train and give up drinking. Nevertheless he failed the tests and was told that his services were no longer required.

At the age of 27 Harry found himself a civilian once more, with no employment, very little money, no friends and nowhere to go. Returning to Newcastle, he got a flat and a job as a security officer. The work was boring and he did not like his employer. After a few months, for reasons that are unclear, he was asked to leave. Attempts to find other jobs proved fruitless so he decided to move to London.

Harry's intelligence, his degree of insight and his motivation were such that the process of assessing his problems was relatively straightforward. Although he was sometimes unaware of what exactly his problems were, he readily accepted the interpretations and formulations presented to him and there were no major discrepancies between his perception of his situation and the CPN's perception.

Neuman's model was chosen as appropriate to Harry's needs.

Fig. 20.9 *Profile: Harry*

The effect of his inability to defend himself against internal and external stressors was a degree of impairment in physical, psychological and social functioning. He experienced physical symptoms of anxiety and constant tension, he felt miserable, worried and frustrated, and he was lonely, unemployed and homeless. Immediate remedial intervention was required to repair his normal lines of defence to enable them to repel stressors. In terms of the model this process is known as *reconstitution* (Neuman, 1980).

An important aim of CPN intervention was to prevent Harry's stress reaction becoming any worse. Nursing action directed towards this end, as well as towards alleviation of immediate distress, is referred to by Neuman as *secondary prevention*. Allied to the aim of reducing the severity and duration of the stress reaction was the aim of *tertiary prevention*. This seeks to reduce the residual effects of the stress reaction and to maintain stability after reconstitution has occurred. Readaptation is promoted through education in methods of increasing the system's resistance to stressors.

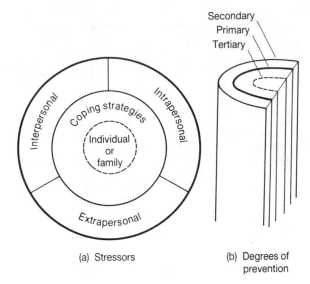

Secondary
Primary
Tertiary

Interpersonal

Intrapersonal

Coping strategies

Individual
or
family

Extrapersonal

(a) Stressors

(b) Degrees of
prevention

Fig. 20.10 *Representation of Neuman's model (with thanks to E.A. Palmer)*

Tertiary prevention in Harry's case was conceptualised separately but carried out in conjunction with the secondary prevention. Harry's problems were inter-related but what he presented was a complex of separate reactions to intrapersonal, interpersonal and extrapersonal stressors. It was therefore necessary to use a number of different therapeutic approaches. The CPN's interventions were largely based on two therapeutic approaches: client-centred therapy and *cognitive therapy*.

The primary aims of therapy were concerned with helping Harry to explore his problems at a time of crisis so that he could decide what to do about them, and providing him with the knowledge and skills necessary for adaptation. The longer term aims were concerned with helping him to anticipate and recognise the cues of future problems, and augmenting his repertoire of coping and problem-solving skills to enable him to prevent problems developing into crises.

Individual client-centred counselling formed the core of the CPN intervention. This approach was originated by Rogers (1951) and recognises the worth and significance of the client, aiming to promote personal autonomy and self-direction. By showing respect, empathy and genuineness, the counsellor establishes a therapeutic relationship in which his role is to listen, ask open questions, balance support and confrontation, encourage specificity and *concreteness*, and help the client

develop strategies for solving problems. Through this process the client is helped to clarify issues and uncertainties, to explore options and alternatives, to develop clear objectives and plans, and, with support, do what needs to be done (Hopson, 1981a).

Along with this form of nursing intervention, Harry was offered a form of cognitive therapy. The CPN explained to Harry that the problems we create for ourselves and the support we give ourselves derive mainly from the same source – our internal dialogue. Harry was taught how to prevent 'thought-chaining', the process by which a negative perception leads, via a chain of other thoughts, to feelings of self-blame and worthlessness. Positive coping statements were formulated to suit every occasion, and Harry was encouraged to use them to 'talk himself out of' feeling bad. He applied the technique conscientiously and, after a month, objective assessment along with Harry's subjective feeling indicated absence of depression.

In addition to alleviating feelings of helplessness and depression, cognitive therapy played an important role in the treatment of Harry's anxiety. Depression and anxiety are often experienced as two sides of the same coin, with both emotional reactions being caused by some fundamental stressor (Wolpe, 1973). In Harry's case the primary stressor was intrapersonal: his loss of self-esteem. He did not have a very strong self-concept to begin with but his career in the Army did much to boost his self-confidence. When he was discharged he lost his home, friends, occupation, income, social role and self-esteem. This multiple loss created a kind of bereavement reaction that manifested as anxiety as well as depression. He worried about everything: how he was going to get through the day, what people thought of him, whether his belongings would be safe in the hostel, what was going to become of him, etc. The only time he did not worry about something was when he was feeling depressed – when he lacked the energy to be anxious.

Much of Harry's anxiety had a realistic basis in the circumstances but it was exaggerated to a pathological degree. During the treatment, he was given an explanation of his anxiety, and told that his anxiety-provoking thoughts and images (stressors) lead to heightened arousal and physical symptoms such as palpitations, tremor and shortness of breath. He was then taught *cognitive restructuring*. In its application to depressive thoughts, this consisted of teaching Harry to become aware of, and to monitor, his anxiety-arousing statements about himself, and to substitute positive, coping statements.

Relaxation training was also carried out during this phase, with special emphasis on the control of breathing. Harry was taught how to apply these coping skills in different anxiety-provoking or stressful situations, first in the clinical setting and then in real life. He was asked to rate his anxiety level and keep a weekly record which showed a marked decrease from the third week until the end of treatment. As he mastered the relaxation technique he reported feeling less tense and better able to get to sleep at night.

A feature of the depressive phase is the occasional high energy periods that people experience before sliding back into feelings of hopelessness (Hopson, 1981b). This high energy often takes the form of anger or frustration caused by the difficulty of knowing how best to cope with new roles, relationships, ways of being, or other changes that may be necessary. Harry's energy periods were characterised by anger that was directed both against himself and towards others. Disinhibited by alcohol, he sometimes felt an urge to smash up the pub he was drinking in, the room he lived in or the shops whose luxury goods he could not afford to buy. On a couple of occasions he thought about taking his own life in a highly spectacular way. The counselling situation provided Harry with an opportunity to vent his feelings of anger, resentment and frustration safely.

The changes in Harry's outlook and behaviour as his therapeutic relationship with the CPN progressed are considered in Fig. 20.11. Harry's self-esteem returned and he developed realistic coping strategies. The final stage of the process was the termination of the therapeutic relationship. This did not present a problem for Harry as he understood clearly that no rejection on either side was implied but that roles which were no longer necessary were being relinquished.

The value of nursing theory

The two profiles of Jack and Harry indicate the uniqueness of the nurse's role in caring for mentally ill people and in promoting mental health.

As Harry's depression lifted and his anxiety abated, he came to accept the reality of his situation for what it was. He became more active and started testing himself and trying new behaviours. A list of areas of his life that were felt to be problematic or in need of change was jointly formulated and an action plan drawn up.

Harry's new found energy and determination to lift himself up from 'rock-bottom' ensured his success in putting the plan into effect. He reduced his intake of alcohol and started going to the pub to meet people rather than to drink. He got a casual job in a hotel kitchen, not so much for the meagre wages as for the increased self-respect it gave him.

Following advice about the relationship between physical fitness and the ability to cope with stress he took up swimming at the local baths every day. Assessment of Harry's eating habits revealed that he had little idea of what constituted a healthy diet. He had never cooked for himself, being used to Army food, and he lived on takeaway foods. A booklet containing an introduction to good nutrition was obtained for him and it was agreed that, at a later date, when he was more settled, he should be referred to a dietician for advice on losing weight, and to a Community Occupational Therapist for instruction in home cooking.

Referral to a hostel resettlement officer was extremely productive: within a month Harry was offered a long-term bedsitter accommodation.

Fig. 20.11 Profile: Harry (2)

One might wonder why, if there are already models in use that determine the medical and nursing approach to mentally ill people, there is a need for nursing models as well.

McFarlane (1986) argues that models designed by other disciplines do not 'reflect the reality or totality of nursing'. Working to a nursing model does not imply that nurses work in isolation from other disciplines, rather that the specific contribution of the nurse is identified and the nature of the relationship with the patient is guided and directed by this. Hall (1963) argued that as the need for medical care decreases, the need for professional nursing care increases and nowhere is this more evident than in psychiatry. Part of the nursing process is using the relationship to help the patient explore his feelings regarding his illness, his future, his relationships and himself, and to harness his motivation and capacity for maturity and self-healing, a process that may continue long after the disease has been treated and the body's wholeness restored. Hall referred to this aspect of nursing as the *core* function while bodily care or nurturing she referred to as the *care* function, and assisting the patient and family through the medical care as the *cure* function.

Primary nursing

One of the essential elements of many nursing models is that of primary nursing (Manthey, 1980). In other words the patient is able to develop a one-to-one relationship with a nurse and to trust that changes in his care will be discussed between him and that nurse, rather than imposed upon him by the other nurses in the team. Any system in which many nurses take responsibility for one patient's care renders the use of many nursing models impractical.

There is, as yet, little research evidence supporting the use of one conceptual model over another, and some nurses are sceptical of the value of 'generic' nursing models (Barker, 1990). Nevertheless, there are advantages in nurses understanding the essence of a nursing model as opposed to a medical model; agreeing a philosophy of nursing care for their clients; articulating the nature of nursing and not underestimating the therapeutic function of the nurse. After all, there is much more to care of patients than the psychiatric treatment, as Hall's model so succinctly illustrates.

Care of a disturbed patient

Provision for disturbed patients varies according to their need for security and observation. Special hospitals like Broadmoor in Berkshire and Ashworth in Liverpool exist for the care of homicidal or extremely aggressive patients, many of whom will be admitted under Section 41 of the Mental Health Act 1983 (see page 591). In the 1970s each regional health authority was required to provide a secure unit which could admit for shorter periods patients who required less security but specially skilled staff and greater facilities for maintaining safety than an ordinary ward could provide.

Some mental hospitals have retained one locked ward for admission of acutely disturbed patients who need less security, but require close observation and therefore a reasonably high ratio of nurses to patients. In other hospitals and units, these patients are admitted to open wards or wards which may be locked in an emergency, and security measures such as one-to-one **specialling** may be adopted. In places where there is insufficient staff to provide the security, seclusion rooms may still be used. Such a room would have nothing in it except a mattress, nothing to stimulate the patient or with which he could hurt himself. Only a small observation window would allow staff to monitor the patient's activities from outside. Seclusion rooms have been misused in the past, for instance to punish a patient.

The Mental Health Act 1983 stipulates maximum times and conditions for the use of seclusion, while a policy regarding seclusion should be available in every hospital, with clear indications and instructions for its use.

The placement of an acutely ill patient in the appropriate ward or unit needs careful consideration, and can take time to organise. Nursing staff need to be involved in decision-making as there are implications for nurse managers concerning manpower and the environment to which the patient is accepted. With quick but careful planning the patient can be admitted by a calm, friendly team of nurses, psychologically prepared to manage whatever behaviour the patient exhibits. Other patients will be affected by a new arrival, especially if they witness a violent incident being badly managed. Insufficient preparation and a lack of consultation between medical and nursing staff can lead to the ward atmosphere becoming disturbed, staff feeling their needs are not accounted for and resentment building up. Staff morale can then deteriorate over time, recruitment to the ward become problematic and turnover of staff rapid – far from ideal conditions in which to nurse mentally ill people.

If the patient is being transferred from another hospital or ward, prior assessment may be possible by the admitting ward staff. This can be useful in a number of ways.

(1) The patient and at least one member of the nursing team will have met beforehand, which can facilitate introductions once the patient is admitted.

(2) An assessment of the patient's priority needs can be made and the initial care plan formulated.

(3) Other members of the team can familiarise themselves with this care plan prior to the patient's arrival on the ward, thereby ensuring a consistent approach by all staff from the outset.

(4) Details, such as the need for a special diet or

medication that is not normally stocked on the ward, can be elicited and ordered in advance. Attention to detail can be important in reducing tension and frustration in the patient, whose tolerance may be reduced by the nature of his illness.

Often, prior assessment is not possible and misleading or scanty information may precede the patient's arrival on the ward. It is therefore essential for one nurse to be allocated to admit the patient, to orientate him to the ward, and introduce him to the staff and patients. Details of his circumstances may be taken from the patient, and relatives if they accompany him. However, if the patient is disturbed it is quite unrealistic to interview him at length as soon as he arrives.

Documentation and planning are not possible prior to the initial intervention since the nurse must relate to the patient immediately, but this first assessment can bring about 'planned action' as opposed to 'spontaneous reaction', the nurse using her knowledge of verbal and non-verbal communication to consider how best to respond to the patient.

Skilled nursing can in itself prevent a patient from **acting out** his feelings in a violent way. However, severe mental disorders will produce in the patient disturbing thoughts and ideas (**delusions**), strange perceptions (**hallucinations**), **compulsive** self-injurious urges or sudden, dramatic changes in mood. **Psychotropic drugs** are often the most effective form of treatment to provide relief from these symptoms. On occasion, it may be necessary to medicate a patient against his will, for his own or others' safety, if persuasion and explanation are unsuccessful. While this may seem to be abuse of a person's freedom of choice, it is important to weigh this against his right to treatment. In a severely disturbed state, a patient will trust nobody and, in a desperate attempt to 'save' himself, will put his and others' lives in jeopardy. This state of mind cannot be likened to freedom.

Restraining a patient requires knowledge and skill on the part of the nursing team. Timing is crucial: too rapid and the patient can feel disadvantaged and bitter, too slow and he will believe it is all a game. Staff judgement is important, and if possible the nurses allocated to carry out this procedure should have a good relationship with the patient.

Not all unacceptable behaviour will be due to the patient's illness. At times it will be to test the limits to which the patient can go before others take control. In these instances, the patient can be helped by staff being consistent in their approach, which itself will depend on the extent to which the patient is seen as being able to take responsibility for his own behaviour. Turning down a frustrated patient's demands too many times without suggesting alternatives or giving explanations is likely to result in him destroying property of some kind, yet this cannot be seen as entirely his responsibility. On the other hand, a patient may break a window having been thwarted in his wish whilst remaining in control of his behaviour. In both cases violence to property has been demonstrated. In the first case, however, little might be made of the destroyed property and attempts stepped up to distract the patient and relieve his frustration, while in the second case the patient may be asked to pay for the broken window, and have it explained to him that such behaviour will not result in him getting his own way.

Ethical dilemmas

By definition, an ethical dilemma is one in which decisions to be made involve moral choices, and thus one can say that there is never one right or wrong decision, but a choice of options about which people will disagree (see Chapter 13). Oft-published examples include euthanasia, abortion and maintenance of confidentiality regardless of the nature of the confidence. Schröck (1980) points out that less emotive issues face nurses daily and include care of patients' property, availing patients of the truth and preserving patients' dignity.

Bearing in mind that psychiatric patients often lack insight into their illness, a few examples of ethical dilemmas are presented for the reader to consider, in the profiles given in Figs. 20.12, 20.13, and 20.14.

Each of the situations in these client profiles involves making decisions about people's freedom to choose. Should we use the Mental Health Act to prevent a vulnerable girl from being sexually abused when otherwise she is deemed not to require formal detention? Should we leave an isolated patient alone as he wishes when we think

Jill is a 27 year old girl who has been in hospital continuously for four years. She has been diagnosed as suffering from chronic schizophrenia and has received treatment in the form of drugs which have minimised but not eradicated her symptoms.

Jill used to be very attractive with a slender figure and long auburn hair. She dressed well and had a lively disposition. She was an intelligent girl and had been studying for an English degree at university when her illness struck. Now she is overweight, takes poor care of her appearance, and is unable to sustain conversation. She is often aggressive, is sometimes incontinent and has little motivation to engage in any constructive activity. She has no insight into her illness and has had to be kept in hospital on Section 3 of the Mental Health Act 1983. For the past year she has been in a locked ward, since at any opportunity she absconds from the hospital and travels, probably by hitch-hiking, to far away towns, having to be brought back by the police or fetched by a nurse at considerable expense.

Sometimes when she is away she is beaten up, and, it is suspected, sexually abused. However, Jill, although occasionally tearful on return to the ward, is never regretful of her escapade and denies being ill-treated. Jill flirts with male patients and has always got a boyfriend in tow, though more for what they can get from her than for an affectionate relationship. She has refused to have a contraceptive device inserted, and is an unreliable drug-taker, so the contraceptive pill is not an efficient way of protecting her from an unwanted pregnancy if she does have intercourse when away from the hospital.

Dilemma: Should Jill be kept in hospital on a section of the Mental Health Act, or allowed to be free to come and go? If the latter, should she be given contraception, and if so by what method, and again, against her will?

Fig. 20.12 *Profile: Jill*

Cecil is 34, married with children. He was admitted to hospital three weeks ago having been referred by his wife, who became concerned about her husband's behaviour. He is withdrawn, isolates himself in his bedroom and does not leave it even to wash himself. He refuses all hospital food, although he does eat what his wife brings him.

The psychiatrist suspects he has schizophrenia and wishes to medicate him, but Cecil staunchly refuses, saying he is perfectly well and does not need any medication. Other than this he offers no information about himself or his behaviour. He denies being unhappy or inconvenienced by his situation, but his family are clearly distressed by his behaviour.

Dilemma: Should Cecil be detained under a section of the Mental Health Act though he presents no immediate danger to himself or others? If not, how long can one leave a patient in this state of unwellness before at least forcing him to have a bath?

Fig. 20.13 *Profile: Cecil*

Marian is a 19 year old girl who has *psychotic depression* following the break-up of a relationship with her boyfriend. For two months she has not eaten properly, with the result that her hair is falling out and she has amenorrhoea. She has *nihilistic* delusions including the belief that she is made of rubber, that she is hollow and that if she eats, the food gradually fills her legs and then her body. Being constipated reinforces this delusion.

In many ways Marian is rational; for instance, she refuses to receive *ECT* because she has read that it may affect her memory. Although this is extremely unlikely if the treatment is administered in moderation, the possibility of temporary memory loss is indisputable.

Marian refuses to be persuaded to receive the treatment and demands instead to have a barium meal 'to prove to the staff that she is hollow'. She claims that if the test shows no abnormality, she will agree to have ECT.

Dilemma: Should Marian be detained under a section of the Mental Health Act and given ECT forcibly if two doctors agree but nursing staff are unhappy about it? Furthermore, should Marian receive a barium meal, although the very act of granting the request may add credence to her belief, and it would be an expensive test to perform on a psychotic patient, who, by the nature of her illness, is unlikely to be convinced by the X-ray showing nothing abnormal?

Fig. 20.14 *Profile: Marian*

this behaviour is a symptom of his illness? Should we force a patient to have a controversial treatment even if the chances are it will greatly reduce the duration of her depression?

You may feel strongly one way or another, or you may hope you never have to make such a difficult decision. In the end it comes down to personal values, but it is essential that the multidisciplinary team takes time to consider the issues and to be as informed as possible about the effects of its decisions. By their very nature, ethical decisions are difficult to make, but it is important that such decisions are made and that all members of the team stand by that decision, once taken, regardless of their individual opinions.

Conclusion

Students often find it difficult to adjust to the pace of the work during the first few days of a placement on a psychiatric ward. Many student nurses remark on the discomfort they feel since there does not appear to be anything to do.

Nevertheless, nurses will feel tired at the end

of a shift, having absorbed some of the tension generated by the patients' disturbed emotional state. They will have been wary of anybody unpredictably acting out some of this emotion in disturbed behaviour, or of disputes occurring between patients, whose tolerance of others is lowered by their illness.

Students visiting patients in their homes may be disturbed by the conditions some people live in. They may feel moved by the plight people find themselves in, and powerless to help them feel better.

Some may find it stressful when patients resist their care or sabotage their own treatment. They may experience difficulty in tolerating abuse or rejection they receive from patients who mistrust the care shown to them. Patients may not show much improvement within the timespan of the placement.

Despite the stresses, nursing people with mental health problems is stimulating and rewarding. Using oneself consciously and with purpose is a constant challenge, and can have positive repercussions within one's own personal relationships. I hope my enthusiasm for it has been communicated in this chapter.

Suggestions for further reading given on page 611 should enable topics addressed here to be explored in greater depth.

Acknowledgements

The author would like to thank the staff on Avondale Ward, St Charles' Mental Health Unit, London W10, and Dennis Parrish, CPN with Bloomsbury Health Authority, both at the time of writing, for allowing Jack's and Harry's care plans and progress notes to be used in compiling the profiles.

Glossary

Acting out: The expression of painful feelings through behaviour – for example, wrist-cutting when feeling self-loathing, breaking windows when feeling angry

Active listening: Observing and interpreting a person's non-verbal behaviour as well as listening to and interpreting the person's verbal messages

Alzheimer's disease: A form of senile dementia, accounting for 60% of cases, characterised by severe intellectual and behavioural deterioration until death, usually 4–5 years

Behaviour therapy: The application of the principles of learning theories to the treatment of mental disorder

Behavioural sciences: Psychology and sociology, pure and applied

Clarifying: Stating the issues that have been talked about in an interaction with another person, so that they may be confirmed by the person and/or elaborated upon

Cognitive restructuring: A technique of *cognitive therapy* whereby the client is taught to manipulate his own thoughts in order to bring about a change in mood

Cognitive therapy: Treatment involving the client's thoughts, perceptions, knowledge

Compulsive: A description of behaviour governed by an irresistible inner force compelling the performance of an act without, or even against, the will of the individual performing it

Concreteness: Type of intelligence manifested in dealing with things and practical affairs as opposed to abstract notions

Counsellor: One qualified in counselling who sees clients on a contractual basis for one-to-one or group counselling

Debrief: Reflect on role play to absorb and analyse the impact of new learning on the players and to draw out new perceptions

Defensive: The use of involuntary or unconscious measures by an individual to protect himself from painful feelings or to avoid exposing something there is a strong desire to conceal

Delusion: A false belief that cannot be altered by contrary evidence or reasoning – for example, Marian's belief that she was hollow and made of rubber (page 605). More common delusions are that a person is Jesus or is being followed by the KGB

Derole: Formally leave a role one has played in order to avoid taking the feelings evoked by the role play out of the context of the session

Desensitisation: A technique used in *behaviour therapy* in which the client experiences anxiety by imagining progressive situations that are increasingly anxiety-provoking. The level of anxiety is rated and counteracted by *relaxation techniques*

Dynamic: Term used in the study of human relations to depict the changing nature of relationships

Electroconvulsive therapy (ECT): A treatment for depression involving the passage of an electric current through the brain while the patient is under general anaesthesia and has been administered a muscle relaxant. The number of sessions is usually six or eight over three to four weeks

Empathy: The skill of understanding another person by (a) getting inside that person's world, getting a feeling for that world and looking at the outer world from the other's perspective; and (b) communicating this understanding to the other person (Egan, 1990)

Experiential learning: Learning through techniques that 'rely for their effect on the student's actual experience of emotions, feelings, communications, situations and other intangibles' (Van Ments, 1983)

Exposure: The term used in *behaviour therapy* for the client being faced with an anxiety-provoking stimulus

Family therapy: The treatment of a client by involving the whole family in a series of group therapy sessions. The therapist aims to help the family members to understand the *dynamics* within their group and how these contribute to the sick member's behaviour

Flooding: A behavioural technique based on the premise that physiological responses to anxiety cannot be maintained for prolonged periods. The client is therefore exposed to the main focus of his anxiety straightaway with the expectation that he will overcome his fears in a much shorter time than with *densensitisation*

Focusing: Drawing a person's attention to a particular idea or non-verbal communication they have initiated in the course of an interaction

Generalised hopelessness: A symptom of depression in which the client experiences lack of hope about every aspect of his life

Grief reaction: 'A broad range of feelings and behaviours that are common after a loss' (Worden, 1983)

Group dynamics: The study of interactions and inter-relationships that take place within groups

Hallucination: A sensory perception without an external stimulus. Any of the senses may be involved, hence hallucinations are usually classified as *auditory* (hearing voices, etc.), *visual* (seeing people, etc. who are not there), *tactile* (for example, feeling insects on the skin), *olfactory* (for example, smelling gas), or *gustatory* (i.e. tasting something that is not in the mouth, although one can never be sure this is not due to a metabolic cause)

Industrial therapy unit: Workshop within a hospital where patients can undertake real work contracted out by firms (packaging, for example) and earn money according to their production

Innate: Present in the individual at birth; generally implies inheritance

Institutional neurosis: The term coined by Russell Barton (1976) for a condition seen in many patients in large mental institutions at that time. The condition was characterised by stooped posture, shuffling gait and submissiveness, and was thought to be induced by excessive use of *psychotropic drugs*, lack of personal belongings, brow-beating and abuse from the staff, and lack of contact with the world outside hospital

Institutionalisation: Adaptation to institutional life to the extent that there are adverse signs such as are present in the condition *institutional neurosis*.

Locus of control: The centre of responsibility for the control of behaviour. Internal locus of control refers to the conviction that one can use one's behaviour to achieve goals. External locus of control refers to the belief that real power resides outside the individual and that forces other than oneself determine one's life

Long-stay wards: Wards in large mental hospitals caring for chronically ill people. They became notorious for the effects of *institutionalisation* brought about in patients and staff. It was not uncommon for patients to be in these wards for 40 years

Microskills teaching: The teaching of skills by breaking complex skills down into their component parts, each of which is practised separately before being practised together

Nihilistic: Type of *delusion* found in *psychotically depressed* patients where they deny existence of all or part of their body

Open question: A question which encourages an informative answer that is also spontaneous rather than prompted, e.g. 'How do you find the course?' rather than a closed question 'Do you find the course interesting?' which demands a 'Yes' or 'No' answer

Organic: Of structural or chemical origin as opposed to stress-related

Paranoid: Characterised by *delusions* and *hallucinations* often of a persecutory nature

Paraphrasing: Rephrasing a person's words in one's own words as a response to their telling their story, as a way of ascertaining and indicating the extent to which one has understood what the person said

Parasuicide: Acts of self-injury and attempts at suicide

Psychiatrist: One who professes and practises *psychiatry*

Psychiatry: The study of mental and nervous disorders, and generally encompassing abnormal psychology

Psychoanalysis: Investigation and treatment of mental disorder by the process of free association and dream interpretation, developed by Sigmund Freud

Psychomotor retardation: A slowing up of all bodily systems including the brain, seen in patients suffering from depression. The patient will move very slowly, his heart rate and respirations will decrease, he may become constipated and his speech and thoughts will slow down

Psychopathology: Mental pathology or pathology of the mind; a study of mental functions and processes, under conditions brought about by disorder or disease, physical or mental

Psychosocial: Term employed with reference to social relations dependent on mental factors and functions

Psychosomatic disorder: A physical disorder precipitated by emotional disturbance

Psychotherapy: The treatment of disorders by psychological methods

Psychotic: Pertaining to psychosis, a mental state in which there is distortion of reality. Personality is usually affected and *paranoid* symptoms present. The patient will lack insight into his state of unwellness

Psychotic depression: Depression accompanied by *delusions* and occasionally *hallucinations*

Psychotropic drugs: Drugs whose action on the central nervous system brings about a change in mental state – for example, major tranquillisers used for control of *psychotic* symptoms, minor tranquillisers for anxiety, and anti-depressants

Reflecting: Responding to a person by referring to the feelings being communicated, rather than the verbal message

Reinforcement: A procedure which strengthens the frequency, speed or magnitude of a response – for example, praising a client for desirable behaviour or rewarding a dog with a biscuit for coming when he is called

Relaxation training: The client is taught methods of inducing a relaxed state in himself. Examples include regulation of one's breathing; listening to a tape instructing one to tense and relax groups of muscles in turn or to let one's thoughts be guided into a fantasy; meditation and massage

Repression: One of the Ego Defence Mechanisms, a concept developed by Sigmund Freud. Ideas are actively or automatically thrust into the unconscious in order to protect the individual from painful thoughts and feelings

Role play: Practising of behaviours associated with an imaginary person, a real person or oneself, not to influence or entertain an audience, but to experience the feelings that are generated, increase one's understanding, and allow ideas to emerge

Rumination: Obsessional thought

Schizophrenia: A group of *psychotic* disorders characterised by *delusions* and *hallucinations*, emotional disturbances, deterioration of personality and intellect, and disorders of volition or drive

Sensitivity group: A group of people meeting to develop self-understanding and awareness of personal attitudes through a combination of cognitive and experiential learning

Socialisation: The process by which the individual is adapted to his social environment and becomes a recognised, cooperating and efficient member of it

Sociotherapeutic: Concerned with the client's functioning within a social setting

Specialling: A form of nursing intervention for patients who are seriously dangerous to themselves or to others. It involves one nurse being allocated for a named period of time to accompany the patient wherever he goes, including to the toilet

Summarising: Drawing together the main points that are talked about during an interaction

Supervision: Support and, where appropriate, guidance and teaching of an individual working with distressed and distressing people

Unconscious: Not having the characteristic of consciousness. Aggregate of the **dynamic** elements of the personality of which the individual is only partially, if at all, aware

Some definitions adapted from Glossary Terms and Tests used in Psychiatric Practice, *Lancaster Moor Hospital* (1973) *and* A Dictionary of Psychology, *Penguin Books* (1964).

References

Altschul, A. (1972). *Patient Nurse Interaction*. Churchill Livingstone, Edinburgh.

Argyle, M. (1981). *Social Skills and Health*. Methuen, London.

Argyle, M. (1988). *Bodily Communication* (2nd ed.). Routledge, London.

Arnetz, B.B., Wasserman, J., Petrini, B. *et al.* (1987). Immune function in unemployed women. *Psychosomatic Medicine*, 49, 3–12.

Atkinson, R.L., Atkinson, R.C., Smith, E.E., Bem D.J. and Hilgard, E.R. (1990). *Introduction to Psychology* (10th ed.). Harcourt Brace Jovanovich, San Diego.

Barker, P. (1988). *Nursing the Patient with Major Affective Disorder*. Unpublished PhD thesis, Dundee College of Technology, Dundee.

Barker, P. (1990). The conceptual basis of mental health nursing. *Nurse Education Today*, 10, 339–348.

Barton, R. (1976). *Institutional Neurosis* (3rd ed.). Wright, Bristol.

Bolton, P. (1984). Management of compulsorily admitted patients to a high security unit. *International Journal of Social Psychiatry*, 30, 77–84.

Bond, M. (1986). *Stress and Self-awareness: A Guide for Nurses*. Heinemann, London.

Bowlby, J. (1980). *Attachment and Loss: Loss, Sadness and Depression (Vol 3)*. Basic Books, New York.

Brenner, H.M. (1979). Mortality and the national economy. *Lancet*, 2, 568–573.

Brooker, C. (1990). A new role for the Community Psychiatric Nurse in working with families caring for a relative with schizophrenia. *International Journal of Social Psychiatry*, 36(3), 216–224.

Brown, G.W. and Harris, T. (1978). *Social Origins of Depression: A Study of Psychiatric Disorder in Women*. Tavistock Publications, London.

Burnard, P. (1990). Stating the case. *Counselling*, 1(4), 114–116.

Burnard, P. and Morrison, P. (1991). Nurses' interpersonal skills: a study of nurses' perceptions. *Nurse Education Today*, 11, 24–29.

Busfield, J. (1986). *Managing Madness: Changing Ideas and Practice*. Hutchinson, London.

Carpenter, L. and Brockington, I.F. (1980). A study of mental illness in Asians, West Indians and Africans living in Manchester. *British Journal of Psychiatry*, 137, 201–205.

Carter, B. and McGoldrick, M. (1989). *The Changing Family Life Cycle* (2nd ed.). Allyn and Bacon, Boston.

Clare, A. (1980). *Psychiatry in Dissent* (2nd ed.). Tavistock Publications, London.

Cohen, S. and Williamson, G.M. (1991). Stress and infectious disease in humans. *Psychological Bulletin*, 109(1), 5–24.

Cormack, D. (1976). *Psychiatric Nursing Observed*. RCN, London.

Cormack, D. (1983). *Psychiatric Nursing Described*. Churchill Livingstone, Edinburgh.

Corey, G. (1990). *Theory and Practice of Group Counselling* (3rd ed.). Brooks-Cole Publishing Co., California.

Dean, G., Walsh, D., Downing, H. and Shelley, E. (1981). First admissions of native-born and immigrants to psychiatric hospitals in South-East England, 1970. *British Journal of Psychiatry*, 139, 506–512.

Department of Health and Social Security. (1966). *Report of the Committee on Senior Nursing Staff Structure*. HMSO, London.

DHSS. (1975). *Better Services for the Mentally Ill*. HMSO, London.

DHSS. (1980). *Report of the Working Group on Organisational and Management Problems of Mental Illness Hospitals*. HMSO, London.

DHSS. (1981). *Care in Action*. HMSO, London.

Dickson, A. (1982). *A Woman in Your Own Right: Assertiveness and You*. Quartet, London.

Dickson, D.A., Hargie O. and Morrow, N.C. (1989). *Communication Skills Training for Health Professionals: An Instructor's Handbook*. Chapman and Hall, London.

Egan, G. (1990). *The Skilled Helper* (4th ed.). Brooks-Cole Publishing Co., California.

English and Welsh National Boards for Nursing, Midwifery and Health Visiting. (1982). *Syllabus of Training Professional Register – Part 3 Registered Mental Nurse*. ENB, London.

Fagin, L. (1981). *Unemployment and Health in Families – Case Studies Based on Family Interviews*. DHSS, London.

Fagin, L. and Little, M. (1984). *Forsaken Families: The Effects of Unemployment on Family Life*. Penguin Books, Harmondsworth.

Field, W. (1985). Hearing voices. *Journal of Psychosocial Nursing*, 23, 9–14.

Freud, S. (1962). *The Ego and the Id*. Pelican Freud Library, London.

Goffman, E. (1967). *Interaction Ritual*. Penguin Books, Harmondsworth.

Hall, L. (1963). A center for nursing. *Nursing Outlook*, 2, 1.

Hargie, O. (ed.). (1986). *A Handbook of Communication Skills*. Croom Helm, Kent.

Heron, J. (1990). *Helping the Client. A Creative Practical Guide*. Sage Publications, London.

Her Majesty's Stationery Office. (1959). *Mental Health Act 1959*. HMSO, London.

HMSO. (1983). *Mental Health Act 1983*. HMSO, London.

HMSO. (1991). *The Health of the Nation: A Consultative Document for Health in England*. HMSO, London.

Hollingshead, A. and Redlich, R.C. (1958). *Social Class and Mental Illness*. John Wiley and Sons, New York.

Holmes, G. (1990). *Alcohol among Young People: Obtaining the Full Measure*. Boys' and Girls' Welfare Society, Cheadle.

Holmes, T. and Rahe, R. (1967). The social readjustment rating scale. *Journal of Psychosomatic Research*, 11, 213–218.

Hopson, B. (1981a). Counselling and helping. In *Psychology and Medicine*, Griffiths, D. (ed.). British Psychological Society/Macmillan Press, London.

Hopson, B. (1981b). Transition: understanding and managing personal change. In *Psychology and Medicine*, as above.

Illich, I. (1977). *Limits to Medicine. Medical Nemesis: The Expropriation of Health*. Penguin Books, Harmondsworth.

Ineichen, B. and Harrison, G. (1984). Psychiatric hospital admissions in Bristol. 1: Geographical and ethnic factors. *British Journal of Psychiatry*, 145, 600–604.

Institute for the Study of Drug Dependence. (1991). *Drug Misuse in Britain*. ISDD, London.

Kelly, G.A. (1955). *The Psychology of Personal Constructs, Vols 1 & 2*. Norton, New York.

Kiecolt-Glaser, J.K., Fisher, L.D., Ogrocki, P. et al. (1987). Marital quality, marital disruption and immune function. *Psychosomatic Medicine*, 49, 13–34.

La Monica, E.L. (1979). *The Nursing Process: A Humanistic Approach*. Addison-Wesley, Reading, Mass.

Laurance, J. (1986). Unemployment health hazards. *New Society*, 75(1212), 492–493.

Lazarus, R.S. and Folkman, S. (1984). *Stress, Appraisal and Coping*. Springer, New York.

Leiba, P. (1990). *Learning from Incidents of Violence in Health Care. An Investigation of 'Case Reports' as a Basis for Staff Development and Organisational Change*. Unpublished MPhil thesis, Institute of Education, London.

Llewelyn, S.P. (1989). Caring: the costs to nurses and relatives. In *Health Psychology: Processes and Applications*, Broome, A.K. (ed.). Chapman and Hall, London.

Luft, J. (1970). *Group Processes: An Introduction to Group Dynamics*. Mayfield, Palo Alto.

Macilwaine, H. (1983). The communication patterns of female neurotic patients with nursing staff in psychiatric units of general hospitals. In *Nursing Research: Ten Studies in Patient Care*, Wilson-Barnett, J. (ed.). John Wiley and Sons, Chichester.

Macleod Clark, J. and Faulkner, A. (1987). Communication skills teaching in nurse education. In *Nursing Education: Research and Developments*, Davis, B. (ed.). Croom Helm, Kent.

Macleod Clark, J., Hopper, L. and Jesson, A. (1991). Progression to counselling. *Nursing Times*, 87(8), 41–43.

Main, T.F. (1968). The hospital as a therapeutic institution. In *Psychosocial Nursing*, Barnes, E. (ed.). Tavistock Publications, London.

Manthey, M. (1980). *The Practice of Primary Nursing*. Blackwell Scientific, Oxford.

McFarlane, J. (1986). Looking to the future. In *Models for Nursing*, Kershaw, B. and Salvage, J. (eds.). John Wiley and Sons, Chichester.

McGovern, D. and Cope, R. (1987). First psychiatric admission rates of first and second generation Afro-Caribbeans. *Social Psychiatry*, 122, 139–149.

Medical Research Council. (1991). *Annual Report April 1990–March 1991*. Medical Research Council, London.

Miles, A. (1987). *The Mentally Ill in Contemporary Society* (2nd ed.). Basil Blackwell, Oxford.

MIND. (1983). *The Mental Health Act 1983: An Outline Guide*. MIND, London.

Neuman, B. (1980). The Betty Neuman Health Care Systems Model: a total person approach to patient problems. In *Conceptual Models for Nursing Practice* (2nd ed.), Riehl, J. and Roy, C. (eds.). Appleton Century Crofts, New York.

Orem, D. (1985). *Nursing: Concepts of Practice* (3rd ed.). McGraw Hill, New York.

Peplau, H.E. (1988). *Interpersonal Relations in Nursing* (2nd ed.). Macmillan Education, Basingstoke.

Powell, D. (1982). *Learning to Relate? A Study of Student Psychiatric Nurses' Views of Their Preparation and Training*. RCN, London.

Reynolds, W. (1986). *A Study of Empathy in Student Nurses*. MPhil thesis, Dundee College of Technology, Dundee.

Reynolds, W. and Cormack, D. (1990). *Psychiatric and Mental Health Nursing Theory and Practice*. Chapman and Hall, London.

Ritter, S. (1989). *The Bethlem Royal and Maudsley Hospital Manual of Clinical Psychiatric Nursing Principles and Procedures*. Harper and Row, London.

Robertson, D. (1981). For richer, for poorer. *Nursing Mirror*, 153, 21.

Rogers, C.R. (1951). *Client-centered Therapy: Its Current Practice, Implications and Theory*. Constable, London.

Rogers, C.R. (1967). *On Becoming a Person: A Therapist's View of Psychotherapy*. Constable, London.

Roper, N., Logan, W.W. and Tierney, A.J. (1980). *The Elements of Nursing*, Churchill Livingstone, Edinburgh.

Rosenhan, D.L. (1979). On being sane in insane places. In *Readings in Sociology: Contemporary Perspectives*, Whitten, P. (ed.). Harper and Row, New York.

Roth, S. and Cohen, L.J. (1986). Approach, avoidance and coping with stress. *American Psychologist*, 41, 813–819.

Royal College of Physicians. (1987). *A Great and Growing Evil*. Tavistock Publications, London.

Scheff, T. (1966). *Being Mentally Ill*. Weidenfeld and Nicolson, London.

Schleifer, S.J., Keller, S.E., Camerino, M. et al. (1982). Suppression of lymphocyte stimulation following bereavement. *Journal of American Medical Association*, 250, 374.

Schröck, R. (1980). A question of honesty in nursing practice. *Journal of Advanced Nursing*, 5, 135–148.

Schwabb, J.J. and Schwabb, M.E. (1978). *Sociocultural Roots of Mental Illness: An Epidemiological Survey*. Plenum, New York.

Selig, N. (1988). Ethnicity and gender as uncomfortable issues. In *Psychiatry in Transition: The British and Italian Experiences*, Ramon, S. and Giannichedda, M.G. (eds.). Pluto Press, London.

Selye, H. (1974). *Stress without Distress*. J.B. Lippincott, Philadelphia.

Shepherd, D.M. and Barraclough, B.M. (1980). Work and suicide: an empirical investigation. *British Journal of Psychiatry*, 136, 469–478.

Smith, P.B. (1980). *Group Processes and Personal Change*. Harper and Row, London.

Towell, D. (1975). *Understanding Psychiatric Nursing: A Sociological Study of Modern Psychiatric Nursing Practice*. RCN, London.

Travelbee, J. (1971). *Interpersonal Aspects of Nursing*. F.A. Davis, Philadelphia.

Trower, P., Bryant, B. and Argyle, M. (1978). *Social Skills and Mental Health*. Methuen, London.

United Kingdom Central Council. (1991). *Report on Proposals for the Future of Community Education and Practice*. UKCC, London.

Van Ments, M. (1983). *The Effective Use of Role-Play: A Handbook for Teachers and Trainers*. Kogan Page, London.

Watkins, M. (1988). Lifting the burden. *Geriatric Nursing and Home Care*, 8(9), 18–20.

Watkins, M. (1992). Personal communication.

Wolpe, J. (1973). *The Practice of Behaviour Therapy*. Pergamon Press, Oxford.

Worden, J.W. (1983). *Grief Counselling and Grief Therapy*. Tavistock/Routledge, London.

World Health Organisation (1975). *International Classification of Diseases*. WHO, Geneva.

Suggestions for further reading

Altschul, A.T. (ed.). (1985). *Psychiatric Nursing*. Recent Advances in Nursing Series 12. Churchill Livingstone, Edinburgh.

Barker, P. (1985). *Patient Assessment in Psychiatric Nursing*. Croom Helm, Kent.

Barker, P.J. and Fraser, D. (eds.). (1985). *The Nurse as Therapist. A Behavioural Model*. Croom Helm, Kent.

Bender, K. (1990). *Psychiatric Medications*. Sage, London.

Bluglass, R. (1983). *A Guide to the Mental Health Act 1983*. Churchill Livingstone, Edinburgh.

Collister, B. (1988). *Psychiatric Nursing: Person to Person*. Edward Arnold, London.

Dexter, G. and Wash, M. (1986). *Psychiatric Nursing Skills*. Croom Helm, Kent.

Fernando, S. (1989). *Race and Culture in Psychiatry*. Routledge, London.

Goffman, E. (1968). *Asylums*. Penguin Books, Harmondsworth.

Gutemag, M. and Belle, D. (eds.). (1980). *The Mental Health of Women*. Academic Press, New York.

Laing, R.D. (1965). *The Divided Self*. Penguin Books, Harmondsworth.

Rogers, C.R. (1951). *Client-centred Therapy: Its Current Practice, Implications and Theory* (reprinted 1991). Constable, London.

Rogers, C.R. (1967). *On Becoming a Person: A Therapist's View of Psychotherapy*. Constable, London. stable, London.

Simmons, S. and Brooker, C. (1986). *Community Psychiatric Nursing: A Social Perspective*. Heinemann, London.

Stuart, G.W. and Sundeen, S.J. (1990). *Principles and Practice of Psychiatric Nursing* (4th ed.). Mosby, St Louis.

Szasz, T. (1962). *The Myth of Mental Illness*. Secker and Warburg, London.

Ward, M.F. (1985). *The Nursing Process in Psychiatry*. Churchill Livingstone, Edinburgh.

Wolff, H., Bateman, A. and Sturgeon, D. (eds.). (1990). *UCH Textbook of Psychiatry: An Integrated Approach*. Duckworth, London.

Wright, H. (1989). *Groupwork: Perspectives and Practice*. Scutari, Harrow.

Useful addresses: support groups and helpful organisations

Alcoholics Anonymous
General Service Office, Great Britain, P.O. Box 1, Stonebow House, York.

Anorexia & Bulimia Nervosa Association
Annexe C, Tottenham Town Hall, Town Hall Approach Road, London N15.

Boys' and Girls' Welfare Society
Schools Hill, Cheadle, Cheshire SK8 1JE.
This organisation offers help for young people with a wide range of problems.

MIND (National Association for Mental Health)
22 Harley Street, London W1 2ED
There are also local associations for mental health (check your local telephone book for addresses)

National Schizophrenia Fellowship
78–79 Victoria Road, Surbiton, Surrey
This organisation is a national support group for relatives of people suffering from schizophrenia

Patients' Association
18 Victoria Square, London E2.

Psychiatric Rehabilitation Association
1 Bayford Mews, Bayford Street, London E8
This association will give advice and guidance on the rehabilitation of mental patients

RELEASE
169 Commercial Street, London E1.
Just one organisation for patients addicted to drugs

21

CARE OF THE PERSON WITH A LEARNING DISABILITY

David Sines

Changes in the care of people with a learning disability have been influenced by political, social and economic factors and by new demands for responsive care and treatment by informed users of public services and carers in the community. This chapter will provide a framework which presents a series of introductory competences for nursing people with a learning disability. It will emphasise the importance of working with people with learning disabilities and their families as partners in care and will describe a range of intervention strategies within the context of holistic and multi-agency care approaches.

The chapter includes the following topics:

- Social policy and political influences

- The context of care provision

- Approaches to learning disability and intervention strategies

- Overview of causation and presentation

- Principles of learning theory

- Consumer advocacy, independence, rights and risk-taking

- Individual programme planning and care management

- Normalisation, independence, social relationships

- Promotion of health

- Management of disturbed and challenging behaviour

- Community care and family support

- Multidisciplinary teamwork

- Evaluation and effectiveness of care practice

- Nursing skills for clinical practice and relevant research

People with a learning disability are similar to many other members of the society within which they live; they have similar **needs**, wants and ambitions; the majority are not ill and all have a basic right to participate in the everyday life of their neighbourhood (Towell and Beardshaw, 1991).

Learning disability has been associated over the years with a number of misconceptions arising from stereotypes which assume that people with learning disabilities are 'all the same', that 'they can do nothing for themselves' and that 'they are unable to learn new skills or to make progress towards independence'.

The titles that have been attributed to this client group (for example, mentally handicapped; subnormal and mentally deficient) reflect, in part, the different perceptions that the general population and professional carers have had towards people with learning disabilities. For example, negative associations are attributed with terms such as 'mental subnormality' or 'handicap'. A challenge therefore exists for students of nursing to consider the actual needs of people as individuals rather than in accordance with subjective stereotypes which may have been produced as the result of negative associations or 'labelling'.

This chapter introduces a rather different approach and emphasises the more positive role that nurses may assume as they work in partnership with people with learning disabilities and their families to promote valued lifestyles for service users in the community.

A range of different perspectives is outlined in this chapter which explores the way in which nursing care has developed in response to the various social, psychological and political influences that have conditioned the development of the present pattern of social and health services. The contribution made by various agencies involved in the provision of care and support for this client group will be critically analysed.

The application of a range of general and specialist intervention strategies will be discussed and the role of the mental handicap nurse will be illustrated through the use of a care management and shared action planning approach (Brechin and Swain, 1987). A brief review of the particular responses required by people with a number of specific conditions will be included.

The nature of learning disability

Learning disability may present in a number of ways but is always associated with difficulties in learning new skills and competences in society. Some users of services have received responses from their families and carers that foster unnecessary dependence and which make assumptions about the limitations that may be made as new learning opportunities are presented. Some members of this client group have also been exposed to a sense of failure in their lives which may be the result of inappropriate learning situations and high expectations by society.

So what is learning disability? The term itself has only recently been acknowledged as an official designation in the United Kingdom. Previously, terms such as 'mental subnormality' and 'mental handicap' have been used. Quite clearly each of these terms or labels reinforces certain views and responses from the general public; they are also imprecise.

Take the term 'learning difficulty', for example. We all have a learning difficulty of one sort or another but when minor difficulties are compounded by a variety of other needs, society prefers to attribute a label that offers some explanation for the way in which its members behave. The need to categorise does not always receive the support of the group in question and consequently when people with learning disabilities are asked, 'How would you prefer to be addressed?', one receives the expected response of 'as Peter' or 'as Mary'.

There is no simple way of explaining or defining learning disability since it is not restricted to any one clinical entity or another. It is a euphemism for a collection of conditions, needs, symptoms and problems that are often lumped together and described as 'clinical types' or 'syndromes', e.g. Down's syndrome. Causes may be linked to genetic defects, birth injury or to a variety of reasons after birth. In many cases it is not possible to offer a firm diagnosis (Clarke and Clarke, 1985).

The definition of learning disability is also culturally determined. In some societies, those considered to be of 'normal' intelligence may include some who would be thought in other societies to lack the functional and social skills required to be identified as core members of a valued social order. In other cases the background of the professional making the diagnosis may influence the label apportioned to the individual. Since people who may be described as having a learning disability are not the responsibility of any one professional group, there may be different interpretations depending on the perceived cause of the disability. Doctors, nurses, social workers, psychologists and paramedical staff may be involved in the diagnosis and definition of each presenting problem and the interdependence on a multidisciplinary approach to **assessment** and planning to meet the needs of people with learning disabilities is emphasised.

This approach is most important when diagnoses are first made. Take, for example, a young child who exhibits speech or language delay and who has demonstrated difficulty in walking. A diagnosis of learning disability might be premature unless a full range of developmental assessments had been carried out to determine the extent, severity and range of disabilities that are actually present. In many cases an isolated area of development such as language delay may be attributed to developmental delay rather than a long term disorder (Craft, Bicknell and Hollins, 1985).

People with learning disability can learn and can look quite normal but the majority do lack some degree of social competence. Perhaps the most important thing to acknowledge (McConkey and McCormack, 1983) is that people with learning disabilities have normal feelings; our task is to ensure that opportunities are presented that allow these feelings to be explored and developed appropriately and to enable people to acquire a range of skills to assist them to function to their maximum ability.

The care context

The concept of learning disability is now accepted as being mainly a social condition associated with social competence and social skill development. The majority of people who fall into this care group will, in fact, live in their own homes with their families and will not require residential support services. Eighty percent of people (DHSS, 1988) who have attended some form of 'special' educational provision fall into this category and of these, very few will need skilled nursing support for anything other than ordinary ailments or illnesses (as for other members of the population).

During the course of their training, students of mental handicap nursing will have the opportunity to develop a number of specific competences which have been identified in response to the needs of people with learning disabilities. Mental handicap nurse practitioners receive in excess of 80% of their training in community and domiciliary family-based settings outside hospital.

During this time they are encouraged to foster close links with the primary health care team, with the local authority Social Services department and with the voluntary and independent sectors. Opportunities to share learning experiences with informal carers, social workers and with other professionals are very important. It is this opportunity for collaboration that provides the mental handicap nurse with the basic tools to develop a clear framework within which she can work in partnership with the local authorities and to develop her own process of coordination at local level between her skills and those of social workers. Nurses may offer nursing skills in a variety of ways but access is usually determined by the actual needs of the person concerned.

No single definition of learning disability covers all of the people who may require access to specialist services at some time in their lives. There is, however, likely to be some degree of accord amongst lay and professional people about what constitutes either more severe or milder forms of learning disability. The number of people in the latter category usually present problems for social scientists and statisticians since the criteria for inclusion are less well defined. Many of their needs may be of a social nature and relate to competence in that area. Examples include those who may have attended schools for people with mild learning disabilities, of whom the majority will be semiliterate and able to seek employment in the ordinary labour market. Most will adjust normally to adult life and may enjoy ordinary social relationships. A minority may require ongoing support to assist in the acquisition of appropriate social skills.

Conversely, for the former group, there may be an associated physical cause with attributes which provide easier diagnosis for both service assessment and for the specification of service responses. The person with severe learning disability will also require more intensive (and often life-long) support which should be offered by a variety of professional (and lay) supporters at different times. The majority will not acquire total independence or competence in a range of basic self-help skills and will require supervision in most areas of daily life. Examples typical of high dependency clients may be witnessed in the form of multiple handicap associated with profound learning disabilities.

The actual needs of people with learning disabilities will often determine the kind of service response that they receive.

Health and social care

Following the publication and introduction of the National Health Service and Community Care Act (HMSO, 1990) local authorities have assumed responsibility for the assessment and coordination of services for people with learning disabilities. For the majority, care will be provided in the community and clients will receive their services from generic health and social care practitioners in health centres and Social Services departments. For many, their needs will be similar to any other member of the population and the approaches required to provide individualised nursing care to meet their specific needs will require minimal (yet sensitive) adaptation.

However, for a small yet significant group of people (between four and six per thousand population in the United Kingdom) (DoH, 1990), health care needs may be present in addition to the social needs mentioned above. Such needs may be physical, behavioural, emotional or psychological in both cause and nature and in most cases, specialist nursing care will be required as part of a multidisciplinary support service. The health context of care usually has a physical or organic origin that demands an intensive and often specialist response from professional staff.

In some cases the requirement for specialist services may be transitory and there may not be a long term need for support (e.g. for people with challenging behaviours who require some intensive support to determine more appropriate coping or learning behaviours, compared to a person who has a severe behavioural problem that persists over time). Most people who fall into this category have accumulated a history or biography that has been influenced by physical or psychological behaviours or needs and in turn these have been influenced by life experiences received in the context of their family, care agency or from the society within which they live. The need for health care may be determined by a variety of factors relating to their social world and the responses that are demanded by society, which are in turn translated in the form of government policies that determine the way in which services are provided.

People with challenging behaviour often require considerable attention and support. The intensity of their behavioural presentation will determine the extent to which services are provided and will differ from person to person. Typical examples may be used to illustrate the problems presented by people who challenge the coping abilities of carers and these excessive behaviours may be summarised as:

- kicking, biting or spitting;
- self-injurious behaviour;
- aggressive outbursts and violent displays;
- shouting and swearing.

To date, the extent to which relevant services have been received has been largely determined by fitting people into services rather than by designing specific services to meet the needs of individuals. The NHS and Community Care Act (HMSO, 1990) advocates a rather different approach – the Care Management Approach.

Care management

Care management places an emphasis on providing individualised services for people and requires that we design systems that are sensitive enough to take account of each person's needs (National Development Team, 1991). The government requires each local authority to have in place by April 1993 an effective, flexible and responsive framework within which individual care needs can be assessed and through which services can be delivered and evaluated to service users.

Care management requires that each person with significant social or health care needs should have access to a named person who will be designated as a care manager. Care managers will usually be social workers, nurses or other community workers and they will be responsible for getting to know each individual consumer and their family, will 'map' their day-to-day needs and requirements, and formulate a clear action or care plan to take account of their needs, wants and ambitions.

The care management system requires that service users and their families are actively engaged in the identification of their needs; it does not necessarily restrict individual choice to the current range of services on offer at the time the assessment is made. Care management is essentially a way of ensuring that individuals are connected to all the services that they require, irrespective of the source. It is a model based on the principle of providing the widest range of choice possible to clients without reliance on any one service agency.

Once the care manager has agreed a package of care to meet the needs of each individual, contracts will be assigned to one or more service providers who may be selected from statutory, voluntary or independent sector agencies. Contracts will identify the exact nature and cost of services to be offered and delivered and will contain clear statements of responsibility and accountability (see Table 21.1).

Table 21.1. *The multi-agency context of care provision*

Social Services

Hostel provision
Home help service
Day services
Home adaptations
Respite care
Social work support

Health services

Community Mental Handicap Teams
Specialist therapy services
Respite care
Specialist residential care
Assessment and intervention services
Acute care
Primary and secondary health care provision

The voluntary sector

Employment schemes
Residential provision
Parent and client support schemes
Respite care
Neighbourhood support
Community relations (e.g. Citizens Advice Bureau)
Social support (clubs and befriending schemes)

The independent sector

Residential provision
Private health care

Each care package will also be costed and paid for from a complex system of allowances which will be coordinated by the local authority Social Services department. Care packages are evaluated against a set of common standards and their effectiveness judged by the extent to which they meet the actual needs of users (Brandon and Towe, 1989).

In order for care management to operate successfully it will be necessary for health and social care agencies to work closely together at both a planning level (where major service decisions and strategic plans are made) and at the point of service delivery. In support of this approach it will also be necessary to demonstrate that multi-agency systems are in place to assess client needs and to measure their effectiveness. Shared training opportunities for nurses and social workers and joint participation in the design of both care packages and service systems will become an important feature of provision for people with learning disability in the future.

The principles of care management rely on the promotion of individually designed packages and as such this replaces traditional models of fitting people into existing services (such as hostels, day services and long-stay hospitals). It requires that a range of opportunities is provided to service users based on the principle of integration within normal communities and that people have the right to adopt and to maintain an ordinary life and to have personal relationships and friendships.

The nature of nursing

The nature of nursing for this client group has undergone major revision during the past ten years in recognition of changes in social and public attitudes about the definition of health and social care referred to above. Mental handicap nurses follow their own branch programme which aims to provide students with a competence-based model of training which includes an appraisal of specialist responses that will be required by users of services in both hospital and the community (ENB, 1989).

Nurses work with individual clients and in groups and adapt their interventions to suit the needs of the people concerned (the versatile nature of the nursing model adopted provides for assimilation into the care management model; this is outlined in the last section of the chapter). The activity of nursing needs to involve different kinds of knowledge, ranging from biological sciences to interpersonal behaviours, which acknowledge the importance of affective and psychomotor responses to need. Other aspects of the nurse's role require more personal knowledge of both the nurse and the client. Such skills involve an appreciation

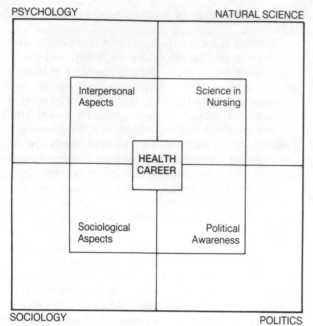

Fig. 21.1 *The health career matrix (simple form)*

of feelings and the development of self-esteem and personal growth. These attributes, from mechanistic to humanistic, may be demonstrated as intersecting continua (Fig. 21.1). The model of mental handicap nursing is made up of scientific aspects, interpersonal aspects, social aspects, and political awareness. Although they may not have equal importance, the contributions of the various quadrants of the model occur in all nursing situations.

An understanding of personal and group psychology (see also Chapter 14) and the application of learning theory (see also Chapter 7) should enhance the quality of care given to people with learning disabilities. Similarly an awareness of the importance of physical and sociological concepts can promote a holistic appraisal and intervention strategy to meet the various needs of clients wherever they live.

Nurses are becoming politically aware as they recognise that essential to our perception of nursing care is a knowledge of the social structures and policies that shape our environment. An understanding of the economic cost and social policy context that determine the way in which health care is delivered would appear to be important.

As one might imagine, there is a range of ways in which nursing care may be delivered to people with learning disabilities. These may be described as being instrumental, interpersonal, educational or organisational.

Instrumental

Instrumental nursing interventions include, for example, the use of instruments, appliances, techniques and schedules that have the potential to be administered impersonally. In this field, we may include the provision and appropriate use of special seating or mobility aids, the use of non-verbal communication systems such as **Makaton**, and the use of toys and equipment to shape and encourage the learning of new skills (Cornforth *et al.*, 1976). Other instruments may be used to screen or test intellectual function and these range from traditional measures of intelligence to more sophisticated and applied tests of cognitive and social functioning.

Interpersonal

Interpersonal nursing interventions form the most important element of care provision for people with learning disabilities. These include therapeutic interventions which range from applied **family** or **personal psychotherapy** to the development of social skills training programmes.

Educational

Educational nursing interventions involve the use of educational opportunities to promote and maintain positive health, to enable people to develop appropriate behavioural responses and to facilitate new learning. Examples include one-to-one teaching in the acquisition of self-help skills or social skills training in the community (teaching somebody to use public transport, for example).

Organisational

Organisational nursing interventions include referral processes which enable advice and specialist skills to be transferred to parents and to other carers. In such situations nurses may not be directly involved with clients but they may teach individuals or groups to respond appropriately to the needs of people with learning disabilities, for example, through the provision of parent teaching sessions or group teaching for day centre staff on the management of people with epilepsy.

Nursing is quintessentially future-orientated and concerned with the person in a social context. Intervention, including counselling, education or information-giving, needs to take account of the physical needs and other attributes that impinge on health. Equally, psychological attributes (in terms of attitudes, beliefs, motivation, personality, cognition, perception, group processes and relationships, the dynamics of the family or network of friends) should also be taken into account.

In respect of social needs, the nurse should be aware of the norms, values and social pressures that relate to such concepts as social class, cultural and subcultural determinants in respect of their influence on the concept of health and well-being. These factors remind practitioners that the delivery of nursing care operates within a framework of politically inspired policies that need to be understood, if not challenged. These social policies construct the systems within which care is provided and determine how clients will access the particular skills of nurses; nurses should therefore acquire skills associated with political awareness. Accessibility of clinics, provision and allocation of resources and the ethics of any intervention all fall within the political arena of policies that shape the human environment.

Biological causes of learning disability

Some refer to this as the 'clinical syndrome' approach and most particularly it refers to a biological cause for slow learning. Developmental screening is undertaken from birth and involves health visitors, doctors and educational psychologists to identify developmental delay as an indication of potential learning disability and to institute further investigations or interventions. This assessment approach is described by Griffiths (1970), Illingworth (1987) and Cunningham and Sloper (1987).

A range of signs and symptoms may be grouped together to form syndromes; there are a large number of syndromes but they actually account for very few definite diagnoses of learning disability. Whilst it is helpful to understand the cause of certain conditions, this knowledge rarely assists in meeting the needs of people with learning disabilities (Sines, 1987).

Down's syndrome

Down's syndrome is the most common syndrome and arises as the result of an extra ***chromosome*** (number 21 on the ***karyotype***) which may be in the form of ordinary ***trisomy*** 21, ***mosaicism***, or translocation of a number 21 chromosome. In mosaicism, the problems have arisen in the mitotic stage of embryo development and as a result some of the cells have an extra chromosome and some have the normal complement, the degree of disability being related to the number of abnormal cells. Down's syndrome currently accounts for one in 900 live births, this being a significant reduction in the incidence (from 1 in 600 in the 1970s) as a result of genetic counselling, screening high-risk pregnancies by amniocentesis, biopsy, testing for alphafetoprotein and selective abortion. There is an increased incidence of trisomy with maternal age: below 20 years, the chances are one in 2300, but at 45 years they are one in 40 (Clarke and Clarke, 1985).

The physical characteristics of Down's syndrome have been well recorded and the social, physical and psychological attributes of the condition do not appear to influence the care provided to any great extent. The typical features are present at birth (Table 21.2). The person is usually shorter in stature, has poor muscle tone that gives hyperflexibility of joints and enables contortions with the tongue. The strong facial resemblance that one person with Down's syndrome has to another enables instant recognition of the condition. The corollary is that the similarities may encourage others to disregard the uniqueness of each person as an individual in acknowledgement of their different needs and wants.

Although there is not a particular heart defect with Down's syndrome, common cardiac anomalies occur with increased frequency. The discoloration (cyanosis) of the face associated with this condition is a common feature and poor peripheral circulation also occurs in many instances.

People with Down's syndrome are predominantly mouth-breathers (Craft, Bicknell and Hollins, 1985) and they appear to have a reduced

Table 21.2. *Features and characteristics of Down's syndrome*

- Short stature
- Poor muscle tone and hyperflexibility of joints
- Tendency to be overweight
- **Epicanthic skin folds** of the eyelids
- Rounded head and facial structure
- Low set ears
- Eye socket typically slopes forward
- Small nose with a poorly developed bridge
- High arched mouth palate
- Long and mobile (occasionally protruding) tongue
- Poor or delayed dentition
- Square-shaped hand with short digits that show deviance in shape and length
- The dermal ridges of the hands and feet have a **pathognomic** pattern
- **Syndactyly** may occur
- Chromosomal abnormality (trisomy 21)
- Possibility of cardiovascular abnormalities and poor immunological response (leading to recurrent infections)

capacity to combat infection as a result of poor immunological response. This sometimes results in frequent and episodic respiratory infections.

Perhaps one particular clinical indication is worthy of note. A significant number of children with Down's syndrome have associated congenital heart disease (Sines and Bicknell, 1985). Not all of these are severely affected. The most common type of congenital heart disease is found in the atrioventricular canal, where they may have a low atrial septal defect or a common (i.e. single) atrioventricular valve. Babies born with this condition may be cyanosed when crying during the first few days of life because there is a mixing of blood between the two sides of the heart. Heart failure may result in severe cases but many young children recover spontaneously so that later in life the problem may be much reduced. However, there is always a risk that the child may develop secondary pulmonary vascular disease as he or she grows older. This may be witnessed in the form of persistent cyanosis which may become most disabling.

The symptoms of cardiac failure in young people with Down's syndrome include poor feeding and breathlessness. The signs are tachycardia, enlarged liver, pallor, sweating and cyanosis. Treatment includes avoidance of exertion, rest and (occasionally) the administration of minor sedatives.

Diuretics may also be used to reduce oedema and medicines such as digoxin are usually successful in regulating the heart rate and as a result myocardial function may improve. In some cases surgical correction may be offered.

Much research has been carried out in relation to the causes and presentational patterns of Down's syndrome but conclusively all point to the need to provide responsive and individual approaches to care provision based on an acknowledgement of the enhanced health risk that may occur from time to time (chest infections, dyspnoea, congestive heart disease) (Cunningham, 1982). In response to these needs, nursing care should be delivered in much the same way as care would be provided for other client groups. When health risks are identified, additional support will be necessary but this rarely intrudes on the pattern of daily living that is to be encouraged for all people with learning disabilities.

The provision of nursing care demands that appropriate (and sensitive) communication is developed with service users in response to their perceived level of intelligence (the level of intelligence may follow a normal distribution although all have degrees of learning disability). Nurses should also have regard to each person's potential for independence in areas where the individual can perform activities of daily living (such as dressing, feeding, washing and shaving) unaided. Through the introduction of sensitive (and discreet) behavioural strategies, e.g. behaviour modification, new skills may be encouraged and others enhanced towards independence (the concept of behaviour modification will be discussed later in this chapter).

Of equal importance will be the need for socialisation and the development of relationships with others. The approach adopted by many nurses is more commonly known as **normalisation** which aims to offer a range of ordinary life experiences and choices which prompt new and appropriate responses from clients. The maintenance of age-appropriate friendships and behaviours underpins the basic philosophy of nursing care practice (Sines and Bicknell, 1985).

Cerebral palsy

Cerebral palsy is a term used to cover a family of conditions that have a multiplicity of causes and a variety of manifestations. The cause may be genetic, the result of birth injury, infection or other injury. Cerebral palsy is characterised by disorders of posture and movement that are highly visible and by perceptual anomalies that may be unnoticed.

A particular challenge exists for nurses in respect of the degree of learning disability that actually exists; in some cases the level of intelligence may even be above normal.

The clinical signs of disorders of the motor system are **spasticity**, uncoordinated movements, tremor and rigidity, dependent on the site of the brain lesion. Spasticity may affect one limb, both limbs on one side (*hemiplegia*), all four limbs (*quadriplegia*) or the legs more than the arms (*paraplegia*). Other manifestations are athetosis characterised by uncoordinated rhythmic movement of the body, in particular the limbs, and ataxia in which the person has a wide-based gait, diminished muscle joint sense and disturbances of speech and eye movements.

The classification of cerebral palsy provides some insight into the multiple ways in which this condition may be manifested. With or without learning disability (43% have an intelligence level of above 70 (Clarke and Clarke, 1985)), it will be necessary to provide responsive (and individual) services to people and their families in accordance with the motor and sensory needs that may result. One of the most commonly associated needs is to enable people to live as independently as possible and for 29% to learn to live with the secondary handicap of epilepsy (Spastics Society, 1991). Epilepsy affects one person in three but there is no consistent pattern to determine when the condition emerges. Some people develop seizures when they are infants and others not until they reach adult life.

Through the use of anticonvulsant medicines it is now possible to provide excellent control for people with epilepsy without necessarily requiring them to alter or to inhibit their lifestyle. The promotion of healthy patterns of living requires that assistance is provided to enable the person to assess the degree of risk that they encounter in their environment, and like others with epilepsy, common sense is required to avoid those situations that might be hazardous during the course of a seizure.

Nursing care will also require that individuals and their carers are skilled in first aid (in particular in managing the actual process of the seizure and

its after effects) and the importance of recording seizure patterns and of taking medicines regularly must be emphasised.

The person with cerebral palsy will require the services and support of a team of specialists. Physiotherapy facilitates coordinated movement, enhancing the capacity to explore and thus to learn through the manipulation of objects, and to become independent in terms of mobility through exercises and adaptations to the environment or appliances. Speech therapy will be essential in most situations to improve communication skills and to facilitate interpersonal relationships. The combined talents of both professionals may also be witnessed in the formulation of feeding programmes that promote growth. Passive movements under the supervision of a physiotherapist and the active encouragement of movement are essential for the promotion of positive health gain.

Recently, much interest has been shown by the profession in the use of a range of alternative therapies such as **reflexology**, **aromatherapy**, **therapeutic massage** and therapeutic touch. For those people who do not appear to respond well to external stimuli through normal channels of communication such as verbal reinforcement, touch, smell and physical contact may be alternative routes for stimulation. Nurses now use a variety of therapies for people with multiple handicaps (such as cerebral palsy) and also with those who require additional assistance to relax (for example, people with hyperactive behaviours).

Other causes

Many theories have been generated to account for the causes of learning disability. So far this chapter has considered two specific conditions, Down's syndrome and cerebral palsy. Whilst they may be very different in respect of their cause, the care that people will require may be very similar and they serve as exemplars of care practice and provision that will be typical of many people with learning disabilities.

There are, however, other conditions that may be caused by environmental factors. These are summarised in Table 21.3.

Learning disability may be caused by a variety of factors before birth, at birth or during infancy.

Table 21.3. *Environmental factors causing or contributing to learning disability*

Prenatal	Natal	Postnatal
Infections: – rubella – cytomegalovirus – toxoplasmosis **Trauma:** – irradiation – rhesus incompatibility	**Trauma:** – hypoxia – anoxia – mechanical damage – cerebral haemorrhage – hyperbilirubinaemia (*arising from rhesus incompatability*) – hypoglycaemia	**Infections:** – meningitis – encephalitis – septicaemia – pneumonia – influenza – pertussis **Trauma:** – anoxia (*near suffocation, near drowning, post status epilepticus*) – head injury (*road traffic accident, cerebrovascular incident*)

Such factors include infections, trauma, malnutrition and understimulation.

Although not directly causal, an increased risk occurs in babies who are small-for-dates arising from unfavourable conditions *in utero*, prematurity, multiple births and low birth weight. Some of these may be attributed to maternal malnutrition, smoking, drug abuse or excessive abuse of alcohol while pregnant. Obstetric hazard is not a major factor.

There also appears to be a relationship between learning disability and poverty (Webb and Tossell, 1991). The incidence of learning disability, particularly mild disability, amongst populations with a low socio-economic status is higher than would be expected from a random distribution. Genetic causes such as Down's syndrome are non-selective in this respect; on the other hand, cerebral palsy and non-specific or undifferentiated disabilities are more prevalent. The situation may thus be the result of biological, psychological, social or political determinants (see Table 21.4).

The remedy may be educational in terms of diet (for young persons with metabolic disorders such as **phenylketonuria**), child development strategies, changes in lifestyle to promote greater use of services or the general raising of living standards. Nurses have a social and professional responsibility to develop awareness amongst members of the community to adopt positive health promotion strategies and need to be aware of factors affecting the health of the population as well as the specific nursing needs of individuals.

Table 21.4. *Social factors contributing to the presentation of learning disability*

- Poor nutrition
- Understimulation (absence of play and parental interaction)
- Social class differences in the pattern of child–parent interaction
- Differential use of health and social resources
- Inequalities in health provision and health promotional activities
- Class bias of school selection
- A combination of these factors

Prevention and intervention

Primary conditions relate to those factors that are an intrinsic component of the condition and are potentially disadvantaging. The restricted movement found in cerebral palsy is an example of this. In most cases the primary conditions are unlikely to respond completely to remedial intervention.

Secondary conditions relate to those factors that arise from the interaction of the primary disability with the environment. In many instances these may be of a social nature and may be experienced in the form of social stigma, such as the inability of some people with learning disability to form personal relationships with members of the general public because of their facial characteristics or behavioural responses. Further examples of secondary handicaps would be the manner in which restricted mobility reduces the opportunity to learn from the environment, or reduced manipulative ability.

Secondary conditions are, by contrast, potentially avoidable. One of the difficulties is that most of the adjustments have to be made by the person concerned, who may have a limited range of coping strategies to choose from. An important nursing function will be in preventing a disability from becoming a handicap.

A consideration of handicapping conditions, those factors that are inhibiting or preventing normal functioning, is more important than the cause of the dysfunction itself. Children with cerebral palsy may have restricted and/or reduced mobility. The problem, however, is the lack of mobility, not the clinical cause. The nursing intervention should concentrate on the possible; on overcoming the functional deficit of lack of mobility.

As in all forms of nursing care, prevention is an essential part of any intervention strategy. Prevention may be described as primary, secondary or tertiary (see also Chapter 3). In the learning disability field, prevention refers to the use of a range of measures or processes that aim to minimise the effects that the disability may have on the person's lifestyle and level of independence.

There are, however, a number of instances when prevention may assume more traditional forms such as in the case of primary prevention. One example relates to the provision of extensive immunisation programmes aimed at protecting mothers and their unborn children (e.g. rubella immunisation programmes) and through the development of awareness amongst pregnant mothers with regard to drinking and smoking. Preconception counselling, genetic counselling, good antenatal care, health education, special diets and improved social conditions are other examples.

Nurses who work with people with learning disabilities and their families will also have a major role to play in the prevention of secondary handicaps. Secondary prevention refers to the identification of conditions in susceptible people before they themselves are aware of the problem and involves making interventions aimed at preventing (or reducing) the effects of the condition on the person's health or lifestyle. Examples include the early diagnosis of phenylketonuria (through the use of universal screening programmes), special diets for people with phenylketonuria, and the use of thyroid supplements for hypothyroidism, a condition that has virtually disappeared, although it was previously a cause of potential learning disability.

Mental handicap nurses most often engage in tasks that aim to limit the effects of existing disabilities (tertiary prevention). Examples are the use of early intervention programmes to facilitate the development of individuals and to assist the family and other carers to provide a stimulating, growth-potentiating environment. Other examples are social training programmes, skills development strategies, educational provision, interpersonal skills awareness training, survival skills, habilitation and rehabilitation. Without doubt, tertiary prevention is the major arena where nurses have a positive contribution to make to the health of individuals and their families.

The social context of care provision

Following the publication of the National Health Service and Community Care Act in 1990, responsibility for the provision of services has been divided between the NHS and Social Services departments. In the past, access to services appears to have been conditional upon the extent to which the needs of service users were met by existing resources. The key to whether services were provided by health or social agencies was usually client ability (or lack of ability, as the case may be) and reliance was placed on assessment schedules to determine the level of dependence (some of which were biased and subjective in their formulation and administration), which often restricted choice for people with learning disabilities (Hogg and Raynes, 1987).

Hogg and Raynes refer to the 'plethora of assessment instruments' available to people working in the field (page 2) and they conclude that disability is increasingly viewed as an outcome of an interaction between a person and the environment in which he or she lives. Consequently a person who has lived a stable life in the family home may find that major changes have to take place when their family dies or when a new home is chosen. Perhaps the most important criterion for change will be the degree of support that the person will require in their new life and whilst parents and informal carers have often learnt to provide a 'tailored' service, professional agencies have tended to differentiate between high and low levels of support.

The latter has usually been seen to be the responsibility of the Social Services department, thus leaving the more dependent person to the health services (and consequently to care practices provided predominantly by nurses). The problem relating to placement has also been linked to unreliability in the assessment phase (Hogg and Raynes, 1987), which may be attributed to bias on the part of the professional administering the tests or to major fluctuations that can occur in the person's behaviour on the day of the assessment.

All of these difficulties point to the need for a radical revision of the way in which nurses, doctors, social workers and psychologists assess people and plan to meet their needs. The care management process mentioned earlier in this chapter has been one attempt to improve the way in which we match services to people's needs. This approach requires that sensitive information is collected about individual choices and wishes and demands that an individual care package is designed in response. This is a very different approach from one which recommends a residential placement on the basis of the person's assessed intelligence level or on the extent to which they 'fit' prescribed criteria for access to health or Social Service facilities.

The needs of people with learning disabilities have never been a great priority within the health and Social Service departments in the United Kingdom (Webb and Tossell, 1991). Services have often been provided in response to crisis situations or may be limited in the extent to which they meet the total needs of clients. The government has attempted to correct this imbalance and during the 1980s some priority was given to providing more money to establish a broader range of comprehensive services for this client group. The extent to which this objective has been achieved has been dependent upon the philosophy that local service providers have used in valuing and acknowledging the actual needs of people with learning disabilities and their families. For example, in 1989 the Royal College of Nursing undertook a survey of all health services in the United Kingdom and found that only 53% of authorities had published

their definition of community care and that 62% had generated an explicit philosophy against which their service aims and outcomes could be measured and evaluated (RCN 1989).

The study concluded that:

'The way in which certain services are being planned and delivered is fragmented and varies in how far the philosophy of community care (as determined by the government) matches practice. There are many examples of excellent practice in the community provided by health and social services and by the voluntary and independent sectors . . . examples have been used in this study to illustrate the wide range and variation of the determinants which effectively provide a high quality of life for people with mental handicaps and their families'

(RCN, 1989; page 68)

It is the wide variation in service provision that led the government to encourage health and Social Service departments to move their services away from institutional bases to the community.

Care in the community

According to government sources, over 30,000 people remain resident in long-stay mental handicap hospitals in the United Kingdom (DHSS, 1988). Fortunately nearly all of these people are now adults and children appear to be able to live either in their family home or in small supported houses in the community.

In an excellent review of social policy development in the community, Walker (1989) argues that the Conservative governments of the 1980s introduced a new (and deliberate) process of decentralisation for service provision for groups such as people with learning disabilities. Walker notes that care initiatives in the community have been sponsored by the government in an attempt to transfer responsibility for care from the NHS to families and the voluntary and private sectors, and in so doing to reduce the actual burden of costs for the Treasury. Political influence cannot, it seems, be distanced from the quality and range of services that people with learning disabilities receive and the organisation of services will depend upon public influence and social policy.

As a result of government policy there is an increasing pattern of change in the way in which residential care is provided for people with learning disabilities. Many of the large, outdated hospitals are closing and over 40% are actively engaged in contracting their numbers as people are transferred to live in community residential facilities (RCN, 1989). These facilities may be provided by a variety of social and health care agencies and together they form what is now regarded as the 'mixed economy of care' (HMSO, 1990). The mixed economy of care refers to the broader context of care by the voluntary and private sectors who are now responsible for the provision of 20% of care for people with learning disabilities (Walker, 1989).

Service provision and its corresponding pattern of nursing care must be viewed in the context of the policies and uses of power that shape the world in which we all live. This includes the legislative framework (the NHS and Community Care Act 1990 is an example), social policy and administration, decision-making on behalf of people with learning disabilities (and the extent to which individuals are involved in discussions that determine their own futures) and power relationships in caring teams that influence care.

Policies may be simple (the way in which staff members respond to a person's physical needs) or complex (relating to the philosophy of care to be provided in a new community home). The way in which these policies are enacted may well be in the hands of the nurse in terms of how much the policy aims are respected or adhered to. Take for example a policy that states 'people with learning disabilities will have the same rights as other members of society'. A statement such as this requires that services are designed in such a way as to enable users to participate in ordinary life experiences and to receive opportunities to make decisions about their lives. However, participation in decisions may be limited (Towell and Beardshaw, 1991) and there are few local service strategies that promote ordinary living experiences to the full.

Nurses should acknowledge the influence and control that they may impose when providing their clients with information about their rights and choices when selecting their support services. Nurses should occasionally reflect upon the use of power afforded to them by the nature of their relationship with their clients. An excellent review of abuse in such power relationships is that of Martin (1984) who offers some explanation for the apparent persistence of poor care practice in some long-stay hospitals for people with learning disabilities during the 1970s, which he attributes to ineffectual management and impoverished resources. The UKCC, in an analysis of cases referred to the Professional Conduct Committee, noted that the majority of cases related to client/patient abuse were associated with the long-stay sector (which includes services for people with a learning disability) (UKCC, 1991). In their analysis they noted the association between unacceptable standards of care practice and the allocation of reduced levels of funding and support services.

Learning disability does not, by itself, attract any particular social legislation but the presence and severity of the condition will determine access to support services and to social security benefits, e.g. attendance allowance, mobility allowance and community living grants. The Disabled Persons (Services, Consultation and Representation) Act (HMSO, 1986) does, however, offer some degree of support to uphold the rights of people who have special needs. As with its counterpart for school-age children, the Education Act (HMSO, 1981), local authorities are empowered to provide service users and their carers with access to information about their rights and services and also to receive regular reviews that determine their future care needs. However, whilst legislation is certainly moving in the right direction the government has failed to offer an independent ***advocacy*** service for those people who require representation when their abilities prevent them from speaking for themselves.

Philosophy of care

The philosophy of nursing care is based on the principle of normalisation (Wolfensberger, 1972). The characteristics of ordinary living underpin this approach, which aims to offer a range of choice and opportunities to people with learning disabilities so that they may be enabled to participate in real life experiences.

Community care is based on this principle and refers to the access to shops, public houses, leisure facilities and opportunities provided for the clients in the context of local neighbourhoods. The proximity of main public transport routes and the presence of community centres and local community groups also influence local perception of the community and its inhabitants.

The Oxford and Chambers dictionaries provide the following definitions of the term 'community':

> 'Joint ownership or liability; state of being held in common fellowship; organizational social body; body of people living in the same locality; body of people with the same needs and interests in common'
>
> (Oxford Concise, 1990)

> 'Common agreement; people having common rights; a body of people living in the same locality'
>
> (Chambers Concise, 1987)

Most local services now confirm that their published definition of community care will be based on the key principles presented above. These can be best summarised in the following government statement on community care policy for people with learning disabilities, published by the National Development Team for People with a Learning Disability:

> 'Community care should be planned as good local services, capable of responding flexibly to differing needs and circumstances and provided by a variety of agencies working together both in the planning and delivery of services. They should be able to identify and to meet both the general and specific needs of people with mental handicaps and their families. We are talking about our relatives, friends and next door neighbours; but the better we know people the more keenly we are aware that they are all different and that standard packages will not do. The only right answers are the relevant ones, flexible enough to change with changing needs – and when necessary to promote change'
>
> (Hansard, 1986)

General principles

Local services should publish a set of general principles which underpin the philosophy and values of their community provision. A common philosophy of care is necessary; the key working principles are summarised in Table 21.5.

In order to achieve these aims nursing staff and client relationships should be developed to maximise the concept of 'life sharing' to:

- diminish rather than accentuate distinctions be-

Table 21.5. *Key principles involved in the formulation of a value statement*

1 People with a learning disability are entitled both to the same range and quality of services as those available to other citizens, and to services designed to meet their special needs

2 Services for younger people should recognise their distinctive needs

3 In order to be effective, the services must be readily available and acceptable to individuals and the families who need to use them

4 Services should be able to adapt to meet the needs of each individual

5 The philosophy must be to provide maximum opportunities for the residents to experience an ordinary lifestyle

6 Emphasis must be on encouraging the development of new skills and staff are expected to allow or assist residents to experience life for themselves, rather than to do things for them

7 Residents are encouraged to integrate within their local communities and neighbourhoods; every opportunity is taken to encourage the use of local facilities for recreation, leisure, education, shopping and employment; people will therefore be supported to contribute to the local community

8 Individuals are encouraged to define their own lifestyle and individuality

9 People will be encouraged to develop friendships and to form personal relationships of their choice in order to enhance the quality of their lives

(Adapted from Sines, 1990; Towell and Beardshaw, 1991)

tween staff and residents (as fellow human beings);
- ensure that staff and residents share space, activities, toilets, meals, recreation, holidays and interests;
- encourage nursing staff to demonstrate appropriate behaviours and attitudes that will promote social acceptance and community integration.

Maintaining valued and integrated lifestyles

All nursing services should aim to develop services which are as fully integrated into local neighbourhoods as possible. Staff care practices should emphasise the importance of involving service users in the planning of their lives and should aim to promote the concept of advocacy to encourage their participation in all decision-making processes.

Essentially most people's lives revolve around their homes, friends, work and families, and the ways in which they choose to spend their time depend on their personal choices and the demands made on their 'free time' by others.

Many nursing staff are also aware of the need to ensure that clients engage in leisure pursuits that are integrated with other members of the community. This contrasts with outdated policies that encouraged segregated activities. Several reasons were given for the provision of segregated resources:

- They were often more accessible;
- They were cheaper;
- Attitudes amongst organisers considered them to be relevant to the needs of the client group 'who preferred their own company';
- There were often considered to be few alternatives.

Wherever possible nursing staff are now discouraging such activities in favour of integrating and sharing leisure time with friends and neighbours. Use may be made of the local swimming pool and riding club, and visits to the local pub and restaurant to celebrate birthdays or to entertain friends are common features of the range of opportunities offered to clients. As a result nursing staff now find that they are receiving positive feedback from neighbours and members of the community regarding the integration of people with learning disabilities in local neighbourhoods. Through the use of shops, cafés and public houses a high profile in the local community may be maintained.

In a research study undertaken by the author (Sines, 1990), the majority of nursing staff interviewed in community settings mentioned the importance of the 'purchasing power' that their clients had in the community. Equipped with real money to spend on goods in local shops and facilities, shopkeepers soon came to accept them as valued customers and thus assisted in their integration in the community as their businesses benefited. Other examples of integration may be witnessed in work placement schemes where some people with learning disabilities are employed in restaurants and garden centres, etc.

Staff are also expected to ensure that people are provided with maximum control over their finances, and although many people still appear to have less money than the average unemployed person, integrated social and leisure activities are now much in evidence. One particularly important contribution made by nurses to encourage integration was that more staff were employed in small houses in the community (compared to the resident/staff ratio in hospitals), which enabled many residents to experience a range of leisure or work pursuits. This in turn required a commitment from their carers to give time, energy and imagination in the design and realisation of local opportunities (Sines, 1990).

Work practices and opportunities

Nursing time and resource allocation is, in most cases, planned flexibly to facilitate the use of leisure activities which did not always fit neatly into ordinary staff shift patterns in hospital. One other important feature of the new services is the recognition that people with learning disabilities have the right to form relationships with others and to have the opportunity to feel valued and needed. Nurses are now noting the need to provide opportunities to form friendships and relationships with people of their choice from within older friendship networks and from within the wider community within which people now live.

The rapid extension of adult education programmes to people with learning disabilities has assisted in the acquisition of new social skills and leisure opportunities. Clients may attend a range of classes in photography, cookery, literacy and design. In some cases the projects have enabled people to form new and varied friendships with members of the local community and the advantages of such activities are obvious to staff. New skills are acquired, new friends made, ordinary members of the local community are demonstrating their willingness to share learning with people with disabilities. Support is provided without undue attention being drawn to the 'special learning needs of the individual'.

Taking risks has formed a central part of the debate and it should be acknowledged that an environment which allows an appropriate degree of personal choice and privacy can never be risk-free. From the author's experience it would appear that staff consider that this was one of the most difficult challenges for them to accept. Life in hospital offered protection from 'risks' and opportunities were restricted to avoid accusations being made against staff. In many services, 'risk-taking' policies have been written to assist staff in calculating the risks that naturally appear to accompany life in the community. Examples of some of the principal risks are:

- Fear of pregnancy;
- 'Bullying' by the 'caring' community;
- 'Getting lost';
- Accidents when encouraging people to acquire new skills, e.g. crossing the road.

Work practices will also be determined by the extent to which staff extend certain rights to service users.

The right to choose

People must be offered the opportunity to receive individually tailored services to meet their needs based on the principle of providing real choices, e.g. where to live, work or where to go on holiday. The right to choose also implies the right to refuse to accept some or all of the facilities on offer.

The right to dignity and respect

Nurses should also aim to present a positive image for their clients by ensuring that they present themselves in an appropriate manner to the general public. Staff must make efforts to signal to members of the general public the respect and dignity that they give their clients in order to encourage the transfer of a valued image to the community.

The right to a home of their own

Services must aspire towards the offer of a tenancy agreement to their clients. Homes should be selected in partnership between staff and residents and should be in ordinary dwellings, in ordinary streets, as close to the residents' family homes as possible. People should also have the right to have a room of their own and and to have their privacy respected.

The right to a meaningful occupation

Evidence of a range of opportunities for daily occupation and leisure is also to be found in many services. Some people are engaged in paid employment (Shearer, 1986), some participate in voluntary activities, thus serving the local community, and others still attend more traditional day centres. It appears that wherever possible people are now being offered choice from a range of available opportunities.

The right to personal and sexual relationships

Each service should publish a policy statement advising clients of their rights to form personal relationships. Some degree of privacy must be afforded to develop personal friendships, and practical assistance and counselling should be available to support people to form and maintain relationships of their choice. (Safeguards will also be necessary to avoid unwanted pregnancy and health-related risks.)

The right to independence

The right to self-assertion and direction is a requirement in all services. Nursing staff should encourage people to participate in all decisions affecting their lives and many provide assistance for residents to become more autonomous in their everyday lives.

The right to advocacy and representation

Services are also encouraging and providing opportunities for people to have a right to speak and to have their point of view taken seriously.

Many services now recognise the possibility that conflicts might occur between the expressed wishes of service users, their families and their carers. On such occasions it may be necessary to acquire the services of an independent advocate or representative to provide an objective opinion of the needs of each person.

The right to make mistakes

Rather than adopt a punitive approach when service users make mistakes or exhibit antisocial behaviour, service staff should provide support and encouragement in order to demonstrate appropriate behaviours for clients to learn new ways of dealing with situations. Staff should respond to such situations as learning opportunities for service users and should offer support to each person and encourage them to 'try again'. This approach is markedly different from the punishment models used in some hospitals where residents were rarely given the opportunity to apologise for their mistakes or encouraged to try again. Rather, they were labelled as difficult and either ignored or rejected.

Views of service users

The following three extracts of consumer views in respect of their new service are presented to illustrate some of the points raised in the last section (these are abstracted from a research thesis; Sines, 1990). They provide a client-focused perspective of the way in which services are provided in the community and reinforce a range of issues raised throughout the chapter.

Illustration One

'I now live in a house with three friends in ****. When I first moved in I enjoyed going out with my staff friends to get the carpets and the TV. My dad provided the furniture for my bedroom and we got some furniture from an old house in the next town. I was really excited when I first moved in. I enjoyed going out shopping and to the launderette and I go to Scrabble classes once a week. On Saturdays I go into town and I have a bus rover ticket for £1.75. On Tuesday nights we go to the local club where I can draw, play darts or enjoy a disco. On Fridays we have a raffle and I won this basket of fruit for the house. I went on holiday to Germany on a coach with my friends and staff, it was great fun. On Sunday I go to church in the town and on Saturdays I have lunch at the British Home Stores. I visit my friend's house sometimes and I also spend some weekends with my parents. It is much better than the hospital. Here people make me feel wanted and I can share things with them.'

Illustration Two

'Let me introduce the "family". There is John, Mary, Peter, Paul, Sharon and me (and the dog). We are proud because we have something to be proud of. We have had our problems, like other people do when they move into a new house. They were not terrible problems, but we got over them and now we are all going along the same path. What have we achieved?

Well! We are all a bit older and wiser, we have all got a bank account at Lloyds Bank and we are learning to understand and to appreciate what it costs to buy things and that sometimes we have to wait for things. We all choose our own clothes with our staff; we have learnt to mix with ordinary people and to be part of crowds of people without fearing them. The luxury of having a bath when we want one and to linger in it if we wish.

We know that we have the right to go to our own rooms if we so wish and to be on our own when we want. We know our possessions are kept safe and respected, as are our views. We are all going to Greece for our holidays next year. We have passports and this summer we voted!

We go out a lot and we are all members of hobby clubs and we go to adult education classes in town. We had a "Tupperware" party in the house last week. I go to sewing and embroidery and two of the men go to pottery and photography. We also have a residents association that we go to. Life has been good to us and for us; some people, not many, seem frightened of us, but they have to learn as we had to learn. There is nothing to be frightened of! There is some rain but there is an awful lot of sunshine!'

Illustration Three

'It is not just the physical surroundings that are different, for example having your own bedroom instead of a dormitory is great, but it is even better to be able to do what you want to. I have my own guinea pig in the garden, I call him "Toby". I used to be locked in a ward because I got angry sometimes. Now I only get cross if they upset me. The staff are OK here, they only make me do things I don't want to sometimes, but not often. I peel the potatoes and weed the garden, I don't like the washing up. The front room's nice, we can all use it, you know? We had one at home before I came into hospital, we were only allowed in it on Sundays. People no longer rush in or out of the house for meetings and the telephone is quieter. There are no real routines here, just some orders for the house. The neighbours are friendly, the man next door cuts the grass. I used to wet the bed, I don't now.

I like Janet, she is my girlfriend. She and I want to get married, John (a member of staff) said maybe one day!'

People with learning disabilities now increasingly receive their care in accordance with the principle of 'normalisation' and efforts have been made to enable service users to enjoy ordinary lives. This aim requires some degree of commitment from staff to enter into contracts with service users to provide specific services in respect of their individual needs. A partnership in care is beginning to emerge in the services, based on a genuine concern for the interests of individuals.

Service users are now offered a range of choice (although this is limited in some areas by outdated management responses and inadequate resources) and for those persons who require the provision of specialist support, the National Health Service still has a responsibility to make provision in accordance with government aims and philosophy:

'The Government's overall objectives are to develop a comprehensive range of coordinated health and social services for mentally handicapped people and their families, including assessment, day services and long-term and respite care in each locality; and to achieve a major shift from institutional care for mentally handicapped people to a range of community care according to individual needs, with a corresponding shift of resources. This will go along with a continued run-down of large mental handicap hospitals, but specialised residential health provision, which may be in small units in the community, will continue to be needed for people with special medical or nursing needs, as well as specialist support for those in other settings'

(Hansard, 1987)

Nursing people with a learning disability

Nursing care for people with learning disability may be categorised in much the same way as for general nursing: instrumental, educational, interpersonal and organisational.

Instrumental activities involve doing things for people. With people with more severe disabilities, nurses may undertake the daily living activities that the person would do unaided if they were able: basic hygiene, dressing, prevention of pressure necrosis by changing position, feeding or the monitoring of medicines for people with epilepsy, for example. For some people the presence of secondary handicaps may necessitate continued nursing care to prevent recurrent infections from causing irreparable damage or, in the case of people with multiple disabilities, to ensure that nutritional needs are balanced and met (these needs have often been neglected, as witnessed in research studies undertaken by Mamel (1989) and Patrick et al. (1986)).

One of the primary goals of nursing will be to assist the person to care for him or herself or to teach the primary carer to carry out these simple nursing activities and procedures. The educational role of the nurse is of major importance in the encouragement of independence in all activities of daily living and the development of functional skills. These range from personal safety, maintenance of continence and personal hygiene to the learning of socially acceptable behaviour and reducing inappropriate behaviours; learning social survival skills such as cooking, cleaning, budgeting, shopping and promoting personal growth.

Interpersonal relationships may pose particular problems for people with learning disabilities as interpersonal skills are usually learnt through modelling. The difficulties surround the inherent learning disability and the shortfall in role models arising from the segregation of schooling and recreational activities. The nurse has an important role in the development of interpersonal skills, the promotion of advocacy, self-awareness, self-assertion and the promotion of positive health.

The nurse may also have a useful role to play in the organisation and mobilisation of a range of various support services for the individual and the family. The support of various community groups may also be enlisted and opportunities extended for collaboration with other nurses and members of the multidisciplinary team.

The role of the mental handicap nurse is more concerned with education and social functioning than with clinical aspects of care but the mental handicap branch programme for Project 2000 ensures that the mental handicap nurse is proficient and competent to provide holistic care in response to a multiplicity of needs.

Planning to meet individual needs

The problem-solving approach associated with the profession of nursing is incorporated within a framework known as *individual programme planning*. Wilcock (1987) emphasises the importance of planning for people within the context of service management structures and supports:

'The increasing emphasis on providing individualised services for people with a mental handicap demands the development of service systems that will help identify the person's needs and plan to meet them . . . approaches are designed to ensure that staff make decisions that are relevant to a person's life and which emphasises the need to relate the process of individual life planning to service management'

(Wilcock, 1987; page 57)

The individual programme planning (IPP) system has become as much a part of care for nurses working with people with a learning disability as the nursing process has for their colleagues working in other specialties. There are many parallels between the two systems. Both require:

- a systematic framework and approach;
- a detailed method to assess and identify needs;
- the involvement of clients and their carers in the planning and implementation of care programmes;
- a method of recording and evaluating outcomes.

Perhaps the most appropriate place to start is to consider the work of Houts and Scott (1978) who described the process of goal planning with this client group. They presented their work in a format which lent itself to adaptation by parents and carers from which it was possible to construct teaching plans which used the principles of behaviour modification. One adaptation of these principles was the Portage Home Teaching Project (Blunden, 1978) which provided parents and carers with a systematic teaching package for children which required an accurate assessment of skills and needs to identify a baseline. From the baseline it is possible to plan teaching programmes and evaluation techniques. This then was the start of a process which was to be adapted and further refined.

The following principles underpin the IPP system:

- People with learning disabilities should be involved in planning their own futures;
- Desirable futures should be planned for people with learning disabilities;
- All relevant people should be involved in the planning process;
- Services should be coordinated to meet people's real needs;
- Service deficiencies should be identified and used in the planning of future services.

Mansell *et al.* elaborated on these principles and devised a specific teaching and training package for adult service users which they named the *Bereweeke Skills Teaching System* (Mansell *et al.*, 1983). This approach forms the basic system for individual programme planning and is described in operational detail by Jenkins *et al.* (1988). The system offers a mechanism for ensuring that members of the multidisciplinary team share with their clients aspects of decision-making and the implementation of care plans. Within the system professional workers meet with the person, their family, carer or advocate in order to:

'determine objectives, coordinate activities, and find out who is already involved with the individual. The meetings are held on a regular basis, so that the progress towards the goals or objectives set with the individual at one meeting with a defined timescale, can be reviewed at a subsequent meeting. In this way plans to meet the individual's future needs can be drawn up and services from different agencies can be made available when required'

(page 5)

Whilst these systems were admirable and enabled coherent thought about people's needs, they failed to provide a holistic framework in respect of the importance of considering relationships between clients, their friends and carers.

Brechin and Swain (1987) provide an opportunity to address this imbalance and introduce the concept of ***shared action planning*** which emphasises the importance of relationships. They start their analysis of shared action planning with the following quote:

'Let us start from where you are: you are already a skilled person. The skills discussed and explored in this book are not just for "experts", though many professionals would see them as crucial to their work. These skills are part and parcel of day to day living. They are used in friendships, family living, relationships at work and in mutual helping and caring. Such skills grow and develop through and within personal relationships. Relationships are, in this sense, the heart of the matter'

(Brechin and Swain, 1987; page 3)

They introduce a new dimension into the personal planning process which is based on the principle of the importance of the interactions that take place between the client and the carer (and his or her friends). They talk of compassionate and supportive caring relationships with reference to their place in determining the context of successful care planning and life experiences. They describe the shared action planning approach as having a focus on communication and relationship building, which are central to the process of growth and human development. It involves the sharing of key relationships, joint decisions and the pooling of ideas with the service user in order to challenge their environment by constructing an agenda of positive action. This agenda involves the formulation of shared plans of action about identified needs and includes safeguards to ensure that action plans are actually carried out:

'Shared Action Planning happens when there is coordination, organisation and people know who is responsible for doing what'

(ibid, page 131)

Consequently, individualised approaches to care should provide a framework for people to express their wishes and desires through a shared process with named workers which in turn should lead to valued outcomes for the individual. Individual programme planning uses the same four stages as the nursing process (assessment, planning, action and evaluation) but it is not a purely nursing method as it includes inputs from every relevant discipline and carer on the basis of equality. It pays particular attention to clarifying the client's unique needs as he or she sees them.

Shared action planning, like all other intervention techniques, will only be successful if the principles underpinning the approach are understood and practised to a proficient standard by the workforce. Perhaps one criticism is that it reads as a 'DIY manual' and there is an inherent danger that people will be enthused by its readable style and cartoon illustrations. As a teacher, one must ensure that such systems are introduced within the context of a structured teaching programme which must commence with a foundation course on the principles of individualised approaches to care and goal planning.

Application of nursing models

Any of the nursing models, suitably adapted to meet the needs of clients, may be applied to the provision of nursing care for people with learning disabilities. Roy's adaptation model (Roy, 1976), for example, would appear appropriate as people in this category may have problems in adapting to their physical and social world. Orem's self-care model (Orem, 1980) may also be useful in some situations as the person will have therapeutic self-care deficits and may need to learn to become proficient in self-care activities. Roper, Logan and Tierney (Roper *et al.*, 1983) also provide a useful model as the problems experienced by people with learning disabilities may manifest themselves with problems of daily living (nursing models are also examined in Chapter 12).

Whatever model is used, the importance of application within a shared action planning framework will be paramount and the use of holistic models of nursing will be of great assistance to nurses involved in the assessment of need and in the design of responsive packages of care.

The premise has to be the fact that all people with learning disabilities are first, foremost and forever individuals. The various problems, difficulties or needs relate to their humanity and as such, any of the nursing models may be used in the provision of nursing care. The desire of nurses working in this specialty to distance themselves from the medical model of care sometimes witnessed in general nursing and the medical or psychiatric model sometimes seen in the mental health fraternity resulted in a practical approach which is known as 'behaviourism'. The great advantage of these approaches is that they often achieve results, giving in addition a specific task for nurses to undertake.

Intervention strategies

The intervention strategy adopted will depend on the assessment of the person in their social context. Nurses must ask two questions:

(1) What intervention will enhance the health potential of the individual?
(2) What knowledge would support this intervention?

This requires an examination of those factors that impinge upon a person's needs and lifestyle from natural science, social, interpersonal and political domains. This involves a retrospective examination of the person's biography and speculation about future health needs which should aim to provide for maximum independence.

Behavioural approaches to caring

Behavioural approaches to caring are based upon the principle of learning theory, in particular classical and operant conditioning. In *classical conditioning* (Clarke and Clarke, 1985) behaviour is influenced by cues from the environment (as in people preparing to go home five minutes before the factory whistle blows). Cues and physical prompts are important teaching mechanisms whereby people with learning disabilities may learn new skills. Physical and verbal prompts are reduced as people become progressively competent in the required behaviour being taught.

Operant conditioning (Clarke and Clarke, 1985) relies on the rewarding of appropriate behaviour when it occurs, whatever prompted the behaviour, thereby reinforcing that positive behaviour and increasing the likelihood of its recurrence. In behavioural terms, if behaviour exists then something somewhere must be reinforcing it. Rewards may be physical (for example, food or drink), social (in the form of praise) or intrinsic as in simple mastery of a task. The intention in teaching is to progress

from physical to social to self-fulfilment although such a progression may be hard for any human being!

Behavioural shaping

Behavioural *shaping* involves a progressive rewarding of behaviour that approximates to the required behaviour. If the intention is that a person should learn to eat with a spoon, then a system could be devised by which a reward is given whenever the spoon is grasped, with no reward being given whenever the spoon is rejected. This may progress to rewards being given for touching the spoon for a split second, to one second, to five seconds and so on until the spoon is grasped. The rewards continue in the form of verbal praise until the spoon is eventually moved to the mouth, loaded with food, and the food is swallowed. The establishment of the behaviour depends on the *reinforcer* – what the student finds rewarding – and the skill of the teacher in breaking the task down into discrete and small steps that can be taught incrementally at the level required.

The whole process of behavioural change and modification requires skill, patience and perseverance. A series of skills-based teaching packages have been introduced to assist potential teachers in this process and the Bereweeke Skills Teaching System mentioned in the last section is one such example. This system provides the opportunity to break tasks down into short term goals and offers a systematic approach to writing weekly teaching targets through the use of activity charts or plans (see Fig. 21.2).

The common approach to the teaching of new behaviours is to model the behaviour to be learned. This also applies to reducing those behaviours that we find to be either challenging or undesirable.

The term 'challenging' is sometimes attributed to behaviours that we regard as being antisocial or 'disturbing' in respect of the pattern of our everyday lives. Screaming, hitting or self-mutilation are examples. Rather than aiming to encourage total conformity in our world, nurses must respond positively to people who exhibit these forms of expression since they may be an indication that other means of communication have failed.

The principles of operant conditioning suggest that any behaviour that is reinforced is likely to

INTERPERSONAL ASPECTS OF NURSING	SCIENTIFIC ASPECTS OF NURSING
Challenging behaviours Solitary Limited speech Speak if prompted Attention span Frequency Boredom Absence of interpersonal skills Manipulative Will work when in a group Disrupted family life Inconsistency of management	12 years Male Epileptic – major seizures – increasing – treatment: carbamazepine 2 × 400mg
Secondary gain Stigmatism Treated age inappropriately Patient career Life chances Council house	Epilepsy – complacency of the doctor about treatment Respite care Play area: fencing Benefits – Attendance Allowance Funding from Rowntree Trust Individual Programme Plan School
SOCIOLOGICAL ASPECTS OF NURSING	POLITICAL ASPECTS OF NURSING

Fig. 21.2 *David Snow: case history set out in the form of the health career matrix*

occur again given the same opportunity and circumstances (see also Chapter 7). Consequently people who learn that to behave in an unsociable manner gains them a reward are likely to repeat that behaviour again. The application of behaviour modification as a response to such problematic situations may be effective in reducing the association that occurs between the action and the subsequent attention the person experiences. Take, for example, a person who screams for attention. If a positive response is received every time then it is likely that screaming will become associated with attention. However, if attention is not given on every occasion it is likely that the association will be weakened and the behaviour may reduce in frequency or intensity.

Since most behaviours signify some form of communication with the world it is important that new, appropriate behaviours are taught at the same time as we aim to reduce undesirable ones. This technique is known as *differential reinforcement* and offers an excellent opportunity for nurses to promote appropriate learning for people with learning disabilities.

A consistent approach to care (which is so im-

portant in all aspects of care for people with learning disabilities) is facilitated by the meticulous keeping and use of objective records, a point emphasised by the Health Service Ombudsman Report (Health Service Commissioner, 1991).

The multi-agency context of care

Following the publication of the NHS and Community Care Act in 1990, health and social care agencies have been charged with responsibility to work together to assess, plan, provide and evaluate services for people with learning disabilities.

Mental handicap nurses have been preparing themselves for the emergence of a new partnership in care and many nurses work as integral parts of community teams. The concept of the Community Mental Handicap Team developed in the 1970s with the explicit aim of providing a coordinated range of support to people and their families in the community. These teams have gradually permeated every health district and board throughout the United Kingdom and may consist of community mental handicap nurses (trained to an advanced practitioner level, following attendance at a one year post-qualifying Diploma course), social workers, psychologists, psychiatrists and other paramedical staff working together to provide comprehensive packages of care for people with learning disabilities and their families.

Following the success of domiciliary support for users of services, nurses and social workers have also confirmed their intention to train together wherever the opportunity facilitates shared training. Each of the National Boards for Nursing, in association with the Central Council for the Education and Training of Social Workers (CCETSW), has established a joint or shared training committee to coordinate and to stimulate the development of interdisciplinary training initiatives.

In Wales a comprehensive strategy was introduced in 1983 which effectively united all major care providers across the Principality (Welsh Office, 1983). The county councils in Wales have been given lead responsibility for the development of local plans and strategies for this client group which are scrutinised by the Welsh Office against a set of core principles that promote ordinary living and valued lifestyles.

Throughout the United Kingdom, health and Social Service departments are actively engaged in the formulation of joint strategies to provide a 'seamless' service for people with learning disabilities and their families. The service of the future will cease to be dependent on outdated service structures such as the adult training centre, the mental handicap hospital and the Social Service hostel. In their place will be a comprehensive local network of services, designed to promote ordinary living in local neighbourhoods.

Integration will demand that people with learning disabilities access further education colleges, leisure centres and live in ordinary houses. One might well wonder whether all of this will be possible and if so, how might it happen and what role will nurses play in this new 'world'?

In 1991 the four Chief Nursing Officers of the UK published the Cullen Report, which offered a new future for mental handicap nursing practice (DoH, 1991). In this report Cullen recommended that mental handicap nurses would be most useful in the context of the emerging community model of care identified in this chapter. He saw their skills as being independent of buildings or facilities and recommended that mental handicap nurses should deploy their skills flexibly in the community.

The 'facility independent' model that followed suggests that mental handicap nurses will provide specialist care to people with special needs (people who have multiple handicaps, people whose behaviour requires specific attention and intervention, people with superimposed mental health needs, people with medical and sensory impairments and others who require intensive nursing care). Nurses will offer their skills on a contractual basis to their clients either through domiciliary support teams or by working with them in their new homes in the community. New opportunities for people with learning disabilities therefore offer nurses a range of fresh challenges to provide appropriate nursing care in integrated settings in the community.

A new partnership with social workers will also emerge. Social workers will be particularly involved with the provision of social care for people, thus leaving nurses to meet the health requirements of their clients. The context within which care will be provided may be different in the future (for example, many nurses and social workers will work with people who live in accommodation managed and owned by the independent and voluntary sectors) and in some cases people may receive intensive care in homes of their own. Care management processes (mentioned earlier in this chapter) will determine the skills that mental handicap nurses will be expected to provide for their clients. Care managers (mental handicap nurses may be ideal applicants for these positions) will coordinate the assessment of needs and will assist nurses and social workers to differentiate between their unique contributions to meeting the needs of individual clients and their carers.

Access to generic health care services

The government has recommended that for the major part, people with learning disabilities should have access to generic health care services through primary health care teams and in general hospitals. People with learning disabilities are not immune from the trials and tribulations of day-to-day life, and as such are as likely as the next person to require access to general health services. In certain circumstances two areas might require specific attention whenever people with learning disabilities are admitted to hospital: the person as a patient may have anxieties and the family at home may be concerned that the nurses will not be able to provide appropriate care.

People with learning disability often like consistency and order and may become anxious when confronted with changes in their routine (even minor ones). The problems raised will be much more to do with the shortfall in the coping mechanisms of the nurse than in the nature of the disturbed behaviour. A noisy or distressed person may be an unfamiliar sight or experience for some nurses. At times of crisis an increase in attention is sought by all of us, and avoidance of people in distress is seldom helpful. Like any person in a situation of acute stress, the individual may exhibit behaviour usually associated with an earlier age, and this needs to be recognised with warmth and understanding. The situation needs to be responded to tactfully, firmly and with compassion. The client's behaviour may be unintelligible to the uninitiated but it is likely to follow a particular pattern. Violence very rarely occurs but aggressive outbursts are occasionally witnessed.

Avoidance of many of these problems can be

achieved if time is allowed to take a full history from family members or carers. Normal patterns of behaviour can be predicted and if nurses are prepared in advanced, precautions can be taken to ensure that the patient is settled in a manner that minimises anxiety and uncertainty. In particular, nurses should understand any form of communication system that the person uses. Communication will often be the most important aspect of care and people with learning disability may have developed elaborate systems of communication in the absence of verbal reasoning or speech. In such situations reassurance and positive body language may be most helpful and may reduce anxiety. Conversely vacillation and ambiguity on the part of the nurse are unhelpful and the situation needs to be managed with confidence, decisiveness and sensitivity.

Conclusion

Pratt *et al.* (1980), in a research paper relating to the quality of life experienced by people with learning disabilities, suggest that community care offers tremendous advantages to people with learning disabilities in respect of their perception of life experience. However, in their conclusion they offer a salutary warning that the provision of a small, integrated environment offers no guarantee that people will be treated with dignity or that all of their needs will be met.

Margaret Flynn (1986), in a report on interviewing people with learning disabilities, suggests that it is possible to encourage people to speak for themselves and this is the challenge that now faces the mental handicap nursing profession.

The English National Board's branch outline criteria for the specialty (ENB, 1989) offers explicit criteria against which the competences possessed by mental handicap nurses may be measured at the end of their training. With an increasing move to the community, Project 2000 appears to offer new opportunities for nurses to share both general and specialist skills within the family of nursing.

Care for this client group is essentially a multi-agency and interdisciplinary responsibility and as such the future of mental handicap nursing will depend on the extent to which it responds to meet the actual needs of service users in partnership with other professionals.

Mental handicap nursing must continue to evaluate the extent to which it meets the needs of people with learning disabilities and the ordinary life philosophy referred to in this chapter provides valuable criteria against which to assess effectiveness of care delivery. Towell and Beardshaw (1991) suggest that through the provision of advocacy for service users, new opportunities and partnerships may be developed to improve the quality of life of people. There are seven key accomplishments which will be necessary if nurses are to achieve high quality care for their clients. The extent to which nurses are successful in providing high quality services to their clients may be evaluated by the extent to which they provide opportunities for people to receive and to experience:

* integration
* choice
* relationships
* image and status
* participation
* rights and responsibilities
* skill enhancement.

Towell and Beardshaw comment on the need to translate these value principles into real action if improvements are to be experienced and introduced into people's lives. Using the care management framework and the process of shared action planning, nurses are ideally placed to respond to this challenge. They have been able to demonstrate their versatility in responding to needs in a variety of settings and as they assist people to move from large hospitals to the community, their skills and competences adapt to meet new demands and responses from their client group.

Learning disability is not a diagnostic category but reflects a range of conditions that require a multiplicity of responses, most of which will affect other people. It is marked by slower responses to learning but also by genuine optimism in respect of what can be achieved if people empower their client group to share in ordinary life experiences. Because learning disability does not fall into the domain of any one care group or agency, a range of complementary and sometimes competing service responses have arisen, namely medicine, social work education and nursing. The changing values of society have resulted in a situation whereby ordinary people are more willing to accept people with learning disability into their midst. The multiplicity of services and the difficulties of categorisation merely reinforce the fact that people with learning disabilities are ordinary people!

The ordinary life framework presented in this chapter complements the role of mental handicap nursing and offers opportunities for nurses to regard people as ordinary citizens who require a range of interventions designed to maximise their integration in the local community. Such interventions should accord with the wishes, desires and beliefs of the person with whom they are working and should facilitate the development of a reflective and competent practitioner. Nurses are certainly able to apply their skills wherever people live and are not reliant on a hospital or other NHS facility within which to practise. In this respect they might be regarded as 'facility independent' (DoH, 1991); their future relies on the empowerment of their clients and on the relationship and partnership that follow.

Glossary

Advocacy: This term is used in three forms: (1) To speak or act on behalf of another person; the nurse as advocate, for example. (2) Citizen advocacy, of which several schemes exist, whereby an especially recruited volunteer ordinary citizen speaks on behalf of a person with learning disability. (3) Self-advocacy expressed in terms of 'We can speak for ourselves'. The encouragement of people with learning disability to be assertive and self-determining

Aromatherapy: A form of therapy in which disorders are treated by body massage using aromatic oils; sometimes described as an 'alternative therapy'

Assessment: Involves acquiring information about a person or situation that may include a description of the person's wants, needs, wishes and ambitions. Part of a larger procedure and service to support planning towards goals which have been separately identified

Bereweeke: A system of teaching skills which is accompanied by two checklists, one for children and one for adults. It should be used as an integral component of the *IPP* process. Areas covered include language, self-care, motor skills, social skills and cognitive skills. The main purpose is to develop individual teaching programmes

Care management: A process introduced in the NHS and Community Care Act (1990) that provides a consistent approach for matching individual needs to services (rather than the other way around). The process depends upon the holistic assessment of individual needs and the appointment of a care manager who is responsible for the design and costing of a care package that will be systematically evaluated in respect of its effectiveness in meeting the identified needs of the client concerned

Chromosome: The threadlike bodies in the cell composed of genetic material of heredity. Normal complement in humans is 22 matched pairs of autosomes and a pair of *sex chromosomes*

Classical conditioning: The construction of reflex responses by the presentation of paired stimuli. Theory devised by I.R. Pavlov (1927)

Epicanthic skin folds: A fold of the upper eyelid over the lower eyelid at the inner corner

Family psychotherapy: The application of psychotherapeutic techniques within a family context (see *Personal psychotherapy* below)

Individual programme plan (IPP): A system for making plans for one person based on the strengths and needs of that person as an individual with the assistance of people who are well known to him/her. A meeting is held to formulate the IPP, at which objectives are set to be achieved within a specific time span. The person responsible for each of their needs is identified. Any service deficits which prevent the need from being met are also identified and managers are informed. In this way service provision can be based on the needs of clients

Karyotype: The genetic map comprising an electron microscope picture of the matched chromosome pairs arranged in order of size. Commonly used to show the existence of chromosomal anomalies such as *trisomy* 21

Makaton: A manual signing or communication system designed for use with people with severe learning disabilities

Needs: Things that can be identified or assigned. They are presented as statements of fact which can be deduced by someone else

Normalisation: In short, 'valued means for valued lives', or like ordinary people. A concept forming the basis of care that postulates that any special provision is discriminatory. A non-devaluing approach to care; a denial of deviance

Operant conditioning: A method used widely in behaviour modification, in which behaviours are altered by changing their consequences. It is a process of training behaviour using reinforcement techniques which involves four types of conditioning – positive reinforcement, negative reinforcement, punishment and extinction

Pathognomic: A characteristic that positively identifies a condition, e.g. Koplik's spots on the buccal membrane in measles and the palm print of people with Down's syndrome

Personal psychotherapy: Treatment of emotional or psychosomatic disorders based on the application of psychological knowledge rather than on physical forms of treatment. Explores inner feelings and encourages the exploration of 'inner' coping strategies to deal with stress and life events

Phenylketonuria: A condition caused by a deficiency of an enzyme (phenylalinine hydroxylase) in the body. Phenylalanine cannot be converted to tyrosine, an amino acid, and as a result phenylalanine builds up in the body causing damage to the brain. Phenylpyruvic acid is excreted in the urine. The degree of learning disability may be severe unless detected and treated early in life. Untreated children have blue eyes, fair hair and dry (and sometimes eczematous) skin. This deficiency is routinely tested for in the UK and early treatment results in total recovery. The Guthrie test is generally used. Treatment is with a low phenylalanine diet. Blood screening for the measurement of phenylalanine is also necessary

Reflexology: Reflexology is based on the principle that particular parts of the feet relate directly to various systems or organs of the body, and by gently stimulating specific areas, disorders can be alleviated or relieved

Sex chromosomes: The chromosomes responsible for the determination of sex (amongst other things). XX is female, XY is male

Shaping: A behaviour modification teaching technique in which existing behaviours are built on and expanded. Initially a response similar to the desired one is reinforced so that it occurs more frequently. The next stage is to reinforce it selectively when it is a closer approximation to the required response

Shared action planning: A system based on the IPP approach which emphasises the importance of relationships and friendships as the core principle for the development of care plans. It ensures that service users share in all aspects of the process as joint decision-makers. It involves goals, aims and assessment and provides strategies and actions to ensure that outcomes are evaluated in accordance with prescribed action plans

Syndactyly: Webbing of the fingers and toes

Therapeutic massage: The rubbing or kneading of different parts of the body, as to aid circulation or to relax the muscles

Trisomy: The existence of three chromosomes in place of the more usual matched pair. Down's syndrome is the result of an extra number 21 chromosome

References

Blunden, R. (1978). *Individual Plans for Mentally Handicapped People: Draft Procedural Guide*. Mental Handicap in Wales Applied Research Unit, Cardiff.

Brandon, D. and Towe, N. (1989). *Free to Choose – An Introduction to Service Brokerage*. Good Impressions Publishing Ltd, London.

Brechin, J. and Swain, A. (1987). *Changing Relationships – Shared Action Planning for People with a Mental Handicap*. Harper and Row, London.

Chambers Concise English Dictionary. (1987). Chambers, London.

Clarke, A.M. and Clarke, A.D. (1985). *Mental Deficiency – The Changing Outlook*. Methuen, London.

Cornforth, A.R.T., Johnston, K. and Walker, M. (1976). *The Revised Makaton Vocabulary*. Makaton Vocabulary Project, Farnborough.

Craft, M., Bicknell, J. and Hollins, S. (1985) *Mental*

Handicap – A Multi-Disciplinary Approach. Baillière Tindall, London.

Cunningham, C. (1982). *Down's Syndrome: A Guide for Parents*. Souvenir Press, London.

Cunningham, C. and Sloper, P. (1987). *Helping Your Handicapped Baby*. Souvenir Press, London.

Department of Health. (1990). *Statistical Bulletin 2/90*. HMSO, London.

DoH. (1991). *Mental Handicap Nursing in the Context of the White Paper 'Caring for People in the Next Decade and Beyond' (The Cullen Report)*. HMSO, London.

Department of Health and Social Security. (1988). *Health Service Development – Resource Assumptions and Planning Guidelines*, HC(88)43. HMSO, London.

English National Board of Nursing, Midwifery and Health Visiting. (1989). *Project 2000: Mental Handicap Nursing Branch Programme*. ENB, London.

Flynn, M.C. (1986). Adults who are mentally handicapped as consumers: issues and guidelines for interviewing. *Journal of Mental Deficiency*, 30, 369–377.

Griffiths, R. (1970). *The Abilities of Young Children*. London University Press, London.

Hansard. (1986). *Session 1985–6, Vol. 106, Col. 246*. HMSO, London.

Hansard. (1987). *Session 1986–7, Vol. 108, Col. 530*. HMSO, London.

Health Service Commissioner. (1991). *3rd Report for the Session 1990–1991. Annual Report for 1990–1991*. HC536. HMSO, London.

Her Majesty's Stationery Office. (1981). *Education Act – An Act to Make Special Provision for Children with Special Needs*. HMSO, London.

HMSO. (1986). *Disabled Persons (Services, Consultation and Representation) Act*. HMSO, London.

HMSO. (1990). *National Health Service and Community Care Act*. HMSO, London.

Hogg, J. and Raynes, N (1987) *Assessment in Mental Handicap – A Guide to Assessment Practices, Tests and Checklists*. Croom Helm, London.

Houts, P.S. and Scott, R.A. (1978). *Planning for Client Growth: A Guide to Selecting Meaningful Goals for Developmentally Disabled Persons*. University of Pennsylvania Press, Philadelphia.

Illingworth, R.S. (1987). *The Development of the Infant and the Young Child*. Churchill Livingstone, Edinburgh.

Jenkins, J., Felce, D., Toogood, S., Mansell, D. and de Kock, U. (1988). *Individual Programme Planning*. BIMH Publications, Kidderminster.

Mamel, J.J. (1989). Percutaneous endoscopic gastrostomy. *American Journal of Gastroenterology*, 84(7), 369–377.

Mansell, J., Felce, D., Flight, C. and Jenkins, J. (1983). *The Bereweeke Skill Teaching System: Programme Writers Handbook*. NFER-Nelson, Windsor.

Martin, J. (1984). *Hospitals in Trouble*. Blackwell Scientific, Oxford.

McConkey, R. and McCormack, B. (1983). *Fact Sheets*. St Michael's House Research, Dublin.

National Development Team. (1991). *The Andover Case Management Project*. National Development Team, London.

Orem, D. (1980). *Nursing: Concepts of Practice*. McGraw-Hill, New York.

Oxford Concise English Dictionary. (1990). Oxford University Press, Oxford.

Patrick, J., Boland, M., Stoski, D. and Murray, G. (1986). Rapid correction of wasting in children with cerebral palsy. *Developmental Medicine and Child Neurology*, 28, 734–739.

Pratt, M.W., Luszcz, M.A. and Brown, M.E. (1980). Measuring dimensions of the quality of care in small community residences. *American Journal of Mental Deficiency*, 85(2), 188–194.

Roper, N., Logan, W. and Tierney, A. (1983). *Using a Model of Nursing*. Churchill Livingstone, Edinburgh.

Roy, C. (1976). *Introduction to Nursing – An Adaptation Model*. Prentice-Hall, New Jersey.

Royal College of Nursing. (1989). *An Objective Review and Survey of the Implementation of Care in the Community Initiatives Provided by Health Authorities/Boards within the UK*. Society of Mental Handicap Nursing/Royal College of Nursing, London.

Shearer, A. (1986). *Building Community with People with Mental Handicaps, Their Families and Friends*. Campaign for People with Mental Handicaps/King's Fund, London.

Sines, D.T. (ed.). (1987). *Towards Integration – Comprehensive Services for People with a Mental Handicap*. Harper and Row, London.

Sines, D.T. (1990). *Valuing the Carers: an Investigation of Support Systems Required by Mental Handicap Nurses in Residential Services in the Community*. PhD thesis, University of Southampton.

Sines, D.T. and Bicknell, J. (eds.). (1985). *Caring for Mentally Handicapped People in the Community*. Harper and Row, London.

Spastics Society. (1991). *What is Cerebral Palsy?* The Spastics Society, London.

Towell, D. and Beardshaw, V. (1991). *Enabling Community Integration – The Role of Public Authorities in Promoting an Ordinary Life for People with Learning Disabilities in the 1990s*. King's Fund, London.

United Kingdom Central Council for Nursing, Midwifery and Health Visiting. (1991). *Statistical Analysis of the Council's Professional Register 1 April 1990–31 March 1991*. UKCC, London.

Walker, A. (1989). Community care. In *The New Politics of Welfare – An Agenda for the 1990s?* McCarthy, M. (ed.). Macmillan, London.

Webb, R. and Tossell, D. (1991). *Social Issues for Carers*

– *A Community Care Perspective*. Edward Arnold, London.

Welsh Office. (1983). *The All Wales Strategy*. HMSO, Cardiff.

Wilcock, P. (1987). Life planning. In *Towards Integration – Comprehensive Services for People with a Mental Handicap*, Sines, D. (ed.). Harper and Row, London.

Wolfensberger, W. (1972). *The Principles of Normalisation in Human Services*. National Institute on Mental Retardation, Toronto.

Suggestions for further reading

Abbott, P. and Sapsford, R. (1987). *Community Care for Mentally Handicapped Children: The Origins and Consequences of a Social Policy*. Open University Press, Milton Keynes.

Clarke, D. (1986). *Mentally Handicapped People: Living and Learning*. Baillière Tindall, London.

Hattersley, J., Hosking, G.P., Morrow, D. and Myers, M. (1987). *People with Mental Handicap*. Faber and Faber, London.

Korman, N. and Glennerster, H. (1990). *Hospital Closure: A Political and Economic Study*. Open University Press, Milton Keynes.

Mansell, J. (1989). Evaluation of training in the development of staffed housing for people with mental handicaps. *Mental Handicap Research*, 2(2), 137–151.

McGrath, M. and Grant, G. (1989). *Supporting 'Needs-led' Services: Implications for Planning and Evaluating Services*. Centre for Social Policy Research, Bangor.

O'Brien, J. and Lyle, C. (1987). *Framework for Accomplishment*. Responsive Service Systems Associates, Georgia.

Personal Social Services Research Unit. (1990). *Care in the Community: Lessons from a Demonstration Programme*. PSSRU, Canterbury.

Shanley, E. (1986). *Mental Handicap: A Handbook of Care*. Churchill Livingstone, Edinburgh.

Sutcliffe, J. (1991). *Adults with Learning Difficulties – Education for Choice and Empowerment*. Open University Press, Milton Keynes.

Welsh Office. (1988). *Residential Services for Mentally Handicapped People in Wales: Standards Matrix*. Welsh Office, Cardiff.

Winkler, F. (1991). *Who Protects the Consumer in Community Care?* Greater London Association of Community Health Councils, London.

22

INITIAL CARE OF THE ACUTELY ILL

Marion Richardson

The aim of this chapter is to help prepare the nurse for giving effective care, appropriate to her level of experience, to those with whom she is likely to come into contact in the Accident and Emergency department. (N.B. The patient with diabetes mellitus, whose care is described in this chapter, will be followed up in Chapter 23.)

This chapter covers the following topics:

- Introduction to the work of the A and E department
- The organisation of the A and E department
- Triage
- The scope of practice of the A and E nurse
- Working as a team
- Patients who may present problems
- Violence and aggression
- Legal aspects of A and E care

- Stress
- Reception of clients
- Specific care of the acutely ill
- The patient with:
  —myocardial infarction
  —cerebrovascular accident
  —chest wounds following stabbing
  —diabetes mellitus
  —drug overdose
  —asthma
  —acute abdominal pain

The doors of the Accident and Emergency department flew open and two ambulance personnel rushed through them guiding a stretcher on which lay a young man. They were closely followed by several policemen. The youth was taken immediately to the emergency treatment area and transferred from the stretcher to a trolley. He was clearly unwell – he looked pale and was moaning to himself. The ambulance crew said that he had been involved in a fight and had been stabbed in the chest. They stated that his condition had deteriorated since they arrived at the scene of the incident. The young man became increasingly breathless and began to sweat. His speech became incoherent and barely audible. Within minutes a team of nurses and doctors had surrounded the trolley; the young man's clothes were removed, oxygen was being administered and a cannula had been inserted into his pleural space and connected to an underwater seal drainage system. (An account of this man's continued care will be found on page 665–667.)

This is the generally held view of the type of work which forms the basis of Accident and Emergency (A and E) nursing and it is certainly the sort of situation which every nurse new to this specialty fears and yet hopes to become competent in dealing with. It is precisely this kind of incident which makes A and E nursing so different from other areas of hospital nursing, but it is by no means definitive of the work of the department. A and E work is very varied. Large numbers of clients and their relatives pass through the department and all types of problems are dealt with. The variety of the work is endless. It is possible to be comforting a frightened child who has a dried pea stuck up his nose one minute and caring for a client who has suffered severe burns in an accident the next. It is impossible to know at the start of a shift what will be achieved by the end of it. Sometimes the work is exciting and provides a sense of achievement while at other times it can be mundane or involve situations which leave the staff feeling sickened or wishing that they could have done more. Some nurses thrive in this type of atmosphere and work at their best when faced with the sort of challenge that A and E provides; others find the lack of continuity and the inability to plan their day extremely frustrating. It is natural to feel some trepidation when beginning A and E nursing but the area will have a good complement of qualified and experienced staff who will always be close by. The biggest challenge may be finding something useful to do when a very sick patient arrives as the room suddenly fills with a competent, busy team of nurses and doctors.

A written philosophy of care will generally be available within the department so that staff, clients and visitors are clear as to the rationale of care within the area. The philosophy will reflect the beliefs of the nursing staff as to the needs and rights of their clients and of their own approach to caring for clients and their relatives or friends. It may also reflect the importance placed on the role of the nurse as a health educator and of the department as a learning environment. Such a philosophy will underpin the approach to clients and their care which is demonstrated in the department.

Aspects of A and E nursing

Learning to nurse clients in some specific emergency situations is important but will not form the bulk of the A and E nurse's work. She must learn how to do things quickly but without taking dangerous short cuts. She must be able to deal sensitively and competently with a wide range of people, some of whom will speak no English and many of whom may come from a totally different ethnic and cultural background to her own. Not all of the clients will be polite, clean and friendly and the importance of interpersonal skills and means of communication other than the spoken word will soon become apparent.

There are new skills to learn, new techniques to master and the pressure of the work may reveal facets of the nurse's character and coping mechanisms of which she was previously unaware.

Accident and Emergency departments exist primarily to provide care for the acutely ill or injured. This category includes those with acute medical conditions such as myocardial infarction, cardiac arrest, cerebrovascular accident, hypoglycaemia, asthma and pneumothorax. It also includes those who have suffered traumatic injury, for example burns, fractured bones, head injuries, stab wounds or severe lacerations. There may also be clients who are acutely mentally ill and who may be deluded or hallucinating. Whilst the nurse may have had experience of nursing clients with these conditions, she may never before have seen a client in the acute stage of their illness – actually experiencing the pain of a myocardial infarction or in the acute phase of an asthmatic attack. Many nurses assist at their first cardiac arrest during their allocation to A and E and most find it rewarding to help establish a diagnosis and initiate effective care when a client is brought in unconscious.

Hospitals in inner cities tend to receive fewer clients with major traumatic injury because of the relatively slow traffic speeds in such locations but any department situated near a major road will frequently receive the victims of road traffic accidents. Such clients can sustain severe and multiple injuries which sicken even the most experienced staff members.

The mentally ill client may pose particular problems, especially if none of the staff members on duty is qualified in this aspect of nursing. One such client can quickly disrupt the entire department if not managed appropriately. (The nursing care of clients with acute psychiatric disorders will not be covered in this chapter – the reader is referred to Chapter 20 for further information.)

With all acutely ill clients, assessing priorities of care is vitally important. The nurse will need to work quickly and accurately and must monitor her client's condition constantly so that any deterioration is noted early, reported and dealt with at once.

The acutely ill are not, however, the largest group of clients seen in most A and E departments. Most clients will have sustained minor injuries such as sprains, small burns or lacerations which will not necessitate their admission to hospital. Some may require treatment under local anaesthetic, for example to suture a wound or drain an abscess; others will be X-rayed or have their injuries cleaned and dressed or be given an antitetanus injection. Some A and E departments will have follow-up clinics where clients are seen again to check healing, re-dress wounds, remove sutures or re-apply bandages or plaster casts. Caring for these clients forms the bulk of the A and E nurse's work in most departments. For some nurses, these relatively simple treatments are a disappointment and can appear less than rewarding. It is important to remember that what appears to the professional carer to be just another cut finger needing a suture is a painful, perhaps frightening injury to the client and one which may affect his life substantially for the next few days or weeks.

Some people visit or telephone their local casualty department to seek help and advice. Many people, particularly in large towns and cities which attract visitors and people seeking work, are not registered with a general practitioner and use the A and E department as a substitute. These are one section of a much larger group of clients who might be termed 'inappropriate attenders'. These include clients who use the A and E department because it is convenient to their home or work or because they think they will be seen by a doctor without the need to make an appointment or at whatever time of day or night they choose to present themselves. Many of these clients would be more appropriately dealt with elsewhere. Seeing and treating them in such a specialist department may mean that waiting times for treatment may be delayed for others with more acute problems.

Many A and E departments now have a policy to which they adhere strictly with regard to which client groups will be seen and treated. Those whom they consider to be attending inappropriately are urged to visit a general practitioner or are directed to other applicable agencies such as the Samaritans or a pregnancy advisory service (a list of such agencies is provided at the end of the chapter). In general, clients who have been suffering with a complaint for more than 48 hours will not be seen in an A and E department unless they have been referred there by another agency such as a general practitioner, health visitor or occupational health unit. Other hospitals do not have such a policy and maintain that the hospital is there to serve the local population and that anyone who feels they need to be seen in the A and E department should be seen. This policy is clearly open to abuse and there should be some mechanism to ensure that those with non-urgent complaints do not delay the treatment of those who are seriously ill or injured or who are in the most appropriate place for the care they require. Some of these methods will be looked at in the following sections of this chapter.

The organisation of the A and E department

Layout

Every A and E department is different in terms of layout but all have some features in common whether they are modern, purpose-built departments or old units which have been altered and adapted over the years.

An emergency treatment area or 'resus' (resuscitation) room will be identified. This area is used for caring for the acutely ill and injured requiring, or likely to require, resuscitation and will contain equipment necessary to monitor the condition of the seriously ill and to save and sustain life if necessary. The area may be a room or rooms with several trolleys or simply a designated bay within the unit. In areas where more than one room is available, it is customary to specify the client groups that will be cared for in each room; for example, those with acute medical problems in one, trauma victims in another, or adults in one area, children in the other. The A and E nurse must familiarise herself with the location and working methods of the equipment within this area to ensure that she is ready to care for the clients who are nursed there.

In recent years, some A and E departments have provided special facilities for the care of trauma victims and have been designated as trauma units. Such units generally have a helicopter and crew available on site which can be called upon to facilitate the speedy transfer of trauma victims. Within these departments a strict protocol for trauma care is adhered to so that everyone is familiar with their role and prescribed actions. The A and E nurse can prepare herself for this type of work by undertaking a course in trauma nursing such as the Advanced Trauma Nursing Course or the Trauma Nursing Care Course. These courses are run independently of the various National Boards' Accident and Emergency Nursing courses. (Details of all these and other A and E nursing courses are available through the A and E Nursing Forum at the Royal College of Nursing.)

Most A and E clients are seen and treated not in the emergency room but in the cubicles or bays within the department which enable them to sit or lie down. The bays may be divided by curtains or may be rooms with doors to afford greater privacy. Bays may be designated for the care of specific client groups such as children, or those with eye problems or gynaecological complaints. This means that specific equipment can be appropriately stored and readily available.

One or more theatres is generally available and may be used for the administration of treatment under local, regional or general anaesthesia. Wherever possible, one theatre will be kept for 'clean' procedures such as suturing and another for 'dirty', for example draining abscesses or applying plaster casts.

Many departments have an observation or short-stay ward attached to them where clients who require observation for around 48 hours may be made comfortable and cared for without being admitted to other ward areas unless this becomes necessary. Examples of clients who might be admitted to a short-stay ward are those who have suffered head injuries causing a period of unconsciousness and who require observation for 24 hours to ensure there is no concussion. Patients who have taken a drug overdose may be admitted

to the short-stay ward following treatment so that they can be monitored and any adverse drug effects noted and promptly treated. Others might include those who have been given a general anaesthetic, perhaps to reduce a fracture, and who are unfit to go home. This type of unit is advantageous in that it allows clients to be cared for by the same group of nurses throughout their stay and it does not 'block' the longer-stay beds on the other hospital wards.

The waiting room is the area of A and E where many clients and their relatives spend most of their stay within the department. It is an excellent place for passing on information to the clients about the management of care within the department and on health education matters. Some waiting areas house a television or video for the use of waiting clients.

Nurse triage

Nuttall (1986) demonstrated that waiting times in A and E are universally lengthy and this may prove dangerous for the severely ill. It also means that a poor service is provided for those with more minor injuries (Blythin, 1988). In an attempt to rectify this situation, nurse triage is being widely implemented in A and E departments. The system of triage was developed in war time as a means of categorising the wounded into priority order for treatment. It was not until 1960 that the system was adopted in a wider context in the USA and it was not formally introduced into the UK until the 1980s. Each department will have a specific system but all aim to provide a safer environment for the ill and injured.

All clients presenting in the department will be seen as soon as possible by the triage nurse who will have received guidance and training in this aspect of A and E management. Her role is to elicit the relevant history, give any first aid treatment required and to give the client a priority rating before asking him to wait to be seen. Differing numbers of categories are used in different departments (usually between three and five). An example of the triage categories which may be used is given in Table 22.1. Usually guidelines and protocols are formed and adhered to to ensure uniformity of categorisation. The client is then informed of the likely waiting time and the fact that others who arrive after him, but are given a higher priority weighting, will be seen and treated before him. If their attendance is felt to be inappropriate,

Table 22.1 *Suggested triage categories*

1	**Life-threatening**	Over-rides all other categories
2	**Urgent**	e.g. profuse haemorrhage, unconscious, unstable myocardial infarction
3	**Semi-urgent**	e.g. haemorrhage, fracture, great pain, drug overdose
4	**Non-urgent**	Injuries or illnesses which do not require detailed investigation or treatment
5	**Delay acceptable**	Injuries or illnesses requiring minimal investigation or treatment

they may be given advice as to how to seek help. Mallett and Woolwich (1990) demonstrated that whilst overall waiting times within the department were not reduced, the time for which clients waited before being clinically assessed was significantly reduced and those clients who were given high priority ratings were seen and treated more quickly. In addition, the triage nurse is able to communicate with clients and their relatives within the department and constantly reassess the needs of clients within the waiting area.

Telephone triage has been adopted in some areas so that clients who are uncertain as to whether they need to attend an A and E department may be given guidance over the telephone and, if necessary, advised to attend at a specific time.

All information gleaned and advice given by the triage nurse is documented in the client's notes.

Emergency nurse practitioners

Recent years have seen the emergence of the role of clinical nurse practitioner to whom clients may be referred (Jones, 1990). Lee (1988) describes her as having the knowledge, skill and authority to make professional, autonomous decisions about the initial assessment of the client. She may initiate primary management for that client and, if necessary, client care. The nurse practitioner may initiate certain diagnostic tests and may prescribe some treatments within agreed policies. Her remit may include treating those with minor injuries, requesting X-rays, plastering, suturing and referring clients to other agencies. Again, protocols and guidelines are drawn up and adhered to and appro-

priate training and education must be available to the A and E nurse who wishes to specialise in this way. The system is open to abuse by clients who regard this as an alternative to attending their GP surgery and the nurse practitioner must beware of seeing only those clients whose attendance in A and E is regarded as inappropriate.

The scope of practice of the A and E nurse

One of the solutions to reducing the waiting time for clients in A and E is to allow the nurse to expand her traditional role to include some of the aspects of client care that have historically been regarded as the work of the medical staff or of technicians. Normal staff ratios in A and E mean that there are relatively more nurses than doctors and in this way medical staff can be freed to see other clients. This can be rewarding for the nurse because it increases the scope of her client care and extends her field of skill and knowledge. By undertaking further training and expanding her role, the nurse's practice may include administering Entonox, suturing, applying plaster casts, venepuncture, recording electrocardiograms, etc. As always, protocols and guidelines should be set and local policies adhered to. The nurse should not feel pressured to take on these roles without adequate planned education and training. The UKCC *Scope of Professional Practice* (1992) document makes it clear that the nurse is responsible for her own actions and for ensuring her own competence when extending the scope of her practice. She must also acknowledge her own limitations.

Working as a team

Team work is vital if care of the acutely ill is to be carried out expertly and efficiently. The A and E team consists not only of doctors and nurses but also many other personnel from both within and outside the hospital (Fig. 22.1). Liaison and effective communication within this team is essential to ensure optimum client care.

Hospital staff

A and E nurses are trained to cope with emergency situations and will be able to assess priorities of need, plan and give care to meet those needs almost without thinking – there is no time for writing detailed care plans in an emergency! A

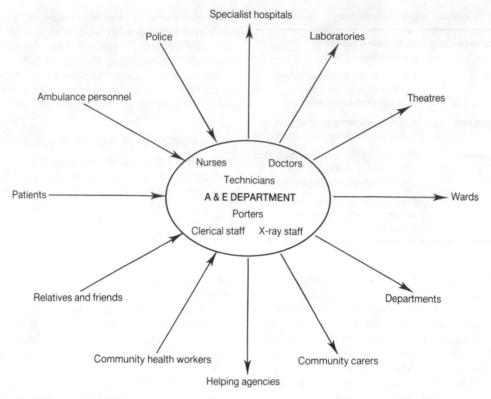

Fig. 22.1 *Working as a team*

doctor will usually direct the team caring for a particular client. This may be the casualty consultant or one of his team or another senior doctor if he has been asked to attend. An anaesthetist may also be present if needed. Normally the most senior doctor will make decisions about treatment in consultation with his medical and nursing colleagues. Other hospital personnel who are likely to be involved in a client's care are listed in Table 22.2.

The ambulance service

The ambulance service provides a remarkable link between the community and the A and E department. Ambulance crews are highly skilled and many have now undertaken intensive paramedical training and can stabilise a client by giving drugs on medical advice, interpreting cardiac rhythms, defibrillating, intubating and setting up intravenous infusions. They are expert at administering first aid in the most awkward and dangerous situations and the care which they provide for the

client before he arrives at the hospital may well save his life and prevent further injury or deterioration. In most areas the local crews are well known to the departmental staff and may be involved in the emergency care of the client within the department. Their information and history sheets provide important information about the client's condition since the time of the incident and they often provide vital details about how an incident occurred. They provide an essential link in the client care chain and every effort should be made to maintain their friendly cooperation.

The police force

The police also liaise closely with emergency department staff and will usually attend the hospital following any road traffic accident. They will provide assistance in identifying individuals, will check details such as whether a given address is correct and will convey information to the next of kin if requested to do so. They will provide an escort if a rapid ambulance transfer of a client to

Table 22.2. The caring team

- Reception clerks who ensure that the patient's details are documented and any previous hospital notes and X-rays located

- X-ray staff. Many large A and E departments have X-ray facilities with radiographers available at all times; others will have trained staff available 'on call'

- Theatre staff – who must be prepared to receive emergency cases within minutes

- Staff in the intensive care unit (ICU) who must be prepared to do likewise

- Technicians and laboratory staff who may be required to perform electrocardiograms (ECGs), analyse specimens of body fluids and cross-match blood

- Security officers and porters

- Chaplains and priests who may be asked to say the last rites for a dying patient or talk to distressed relatives

another specialist hospital is needed and will remove clients from the department at the request of staff or give assistance in difficult or violent situations. Again, maintenance of friendly relations with members of the police force will enhance the effective, all-round care of the client.

The primary health care team

General practitioners, district nurses, practice nurses, health visitors, social workers, etc. have important links with the A and E department. Many clients are referred by them and will return to their care once they leave the hospital. Communication with them is essential if continuity of client care is to be achieved.

The special needs of children in A and E

Research by the British Paediatric Association (1985 and 1987) has shown that between 20% and 25% of the child population of the UK will attend A and E departments each year (a total figure of 2–2.5 million). Most of them have little or no experience of hospitals and particularly of the emergency care areas. Caring for children in A and E can present problems for all concerned unless forethought is given to their special needs.

Several studies have looked at the effect of school-based education programmes to prepare the children for the possibility of hospital admission. McGarvey (1983) and Elkins and Roberts (1984) reported fewer fears, improved understanding and easier adjustment to hospital admission in the children they studied. This increasing awareness of the effect of information and preparation has led to nurses being invited, or asking, to speak to groups of school children, and has also included the setting up of relevant hospital play corners in classrooms and to organising visits by groups of children to their local A and E department.

There is usually very little time to prepare the ill or injured child for the fact that he is going to A and E and inappropriate handling of such a child can heighten his fear. Laing (1988) argues that all children should be given a higher priority rating at the point of triage so that their waiting time is minimised. Others have found this to be unacceptable within their departments, particularly in inner city areas.

Many departments have part of the waiting area specially adapted to provide facilities for children. This may involve decorating the walls with colourful posters or providing suitable toys for the children to play with or a selection of videos which they may watch. Such an area should be within clear view of the staff since the condition of small children is prone to rapid change. It is now common practice to have a treatment area which is suitable for children within the department. Again this could be appropriately decorated so as not to look too clinical and unfamiliar.

The benefits are well recognised of allowing a parent or guardian to remain with a child whenever possible. This can provide a familiar face and comfort in an otherwise unfamiliar setting. If appropriate, the accompanying adult should be encouraged to help as much as possible in caring for the child. Explanations of any necessary treatments should be given in terms that both can understand and such treatments carried out efficiently and quickly. The child may be given a 'bravery award' of some sort when treatment is concluded – perhaps a sticker or badge or a certificate to keep.

Unless emergency care is required, the child should be given time to settle into the new surroundings before treatment is carried out. This should be done quickly and efficiently by a skilled nurse. Examinations should be made as much fun as time permits, allowing the child to hold or use equipment if applicable. Any equipment needed should be prepared out of the child's sight and explanations about what will happen should be brief and given immediately prior to the event so that the child does not have time to worry. If possible, the child should sit on her parent's or a nurse's knee though sometimes restraint will be necessary. Wrapping babies or small children securely in a blanket whilst treatment is carried out can save time and tears in the long run.

There has been extensive debate about who should care for children in the A and E department. Should it be a nurse whose name appears on Part 8 of the UKCC Register and who is recognised as a sick children's nurse, or is an experienced A and E nurse best? It would clearly be ideal if the child could be cared for by a nurse appropriately qualified and expert in both areas of expertise but such nurses are not always available. Many departments now have a children's nurse among their complement of staff and make use of her expertise in a variety of ways. Webb and Cleaver (1991) argue that the presence of a paediatric nurse in A and E should be considered a necessity rather than a luxury. Her primary responsibilities would be to assess the needs of chidren and their families following their arrival in the department and to ensure that good practice continues in her absence through an agreed philosophy and written standards of care.

Whether there is a designated nurse within the department or not, there are certainly some nurses who are naturally adept at dealing with children and others who are not. The choice of the correct nurse to deal with a child may help to make them less fearful during their stay and in the future.

The condition of a sick child can deteriorate very quickly and many who are brought in are acutely ill on arrival. Speed, calm and efficiency are essential when dealing with such children. They will have no wish to play games or look at posters until they feel better. Again, the carer's help should be enlisted wherever practical though the nurse must be constantly aware of the concern the carer will feel for the child's welfare and of the fact that there may be other pressing factors which need to be dealt with (other siblings at home, for example). Both child and carer should be encompassed in the nurse's care perspective.

Caring for the client's relatives and friends

Many clients will be accompanied to the A and E department by a relative or close friend. The relative may be able to provide useful information about what has happened to the client, particularly if the latter is drowsy, confused or unconscious. It is all too easy to forget waiting relatives in the hustle and bustle of caring for or treating casualties but the nurse must make every effort to keep them informed of what is happening to the client. Whenever possible, relatives should be allowed to sit with clients or, if this is inadvisable, they could be informed of the likely wait and advised to go for a cup of tea or a meal in the interim.

Imparting information to visitors is particularly important if the client is seriously ill or gravely injured. It is unfair to be other than truthful about the client's condition. Whenever possible, such relatives should be allowed to remain in the department, in a separate room if one is available, where they can talk together and make tea or coffee. If the client is likely to die, every effort should be made to warn the relatives in advance. Parkes (1985) and Pisarick (1981) concluded that even the shortest period of warning of the impending death of a loved one is better than none at all. It is not always possible to allow relatives to be with a dying client and some may not wish to be present. Relatives should always be warned about how the client will look when they are taken to see him, whether he is alive or dead, and special mention should be made of any intravenous infusions, monitors or other equipment attached to or beside him.

In the event of a client's death

If a client dies, either in the department or before his arrival there, the family and friends should be taken to a quiet room away from the main working area. The news will be broken by a doctor or a qualified nurse and ambiguous terms such as 'passed over' or 'left us' should be avoided since they are open to misinterpretation. The words 'died' or 'dead' should be used so that there can be no misunderstanding. Studies by Lenaghan (1986) and Wright (1989 and 1991) have identified the provision of a private waiting area as one of the most helpful activities following the death of a loved one.

Wright's 1989 study showed that the nurse who stays with the relatives is always remembered, especially if she deals with the situation skilfully and sensitively. Sitting down with relatives and showing empathy with them are seen as highly significant and contribute to the quality of support.

Relatives who have had no time to prepare for the sudden death of a loved one will need to talk and ask questions about exactly what happened and about the last minutes of their loved one's life. This is recognised as a normal part of adjustment to the news of sudden death and every attempt should be made to answer honestly and truthfully, stressing any positive aspects such as the fact that death was instant and probably without pain or that all the correct things were done.

Reactions to sudden bad news vary widely and the nurse should be prepared for any reaction from verbal abuse through uncontrolled weeping to hysterical laughter. Occasionally relatives will refuse to believe the truth and may even deny it once they have seen the body. A nurse should remain with the family to offer comfort and to answer their questions. A cup of tea or coffee may be appreciated. The nurse should aim to accept reactions to shock and to allow the grieving process to begin.

If the dead client is a child, the experience may be a particularly traumatic one for all concerned and the nurse may find herself weeping openly with the parents. This is a natural reaction to a tragedy and should not be thought of as unprofessional.

Viewing the body as soon after death as possible was shown by Wright to be of positive benefit to grieving relatives. This was valuable not only so that they could say goodbye but so that they could see the reality of the situation. There are clearly instances when this is not possible or advisable, but it should be allowed whenever possible. The relatives must always have the final right of choice as to whether or not to view the body but sensitive

guidance from the A and E staff may help them in their decision.

The nurse who has spent time with grieving relatives who were previously total strangers to her will need time to recover her own thoughts and emotions once they have left and should try to talk over the event with a trained staff member as soon as possible (see also Chapter 11). A counselling service may be available within the hospital or locality, of which the A and E nurse can avail herself.

Clients who may present problems

Not all clients who attend the emergency department are pleasant or polite and the nurse may be exposed to a number of groups of people with whom she has had no previous contact.

Alcohol abusers

Many road traffic accidents, muggings and other violent incidents are alcohol-related and the A and E nurse will regularly find herself dealing with clients who have had too much to drink.

Alcohol affects people differently and some clients may be very happy and eager to laugh at anything, including the injuries they have sustained. They usually feel little or no pain because of the analgesic effect of the alcohol and are only too keen to oblige with any necessary treatments. The best policy is usually to laugh along with them whilst trying to keep them on the couch or in the cubicle. The problem is more likely to be one of convincing them that something is wrong, particularly if surgery or hospital admission is indicated.

Other clients who have abused alcohol will be aggressive or perhaps even violent. If allowed to remain in the general waiting area they may quickly disrupt the entire department, hurling abuse and sometimes furniture at anyone within reach. Many feel 'trapped' in the hospital and are anxious to escape, particularly if they think the police are likely to arrive to interview them. These clients are usually male and if possible should be dealt with by males who should be firm and persuasive. In general, whilst queue-jumping is not to be advocated, such clients are best dealt with promptly and ushered off the premises as soon as possible. Dealing with those who become violent will be discussed later in the chapter.

Some persistent alcohol abusers will be well known to the staff as regular visitors. These people will drink anything alcoholic and it is vital to ensure that any suitable substances, particularly methylated spirit, are locked away securely. It is not uncommon for these visitors to arrive in pairs so that one can keep the staff occupied whilst the other seeks out any unlocked cupboards in out-of-the-way areas. Such clients can be very devious and may become verbally or physically abusive if challenged.

Drug abusers

Drug addicts are also frequent visitors, particularly in large towns and cities, and many will be known to the staff by name. They are often found unconscious by a member of the public, often in a public convenience, following their latest 'fix' and are brought in by ambulance. Most departments have their own policy guidelines for dealing with drug addicts which usually entails placing them in the recovery position on a mattress on the floor and allowing them to 'sleep it off'. Naloxone (Narcan) is not used to reverse the effect of the opiates unless there is cause for concern about the client's condition or any doubt as to the cause of their unconsciousness. Two nurses should check the pockets of these clients' clothes for any other drugs which should be labelled and correctly stored until the client wakens. The drugs are the property of the client and should be returned to him. When they waken, drug addicts are usually eager to leave and go out to find their next 'fix'. They may insist that they had drugs on them when they arrived and that these have been 'stolen' whilst they were asleep – for this reason a careful record should always be kept. It is also essential to ensure that all hospital drugs are kept locked in appropriate cupboards since such clients will not hesitate to help themselves.

The nurse dealing with drug addicts should bear in mind that many of them are carriers of hepatitis B or the human immunodeficiency virus (HIV) and she should take all necessary precautions when caring for them (see Chapter 16).

These people often spend night after night in various A and E departments and little can be done for them in the long term unless they decide to seek help for themselves.

Solvent abusers

The sniffing of solvents used in glues and cleaning agents, lighter gas and gas from aerosol cans tends to occur in the younger age groups (12 to 16). McGrath and Bowker (1987) describe two phases of mood which follow glue solvent inhalation: first, intoxication with euphoria and exhilaration and sometimes hallucination, and then a period where cerebral depressant effects are noticeable as slurred speech, ataxia and drowsiness. These effects are achieved quickly and fade quickly but bizarre behaviour may occur and lead to accidents or render the inhaler unconscious. Care consists of ensuring that a clear airway is maintained and of treating any other symptoms which arise. The client should be detained in the department until the intoxicating effects of the substance have worn off (unless admission to a ward is indicated). An interview with a social worker may be offered if this seems appropriate but, sadly, it is often impossible to help these young people as they commonly resent all forms of authority including that of their parents.

Munchausen's syndrome

Clients with this condition present in A and E with fictitious disorders in an attempt to gain either drugs or hospital admission or both. McGrath and Bowker (1987) list the most common presenting complaints as abdominal pain, usually colic, haemorrhage, neurological symptoms, myocardial infarction or pulmonary embolus. The client will generally give an extremely convincing performance. Others will swallow objects suchs as coins or open safety pins in order to obtain surgical treatment.

These clients are often difficult to identify and assess since they tend to travel all over the country visiting different A and E departments and may only visit a particular area once a year or so. Something in their behaviour or medical history may arouse the suspicions of the staff and analgesic drugs should be withheld until further enquiries are made. Such clients may become aggressive if questioned in detail and most will leave the department quickly if they realise they are suspected. Many departments have a list of such clients with description, names used (they usually have a number of aliases) and presenting symptoms. Other hospitals in the area should be contacted and given relevant details so that as little time as possible is wasted in dealing with these people.

Vagrants

Vagrants and other persons of no fixed abode will also be regular visitors to inner city A and Es, particularly in winter when nights are cold and sleeping rough is difficult. It is not uncommon to find them sleeping on chairs in a quiet corner of the department in the middle of the night. Heartless as it may seem, they must be removed, by the security staff or police if necessary (it rarely is), or word will soon spread that a blind eye is being turned and the department will be full.

Obviously those who are ill must be seen and treated. Many vagrants do not wash themselves or their clothes and are infested with lice. It is wise to wear protective clothing when caring for these clients and to be alert for head lice, body lice and pubic lice ('crabs'). The use of protective clothing should be explained sensitively to the client and he should be accorded the same dignity and respect as every patient.

Many are extremely apologetic and embarrassed about their state; others will be rude and abusive. It is important if these clients are undressed that their clothing and property are searched carefully before being tied securely in a plastic bag or bin sack as they often carry large amounts of money. If clients are to be admitted to the ward, it is usual to bathe them and wash their hair with appropriate disinfectant solutions in the A and E department, some of which have special bath or shower rooms for this purpose. If possible, the clothes should be sent for incineration once the client's written consent has been obtained. New clothes will be supplied by the social work department prior to the client's discharge.

The cubicle in which they have been examined will require fumigation once the client has left the department and, for this reason, a room with a door should be used in preference to a curtained cubicle.

Violence and aggression

A number of factors lead to aggressive behaviour in the acute care environment and aggression, if mishandled, can soon turn to violence. It is not always the client who becomes aggressive but often the relatives or friends who accompany him. Long waiting times, lack of information about what is happening, fear, alcohol or drugs and a wish to look 'big' in front of others are some of the reasons identified as precipitating aggressive behaviour. What begins as verbal abuse may quickly turn into disruptive or physically violent behaviour if not rapidly defused. With experience it is possible to identify those persons who are likely to become aggressive before the situation actually arises. Communication is vital, whether it be a general announcement in the waiting room about the cause of any delay or individual explanations to clients and their relatives about what is happening and how much longer they are likely to have to wait. The triage nurse is usually in an ideal position to disseminate information of this sort as she is aware of who is waiting to be seen and of the overall workload of the department.

The guidelines for dealing with aggression in the A and E department produced by the Accident and Emergency Nursing Forum (1989) of the Royal College of Nursing stress the importance of preventing violence from occurring by all means possible.

If an individual begins to get aggressive or argumentative, every effort should be made to find the cause of his discontent so that the problem can be addressed. If he is sitting, the nurse should sit beside him and not remain standing as he may perceive this as a threatening posture. It is inadvisable to touch an angry client since it may provoke physical violence in return. Help should be sought if the client refuses to calm down once explanations have been given. He should be removed from the department if this is appropriate or 'guarded' by a security officer or police officer if he requires medical attention.

Groups of youths may accompany an injured friend and become rowdy and disruptive. They should be approached at once with a friendly but firm warning that their behaviour is unacceptable. If this tactic fails, the ringleader should be identified and isolated as the other group members will often calm down when leaderless. The situation must not be allowed to get out of hand before the hospital security officers or the police force are called to remove them – it is not unknown for violent fights to occur inside an A and E department.

Should violence erupt within the department, help must be summoned immediately. In many inner city hospitals nurses carry alarms and have emergency call bells to summon security or police officers. In places renowned for their violent clients, security officers will be on duty within the department. Nurses should aim not to become involved in the fighting and not to become the victim of an attack. It is advisable to remain in the main well-lit area of the department at night and certainly not to leave this area without a colleague.

If the aggressive client is in a room or cubicle for observation, the nurse should ensure that she does not become trapped inside with him. She should always make sure she has an escape route and that the client cannot place himself between her and the door. Someone who is angry can display extreme strength and if physical restraint is necessary it is advisable to wait until sufficient help (preferably male) arrives. When restraint is attempted, the client's fists, feet and head should be avoided.

Self-defence

Attacks do sometimes happen in spite of all preventive measures being employed and in these circumstances the nurse has no choice but to defend herself. More injuries than necessary may be inflicted if the nurse is unable to put aside her caring role immediately and consider her own safety first. The following simple guidelines are recommended for those who find themselves in the position of being attacked:

(1) Shout loudly for help.

(2) Attempt to release the attacker's grip by causing him acute pain in one or more sensitive areas (see below).

(3) Run away as soon as his grip is released.

If attacked from the front, any of the following may help to secure the victim's release: kneeing the assailant in the groin with maximum force, pushing fingers up his nostrils, pinching the inside of his thigh as hard as possible, kicking his shins. Aim should be made for any vulnerable areas within reach – this will, in part, be dictated by the position in which the victim is held.

If attacked from behind it is best to aim for the assailant's shins. He should be kicked hard with the heel of the victim's shoe which can then be scraped down the lower part of his leg.

There is no place in such a situation for gentle action. The first attack should be intended to secure release from the assailant and strength, speed and surprise will all help to achieve this. As soon as the grip is released, the victim must run. No attempt should be made to try and reason with the client.

Following the occurrence of any violent incident a detailed account should be written and signed by victim and witnesses and any appropriate hospital documentation completed. The police force, if called to the incident, will advise on any further steps to be taken.

Legal aspects

The nurse working in A and E should be aware of certain legal aspects and implications of her work.

Patients' property

In the rush and excitement of emergency care, it is vital not to neglect or mislay any client's property. Often the client does not realise something is missing until he is ready for discharge some weeks later and difficulties can arise unless accurate records are kept. It is always wise to keep together all the property of a client and to search through it as soon as possible, listing it in detail. This is particularly important if there are valuables such as money or jewellery. Note, too, if a client is *not* wearing a watch or carrying any money so that there is a written record should any confusion arise. If the client is unfit to make a decision, his valuables should be stored in a safe place in accordance with hospital procedure. Otherwise he should be advised that the hospital authorities disclaim responsibility for his property and that he should deposit it in the hospital safe. The client should always be given a receipt for anything that is taken from him. Property should not be handed to relatives other than at the client's specific request and written documentation of this should be kept. When a client leaves the department, all his property, including receipts for articles taken into safe custody, should go with him, preferably in one large bag clearly labelled with his name and destination.

Consent to treatment

A person is regarded in law as able to give consent if he is able to understand what is being said to him and to make a decision based on that information. There is no predetermined age limit but, in practice, 16 years is generally regarded as the minimum age for consent to hospital treatment.

The procedure(s) involved should be explained to the client by a doctor, whose responsibility it is to ensure that written, informed consent is obtained. In the case of those under the age of 16, consent is generally obtained from the parent or guardian who should be contacted and asked to come to the department as soon as possible. In an emergency a doctor may decide to treat a minor having received verbal consent over the telephone from a responsible adult or may accept the child's own consent.

A nurse should not accept, nor take responsibility for accepting, verbal consent.

The medical team may assume the consent of an unconscious client to any treatment necessary to save life or limb or to alleviate great pain. They may also act despite refusal of consent from a client's relative in these circumstances (Young, 1991).

Telephone enquiries

A number of people will telephone the A and E department seeking advice or information. It is advisable, without being rude or abrupt, not to give advice but to suggest that the individual seek help from the most appropriate source. This may be the A and E department, his GP or some other agency.

Information should never be given to anyone about the condition of a client without first checking that this is acceptable to him. Details should never be disclosed over the telephone. It is generally best not to break sudden, unexpected bad news over the telephone but to ask relatives to attend the department or the police to go to their home to inform them in person.

Informing the police

Often police officers will arrive with the casualties of a road traffic accident and will be aware of the circumstances and of the injuries sustained. The police do not normally have the right to medical information contained in the client's notes without his permission. They have no right to interview a client unless they wish to arrest him and may only do so when he is medically fit to be seen. Most clients will, however, agree to be interviewed by a police officer and relevant information will normally be made available to them. In general, friendly relationships with the police force are easily maintained.

Medical and nursing records

The medical and nursing notes of a client may be used as legal evidence if necessary. This should be borne in mind when making any entries to these documents. Abbreviations should be avoided and any observations made should be accurately recorded and timed. Any extra sheets of documentation, such as fluid balance sheets, head injury charts and drug charts, must be clearly marked with the client's name and kept together with his notes. It is all too easy to lose loose pieces of paper when a client is being transferred around the hospital.

Confidentiality

It is the nurse's duty to maintain her client's confidentiality (UKCC, 1987 and 1992) and this must always be borne in mind. There may, however, be times when the nurse has information which she feels she must pass on – for example, if she feels that her client presents a danger to himself or others. In such circumstances the nurse must weigh her professional duty of confidentiality against her duty as a citizen in making a decision about her actions.

Stress

The stress experienced by those working in an A and E department can be intense. Anyone can present through the doors including the severely injured, the dead and the dying and the nurse has only seconds to prepare herself to deal with the situation. Fear of the unknown is recognised as a potent stress agent (Thompson, 1983). Sudden, tragic death is commonly encountered and comforting bereaved relatives can be one of the most difficult duties of a nurse. The department can become extremely crowded and busy, resulting in long waits to see the doctor so that the nurse feels she has no time to do anything properly and little time to spend getting to know her patients. There is little continuity of care in the long term and unless one makes an effort to find out how a particular patient is progressing there is not the reward of seeing him improve. Violence and aggression are frequent occurrences in many departments and the nurse may feel very threatened, particularly during the night. The rewards, though, can be immense and the excitement of assisting in an emergency, and of helping to save life or initiate treatment for an acutely sick person, can provide particular satisfaction. Most trained staff are aware of the situations that cause stress and will be prepared to talk them through, either at the time or soon afterwards in order to alleviate any feelings of tension or worry. However, it should be remembered that not everyone will enjoy Accident and Emergency work, though most will find some aspects of it enjoyable in the extreme.

Reception of patients

The Accident and Emergency department has been described as the 'shop window of the hospital'. For some patients it will be the only time they have been in a hospital and for others first impressions of the hospital are gained in the department. This means that the maintenance of high standards of care is particularly important since the rest of the hospital's nursing staff may be judged by the standards of those in this small area.

(1) The nurse working in the A and E department must learn to hide her feelings of fear, horror or uncertainty from her patients. If these are allowed to surface she may fail to win her patient's confidence and trust. It behoves her to remember always that the patient's feelings are usually far stronger than her own.

(2) The reception of patients must be carefully managed. An impression of quiet, friendly efficiency must be conveyed in the first few seconds of the encounter with each new, strange patient. The client who feels at once that he is in safe, caring hands is far more likely

to cooperate with and respond to any treatment.

(3) Standards of appearance are important and the sight of a well-groomed, neatly attired nurse can bring great comfort and relief to the acutely injured.

Specific care of the acutely ill

The remainder of this chapter is devoted to seven patient care studies which are representative of Accident and Emergency nursing. They have been chosen to include both medical and surgical conditions, a wide age range encompassing sudden unexpected illness or accident, and the acute presentation of longer term 'illness. Each study highlights different aspects of care which the A and E nurse will be required to give.

Care plans have been included for some patients. These are based on Roper's Activities of Daily Living model (Roper *et al.*, 1985). The appropriate activity is indicated in a box beside each problem.

The use of this model should enable the reader to become familiar with the priorities and concepts of A and E nursing. Such familiarity will make it easier for her to adjust her thinking to other models of care. The Roper model is not universally regarded as suitable for A and E care and the learner may be faced with using a model with which she is unfamiliar and which is not used in other areas of the hospital. For this reason care plans are not given in all the following studies but rather priorities are stressed and major areas of nursing concern indicated.

The writing of lengthy care plans in A and E is inappropriate for many patients with minor injuries. In an emergency there is no time to write down other than essential details until the patient's condition is stable. It is, however, crucial to the administration of effective nursing care that the A and E nurse is able to think in terms of her patient's problems or deficits, and how she will attempt to solve or remedy them. Constant evaluation of the effectiveness of care and re-adjustment of plans is vital if the nurse is to respond effectively and rapidly to changes in her patient's condition. There should be no presumption as to the care that might be required by a particular patient and the A and E nurse must, at all times, be flexible and open-minded so that she is constantly able to re-appraise her patient's condition and adapt her care to fit his changing needs.

Mr Frederick Davies who suffered a myocardial infarction

The profile given in Fig. 22.4 shows a 52 year old man who had suffered a *myocardial infarction* – what he would describe as a 'heart attack'.

Related structure and function

The heart is a hollow muscular structure about the size of the owner's clenched fist, lying in the thorax. It is made of specialised striated muscle which contracts and relaxes constantly and rhythmically in response to electrical impulses, to keep blood flowing around the body. Cardiac muscle, or the myocardium, has fibres which branch and re-branch to form a meshlike sheet of muscle in which it is difficult to see where one fibre ends and the next begins. This arrangement allows electrical impulses and subsequent waves of muscle fibre contraction to spread evenly throughout the entire heart. The heart beat is generated in the pacemaker cells of the sino-atrial node in the right atrium and spreads throughout the atria (Fig. 22.2). The impulse cannot pass straight through to the ventricles

because of the insulating effect of the fibroten-donous ring of tissue at the junction between the atria and ventricles. The impulse is picked up at the atrio-ventricular node and passes down the fibres of the bundle of His to spread through the ventricular myocardium from the base of the heart upwards via the Purkinje fibres (Fig. 22.2). Myocardial contraction follows the wave of electrical impulse so that the atria contract from the top to complete filling of the ventricles. The ventricles contract from their bases to push blood up and out to the lungs (pulmonary circulation) and the rest of the body (systemic circulation). The thickness of the myocardium is related to the amount of work it does and that of the left ventricle is much thicker (approximately five times) than the right to enable it to pump blood with sufficient force to circulate around the body.

In order to maintain this constant activity, the myocardium requires a rich blood supply to provide it with oxygen and nutrients. This need is met by the two *coronary arteries* which branch from the aorta just as it leaves the heart, slightly distal to (i.e. away from) the cusps of the aortic valve. The right coronary artery branches supply the muscle of the right atrium and right ventricle and the diaphragmatic surface of the left ventricle. The left coronary artery is larger and its branches supply the left atrium and the remainder of the left ventricle, as may be seen in Fig. 22.3. The left coronary artery has two main branches – the anterior descending artery and the circumflex artery. Blood circulates through the complex capillary network of the coronary circulation carrying oxygen and nutrients to the heart muscle and re-

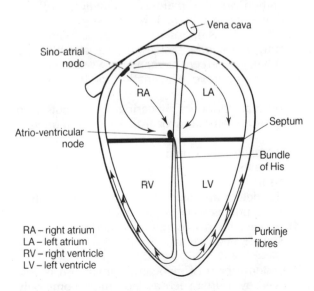

Fig. 22.2 *The conducting systems of the heart*

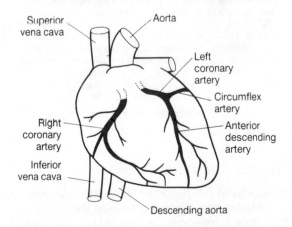

Fig. 22.3 *The coronary arteries*

moving the waste products of metabolism. The blood is drained via the coronary capillaries to a large vein, the coronary sinus, which empties into the right atrium.

If the coronary arteries become obstructed or narrowed, the blood supply and therefore oxygen supply to the heart muscle will be reduced and the heart will function less well. Narrowing is usually caused by a build-up of cholesterol and other fatty deposits in the vessel walls (atherosclerosis) and may become severe when combined with a degenerative hardening of the arteries (arteriosclerosis). Inadequate blood supply to an area of myocardium will result in the pain of *angina pectoris*. The pain is usually felt centrally in the chest, though it may radiate to the back, arms or neck and it is often brought on by physical exercise which increases the oxygen requirement of the myocardium.

Sometimes a small piece of the fatty plaque breaks off and blocks a tiny coronary artery, thus cutting off the blood supply to the area of muscle supplied by it. Such an area of myocardium dies and the patient suffers a myocardial infarction or 'heart attack'. The damage is irreparable and 40% of patients will die from their myocardial infarction (Fry, 1968).

Myocardial infarction is thought to be associated with cigarette smoking, diets high in saturated fats, especially cholesterol, and stress. A familial history of myocardial infarction is perhaps the most important factor.

Mr Frederick Davies, a 52-year-old business executive, was walking back to his office following a working lunch with some clients when he experienced severe central chest pain which he described as 'crushing'. The pain spread to his left shoulder and down his left arm. He was unable to walk further and his companions telephoned for an ambulance which brought him to hospital within minutes. On arrival he was smartly dressed but looked sweaty, pale and greyish in colour. He was still in considerable pain and finding breathing difficult.

Fig. 22.4 *Profile: Mr Frederick Davies*

Nursing care for Mr Davies

On arrival at the hospital, Mr Davies was greeted by the triage nurse who recognised the seriousness of his condition and accompanied him to the emergency room before handing over his care to a col-

league. The ambulance crew transferred him from their stretcher to a hard-based trolley in the emergency room. A hard-based trolley is important when caring for patients following myocardial infarction since it may be necessary to perform external cardiac massage and this cannot be carried out effectively on a soft trolley. It is also necessary to nurse the patient in an area where resuscitation equipment and emergency drugs are readily available should they be needed.

The nurses assigned to his care explained what they wanted to do and helped Mr Davies to undress – they asked him to do as little as possible since stress to the damaged heart should be minimised. He was helped into a hospital gown. All his clothes were folded and put into a polythene bag which was secured and labelled with Mr Davies' name. He had numerous credit cards, a cheque book, travellers' cheques and £73 in cash in his pockets in addition to some gold cufflinks and an expensive watch. One nurse began to collect relevant information about Mr Davies and his condition whilst the other made arrangements for the safe storage of his valuables following hospital policy.

Mr Davies' temperature was recorded (37.4°C) and the nurse assessed and recorded his pulse rate (88 beats per minute and slightly irregular), respirations (28 per minute and shallow) and blood pressure (130/85 mmHg). These initial observations are important since any future improvement or deterioration in the patient's condition will be measured against them. The nurse also noted that Mr Davies was in pain, looked pale and felt clammy and said he thought he was about to die. Twenty-eight percent oxygen was given via a ventimask to improve oxygenation of the myocardium.

The main priorities in caring for patients who have just suffered a myocardial infarction are:

(1) To relieve their pain;
(2) To avoid undue exertion in order to rest the heart;
(3) To detect any signs of deterioration in their condition as soon as possible;
(4) To keep the patient informed and respond sensitively to questions.

The intense pain of myocardial infarction is best relieved by a drug such as morphine, commonly given intravenously by a doctor. The nurse can help to relieve pain by caring for her patient in a calm and efficient manner. It is also known that information about what is happening, and why this is so, helps to reduce pain and fear (Hayward, 1975). Since pain and fear are two important symptoms of myocardial infarction, the nurse should take extra care to explain as much as she is able to her patient. The risk of death following MI decreases markedly with time, the first hours being the period of greatest risk (Colling *et al.*, 1976). Again, explanation is necessary if patient cooperation is to be achieved. Many patients who suffer MI are at the peak of their careers and are unused to resting or having things done for them and will be most reluctant to be undressed or use a urinal instead of the lavatory unless they are apprised of the reasons for so doing.

Mr Davies was seen briefly by the Casualty Officer and was given an intravenous injection of diamorphine (heroin) 5 mg. Stemetil 12.5 mg was also given intramuscularly to counteract the common side effect of nausea caused by opiate drugs. The intense pain subsided after only a few minutes, Mr Davies relaxed noticeably and his face looked less drawn. Further details of Mr Davies' history could now be obtained.

It is poor nursing practice to ask irrelevant and unnecessary questions of an acutely distressed patient and only vital details should be obtained before acute pain is relieved. Such details should include: full name, date of birth, home address and telephone number and name, address or telephone number of the patient's next of kin.

On further questioning it became apparent that Mr Davies had a long family history of heart trouble and he had been experiencing mild angina for several months whenever he indulged in physical exertion. He had not consulted his GP since the pain passed quickly if he rested and he had been extremely busy in recent weeks, often working until late in the evenings. His father and elder brother had both suffered 'heart attacks' and he was not surprised to learn that he had probably experienced one himself. An electrocardiograph (ECG) recording was made to assist in confirming the diagnosis.

An ECG records electrical impulses passing through cardiac muscle in various planes and indicates not only any disturbance to the passage of electrical waves but also the location of the problem. The procedure is painless but the patient should be relaxed with legs uncrossed and his arms

at his sides in order to minimise the electrical activity of muscles impinging upon the trace. Leads are attached to both wrists and both ankles and a further lead is placed at various points on the chest. Certain changes occur in the ECG pattern following myocardial infarction though they are not always immediately apparent, as was the case with the recording taken of Mr Davies. (An ECG taken the following morning, however, did show changes and that the damage was located anteriorly.) The doctor also took a sample of Mr Davies' venous blood so that it could be examined for evidence of raised levels of cardiac enzymes including AST (serum aspartate aminotransferase) and LDH (lactate dehydrogenase). These enzymes are released by necrotic muscle tissue and raised levels are diagnostic of myocardial infarction. Cardiac monitor leads were connected to Mr Davies' chest so that any further irregularities in electrical transmission could be noted and corrected at once. Arrhythmias are common following myocardial infarction and may be fatal if left untreated. Mr Davies' heart beat had returned to a regular pattern unaided. A registered nurse, familiar with the use of cardiac monitors, assisted in Mr Davies' care throughout his stay in A and E.

Now that his pain had subsided, Mr Davies' main concern was that he was supposed to be at a board meeting and had an important evening dinner engagement. He was fully aware that he would need to remain in hospital but was extremely anxious to inform his colleagues. A portable telephone was made available so that he could speak to his secretary and ask her to deal with the important matters. This done, he became much less anxious and began to joke with the nursing staff. In many instances the nurse may be able to pass on a message over the telephone but, wherever possible, the patient should be allowed to make the calls himself. The importance of business commitments should never be underestimated and it is generally much quicker and easier for the executive to speak with his secretary for a few minutes than for him to explain things to a third party and then worry whether facts have been passed on accurately.

Mr Davies' wife had been contacted, with his permission, when he arrived in the department, and she arrived about half an hour afterwards. She was allowed to see her husband at once and was able to sit with him while arrangements were made for his admission to the ward. They were both shocked by the suddenness of Mr Davies' illness but Mrs Davies was calm and supportive and re-assured him that she would contact their children and cancel their social engagements. The under-standing support of a patient's next of kin can help to alleviate many of his worries and hasten his recovery.

Mr Davies was transferred by trolley to a bed on a coronary care unit with facilities for cardiac monitoring 40 minutes after his arrival in the A and E department. He was accompanied by his wife and a nurse who had cared for him in A and E. His clothes and valuables were given to his wife at his request and she signed a proforma indicating that she had received them. He left the department pain-free and relatively relaxed though still stunned by the suddenness and seriousness of his illness and the impact it would have on his future.

Mr Davies' case highlights a number of important points for the Accident and Emergency nurse.

(1) It is vital when caring for any acutely ill patient that the staff are not only aware of the patient's present condition and are acting to aid his recovery but also that they are prepared to deal with any sudden deterioration which might occur. The use of a hard-based trolley, proximity of emergency drugs and resuscitation equipment, and use of a cardiac monitor were not essential to care adequately for Mr Davies, but had his condition worsened rapidly then nursing actions would have been facilitated by this forethought.

(2) Constant explanation to the patient of what is happening and why actions are necessary is par-ticularly important in the emergency setting. The nurse must ensure that she speaks in terms which the patient can understand and that she repeats herself as often as necessary. Fear and the shock of an emergency admission readily block the indi-vidual's ability to comprehend or retain infor-mation and the nurse should never assume that because she has told her client something he has either understood or taken in the information.

(3) Psychological aspects of patient care must not be forgotten in the intense endeavour to correct the client's physical deficits. Once his physical condition is stable, it is possible that dealing with his immediate worries and fears will improve his progress more than physical care. In Mr Davies' case, he became visibly more relaxed once he had

spoken to his secretary and spent a few minutes with his wife. A and E is not the place to deal with long term psychological problems but the nurse must aim to relieve the natural anxieties which her patients will feel. This will require a flexible and sensitive approach to each individual.

Mr Victor Adams who suffered a cerebrovascular accident

The profile in Fig. 22.6 introduces an elderly man who has had a cerebrovascular accident (CVA).

Related structure and function

Blood is supplied to the brain via the two internal carotid arteries and the two vertebral arteries. The two sets of arteries are linked together by a circular anastomosis – the circle of Willis (Fig. 22.5) – at the base of the brain. The brain receives approxi-mately 15% of the resting cardiac output (i.e. about 800 ml per minute at rest). If the blood supply is cut off the individual will become uncon-scious after about five seconds and there will be irreversible brain damage after three or four minutes. Tissue death (infarction) will occur if the oxygen supply to an area of the brain is decreased because the blood flow is impeded in some way – either by haemorrhage, thrombosis or embolism. These incidents are termed *cerebrovascular acci-dents* (CVA) or 'strokes'.

Haemorrhage may occur where degenerative changes have weakened an artery or following trauma or chronic inflammation. Hypertension may predispose to brain haemorrhage. The haema-toma formed presses on the surrounding brain tissue, decreasing its blood supply. The affected

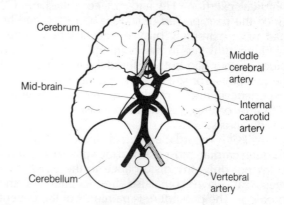

Fig. 22.5 The circle of Willis

Mr Victor Adams, an 81-year-old gentleman, was brought to hospital by ambulance. He was accompanied by his elderly, frail-looking wife. They had been at home and had gone to sleep in armchairs after lunch, as was their custom. Mrs Adams had woken first and noticed that her husband's face looked odd. She was able to rouse him but he was unable to speak coherently and his right arm and leg seemed to be paralysed.

Mr Adams was transferred to a trolley in the A and E department. The nurse allocated to care for Mr Adams greeted him and his wife, giving her name and status, and explaining to Mr Adams where he was. Mrs Adams was allowed to stay with her husband whilst he was made comfortable, undressed and helped into a hospital gown. Since Mr Adams was unable to express himself, the A and E team relied heavily on his wife to give information not only about the incident which had just occurred but about his previous medical condition. He was apparently generally very fit for his age and able to do most of the heavier tasks in the house. He was a keen vegetable gardener and had been digging only a day or two previously. He had complained of feeling unwell that morning and had taken a paracetamol tablet for his headache – something he very rarely did. His younger brother suffered with **hypertension**, but Mr Adams had not seen a doctor for five years and there had been no mention of blood pressure problems previously.

Fig. 22.6 *Profile: Mr Victor Adams*

individual will experience a sudden, violent headache and will lapse into unconsciousness, often following an epileptic-type seizure. The prognosis is poor.

Thrombosis is often associated with degenerative arterial disease (arteriosclerosis) combined with the laying down of atheromatous plaques which narrow and eventually block the vessel lumen. It may also be associated with a tumour pressing on the vessels. The internal carotid and middle cerebral arteries are those most commonly affected (see Fig. 22.5). These arteries supply the sensory and motor areas of the cerebrum and their blockage will result in *hemiplegia* of the side of the body opposite to the thrombosis. Speech may be affected if the damage occurs in the dominant hemisphere (usually the left in right-handed individuals).

Embolus is a less common cause of CVA. The embolus may be formed of blood clot, fat, tumour cells or bacteria which circulate from other parts of the body. The onset of symptoms is sudden and usually results in hemiplegia.

The majority of individuals who suffer a cerebrovascular accident are over the age of 65 and about half of them die as a result. The signs and symptoms are very varied depending on the site and severity of the brain damage. Some CVAs go almost unnoticed while others cause rapid death. Conscious patients may complain of headaches or vomiting if the vomiting centre in the medulla is stimulated. Convulsive movements similar to an epileptic seizure will occur if the neural pathway is compressed. *Hemiplegia* (paralysis of one side of the body) is common with decreased muscle tone and loss of reflexes on the affected side. *Aphasia* (loss of speech) or *dysphasia* (difficulty with speaking) may occur if the dominant hemisphere is affected. Raised **intracranial pressure** will cause the pupils of the eye to contract and the condition of **papilloedema** may be present. The intellect may be affected so that the patient is unaware of his condition but in many instances the individual will be shocked and terrified to find himself paralysed and unable to express himself.

Nursing care for Mr Adams

Once the nurse caring for Mr Adams had introduced herself, helped him to undress and made him comfortable, and had taken a history, she then measured and recorded Mr Adams' blood pressure, temperature, pulse and respiratory rate, noting that they were all slightly higher than expected: blood pressure, 150/110; temperature, 37.6°C; pulse, 92; respirations, 24 and shallow. She noted that he was unable to move his right arm and right leg though there was a small amount of movement in his right hand when she asked him to squeeze her fingers. He seemed unaware of his right side and appeared not to notice if he was approached from that side. Great care was taken to ensure that the **flaccid** limbs were supported in a natural position. Mr Adams replied 'No' to everything he was asked and was clearly distressed and frustrated to hear himself saying the word.

The medical examination performed on Mr Adams confirmed that he had suffered a cerebrovascular accident in the left hemisphere of his brain leaving him with a right hemiplegia and dysphasia. The medical staff explained his condition to Mr Adams, pointing out the fact that he could speak and had some movement in his right hand were good signs and that he had a good chance of recovering from his stroke. They spoke similarly to Mrs Adams, explaining that the outcome was impossible to predict at this early stage. Mrs Adams

Fig. 22.7 Care plan for Mr Adams

Name: *Victor Adams*
Age: 81
Date: 17.8.92

Next of Kin: *Wife*
Informed: *Present*
Religion: *C/E*

Time: 15:15
Medical Diagnosis *Cerebrovascular accident*

Problem	Aim	Intervention	Evaluation
(1) Condition necessitates hospital admission *Working and playing*	Prepare patient mentally and physically ensuring adequate information is given	(a) Explain clearly the need for admission (b) Advise about the ward as soon as known (c) Assure that the hospital will provide pyjamas, etc., until wife can bring his own (d) Ensure nursing notes and observation charts accurate and up-to-date (e) Make patient comfortable and ensure he is well covered before transfer to ward (f) Accompany the patient and his wife to ward to ensure continuity of care and informed hand-over to ward staff	
(2) Unable to move right arm and right leg *Mobilising*	i) Avoid further damage to limbs from: – poor positioning – ***contractures*** developing	(a) Position comfortably in natural position with affected limbs well supported by pillows (b) Ensure environment is safe – trolley sides up at all times – nurse to stay with patient (c) Encourage patient to move affected limbs if possible (d) Perform passive exercises hourly to prevent contractures occurring. Ensure foot is supported to avoid **foot drop**	
	ii) Avoid development of pressure sores	(a) Change position hourly (b) Sheepskin under buttocks to reduce pressure from hard trolley base	
(3) Unable to express himself – says only 'no' *Communicating*	Encourage self-expression by all means available	(a) Give patient time to reply to questions (b) Ensure patient feels able to try to respond – ensure that staff know he is aware what he *wants* to say	

Problem	Aim	Intervention	Evaluation
		(c) Anticipate needs where possible	
		(d) Offer pencil and paper – Mr Adams may be able to write	(d) Writing indecipherable
		(e) Ask questions which require 'yes' or 'no' answers wherever possible. The patient may be able to nod/shake head, or squeeze the nurse's hand in response	(e) Sometimes responds appropriately
		(f) Be alert for non-verbal responses such as facial or hand movement	
(4) Unable to ask for toilet facilities Eliminating	Assess continent state Avoid catheterisation if possible	(a) Offer urinal half-hourly and help to position it	(a) Passed a good amount of urine when offered bottle at 15:45
		(b) Place urinal within sight and easy reach on 'good' side	
		(c) Offer bed-pan two-hourly	
		(d) Explain to Mr Adams the importance of maintaining fluid intake	
		(e) Commence fluid balance chart for accurate assessment of intake and output	
		(f) Determine which fluids are most acceptable	(f) Wife says Mr Adams dislikes coffee but likes milky drinks and tea
(5) Unable to feed himself Eating and drinking	Maintain adequate fluid (2000 ml/24 hrs) and calorie intake	(a) Offer frequent small amounts of fluid – 20 ml every half hour	(a) Drinking as offered
		(b) Ensure fluids at suitable temperature	
		(c) Unable to manage glass – try feeder beaker or give help with glass	(c) Manages feeder beaker
		(d) Order meal in A and E if necessary and assist as required	
		(e) Record all food and fluid intake	
(6) Potential for further deterioration in condition Maintaining a safe environment	Prevent if possible or detect early any change in vital signs which may indicate deterioration	(a) Half-hourly observations of conscious level, pulse, blood pressure, temperature and respirations to detect signs of haemorrhage or raised intracranial pressure	

Problem	Aim	Intervention	Evaluation
		(b) Constant visual evaluation of patient's condition including skin colour, facial and limb movements	
		(c) Report any changes noticed	
(7) Loss of self-respect and dignity Communicating	Maintain and restore self-esteem	(a) Display understanding, caring attitude at all times	
		(b) Explain to Mr Adams that the staff understand how he feels	
		(c) Do not treat him as though he is stupid because he cannot speak properly	
		(d) Involve Mr Adams in decision-making as much as possible	
		(e) Reassure him that improvement is likely	
(8) Worries regarding his wife's welfare	Ensure adequate provision for Mrs Adams	(a) Contact the Adams' son and daughter-in-law who live nearby. They will take Mrs Adams to stay with them for the present	(a) Contacted – on the way. Are quite happy to take Mrs Adams to stay with them
		(b) Mrs Adams to stay with her husband in A and E as much as possible	

was allowed to stay with her husband until his transfer to the ward.

A synopsis of Mr Adams' care has been included in this chapter to illustrate a number of points.

(1) The importance of assessing each client individually and planning care to meet his needs cannot be overstressed. Cerebrovascular accident affects each sufferer differently and care which is suitable for one individual may be totally inappropriate for another. Each patient responds differently to care and constant re-appraisal of the patient's condition and the effectiveness of care given will ensure that necessary changes can be made.

(2) Goals and aims of nursing care should be short term if they are to be achieved during the patient's stay in A and E. Normally patients are discharged home or transferred to other wards or departments within an hour or two and nursing care in A and E should be directed in the first instance to helping the patient through the acute stage of his condition. However, many of the nursing activities begun in the department will be continued by nurses on the ward to which the patient is transferred and failure to consider basic points of nursing care (such as maintaining the skin's integrity) whilst the patient is in A and E may adversely affect his future recovery.

(3) Allowing relatives, particularly partners, to spend time with the patient whilst he is in A and E is generally of benefit to all. For the patient it provides a link with the 'real' world – particularly important for those who are elderly or confused. Relatives benefit because they are able to see what is being done for their loved one and may be able to assist with his care. Staff in A and E also benefit because a relative is often able to give much information about the patient and his previous con-

dition which would not otherwise be forthcoming, (Encouraging parents to stay with their children has been discussed earlier in the chapter.)

(4) It is important not to allow a deficit in one area of the patient's abilities to affect other areas. For example, the fact that Mr Adams was unable to speak coherently might have led to his being incontinent since he was unable to ask for a urinal. In fact the potential problem was overcome by asking him every half hour whether he would like to pass urine and by leaving the urinal where he could see and reach it – i.e. on his unaffected side.

Peter Edwards who was stabbed in the chest

The profile of a young man who has been stabbed in the chest is given in Fig. 22.11.

Related structure and function

The respiratory system is concerned with:

(1) The intake of atmospheric air to supply oxygen to all cells via the blood;
(2) Ridding the body of carbon dioxide, a waste product of metabolism.

Air is drawn in through the nose and mouth where it is warmed, moistened and filtered before being sucked via the pharynx and larynx into the trachea. The trachea divides into two bronchi which each supply a lung and the bronchi then divide and subdivide many times into smaller and smaller

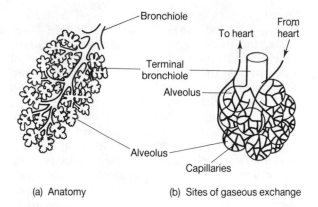

(a) Anatomy   (b) Sites of gaseous exchange

Fig. 22.8 *The terminal airways*

bronchioles terminating in alveoli (Fig. 22.8). These branches of the bronchial tree form the framework of two elastic, spongy organs, the lungs, situated in the thoracic cavity. Oxygen passes from the air in the terminal bronchioles and alveoli into the capillaries surrounding them and carbon dioxide passes from the capillaries into the lungs to be exhaled (expired). A constant and adequate supply of oxygen in the blood is essential for normal cell metabolism.

Normal respiration is under voluntary control to some extent (for example, when talking or singing) although the respiratory centre in the medulla of the brain provides the ultimate involuntary control. Its main action is to stimulate the muscle fibres in the diaphragm which separates the thorax from the abdomen. As the muscle fibres contract and shorten, the diaphragm flattens (Fig. 22.9), the volume of the thorax is increased (with a conse-

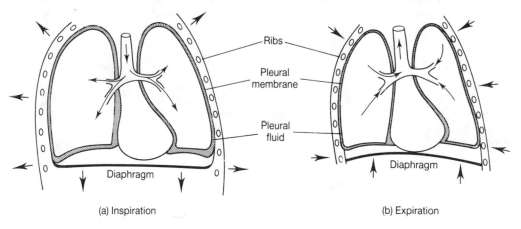

(a) Inspiration   (b) Expiration

Fig. 22.9 *Mechanics of respiration*

quent drop in intrathoracic pressure) and air is drawn into the lungs. When the muscle fibres relax, the diaphragm moves upwards, intrathoracic pressure increases and air is pushed out of the lungs. At the same time the respiratory centre stimulates the intercostal muscles to increase and decrease the diameter of the thoracic cavity and hence of the lungs. Accessory muscles hold the lung apices in position and pull them upwards if necessary during any respiratory exertion, and the abdominal muscles can aid expiration by pushing the abdominal contents up against the diaphragm.

The pleurae are formed of fine membranous tissue and line the outer surface of each lung. There are two layers – the *visceral pleura* adherent to the lung and the *parietal pleura* which adheres to the inner chest wall and ribs (see Fig. 22.9). The two layers are normally apposed and held together with a small amount of pleural fluid between them. The pressure between the two pleural layers is negative compared with atmospheric pressure and a potential space is said to exist. The pleurae hold the lungs in shape. During inspiration the intrapleural pressure decreases (i.e. becomes more negative) and this helps to expand the lungs. If either layer of the pleurae is torn, air will enter the space, destroying the negative pressure and so causing the lung to collapse. This is termed *pneumothorax*. The pleurae may be ruptured from the outside by a penetrating wound – such as a stab wound – or internally, for example by a fractured rib or, more commonly, the rupture of a tiny air sac in the lung (spontaneous pneumothorax). This latter type of pneumothorax is often preceded by a chronic lung condition such as emphysema. It can also occur in otherwise healthy individuals, commonly in tall, thin, athletic young men.

In some instances the hole seals itself (*closed pneumothorax* – Fig. 22.10a) and the small amount of air between the pleural layers is absorbed spontaneously. In an open pneumothorax (Fig. 22.10b) the hole between the lung and the pleural space remains open and air passes in and out. The intrapleural pressure is equal to atmospheric pressure and the affected lung remains collapsed.

A more serious situation arises when a flap of pleura acts as a one-way valve opening during inspiration to allow air into the pleural space and closing during expiration, trapping the air. Intrapleural pressure rises steadily above atmospheric pressure. The affected lung will collapse quickly, and the rising pressure will push the mediastinum and its contents across to begin compressing the other lung (Fig. 22.10c). This is termed a *tension pneumothorax* and if it is not treated *at once*, respiratory failure and death will occur.

Patients who develop pneumothorax usually experience sudden sharp one-sided chest pain which persists and is worse during inspiration. Depending on the severity of the incident they may appear pale or **cyanosed**; the pulse rate is generally accelerated and respirations are rapid and shallow. Chest movements on the affected side are reduced or absent. The patient may become clammy or sweaty as adrenaline levels in the blood begin to rise and will, naturally, be frightened about what is happening. Those patients with tension pneumothorax will become confused and then unconscious since poor lung expansion means that the blood receives insufficient oxygen to maintain normal brain function.

The intrapleural air must be removed in order to restore normal lung function. A small, closed

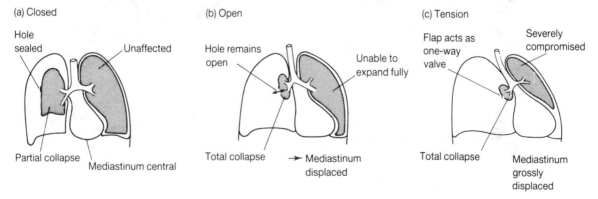

(a) Closed

Hole sealed

Unaffected

Partial collapse

Mediastinum central

(b) Open

Hole remains open

Unable to expand fully

Total collapse

→ Mediastinum displaced

(c) Tension

Flap acts as one-way valve

Severely compromised

Total collapse

Mediastinum grossly displaced

Fig. 22.10 Pneumothorax

pneumothorax may be left to resolve spontaneously over a few weeks but more serious pneumothoraces will be treated by the insertion of an intercostal catheter connected to an underwater seal drainage system. If recurrent spontaneous pneumothorax occurs, surgical intervention may be necessary in order to induce adhesions between the two layers of pleura as these will make further episodes of pneumothorax unlikely.

Peter Edwards was brought to hospital late one Saturday night (an account of his arrival began this chapter). He was only sixteen, though he looked older, and had spent the evening drinking with his friends in a local public house. Shortly before closing time another group of youths had arrived and several unpleasant verbal exchanges took place. The landlord managed to empty the pub at closing time but a scuffle had broken out between the rival groups during which four other people received superficial knife wounds to their faces and arms. Peter was stabbed with a knife in the right side of his chest during the fight. A passer-by called the police and ambulance service and the injured youths were brought to the A and E department accompanied by several policemen. The other injured youths were shouting at one another and keen to continue the fight — they were separated and taken to await treatment. Peter was clearly unwell and was taken immediately to the emergency treatment area. Two nurses were assigned to look after him and the Casualty Officer was asked to see him at once.

Fig. 22.11 *Profile: Peter Edwards*

Care of Peter Edwards

On arrival at the hospital, the ambulance crew transferred Peter to the A and E trolley and assisted the nursing staff with the removal of his clothes. His leather jacket was removed over his head — this is often easier than manoeuvring the patient to remove it in the conventional manner. His tight teeshirt was covered in blood and was cut off to save time and effort on his part. The wound on his chest had been covered with a dressing by the ambulance crew and this was left undisturbed but covered with impermeable waterproof adhesive tape to prevent any further air entry. The back rest of the trolley was raised so that Peter was sitting as upright as possible since he was clearly experiencing difficulty breathing. He was well supported with pillows. Oxygen was administered via an MC mask in order to maximise the oxygen content of the blood. Once Peter's clothes were removed it was plain that only the left side of his chest was moving when he breathed and a provisional diagnosis of right pneumothorax was made. His respiration rate and depth were noted (40 per minute and shallow), his pulse rate was 104 bpm. Peter

was sweating profusely and mumbling to himself. He would not answer questions but would respond to repeated commands. The ambulance crew commented that his condition had considerably deteriorated since they had arrived at the scene of the incident when he had been able to give his name and address. He was now cyanosed — his lips and fingers were blue — and he was becoming progressively less coherent. A decision was made to insert a catheter attached to an underwater seal drain to relieve the presumed pneumothorax without waiting for an X-ray to confirm the diagnosis.

When assessing a patient who has been stabbed it is essential to consider all the possible damage which could have occurred to internal organs. The exact direction of the injury and the length of the weapon are generally unknown and an apparently small entry wound may belie the extent of internal damage. In Peter's case the wound was in such a position that the diaphragm, liver and heart were unlikely to have been touched — though the possibility of damage to one of the great blood vessels was considered. Constant observation of the patient's condition is essential so that any deterioration is noted at an early stage and corrective measures can be taken.

Consent to the insertion of the intercostal drain under local anaesthetic was not obtained. Peter was unable to give even verbal consent because of his condition even though, as he had stated to the ambulance crew, he was sixteen and thus considered able to consent to his own treatment. The police were trying to contact his parents but thus far without success, so consent from them was not available. His condition was considered sufficiently life-threatening for the medical staff to proceed regardless. The decision was later documented in the medical notes.

The nursing staff hurriedly prepared the necessary equipment and helped to position Peter with his right arm raised so that the catheter could be inserted into the apex of the lung under the axilla (air trapped between the pleural layers generally rises to the top of the lung; blood or pus fall to the base of the lung and are drained from there).

Peter's care highlights the need for all the A and E nursing team to know what will be needed for any emergency situation and exactly where it is to be found. Minutes spent searching for equipment, either because of poor stock-keeping or through lack of knowledge, may cost the patient his life.

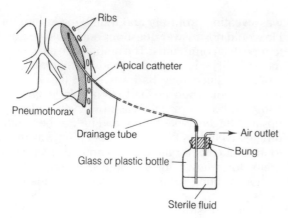

Fig. 22.12 *Underwater seal drainage system*

Once the catheter was in position it was connected to the prepared underwater seal drainage system (Fig. 22.12). Air immediately began to bubble through the saline solution in the attached bottle – this confirmed that there was a pneumothorax and that the catheter was in the correct position to drain it. Peter was almost unaware of what was happening during the procedure. Oxygen was still being administered via an MC mask but his respirations were so shallow and gasping that very little oxygen was actually reaching his lungs. A nurse had explained throughout what was happening and she now encouraged Peter to take slower, deeper breaths. This not only aids ventilation of the undamaged lung but helps to drain the air from and re-inflate the affected lung. Peter's cyanosis improved noticeably over the next few minutes as more and more air bubbled out of his pleural space and he became a little less breathless and more coherent.

The catheter was sutured in place and a 'purse string' suture inserted around it so that the hole could be easily closed when the catheter was removed. The dressing over Peter's stab wound was then removed and the wound cleaned, explored under local anaesthetic and sutured to prevent air entry through it.

Peter's position was adjusted so that he was as comfortable as possible and sitting almost upright in order to aid his lung expansion. A portable X-ray was taken which showed a large pneumothorax and indicated that the drainage catheter was in the correct position. Two clamps were attached to one of the pillows in case of any accident which might allow air entry via the drainage system. The intercostal catheter must be immediately clamped in

such an incident or atmospheric air will rush into the pleural space. The clamps must also be applied if it is necessary to raise the drainage bottle above the level of the catheter's entry into the chest. Failure to do this will mean that the fluid in the drainage bottle pours into the patient's pleural space. The drainage bottle was placed in a carrying basket which was hooked onto the side of the trolley.

Although the immediate danger to Peter's life seemed to be over, constant observation of his condition remained vital. It is difficult to detect internal bleeding until a large amount of blood has been lost unless a constant and accurate check is kept on the patient's condition. Bleeding may be presaged by a change in the patient's skin colour and appearance before it can be detected by changes in his pulse rate and blood pressure (pulse rate will rise and blood pressure will fall). Peter had been given no analgesic, partly because it was feared that this may mask his symptoms and partly because he was known to have consumed several pints of beer which would have its own analgesic effect.

The several pints of beer had a further effect and Peter, unable to ask for a urinal, had emptied his bladder during the insertion of the chest drain. Earlier consideration of this aspect of alcohol consumption by the nursing staff might have prevented this and saved unnecessary discomfort, embarrassment, time and effort. The linen was changed, Peter's skin washed and dried and a urinal was left in an appropriate position so that Peter could urinate whenever he needed to.

Arrangements were made to transfer Peter to a medical ward. The police wished to interview him as soon as possible but were asked not to do so in A and E since he was medically unfit. They therefore arranged that an officer should be allowed to wait on the ward until Peter was able to cooperate. Peter was told what was happening, though it was impossible to tell whether he understood. The oxygen tubing was attached to the oxygen cylinder beneath the trolley, Peter's bloodstained clothes were put in a bag, labelled and placed on the trolley; his notes and X-rays were gathered and he was covered with several blankets before being moved. Great care was taken not to disturb the drainage system during the transfer.

Once Peter was positioned comfortably in bed on the ward, the nurse who had cared for him in A and E handed over his care to the ward staff. A brief outline of the events prior to Peter's arrival at the hospital was given and the nurse explained that his deteriorating condition had necessitated the emergency insertion of a chest drainage system. The ward nurse was shown the entry site in Peter's chest and assured herself that the system was functioning adequately. Observation charts were handed over and it was explained that Peter's condition had improved during his stay in A and E but that it was thought necessary to record his pulse and respiration rate every fifteen minutes at present.

Peter had been in A and E for less than an hour and his position had been changed several times during that period. He had now been positioned lying towards his right side, well supported with pillows. Care had been taken to ensure that his drainage tube was not kinked, nor causing him discomfort. The nurses decided that hourly changes of position would probably be appropriate at this stage.

The ward nurse was advised of Peter's alcohol consumption and the fact that he had been unable to ask for a urinal. One had been appropriately positioned in Peter's bed and this would be checked frequently until Peter was able to take care of this activity for himself.

Peter did not appear to be in pain but the A and E nurse pointed out that he had received no analgesics since his admission.

It was further explained that consent to insertion of the intercostal drain had not been obtained (this was documented in both medical and nursing notes) and that the police had as yet been unable to contact Peter's parents though this was in hand. The police officer accompanying Peter had been asked to wait outside his room to avoid causing him any worries which might aggravate his condition. The medical staff would indicate when Peter was fit to be interviewed.

Peter's belongings were handed over. The clothes were bloodstained and torn and he had only 76 pence in cash with him. This was handed to the ward staff and a receipt for the amount put with Peter's clothing. Mention was made that he had not been wearing a watch – a fact that had been documented in the nursing notes.

Having assured herself that Peter's care had been handed over accurately and adequately, the A and E nurse explained once more to Peter where he was, wished him well and said good-bye. She was rewarded with a mumbled expletive.

Margaret Parfitt was brought to hospital by ambulance accompanied by her fiancé, Robert Green. He had returned after work to the flat which they shared and had found her, still in her dressing gown, asleep on the settee. Her half-eaten lunch was on the table. He had managed to wake her but she was confused and incoherent and kept going back to sleep. Robert was extremely worried and telephoned to request an emergency ambulance. He said that Margaret had been feeling unwell for the past two or three weeks and had been very tired and lethargic. She seemed to have lost all her enthusiasm and interest in life and had missed a number of lectures at the local university where she was taking a social sciences course. He had no knowledge of any previous problems or of her family medical history.

Robert was shown to the waiting room, thanked for his help and told that he would be kept informed of Margaret's condition. He was asked about Margaret's next of kin and offered to telephone her parents to inform them. As they lived a considerable distance away he was advised to wait for a short while until a provisional diagnosis had been made as this might be less alarming for them.

Meanwhile Margaret was transferred to a hard-based trolley in the emergency area where any equipment which might be needed was readily accessible. Her nightdress and dressing gown were removed to facilitate medical examination and were placed in a labelled bag beneath the trolley. Margaret was helped into a hospital gown and she was placed in a semi-prone position on the trolley with a pillow under her head and a blanket to cover her. The trolley sides were raised so that she could not fall.

Fig. 22.13 *Profile: Miss Margaret Parfitt*

Margaret Parfitt, who was unconscious

The profile in Fig. 22.13 concerns a young woman, found unconscious at home by her fiancé, and brought into the A and E department by ambulance.

In the absence of any known medical condition which might cause a patient to become unconscious, the nursing staff have a vital part to play in helping to establish a diagnosis. The first priority must always be to maintain a patent airway but there should also be careful, close, continuous observation of the patient, bearing in mind the possible causes of semi-consciousness will mean that medical treatment can begin sooner.

Possible causes which must be borne in mind are head injury, drug or alcohol overdose, cerebrovascular accident (unusual in young patients), epilepsy, hypoglycaemia and ketoacidosis (a sign of hyperglycaemia). The patient should be examined quickly from head to foot for any helpful signs. Bleeding or bruising may indicate trauma as a cause, particularly when found on the head. Needle marks may indicate a diabetic patient (usually on the abdomen or thighs) or a drug addict (marks often on forearms close to veins). Any limb flaccidity or weakness should be noted (this may indicate cerebrovascular accident as a cause). It may be possible to smell alcohol or ketones on the patient's breath, again indicating a likely cause. A pinprick of blood from the patient's finger applied to a reagent test strip for blood glucose will give an approximate blood glucose level and will indicate whether hypo- or hyperglycaemia is a possible cause. Observations of the patient's general condition, conscious level, pupil reactions, pulse, blood pressure and respirations should be made and recorded every 15 to 30 minutes until a provisional diagnosis is established. This will ensure that any significant changes are noted promptly and treatment or care adjusted accordingly.

A problem-solving approach to care should be utilised in the absence of medical diagnosis. Nursing care given will need constant evaluation and re-appraisal as problems are dealt with and new ones arise and the nursing staff must be alert, flexible and able to adjust their care quickly in the light of new information. The reader should refer now to Margaret Parfitt's care plan (Fig. 22.14) to see how this has been achieved for one particular patient.

Diabetes

Margaret's fiancé, Robert, was understandably shocked when told that Margaret may be diabetic. He knew very little about the disease and was anxious to know about its long term course. He and Margaret were due to marry soon and he wished to be fully conversant with her condition so that he could share the problem with her. Robert was reassured that her life was not in danger and informed of what had been done for Margaret in the A and E department. It was felt that this was not the right time to discuss long term prospects but Robert was assured that he and Margaret would be able to discuss the situation fully with an endocrinologist before she was discharged from hospital. A note was made in the nursing records to ensure that this was arranged. Robert was allowed to see Margaret as soon as the urgent treatment was completed and accompanied her to the ward. She had been in the department for only 30 minutes.

Related structure and function

The pancreas lies in the abdomen behind the stomach. It produces digestive enzymes (its exocrine function) and is also an endocrine organ. Scattered throughout the pancreas are groups of cells called the islets of Langerhans. These contain at least three different types of cell, of which the α and β cells are concerned with maintaining blood glucose levels via hormone secretion. The central nervous system, including the brain, must have a constant glucose supply in order to function properly.

The α cells in the islets of Langerhans produce *glucagon* in response to low blood glucose levels. Glucagon acts by releasing glycogen stored in the liver so that it can be converted to glucose. The β cells produce insulin in response to a rise in blood glucose levels, for example after a heavy meal. Insulin acts to remove glucose from the bloodstream by:

(1) Allowing it to enter cells throughout the body for use as a metabolic fuel; and
(2) Promoting its entry into the liver where it is stored as glycogen.

Insulin and glucagon together with other hormones (for example, cortisol, adrenaline) maintain the delicate balance of blood sugar levels that the body requires to function at its best.

If insulin is lacking or insufficient, the condition of diabetes mellitus will occur. Blood glucose levels rise until the kidneys cannot reabsorb all the glucose, when it will appear in the urine. Glucose attracts water by osmosis and large quantities of urine will be passed (*polyuria*) causing the individual to become dehydrated and thirsty. He will drink large amounts (*polydipsia*) to try to compensate. Because glucose cannot enter the cells for use, the body will start to break down proteins to use as fuel. Breakdown products of this will appear in the urine as urea and weight loss will occur. Fats will also be broken down and their by-products, ketones, will appear in the urine and blood. Ketones are toxic acids and the individual will exhibit a metabolic acidosis. If the condition is untreated, dehydration and acidosis will result in coma and eventually death.

Diabetes mellitus occurs in individuals of either sex and at any age. Its precise cause is unknown but the disease is more prevalent in the Western

Fig. 22.14 Care plan for Margaret Parfitt

| **Name:** *Margaret Parfitt*
Age: 24
Date: 28.4.92 | **Religion:** *Non-conformist*
Time: 17:45 | **Next of kin:** *Parents*
Fiancé
Informed: *Fiancé present*
Parents telephoned | **Medical diagnosis:**
Unconscious
? cause |

Problem	Aim	Intervention	Evaluation
(1) May be unable to maintain own airway due to semi-conscious state Breathing	Prevent airway obstruction	(a) Position the patient so she is lying flat on her side with one pillow under her head to ensure drainage of any oral secretions	
		(b) Clear mouth of any vomitus. Remove any dentures	(b) Teeth all patient's own
		(c) Suction equipment readily available in case required	
		(d) Call anaesthetist to intubate if condition worsens	
(2) Unable to maintain safe environment Maintaining a safe environment	Ensure Margaret does not injure herself	(a) Trolley sides to remain up	
		(b) A nurse to stay with the patient at all times	
		(c) Pad any hard or sharp objects to avoid traumatic injury	
		(d) Ensure limbs are in their natural position	
(3) Cause of condition not known Communicating	Try to determine cause of unconsciousness while caring for patient	(a) Half-hourly observations to determine level of consciousness	
		(b) Record pulse, blood pressure and respirations half-hourly	(b) Resps. 30 per minute and gasping ('air hunger'). Record every 15 minutes
		(c) Examine skin for bleeding, bruising, injection marks, sweating	(c) Skin noted to be dry and inelastic – see Problem (5)
		(d) Reagent stick test for blood glucose	(d) 40 mmol/litre (normal 3.5–5.8 mmol/l) venous blood Sample sent for accurate estimation (38.7 mmol/l) – see Problem (6)

Problem	Aim	Intervention	Evaluation
(4) Unable to control bladder emptying *Eliminating*	Prevent problems associated with urinary incontinence	(a) Wash and dry skin if incontinent	
		(b) Offer bedpan half-hourly	(b) Unable to use
		(c) Catheterise in view of need to maintain accurate fluid balance	(c) Catheterised. 500 ml urine drained
(5) Skin dry and inelastic – seems dehydrated *Eating and drinking*	Maintain adequate fluid intake to restore normal skin texture	(a) Oral fluids as tolerated	(a) Drinking sips occasionally
		(b) Commence intravenous infusion of isotonic saline (154 mmol/l) (0.9%) to ensure adequate fluid intake – 1 litre in two hours, as per doctor's orders	
		(c) Keep accurate record of fluid balance including hourly urine measurement	
(6) Hyperglycaemic *Maintaining a safe environment*	Reduce blood sugar levels	(a) Soluble insulin 10 units given I/M at 17.50 hrs	
		(b) Insulin pump set up – dose to be regulated on a sliding scale depending on hourly reagent stick glucose test. See doctor's instructions	
		(c) Watch for signs of hypoglycaemia including sweating, tachycardia, restlessness	
(7) Vomiting *Eating and drinking*	Reduce unpleasantness as much as possible	(a) Ensure tissues and a clean vomit bowl are readily available	
		(b) Support head when vomiting	
		(c) Ensure airway remains clear	
		(d) Wash face and change bed linen as necessary	
		(e) Explain that vomiting will stop when treatment starts to work	
		(f) Ensure suction readily available if patient unable to empty mouth	
		(g) Offer mouthwash as appropriate	
		(h) Maintain accurate fluid balance chart	

Problem	Aim	Intervention	Evaluation
(8) Unprepared for admission Working and playing	Provide reasoned information	(a) Ensure that Margaret knows where she is. Repeat information if necessary	(a) Margaret says she is in hospital
		(b) Explain that she needs to stay in for treatment	
		(c) Encourage her to ask any questions and answer them	
		(d) Allow fiancé to talk to her and arrange to bring in her things	
(9) Parents (next of kin) unaware of Margaret's condition	Inform them – Margaret's fiancé says she would wish this	Staff nurse to telephone Mr and Mrs Parfitt. Fiancé to speak to them to make any necessary arrangements	Parents informed (Margaret's paternal grandfather – long dead – had diabetes mellitus)
(10) Fiancé worried	Ensure he is kept informed	(a) Staff nurse to speak to him about immediate plans	(a) Done. He will stay to accompany Margaret to the ward
		(b) Answer any queries he may have	
		(c) Ensure ward staff are aware of his concern and of the need for counselling	

world. A family tendency to diabetes and obesity seem to predispose to the disease. Treatment is either by diet alone and/or hypoglycaemic drugs, or diet and insulin, depending on the type and severity of the disease.

Patients who are treated with insulin must take great care to balance the amount of food they eat, and the amount of exercise they take, against their insulin requirements. Too little carbohydrate, too much exercise, or too much insulin can all lead to hypoglycaemia and the risk of hypoglycaemic coma.

Table 22.3 will help the A and E nurse differentiate between hyperglycaemia and hypoglycaemia.

Mrs Mary Barnfield who had taken a drug overdose

The profile given in Figs. 22.15 and 22.16 concerns a woman who has taken a drug overdose – in this instance, diazepam, paracetamol and alcohol.

Related structure and function

The gastro-intestinal tract is a muscular tube stretching from the mouth to the anus. It is responsible for rendering ingested food into a form suitable for absorption and use by cells throughout the body. The process is highly efficient and of the two kilos or so of food eaten each day only about 150 grams are passed as faeces.

Food is taken in via the mouth where it is chewed by the teeth and moistened, softened and formed into a bolus by saliva. The bolus of food is swallowed by a voluntary action until the food reaches the back of the pharynx when an involuntary reflex takes over. It passes down the oesophagus, its speed depending on the individual's position and the consistency of the food (liquids take about one minute, solids about three), into the stomach.

The stomach is the widest part of the gut with a capacity of about one litre. Food is diluted in the stomach with gastric juices secreted by cells in the

Table 22.3. *Differences between hypo- and hyperglycaemia*

	Hypoglycaemia	Hyperglycaemia
Onset	Rapid (usually minutes)	Slow (several days)
Skin	Profuse sweating	Dehydrated, dry and hot
Other reactions	Tachycardia	'Air hunger'
	May be irrational, abusive or disorientated	Smell of ketones on breath
	BP, pulse and respirations usually normal	Glycosuria
		BP ↓ P ↑ + rapid

Both conditions will lead to coma and death if left untreated. Careful, thoughtful observation by the A and E nurse will be valuable in reaching an accurate diagnosis and commencing the appropriate therapy

---

Mrs Mary Barnfield was well known to the A and E staff. She often presented in the department with minor problems and worries. She had no GP as several doctors had asked for her to be removed from their lists and the others she 'did not trust'. She looked much older than her 35 years and took little care of her appearance or personal hygiene. She had been an inpatient in the psychiatric unit of the hospital on a number of occasions, being treated voluntarily for depressive illness.

Both Mary and her common-law husband Jack were known to abuse alcohol and Jack often became violent following extended drinking bouts. He frequently damaged furniture in their council flat and would occasionally hit Mary as well. It was usually a day or two after such an incident that Mary was brought in by ambulance having taken an overdose of drugs.

On this occasion she was brought in during the early evening having consumed an unspecified quantity of cider, twenty 5mg tablets of diazepam and, unusually for Mary, ten paracetamol tablets. She said she had taken them about 40 minutes previously because she was worried Jack would hit her again. She was extremely tearful and verbally abusive when she arrived but quietened down as soon as she saw a staff nurse whom she recognised.

Fig. 22.15 *Profile: Mrs Mary Barnfield*

stomach wall. Gastric acid, secreted by parietal cells, inhibits the reproduction of bacteria in the food and begins to break down proteins into a form suitable for absorption. Very little is absorbed from the stomach, the notable exceptions to this being alcohol, some water and certain drugs such as aspirin (acetyl salicylic acid).

The stomach empties its contents into the duodenum. The rate at which it empties will depend on the amount and type of food it contains. As a general rule, the greater the volume of food in the stomach, the more rapidly it will empty. The process will be slowed if the individual is lying down since gravity plays a part in the process. The presence of fat, protein and starch all slow gastric emptying as the duodenum needs more time to cope with them. Fear and the presence of narcotics or barbiturates will also slow emptying of the stomach.

Food is squirted into the duodenum where it is mixed with bile and pancreatic secretions and propelled by peristalsis into the jejunum. Calcium, magnesium, copper and iron are absorbed from the duodenum. The jejunum and ileum are the main site of absorption in the gut. Food is mixed with 'intestinal juice' and its final breakdown into products suitable for absorption occurs. The large intestine is an important site of water absorption but most other substances are absorbed in the small intestine.

The liver is the most important single organ in the metabolism of all dietary constituents (fats, proteins and carbohydrates). It either converts the food products into forms suitable for cellular use or into their storage form. Most drugs and alcohol are metabolised and detoxified in the liver by specific enzymes. Drugs are made water-soluble in the liver and excreted.

Waste products of digestion consisting of cellulose, bacteria, fats, calcium, desquamated cells and water (75%) will be passed as faeces.

Care of Mary Barnfield

Mary was taken to a cubicle where oxygen and suction were available. She was placed on a hard-based trolley which could be tipped to a head-down position (this would be necessary if gastric lavage were to be performed). Her own clothes were removed and placed in a labelled bag – she had no valuables and no means of identification but gave her name and address willingly. She was helped into a hospital gown. A vomit bowl was placed within her reach and she was offered a bedpan. Her temperature, pulse, blood pressure and respiration rate were recorded and all were noted to be within normal limits. She was fully conscious.

Two possible courses of care for Mary are outlined and discussed in the following section.

Scenario 1

The Casualty Officer was asked to see Mary as soon as possible. He examined her briefly, ascertained what she had taken and when she had taken it, and asked for a stomach washout to be performed in order to remove as many of the tablets as possible from Mary's stomach. Mary was asked if she had vomited since taking the tablets and replied that she had not.

Mary had had stomach washouts before and knew what to expect. At first she refused to allow the procedure to be carried out but agreed when the staff nurse whom she knew said that she would perform the procedure. Patient cooperation in this rather unpleasant task is highly desirable and time spent by one nurse gaining the individual's confidence and trust is usually well rewarded. A brief explanation of what is to be done must be given and the patient assured that the procedure is uncomfortable but not painful. The need for removing the tablets whilst they remain in the stomach should be stressed. Verbal or written consent to the procedure should be obtained – it constitutes criminal assault to perform a washout on an unwilling patient.

The necessary equipment was prepared out of Mary's sight though she was not left unattended. A wide-bore stomach tube (at least 35 FG) should generally be used since tablets easily become lodged in and block a smaller tube. Once the equipment was prepared the nurse in charge ensured that powerful suction apparatus was close by and switched on.

Mary was asked to lie flat on her right side, the trolley sides remained raised, her pillow was removed and the trolley tilted head down. She did not have her dentures in but they would have been removed at this stage and placed in a labelled container with her other personal possessions. Mary's hands were firmly held by a second nurse so that she would be less likely to try to pull out the tube. A padded gag was placed between Mary's teeth to prevent the tube being bitten during the procedure and the staff nurse passed the tube through the mouth and into the stomach asking Mary to swallow as she did so. The patient must be carefully observed at this stage to ensure that the tube has not passed into the larynx thus obstructing the airway, though this is highly unlikely. Fluid and partly dissolved tablets came through the tube when it was lowered below the level of Mary's stomach and a specimen of this fluid was taken in a universal container labelled with Mary's name. This would be kept for two weeks in case evidence of what she had taken should be needed. About 100 ml of water at 37°C was poured through the funnel and tubing into Mary's stomach, the funnel was then lowered over a bucket and the fluid, together with more stomach contents, allowed to flow out. The procedure was continued using 200–400 ml of fluid at about 37°C each time until only clear fluid returned. It was assessed that at least as much fluid had returned as had been used in the procedure, making it unlikely that excess fluid remained in Mary's stomach. Intermittent bouts of suction had been necessary during the procedure as Mary had vomited around the tube. The tube was allowed to drain and then removed. The equipment was cleared away and a nurse remained with Mary, washed her face, sat her up on the trolley and made her feel as comfortable as possible.

Scenario 2

The Casualty Officer was asked to see Mary as soon as possible. He examined her briefly, ascertained what substances she had ingested and when, and asked for her to be given 50 ml of Paediatric Ipecacuanha Emetic Mixture followed by two glasses of strong orange juice. It was explained to Mary that the mixture would make her vomit and so empty her stomach of the noxious concoction of tablets and alcohol which she had taken. This would avoid the need for a stomach washout to be performed. Mary drank the mixture and juice as she was requested and within 20 minutes had vomited copious amounts of fluid containing tablet debris. Following the treatment, Mary was helped to wash her face and hands and was positioned on the trolley as comfortably as possible.

Mary was seen again by the Casualty Officer following her stomach washout and agreed to remain in the short-stay ward overnight to ensure that her condition did not deteriorate. Although many fragments of tablets had been removed it was felt wise to ensure that any remaining did not affect Mary adversely. A specimen of venous blood was taken to assess the level of paracetamol in Mary's blood. Mary had thought this a harmless drug and was shocked to hear that the lethal dose could be as few as ten tablets.

Mary spent a comfortable night in the short stay ward where she was seen by the duty psychiatrist the following morning and declared medically and psychologically fit for discharge. She was given an outpatient appointment to see her psychiatrist the following week.

Fig. 22.16 *Profile: Mary Barnfield (2)*

Stomach washout (or gastric lavage) is an unpleasant procedure for both the patient and the nursing staff who are required to perform it. The unwary nurse can easily fall into the trap of making the experience a punishment for the patient, particularly if she is uncooperative and abusive. Many of the patients who require this treatment will have taken an overdose of drugs in order to gain attention in some form and it can be difficult in a busy department, full of acutely ill patients, to spend the necessary time talking to the individual, gaining her trust and coaxing her through the experience. This is especially so when the patient is a 'regular' who may be considered by some to be wasting the staff's time. The nurse should make every effort to care compassionately and without prejudice for such patients.

Blake *et al.* (1978) and Proudfoot (1984) suggest that many patients are subjected to the trauma of gastric lavage unnecessarily. Gordon (1985) concluded from his study that 'emesis induced by correctly administered Paediatric Ipecacuanha Emetic Mixture (BP) (adequate dose accompanied by adequate fluid) is safe, less traumatic for the patient, at least as effective as gastric lavage, considerably less time-consuming for the Accident and Emergency staff and can be administered within minutes of the patient being seen by the medical staff.'

Forced emesis has been used for treating children for many years as gastric lavage is avoided if possible. It has become increasingly popular in recent years for the treatment of adults who have ingested poisons. Its use is contra-indicated in those clients whose consciousness is impaired and in those whose poisoning is due to corrosive fluids, petroleum distillates and iron. It should be induced as soon as possible following the ingestion of the poisons for maximum efficacy. The dosage of ipecacuanha may be repeated if the client has not vomited within 30 minutes.

Overdose in children

Overdose in children is almost always accidental and the variety of ingested substances is enormous – from poisonous berries and garden debris to household cleaners and any brightly coloured tablets. The child rarely understands why he has been brought to hospital and usually feels quite well. It is often difficult to ascertain precisely what quantity of poisonous substance has been consumed or even when it was taken. The regional poisons centre (the telephone number will be available in every A and E department) will give information as to the constituents of most proprietary brand substances and the advised treatment. Induced vomiting should not be undertaken if any form of corrosive substance has been swallowed. If a stomach washout is essential it is best done quickly with the child held tightly wrapped in a blanket. Experience suggests that it is usually best if the child's already guilt-ridden mother is not present during this procedure but is allowed to comfort her child *immediately* afterwards.

Overdose: general points

Some substances have specific antidotes but for the most part the rule is to treat the symptoms as they arise. Each region in the UK has a poisons centre which may be consulted regarding the contents of a particular substance or any specific antidote or treatment available. They will also advise of any likely effects that should be observed for.

Mary Barnfield's care has been included as a reminder that not all A and E nursing is glamorous and exciting and the learner will find herself faced with many unpleasant duties. Very little was done for Mary during this admission, apart from treating her presenting symptoms and providing a little of the time and attention which she so desperately needed. For patients such as Mary there is often little of lasting value that can be done until the patient is, herself, ready to receive help with her problem. Accepting this fact can be one of the most difficult aspects of A and E nursing.

Claire Richards who was finding breathing difficult

A little girl suffering from an asthma attack is the subject of the profile in Fig. 22.17.

Related structure and function

The respiratory pathway and its function have been discussed earlier in the chapter (see pages 663–664). Asthma is a respiratory disease characterised by bouts of dyspnoea and wheezing. An allergic reaction occurs in the bronchioles of the lungs when substances, including histamines, are released in response to the inhalation of allergens such as pollen. Histamines cause the smooth muscle around each bronchiole to constrict. They further cause swelling of the bronchial mucosa and thick mucous secretions are produced. Wheezing tends to occur during expiration as the individual tries to force air through the constricted bronchioles and air becomes trapped in the alveoli, adding to respiratory difficulties.

Childhood asthma usually occurs in individuals who are allergic to certain substances, such as pollen, feathers, or house-dust mites. It is an inherited tendency and sufferers may have other allergic disorders such as eczema or allergic rhinitis. The symptoms may be aggravated by irritation from smoke, cold air and dust. Chest infections, emotional stress and strenuous exercise may also provoke an asthmatic attack.

Nursing care for the child who has difficulty in breathing

The use of standard care plans can save time in a busy A and E department and such a plan was used for Claire. The basic care plan in Fig. 22.18 outlines the care that is likely to be needed by all children with this problem. Problems 1 to 5 were already listed along with the aims of care and the proposed nursing intervention. Problems 6 to 9 were additional problems pertinent to Claire's condition and were added to the standard care plan as her needs were assessed.

Claire Richards was brought into the A and E department by her mother soon after midnight one February evening. She was four years old and had suffered with asthma since she was five months old. That afternoon she had been to her closest friend's birthday party and had returned well and excited. She had gone to bed as usual at about seven o'clock but had woken at eleven finding it difficult to breathe. Claire's mother, Ann, had tried to get Claire to use her inhaler but it proved ineffective. A dose of salbutamol administered in the nebuliser Claire had at home gave temporary relief but the wheezing soon began again. Mrs Richards had telephoned their GP who had advised her to take Claire straight to the hospital.

Claire looked pale and very frightened. She was clearly having great difficulty breathing and a marked expiratory wheeze was noted. She and her mother were greeted by the nurse allocated to care for Claire and shown without delay to a cubicle with piped oxygen available. Claire was placed on a trolley sitting upright and well supported with pillows but she immediately wriggled around and dangled her legs over the side of the trolley. A table was placed in front of her and her mother stood beside it to ensure that Claire did not fall. Claire leaned forward and rested her arms on the table – this pose is typical in individuals experiencing an asthmatic attack and is the position in which best use may be made of the accessory muscles of respiration. The staff nurse noted that Claire appeared cyanosed and decided to administer oxygen.

Bronchodilator drugs were administered in a nebuliser attached to the oxygen circuit but provided minimal relief for Claire and the Casualty Officer requested an intravenous infusion to be prepared so that aminophylline (a strong bronchodilator) and a steroid drug (hydrocortisone) could be administered intravenously. Intravenous fluids help to counter the dehydration which is a common feature of acute asthmatic attacks.

Claire's wheezing became less pronounced and her breathing noticeably easier a few minutes after the intravenous drugs had been given. It was clear that admission was necessary since this was a more severe attack than Claire had experienced for many months and her condition was liable to deteriorate again if treatment was stopped too soon.

A paediatrician saw Claire in A and E and arranged a bed for her on the children's ward. The nursing staff made arrangements for Mrs Richards to stay with Claire. She was transferred to the ward as soon as her breathing had eased and was accompanied by the nurse who had cared for her whilst she was in the department. She was lifted into bed and made comfortable, sitting at an angle of 45° propped up on pillows, and fell asleep within a few minutes.

***Fig. 22.17** Profile: Claire Richards*

The reader is referred to the discussion earlier in this chapter on the special needs of children in A and E.

Fig. 22.18 *Care Plan for Claire Richards*

Name: *Claire Richards* **Next of Kin**: *Mother/*
Ann Richards **Time**: 00.20 hours
Age: 4 **Informed**: *Present* **Medical Diagnosis**: *Acute asthmatic attack*
Date: 16.2.92 **Religion**: *C/E*

Problem	Aim	Intervention	Evaluation
(1) Difficulty breathing Breathing	Reduce difficulty and observe for signs of deterioration	(a) Position the child sitting upright on trolley, well supported by pillows (b) Reduce anxiety by calm, unhurried but efficient approach (c) Do not ask unnecessary questions – if possible phrase questions so that the child may reply by nodding or shaking head (d) Give drugs as prescribed	(a) Not comfortable. Try legs over side to aid use of accessory muscles of respiration 00:40 hours. Prefers this position (d) Needs intravenous infusion for drugs – see Problem (7)
(2) Frightened Communicating	Reduce fear	(a) Allow parent/carer to stay throughout if possible (b) Explain everything to the child (c) Calm approach in manner and voice	
(3) Unable to maintain own safety Maintaining a safe environment	Ensure safe environment	(a) Stay with the child at all times (b) Trolley sides securely up whenever possible (c) Remove any sharp or dangerous objects from the vicinity	(b) Trolley side down to enable Claire to sit comfortably – ensure that the table will not move and allow her to fall
(4) Potential for deterioration in condition	Recognise any change in condition as soon as possible so that prompt action may be taken	(a) Assess and record level of consciousness, skin colour, respiration rate and pulse every 15–20 minutes (b) Note any changes in condition and report at once	(a) 00:40 hours – observe every 15 minutes
(5) Anxious parent Communicating	Reduce anxiety by all means	(a) Allow the parent to assist with care as much as possible (b) Explain fully what is being done (c) Allow access to telephone to organise home situation – if necessary	(c) Mother not worried – husband is at home with two older children

Additional problems	Aim	Intervention	Evaluation
(6) Blue fingers and lips – Claire feels cold Breathing	Increase oxygen supply to lungs, blood and tissues in order to reduce cyanosis	(a) 36% oxygen via a paediatric mask (b) Mother or nurse to hold the mask for Claire until she can tolerate it (c) Constantly explain need for oxygen therapy to Claire	(a) Mask not tolerated so try (b)
(7) Claire needs an intravenous infusion. Potential problems of fear, infection and overloading circulation with too much fluid Eating and drinking Breathing	Ensure safe and accurate delivery of IV fluids and drugs	(a) Explain to Claire the need for IVI (b) Prepare equipment out of sight to reduce anxiety (c) Ensure cannula and tubing securely sited and not able to be pulled out (d) Strict aseptic technique to ensure infection avoided at cannula entry site and in IV solution (e) Ensure fluids and drugs are administered as directed	(e) Infusion commenced 00:40 hours
(8) Feels there is 'no air to breathe' Breathing	Increase air flow around Claire	Too cold to open windows. Try fan in room on low setting. Ensure Claire is warmly wrapped and does not get cold	00:50 hours. Feels better Fan switched off
(9) Is unprepared for hospital admission Working and playing	Prepare as well as possible in time available	(a) Explain the need to go to the ward (b) The nurse to accompany Claire and her mother (c) Arrange for Mrs Richards to stay if she wishes	(a) Claire is happy to go to the ward. She wants to 'get better' (c) Arranged with ward 01:00 hours

Claire's care in the A and E department illustrates the need for the nurse constantly to evaluate her care and to update her plans and their implementation whenever necessary. This is particularly important when caring for children as their condition is susceptible to particularly rapid change.

It further illustrates the importance of extending care not only to the child but to the family group to which she belongs, and particularly to any family members who are present.

Caroline George suffering acute abdominal pain

The profile in Fig. 22.19 concerns a young woman admitted to the A and E department with acute abdominal pain.

Related structure and function

The abdomen contains a number of structures which are susceptible to inflammation, obstruction, vascular disorders or haemorrhage. Because none of the organs is externally visible, diagnosis in the early stages of an episode of acute abdominal pain can be difficult and the patient may be severely shocked before decisive action is taken. Necessary surgical intervention should begin as soon as possible but unnecessary surgical intervention may exacerbate the patient's condition or put his life at risk. Accurate history taking and careful, constant observation and assessment of the patient's condition are essential if appropriate and effective treatment is to begin at the earliest possible stage. The A and E team must also be

Caroline George, aged 29, was brought to the A and E department by ambulance from her office in town. She had felt vaguely unwell all morning and about an hour previously had felt intense lower abdominal pain which persisted. She was unable to continue her work and could not find a comfortable position. Her colleagues thought she looked extremely unwell and had called for an ambulance. A female colleague accompanied her.

On arrival in the department Caroline appeared to be in considerable pain and was constantly changing her position in an attempt to ease the discomfort. She looked pale and her skin was clammy to touch. She was transferred to a hard-based trolley and two nurses helped her to remove her clothes and put on a hospital gown. Whilst doing this the nurses were able to ask relevant questions about Caroline's personal details (name, age, address, next of kin) and her history related to abdominal pain. They ascertained that her appendix had been removed several years previously; she had never experienced similar pain before, and she thought she could be pregnant as her menstrual period was two weeks late. The nurses took and recorded Caroline's pulse, blood pressure, temperature and respiration rate as soon as she was undressed. Her temperature, pulse and respiration rate were all raised above the expected normal levels (temperature, 38.4°C; pulse, 104; respirations, 28). Her blood pressure was lower than expected (85/55 mmHg). They asked the Casualty Officer to see her at once since they were unhappy about her condition.

The doctor's examination revealed acute lower abdominal pain with accompanying rigidity of the abdomen in that area. In view of her history and the fact that she was clearly very unwell, he suspected a ruptured **ectopic pregnancy**. He requested that a gynaecologist see her at once, that blood be taken and cross-matched as an emergency and that an intravenous infusion be set up to replace lost fluid until the blood was ready.

Fig. 22.19 *Profile: Mrs Caroline George*

aware of the possible causes of acute abdominal pain and the relevance of specific signs and symptoms.

Pain is a feature of all acute abdominal conditions and its exact location, intensity and type may give vital clues as to the organ involved.

(1)   *Central abdominal pain* which moves to the right iliac fossa commonly indicates appendicitis, while central pain moving to the left iliac fossa may be caused by acute diverticulitis.

(2)   *Generalised abdominal pain* may indicate an intestinal obstruction or pancreatitis if it is constant, or a perforated peptic ulcer if it is 'wave-like' and radiating.

(3)   Pain from the liver, bile ducts, gall bladder, stomach, spleen and duodenum tends to be felt in the *upper portion of the abdomen*, while pain in the *lower third of the abdomen*, the hypogastrium, is more probably indicative of problems with the colon (usually in elderly people) or of a gynaecological emergency in a female of child-bearing age.

(4)   If an abdominal organ ruptures and fluid or blood is spilled into the abdominal cavity, acute generalised abdominal pain will result.

Vomiting is sometimes associated with acute abdominal conditions.

(5)   *Pain generally precedes vomiting* when the cause is acute appendicitis, intestinal obstruction or acute cholecystitis.

(6)   If *vomiting precedes pain* and is the more dominant feature of the episode the cause is more likely to be gastro-enteritis, pancreatitis, pyelitis or severe constipation.

(7)   The abdomen is usually *tender and rigid near the site of the affected organ*, particularly when an organ has perforated or ruptured.

Abdominal distension may indicate the presence of gas or fluid in the abdominal cavity or acute intestinal obstruction. Measuring and recording the patient's girth measurement may indicate any increasing distension. However, these recordings are often inaccurate and should be interpreted only in conjunction with other observations of the patient's condition.

Shock and collapse are likely if internal haemorrhage or fluid leakage remain untreated. *Hypovolaemic shock* will occur when there is insufficient circulating blood volume to supply the oxygen requirements of the body's tissues. The patient will look pale and unwell. The skin often looks grey and peripheral or central cyanosis may be apparent; the skin is usually cold and clammy to the touch. This is because circulation to the heart and brain is maintained at the expense of blood supply to the skin and other less vital organs. The patient may be restless, confused and disorientated if the oxygen supply to the brain is inadequate and coma and death will result if hypovolaemia remains untreated. The heart rate will increase to compensate for the loss of blood volume and the pulse will be rapid, shallow and often irregular. Blood pressure will be lowered. Respirations will generally be rapid but shallow because of the patient's **hypoxic** state. Urinary output will fall as the kidneys re-absorb fluid in an attempt to compensate for lost blood volume. The patient may be thirsty.

If fluids are not replaced and the loss arrested, the patient will become acidotic and comatose and death will quickly ensue. Early diagnosis of shock is thus essential.

Care of Caroline George

Caroline's observations 20 minutes after her arrival revealed: respirations, 32; pulse, 108; and blood pressure, 80/50 mmHg. Her skin was grey, pale and cold and clammy and she was moaning to herself. She was reluctant to answer questions. An intravenous infusion was set up with one litre of normal saline (154 mmol/l-0.9%) to run over four hours. Caroline was laid flat on the trolley with one pillow under her head to maintain adequate blood circulation to her heart and brain. The staff explained to her what was happening and tried to appear relaxed and calm.

The nurses began to prepare Caroline for emergency surgery since it seemed that this may be necessary. Mental preparation of the patient is an important part of the patient's care though most people who are in acute pain are happy to accept any treatment which will relieve it. Whilst it is the surgeon's job to ensure that he obtains the patient's informed consent to surgery, the nursing staff frequently spend more time with the patient and are able to reinforce his comments and answer any questions the patient may wish to ask.

Caroline had had nothing to eat or drink for five hours because she had felt unwell, so it was deemed unnecessary to pass a nasogastric tube to remove the stomach contents. She was helped to use a bed-pan since she was unfit to move from the trolley. Her nail polish was removed and she was asked if she had any dentures, contact lenses or other prostheses. She was able to remove her own contact lenses and these were stored in the special case found in her handbag. She was informed that her husband had been contacted and was on his way to the department.

The gynaecologist rapidly agreed with the provisional diagnosis of ruptured ectopic pregnancy, and arranged for Caroline's transfer to theatre for surgery ten minutes later. Her observations were stable but she continued to look unwell and in pain. Final pre-operative preparations were made

(see Chapter 24). There was not time for a premedication to be given and analgesics had been withheld since they can mask the patient's symptoms and increase the rate at which shock develops. Caroline's wedding ring was covered with adhesive tape, her jewellery was removed and kept in safe custody, along with her other valuables, in accordance with the hospital policy. A nameband was completed with Caroline's name, age, casualty notes number and home address (no decision had as yet been made as to which ward she would be admitted) and these details were checked with Caroline before the name-band was attached to her wrist.

All relevant documentation was completed including nursing notes, fluid balance chart and observation charts and these were clipped together with her medical notes, consent form and receipt for valuables. Her belongings were placed in a polythene bag, tied and clearly labelled with her name. The intravenous fluid bag was hung on a pole attached to the trolley. Brief explanations of what was being done were given to Caroline throughout and the colleague who had accompanied her was informed that she needed immediate surgery and that her husband had been contacted. She was allowed to see Caroline briefly, thanked for her help and advised to telephone later for further information.

Caroline was accompanied to theatre by the nurses who had cared for her in the department. They stayed with her until she was fully anaesthetised and ensured that her property was handed over to the theatre staff before leaving.

The gynaecologist later confirmed that he had found a ruptured uterine tube suggesting an ectopic pregnancy. There had been almost a litre of bloody fluid in Caroline's abdominal cavity but haemostasis had been quickly achieved and her condition was stable. She was expected to make a good physical recovery.

Caroline's care illustrates many aspects of Accident and Emergency nursing:

(1) The importance of team work is essential if acutely ill patients are to be cared for optimally;

(2) The nurse must not only record observations but interpret them and ask for immediate medical help if she is unhappy about her patient's condition;

(3) Establishing a rapport with each patient and so gaining his confidence and cooperation will mean that care can be delivered efficiently and quickly;

(4) Many patients are in the department for less than an hour and the A and E nurse must do her best to prepare them for a totally unexpected admission to hospital;

(5) A great deal of time can be saved if the A and E nurse is familiar with preparations required prior to emergency surgery and other emergency procedures.

Conclusions

This chapter has covered, very briefly, some of the many facets of nursing care as practised in an A and E department. The care studies have aimed to illustrate various aspects of that care and to highlight, above all, the need for assessing each patient and his needs *on an individual basis*. The need to be prepared for possible deterioration in the patient's condition has been stressed, as has the importance of interpreting any observations in the light of the patient's overall condition. Helping the patient and his relatives to come to terms with acute illness without feeling they have lost control of the situation is an important skill for all Accident and Emergency nurses to learn.

It is hoped that the chapter will help to prepare the nurse for the many individuals with whom she is likely to come in contact during her experience of Accident and Emergency nursing.

Glossary

Contracture: A permanent contraction of a muscle or group of muscles caused by shortening and fibrosis of the muscle fibres, and leading to the loss of, or alteration in, function

Cyanosis: The appearance of blueness of the skin and mucous membranes caused by inadequate oxygenation of the tissues – for example, in patients with respiratory disease. Cyanosis is evident when more than 5g of haemoglobin per decilitre is in the reduced state

Ectopic pregnancy: Occurs when the products of conception implant outside the uterus, most commonly in the uterine tubes which rupture when the embryo becomes too large

Flaccid: Soft, without tone. *Flaccid paralysis* is the term applied to limbs where muscle tone and reflexes are absent

Foot drop: A condition in which the patient is unable to maintain his foot in the correct position because of paralysis of the ankle muscles

Hypertension: Abnormally high blood pressure (a diastolic pressure persistently above 90 mmHg). 90% of cases have no known cause, the remaining 10% are secondary to other diseases, particularly renal and cardiovascular diseases

Hypoxia: Reduced oxygen supply to the tissues, which affects their metabolic needs

Intracranial pressure: The pressure within the cranium. The pressure is measured by carrying out lumbar puncture and may be raised following head injury, when there is a space-occupying lesion in the cranium, or when a cerebral haemorrhage has occurred

Papilloedema: Oedematous swelling of the optic disc seen on ophthalmoscopy. Indicates raised intracranial pressure

References

Accident and Emergency Nursing Forum. (1989). *Guidelines for Dealing with Aggression in the Accident and Emergency Department*. RCN, London.

Blake, D.R., Bramble, M.G. and Grimley Evans, J. (1978). Is there excessive use of gastric lavage in the treatment of self-poisoning? *Lancet*, ii, 1362–1364.

Blythin, P. (1988). Triage in the UK. *Nursing*, 3(31), 16–20.

British Paediatric Association/British Association of Paediatric Surgeons. (1985). *Children's Attendances at A*

& E Departments. *A Report by the Joint Committee of the BPA and BAPS*. British Paediatric Association, London.

British Paediatric Association/British Association of Paediatric Surgeons and Casualty Surgeons Association. (1987). *A Joint Statement on Children's Attendances at Accident and Emergency Departments*. British Paediatric Association, London.

Colling, A., Dellipiani, A.W., Donaldson, R.J. and McCormack, P. (1976). Teeside Coronary Survey. *British Medical Journal*, 2(6045), 1169–1172.

Elkins, R. and Roberts, M. (1983). Psychological preparation for paediatric hospitalisation. *Clinical Psychology Review*, 3, 275–295.

Fry, J. (1968). Acute myocardial infarction. In *Cardiology*, Julian, D.G. and Oliver, M.F. (eds.). Churchill Livingstone, Edinburgh.

Gordon, G. (1985). Ipecacuanha induced emesis in the treatment of self-poisoned adults. *Archives of Emergency Medicine*, 2, 203–208.

Hayward, J. (1975). *Information: A Prescription against Pain*. RCN, London.

Jones, G. (1990). A & E nursing: today and the future. *Nursing Standard*, 4(27), 51–52.

Laing, G.S. (ed.). (1988). Children in the A and E department. *The A and E Letter*, 3, 1–7.

Lee, M. (1988). The nurse practitioner in the Accident and Emergency department – a possible way forward. *Emergency Nurse*, 3(1), 2.

Lenaghan, P. (1986). *Nursing Interventions after Sudden Death in the Emergency Department*. Presented at Emergency Nurses Association Scientific Assembly.

Mallett, J. and Woolwich, C. (1990). Triage in Accident and Emergency departments. *Journal of Advanced Nursing*, 15, 1443–1451.

McGarvey, M.E. (1983). Pre-school hospital tours. *Children's Health Care*, 11, 122–124.

McGrath, G. and Bowker, M. (1987). *Common Psychiatric Emergencies*. Wright, Bristol.

Nuttall, M. (1986). The chaos controller. *Nursing Times*, 82(20), 66–68.

Parkes, C.M. (1985). Sudden death prolongs mourning period. *Nursing Mirror*, 161(14), 10.

Pisarick, G. (1981). Psychiatric emergencies and crisis intervention. *Nursing Clinics of North America*, 16, 85–94.

Proudfoot, A.T. (1984). Abandon gastric lavage in the Accident & Emergency department? *Archives of Emergency Medicine*, 2, 65–67.

Roper, N., Logan, W. and Tierney, A. (1985). *The Elements of Nursing* (2nd ed.). Churchill Livingstone, Edinburgh.

Thompson, J. (1983). Call Sister – stress in the Accident and Emergency department. *Nursing Times*, 79(31), 23–27.

United Kingdom Central Council for Nursing, Midwifery and Health Visiting. (1987). *Confidentiality. An Elaboration of Clause 9 of the Code of Professional Conduct*. UKCC, London.

UKCC. (1992). *The Code of Professional Conduct* (3rd ed.). UKCC, London.

UKCC. (1992). *The Scope of Professional Practice*. UKCC, London.

Webb, J. and Cleaver, K. (1991). The child in Casualty. *Nursing Times*, 87(15), 27–29.

Wright, B. (1989). Sudden death. Nurses' reactions and relatives' opinions. *Bereavement Care*, 8(1), 2–4.

Wright, B. (1991). *Sudden Death: Intervention Skills for the Caring Professions*. Churchill Livingstone, Edinburgh.

Young, A.P. (1991). *Law and Professional Conduct in Nursing*. Scutari Press, Harrow.

Suggestions for further reading

Awoonor-Renner, S.(1991). I desperately needed to see my son. *British Medical Journal*, 302, 356.

Bache, J.B., Armitt, C.R. and Tobiss, J.R. (1985). *A Colour Atlas of Nursing Procedures in Accidents and Emergencies*. Wolfe Medical, London.

Chaney, P.S. (1976). *Dealing with Death and Dying*. Intermed, Pennsylvania.

Dimond, B. (1990). *Legal Aspects of Nursing*. Prentice Hall, Hemel Hempstead.

Hogg, C. and Rodin, J. (1989). *Setting Standards for Children in Health Care*. National Association for the Welfare of Children in Hospital, London.

Huber, P. (1980). *Nurses' Guide to Cardiac Monitoring* (3rd ed.). Baillière Tindall, London.

Jones, G. (1988). Top priority. *Nursing Standard*, 3(7), 28–29.

Orr, J. (1984). Violence against women. *Nursing Times*, 80(17), 34.

Parkes, C.M. and Weiss, R.S. (1983). *Recovery from Bereavement*. Basic Books, New York.

Rock, D. and Pledge, M. (1991). Priorities of care for the walking wounded. *Professional Nurse*, May, 463–465.

Royal College of Nursing Accident and Emergency Nursing Forum and Society of Paediatric Nursing. (1990). *Nursing Children in the Accident and Emergency Department*. RCN, London.

Royal College of Nursing Association of Nursing Practice, Accident and Emergency Nursing Forum. (1987). *Guidelines for Dealing with Aggression in the Accident and Emergency Department*. RCN, London.

Skinner, D., Driscoll, P. and Earlam, R. (eds.). (1991). *ABC of Major Trauma*. BMJ, London.

Walsh, M. (1985). *Accident and Emergency Nursing: A New Approach*. Heinemann, London.

Westaby, S. and Thorn, A. (1985). Treatment of wounds in the Accident and Emergency department. In *Wound Care*, Westaby, S. (ed.). Heinemann, London.

Relevant support groups and organisations

The following groups and organisations may provide help for some Accident and Emergency patients who do not require hospital admission. Most have local groups – the addresses may be kept in your A and E department or may generally be found in the local press or telephone directories.

Age Concern

Al-Anon
(For relatives of people with drink problems)

Alcoholics Anonymous (AA)
(For those with drink problems)

British Diabetic Association
10 Queen Anne Street, London W1M 0BD

British Epilepsy Association
New Wokingham Road, Wokingham, Berks RG11 3AY

British Pregnancy Advisory Service

British Red Cross

Chest, Heart and Stroke Association
Tavistock House North, Tavistock Square, London WC1N 9JE

Foundation for the Study of Infant Deaths
35 Belgrave Square, London SW1X 8QB

Gingerbread
(For one-parent families)

Relate
(Formerly the Marriage Guidance Council)

Salvation Army

Samaritans

Terrence Higgins Trust
38 Mount Pleasant, London WC1
(For patients and their partners with AIDS or HIV antibodies)

There may also be a local hostel for *battered wives*, day centres for the *lonely* or *homeless*, and support groups for women who have been victims of *rape* or have suffered a *miscarriage*.

23

CARE OF THE ACUTELY ILL ADULT

Kim Manley

This chapter focuses on the biological, psychological and social aspects of caring for the acutely ill adult. Throughout, attention is directed towards helping the sick individual towards growth and self-actualisation, taking a holistic approach and encouraging a return to self-care.

This chapter will include the following topics:

- Self-care concept
- Sympathetic nervous system arousal
- The nurse's role in the care of the acutely ill adult
- The use of Orem's model
- Biological factors in the acutely ill adult
  - stress
  - measurement and monitoring of physical/biological parameters
  - metabolic considerations

- Psychological factors in the acutely ill adult
  - communication and memory
  - sleep
  - sensory deprivation
- Social factors in the acutely ill adult
  - stressful life events
  - the role of the family
- Assessment tools for use with the acutely ill adult
- Planning care

The person who is acutely ill is someone suffering a temporary physiological crisis resulting in partial or total loss of independent function. The nurse's role therefore involves:

— supporting both the patient and those people closely involved with and important to the patient;
— acting for and doing temporarily those activities that the patient (or family) is unable to do for himself;

— facilitating and encouraging the patient's recovery and return to self-care;
— monitoring the patient's progress physiologically, psychologically and socially.

It is believed that physical well-being is closely inter-related with both psychological and social well-being, and that disruption of any one of these aspects will have implications for the others (Dohrenwend and Dohrenwend, 1974; Monat and Lazarus, 1985). It is for this reason that a large component of this chapter addresses psychological and social influences on nursing care.

Biological aspects are also considered in depth because a sound understanding of underlying principles is essential for accurate measurement and interpretation of biological parameters.

Self-assessment questions are included to assist with learning, and are identified by grey boxes.

Finally, in the last part of the chapter, some assessment tools which aid comprehensive assessment in the acute setting are considered and the chapter concludes with a focus on care planning. A care plan for Margaret Parfitt, the young woman with diabetes introduced in Chapter 22, is presented, bringing together many of the principles introduced throughout the chapter.

Before proceeding to these principles, the values and beliefs concerning the nature of the individual person which underlie the chapter are first stated. These values are encompassed by humanistic psychology, existential philosophy and holism.

(1) *Humanistic psychology*: where the person is considered as a complex human being who is forever changing and developing towards growth and self-actualisation. This view differs from preceding schools of thought in psychology where either individuals are considered a product of their past – as in the *psychoanalytical* theory of Freud – or they are considered as mechanistic, learning only through positive and negative reinforcement – as in the *behaviourist* theory of Watson and Skinner (see also Chapter 7).

(2) *Existential philosophy* stresses the uniqueness of the individual human being, the meaning and purpose of human lives and, finally, the freedom of the individual to choose, rather than comply with the dictates of others.

(3) **Holism** where the focus is on the whole person rather than on the constituent parts as in *reductionism* (the opposite of holism). The underlying beliefs are that individuals always respond as a unified whole and that individuals as a whole are more than a sum of their individual parts.

Two themes run throughout the chapter: one relates to the self-care concept, and the other to sympathetic nervous system arousal. These concepts will now be considered in more detail.

(1) Increased concern with active improvement and maintenance of health rather than curing disease

(2) Increased individual responsibility for meeting present and potential health needs

(3) Increased personal control of health and more information pertaining to health as a result of:

    (a) consumerism

    (b) increased media coverage of health topics

    (c) increased *medicalisation* and *iatrogenic disease*

(4) Evidence that psychosocial factors and lifestyle are increasingly connected to mortality and morbidity (for example, environmental hazards, alcoholism)

(5) Increased recognition of the psychological aspects in health and disease as demonstrated by placebo effects

(6) Economic and political factors (for example, costly health care provision can be paid for by the individual rather than the state)

(7) Increased dissatisfaction with health care provision by users

Fig. 23.1 *Factors influential in the developing self-care movement*

Self-care concept

During the past few decades there has been an increased emphasis on the individual's responsibility for his own health. Many of the factors influential in this growing movement are listed in Fig. 23.1.

Encompassed within this concept are the functions of health maintenance, disease prevention, self-diagnosis, self-medication and participation by the patient within the health services.

Orem (1991) defined self-care as 'the practice of activities that individuals initiate and perform on their own behalf in maintaining life, health and well-being'. For the acutely ill person many, if not most, of the activities normally performed by the individual cannot, temporarily, be carried out because of their changed health status. Where such an individual is unable *wholly* or *partially* to perform his own daily health-related care, Orem specifies that nursing assistance will be required.

Sympathetic nervous system arousal

An understanding of the autonomic nervous system and, in particular, the sympathetic nervous system is vitally important for any nurse wishing to care for the acutely ill person. This understanding is necessary for three reasons.

(1) Biological, psychological and social **stressors** have the same outcome in stimulating the sympathetic nervous system.
(2) Acutely ill medical and surgical patients are particularly vulnerable to biological stressors and, to a lesser degree, psychological and social stressors.
(3) Stimulation of the sympathetic nervous system is a well-recognised state which can be easily monitored by the nurse and which provides a valuable indicator of improvement or deterioration.

Autonomic nervous system

The autonomic nervous system has two subdivisions; the *sympathetic nervous system*, active in response to stressors and termed the 'fight and flight' system, and the *parasympathetic nervous system*, most active during sleep and rest, which has a 'conserving' effect on body resources.

Within the body, it is the autonomic nervous system which is responsible for controlling the

- Digestive tract
- Bronchi and bronchioles
- Blood vessel walls
- Bladder
- Eye

Fig. 23.2 *Involuntary muscle sites*

function of the heart, secreting glands and involuntary muscle (involuntary muscle is found at the sites listed in Fig. 23.2). Most of these tissues are supplied by a double motor nerve supply (i.e. both parasympathetic and sympathetic). One set of neurones will be responsible for stimulating smooth muscle fibres to contract (i.e. *excitation*), the other set inhibits fibres, thus causing relaxation (i.e. *inhibition*). For some tissues it is the sympathetic nerves that produce excitation and the parasympathetic nerves which produce inhibition: in other tissues the reverse is so. When both sets of neurones are activated, then the muscle fibre will exhibit a state of partial contraction and partial relaxation. It is this concept of control achieved by the balance between sympathetic and parasympa-

Table 23.1. *Effects of sympathetic and parasympathetic stimulation on various organs and tissues.*
(a) Organs and tissues with both sympathetic and parasympathetic nerve supplies

Organ	Effect of sympathetic stimulation (or parasympathetic inhibition)	Effect of parasympathetic stimulation (or sympathetic inhibition)
Eye	Pupil dilates	Pupil constricts
Salivary glands	Viscous saliva	Thin watery saliva
Bronchial tree	Dilates	Constricts and increases mucus production
Heart		
– Rate	Increases	Decreases
– Atrial excitability/ conductivity	Increases	Decreases
Gut		
– Tone	Decreases	Increases
– Motility	Decreases peristalsis	Increases peristalsis
– Sphincters	Constriction	Relaxation
Bladder		
– Tone	Relaxation	Contraction
– Internal sphincters	Increased tone	Decreased tone

(b) Organs with predominantly sympathetic innervation

Organ	Minimum or no sympathetic activity	Maximum sympathetic activity
Heart		
– Ventricular excitability	Decreases	Increases
– Ventricular contractility	Decreases	Increases
– Coronary arteries	Constriction	Dilation
Blood vessels		
– Systemic	Dilation	Constriction
– Skin	Dilation	Constriction
– Skeletal muscles	Constriction	Dilation
Sweat glands	No sweating	Increased sweating
Liver	–	Glucose release
Kidney	Normal urine formation	Decreased urine output
Blood glucose	Normal	Increased
Basal metabolic rate	Normal	Increased by up to 50%
Adrenal medullary secretion	–	Increased
Mental activity	–	Increased

(c) Organs with predominantly parasympathetic innervation

Organ	Increased parasympathetic activity
Exocrine glands	
– Stomach	Increased secretions
– Pancreas	Increased secretions

NB: *Sympathetic effects may occur indirectly due to reduced blood supply to secreting glands during excessive sympathetic stimulation*

thetic nervous activity that contributes to **homeostasis** (Table 23.1a). Exceptionally, some tissues have only a single motor nerve supply; for example, there is only a sympathetic nerve supply to the sweat glands and blood vessel walls and a predominantly parasympathetic nerve supply to the salivary, gastric and pancreatic glands and the external genitalia (Table 23.1b and c). In these instances, it is the degree of stimulation which determines the level of relaxation, contraction or secretion.

In the context of this chapter, sympathetic nervous system arousal will be further considered.

Once aroused, the sympathetic nerves stimulate the adrenal medulla to release the hormones adrenaline and noradrenaline. These hormones circulate in the blood and further augment and sustain the action of the sympathetic nervous system. Recognition of increased sympathetic activity in the acutely ill person can often alert the nurse to impending deterioration from physiological stressors such as hypoxia or haemorrhage. By working through learning check 1 (Fig 23.3) the essential signs of increased sympathetic activity can be derived.

Self-assessment question one

What are the signs of increased sympathetic drive?

You may find that considering your own body when you are frightened may help you to list them

Answer

- Increased pulse rate/heart rate
- Increased blood pressure
- Peripheral shut down so the limbs feel cool to the touch
- Sweating
- Dilated pupils
- Reduced urinary output
- Dry mouth
- Contracted muscles (increased muscle tone)

Self-assessment question two

When considering a patient who is stressed physiologically, e.g. following haemorrhage, following major surgery or myocardial infarction, which signs of increased sympathetic drive may be reversed and why?

Answer and rationale

Blood pressure and heart rate.
The *blood pressure* may be low following large blood loss resulting in reduced circulating volume which cannot be compensated for by the body. The blood pressure may also be low if a patient has had a large left ventricular myocardial infarction, the ventricle having insufficient functioning muscle to eject the volume of blood necessary to maintain the cardiac output and blood pressure.
The *heart rate* may be reduced because of interruptions or blockages in the heart's conduction system following inferior myocardial infarction which can subsequently also produce a drop in blood pressure.
Three other important exceptions to the typical stressor response of increasing blood pressure also exist and these relate to the following situations:

- Patients receiving *beta-blocking* drugs which inhibit the actions of the sympathetic nervous system

- Drugs which affect the muscle tone of blood vessels, producing vasodilation which causes a subsequent drop in blood pressure

- Septicaemia, which also affects the tone of peripheral blood vessels, causing vasodilation and hence reduced blood pressure, even when other signs of increased sympathetic drive are evident

Self-assessment question three

If increased sympathetic arousal is sustained and large amounts of noradrenaline and adrenaline are continually circulating in the body, what changes may occur other than those identified in self-assessment question one?

(Studying Table 23.1 may help you)

Answer

- Decreased peristalsis potentially leading to paralytic ileus
- Hyperglycaemia
- Perceptual inaccuracies
  - memory alterations
  - communication difficulties

Fig. 23.3 *Learning check one*

The nurse's role in caring for an acutely ill patient

Using Orem's model as a guide, the nurse's role will depend on how able or to what extent the patient can, or should, meet his own self-care needs. Three different nursing systems have been identified by Orem – a system in general terms being considered as the combined actions and interactions of nurses and patients in nursing practice situations.

The 'wholly compensatory' system

The system most pertinent to acute situations is termed the 'wholly compensatory' system because the nurse needs to compensate for the patient's inability to fulfil self-care activities requiring movement. The following patients may require the use of this system:

(1) Unconscious and/or paralysed patients;

(2) Patients who have to limit movement because of their health status. For example, those who have angina pectoris; intermittent claudication; multiple fractures;

(3) Patients who lack the knowledge and skills or who are psychologically unready to perform self-care actions requiring controlled movement; or who require continuous support and supervision (for example, rehabilitation following a head injury if there is residual paresis/plegia of the limbs).

The 'partly compensatory' system

The second system is the 'partly compensatory' system which exists when both nurse and patient perform care involving movement and manipulations.

The supportive–educative system

The third system is the 'supportive–educative' system. Here the nurse would act as a resource and teacher but would also provide psychological and social support.

Table 23.2 summarises these nursing systems and identifies appropriate nurse and patient actions.

Acutely ill patients would normally be expected to progress through these systems as they become increasingly able to care for themselves again. However, the supportive–educative system may

Table 23.2. *Orem's three nursing systems applied to the acutely ill patient and his family*

Nursing system	Nurse's action	Helping method	Patient's action
Wholly compensatory	Identifies needs and goals. Performs self-care for patient. Supports and protects patient	Doing and acting for	Patient does not perform any self-care or is unable to identify needs and goals
Partly compensatory	Identifies with the patient's needs and goals to achieve self-care. Assisting some self-care where the patient is unable to do so himself	Supporting physically and psychologically, teaching. Some doing. Providing a developmental environment	Identifies some needs and goals independently and some with help from the nurse. Needs assistance in some areas
Supportive–educative	Consultant/resource for patient on request	Teaching, guiding, supporting psychologically. Providing a developmental environment	Accomplishes self-care. Identifies own needs and goals. Seeks out resources necessary to meet goals

be the appropriate nursing system for the patient's family and close friends during the acute period.

Helping activities

Five helping activities have been identified and described by Orem (1991): acting or doing for, guiding, supporting, providing a developmental environment, and teaching. These helping activities are related to each of the nursing systems in Table 23.2.

Acting or doing for

This activity would be one of the most frequently used methods for helping patients in acute care settings, especially where the patient is unconscious, unable to participate in decision-making or should not perform a function because of medical treatment. Where the patient is conscious, then the nurse would try to help the patient become involved in making decisions and plans.

Examples of situations where this would be the most appropriate helping activity include:

(1) Positioning an unconscious patient;

(2) Performing tracheal suction on a patient with a newly formed tracheostomy who cannot clear his own secretions;

(3) Measuring blood sugar and administering insulin to a person in diabetic ketoacidotic coma.

Guiding

This helping method is appropriate when the patient must either make a choice or pursue a course of action. It is, however, dependent on the patient's level of motivation and ability to perform the activities required.

For example, a patient recuperating from thoracic surgery may be asked when he would like to sit out of bed during the day. The nurse may guide the patient in his choice by raising considerations such as the time that lunch will arrive or when his visitors and the physiotherapist are expected.

Another example of guiding occurs when the nurse suggests that supporting a surgical wound would reduce a patient's pain when coughing. The patient, assuming he has the physical ability, would probably be motivated to follow such a suggestion if he thought the pain would be reduced.

Other examples of guiding actions include suggestions about the types of food that would be suitable for the patient with a new colostomy to try when eating for the first time. Keywords associated with these guiding activities include:

(1) Suggestions
(2) Instructions
(3) Directions
(4) Supervision.

Supporting

This activity includes the giving of verbal or non-verbal encouragement and physical help to a patient faced with something unpleasant or painful to do.

For example, helping a patient with pain on movement to sit in a chair or walk for the first time following a period of bedrest. Or, alternatively, supporting a patient who is changing his own colostomy bag for the first time, or self-administering his first insulin injection.

Important considerations when using this helping method are, firstly, that once psychological and/or physical support has been received, the patient *must* be capable of controlling and directing the action. Secondly, the nurse must know how much the patient can do for himself without help and when it is appropriate to intervene.

Providing a developmental environment

This helping method involves providing the psychosocial and/or physical environment necessary to motivate the individual to establish appropriate goals. For example, this may involve changing attitudes and values and improving a patient's self-concept.

Physically, this helping method may involve providing resources and demonstrating their use – for example, a patient who cannot speak may be given a communication board which he will also need to be shown how to use.

Teaching

This involves helping a patient who needs to develop new knowledge and skills. For example, a patient following myocardial infarction will need to understand what the predisposing factors to ischaemic heart disease are and how to change his lifestyle to reduce them.

Questions for the nurse delivering acute care

Mullin (1980) has identified two important questions for the nurse to consider when using any helping activity:

(1) Why am I doing this (activity)?

(2) How does this activity assist the individual to increase his ability to care for himself?

Mullin considered these questions important to ask because:

> 'they change the nurse's focus from the illness to the individual and from the tasks to the assistance provided to the individual'
>
> (Mullin, 1980)

Answers to such questions also help the nurse to define the purpose of the task (assisting the individual), clarify issues of **accountability** and consider the rights and responsibilities of the ill person.

Biological factors in the acutely ill adult

This section first considers stress from a biological perspective. The theme of increased sympathetic nervous system arousal (introduced earlier) continues throughout; and the relationships of psychological and social factors to biological factors and stress are introduced. The measurement and monitoring of biological parameters are then considered, followed by metabolic aspects in the acutely ill person.

Stress (see also Chapter 9)

As an acute physiological event, stress has been defined by Hans Selye (1976) as the non-specific, stereotyped response of the body to any demand which is interpreted as a threat to physical or emotional homeostasis.

Acute illness itself may precipitate or result from such a response.

Normally, the first response to a local stressor such as trauma or infection is termed the 'local adaptation syndrome' and this results in the classic features of inflammation; redness, swelling, heat, pain and loss or decrease in function (see Chapter 16). This local adaptation syndrome serves to attack the stressor, repair the tissue and return it to its previously balanced and functioning state. If, however, the tissue damage involved is more extensive, or the local adaptation response is unable to contain the stressor, then a more general widespread response occurs. This is called the **general adaptation syndrome** and represents the culmination of Selye's extensive work into stress.

The general adaptation syndrome reflects the whole body's reaction to the stressor and consists of three distinct response phases. The first phase is termed the *alarm reaction* and consists of a widespread physiological response which includes a large outflow into the bloodstream of the adrenal hormones and the activation of the sympathetic nervous system in an attempt to defend the body from the stressor.

If the stressor is extremely damaging, then continued exposure will be incompatible with life. If the individual survives then the second phase is entered, the stage of *resistance* or *adaptation* where an attempt is made by the body to re-establish equilibrium.

The reserves of hormones are built up again in the adrenal gland and the parasympathetic nervous system tries to regain control to maintain homeostasis.

If the body is unable to re-establish homeostasis because of persistent exposure to the stressor, then the third phase of *exhaustion* will result with similar responses to the alarm phase, ending in death.

The three phases of the general adaptation syndrome are illustrated in Fig. 23.4.

The causative agents producing this response are termed 'stressors' and may be physical, psychological or social in nature. For the acutely ill person possible stressors are identified in Table 23.3.

Greater insight into such stressors can be obtained by considering the Hospital Stress Rating Scale (Table 23.4) which is the result of an American study by Volicer, Isenberg and Burns (1977) to assess the degree of stress associated with

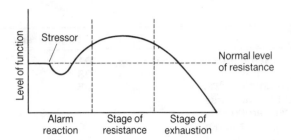

Fig. 23.4 *The three phases of the general adaptation syndrome*

Table 23.3. *Stressors (after Selye, 1976)*

Biorhythm disruption	Noise
Chronic illness	Physical dependency
Crowding	Poor ergonomics/ non-anatomic position
Drugs, including nicotine, caffeine, and alcohol	Poor illumination
Food excess	Restraints
Hypoxia	Sensory overload or deprivation
Inability to earn a living	Separation from social support
Inactivity	Sleep deprivation
Infection	Toxins in air and water
Injury	Ultraviolet light
Lack of information or misinformation	Unfamiliar environment
Loss of control	Vibration
Loss of social position	

different aspects of hospitalisation. This scale was devised from the perceived 'stressfulness of hospital events' for medical and surgical patients.

Monat and Lazarus (1985) consider the role of perception in stress in their definition:

'Stress is a perceived imbalance between demand and resources'.

This definition explains why some people react to a given situation differently to others depending on how they have perceived a stressor. Perception itself is an intricate concept which may in turn be affected by past experiences, genetic predisposition, values and beliefs, self-concept and the level of anxiety at the time the stressor is perceived.

Although it is well recognised that some stress is necessary for normal healthy living and optimal

functioning, the acutely ill individual is exposed to many stressors simultaneously. These act **synergistically** rather than cumulatively. Continued exposure to stressors, whether physiological or psychosocial, can result in the development of stress ulcers, reduced wound healing and reduced cardiac function, amongst other physiological and psychological sequelae.

Measurement and monitoring of physical/biological parameters

The measurement and monitoring of vital signs in the acute setting forms a large part of the nurse's role. The parameters of temperature, pulse, central venous pressure, electrocardiogram, blood pressure and respiration are now considered in detail, as a sound understanding is vital for their correct measurement and interpretation.

Temperature

Temperature measurement may seem a simple procedure, but it is in fact fraught with problems which may lead to inaccurate recordings. Nursing and medical interventions are commonly based on temperature recordings which, if erroneously made, can lead in extreme instances to an elevated temperature being unrecognised. A sound understanding of temperature measurement and influencing factors is essential for nurses who care for acutely ill patients.

Temperature usually fluctuates within a **circadian rhythm** being highest in the evening and lowest at about 6 am. Ganong (1983) cites a large study where 95% of young adults demonstrated an early morning oral temperature range of 36.3°–37.1°C. Normal circadian fluctuations of the core temperature can vary between 0.5°–0.7°C.

Since the rectum is well insulated from the external environment, rectal temperature is considered most representative of the core temperature when using conventional methods of temperature recording. Rectal temperatures will, therefore, be consistently higher than oral temperatures and Durham et al. (1986) cite that the difference is usually in the region of 0.3°–0.65°C. Rectal temperatures, however, take longer to respond to changes in core temperature than other methods.

Durham et al. (1986) reviewed the literature on temperature measurement and summarised a variety of factors which will affect the accuracy of

Table 23.4. *Hospital stress factors*

Factor	Stress-scale events	Assigned rank
(1) **Unfamiliarity of surroundings**	• Having strangers sleep in the same room with you	01
	• Having to sleep in a strange bed	03
	• Having strange machines around	05
	• Being awakened in the night by the nurse	06
	• Being aware of unusual smells around you	11
	• Being in a room that is too cold or too hot	16
	• Having to eat cold or tasteless food	21
	• Being cared for by an unfamiliar doctor	23
(2) **Loss of independence**	• Having to eat at different times than you usually do	02
	• Having to wear a hospital gown	04
	• Having to be assisted with bathing	07
	• Not being able to get newspapers, radio or TV when you want them	08
	• Having a roommate who has too many visitors	09
	• Having to stay in bed or the same room all day	10
	• Having to be assisted with a bedpan	13
	• Not having your call light answered	35
	• Being fed through tubes	39
	• Thinking you may lose your sight	49
(3) **Separation from spouse**	• Worrying about your spouse being away from you	20
	• Missing your spouse	38
(4) **Financial problems**	• Thinking about losing income because of your illness	27
	• Not having enough insurance to pay for your hospitalisation	36
(5) **Isolation from other people**	• Having a roommate who is seriously ill or cannot talk with you	12
	• Having a roommate who is unfriendly	14
	• Not having friends visit you	15
	• Not being able to call family or friends on the phone	22
	• Having the staff be in too much of a hurry	26
	• Thinking you might lose your hearing	45
(6) **Lack of information**	• Thinking you might have pain because of surgery or test procedures	19
	• Not knowing when to expect things will be done to you	25
	• Having nurses or doctors talk too fast or use words you can't understand	29
	• Not having your questions answered by the staff	37
	• Not knowing the results or reasons for your treatments	41
	• Not knowing for sure what illnesses you have	43
	• Not being told what your diagnosis is	44
(7) **Threat of severe illness**	• Thinking your appearance might be changed after your hospitalisation	17
	• Being put in the hospital because of an accident	24
	• Knowing you have to have an operation	32
	• Having a sudden hospitalisation you weren't planning to have	34
	• Knowing you have a serious illness	46
	• Thinking you might lose a kidney or some other organ	47
	• Thinking you might have cancer	48

Factor	Stress-scale events	Assigned rank
(8) **Separation from family**	• Being in the hospital during holidays or special family occasions	18
	• Not having family visit you	31
	• Being hospitalised far away from home	33
(9) **Problems with medication**	• Having medications cause you discomfort	28
	• Feeling you are getting dependent on medications	30
	• Not getting relief from pain medications	40
	• Not getting pain medication when you need it	42

Source: Volicer, B.J., Isenberg, M.A., and Burns, M.W. Medical-surgical differences in hospital stress factors. *Journal of Human Stress*, 1977, 3, 7. Reprinted from *Journal of Human Stress*, vol. 3, no. 2, June, 1977, page 7, by kind permission of the publisher.

Table 23.5. *Factors affecting the accuracy of oral and rectal temperature measurement (Durham et al., 1986)*

Oral temperature	Rectal temperature
Mouth breathing	Presence of stool
Smoking	Placement of thermometer at different sites in the rectum
Recent ingestion of hot or cold liquids	
Local inflammatory processes	
Placement of thermometer at different sites in mouth	
Time left in position	
Oxygen administration	
Tachypnoea	

oral and rectal temperature measurement. These are summarised in Table 23.5.

Because of the embarrassment and psychological effects of measuring temperature rectally, this method would only be performed in an acutely ill person where consciousness is impaired or the use of a glass thermometer in the mouth is contraindicated.

Effective oral temperature measurement involves placing the thermometer in either the left or right posterior sublingual pockets since recorded temperatures are significantly higher in these positions than in the sublingual area at the front of the mouth.

Nichols and her colleagues (cited by Baker et al., 1984) investigated how long an oral glass thermometer should be inserted for different groups in varying environmental temperatures. Their results are summarised in Table 23.6.

Hyperpyrexia is defined as a core temperature between 41° and 43°C. Prolonged temperatures of 41°C and over lead to unconsciousness, brain damage, acute multisystem failure and haemorrhage.

Hypothermia is defined as a core temperature below 35°C. Progressive temperature reduction below this level will result in reduced metabolic rate and risk of cardiac arrest. At 28°–30°C, loss of consciousness will ensue.

Table 23.6. *A summary of insertion times when measuring oral temperature*

Minutes	Group	Environmental temperature
8 mins	Men	18–24°C
9 mins	Women	18–24°C
7 mins	Adults	24.5–30°C
6 mins	Febrile adults	Not noted

Pulse

The rhythmic contraction of the left ventricle results in transmission of a pressure impulse through the arteries. This impulse is customarily palpated at the radial artery in the wrist as the *pulse*. Other pulses of significance include the *femoral* and *ca-rotid pulses* which are important when establishing the adequacy of cardiac output, for example in someone who has suddenly lost consciousness due to possible cardiac arrest; the *brachial pulse* which is used to measure blood pressure; and the pulses of the *lower limbs*, important in determining adequacy of perfusion to these parts. Such pulses

Self-assessment question four	Answer	Rationale

List some possible causes of an increased core temperature in an acutely ill person	(1) Infection:
	  – wound
	  – urinary tract
	  – intravenous cannula site
	  – chest infection
	  – septicaemia
		The temperature regulating centre in the hypothalamus is 'reset' at a higher level due to the effects of pyrogens

	(2) Reduced cardiac output due to
	  – myocardial failure
	  – *hypovolaemia*
		Increased sympathetic activity produces severe peripheral vasoconstriction which then prevents the dissipation of heat produced from *metabolism*. Heat is, therefore, retained within the core circulation. Adrenaline release also increases the metabolic rate which results in greater heat production

	(3) Tissue damage/destruction or inflammation (for example, deep vein thrombosis, myocardial infarction)	Local inflammatory responses produce heat
	(4) Atropine poisoning	Atropine blocks the sympathetic nerves to the sweat glands, therefore preventing heat loss via sweating
Self-assessment question five		

What examples can you think of that are likely to cause hypothermia in patients admitted to acute care areas ?	(1) Accidental exposure to cold	For example:
		  – elderly people due to poor socio-economic conditions
		  – accidental immersion in cold water

	(2) Prolonged anaesthesia	– due to reduced metabolic rate
	(3) Elective cooling	– for example, for the purposes of reducing metabolic demands in patients undergoing cardiac surgery and neurosurgery

	(4) Endocrine disorders
	  – myxoedema
	  – hypopituitarism
		People with these medical problems are unable to increase their metabolic rate in response to exposure to cold

	(5) Barbiturate overdose/acute alcohol poisoning	These drugs cause gross vasodilation and, therefore, excessive heat loss
	(6) Spinal cord injury	Loss of vascular tone can result in gross vasodilation of peripheral vessels with corresponding heat loss

Fig. 23.5 Learning check two

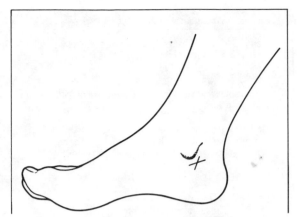

Fig. 23.6 *Region where the posterior tibialis pulse can be palpated (i.e. just behind and slightly below the medial malleolus)*

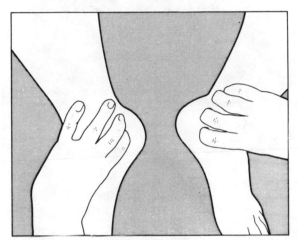

Fig. 23.7a *Palpation of the posterior tibialis pulse*

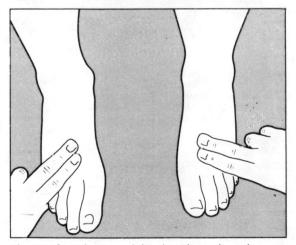

Fig. 23.7b *Palpation of the dorsalis pedis pulse*

include the *popliteal pulse* located behind the knee and the *dorsalis pedis* and *posterior tibial pulses* in the feet (see Fig. 23.6).

Suggested methods of palpating these foot pulses are illustrated in Fig. 23.7 as they can often be difficult to locate – especially when perfusion to limbs is severely reduced (for example, in peripheral vascular disease or where there is extreme vasoconstriction due to the increased activity of the sympathetic nervous system).

Important factors to consider in relation to the radial pulse are:

(1) Rate
(2) Rhythm
(3) Pressure (volume)
(4) Deficits with apex rate.

Pulse rate (usually equivalent to heart rate) is an important component of cardiac output.

> *Cardiac Output* is equal to *Heart Rate (Pulse Rate)* multiplied by *Stroke Volume* (volume of blood ejected by each ventricle with each beat).

Fluctuations of pulse rate in the well individual normally occur together with fluctuations in **stroke volume** to maintain optimum cardiac output for the activity being performed, for example, rest or exercise. In the resting adult, the pulse rate would normally be about 70 beats per minute but in the athlete it can be considerably lower. A rate greater than 100 beats per minute is by definition termed a *tachycardia*, and a rate less than 60 beats per minute is termed a *bradycardia*. Learning check three (Fig. 23.9) asks you to consider why the heart rate (pulse) may deviate from the norm in an acutely ill person.

The *rhythm* of the pulse may vary normally with respiration especially in young adults, so that the pulse is irregular, speeding up at the peak of inspiration and slowing down with expiration. This is termed *sinus arrhythmia*.

Irregular pulses are commonly categorised into the following rhythms:

(1) Regularly irregular
(2) Irregularly irregular.

Regularly irregular pulses are most likely to be caused by *ectopic beats* which occur prematurely. (An ectopic beat is one that originates from a site other than the sino-atrial node.) Occasionally odd ectopic beats may occur in healthy individuals. If, however, they are found to persist in an acutely ill person, the medical staff will require notification as they could be indicative of increased cardiac irritability due to ischaemia or drugs (such as digoxin), increased sympathetic activity as a result of stressors (for example, hypoxia), or they may be related to potassium imbalance, all of which require further investigation.

Irregularly irregular pulses usually indicate **atrial fibrillation** where, because atrial behaviour is chaotic and disorganised, the transmission of impulses to the ventricles is irregular.

The *pulse pressure* determines the strength or force of the pulse and it can be defined as the difference between the systolic and diastolic blood pressures.

The force can be recorded using the scale shown in Fig. 23.8.

```
      0 = impalpable
     +1 = feeble, thready, barely palpable
     +2 = decreased
     +3 = full
     +4 = bounding
```

Fig. 23.8 *Scale for recording pulse pressure*

When the pulse pressure is low, the strength of the pulse may be feeble and thready. This may occur when hypovolaemia exists, because the stroke volume ejected by the left ventricle into the circulation is greatly reduced.

When the pulse pressure is high, the pulse strength may be bounding and the person experiencing this may feel palpitations or hear his heart pounding. You may also have experienced this phenomenon when your sympathetic nervous system is activated – when you are anxious, for example – since this results in your heart contracting more forcibly, causing the systolic blood pressure to increase with subsequent expansion in the pulse pressure.

A *pulse deficit* is the difference between the heart rate counted at the apex of the heart using a stethoscope and the pulse rate counted simultaneously at the wrist. For the majority of patients the heart rate and pulse rate will be the same but, for those who are in atrial fibrillation, or who are having multiple ectopic beats, there will be a

---

Self-assessment question six

Can you think of reasons why the heart rate may deviate from its norm in an acutely ill person?

Answer

Causes of *tachycardia* (i.e. pulse rates higher than 100 beats/min) include:

(1) Increased sympathetic activity due to stressors, whether biological (for example, hypoxia) or psychological (for example, pain, anxiety)

(2) Infection

(3) Cardiac failure
   (The stroke volume is limited and so the heart rate increases to maintain cardiac output)

(4) Cardiac *arrhythmias* (i.e. abnormal rhythms) resulting from electrolyte imbalance or myocardial ischaemia following infarction

(5) Thyrotoxicosis

(6) Drugs
   – particularly those that mimic the sympathetic nervous system, such as inhaled, nebulised salbutamol

(7) Anaemia

Causes of *bradycardia* (i.e. pulse rates below 60 beats/min) include:

(1) Increased parasympathetic activity due to anaesthesia or excessive vagal stimulation (for example, following myocardial infarction, spinal shock, surgery)
   – also vaso-vagal attacks/fainting

(2) Hypothermia
   – accidental or elective

(3) Dysfunction or disease of the cardiac conduction system

(4) Intermittent or continuous interruption of the conduction system of the heart (i.e. atrio-ventricular block), or damage to the sino-atrial node (following myocardial infarction, for example)

(5) Raised intracranial pressure when associated with an increase in blood pressure

(6) Drugs
   – for example, digoxin or beta-blockers (which inhibit receptors in the sympathetic nerve pathway) e.g. propranolol, labetalol, atenolol

Fig. 23.9 *Learning check three*

deficit which it is important to monitor by recording both apex and radial rates.

For an individual who is in atrial fibrillation, the effectiveness of medical treatment, for example with medications such as digoxin, can be judged by a slower irregularly irregular pulse rate of approximately 60–80 beats per minute with minimal or no deficit when compared with the heart rate.

Electrocardiogram (ECG)

The ECG is a record of the changes in electrical activity occurring within cardiac muscle prior to mechanical contraction.

Cardiac cells, in common with other cells within the body, are polarised in the resting state, i.e. the inside of the cell is predominantly negatively charged and the outside predominantly positively charged as shown in Fig. 23.10a. If an electrode were placed within a resting cardiac cell then the potential difference (i.e. the potential for an electrical current to flow) measured would be in the region of −90 millivolts (Fig. 23.10c). When a car-

diac cell is stimulated, the cell depolarises for a few milliseconds and the charges reverse (Fig. 23.10b). This is due to a temporary change in the permeability of the membrane before it returns again to the resting polarised state (repolarisation).

During depolarisation the potential difference across the cell membrane changes so that it becomes +20 millivolts. This change in potential difference is called an **action potential** and if recorded would appear as in Fig. 23.10c.

As a depolarisation wave passes through the heart, a string of action potentials occurs, each cell acting as stimulus to the next. The ECG depicts these electrical changes within the heart and each part of the ECG represents the depolarisation wave at certain stages on its path through the myocardium (Fig. 23.11).

The term *inherent property of rhythmicity* is often used to describe cardiac muscle and its depolarisation. This term means that cardiac muscle can spontaneously depolarise on its own at regular intervals without the need for external stimuli.

This property is most highly developed in the sino-atrial node because the sino-atrial node can depolarise *more quickly* than other potential pacemakers within the heart.

Although cardiac muscle has this special property, external stimulants are important in producing the finer control of the heart in the maintenance of homeostasis.

Where cardiac cells become more excitable and therefore more vulnerable to depolarisation, there is an increased risk of *ectopic* beats occurring (i.e. instead of depolarisation originating in the sino-atrial node, it may originate from any focus in the atria or the ventricles).

Atrial ectopics, or arrhythmias if they arise, may occasionally affect the patient's cardiac output and blood pressure because the atria no longer fulfil their function of completing ventricular filling. Ventricular ectopics and arrhythmias are however more serious as the heart's ability to eject blood into the systemic circulation may be severely affected.

Both atrial and ventricular ectopics occur prematurely (i.e. before the next sinus beat is expected). Atrial ectopics usually have normal QRS complexes, and ventricular ectopics have bizarre complexes (Fig. 23.13) because the depolarisation wave passes through the ventricles in an abnormal, round-about and therefore more time-consuming way.

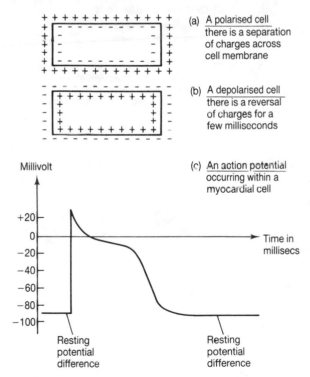

Fig. 23.10 a, b, c.

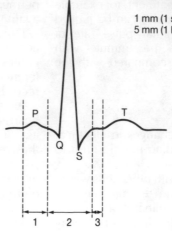

PAPER SPEED

When recording ECGs the paper speed
should be set at 25 mm/s then:

1 mm (1 small square) = 0.04 s
5 mm (1 large square) = 0.20 s

IMPORTANT LANDMARKS

Baseline between T wave and P wave	: iso-electric line indicating no electrical activity
P wave	: atrial depolarisation
QRS complex	: ventricular depolarisation
T wave	: ventricular repolarisation

ECG TERMS

Sinus rhythm	Normal ECG where the impulse originates in the sino-atrial node
	All waves are present. All intervals are normal Rate 60 – 100 per minute Complexes are regular (ie distances between consecutive R waves are constant)
Sinus tachycardia	Complexes are normal but occurring 100/min to 160/min
Sinus bradycardia	Complexes are normal but occurring more slowly than 60/min

IMPORTANT INTERVALS/SEGMENTS

(1) P – R Interval   0.12 – 0.20 s

Represents time taken for impulse
to reach the ventricular
myocardium from the sino-atrial node

(2) QRS Interval   0.08 – 0.12 s

Represents time taken to
depolarise the ventricles

(3) S – T segment

Deviation of this segment above
or below the iso-electric line
may indicate myocardial ischaemia
or injury

Fig. 23.11 *The electrocardiogram*

Fig. 23.12 *Learning check four*

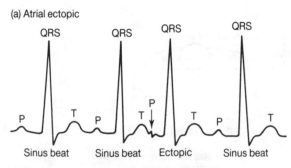

(a) Atrial ectopic

- Premature i.e. occurs earlier than expected
- P wave usually of a different shape
- P – R interval normal/long/short
- QRS normal
- An incomplete compensatory pause following the ectopic

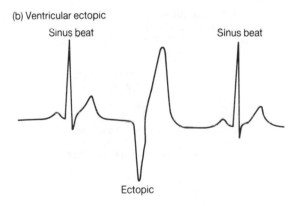

(b) Ventricular ectopic

- No P wave
- QRS wave – premature
  – wide and bizarre looking compared with normal sinus beats
  – > 0.12s
- T wave – usually in opposite direction to QRS
- A complete compensatory pause following the ectopic

Fig. 23.13 *Characteristics of an atrial ectopic and a ventricular ectopic*

Central venous pressure (CVP)

Central venous pressure (CVP) is the pressure of blood in the right atrium or vena cava and measuring it can provide information about:

(1) Blood volume in relation to circulatory capacity;
(2) Vascular tone;
(3) Effectiveness of the right side of the heart as a pump;
(4) Pulmonary vascular resistance.

The venous system contains approximately three fifths of the total circulating volume at any one time, but its capacity can alter with changes in venous tone, so that the greater the tone the smaller the capacity and vice versa. The venous system can be considered as analogous to a reservoir which fills the heart under low pressure, while the heart ejects blood into the arteries under high pressure.

If the reservoir becomes bigger due to reduced venous tone, then even if the circulating volume is normal, the volume of blood returning to the heart subsequently drops and so the pressure in the right atrium also falls.

It is not the single CVP reading that is important but the *trend* demonstrated by a series of readings over time. Therefore, each time a CVP measurement is made, it is essential that it is made under identical conditions so that all possible variables (such as patient position) remain constant.

Measurements are usually made using a water manometer (Fig. 23.14) which is connected to a venous cannula usually placed within the subclavian vein or internal jugular vein.

The water manometer's zero point is then aligned (using a spirit level) with a point on the patient's chest which corresponds to the right atrium.

Two points are widely used as reference points for the right atrium:

(1) *The sternal angle* which is directly above the right atrium when the patient is lying flat

(2) *The 4th intercostal space mid-axilla* which is anatomically in line with the right atrium.

It is imperative to use the same reference point for consecutive recordings, as normal ranges vary according to the reference point selected (Fig.

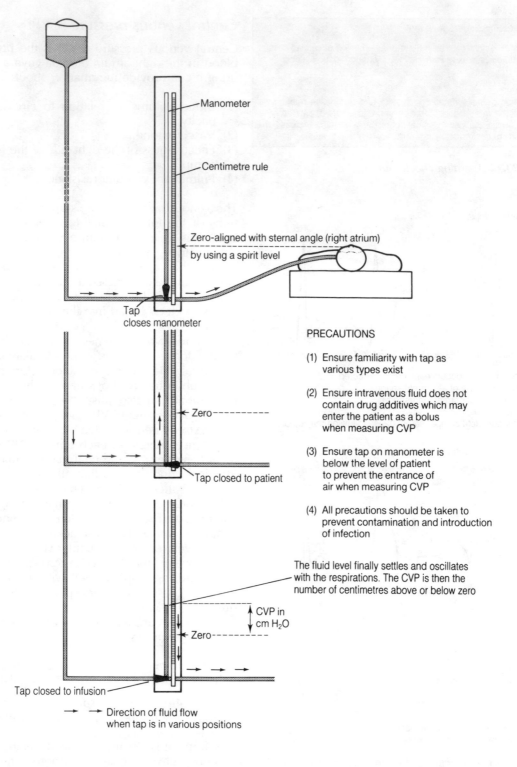

Manometer

Centimetre rule

Zero-aligned with sternal angle (right atrium)
by using a spirit level

Tap
closes manometer

Zero- - - - - - - - -

Tap closed to patient

CVP in
cm H₂O

Zero- - - - - - - -

Tap closed to infusion

→ → Direction of fluid flow
when tap is in various positions

PRECAUTIONS

(1) Ensure familiarity with tap as
various types exist

(2) Ensure intravenous fluid does not
contain drug additives which may
enter the patient as a bolus
when measuring CVP

(3) Ensure tap on manometer is
below the level of patient
to prevent the entrance of
air when measuring CVP

(4) All precautions should be taken to
prevent contamination and introduction
of infection

The fluid level finally settles and oscillates
with the respirations. The CVP is then the
number of centimetres above or below zero

Fig. 23.14 *Measuring CVP using a water manometer*

	Normal CVP ranges
Sternal angle	0 – 5 cm H₂O
Mid-axilla	5 – 10 cm H₂O
4th intercostal space	

Fig. 23.15 Normal CVP ranges

23.15). For either reference point, the patient needs to lie flat but in exceptional circumstances, if breathlessness results when lying flat, the CVP readings may need to be taken with the patient lying at an angle of 45°, in which case this should always be indicated alongside the recorded CVP measurement.

How to perform a CVP measurement is illustrated in Fig. 23.14, and some important precautions are identified.

All lines used to measure CVP are central venous lines and thus present the inherent danger of air embolism. All intravenous administration equipment should, therefore, possess **luer lock** connections to minimise accidental disconnection. Additionally, if the cannula does not possess an on/off switch, then the patient will need to be 'tipped' head down to facilitate the safe changing of intravenous administration sets. Advice will need to be sought if the patient has a tendency to breathlessness in this position.

Another hazard pertinent to subclavian and internal jugular intravenous lines is damage to anatomical structures, e.g. the arteries or the apices of the lungs leading to **pneumothorax**.

In common with all intravenous lines the risk of infection and subsequent septicaemia is high and so the cannula site should be treated as a minor surgical wound requiring the meticulous maintenance of asepsis.

It is important to remember that it is the *trend* in CVP readings which is significant, together with the overall clinical picture of the patient. Table 23.7 gives examples of raised and lowered CVP.

Table 23.7. Causes of raised and lowered CVP

Raised CVP	Rationale
OVERTRANSFUSION	The blood volume has increased in relation to the size of the circulation, so more blood is returning to the right atrium
CARDIAC FAILURE	The heart is impaired in its function as a pump and cannot cope effectively with the blood returning to the heart
PULMONARY EMBOLUS	The right side of the heart has to pump against a greater resistance due to thrombus occluding part of the pulmonary circulation
TAMPONADE	Due to fluid/blood in the pericardial sac the ventricles cannot fill properly. The back pressure is transmitted to the atria

Lowered CVP	Rationale
HYPOVOLAEMIA – Burns – Pancreatitis – Diabetes mellitus HAEMORRHAGE	The circulating volume is reduced so once the venous reservoir is filled there is little blood left to return to the heart
GROSS VASODILATION – Septicaemia – Vasodilatory drugs	Vasodilation increases the capacity of the circulation (or the size of the reservoir) so that the circulating volume is no longer adequate both to fill the veins and provide enough volume to return to the heart.

Blood pressure

By definition, blood pressure is the force exerted by the blood on the walls of the vessels in which it is contained. The maximum pressure is the *systolic*, and the minimum the *diastolic* pressure. Both are currently measured in millimetres of mercury.

Monitoring blood pressure is an important facet of the nurse's role as systolic pressure reflects the adequacy of cardiac output, and diastolic pressure reflects the peripheral resistance exerted by the arterioles.

Maintenance of an adequate blood pressure is essential to permit perfusion of the brain and the coronary arteries and the production of urine by the kidneys.

The blood pressure is maintained at optimum levels in the healthy adult by various mechanisms which finely control the cardiac output and peripheral resistance, so that a constant internal environment can be maintained.

However, in the acutely ill person, the homeostatic mechanisms responsible for maintaining optimum blood pressure may be stretched to their limit, fail to function, or be interfered with by drugs. The consequences of not maintaining an adequate blood pressure can lead ultimately to cerebral hypoxia, cardiac failure, acute renal failure and multi-system failure.

Having discussed low blood pressure it is important not to forget hypertension. This can be equally harmful in the acute setting, especially if it results in the breakdown of a recent surgical anastomosis or increases the work of a damaged myocardium.

Increasing hypertension can also be indicative of raised intracranial pressure (when combined with a simultaneous decrease in pulse rate). The increasing blood pressure in this instance is a protective measure to maintain the cerebral perfusion pressure if the intracranial pressure increases (Fig. 23.16) following head injury or anoxia.

Respiration

Respiration is an essential body function necessary for the diffusion of gases between the alveoli and blood, as well as the maintenance of blood pH.

Effective respiration is dependent on many factors both nervous and chemical in nature. The structures involved in respiration are illustrated in

Cerebral perfusion pressure is the difference between the mean arterial blood pressure and the intracranial pressure and represents the pressure necessary to perfuse the brain. Normally the cerebral perfusion pressure lies between 75–90 mmHg; if it should fall below 50 mmHg then the cerebral blood flow is severely affected.

A rise in intracranial pressure will reduce the cerebral perfusion pressure unless there is a subsequent increase in blood pressure.

CEREBRAL	=	MEAN ARTERIAL	−	INTRACRANIAL
PERFUSION		BLOOD		PRESSURE
PRESSURE		PRESSURE		

Normal intracranial pressure

= 12–15 cm of cerebral spinal fluid (measured at lumbar puncture)

OR = 3–15 mmHg measured using an intracranial pressure monitor

Fig. 23.16 *Cerebral perfusion pressure*

Fig. 23.18, together with possible causes of malfunction.

When assessing respiration there are other important observations to make (in addition to rate) which will help identify the effectiveness of breathing.

Observation of respiration itself can be considered in terms of quality, rate, pattern and depth.

The *quality* of normal, relaxed breathing in any position is effortless, automatic, regular and quiet except for occasional sighing, yawning and coughing.

Noisy, gurgling and wheezing respirations are abnormal and imply an obstruction in the upper respiratory tract. The louder the noise heard at the mouth during inspiration, the greater the degree of airway obstruction present.

Noisy breathing must, however, be separated from other sounds superimposed on a normal breathing pattern which are usually heard through a stethoscope. The noises are termed **crackles** (or **rales**) and **wheezes**. Crackles are heard as 'crackling' or 'popping' sounds and result from the explosive opening of collapsed alveoli in deflated parts of the lungs. Wheezes are musical sounds often associated with asthma which result from opposing bronchial walls oscillating or rapidly opening and closing (Harper, 1981).

The respiratory *rate* in adults is normally between eight to 18 breaths per minute. Counting should be over a minute and take place when the patient is resting and unaware of the observation,

Self-assessment question eight	A low blood pressure in the acute situation is usually the result of a low cardiac output resulting from hypovolaemia. What other signs would indicate that cardiac output was low in this instance?
Answer	**Rationale**
(a) Reduced peripheral perfusion	Peripheral vasoconstriction will occur secondarily to the increased sympathetic arousal found in hypovolaemia, so that the circulating volume is available for the vital organs. As circulating volume increases from transfusion of blood or blood products, cardiac output and blood pressure will improve. Perfusion to the limbs will subsequently increase; this can be felt by the nurse as the warming up of previously cold limbs.
(b) Reduced urinary output	The urinary output will fall to below 1/2 ml/kg body weight/hour for more than two consecutive hours. If the blood pressure is persistently too low to perfuse the kidneys (for urine formation) then *acute tubular necrosis* can result.
(c) Angina pectoris or ECG changes	If cardiac output is persistently low then the blood pressure will be inadequate to perfuse the coronary arteries with oxygenated blood and so ischaemia can result, presenting as angina and/or changes in the S–T segment on the ECG (Fig. 23.11).
(d) Other signs of increased sympathetic arousal	Refer to Fig. 23.3.

Fig. 23.17 *Learning check five*

since conscious awareness of breathing can lead to alterations in rate and pattern.

Closely related to rate is respiratory *pattern*. Many terms are used to describe various patterns and rates; the common ones are defined in Table 23.8 together with possible causes.

The *depth* of respiration relates to the tidal volume, i.e. the volume of air moving in and out with each breath. The depth of respiration can be specifically measured using a spirometer, or observed by inspecting chest expansion for depth or shallowness at the same time as observing for equality and uniformity of movement.

Metabolic considerations in the acutely ill

A consideration of metabolic aspects now follows to complete the section on biological influences relevant to the acutely ill.

Following major injury, whether in the form of accidental trauma, burns, severe illness or major surgical intervention, the body responds with specific endocrine and metabolic changes designed to protect it. These include preparing for volume loss by conserving sodium and fluids, enhancement of the clotting mechanism, and the mobilisation of immediate sources of energy. The duration of this response relates to the severity and extent of the injury. A summary of the main endocrine changes (excluding those due to sympathetic arousal discussed earlier) is given in Fig. 23.20.

Metabolism refers to the sum of all reactions that may occur within the cells of the body. It consists of two components: **degradation** (catabolism) and **biosynthesis** (anabolism).

Biosynthesis is the process of building small organic molecules into complex molecules, for example, proteins, nucleic acids. Such processes consume energy.

Degradation, on the other hand, involves the breakdown of large molecules into smaller ones and this process tends to produce energy which, in turn, can be used for processes such as biosynthesis.

The major energy source in the body is *glucose*, which is degraded through a complex cycle of chemical reactions to release energy. Fats and proteins too can be degraded to produce energy.

In the acutely ill person, not only are the demands for energy increased but often, due to periods of reduction or cessation of nutritional intake, the supply of energy-containing nutrients is reduced. As a result, the stores of glycogen in the liver are used up rapidly, being converted to glu-

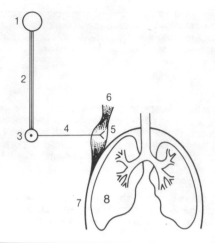

KEY NOS	STRUCTURE	CAUSES OF MALFUNCTION
1.	Respiratory centre	Direct trauma Raised intracranial pressure Drugs; Hypoxia; *Hypercapnia*
2.	Spinal cord	Trauma
3.	Anterior horn cell	*Poliomyelitis*
4.	Peripheral nerve	*Polyneuritis*
5.	Neuromuscular junction	*Botulism* Muscle relaxant drugs
6.	Respiratory muscles	*Tetanus*
7.	Chest wall	Trauma Pneumothorax
8.	Lungs & airways	Pneumonia

(Adapted from Sykes, McNichol and Campbell, 1976)

Fig. 23.18 *Structures involved in respiration (reproduced by permission of the publishers, Blackwell Scientific Publications)*

Self-assessment question nine

How would you recognise that breathing was ineffective in an acutely ill person?

Answer

(1) Central cyanosis of the lips and tongue
  – in persons with normal haemoglobin levels (NB. Peripheral cyanosis only indicates local perfusion problems – for example, cold or local ischaemia)

(2) Pallor of the skin
  – particularly in patients who are anaemic

* (3) Increased respiratory rate (or decreased rate)

* (4) Use of accessory muscles of respiration, laboured breathing and flaring of the nostrils

(5) Anxiety, restlessness and confusion and loss of consciousness in extreme cases

(6) Evidence of increased sympathetic activity i.e. tachycardia and irregularities in pulse
  – increased blood pressure (if patient is not hypovolaemic or in left ventricular failure)
  – sweating
  – peripheral shutdown

(7) Changes in posture and facial expression (for example, hunching over a bedtable, furrowed brow, tired and drawn expression)

* *Points (3) and (4) would only apply if breathing had not been affected by damage to nerves or by drugs which suppress respiration*

Fig. 23.19 *Learning check six*

---

cose to maintain the blood sugar. Maintenance of the blood sugar is essential for brain function. The brain is unable to store glucose or use alternative energy sources, with the exception of ketones.

Once glycogen stores in the liver and muscles have been exhausted, the energy necessary to fuel body processes will be derived from reserves of fat and protein.

Breakdown of plasma proteins and skeletal proteins result in the freeing of amino acids, which can be used to produce energy when their nitrogen-containing part has been removed (deamin-

ation). This nitrogen-containing part is then excreted in the urine as urea. This accounts for the increased urinary and plasma urea levels found immediately following surgery or injury, the loss of muscle mass, and the subsequent negative nitrogen balance. The increased use of amino acids for energy production in turn reduces their availability for tissue and wound repair. This, together with the suppression of the immune response found with high cortisol levels, can predispose the acutely ill person to infection.

Table 23.8. *Variations in respirations with possible causes found in acute hospital settings*

Name	Definition	Possible cause
Tachypnoea	Normal respiratory pattern with a rate greater than 20/min	Fever Hypoxia associated with cardiac/ respiratory failure
Bradypnoea	Normal respiratory pattern with a rate below 8/min	Metabolic disorders (for example, drug overdoses, alcohol, intoxication, abnormal brain function)
Dyspnoea	A feeling of shortness of breath (a subjective sensation)	Cardiac, neurological or respiratory dysfunction Anxiety
Hyperventilation	An increase in respiration rate and depth over and above the body's actual metabolic requirements	Pharmacological Nervous Metabolic } origins Pulmonary Psychological
Hypoventilation	When respirations are unable to match the body's metabolic demands	Any damage or malfunction in the structures involved in breathing. See Fig. 23.18
Cheyne-Stokes	Period of apnoea alternating with shallow, progressively deeper, and then shallow respirations	Congestive heart failure, uraemia, brain disease
Kussmaul's respiration	Deep rapid respirations associated with diabetic ketoacidosis ('air-hunger')	Diabetic ketoacidosis
Apneustic respirations	Uncontrolled gasping respirations with pauses at full inspiration and full expiration	Damage to the pons

Psychological factors in the acutely ill adult

Three topics have been selected for consideration in this section as relevant to the acutely ill person: communication and memory, sleep, and sensory deprivation.

Communication and memory

Communication is an essential activity of living, which is as important as physical support.

Many investigators (Cartwright, 1964; Spelman, 1967; Ley, 1988) have identified patients' dissatisfaction with communication during their hospital stay. This dissatisfaction relates to the quality and amount of information received (Ley, 1988). Many of these studies, however, occurred during the 1960s, 1970s and early 1980s, Ley having collated them. Since that time, little more significant work has been undertaken and so it would be interesting to know how much dissatisfaction with communication still exists. Problems relating to insufficient, confusing and contradictory information have also been identified by the Health Service Commissioner, and various consumer organisations, as an area of complaint.

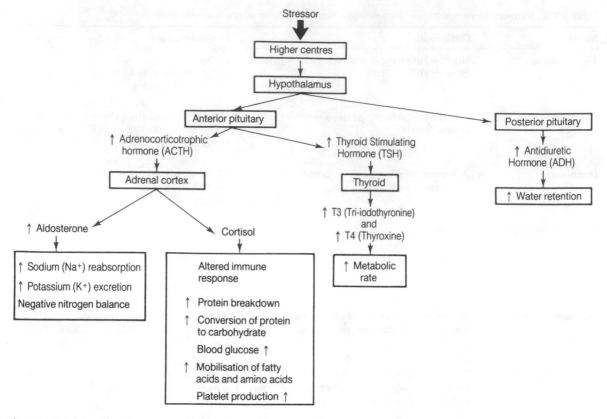

Fig. 23.20 *The endocrine response to a stressor*

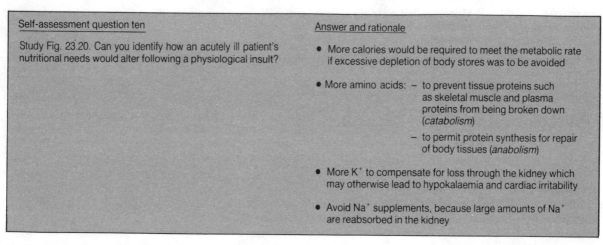

Self-assessment question ten

Study Fig. 23.20. Can you identify how an acutely ill patient's nutritional needs would alter following a physiological insult?

Answer and rationale

- More calories would be required to meet the metabolic rate if excessive depletion of body stores was to be avoided

- More amino acids: – to prevent tissue proteins such as skeletal muscle and plasma proteins from being broken down (*catabolism*)

    – to permit protein synthesis for repair of body tissues (*anabolism*)

- More K$^+$ to compensate for loss through the kidney which may otherwise lead to hypokalaemia and cardiac irritability

- Avoid Na$^+$ supplements, because large amounts of Na$^+$ are reabsorbed in the kidney

Fig. 23.21 *Learning check seven*

In a positive light, nurse researchers such as Hayward (1975), Boore (1978), and Wilson-Barnett (1979) have demonstrated how active information-giving by the nurse can speed up recovery, reduce the number of complications and the need for pain relief, particularly in postoperative patients.

Communication can be defined as all the processes, verbal and non-verbal, conscious or unconscious, by which one mind may affect another (Blattner, 1981). In the acute care setting, the development of verbal skills, the giving of information and the use of listening skills – although they improve the quality of care given – are insufficient on their own.

The nurse in the acute setting needs to increase her proficiency at monitoring and interpreting non-verbal cues from physically dependent patients who are often unable to communicate verbally, due to speech loss or factors affecting speech such as breathlessness, pain, etc.

Non-verbal communication can be used therapeutically by nurses. Stress in acutely ill patients can be actively reduced, using relaxation and soothing techniques, and caring can be conveyed through touch. The components of non-verbal communication are illustrated in Fig. 23.22.

Barnett (1972) made some interesting observations with regard to the use of touch in general hospital settings. In her study patients in good or fair condition were touched 70% more often than acutely ill patients. She suggested that this was partly because 'health team members have a fear of death and find it difficult to provide the emotional support necessary' and partly because 'personnel are often so busy with the technical aspects of stabilising the patients' condition that there is not enough time to provide the emotional support necessary.'

However, Rubin (1963) noted that in situations where patients were under intense personal stress feeling isolated and vulnerable, no other method of communication compared in immediacy to the comforting and quieting effects of touch.

The communication process (Fig. 23.23) itself comprises five elements:

(1) The sender or encoder of the message;
(2) The message itself;
(3) The receiver or decoder of the message;
(4) Feedback that the receiver conveys to the sender;

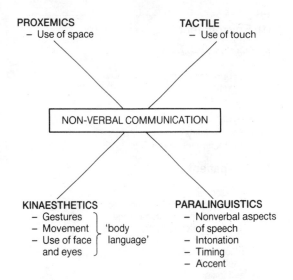

Fig. 23.22 *Components of non-verbal communication*

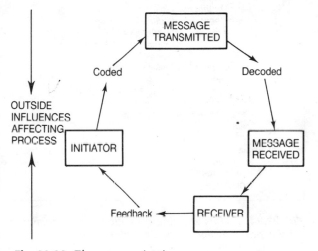

Fig. 23.23 *The communication process*

(5) The environment in which the message is transmitted.

Barriers to and interference with communication can occur at any point in the process. A summary of potential problems relating to the patient's reception of messages from the nurse in acute hospital settings is given in Fig. 23.24.

When planning to meet patients' communication needs, Ashworth (1979) has identified six essential areas in relation to the intensive care

---

(1) Environment

(a) Distortion of message
- noise
- poor/bright light
- vibration
- temperature

(b) Distractions
- other activity
- competing messages

(2) The patient

(a) Psychological
- perception altered by drugs and/or pathology
- motivation/interest in message
- attitudes/values/beliefs
- anxiety/fear
- emotions/mood
- intelligence
- self-image

(b) Physical
- conscious level
- sensory deficits
  - e.g. *hearing impediments/tinnitus*
    - *sight*   (short/long sighted diplopia, hemianopia, blindness)
    - *movement* (paralysis/paresis)
    - *sensation* (loss)
    - *speech*   (dysarthria/dysphasia/ aphasia)
- constraints to movement (position/infusions/equipment)
- pain

(c) Social
- language
- culture/lifestyle
- isolation

Fig. 23.24 *Factors affecting the patient when receiving information/messages in acute settings*

patient. These are equally valid in any acute setting:

(1) Orientation to the time, day, date, place, people, environment and procedures;

(2) Specific patient teaching on any aspect of care;

(3) Adopting methods to overcome patients' sensory deficits;

(4) Comforting patients who are confused or hallucinating;

(5) Communications which maintain the patient's personal identity;

(6) Helping the communications of voiceless patients.

Resources, nursing actions and aids which can be used in connection with these six areas are given in Fig. 23.25.

Having communicated information to patients and with patients, it is important to remember that the information may not be remembered, especially by acutely ill patients whose drugs may interfere with information processing and storage.

Memory disorders can be divided into:

(1) Inadequate acquisition of information
(2) Inadequate recall of information
(3) Inadequate retention of information
(4) Complex-determined forgetting.

It is the first two categories that are particularly relevant to the acutely ill.

Inadequate acquisition usually relates to the circumstances at the time the information was acquired. If the patient has a general debilitating illness involving fatigue, reduced responsiveness, poor concentration and/or exposure to infective toxins, then registration of experiences and communications will be interfered with, leading to poor acquisition. In addition, if the patient is unable to assign meaning to, or organise the information at the time of exposure to it, confusion and lack of memory with regard to the event will also result.

Recall of events and information that has been acquired and stored is dependent on providing the right cues to trigger information retrieval.

The cues used may be distorted for sick individuals in unusual surroundings and circumstances. Emotions and mood also affect the cues used. For example, the prevailing mood at the time will determine which cues will be used and therefore, which experiences will be recalled.

A patient who is depressed is more likely to recall unpleasant matters. It is very important to remember this point when trying to motivate patients who have been acutely ill for a long time and are depressed, since it may be difficult for them to focus on happier and more pleasant feelings and memories.

Amnesia is the inability to recall events which

Essential areas of planning	Resource/aid/nursing action

Orientation in time, place, person, people, environment and procedures	• Information regarding
	  – treatment
	  – care
	  – progress
	  – how patient can help himself
	• Visible clock and calendar
	• Daily newspaper
	• Day and night lighting
	• Positioning near windows
	• Use of glasses, hearing aids (if needed)

Communication which maintains patient identity	• Talking about normal life, home, family interests, preferences, concerns • Offering as many choices affecting the environment as possible • Enable the patient to maintain control of his own body – choices, decisions
Special patient teaching	• Rehabilitation programmes following myocardial infarction • Patient information booklets • Breathing/limb exercises
Overcoming sensory deficit	• Has aids he usually needs • Aids are functioning and effective • Verbal descriptions of environment if the patient can't see • Tactile manipulation of equipment
Comforting patients who are confused or hallucinating	• Acknowledge and accept the patient's delusions or hallucinations while stating that you do not see or believe the same thing
Helping communication of voiceless patients	• Communication bells to attract attention • Communication cards • Pen and pad • Alphabet cards • Work out a system with patient and ensure continuity • Speaking appliances for tracheostomy tubes

have occurred within an individual's waking experience. Amnesia may be *retrograde* relating to events prior to a particular event, or *ante-retrograde* relating to events following it. Head injury and conditions involving loss of consciousness (even though the patient may appear to be conscious and aware of his surroundings) often give rise to an inability to retain current events. This characteristic also applies to many drugs used to sedate patients during unpleasant procedures and investigations.

Sleep and the acutely ill person

Sleep can be defined as an altered state of consciousness from which a person can be aroused by stimuli of sufficient magnitude (Hill and Smith, 1985). The function of sleep is far from clear. Historically it has been considered as restorative and energy conserving although little evidence exists to support these views (Canavan, 1984). If these functions are correctly assumed then sleep deprivation in the acutely ill person could be considered as an additional stressor over and above those physical and emotional traumas already suffered.

During an average night's sleep individuals pass through four or five sleep cycles, each cycle lasting about 90 minutes. Within the sleep cycle, five successive stages have been defined by their distinctive characteristics (which the nurse may learn to identify) and electroencephalographic (EEG) patterns (Fig. 23.26). The first four stages of sleep are called collectively *non rapid eye movement sleep* (NREM) and demonstrate a progressive increase in the depth of sleep. Stage five is called *rapid eye movement sleep* (REM) or *paradoxical sleep* and is associated with dreaming and, in the head-injured patient, increases in intracranial pressure. Following stage five and, therefore, on completion of the first cycle, stage two is entered again, marking the beginning of subsequent cycles, all of which omit stage one.

During non-REM sleep parasympathetic nervous activity predominates, producing a reduction in heart rate, respiratory rate and initially a decrease in blood pressure. During REM sleep sympathetic dominance pervades with a resulting increase in

Fig. 23.25 Resources, aids and nursing actions when planning to meet the communication needs of acutely ill patients

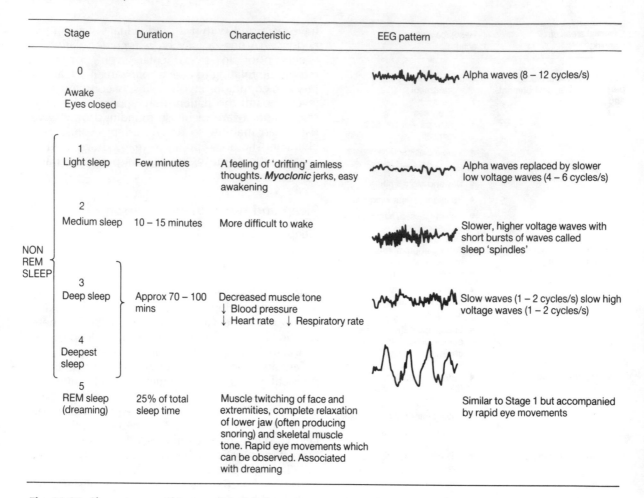

Stage	Duration	Characteristic	EEG pattern
0 Awake Eyes closed			Alpha waves (8 – 12 cycles/s)
1 Light sleep	Few minutes	A feeling of 'drifting' aimless thoughts. *Myoclonic* jerks, easy awakening	Alpha waves replaced by slower low voltage waves (4 – 6 cycles/s)
2 Medium sleep	10 – 15 minutes	More difficult to wake	Slower, higher voltage waves with short bursts of waves called sleep 'spindles'
3 Deep sleep	Approx 70 – 100 mins	Decreased muscle tone ↓ Blood pressure ↓ Heart rate ↓ Respiratory rate	Slow waves (1 – 2 cycles/s) slow high voltage waves (1 – 2 cycles/s)
4 Deepest sleep			
5 REM sleep (dreaming)	25% of total sleep time	Muscle twitching of face and extremities, complete relaxation of lower jaw (often producing snoring) and skeletal muscle tone. Rapid eye movements which can be observed. Associated with dreaming	Similar to Stage 1 but accompanied by rapid eye movements

NON REM SLEEP (Stages 1–5)

Fig. 23.26 *Sleep stages within one sleep cycle*

systolic blood pressure, heart rate and respiratory rate.

During the second part of the night, the period of non-REM sleep reduces and REM sleep predominates. This point has tentatively been related to the early hours as being the time most commonly associated with death, some studies having linked the occurrence of nocturnal angina to REM sleep (Hemenway, 1980).

Prolonged REM sleep deprivation is considered by some authors as exerting no adverse psychological effects (Ganong, 1983; Canavan, 1984). On the other hand perpetual awakening and sleep interruption has been associated with increased anxiety, irritability and disorientation. Anxiety has already been indicated as a cause of increased sympathetic action which may then have a nega-

tive influence on recovery. The reported problems of irritability and disorientation are also cited as resulting from sensory deprivation and bombardment, conditions which commonly co-exist with those of sleep deprivation. In the acutely ill person sleep deprivation and sensory bombardment or deprivation are often difficult to separate due to their inter-relationship.

Fabijan and Gosselin (1982) have made several recommendations for minimising sleep interruption in patients in an intensive care unit. Such recommendations (listed in Table 23.9) are equally applicable to any acute care area.

Sensory deprivation

Studies in sensory deprivation show that when

Table 23.9. *Recommendations for reducing sleep interruption in acutely ill patients*

(1) Turn off maximum number of lights especially at night

(2) Keep noise to a minimum (for example – switch off suction equipment following use; reduce talking and whispering)

(3) Offer cotton wool balls for patients' ears

(4) Continually re-assess the need to interrupt patients' sleep to perform observations

(5) Perform as many nursing interventions as possible together

(6) Chart amount of uninterrupted sleep per shift and evidence of sleep stages

(7) Communicate the patients' need to sleep to other professionals

(8) Use knowledge of
  (a) patients' normal sleeping patterns and
  (b) supportive family relationships
  to optimise environment for sleep

(9) Administer analgesics and sedatives according to patients' felt needs and monitor events. (Care is necessary with some drugs that may interfere with sleep patterns)

(Adapted from Fabijan and Gosselin, 1982)

normal healthy individuals are deprived of all sensory input (i.e. auditory, visual and touch), there is a detrimental effect on the functioning of the individual (Atkinson *et al.*, 1990). Such individuals become bored, restless, irritable and emotionally upset. Visual hallucination, poor concentration and problem-solving difficulties also result.

The reticular activating system in the brain is responsible for producing the conscious alert state which makes perception possible. Ascending sensory information is received by the reticular formation in the brainstem before being sorted, filtered and passed on to the cortex – for example, the sound of a ticking clock is not usually heard because the reticular formation has filtered it out as being unnecessary for our attention. If, however, a conscious effort is made to listen to the clock

ticking, we then become aware of it.

The normal conscious state requires a minimum level of sensory stimulation and/or variation in type of stimuli received. The normal type of sensations received by the reticular activating system would include auditory, visual, olfactory, tactile and *kinaesthetic* stimuli (i.e. stimuli that relate to the position of joints in space and the degree of contraction of muscles). Sensory deprivation itself is not a syndrome associated merely with a reduction in these stimuli but is a more complex concept.

Goldberger (1966) classified five areas for investigation in association with sensory deprivation. These five categories are identified in Fig. 23.27, which demonstrates the diverse aspects of this phenomenon.

Zukerman (1969; cited by Ashworth, 1979) pro-

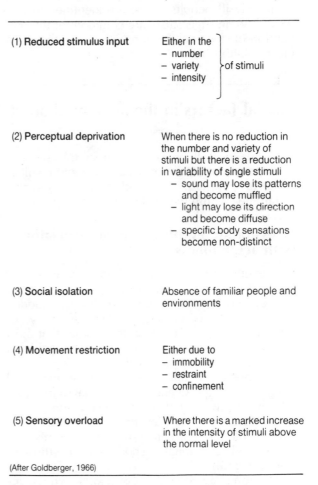

(After Goldberger, 1966)

Fig. 23.27 *Classification of types of sensory deprivation*

duced some interesting findings when investigating Goldberger's five areas. These findings are particularly relevant to acute clinical nursing and include the following points:

(1) *Confinement alone* will produce most of the verbally reported stress effects and the subsequent sympathetic responses.
(2) *Social isolation* produces more dreams, memories and inefficiencies in thinking than confinement with sensory stimulation.
(3) More dreams, visual and auditory hallucinations, and feelings of unreality seemed to be produced by *sensory deprivation* than by social isolation.

Worrell (1977) suggested seven points which it is useful to consider for reducing sensory deprivation in acutely ill people. These are identified in Fig. 23.29. Some suggestions are common for the prevention of sleep deprivation with which there is a close relationship.

Social factors in the acutely ill adult

Two factors will be considered in this section: firstly, stressful life events as a cause and result of acute hospital admission and, secondly, the role of families within the acute care setting.

Stressful life events and their association with acute illness

Life events are significant changes which may occur through choice (such as marriage or divorce) or they may be totally unforeseen (such as sudden bereavement, redundancy, accidental injury, or long term illness). Sociologists consider that most people will undergo at least one such significant event and probably more within a lifetime.

Previously, significant events were identified from outside the event from a behaviourist perspective (Brown, 1989). Currently, the significance and relevance of any event is 'reflected by the event's internal representation and a person's cognitive and emotional responses to it' (Brown, 1989; page 8).

Emerging agreement now exists which recognises that it is the 'meaning' of the event to the individual which is the significant influence (Brown, 1989).

Brown and Harris (1989) have further investigated the relationships between life events and both psychiatric and physical illness and illustrate the complex factors involved. The effects of personal status and social circumstances on physical health are now receiving increasing attention.

Self-assessment question eleven

Can you identify possible contributory factors to sensory deprivation in acutely ill patients using Goldberger's five categories?

Answer

(1) Reduced variety and intensity of stimuli
  - impaired sight, hearing, sensation, taste or smell due to trauma, pathology, drugs
  - inability to communicate verbally e.g. if unable to speak English; dysphasia

(2) Perceptual deprivation
  - sedatives, analgesics
  - reduced conscious level
  - not having hearing aids/glasses
  - pathology

(3) Social isolation
  - barrier nursing
  - the 'unpopular patient' (Stockwell, 1972)
  - cubicles
  - language barrier

(4) Confinement/immobility
  - bedrest
  - traction/plaster casts
  - pain
  - paralysis

(5) Increased sensory input/overload
  - alarms/monitors
  - frequent neurological/other observations
  - persistent disturbance
  - telephone ringing
  - smells

Fig. 23.28 *Learning check eight*

(1) Create an environment with a minimum of sensory deprivation or overload

- Maintain diurnal rhythm, by orientating the patient who is confused to day and night
- Limb exercises to maintain proprioceptive feedback (i.e. information from the joints to the brain relating to position in space)
- Reduce unnecessary noise, disturbance
- Disperse unpleasant odours as soon as possible
- Reduce 'crowding' of patient

(2) Familiarise the environment for the patient

- Photographs of family members or favourite scenes
- Position the patient to look out of a window
- Radio and television
- Encourage family visiting
- Tapes of favourite music and programmes

(3) Assist the patient to interpret incoming stimuli

- Wearing of glasses and hearing aids
- Explain all nursing procedures and interventions beforehand
- Explain unfamiliar alarms and sounds
- Explain effects of drugs which alter sensory perception
- Prepare patient for situations/treatments which may result in sensory deprivation

(4) Orientate the patient to the reality of the moment

- Orientate in time, place and person
- Orientate to physical condition
- Give patient access to a watch, clock or calendar
- Dim lights at night
- Use touch to assure the patient that the nurse cares

(5) Provide the patient with an active role in his care

- Encourage patient to make decisions about his environment
- Ask patient's permission prior to invading his privacy
- Ensure maximum privacy
- Spend time communicating with patient

(6) Encourage patient to use the highest form of cognitive functioning possible

- Encourage questioning and discussion
- Ascertain patient's perception of situation
- Involve him in care planning and decision making

(7) Provide the patient with uninterrupted rest periods

- Make a contract with patient for specific rest periods
- See recommendations for encouraging sleep

(After Worrell, 1977)

Fig. 23.29 *Suggestions for reducing sensory deprivation*

Specific studies of the effects of stress on health

Harvey Brenner, an American economist (cited by McAvinchey, 1984), looked at the effects on health of unemployment. He claimed that the life event of unemployment can be measured throughout the whole population as an effect on the health of a nation. Brenner claimed to show a close association between unemployment rates and the first admission to psychiatric hospitals in New York. As the unemployment rates increased, so did the admission rate, and vice versa. Brenner then examined cardiovascular mortality rates and found that these tended to increase two to three years after an increase in unemployment. In 1979, he investigated unemployment in Britain and was, again, able to demonstrate a positive correlation between unemployment and mortality rates in all age groups. From these studies, Brenner advanced the hypothesis that unemployment, or the fear of unemployment, is a 'life event' which creates stressful effects leading to increases in morbidity and perhaps mortality after several years. He subsequently drew parallels between the life events of divorce, widowhood and unemployment.

Harvey Brenner's work has been replicated by Iain McAvinchey (1984) in Scotland, who demonstrated similar findings.

Creed (1981), a British psychiatrist, considered the relationship between life events and appendicectomy. He stated:

'It has been suggested that stress may precede the operation of appendicectomy whether the appendix is normal or inflamed'

Two authors, Harding (1962) and Paulley (1955), had previously related life events to the onset of pain that leads to appendicitis. Harding (1962) noted that 62% of appendix specimens removed from girls aged 11–20 were histologically normal, and he believed that a large psychological element may exist because of the important changes that occur in the lives of girls at that age. Paulley (1955) had reported that even true appendicitis might occur within hours of an emotional upset or at a time of considerable stress.

Creed (1981) investigated this apparent relationship by studying 119 appendicectomy patients and interviewing them a few days post-operatively. The interview focused on recent experience of any severely distressing events (for example, a serious illness, a death in the family, the break-up of a long term relationship, or a court appearance for a major offence). Creed then compared the results with the control group and previous research into the relationship between life events and the onset of depression conducted by the sociologists George Brown and Tirril Harris (1978). To verify that the accounts given regarding life events were accurate, he talked to siblings of the subjects. A further precaution was taken by Creed, who only permitted the pathologists to examine the appendixes after the research had been completed into the life events. This enabled the research to be 'blind' so that neither the researcher nor the patient knew whether the appendix was diseased or not.

Creed then compared the incidence of acute inflammation with the incidence of severe life events. Of those appendicectomy patients who had an acutely inflamed appendix, just over 10% had experienced severe life events in the nine weeks preceding operation (i.e. there was little difference between these patients and the control group). However, of those patients with a 'lily-white appendix' (i.e. normal uninflamed appendix) nearly one third had experienced a severe life event in the nine weeks preceding operations. In this respect, the results closely resembled the number of people suffering depression in Brown and Harris' study.

Creed (1981) was therefore able to conclude that life events played a greater part in the aetiology of the condition when the appendix was not inflamed than in acute appendicitis. He was also able to suggest that the events associated with acute appendicitis were those which were upsetting in the short term – for example, a short-lived argument or taking an exam; and that events associated with operations when the appendix was *not* acutely inflamed were those which carried lasting threat and unpleasantness to the individual – for example, separation from a spouse. It was these latter events which also resulted in depression in Brown and Harris' study (1978).

The onset of psychiatric illness following a significant loss, a life course transition or an unusually high incidence of disorientating life events has been identified by other researchers too. Paykel *et al.* (1975) found that the incidence of significant life events in a previous period of six months was four times greater in suicidal patients than in matched non-suicidal controls. Maguire *et al.* (1980), in their work with patients with cancer, found that one in five patients required psychiatric treatment within a year of diagnosis, where the diagnosis was considered the significant life event by the researcher. The morbidity is even higher among individuals who undergo disfiguring or disabling surgery such as amputation, mastectomy or colostomy formation (Open University, 1985).

A study by Stein and Charles (1971) claimed to reveal a significantly higher incidence of loss in the family backgrounds of adolescent diabetics (mainly bereavement or parental separation) than in a matched group of adolescents suffering from other types of chronic conditions. However, retrospective studies such as this are open to the criticism that a gradual deterioration of health before an illness was clinically diagnosed may have precipitated the life event, rather than the life event precipitating the illness.

Further support to this argument is given by Tew et al. (1977) and Gath (1977) who have both illustrated that chronic illness in a child is associated with increased incidence of family breakdown.

Marital breakdown and divorce (as a life event) has been studied in terms of its effect on health. Morgan (1980) and Fox and Goldblatt (1982) have shown that divorced people suffer more ill health and a higher than average mortality rate than married counterparts. A similar loss in the form of widowhood has been studied by Parkes et al. (1969). Over a period of nine years, they monitored the health of 4486 widowers aged 55 years or over when their wives died in 1957. They found that the number of widowers who died within six months of their wives was 40% greater than expected for non-bereaved married men, matched for age and social class. The increased mortality was accounted for in two thirds of cases by diseases of the heart and circulatory system.

Implications for the nurse in acute care

Understanding the relationship between major stressful life events and acute illness therefore has several implications for the nurse:

- Assessment of recent and current major life events and/or crises, as these may have predisposed the acute illness.
- Assessment of the individual's normal coping mechanisms and support networks, so that they can be enhanced, reinforced and/or improved.
- Recognition that the present acute illness may act as a stressful life event in itself, particularly with regard to:
  —potential impact on employment;
  —dependent family members;
  —financial insecurity;
  thus making the patient more vulnerable to infection, depression and slower recovery.
- The need to assist the patient's family members with positive coping mechanisms in what may be perceived as a stressful life event for them.

The role of families within acute care settings

A family can be defined, in the broadest sense, as a group of persons either related by birth or who are significant to one another and who share intimate and routine day-to-day living.

Almost every patient has been, or is, a member of a family and a change in one family member has the potential to affect other family members.

If the patient is to be viewed from a *holistic* perspective, it is important to understand the immediate social context in which he is placed. For most individuals that social context is the family.

Wright and Leahey (1984) argue that, in order to foster health care at family level, it is useful for nurses to consider two functions:

(1) The impact of illness on the family;
(2) The influence of family interactions on the 'cause' or 'cure' of problems.

These factors are important for consideration regardless of whether problems are developmental, emotional or organic in nature. Further, support for this statement has been considered above, in the discussion on stressful life events.

Every family will vary in its behaviour and reactions to acute illness in one of its members, and it is important to remember that a crisis for one family would not necessarily be a crisis for another family. Regardless of the family response, there will be a significant effect on the nursing situation which needs to be recognised by the nurse.

Breu and Dracup (1978) found that spouses of patients who had undergone a myocardial infarction frequently experienced feelings of loss because of the potential threat of their partner's death. These spouses were found to have a need for the following:

(1) Relief of initial anxiety
(2) Information
(3) To be with the patient
(4) To be helpful to the patient
(5) Support.

Naismith et al. (1979) have also shown the benefit of including spouses in rehabilitation programmes following myocardial infarction where the psychological recovery of the patient was enhanced. Psychological problems to re-adjustment may often be more retarding than physical problems.

Several studies consider how relatives of acutely and critically ill patients perceive their needs. These studies suggest that some factors are per-

Most important needs	Least important needs
Need for hope (Molter, 1979; Norris and Grove, 1986)	To talk about negative feelings (Norris and Grove, 1986)
To feel that hospital personnel cared for patient (Molter, 1979; Norris and Grove, 1986)	To talk about own feelings (Norris and Grove, 1986)
To be assured that the best possible care is being given to the patient (Irwin, 1973; Norris and Grove, 1986)	To change visiting hours for special conditions (Norris and Grove, 1986)
To have questions answered honestly (Irwin, 1973; Norris and Grove, 1986)	To talk about the possibility of the patient's death (Norris and Grove, 1986)
To receive as much information as possible about the patient (Hampe, 1979)	Personal concerns (Hampe, 1979)
To receive information which would alleviate anxieties (Hampe, 1979)	
The need to be with the patient (Hampe, 1979)	

Fig. 23.30 *The least and most important needs of relatives of acutely ill patients as perceived by the relatives themselves (Manley, 1988)*

ceived to be more important than others (Manley, 1988). The factors considered most and least important to relatives are illustrated in Fig. 23.30.

Information useful to the acute care nurse about the family can therefore be listed under the following headings:

(1) Structure and function of the family;
(2) Roles fulfilled by the patient within the family unit;
(3) Expectations of family members;
(4) Coping abilities of family members.

The assessment tool designed by Campbell *et al.* (1985) and described below specifically addresses some of these issues. It suggests questions that the nurse may ask on admission, to obtain greater insight into family strengths and problems relevant to the care of an acutely ill individual. By having a family meeting from the start, the nurse can set a precedent for the future, contributing to holistic family care instead of fostering splintered family involvement.

Other benefits from increased family involvement include a greater insight into the patient's personality and character, enabling staff to have an opportunity to know the patient better and, secondly, the use of the family as the natural support system for the patient.

To understand the family's boundaries and composition, several simple tools exist which can convey a great deal of information visually. Examples of these include the **genogram** and the **ecomap**.

A genogram is particularly helpful in outlining a family's internal and external structure. The symbols used are illustrated in Fig. 23.31. Family members are placed on horizontal lines according to generation. An example of a blank genogram is included in Fig. 23.32.

An ecomap is a diagram portraying important connections between the family and others outside the family.

Assessment tools for use with the acutely ill adult

Preceding sections have considered biological, psychological and social principles and influences relevant to the acutely ill person. In this section, some of those principles are used as the basis of assessment tools which the nurse may use to improve comprehensive patient assessment.

A tool can be defined as an implement or instrument used to do a job. To use an analogy: when the garden has to be dug, the tool used to do this job may be a spade or a fork or even a mechanical rotavator. It does not really matter which tool is

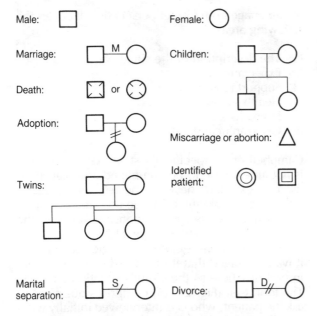

Male: ☐   Female: ○

Marriage: ☐—M—○   Children: ☐—○

Death: ⊠ or ⊗

Adoption: ☐—○

Miscarriage or abortion: △

Twins: ☐—○

Identified patient: ◎ ▣

Marital separation: ☐—S—○   Divorce: ☐—D—○

From Wright L. and Leahey M. (1984). Nurses and Families: A Guide to Family Assessment and Intervention. F.A. Davis, Philadelphia

Fig. 23.31 Symbols used in genograms

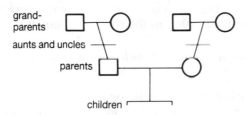

grand-parents ☐—○ ☐—○

aunts and uncles

parents ☐—○

children

Fig. 23.32 Blank genogram

used as long as the job is done; that is, of course, assuming that the user can use all three tools equally as well.

This analogy raises two questions about tools:

(1) Is the tool appropriate for the job to be performed?
(2) Can the person use the tool to perform the job?

For example, with regard to the first question, one wouldn't use a hoe to dig the garden as a hoe is a tool designed to remove weeds.

With regard to the second question, and taking the analogy further, there may be considerable benefit in using a rotavator to dig the garden in terms of time and effectiveness but that assumes that the area to be covered is big enough to turn the rotavator around, and that the user has been taught to drive the rotavator, otherwise the lawn may be dug up as well!

Assessment tools are instruments used to guide patient assessment. Certain points have to be considered when using any tool and these are listed in Fig. 23.33.

---

(1) Does the person using the tool understand it?
(2) In what context was the tool designed and for what purpose?
(3) When should the tool be used?
(4) Is it realistic to use?
(5) Is the tool being properly used?
(6) Does the person need training to use the tool?

Fig. 23.33 Points to consider when using any assessment tool

Campbell *et al.* (1985) identified the need for instruments based on theory to assist nurses in the identification of human responses.

The use of assessment tools encourages us to be organised and systematic in our approach to assessment. Such tools also have benefits for patients and students in that they can be used as teaching aids. Finally, if they are reliable and valid, they can increase objectivity and facilitate precise measurement, accurate record-keeping and evaluation, all of which are potential benefits.

Two general categories of assessment tools exist. These focus either on the broader functions of patient assessment or on more specific areas.

Broader assessment tools are more holistic and would be appropriate in acute care areas when assessing a patient on admission or at the beginning of a span of duty.

More specific tools focus on a single area (such as pain or neurological function) and are therefore reductionist in approach – i.e. they consider parts of a person only, and must always be used with this in mind.

A range of tools which could be used in acute care areas will be considered below.

Assessment man

The assessment man is a simple visual head-to-toe guide designed to assess a patient on admission

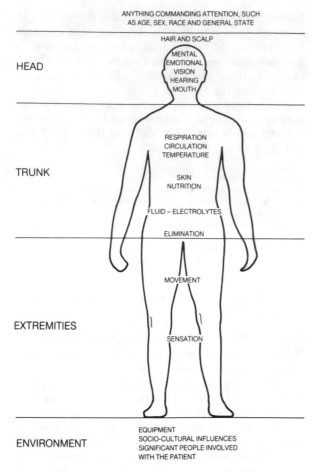

ANYTHING COMMANDING ATTENTION, SUCH
AS AGE, SEX, RACE AND GENERAL STATE

HAIR AND SCALP

HEAD

MENTAL
EMOTIONAL
VISION
HEARING
MOUTH

TRUNK

RESPIRATION
CIRCULATION
TEMPERATURE

SKIN
NUTRITION

FLUID – ELECTROLYTES

ELIMINATION

MOVEMENT

EXTREMITIES

SENSATION

ENVIRONMENT

EQUIPMENT
SOCIO-CULTURAL INFLUENCES
SIGNIFICANT PEOPLE INVOLVED
WITH THE PATIENT

Fig. 23.34 The assessment man (reproduced by permission from Castledine and Macfarlane, 1982)

(Fig. 23.34). Because of its simplicity it can also be used to assess an acutely ill person quickly, at the beginning of a span of duty, as it provides a comprehensive physical, psychological and social *aide-mémoire* suitable for carrying around in a pocket.

Health status (Campbell et al., 1985)

This tool was developed out of the need recognised by Campbell *et al.* for 'instruments based on theory to assist nurses in the identification of human responses'. It was designed to provide the nurse with the basic data necessary to plan holistic care, as well as enabling the nurse to model the client's world, i.e. to interpret relationships and develop a

mirror image from his/her perspective. It covers the following areas:

(1) The description of the situation
(2) Expectations
(3) Support resources
(4) Health status
(5) Strengths
(6) Geographical data.

Campbell *et al.* specifically state that 'assessment is not an exercise to be completed and placed on the client's chart, never to be referred to again, rather it is a tool which can be used to develop or maintain a therapeutic relationship between the nurse and client' (1985, page 112).

This tool was developed in a surgical area where it was envisaged that it may need repeating either in part or whole as the client's situation changes. The tool itself (Fig. 23.35) comprises questions to ask the patient, who is is interviewed initially without the presence of his family; and questions to ask the family (or for the nurse to consider about the family) when interviewing them with the patient, unless the family/patient request otherwise. The responses from the client are recorded in the left-hand column exactly as they are conveyed. The information collected from and about the family is recorded in the right-hand column.

Using a nursing model as an assessment tool

A nursing model can also be used as an assessment tool, providing a structure to aid client assessment both on admission to an acute care area and in later situations.

Unlike other assessment tools, a nursing model will guide what is assessed and how it is assessed from the perspective of what values and beliefs are held about the following four major concepts:

- the nature of health;
- the nature of the individual:
- the nature of the environment or society;
- the nature of nursing.

The key concept in Roy's model of nursing (Roy, 1984) is adaptation. Health is seen to be a state of successful adaptation and the individual person is viewed as an adaptive system. The environment – both internal and external – produces stressors

Fig. 23.35 *Health status of clients (reproduced from the* Journal of Advanced Nursing, *Volume 10, by kind permission of Blackwell Scientific Publications)*

Primary source (patient)	Secondary source (nurse and family)
Description of situation	**Nursing observation analysis**
In your own words, can you tell me how you see your situation?	Describe the patient and the situation
What do you think caused the situation to occur?	**Family:** How does the family view the situation? Do they feel drained or have the energy to handle the situation?
What do you think will improve the situation?	**Family:** What does the family think will improve the situation?
Expectations	
What do you think will happen over the next few days?	**Nurse:** What is patient's feeling state? Are there incongruences between what the patient says and non-verbal data?
What do you expect to accomplish in this hospitalisation? What is important to you at this time in your life?	**Family:** What do they expect to occur over the next few days? During this hospitalisation?
Is this hospitalisation affecting your long term goals?	
Support resources	
Who do you usually talk things over with?	**Nurse:** Does the family appear supportive? Does the patient need help interacting with health team members?
Are they available to you while you are in the hospital? How often? How is the hospitalisation affecting the people who are important to you?	**Family:** How is the patient's hospitalisation affecting the family?
Health status	
How do you describe your general health?	**Nurse:** Describe patient's general appearance. Describe any pertinent alteration in physical systems.
Previous health problems? Current health problems? How do you usually handle stress?	**Family:** How does the family describe the patient's health?

Strengths

What do you see as the healthy or positive aspects of yourself? Is there anything that you will need help with in caring for youself?

Is there anything else you would like us to know about you?

Nurse: Additional strengths identification by the nurse.

Family: What does the family see as the patient's strengths? Anything they will need help with? Anything they would like us to know?

Demographical data

Age   Religion   Allergies/sensitivities

Contact in case of emergency

Patient's report of use of medications

Name	Dose	Frequency	Last dose	Patient's reason for taking medication
Date	Time	Unit	Signature	

(From Campbell *et al.*, 1985).

which can potentially influence adaptation, and nursing is seen as assisting individuals to adapt, by reducing stressors and helping patients to develop and enhance their own coping mechanisms. These values then guide the assessment process, so in Roy's model assessment is focused on establishing whether adaptation exists in four adaptive modes:

- physiological mode;
- self-image mode;
- role mastery mode;
- interdependence mode.

Roy then provides example questions useful to ask when assessing each mode. Roy's model provides therefore a very comprehensive assessment tool, one that gives as much focus to psychosocial assessment as it does to physiological assessment.

Any nursing model can be used as an assessment tool depending firstly on whether it is appropriate to the situation in which it is being used, secondly, on whether the assessor feels it will work by providing cues which are both effective and comprehensive in eliciting information about the areas being assessed, and thirdly on whether it is congruent with a team's philosophy (values and beliefs) about what nursing is.

In Orem's model (1991), self-care is the central theme and Orem identifies three groups of requisites that individuals need to fulfil. It is these three groups that provide the broad structure for determining whether any deficits exist on assessment. The three groups are termed: universal requisites; developmental requisites; and health deviation requisites.

(1)   *Universal requisites* encompass basic human needs fundamental to all individuals (for example, air, food, water, elimination, activity and rest, solitude and social interaction, prevention of hazards and the promotion of human functioning).

Many of these requisites cannot be fulfilled by the client while he is acutely ill.

(2)   *Developmental requisites* focus on those requisites associated with development and maturation during various stages of the life cycle such as adolescence, young adulthood, parenthood, etc. They would be very important to consider in relation to the stage in life at which an individual was admitted to an acute care area.

(3)   *Health deviation requisites* relate to those requisites which develop due to ill health or disability (for example, the need for relief from pain, the prevention of the consequences of immobility, the prevention of iatrogenic infection via invasive equipment). The determination of these requisites in the acutely ill person would focus on two areas – firstly, the felt and perceived effects of ill health on the individual and, secondly, the nurse's knowledge of the potential effects of ill health, medical treatment or invasive equipment.

These three groups of requisites can be simply listed on a card to act as an *aide-mémoire* for on-going assessment. For more formal assessment (as on admission) documentation of the requisites identified may make use of an assessment form as illustrated in Fig. 23.37.

Pain assessment tool (Bourbonnais, 1981)

Bourbonnais devised two pain assessment tools designed to complement each other, one for the patient and one for the nurse. Both tools are suitable for using with acutely ill people.

The nurses' pain assessment tool was developed as a concise and systematic guide which was intended to be 'concise enough that the data could fit on a small card to be kept in "the nurse's pocket"'. The tool (Fig. 23.36) includes five sections. The first two focus on visual observations which may

---

1. **Observe for skeletal muscle response**

(a) Body movements
   – immobility
   – purposeless or inaccurate body movements
   – protective movements including withdrawal reflex
   – rhythmic or rubbing movements

(b) Facial expression
   – clenched teeth
   – wrinkled forehead
   – biting of lower lip
   – widely opened or tightly shut eyes

2. **Autonomic nervous system response**

(a) Sympathetic nervous system activation
   – increased pulse
   – increased respirations
   – increased diastolic and systolic blood pressure
   – cold perspiration
   – pallor
   – dilated pupils
   – nausea
   – muscle tension

(b) Parasympathetic activation in some visceral pain
   – low blood pressure
   – slow pulse

   For example: in pain involving the bladder, colon or rectum
   Remember: patients with chronic pain usually do not display the intensive skeletal muscle and autonomic nervous system responses

3. **Verbal report of the patient**

   Questions to ask the patient
   – location of pain
   – intensity of pain
   – onset and duration
   – precipitating and aggravating factors
   – nature of pain (e.g. sharp, dull)

4. **Questions the nurse should ask herself**

(a) How long has it been since the immediately post-operative patient was medicated for pain?
(b) How fatigued is the patient?
(c) Is the patient in an environment of sensory restriction?
(d) Are you reaching the true cause of the patient's pain?
(e) Are you aware of your biases?
(f) Is the patient anxious?
(g) What is the patient's past experience with pain?
(h) Does the patient have an altered level of consciousness?

5. **Nursing history questions (Mayers, 1972)**

(a) Have you had pain or discomfort recently?
(b) If yes, what did you do to relieve the pain or discomfort?
(c) If you have pain or discomfort while in the hospital, what would you like the nurse to do to relieve it?

(From Bourbonnais, 1981)

Fig. 23.36   *A pain assessment tool for nurses (reproduced from the* Journal of Advanced Nursing, *Volume 6, by kind permission of Blackwell Scientific Publications)*

NAME:	D.O.B.	M.S.W.	NOK	OTHER PERSONS IMPORTANT TO PATIENT	WHO IS TO BE CONTACTED IN EMERGENCY
ADDRESS:	Prefers to be addressed as:				

Tel:

ASSESSMENT — OF SELF-CARE DEFICITS

DOCTOR:

1. HEALTH DEVIATION SELF-CARE REQUISITES

2. UNIVERSAL SELF-CARE REQUISITES

PRIMARY NURSE:

MEDICAL INFORMATION

BASE LINE FUNCTIONS

REASON FOR ADMISSION

RELEVANT PAST MEDICAL HISTORY

	Rate	Rhythm	Cough
Breathing			
Circulation			
Pulse Rate	Rhythm	B/P	

MEDICAL DIAGNOSIS

DRUGS TAKEN AT HOME

ALLERGIES

Colour   Skin Lips;

PATIENT'S UNDERSTANDING OF ADMISSION

PATIENT'S FEELINGS & EXPECTATIONS RELATED TO PRESENT ILLNESS

TEMPERATURE   WEIGHT
USUAL PATTERNS CONCERNING DAILY FLUID INTAKE

ORAL
LIKES
DISLIKES
FOOD INTAKE — TYPE, TIME, REGULAR APPETITE, LIKES, DISLIKES

NURSE'S INITIAL IMPRESSION PHYSICAL AND SOCIAL

FAMILY'S UNDERSTANDING OF ADMISSION

KNOWLEDGE/INFORMATION/SKILLS NEEDED FOR CONTINUED SELF-CARE AFTER DISCHARGE

SOURCE OF ASSESSMENT

SPECIAL DIET (WHY?)
IS PATIENT THIN/OBESE/NORMAL?
Teeth
Mouth

SERVICES PROVIDED BEFORE ADMISSION/SERVICES AFTER DISCHARGE

DISTRICT NURSE —	HEALTH VISITOR —	SOCIAL WORKER —	HOME HELP —
CARE ASSISTANT —	MEALS ON WHEELS —	ANY OTHER —	

UNIVERSAL SELF-CARE REQUISITES CONT'D

PERSONAL CHARACTERISTICS

ELIMINATION: CONTINENCE, FREQUENCY, TIMING, COLOUR, AMOUNT, REGULARITY, AIDS NEEDED

BIOLOGICAL RHYTHM BEST TIME/WORST TIME OF DAY

URINE

WHAT PATIENT IS ABLE TO DO HIM/HERSELF, WANTS TO DO WITHOUT HELP

FAECES

WHAT PATIENT WOULD EVENTUALLY LIKE TO DO INDEPENDENTLY

SELF-CONCEPT: BODY IMAGE AND SELF-ESTEEM

URINALYSIS

PAINS OR OTHER SENSATIONS

CONDITION OF SKIN, NAILS AND HAIR

BALANCE BETWEEN SOLITUDE AND SOCIALISING

COMMUNICATION

FAMILY, FRIENDS, RELATIONSHIPS AND RESPONSIBILITIES

USUAL PATTERNS OF HYGIENE

SEXUALITY: INFORMATION ABOUT MARITAL STATUS, RELATIONSHIPS

SLEEP AND REST, BEDTIME ROUTINE, AIDS TO SLEEP

OCCUPATION AND LIVING ACCOMMODATION

DEVELOPMENTAL SELF-CARE REQUISITES: NOTE THE MAJOR LIFE CHANGES, DEVIATION FROM GROWTH AND DEVELOPMENT NORMS: HOW THE PATIENT COPES WITH THEM, WHAT OR WHO HELPS HIM/HER (CULTURE, RELIGION, BELIEFS, VALUES)

DAILY ACTIVITIES, RECREATION & BODY MOVEMENT

be exhibited by a person experiencing pain. These include non-verbal signs and evidence of any autonomic response, either sympathetic or parasympathetic. The remaining three sections focus on questions which the nurse can ask the patient and questions she should consider herself.

The patient assessment tool has been tried by Bourbonnais on a limited number of patients in a variety of acute settings ranging from a coronary care unit to an orthopaedic ward. She found that patients were able to use the tool easily and that it helped them to tell the nurse about the pain they were feeling. An additional benefit was that patients found it less tiring to point to numbers on a scale than to try to describe the pain they felt.

The tool (Fig. 23.38), a 'pain ruler', consists of two parts: a scale ranging from nought (reflecting no pain) to ten (reflecting excruciating pain), and a list of adjectives which describe different perceptions of pain. The person experiencing pain is then asked to match the word or words that describe their pain to the number which corresponds to the intensity of the pain.

This tool, therefore, enables patients to communicate their pain, which allows for easier evaluation of the effectiveness of relief, and has the further benefit of allowing continuity of pain assessment from one set of staff to another when shifts change.

Other pain assessment tools are considered in Chapter 15.

Glasgow coma scale (Teasdale and Jennett, 1974)

The Glasgow coma scale is an example of a specific tool designed to produce a uniform method of determining and recording conscious level. It was developed in 1974 and based on a study of 700 patients with severe head injury.

The advantages of using this tool are that it increases the objectivity and reliability of neurological assessment, reducing the use of ambiguous descriptions of conscious level and it is also quick and easy to use.

The Glasgow coma scale focuses on the evaluation of three parameters: eye opening, motor response and verbal response. The person's *best* achievement is recorded for each parameter from a predetermined choice of options.

(1)   *Eye opening* is divided into four different

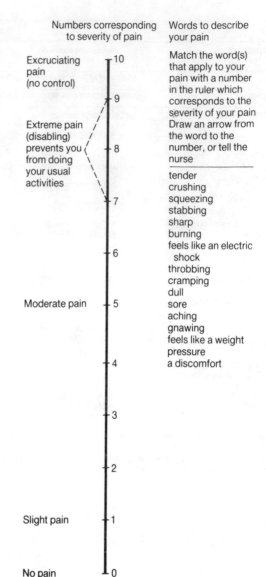

Fig. 23.38 *Patient pain assessment ruler (reproduced from the* Journal of Advanced Nursing, *Volume 6, by kind permission of Blackwell Scientific Publications)*

options: *spontaneous* opening; opening *to speech*; opening *to pain*; and *no eye* opening.

(2)   *Verbal response* is described from a choice of five options: *orientated* in time, place and person; *confused* conversation; *inappropriate* words; *incomprehensible* sounds (for example, groans); no verbal response.

(3)   *Motor response* is described using one of six

options: *obeys* command; *responds* to pain; *localises* to pain; *flexion* response; *extension* response; *no* response to pain.

These motor responses are further illustrated in Fig. 23.39. Each of the parameters can be recorded as in Fig. 23.40 to give a graph which will demonstrate changes visually. Alternatively, each parameter can be scored separately and then totalled to give an overall numerical value which can be used as a baseline against which later changes can be compared. The total can range from a maximum score of 15 – where a person is fully alert and orientated – to a minimum score of three – where a person is completely unresponsive.

Scores over eight are considered high and scores below six are considered low.

Where scores are low, the patient will also be totally dependent on the nurse for all basic needs,

i.e. the total compensatory system would be employed. In addition to providing a neurological assessment therefore, this tool might also have the benefit of indicating the level of patient dependency and, possibly, the subsequent need for nursing.

Planning care

In this final section the care of Margaret Parfitt, introduced in Chapter 22, will be considered. Following a summary of the appropriate disordered physiology, the biological, psychological and social principles introduced throughout the chapter will be used to identify goals and nursing interventions, therefore applying them to care. A detailed assessment has been completed and in the light of this a care plan has been written.

Margaret Parfitt: a 24 year old admitted in diabetic ketoacidotic coma

Margaret was admitted unconscious to the Accident and Emergency department in a diabetic ketoacidotic coma before being transferred to an acute ward conscious but extremely drowsy and rousable only to persistent verbal and tactile stimuli.

Diabetic ketoacidosis

Margaret had become ketoacidotic because of her underlying diabetes mellitus which had been previously undiagnosed.

Diabetes mellitus is a condition where there is a severe insulin deficiency. Insulin is the hormone primarily responsible for lowering the level of glucose in the blood. If there is an absence of insulin, the blood sugar rises making the blood hyperosmotic. Water from the cells and tissues is then attracted into the intravascular compartment. A diuresis then ensues which can ultimately lead to serious volume depletion and electrolyte loss via the kidneys.

Since glucose cannot enter the cells for metabolism, fats are used as an energy source instead. However, fats cannot be completely broken down in the absence of glucose and so ketone bodies are

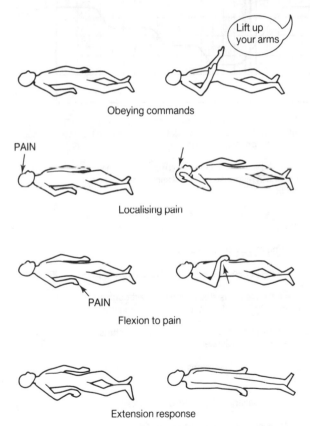

Fig. 23.39 *Motor responses (reproduced by kind permission of the* Nursing Times, *in which this figure first appeared in an article by Teasdale on 12th June 1975)*

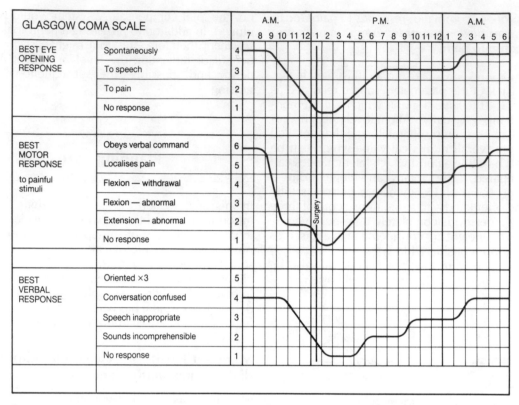

GLASGOW COMA SCALE			A.M. 7 8 9 10 11 12	P.M. 1 2 3 4 5 6 7 8 9 10 11 12	A.M. 1 2 3 4 5 6
BEST EYE OPENING RESPONSE	Spontaneously	4			
	To speech	3			
	To pain	2			
	No response	1			
BEST MOTOR RESPONSE to painful stimuli	Obeys verbal command	6			
	Localises pain	5			
	Flexion — withdrawal	4			
	Flexion — abnormal	3			
	Extension — abnormal	2			
	No response	1			
BEST VERBAL RESPONSE	Oriented ×3	5			
	Conversation confused	4			
	Speech inappropriate	3			
	Sounds incomprehensible	2			
	No response	1			

Scoring of best eye opening

4 = if the patient opens his eyes spontaneously when the nurse approaches

3 = if the patient opens his eyes in response to speech (spoken or shouted)

2 = if the patient opens his eyes only in response to painful stimuli such as digital pressure around nail beds of fingers

1 = if the patient does not open his eyes in response to painful stimuli

Note: record a C if the eyes are closed by swelling

Scoring of best motor response

6 = if the patient can obey a simple command such as 'squeeze my hand'

5 = if the patient moves a limb to locate the painful stimuli applied to the head or trunk and attempts to remove the source

4 = if the patient attempts to withdraw from the source of pain

3 = if the patient flexes only his arms at the elbows and wrist in response to painful stimuli to the nail beds (*decorticate rigidity*)

2 = if the patient extends his arms (straightens his elbows) in response to painful stimuli (decerebrate rigidity)

1 = if the patient has no motor response to pain on any limb

Scoring of best verbal response

5 = if the patient is oriented to time, place and person

4 = if the patient is able to converse although not oriented to time, place or person (e.g. 'Where am I?')

3 = if the patient speaks only in words or phrases that make little or no sense

2 = if the patient responds with incomprehensible sounds such as groans

1 = if the patient does not respond verbally at all

Note: Record a T if a tracheostomy tube or an endotracheal tube is in place

Fig. 23.40 *Glasgow coma scale*

Fig. 23.41 Margaret Parfitt's assessment

DATE OF ADMISSION: 28-4-92

NAME: *Margaret Parfitt*   D.O.B. *01.05.66*   M.S.W.   NOK: *Parents*
18 The Drive
Beaconsfield
B/field 3210

ADDRESS: *24 A Grove Park Ave.*
London
Prefers to be addressed as: *Maggie*

Tel: *071 - 111 2222*

DOCTOR: *Dr P. Jones*

ASSESSMENT – OF SELF-CARE DEFICITS

1. HEALTH DEVIATION SELF-CARE REQUISITES

OTHER PERSONS IMPORTANT TO PATIENT
Robert Green
(Fiancé)

WHO IS TO BE CONTACTED IN EMERGENCY
Parents and Robert Green

2. UNIVERSAL SELF-CARE REQUISITES

PRIMARY NURSE:
K. Manley

REASON FOR ADMISSION

*Became unconscious after
a period of feeling unwell
and increasingly drowsy*

PATIENT'S UNDERSTANDING OF ADMISSION

*Unable to determine
due to unconsciousness*

FAMILY'S UNDERSTANDING OF ADMISSION
Diabetes

SOURCE OF ASSESSMENT
Robert Green

MEDICAL INFORMATION

RELEVANT PAST MEDICAL HISTORY
Nil

MEDICAL DIAGNOSIS *Diabetic Ketoacidosis*

DRUGS TAKEN AT HOME *Contraceptive pill*

ALLERGIES *None*

PATIENT'S FEELINGS & EXPECTATIONS RELATED TO PRESENT ILLNESS
*Unable to assess due to
unconsciousness*

NURSE'S INITIAL IMPRESSION PHYSICAL AND SOCIAL
*Physically fit, well adjusted young
woman with lots of friends*

KNOWLEDGE/INFORMATION/SKILLS NEEDED FOR CONTINUED SELF-CARE AFTER DISCHARGE
*(1) Diabetes and how it affects the body
(2) Insulin therapy and administration
(3) Factors affecting body's need for glucose
(4) Emotional, sexual and social implications*

BASE LINE FUNCTIONS

	Rate	Rhythm	Cough
Breathing	*32/min*	*Kussmaul's*	*Nil*
Circulation	*Warm and well perfused limbs*		
Pulse Rate		Rhythm	B/P
128/min	*Sinus tachycardia*		*90/75*

Colour *Pink*   Skin/Lips *Pink*

TEMPERATURE *38°C*   WEIGHT *8½ st*

USUAL PATTERNS CONCERNING DAILY
FLUID INTAKE *one peripheral I.V. cannula : insulin
one central cannula - CVP measure*

ORAL *2000-3000*
LIKES *Tea, coffee, wine*
DISLIKES *milk*
FOOD INTAKE – TYPE, TIME, REGULAR APPETITE, LIKES, DISLIKES

*Breakfast: cereals and toast
Lunch: roll and fruit
Dinner: two course meal. No dislikes*

SPECIAL DIET (WHY?)
IS PATIENT THIN/OBESE/NORMAL?
Teeth *Own*
Mouth *clean and dry*

UNIVERSAL SELF-CARE REQUISITES CONT'D

ELIMINATION: CONTINENCE, FREQUENCY, TIMING, COLOUR, AMOUNT, REGULARITY, AIDS NEEDED.

URINE *Catheterised
Large volumes passed hourly
(100-150 mls/hr)*

FAECES *Bowels not opened
Pattern not assessed*

URINALYSIS
*Ketone +++   Protein ++
Sugar 2%*

CONDITION OF SKIN, NAILS AND HAIR
*Skin and nails: clean and
healthy. Evidence of dehydration
Hair: well groomed*

USUAL PATTERNS OF HYGIENE
*Bath every evening before going
to bed*

SLEEP AND REST, BEDTIME ROUTINE AIDS TO SLEEP
*Goes to bed at midnight
Up at 6.30 am except weekends*

DAILY ACTIVITIES, RECREATION & BODY MOVEMENT
*Tennis twice weekly
Swims once weekly
Enjoys socialising and entertaining
friends*

PERSONAL CHARACTERISTICS

BIOLOGICAL RHYTHM BEST TIME/WORST TIME OF DAY
*Best in morning
Worst in afternoon*

WHAT PATIENT IS ABOUT TO DO HIM/HERSELF, WANTS TO DO WITHOUT HELP
'Very independent normally'

WHAT PATIENT WOULD EVENTUALLY LIKE TO DO INDEPENDENTLY
'Everything'

SELF-CONCEPT: BODY AND SELF ESTEEM
'Outgoing, confident and fun-loving'

PAINS OR OTHER SENSATIONS
Unable to assess

BALANCE BETWEEN SOLITUDE AND SOCIALISING
Unable to assess

COMMUNICATION
*Unable to assess as currently conscious level
is fluctuating*

FAMILY, FRIENDS, RELATIONSHIPS AND RESPONSIBILITIES
*Lives away from home. Very good relationship with
parents and siblings*

SEXUALITY: INFORMATION ABOUT MARITAL STATUS, RELATIONSHIPS
*Lives with boyfriend
Stable relationship for two years*

OCCUPATION AND LIVING ACCOMMODATION
*Two bedroomed flat - owner occupier
(Estate agent)*

DEVELOPMENTAL SELF-CARE REQUISITES: NOTE THE MAJOR LIFE CHANGES, DEVIATION FROM GROWTH AND DEVELOPMENTAL NORMS: HOW THE PATIENT COPES WITH THEM, WHAT OR WHO HELPS HIM/HER (CULTURE, RELIGION, BELIEFS, VALUES)
Wants to set up own business

Fig. 23.42 Care plan for Margaret Parfitt

Problem	Goal	Nursing Action	Rationale
1. Unconsciousness due to diabetic ketoacidotic coma leading to the potential problems of: (a) Obstructed airway	Maintenance of clear airway and oxygenation	Position Margaret on her side Maintain Guedel airway in mouth until consciousness and swallowing reflexes return. Oropharyngeal suction to remove secretions. Monitor respiratory function continually – i.e. respiratory quality, rate, pattern, depth, colour and for evidence of increased sympathetic arousal. Monitor pulse, blood pressure, respirations half hourly	Until consciousness returns Margaret is very vulnerable to obstruction of her airway and inadequate oxygenation
(b) Vulnerable to external hazards	Prevent Margaret from harming herself	Position Margaret's limbs so that they do not lie on intravenous lines, or become harmed by other equipment. Protect Margaret's eyes particularly when changing her position. Turn Margaret and reposition her two-hourly. Maintain quiet, restful environment which is warm. Check emergency equipment is in working action and nearby	Margaret is unable to control her environment and would not be familiar with equipment that may cause her harm or be aware of other potential hazards
(c) Loss of orientation and control resulting in increased anxiety on returning consciousness	Orientate Margaret to time, place and person	Orientate Margaret in time, place and person hourly until consciousness returns completely. Repeatedly explain what has happened to her. Touch Margaret's arm when communicating with her. Explain her family and boyfriend are nearby. Explain any disturbances, unusual sounds, sensations and the purpose of equipment. Maintain diurnal rhythm. Monitor Margaret for evidence of overt anxiety such as sweating, tachycardia. Encourage family and boyfriend to talk and comfort Margaret and to touch her and hold her hand	Margaret will be waking up in a strange environment not knowing what has happened to her. She will not be in control of her body and environment and will not be able to make sense of the stimuli she is perceiving

Problem	Goal	Nursing Action	Rationale
2. Unable to maintain a safe internal environment due to diabetic ketoacidosis leading to the problems of:			
(a) Unstable blood sugar	Gradually re-establish a stable and normal blood sugar	Measure Dextrostix levels hourly. Maintain insulin infusion according to sliding scale prescribed by doctor. Measure urine sugar and ketones two-hourly and chart trends. Monitor Margaret's breath for acetone	The blood sugar levels previously high will gradually drop under the influence of the insulin. There is however a danger that either inadequate amounts of insulin may be administered or too much, leading to hypoglycaemia
(b) Dehydration	To rehydrate Margaret so that she can drink and eliminate urine naturally	Administer normal saline infusion to keep central venous pressure at level indicated by doctor. Monitor CVP half-hourly. Inform doctor when blood glucose is within normal limits so that infusion can be changed to 5% dextrose. Monitor urinary output hourly. Inform doctor if it falls below ½ ml/kg body wt/per hour for more than two hours or remains excessively high	Saline is administered to rehydrate Margaret until blood sugar nears normal when dextrose will be administered to prevent hypoglycaemia occurring. Over-hydration must also be observed for
(c) Electrolyte and acid base imbalance	Regain electrolyte balance and monitor for effects of electrolyte anc acid base imbalance	Administer potassium supplements when plasma levels fall according to doctor's prescription. Monitor for irregularities in pulse half hourly. Monitor ECG continuously for ventricular ectopics. Monitor respirations continuously for Kussmaul's respiration	Potassium may be low or high. Sodium may be low, normal or high depending on degree of dehydration. Potassium abnormalities and acidosis can lead to dangerous cardiac rhythms
(d) Gastric dilation and possible aspiration of contents into lungs	Maintain an empty stomach until normal intestinal functon returns	Insert nasogastric tube and aspirate hourly. Listen for bowel sounds, two-hourly. Position as 1(a)	Electrolyte disturbances can produce paralytic ileus and gastric dilation. If secretions collect in the stomach there is a danger of aspiration
(e) Further neurological impairment	Monitor neuro ogical status	Perform neurological assessment hourly until consciousness returns fully	Conscious level will be affected by dehydration and ketosis. Blood sugar is main energy source for the brain

Problem	Goal	Nursing Action	Rationale
3. **Infection which may have precipitated diabetes or may result from invasive equipment**	To keep Margaret infection free	Monitor Margaret's skin for any evidence of infection. Monitor temperature two-hourly. Send a specimen of urine for microscopy culture and sensitivity. Monitor Margaret for evidence of a chest infection. Meticulous aseptic care to intravenous cannula sites and infusions. Monitor urinary catheter four-hourly for evidence of infection. Keep urethral orifice clean and dry. Monitor for any evidence of throat, vaginal, ear or eye infections. Clean teeth and gums four-hourly with a mini toothbrush and chlorhexidine gel until Margaret can perform her own mouthcare	An infective focus may have precipitated Margaret's diabetes. Invasive equipment predisposes Margaret to an increased infection risk which in turn will make Margaret's diabetes difficult to stabilise
4. **Anxiety and concern relating to the future due to the sudden change in health status**	To reduce anxiety and allow Margaret to voice concerns	Inform Margaret about her condition and the expected outcome. Inform Margaret and her family of the planned teaching programme organised for her once her diabetes has been stabilised and she feels better	Margaret's previously stable and happy lifestyle would have been overturned. Many feelings and fears for the future may exist which will need to be discussed and come to terms with
5. **Lack of information about diabetes**	To help Margaret understand diabetes and its management	Help Margaret's family and fiancé to understand diabetes and identify how they can help Margaret	Margaret needs to understand about diabetes to become self-caring again

Signed: *K. Manley*

Date: 28.4.92

formed. These accumulate in the blood, reducing the plasma pH, making it acidotic.

The acidosis stimulates compensatory mechanisms in the body in an effort to return the blood pH to normal.

These mechanisms primarily include an increased depth and frequency of breathing, classically recognised as Kussmaul's respiration, in an attempt to rid the body of carbon dioxide which forms carbonic acid in solution in the blood. Coma results when dehydration and ketosis are severe.

Certain infections can precipitate the development of diabetes mellitus in genetically vulnerable groups of people. Infection, too, can precipitate a diabetic ketoacidotic coma in a (previously diagnosed) well-controlled diabetic.

Margaret's assessment is summarised in Fig. 23.41, and her resulting care plan on admission to an acute care area together with the rationale for actions are illustrated in Fig. 23.42.

Conclusion

In this chapter, influences relevant to the care of the patient who is acutely ill have been introduced. These influences include the often neglected psychological and social factors in addition to the biological ones that usually predominate in the acute setting. The biologically related aspects of monitoring parameters have, however, been considered in some detail, as accuracy in measurement and interpretation is an essential prerequisite for any nurse caring for an acutely ill patient.

The principles introduced in the first half of the chapter have been used as a basis for the second half which then focuses on assessment and planning. Hopefully, after reading this chapter, the needs of an acutely ill patient will be more easily and accurately identified, both in breadth and depth.

Glossary

Accountability: Being answerable for one's own actions

Action potential: (Of a nerve impulse) a localised change in electrical potential between the inside and outside of a nerve fibre, which marks the path of an impulse as it travels along the fibre

Acute tubular necrosis: Death of the renal tubular epithelium leading to acute renal failure

Arrhythmias: Any deviation from the heart's normal rhythm

Atrial fibrillation: An atrial arrhythmia occurring at an extremely rapid atrial rate, lacking coordinated activity

Beta-blockers: A class of drugs which block the beta receptors in the sympathetic nervous system therefore reducing sympathetic activity either generally or selectively

Biosynthesis: The building of complex molecules from small organic molecules

Botulism: A rare form of bacterial food poisoning due to ingestion of the toxin produced by *Clostridium botulinum*

Circadian rhythm: Rhythm with a periodicity of 24 hours

Crackles (rales): The sounds heard via a stethoscope when collapsed alveoli open explosively

Decorticate rigidity: A posture characterised by the upper arms being held tightly to the sides with elbows, wrists and fingers flexed and the feet plantarflexed. Implies a destructive lesion of the corticospinal tracts within or very near the cerebral hemispheres

Degradation: The breakdown of large organic molecules into smaller ones

Ecomap: A diagram portraying important connections between the family and others outside the family

General adaptation syndrome: The manifestation of stress in the whole body, encompassing all non-specific changes as they develop throughout time of continued exposure to a stressor

Genogram: A diagram outlining a family's internal and external structure

Holism: An approach where a person is considered to be more than the sum of that person's parts

Homeostasis: The maintenance of a constant internal environment (see Chapter 5)

Hypercapnia: A higher than normal level of carbon dioxide in the blood

Hypovolaemia: Diminished circulating volume of blood in the circulation

Iatrogenic disease: A secondary condition arising from treatment of a primary condition

Luer lock: A screw type connection fitted to intravenous administration sets and accessories to prevent accidental disconnection

Medicalisation: The extension of the influence of medicine over people's lives

Metabolism: The combined actions of *biosynthesis* (anabolism) and *degradation* (catabolism)

Myoclonic: Intermittent muscular contractions

Pneumothorax: Air in the pleural cavity

Poliomyelitis: A disease involving a virus which affects the grey matter of the spinal cord, brain stem and cortex

Polyneuritis: Destruction and/or inflammation of neurones, particularly the myelin sheaths

Stressors: Those factors which produce stress

Stroke volume: The volume of blood ejected from each ventricle at each beat of the heart

Synergistic: One agent facilitates the action of another, i.e. *potentiates* it

Tachypnoea: A respiratory rate greater than 20 breaths per minute

Tetanus: A disease resulting from infection with *Clostridium tetani*. The endotoxin produced affects motor nerve endings and motor nerve cells producing rigidity and spasm, often involving the respiratory muscles

Wheezes: Musical sounds heard from the airways either with or without a stethoscope

References

Ashworth, P. (1979). Sensory deprivation 2. The acutely ill. *Nursing Times*, 75(7), 290–294.

Atkinson, R.L., Atkinson, R.C. and Hilgard, E. (1990). *Introduction to Psychology* (10th ed.). Harcourt Brace Jovanovich, New York.

Baker, N.C., Cerone, S.B. and Gaze, N. (1984). The effect of type of thermometer and length of time inserted on oral temperature measurements of afebrile subjects. *Nursing Research*, 33(2), 109–111.

Barnett, K. (1972). A survey of the current utilisation of touch by health team personnel with hospitalised patients. *International Journal of Nursing Studies*, 9, 195–208.

Blattner, B. (1981). *Holistic Nursing*. Prentice-Hall, New Jersey.

Boore, J.R.P. (1978). *Prescription for Recovery*. RCN, London.

Bourbonnais, F. (1981). Pain assessment: development of a tool for the nurse and the patient. *Journal of Advanced Nursing*, 6, 277–282.

Breu, C. and Dracup, K. (1978). Helping the spouses of critically ill patients. *American Journal of Nursing*, 78(1), 50–53.

Brown, G. (1989). Life events and measurement. In *Life Events and Illness*, Brown, G. and Harris, T. (eds.). Unwin Hyman, London.

Brown, G. and Harris, T. (1978). *Social Origins of Depression: A Study of Psychiatric Disorder in Women*. Tavistock Publications, London.

Brown, G. and Harris, T. (1989). *Life Events and Illness*. Unwin Hyman, London.

Campbell, J., Finch, D., Allport, C. and Erickson, H. (1985). A theoretical approach to nursing assessment. *Journal of Advanced Nursing*, 10, 111–115.

Canavan, T. (1984). The psychobiology of sleep. *Nursing*, 2(23), 682–683.

Cartwright, A. (1964). *Human Relations and Hospital Care*. Routledge and Kegan Paul, London.

Castledine, G. and McFarlane, J.K. (1982). *A Guide to the Practice of Using the Nursing Process*. Mosby, St Louis.

Creed, F. (1981). Life events and appendicectomy. *Lancet*, 1(8235), 1381–1385.

Dohrenwend, B.S. and Dohrenwend, B.P. (1974). *Stressful Life Events*. John Wiley and Sons, New York.

Durham, M.L., Swanson, B. and Paulford, N. (1986). Effect of tachypnoea on oral temperature estimation: a replication. *Nursing Research*, 35(4), 211–214.

Fabijan, L. and Gosselin, M. (1982). How to recognise sleep deprivation in your ICU patient and what to do about it. *Canadian Nurse*, April 21, 20–23.

Fox, A. and Goldblatt, P. (1982). *OPCS Longitudinal Study: Sociodemographic Mortality Differentials 1971–1975*. Series LS1. HMSO, London.

Ganong, W.F. (1983). *Medical Physiology* (11th ed.). Lange Medical Publications, California.

Gath, A. (1977). The impact of an abnormal child upon the parents. *British Journal of Psychology*, 130, 405–410.

Goldberger, L. (1966). Experimental isolation: an overview. *American Journal of Psychiatry*, 122, 774–782.

Hampe, S.O. (1979). Needs of the grieving spouse in a hospital setting. *Nursing Research*, 24, 113.

Harding, H.E. (1962). A notable source of error in the diagnosis of appendicitis. *British Medical Journal*, 2, 1028–1029.

Harper, R. (1981). *A Guide to Respiratory Care*. J.B. Lippincott, Philadelphia.

Hayward, J.C. (1975). *Information: A Prescription Against Pain*. RCN, London.

Hemenway, J. (1980). Sleep and the cardiac patient. *Heart and Lung*, 9(3), 453–462.

Hill, L. and Smith, N. (1985). *Self-Care Nursing: Promotion of Health*. Prentice-Hall, New Jersey.

Irwin, B.L. (1973). Supportive measures for relatives of the fatally ill. *Community Nursing Research*, 6, 126.

Ley, P. (1988). *Communicating with Patients*. Croom Helm, London.

McAvinchey, I. (1984). Economic factors and mortality: some aspects of a Scottish case 1950–1978. *Scottish Journal of Political Economy*, 31(1), 1–27.

Maguire, P., Tait, A., Broke, M., Thomas, C. and Selwood, R. (1980). Effect of counselling on the psychiatric morbidity associated with mastectomy. *British Medical Journal*, 281, 1454–1456.

Manley, K. (1988). The needs and support of relatives. *Nursing*, 3(32), 19–22.

Mayers, M.G. (1972). *A Systematic Approach to the Nursing Care Plan*. Appleton Century Crofts, New York.

Molter, N. (1979). Needs of relatives of critically ill patients: a descriptive study. *Heart and Lung*, 8, 332.

Monat, A. and Lazarus, R.S. (1985). *Stress and Coping: An Anthology* (2nd ed.). Columbia University Press, New York.

Morgan, M. (1980). Marital status, health, illness and service use. *Social Science and Medicine*, 14A, 633–643.

Mullin, V. (1980). Implementing the self-care concept in the acute care setting. *Nursing Clinics of North America*, 15(1), 177–190.

Naismith, L.D., Robinson, J., Shaw, G. and Macintyre, M. (1979). Psychological rehabilitation after myocardial infarction. *British Medical Journal*, 1(439), 41.

Norris, L. and Grove, S. (1986). Investigation of selected psychosocial needs of family members of critically ill adults. *Heart and Lung*, 15(2), 194–199.

Open University. (1985). *Health and Disease. Books I–VIII*. Open University Press, Milton Keynes.

Orem, D. (1991) *Nursing: Concepts of Practice* (4th ed.). Mosby, St Louis.

Parkes, C.M., Benjamin, B. and Fitzgerald, R. (1969). Broken heart: a statistical study of increased mortality among widowers. *British Medical Journal*, 1, 740–743.

Paulley, J.W. (1955). Psychosomatic factors in the aetiology of acute appendicitis. *Archives of the Middlesex Hospital*, 5, 35–41.

Paykel, E.S., Prusoff, B.A. and Myers, K.L. (1975). Suicide attempts and recent life-events. *Archives of General Psychiatry*, 32(3), 327–333.

Pearson, A. and Vaughan, B. (1986). *Nursing Models for Practice*. Heinemann, London.

Roy, C. (1984). *An Adaptation Model* (2nd ed.). Prentice Hall, New Jersey.

Rubin, R. (1963). Maternal touch. *Nursing Outlook*, 11, 828.

Selye, H. (1976). *The Stress of Life* (2nd ed.). McGraw-Hill, New York.

Spelman, M.S. (1967). How do we improve doctor-patient communication in our hospitals? In *Communicating with the Patient*, Ley, P. and Spelman, M.S. (eds.). Staples Press, London.

Stein, S.P. and Charles, E. (1971). Emotional factors in juvenile diabetes mellitus: a study of early life experiences of adolescent diabetes. *American Journal of Psychiatry*, 128(6), 700–704.

Stockwell, F. (1972). *The Unpopular Patient*. RCN, London.

Sykes, M.K., McNicol, M.W. and Campbell, E.J.M. (1976). *Respiratory Failure* (2nd ed.). Blackwell Scientific Publications, Oxford.

Teasdale, G. (1975). Assessing 'conscious level'. *Nursing Times*, 71(24), 914–917.

Teasdale, G. and Jennett, B. (1974). Assessment of coma and impaired consciousness: a practical scale. *Lancet*, 2, 81–84.

Tew, B.J., Lawrence, K.M., Payne, N. and Rawnsley, K. (1977). Marital stability following the birth of a child with spina bifida. *British Journal of Psychiatry*, 131, 79–82.

Volicer, B.J., Isenberg, M.A. and Burns, M.W. (1977). Medical-surgical differences in hospital stress factors. *Journal of Human Stress*, 3(2), 7.

Wilson-Barnett, J. (1979). *Stress in Hospital*. Churchill Livingstone, Edinburgh.

Worrell, J.N. (1977). Nursing implications in the care of the patient experiencing sensory deprivation. In *Advanced Concepts in Clinical Nursing*, Kintzel, K.C. (ed.). J.B. Lippincott, Philadelphia.

Wright, L. and Leahey, M. (1984). *Nurses and Families: A Guide to Family Assessment and Intervention*. F.A. Davis, Philadelphia.

Suggestions for further reading

Burnard, P. (1985). *Learning Human Skills*. Heinemann, London.

Chernin, D. and Manteaffel, G. (1984). *Health: A Holistic Approach*. Wheaton, USA.

Cooper, C. (ed.). (1983). *Stress Research: Issues for the Eighties*. John Wiley and Sons, Chichester.

Cox, T. (1983). *Stress* (2nd ed.). Macmillan, London.

Harris, J.S. (1984). Stressors and stress in critical care.

Critical Care Nurse, Jan/Feb, 84–97.

Kappeli, S. (1986). Nurses' management of patients' self-care. *Nursing Times*, 82(11), 40–43.

Kim, H.S. (1983). *The Nature of Theoretical Thinking in Nursing*. Appleton Century Crofts, Connecticut.

Marriner, A. (1989). *Nursing Theorists and Their Work* (2nd ed.). Mosby, St Louis.

Perry, A. and Jolley, M. (1990). *Nursing: A Knowledge Base for Practice*. Edward Arnold, London.

Synder, C. and Ford, C. (1987). *Coping with Negative Life Events: Clinical and Social Psychological Perspectives*. Plenum Press, New York.

Webb, W.B. (1981). Some theories about sleep and their clinical implications. *Psychiatric Annals*, 11(12), 11–18.

24

CARE OF THE PATIENT REQUIRING SURGICAL INTERVENTION

Carol Blake

The aims of this chapter are: to give the reader some insight into the environment in which she will be working; to outline some of the skills she will gain and have the opportunity to practise; to determine the different problems which may arise with planned and emergency surgery; and to identify, through individual care profiles, the needs and problems common to patients undergoing surgery and some specific needs and problems related to particular types of surgery.

The chapter includes the following topics:

- The surgical environment and contributing personnel
- Nursing skills and knowledge required
- The differing needs of individuals
- Pain – affecting factors

- Wound healing
  – process
  – affecting factors
- Pre-operative care
  – core elements
  – some individual needs
- Post-operative care
  – core elements
  – some individual needs

Figures for the 15 years up to 1986 show the time spent as an inpatient for both preparation and recuperation has been reduced (Table 24.1). Although the nature of the surgery remains largely unchanged, moves towards earlier mobilisation and the introduction of the nursing process have led nursing care to become increasingly geared towards meeting short term needs and problems created by surgery whilst in hospital. Greater em-phasis is also given now to preparing and educating the patient to meet any needs created by long term changes once he is home.

Any individual undergoing surgery – be it planned or emergency – will see himself as facing a physically and mentally traumatic event, even though the operation may be described as 'minor' by health care professionals.

Table 24.1. *Bed occupancy statistics*
(*Source:* Social Trends, 18, *Central Statistical Office,* 1988)

Average length of stay for surgical inpatients.
Number of days:

1971	1982	1986
9.1	7.6	6.5

Environment and personnel

The majority of patients entering a surgical ward are fully able to meet all their own needs. The ward staff should attempt to create a warm, friendly environment, to welcome patients and to enable them to express any anxieties whilst allowing the individual to remain in control. On the other hand the nursing staff must demonstrate and maintain a high level of care to meet the needs of those who have undergone surgery or those re-quiring surgery who are unable to meet their own needs. Patients' relatives and friends should be confident that individual needs will be met before, during and after surgery.

The surgical ward has peaks and troughs of activity governed by routine operating and admission days. Most wards have more than one consultant and this, together with a rapid turnover rate and being on call for emergency admissions, results in an environment which can be very stressful.

Preparation for a learner about to be allocated to a surgical ward should include being given some insight into the roles of other members of the team with whom she may be working. Those she is most likely to meet are shown in Table 24.2.

Skills and knowledge required

The nurse must have some insight into the skills and knowledge required on a surgical ward, many of which will be considered in more detail below.

Table 24.2. *Other health care professionals in the surgical team*

Health care professional	Role	Comment
Physiotherapist	– teaches and assists with pre- and post-operative exercises to prevent deep vein thrombosis and chest infection – meets specific post-operative needs related to the surgery performed	These three often work as a team *within* the team
Occupational therapist	– assists patients to adapt to changes that may later affect their activities of living (e.g. amputation, colostomy)	
Medical social worker	– gives practical and supportive care to meet financial and social needs which may be created by the need for surgery	
Stomatherapist	– usually an RGN in a district post, with specialist training. Will visit the patient with a stoma in hospital and at home giving practical and moral support	
Appliance clerk	– provides practical help when a prosthesis is required following surgery (e.g. amputation, mastectomy)	
District nurse	– usually contacted via the liaison sister. Provides continuity of care for early discharge patients (e.g. removal of sutures)	

She should be able to initiate open communication; be able to speak to the patient in language he will understand; give clear explanations of procedures together with reasons for carrying them out; discuss their after effects and prepare the patient for what he may see and feel.

The nurse must be able to administer the pre- and post-operative care that will ensure the patient's physical safety. Similarly she must meet the psychological needs that surgery may create. She should also be able to understand the reasons for all of these actions.

The nurse must be able to assess physical, verbal and non-verbal cues and react to them in an appropriate way. Sometimes this will involve rapid and immediate action to save a life.

Having given care she must be able to evaluate the results.

The nursing process is a valuable decision-making tool in the surgical area but it must be remembered that there are times when the patient will be neither willing nor able to participate in his care and will rely totally on the skill and expertise of the team around him. The nurse then needs to assess how and when to hand back responsibility to the patient for meeting his own needs and what information he requires in order to respond effectively.

The nurse requires a sound working knowledge of body structure and function in order to identify problems that might occur when function becomes disordered. She needs to understand the process of healing and which factors will promote or delay it (see pages 743–745). She needs to understand that a wound may be closed or left open to heal. If it is closed, she needs to know how and why various types of drainage appliance may be used (see page 759). She will require technical skills, many of which necessitate the use of an **aseptic technique**. The skills need to be used with an understanding of their importance and significance for all concerned. In addition, the nurse will need to meet specific needs created by specific operations.

Above all, she must be empathic. Empathy is 'the ability to understand the world through the eyes of another and convey that understanding to him or her' (Egan, 1990). Nurses generally adapt quickly to new environments and situations. They rapidly accept surgery, its traumatic physical and mental effects, the accompanying pain, nausea and general debilitation as part of the normal process towards healing. The majority of patients, however, have only one operation in their lifetime. They approach this new and sometimes frightening experience with some anxiety.

This anxiety on admission can be a significant problem. Research in the mid-seventies (Hayward, 1975; Boore, 1976) and studies since (McCaffrey, 1983; Carr, 1990) continue to show that patients respond better, have a more realistic expectation of post-operative pain and generally a shorter post-operative recovery period when there is a flow of information and an opportunity to voice their anxieties, opinions and questions. It has been suggested, however, through recent studies that nurses, whilst knowing what the stressors are for their patients, often overestimate the anxiety they cause (Biley, 1989). It would seem that most patients have the ability and reserve to cope physically and mentally with surgery but need help to do so.

Carl Rogers, a humanist psychotherapist, describes a 'helping relationship' as 'one in which one of the participants intends that there should come about, in one or both parties, more appreciation of, more expression of, more functional use of the latent inner resources in the individual' (Rogers, 1967; page 40). Through empathic, individualised care with appropriate information being given, the nurse may help her patient to cope with the experience of surgery.

Needs of individuals

If the nurse is to fulfil her role in the helping relationship, she will need to understand the basic needs that exist in all individuals and how these affect their lives. Models of nursing discussed in Chapter 12 are based on these needs. Maslow described individuals as having a *hierarchy of needs* (Maslow, 1970).

Basic needs start with the physiological requisites of the body – the needs for oxygen, food, water, sleep, warmth and the excretion of waste products. These are the physical requirements necessary for life and once they are satisfied the individual can then express needs for physical and mental safety, for a secure environment and lifestyle. Once the needs for security have been satisfied too, the individual can express the need to be needed by other people, to be accepted, wanted and of value. Next follows the need to feel good about oneself, to like oneself and have positive

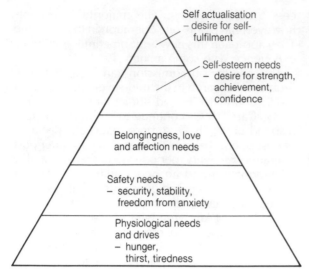

Fig. 24.1 *Maslow's hierarchy of needs (adapted from Maslow, 1970)*

self-regard. Finally Maslow says that some individuals may achieve self-actualisation where they are totally confident about their life, themselves and everything they say and do; in other words, when they are reaching their full potential as individuals. He does say however that very few individuals reach this state and that those who do, do not stay there permanently. As with each of the other levels in the hierarchy, the individual fluctuates depending on the time, place, surroundings, and so forth. Maslow suggests that each level of the hierarchy, starting at the lowest level, must be partially satisfied before the individual can try to meet his needs in the next.

Maslow's work may be used as a guide when assessing individuals' needs and deciding on priorities of care. Roper's model of nursing is based on Maslow's ideas (Roper *et al.*, 1990).

Whilst this chapter looks in detail at the adult patient in a general surgical setting, the reader may like to consider the needs of individuals who fall into specific groups and how that may affect their needs. The following, although not definitive, are examples.

Children

Children undergoing surgery, of necessity, must be admitted to hospital. Their needs and rights are clearly laid down in the National Association for the Welfare of Children in Hospital's (NAWCH) *Charter for Children* (for further information see Useful Addresses). The nurse has an extended client base and must meet the needs of both the patient and the parent(s).

The needs of surgical patients as described in this chapter apply to children but must be met within the context of the developmental stage of the child (see Chapter 19) and any legal requirements. An example of needs assessed within the developmental stage is the need for information which can reduce anxiety (Hayward, 1975). Both parents and children require the information but it may need to be delivered differently.

Child (1981), citing Piaget, suggests that children up to the age of 11 are unable to understand or follow an idea or factual information without concrete tangible evidence in front of them, i.e. they cannot deal in concepts. This would suggest that pre-operative information for children below 11 should be in a form they can see and work with. The use of toys which have intravenous giving sets and drains attached allows the child a mental picture and on returning from theatre they see and feel the nurse was telling them the truth. Truth is important for children in building trust and confidence.

With reference to legal requirements, it should be noted that the age when an individual can sign their own consent to surgery is 16.

Adolescents

Adolescence is a time of confusion, with individuals struggling to find their own identity, when awareness of body changes and body image are at their peak and when not being different is so important. To be hospitalised and operated on at this time can add to the already confusing period of adjustment. Whilst this period is about an increasing independence from the family, adolescents may regress during a period of treatment to wanting and needing their parents close to them. An underlying knowledge of the adolescent developmental stage and skill in assessing each individual can allow the nurse to plan care effectively and help the individual meet his needs.

Elderly people

With projected figures of over 9 million over the age of 65 by the year 2000 as opposed to 7.5

million in 1971 (Central Statistical Office, 1988), the elderly will become an increasingly large percentage of the patients requiring surgery. As with children, their needs pre- and post-operatively remain the same but must be planned for and met taking into account the ageing process (see Chapter 26).

Other groups who have specific needs which should be addressed if they require surgery are: ethnic groups, specific religious groups, e.g. Jehovah's Witnesses, those who are physically and mentally disabled or mentally ill.

Patients admitted for surgery face a new and traumatic event in their lives. Differences in personality will show in their behaviour and attitudes towards the event but there are also outside factors which may affect their needs. Figure 24.7 gives examples of three patients admitted to the ward on the same day. A potted history is given of each patient's stay in hospital. This will be referred to later in the chapter (see post-operative care). The aim in this section is to compare the differing needs that arise depending on which level of the hierarchy the patient is operating on at the time of admission.

Assessment is based on Roper's model of care (Roper *et al.*, 1990) and there is a reminder for learners of Roper's activities of living at the top of each care plan (see also Chapter 12). Although the care plans highlight specific activities of living which are boxed at the top of the care plan, the reader will realise that no activity can be regarded in isolation in the clinical area and that nursing intervention usually involves meeting needs concerned with several activities.

It should be remembered that all care plans used throughout this text are examples only of the subject being discussed. They are not necessarily indicative of what the learner may find in the clinical area.

The profile given in Fig. 24.2 describes a lady admitted from the routine waiting list. She has been well prepared for surgery and fully understands both her diagnosis and the operative procedure she is to undergo. It can be seen from this profile that she has a full, active life both at home and outside. Following assessment, needs and problems are identified.

Figure 24.3 shows a care plan highlighting three activities of living where needs cannot be met totally by the patient. These needs fall into two

---

Mrs Archer is 63 years old, married with two children. She and her husband live in their own home with their youngest daughter. Her eldest daughter lives nearby and has a three month old son. She is a member of the amateur dramatic group and enjoys exercising her two red setters. She has a diagnosed carcinoma of the rectum and has been admitted three days prior to an ***abdominoperineal resection of the rectum*** and formation of a ***colostomy***, in order to prepare the bowel for this surgery. She is fully aware of her condition and understands what the operation will entail. The district stomatherapist has visited her at home. She is admitted, assessed and a pre-operative care plan formulated (Fig. 24.3).

On return from theatre she is physiologically stable although she requires a blood transfusion. She has nylon sutures in her abdominal wound and black silk sutures and a drain in the perineum. On the third day post-operatively her colostomy produces flatus and a programme is drawn up to re-establish her normal eating and drinking habits (Table 24.6). She is mobilised early to prevent complications and the care of her colostomy is gradually transferred from the nurse to the patient.

Abdominal and perineal sutures are removed at ten and 14 days respectively. Mrs Archer is discharged home on the fifteenth day post-operatively. She is now caring fully for her own needs. The stomatherapist will call to follow up with support and advice. Mrs Archer is given an appointment for the outpatient clinic in six weeks' time.

Fig. 24.2 *Patient profile: Mrs Archer*

---

categories. Firstly there are those needs, identified by the nurse using her skill and knowledge, that must be met if the patient's safety is not to be jeopardised. The nurse specifies a dietary regime to meet a set goal but the patient is glad that within the confines of the regime, which is clearly prescribed, she retains control of what she eats and when. Thus with a clear explanation and a set goal she is not reliant upon the nurses to meet this need.

Secondly there are the problems identified by the patient. Because Mrs Archer has been well prepared for her operation, she is confident enough to express needs at a higher level on the hierarchy and is already looking to the future and how this operation may affect her relationships with family and friends. This gives the nurse the chance to initiate care which will form a good nurse–patient–family relationship. The very practical help prescribed at this time enables the nurse to meet recurring needs in this activity of living at a later date, with guidance and support rather than direct intervention (see Post-operative care, work and play).

Fig. 24.3 Care plan for Mrs Archer

Date	Identified needs/problems	Objectives/goals	Nursing intervention	Review
15.1.92	**Maintenance of safety**			
	Needs to be prepared for theatre	(1) To minimise risk of post-operative wound infection from bowel contents and allow surgeon clear access to operation site, i.e. free from faeces	Rectal washout before bedtime for 3 days	Daily
			Purgatives as prescribed	
			Low residue, light diet 15/1	
			Fluids only, including soup and ice cream 16/1	
			Clear fluid only 17/1	
			Nil by mouth from 00.00 hours, 18/1	
		(2) Complete pre-operative care schedule	See standard pre-operative procedure	
	Eating and drinking			
	Potential problem of dehydration due to above	To take 3 litres of fluid orally in 24 hours	Ensure a variety of acceptable drinks	Daily
			Give access to kitchen area	
	Work and play			
	Is anxious about effect of stoma on home and social life	Encourage patient to voice worries	Mrs Potter (ex-ostomy patient) to visit 16/1	16/1
		To involve family members in care	Staff nurse to see Mr and Mrs Archer 17/1 to open discussions on potential practical problems at home	17/1

NAME: Dorothy Archer   **Date of Birth:** 7.4.28   **Signed:** *J. Smith*

Mrs Brown is a widow aged 74 with one son who lives at home. She is admitted as an emergency, accompanied by a neighbour, with a three-day history of abdominal pain, nausea and vomiting. On admission she is pale, shocked, dehydrated and still in pain. History-taking from the patient and the neighbour reveals she is a chronic bronchitic and uses a salbutamol inhaler, as required, to control her respiratory symptoms. She has not eaten for two days and has not defaecated for three. She regularly takes aperients every day.

On assessment her pain is now unremitting. She vomited 450 ml of faecal fluid in the Accident and Emergency department and her breath has a faecal smell. Her baseline observations are temperature 39°C, pulse 104, BP 150/90. Her urine is very concentrated and has a large amount of ketones present. Her skin is very dry and she has red patches on both elbows. The skin of her left heel is broken. She has a dry coated tongue. She is extremely anxious and asking that her son be located.

Peritonitis is diagnosed and she is prepared for theatre within two hours where a left **hemicolectomy** is performed for a perforated diverticulum. **Peritoneal lavage** is done and **functioning and defunctioning temporary colostomies** are formed. Her admission care is formulated (Fig. 24.6).

On return from theatre she has nylon abdominal sutures and a rubber drain. She has a problematic post-operative week and is reliant upon intravenous infusion for hydration and also requires plasma as she is **hypoproteinaemic**. She is given light diet on the tenth post-operative day but is reluctant to eat or drink. Her sutures are removed on the fifteenth day but the wound becomes infected and breaks down at the end of the third week. It is cleaned daily and a week later is resutured.

Her colostomy produces faecal fluid but she shows no interest in its management nor in meeting the needs it creates. She is discharged home six weeks after surgery with a district nurse calling daily. Her abdominal sutures have been removed but the lower end of the wound requires dressing every day. Despite seeing the stoma-therapist she still cannot manage her own colostomy. The necessity for a nourishing diet, before surgery to put the colostomies back can be contemplated, has been emphasised to her and her son.

Fig. 24.4 *Patient profile: Mrs Brown*

Figure 24.4 concerns a lady admitted as an emergency, who is operating at the lowest level of the hierarchy. She has little idea of what is happening to her body and is distressed by the pain which, having been chronic for two days, suddenly became acute and unremitting. She tells the nurse that she thinks it is something she ate. Initial assessment is based on examination by both the nurse and doctor, together with information obtained from the patient and her neighbour. She is distressed both physically and mentally. The needs which are identified and the goals which are set are those of priority for the next two hours and prior to surgery.

The care plan in Fig. 24.6 shows those priority needs and the short term goals. Nursing intervention is total, as the patient has neither the 'necessary strength or will' (Henderson, 1978) to meet her own needs.

Re-assessment after surgery, particularly with additional history from Mrs Brown's son, highlights deeper problems than those identified at the initial assessment. It will be seen later that this patient does not leave the lower levels of the hierarchy, still relying on others to meet some of her needs at the time she is discharged (see Post-operative care, eating and drinking and elimination).

Mr Singh is a nineteen year old Indian who has just commenced a year long visit to his aunt and her family. The main purpose of his visit is to learn English, for which he has enrolled at a private language college, and to see something of Europe before returning to India to help his father run the family business. He is a keen athlete and plays squash at a high level.

Admitted as an emergency with abdominal pain, he vomited 300 ml of undigested food in A and E. His limited English makes assessment very difficult. He is uncooperative and extremely anxious. No contact can be made with his aunt. His baseline observations are temperature 38°C, pulse 100, BP 150/70.

Six hours after admission and having solved his communication problems, he goes to theatre for an **appendicectomy** for an acutely inflamed appendix. On return to the ward, with a member of his family present as translator, he is cooperative and recovers quickly from the anaesthetic. He is eating and drinking within 12 hours after surgery and able to mobilise the following morning.

He is discharged home on the third day to his aunt's house and a district nurse is organised to remove his skin clips on the sixth day after surgery. No follow-up is necessary.

Fig. 24.5 *Patient profile: Mr Singh*

Figure 24.5 gives a profile of a young man who is in some pain but not physically unstable. He would be able to meet his own needs, with the necessary restrictions, if he could understand what was required. His assessment and history are very minimal due to problems of communication, and his lack of understanding is causing him to exhibit very insecure behaviour.

The care plan in Fig. 24.7 highlights the one

Fig. 24.6 *Care plan for Mrs Brown*

Date	Identified needs/problems	Objectives/ goals	Nursing intervention	Evaluation
15.1.92	Eating and drinking/ Elimination	Secure maximum comfort by – position – control of vomiting – rehydration; to have 500 ml in one hour	Sit up with two pillows Give prescribed anti-emetics	
	Pain – cannot have analgesia		Pass nasogastric tube and aspirate stomach contents – hourly	
			Commence prescribed intra-venous infusion	
			Catheterise and record all urine output	
	Maintenance of safety Personal hygiene and dressing			
	Mouth is sore and dry	To make as comfortable as possible Prevent the risk of oral infection	Mouthwashes half-hourly Give ice chips to suck	
	Red, sore elbows. Broken skin on (L) heel	Prevent any worsening of skin condition	Hydration as above (L) heel to be dressed with Op-site. Pressure-relieving bootee to be worn until theatre. Inform theatre staff	
	Prepare for theatre in 2 hours	Perform as much of pre-operative schedule as possible	See standard pre-operative procedure	

NAME: Mary Brown   **Date of Birth**: 10.4.17   **Signed**: J. Smith

need that must be met before any further assessment or preparation for surgery can take place. Although this example is extreme, it does illustrate the need to use language the patient understands and shows how effective communication can have a beneficial effect on recovery time and discharge date (Lane-Franklin, 1974). This example also shows how an individual can move rapidly backwards and forwards through the hierarchy depending on environment and circumstances.

The examples looked at above show that some pre-operative care is common to all patients and the standard pre-operative care plan is looked at later in more detail (see page 746). They also show that there are many variables that affect patients' needs and create problems when those needs are not met. Lastly they highlight the fact that needs and problems can be short or long term and that responsibility for meeting these needs may not always be returned to the patient during his stay in hospital.

Fig. 24.7 *Care plan for Mr Singh*

Date	Identified needs/problems	Objectives/ goals	Nursing intervention	Evaluation
15.1.92	Communication			
	Maintenance of safety			
	Reluctant to undress or undergo preparation for operation as he does not understand what he is being asked	(1) Gain patient's understanding	Keep patient comfortable with nothing by mouth until medical registrar (who is Indian) arrives to translate	
			Inform relatives and ask for an interpreter to be available post-operatively	
		(2) Complete pre-operative schedule	See routine pre-operative care procedure and explain to patient through interpreter	

NAME: Raj Singh   **Date of Birth**: 4.11.72   **Signed**: *J. Smith*

After surgery, the patient's return to independence will be affected by many things. It will be affected by pain and the patient's perception of it; by the healing process; by the skill of the nursing staff in observing for and reacting to potential problems; and by the ability of the nurse to meet the need for psychological comfort and education.

The patient's return to autonomy may also be either beneficially or detrimentally affected by other factors over which the nursing staff have no control. These include the patient's age, social background, religious commitments, personality and any underlying pathological condition.

Pain

Pain is experienced, to some degree, by all patients undergoing surgery. Although the physiological basis for pain can be explained, the subjective experience differs between individuals. Detailed consideration is given to pain in Chapter 15, but this section looks briefly at some of the points that may be taken into account when planning care to meet the pain control needs of surgical patients.

Pain is a functional mechanism. Some patients will be admitted in pain, the pain signalling that all is not well. Occasionally patients will experience pain referred to a functionally unaffected part of the body, for example patients with gall bladder disease may complain of shoulder pain. All surgical patients will experience pain from their wounds. The severed peripheral nerves and tissue and the pressure on these from the subsequent swelling cause local pain (see the section on healing on page 743). When muscles have been cut, the pain is more severe on moving. The body produces its own natural analgesics (*endorphins*) which can control some pain but most patients will require some nursing intervention.

'Pain is what the patient says it is and exists when he says it does' (McCaffrey, 1972). It is *his* pain, it creates needs and problems specific to him, and while nurses must accept that pain control requires a multidisciplinary approach, they hold the key to its effectiveness by being at the bedside 24 hours a day.

In meeting the needs of patients with post-operative pain the nurse may wish to consider the following: the importance of drugs, physical factors, and psychological factors when planning pain control.

Evidence continues to emerge that nurses do not meet the pain control needs of the post-operative patient. In one small study of 16 patients, only one (6.25%) was given the full amount of prescribed post-operative analgesia (Balfour, 1989) This is backed by a later study which also highlighted the difference in patients' pre-operative expectation of pain and their post-operative experience (Carr, 1990). Both pieces of work, although small, make similar recommendations:

- Give the patients information about their access to analgesia and its effects;

- Stress the need not to be in distress;

- Use a pain assessment tool;

- There is the need for further investigation into patient-controlled administration of post-operative analgesia (see below, Administration of drugs).

Administration of drugs

Narcotics, by far the most common method of pain control for the post-operative patient, are usually given intramuscularly. They can induce nausea, so they should be administered with an anti-emetic.

Trials in the early 1980s showed that intravenous morphine administered in solution via a *tekmar* produced good clinical results in giving better pain relief at lower doses than the same drug administered intramuscularly at regular intervals (Rutter *et al.*, 1980). This method has the advantage of maintaining a constant level in the bloodstream, producing not only a continuous local effect but a consistent effect on the central nervous system, reducing anxiety and prompting rest.

Trials in clinical areas are increasingly highlighting the beneficial effect of using syringe drivers and pumps to administer a consistent level of analgesia. In one unit the introduction of a patient-controlled pain relief system resulted in a consistent drop in the amount used, earlier mo-bilisation of the patient and decreased recovery time. The same unit achieved the same result in patient-controlled administration of oral analgesia (Dallison, 1991a and b).

Evidence would suggest that intravenous administration is the most effective way of controlling initial post-operative pain and that when controlled by the patient its effectiveness is enhanced.

Physical factors that exacerbate and temper pain

Physical factors that have an influence on pain include vomiting, position, mobility and temperature control.

Vomiting

Vomiting is a common post-operative problem. It may be induced by anaesthesia and/or post-operative analgesia. The physical action of vomiting is exhausting and psychologically demoralising. If it is uncontrolled, these two factors serve to exacerbate the pain. Administration of an anti-emetic is usually all that is required to control this unpleasant symptom but in cases where a *paralytic ileus* exists following surgery, gastric contents may be aspirated via a nasogastric tube.

Position and mobility

Patients in pain have a tendency to become stiff and not to move the painful area, thus causing a splinting effect. This can be used to advantage when moving a patient by asking him to hold his hand over the wound. However if the patient remains immobile for long periods in an effort to relieve uncontrolled pain, respiratory, cardio-vascular and mobility problems can result.

Temperature control

Patients who are too hot or cold become restless and feel pain more acutely. Some temperature-controlling mechanisms are lost temporarily during anaesthesia, and nursing intervention may be required during post-operative re-adjustment. An increase in local pain accompanied by a rise in temperature from 48 hours post-operatively may be early indications of wound infection.

Psychological factors that exacerbate pain

The patient's experience of pain will not be influenced by physical factors alone: there are psychological aspects, too, to the experience of pain.

Anxiety

Information – A Prescription against Pain (Hayward, 1975), based on data taken from surgical patients, is a piece of research that highlights anxiety as the biggest psychological barrier to pain control. The main cause identified for this anxiety is lack of information.

Attitudes

Attitudes can be described as the sum of a person's beliefs and values. These play a large role both in an individual's perception of pain and in the way he attempts to control it. For example, some indivdiuals find a mantra (a word or phrase used repetitively to focus the mind internally during meditation) is helpful to them.

It should always be remembered that nurses have their own attitudes. Care should always be taken to ensure that pain control is administered according to the patient's actual needs and not to his needs as perceived by the nurse.

Uncontrolled pain in the post-operative patient can make it difficult for him to meet his own needs in many of the activities of living. This may necessitate extended periods of intensive nursing intervention.

Wound healing

The tissue response to trauma is either for cells to regenerate or for **scar tissue** to form. There are four basic types of tissue: epithelial tissue, connective tissue, muscle tissue and nerve tissue (see also Chapter 5).

Epithelial tissue

Epithelial cells form the skin, mucous membranes, the lining of the heart, lungs and gut, and make up some glands, such as the liver and the thyroid. They have the ability to reproduce so long as their basal regenerative layer is intact.

Connective tissue

Connective tissue is found throughout the body. It gives shape, elasticity and support to organs. Adipose tissue, bone, cartilage, collagen and the specialist lymphoid tissue which plays a major role in the healing process are all types of connective tissue. The soft connective tissue cut during surgery does not have the power of regeneration.

Muscle

Muscle cells are so specialised that they are unable to reproduce and are replaced by scar tissue. As long as the damage is not extensive, surrounding muscular tissue compensates and function is maintained. There is, however, a weakness at the site of scar tissue, especially in the weeks and months following surgery, and full tensile strength is rarely recovered.

Nerve tissue

Cells of the central nervous system do not reproduce but regeneration of peripheral nerve fibres can occur if damage has occurred only to the axon of the cell and not to the cell body.

Types of healing

Healing of wounds occurs by either *primary* or *secondary intention*. Healing by primary intention is the most common type of healing following surgery. It occurs when the tissue edges are put into apposition. The lower layers are sutured with a dissolvable suture and the skin is either sutured or clipped together. The wound heals quickly with minimal scarring.

If a wound breaks down superficially due to infection, it may be resutured once it is clean but this leaves a more marked scar. Occasionally, in abdominal wounds, all layers break down and bowel can be seen protruding through the wound. This is called *dehisence* and is a medical emergency (see under 'Complications', page 760).

Secondary intention healing occurs by granulation from the bottom of the wound upwards with the epithelial layer being the last to grow. This is most commonly seen in ulcers but this method of healing is encouraged following some surgical procedures, for example closure of a fistula-in-ano and pilonidal sinus. Secondary intention healing may also be favoured for wound sinuses which result from infection.

The healing process

The healing process occurs as a set of responses brought about by trauma. It produces particular clinical features and by understanding this process the nurse should be able to detect any variance from the normal. Table 24.3 details stages of the process and the reasons for it.

Any deviation from the process described is a sign that healing is not taking place or that the process is being interfered with either at a local level by infection or an underlying disease, or by systemic factors such as pain, poor physical and nutritional status, fluid imbalance, **hypoxia**, or the medication being taken. Pyschosocial factors and poor pre-operative preparation may also have this effect. With the exception of underlying disease and medication, all these factors are discussed in conjunction with activities of living in Post-operative care.

Underlying disease

Breakdown of a wound caused by underlying disease is mainly associated with malignant tumours, some of which undergo rapid proliferation when exposed to oxygen during surgery. Malignant cells invade the wound area, preventing normal healing.

Table 24.3. *The stages of healing*

Stages	Rationale
First stage The area around the injury goes white for a few seconds or minutes	Result of the neuro-endocrine response to stress. Adrenaline is pumped out into the circulation causing peripheral vasoconstriction
Second stage The area rapidly becomes red and warm. An exudate appears and the surrounding tissues become swollen. This occurs in 24–72 hours	The inflammatory response commences with vasodilation at the site of injury and clot formation. Increased permeability of the capillary walls due to histamine release results in the loss of fluid and some protein into the interstitial space. The protein increases the osmolarity of the fluid in the space thus drawing further fluid to it and causing oedema. Some of this fluid is lost through the wound as exudate. Leucocytes are also drawn to the area to ingest bacteria which in turn are liquified and discharged as pus with the exudate
Third stage During the next ten days the area becomes less red but remains warm. A layer of epithelium now covers the wound	Collagen starts to be laid down and the area becomes highly vascular. Regeneration of epithelial cells occurs
Fourth stage From two weeks onwards, up to two or three months, the area returns to its normal colour and underlying muscular strength is largely regained. The scar becomes white and contracts. There is often an accompanying irritation and patients with large wounds may notice the anaesthetic qualities of the scar area, which seldom recovers its full original tensile strength	Collagen tissue is consolidated and the blood supply decreases. The tissue contracts but has no nerve supply

Medication

When a patient is admitted, it is important to find out what medication, if any, he is taking. Two groups of drugs in particular, steroids and anticoagulants, interfere with the healing process.

Steroids, with their anti-inflammatory properties, delay healing. Any patient taking steroids will require an increase in dosage during and following surgery to meet the increasing needs resulting from stress. Long term therapeutic steroid administration prevents the body from meeting its own needs in this respect via the normal physiological feedback mechanism (see Chapter 5). These patients should have their stitches left in longer to allow healing to take place – usually another seven days.

Anticoagulants given prophylactically at the time of surgery or those being taken therapeutically by the patient for a pre-existing medical condition interfere with the formation of a blood clot (see Table 24.3). Close observation is required for signs of uncontrolled bleeding particularly during the recovery stage when blood pressure starts to rise during recovery from anaesthesia.

Pre-operative care

It was Florence Nightingale who reputedly said 'the hospital should do the patient no harm' – a statement which remains true today. Patients being admitted to hospital in her day were exposed to the dangers of overcrowding, deficient sanitation and poor hygiene. Today the patient may still be in danger in a hospital although the nature of the hazards have changed. The majority of pre-operative care, be it routine or specific, is aimed at preventing complications and mistakes of identity, as well as helping the patient to understand what is to happen to him, thus ensuring both his physical and mental well-being.

Examples of specific problems for cold admissions (i.e. those from the planned waiting-list) and non-life-threatening emergencies can be seen in Fig. 24.3 and 24.7. The standard pre-operative procedure and its rationale are shown in Table 24.4; however the following additional material may give the learner a broader understanding.

Pre-operative skin preparation

The skin around the site of operation can be prepared in different ways. The aim of the treatment is to reduce the risk of post-operative infection. Strong evidence suggests now that shaving with a razor increases the risk of post-operative infection, due to the minor abrasions caused during this procedure. Furthermore it has been shown that the more time that elapses between shaving and surgery, the greater the risk (Fairclough *et al.*, 1986).

Evidence is mixed on the uses of depilatory creams to remove hair. Some trials have reported a significant drop in infection rates (for example, Llewellyn-Thomas, 1990) whilst others have found no significant change at all (for example, Winfield, 1986). Depilatory creams may damage the skin if a reaction is induced and a patch test should be conducted first.

Still the most effective method of prevention is the application of an effective antiseptic applied vigorously to the area at the time of surgery. In tests it would appear that chlorhexidine gluconate 4% is the most effective and maintains the longest cover (Kalideen, 1990).

Local policy will determine the extent and type of depilation but whichever method is employed, the utmost care should be taken not to damage the underlying skin.

Restriction of food and fluid pre-operatively

Research in the early 1970s showed that nurses frequently initiated the instruction 'nil by mouth' with very little understanding of how unpleasant this may be mentally and physically for the patient (Hamilton-Smith, 1972). Practice is changing and many areas now assess individual needs for pre-operative withholding of food and fluid. This may be necessary because of the type of surgery (see page 738) or may be guided by the estimated time of surgery. Many units allow a drink of water four hours prior to pre-medication.

Research suggests, however, that patients can still find themselves without food and fluid for longer periods than the recommended 4–6 hours, which Torrance (1991) feels would be better described as 'pre-operative starvation' and 'may be detrimental to a patient undergoing major surgery'. A review of fasting times may alleviate some of the problems encountered, particularly the increased

Table 24.4. *Standard pre-operative care plan*

Problem/need	Goal	Nursing action
Potential wound infection	To minimise risk of wound infection	– Skin preparation as prescribed (page 745) – Bath – Check for, report and cover any broken or infected skin, e.g. ulcers – Remove personal clothing and put on theatre gown
Inhalation of vomitus during or following anaesthesia	Remove potential dangers	– Nil by mouth as prescribed (page 745) – Remove dentures – Note dental caps and crowns
Potential deep vein thrombosis and chest infection	Minimise the risk through education	– Assist physiotherapist in teaching of leg and deep breathing exercises
Potential damage to bladder and/or incontinence	Minimise urinary volume in the bladder	– Ask patient to pass urine directly before premedication
To monitor any changes from normal during and following surgery	To obtain baseline measurements of vital signs and information to safeguard the safety of the patient	– Record temperature, pulse, respiration and blood pressure on admission and immediately pre-operatively – Record weight – Routine urinalysis – Check for allergies – Remove make-up and nail varnish

Potential loss or damage to property and personal injury from property	Be aware of all prostheses and appendages and remove prior to surgery	– Check for glasses
		     contact lenses
		     hearing-aid
		     metal objects (e.g. jewellery,* hairgrips)
		     wigs
		     false teeth
		     any other

Ensure that the patient is aware of what is to happen and that he undergoes the correct operation	The patient gives informed consent and his anxiety is minimised	– Check consent (page 747) – Check surgical area is marked (where necessary) – Two name bands – Explain all procedures (page 747) – Premedication

* Patients may be allowed to wear a wedding band if this is covered with adhesive
N.B. Figures in brackets refer to subsequent pages where a fuller explanation is given

anxiety experienced by some, when something they normally associate, not only with nourishment but also pleasure and comfort, is withheld. It may also reduce those potential problems associated with an increased metabolic rate being met from the body's own resources, for example infection due to poor tissue regeneration (Hamilton-Smith, 1972).

There is increasing evidence of malnutrition in post-operative patients with some suggesting that the figure is as high as 50% (Holmes, 1991; Baughen, 1989). Assessment pre- and post-operatively would not only seem necessary to judge individual need for the withholding of food and fluids but also to identify those patients for whom supplement before and/or after surgery may prevent the complications associated with mal-nourishment.

Although using a small sample, Shireff (1990) shows the most effective measuring tool to be serum albumin which can be easily recorded along with other pre- and post-operative blood levels. It would seem an inexpensive method of assessment and relatively inexpensive to correct a shortfall. Many hours are spent both in hospital and in the community caring for poorly healed wounds. The above would suggest that more attention needs to be paid to prevention rather than using resources to cure.

Consent for operation

The practice of obtaining consent for surgical procedures is firmly in the medical field. Department of Health guidelines lay clear responsibility for obtaining consent, both verbal and written, on the doctor (DoH, 1989).

In reality patients will often turn to nursing staff to allay their fears and check their understanding of the situation. In reviewing the guidelines, John Tingle, a barrister, points out that, 'Nurses who do the doctor's job regarding patient consent should be aware they are entering a very grey legal area' (Tingle, 1990). In accepting that 'Nurses are in a privileged position, if they are willing to recognise and accept advocacy opportunities' (Copp, 1986), the nurse must have a sound knowledge base and be sure of her responsibilities in using it. If unsure of the details, she may have to use her professional judgement by returning to the doctor to ask him to explain the details to the patient again.

'Informed consent is sometimes confused with written consent. Written consent is merely a record that a conversation took place, but is not legally binding. The quality of the conversation and the result of it will, however, be regarded as legally important' (Tschudin, 1989). If this statement is accepted, and Tschudin's premise that 'every treatment' requires informed consent, then the nurse preparing patients for surgery needs to be increasingly aware of her role. For more information on this complex subject see Chapter 13 and the suggestions for further reading at the end of this chapter.

Explanation of procedures

The most important aspect of pre-operative care

> Mrs Janes is 42, a divorcee with two children aged nine and 12. She is admitted routinely for a **partial thyroidectomy** for **thyrotoxicosis** which has not been controlled by medication. She is tense and slightly nervous and has a **tachycardia** of 100. She has good insight into her medical condition and understands the effect it is having on her physically. Her children are being cared for at home by their grandmother and Mrs Janes has three weeks sick leave from her job. She is assessed and her care plan (Fig. 24.9) formulated with explanations for the pre-operative procedure.

Fig. 24.8 *Patient profile: Mrs Janes*

frequently goes undocumented; that is, the communication that occurs as a result of the relationship between nurse and patient. The effects of anxiety from lack of knowledge highlight the need for this communication to occur in order to promote the recovery of the patient (Hayward, 1975). Communication means teaching, showing sympathy and empathy, and above all inducing confidence in the patient. The profile in Fig. 24.8 gives an example of procedural pre-operative care being minimal (see also Fig. 24.9) but the following dialogue – which is not documented – will play a large part in recovery.

Staff nurse:
Now Mrs Janes, I've explained the routine care to you. Is there anything else you would like to know?

Mrs Janes:
Yes . . . what will it be like when I come back after the operation? I've noticed the other patients are lying flat. I get a throbbing headache if I lie flat since having this thyroid trouble.

Staff nurse:
You, in fact, will be sitting upright when you come back – to help you breathe more easily. Your neck may feel very stiff as your head is extended on the operating table, stretching your muscles. (Staff nurse demonstrates to the patient). I'm afraid, too, that you won't get much rest for the first few hours as the nurse will be taking your pulse and blood pressure every quarter of an hour.

Mrs Janes:
Why is that?

Staff nurse:
You may know that your thyroid gland has a good

Fig. 24.9 Care plan for Mrs Janes

Date	Identified needs/problems	Objectives/ goals	Nursing intervention	Evaluation
22.1.92	Maintenance of safety			
	For surgery 10 am 23.1.92	Complete pre-operative schedule	See standard pre-operative procedures	
	Sleeping	Create time and environment to allow maximum rest pre-operatively	Nurse in a side room. Give patient 'do not disturb' sign which she may put on door when resting	
	Tense, does not sleep well but takes short rests during day			

NAME: Alice Janes   **Date of Birth**: 1.5.49   **Signed**: B.Hart

blood supply. In a very small proportion of people, heavy bleeding can follow surgery. We can tell from your pulse and blood pressure whether you are bleeding. If you are one of those rare cases, we remove your stitches or clips to free the clot so that you don't experience any difficulties with breathing. When you come back from the theatre you will have a small drain in the wound to remove any normal amounts of blood and you will notice that we have placed stitch-cutters or clip-removers beside your bed.

Mrs Janes:
You say clips or stitches. Which will it be?

Staff nurse:
That depends on the surgeon – it could be either. They are not in for long, though. We usually take them out three days after the operation.

Mrs Janes:
And the drain?

Staff nurse:
Oh, that comes out 24 hours after the operation as long as everything goes to plan. Now, is there anything else you would like to ask?

Mrs Janes:
No, thank you.

Staff nurse:
There is one more thing I would like to say. After

this operation, many patients worry that movement of their head or neck may cause damage to their wound. This fear is quite understandable, but you cannot damage the area. In fact if you can start to move your head gently as soon as you come back to the ward it will ease the stiffness and help the wound to heal.

If you think of anything else you want to know please just ask me or one of the other nurses.

As this text concentrates on patients undergoing general anaesthesia, the standard pre-operative care plan is designed to meet their needs where their lack of knowledge prevents them from identifying the potential hazards to their activities of living (Roper *et al.*, (1990).

Many patient problems will come to light during assessment or in the process of the delivery of care. However some patients may be at greater risk of developing the potential problems highlighted in the standard pre-operative procedure (Table 24.4) and therefore require more specific care as in Mrs Archer's case (Figs. 24.2 and 24.3) and the example of Mr Allan (Figs. 24.10 and 24.11).

Mr Allan has a greater potential risk of post-operative chest infection because of his personal habits. These also increase the risk of him developing a **subphrenic abscess** if he is unable to breathe deeply and use his diaphragm effectively. Following removal of the gall bladder there is a potential problem of basal consolidation and formation of an abscess in the space left by the organ, particularly if a pool of fluid collects there. This is

Mr Allan, who is 58 years old, has been admitted routinely for a **cholecystectomy** and exploration of the common bile duct to remove gall stones. He is overweight, although he has lost half a stone since being on a low-fat diet, and he smokes 15–20 cigarettes a day. He has a productive cough early in the morning. He has failed to cut down on his smoking despite being warned in the outpatient clinic about his potential problems. On examination by the anaesthetist his operation is deferred for two days and the physiotherapist is asked to give some intensive chest physiotherapy. His pre-operative care plan (Fig. 24.11) reflects his specific problems.

Fig. 24.10 *Patient profile: Mr Allan*

exacerbated by shallow respirations due to pain. To assist with the drainage of this space and encourage lung expansion, the patient is given adequate analgesia and asked to breathe deeply so that the diaphragm pushes down onto the space and any exudate that has collected is expelled through the drain. This is an instance where it is necessary for the patient to formulate his own plan (Fig. 24.11) so that he can understand and accept his care and set himself realistic goals. Figure 24.12 could be used by the nurse to explain the relationships between the various organs to the patient. It may also help learners.

Fig. 24.11 *Care plan for Mr Allan*

Date	Identified needs/problems	Objectives/ goals	Nursing intervention	Evaluation
24.1.92	Breathing			
	Maintenance of safety			
	Surgery deferred until 27.1.92 because Mr Allan is smoking 15–20 cigarettes daily	Reduce smoking to three cigarettes a day	Keep patient's cigarettes (at his request) Give one after each meal	
	Early morning sputum is green/grey colour	Sputum should be clear	Continue deep breathing exercises two hourly – started by physiotherapist	26.1
	Potential post-operative subphrenic abscess and basal consolidation	Minimise risk of post-operative chest infection and sub-phrenic abscess	Give inhalation of tincture of benzoin to assist expectoration (a) early morning (b) before bed	
			Complete standard pre-operative care procedure	
	Eating and drinking			
	Pain when eating fatty foods	Maintain diet as eaten at home	Order 40 g low fat diet	

NAME: Kenneth Allan   **Date of Birth**: 5.12.33   Signed: B. Hart

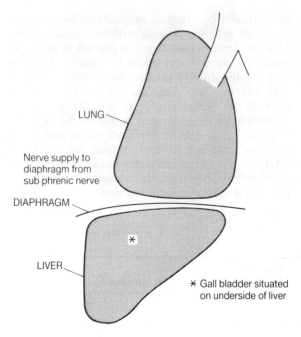

Fig. 24.12 *Diagrammatic representation of the anatomical relationship between the gall bladder and the diaphragm*

All the care described in this section is directed towards ensuring the patient has a smooth post-operative recovery. The basic care necessary for all patients will vary very little but the care specific to certain operations will show local variations. However, the underlying preventive principles remain the same.

Post-operative care

It has been seen that patients arrive on the ward in a variety of physical conditions, and that their psychosocial and spiritual needs also help to determine their total needs in hospital.

Methods of relieving pain during surgery include local anaesthesia, acupuncture and hypnotherapy. The majority of operations are carried out under general anaesthesia, however, and it is with the patients undergoing this procedure that this chapter is primarily concerned.

During surgery under general anaesthesia all patients are rendered unconscious and in some cases paralysed. While they are in this state, the basic physiological and safety needs vital to life become the responsibility of the professional team around the patient. This places him at the lowest point on Maslow's hierarchy (see Fig. 24.1). On the premise that lower needs must be satisfied (at least in part) before higher needs can be expressed, the aim of post-operative care is to assist the patient, by means of intervention, education and support, through the hierarchy of needs, helping him to reach his goals.

Roper's model of care is used to assess needs and plan care. The care plans in this section aim to reflect one particular aspect of care. They do not therefore show the full range of care planned, as they would do in the clinical area. Where a different approach to planning care may be needed, the text and care plan will show this.

In the first 24 hours post-operatively, some patients will require certain elements of care that are common to all. These are primarily concerned with physiological stability and therefore the physical and mental well-being of the patient, with the patient's safety, with his comfort, and with the prevention of complications.

At this point, nursing intervention is total and the patient is fully reliant upon the nurse's skill and knowledge. Some patients may be up and home within 24 hours after 'minor' surgery (vasectomy, for example) while those patients who have undergone major surgery will still require total support after 24 hours. The variation in these needs is governed by factors such as the length and severity of the operation, the individual's response to surgery and anaesthesia, and by the patient's physical condition before the operation.

Evaluation and re-assessment are carried out constantly at this stage and the nurse may need to react quickly to a life-threatening situation. Once physical stability is achieved, the patient may begin to express the next level of needs and require help from nursing staff to meet them.

Specific post-operative problems

This section looks at activities of living as defined by Roper (Roper *et al.*, 1990), the needs common to all patients in that activity and some specific needs and problems related to individual operations. This is by no means a definitive approach to nursing patients who have had surgery but the underlying principles apply whatever nursing model is used.

Breathing and circulation

The majority of patients returning to surgical wards come direct from the theatre recovery unit where their vital signs have been monitored and where they have been judged stable enough to return to the ward. Their normal breathing pattern should be re-established and they should have an effective swallowing reflex. The main potential risk is that of inhalation of vomitus. This can cause a severe inflammatory reaction in the lung lining (*Mendelsohn's syndrome*) on account of the acid gastric juice. Patients who are too weak or drowsy to expel their own vomitus should be laid in the recovery position and suction applied to the naso-oropharynx if vomiting occurs.

Hypoxia occurs when the patient's arterial oxygen tension is lowered. This may be a result either of haemorrhage or of poor ventilation (i.e. defective exchange of gases). The latter is usually caused by an underlying pathophysiological condition such as chronic bronchitis. Observations should include monitoring of the patient's colour for signs of peripheral cyanosis at nail beds and in the mucous membranes, monitoring his skin texture which may be cold and clammy, and being alert for signs of restlessness and/or confusion. Deep breathing is encouraged to expel any remaining anaesthetic agents, to prevent consolidation and possible subsequent infection of lung secretions, and in specific cases to assist in the drainage of the operative site (see Fig. 24.11). Patients, particularly those who have had abdominal surgery, are much better able to cooperate in this exercise if they are given adequate and regular analgesia.

The sudden onset of **dyspnoea**, usually a few days after surgery and accompanied by pain in the chest, is most commonly associated with a pulmonary embolism and is regarded as a medical emergency.

Finally there are specific cases where occlusion of the airway or disruption of the swallowing reflex may be a direct result of surgery (see Fig. 24.13).

As stated above, haemorrhage can be a causative factor for hypoxia. Oxygen is carried on the haemoglobin molecule and blood tests are usually conducted prior to surgery to ensure the patient has a good haemoglobin level. Any blood loss during and following surgery that may compromise the patient's safety is replaced by transfusion.

There are three type of haemorrhage.

(1) *Primary haemorrhage*
This occurs at the time of surgery and haemostasis is achieved with **diathermy** to small bleeding points and by the use of **ligatures** to larger vessels. The normal haemostatic process occurs at the capillary bed (see Chapter 5).

(2) *Reactionary haemorrhage*
This occurs within the first 24 hours after surgery, and may be venous or arterial. Bleeding occurs either at an unsealed vessel or where a ligature slips. In both cases, reactionary haemorrhage is associated with a rise in blood pressure during recovery from anaesthesia.

(3) *Secondary haemorrhage*
This type of haemorrhage occurs approximately ten days after surgery. It is usually associated with a wound infection (either deep or superficial). The breakdown of sutures deep within a wound (for example, in the bowel or kidney) may involve an artery and can cause a rapid and profuse haemorrhage leading to sudden collapse.

Primary haemorrhage is controlled bleeding. Any secondary haemorrhage that occurs is usually sudden. Depending on the size of the vessel involved, it can cause anything from small blood loss to exsanguination.

Patients should be monitored for reactionary bleeding during the first 24 hours. The frequency of observations and their duration will vary according to local policy but will include:

Pulse and blood pressure

Any gradual loss of circulating volume will cause increased peripheral resistance and increased cardiac output, initiated by the vasomotor centre in the medulla, via baroreceptors in the aorta and carotid bodies (see Chapter 5). The vasoconstriction attempts to maintain the blood pressure and the increased heart rate maintains oxygen requirements. As more blood is lost, the body can no longer compensate and the blood pressure begins to fall. In the fit, young patient this latter stage may take some time to occur.

Fig. 24.13 Post-operative care plan for Mrs Janes

Date	Identified needs/problems	Objectives/goals	Nursing intervention	Review	Evaluation
22.1.92	Breathing				
	Potential risk of respiratory distress due to:	– Position to minimise pooling of blood	Sit up in bed with pillows supporting head and neck		
	(1) Occlusion of the airway if haemorrhage occurs	– Detection of excessive bleeding	Record pulse and blood pressure quarter-hourly; check drainage hourly	16.00	Pulse and blood pressure stable–now hourly recordings
	(2) Laryngeal nerve damage	– Relief of pressure if haemorrhage occurs	Have stitch cutters on locker – remove stitches in the event of respiratory distress		
		– Minimise risks of inhalation of fluid	Nil by mouth for 4 hours post-operatively	16.00	Has swallow reflex Is thirsty
			15 ml sterile water hourly for 4 hours	20.00	Well tolerated
			30 ml sterile water hourly for 4 hours	24.00	Is taking fluid with no problems – can commence free fluids

NAME: Alice Janes   **Date of Birth**: 1.5.49   **Signed**: *B. Harb*

Colour and skin temperature

The peripheral vasoconstriction causes the patient's skin to become pale and lose its warmth. He may feel clammy and sweating may result from sympathetic nervous activity. If bleeding remains uncontrolled the patient may start to shiver and signs of oxygen lack will appear.

The wound

The wound should be checked for obvious signs of bleeding but it is not usually left uncovered. Dark red oozing is a sign of venous bleeding; arterial loss is bright red and if the bleeding point is visible, blood can be seen pumping forth. Any wound drainage methods used will allow blood loss to escape and suction drainage apparatus should be checked for excessive loss at the same time as the wound.

Internal haemorrhage

This is more difficult to diagnose and may result in large blood loss before it is detected. Apart from the above observations, signs of internal bleeding may present themselves by some change in the function of the surrounding associated organs – for example, bleeding into the chest wall will result in increasing dyspnoea.

The signs and symptoms of haemorrhage are listed in Table 24.5. It should be remembered, however, that not all of these signs and symptoms will be apparent in every patient who has a haemorrhage, and conversely many of them are exhibited by patients in pain or in neurogenic shock.

Table 24.5. *Signs and symptoms of haemorrhage*

- Rising pulse
- Falling blood pressure
- Cold, damp skin
- Restlessness
- Confusion
- Excessive wound drainage
- Specific signs resulting from internal bleeding

Maintaining body temperature

Four-hourly monitoring of body temperature during the first 24 hours after surgery allows the nurse to assist in maintaining body temperature until the patient's temperature control mechanism returns. As well as the temporary loss of this mechanism, patients lose a considerable amount of body heat through exposure during surgery, exposure of the internal organs and the infusion of cold fluids intravenously. It is frequently the practice to fold patients' bedclothes in packs and on return from theatre the patient is put back into a cold bed. It is advisable to record the patient's temperature before removing the theatre blankets and, if necessary, to leave them under the pack until the patient feels warmer. Where patients are taken to and brought back from theatre in their own beds this problem is reduced.

A core temperature below 35°C requires the patient to have extra insulation.

Any rise in temperature during the first three days is usually a normal response to the inflammation that results from surgery. Any continued fluctuation above the patient's normal temperature may be an early sign of infection. After the first 24 hours, the frequency of temperature recording varies according to local policy.

Eating, drinking and elimination

The activities of eating, drinking and elimination affect the patient's fluid balance and nutritional status as well as his basic comfort.

Fluid balance

Fluid balance and the body's maintenance of it is influenced by the sensation of thirst and affected both mechanically and hormonally.

Fluid balance is affected mechanically by the oral intake of liquid, absorption from the gut and excretion of any excess via the kidneys, the respiratory tract and the skin.

It is affected hormonally by the secretion of anti-diuretic hormone (ADH) and to some extent by aldosterone secretion which affects circulating levels of sodium ions (see Chapter 5).

The average adult requires a daily intake of about two litres of water. He passes 1.5 litres of urine and he loses approximately 500 ml through the skin in 24 hours. The ability of the patient to meet his fluid needs is affected before, during and after surgery, by factors both common and specific which fall into two main categories: the inability to take in and/or absorb fluid, and the inability to produce and/or eliminate urine.

(1)   The inability to take in and/or absorb fluid can result from fasting, from an impaired swallowing reflex or from a paralytic ileus.

Fasting is implemented pre-operatively to minimise risk of post-operative inhalation of vomitus, and post-operatively when surgery has been performed on part of the gastro-intestinal tract. This allows healing at the site of any **anastomosis**. Fasting increases the secretion of ADH which results in a decreased urine output.

An impaired swallowing reflex may occur as a result of surgery. Swallowing is a muscular activity controlled by the laryngeal nerve which is paralysed during surgery when intubation is necessary. On return to the ward the reflex is usually fully recovered but should be checked before the patient is given a drink. Certain operations have the potential to damage or impair the function of the laryngeal nerve and the nursing care should reflect the possibility of this risk. For example, Mrs Janes who was admitted for partial thyroidectomy may have this problem as the care plan drawn up for her (Fig. 24.13) indicates.

Paralytic ileus is a temporary cessation of intestinal **peristalsis**. It occurs in reaction to direct handling of the bowel or indirect contact while gaining access to other organs during surgery. It does not occur in all patients undergoing abdominal surgery and when it does it can resolve itself in a few hours or may take a number of days. Flatus and bowel sounds are indications of the return of peristalsis. A paralytic ileus prevents the absorption of fluid, and gastric contents need to be removed artificially by nasogastric aspiration if the situation does not resolve itself within a few hours.

(2)   Inability to produce and/or eliminate urine can result from a number of causes. The first of these is excessive fluid loss, which can occur with haemorrhage, profuse sweating, **tachypnoea** due to infection, excessive vomiting or profuse diarrhoea. **Oliguria** will result in all these cases.

Another cause is loss of renal function, which may result from actual damage to the renal tract during surgery or poor renal perfusion, usually as a result of haemorrhage. The kidney requires a systolic blood pressure of 70 mmHg to produce urine.

The processes of surgery and anaesthesia themselves can affect the patient's ability to produce and eliminate urine. In specific types of surgery there may be problems with micturition (usually due to an obstruction such as a blood clot following prostatectomy). Atonic bladder is a complication that may arise when paralysis during anaesthesia results in a temporary loss of bladder muscle tone. This usually resolves spontaneously but the patient may require temporary assistance with catheterisation and/or medication.

An increase in the body's requirements can also affect production and elimination of urine. The healing process requires an increased fluid intake and if this is not forthcoming the body will draw from its interstitial and cellular reserves. This results not only in a decreased urine output but also in potential problems in the areas from where the fluid is drawn.

Knowledge of the particular surgery undertaken enables the nurse to assess when the patient is able to recommence fluids. Those unable to take oral fluids will be hydrated by means of intravenous infusion. The volume and type of infusion, as well as any possible additives, are prescribed by the doctor, but this prescription may be based on the nurse's observation and recording of output, urine concentration, skin condition, etc. The nurse's further responsibility lies in maintaining and managing the infusion, and in observing for potential complications.

Nutritional requirements

The average adult requires 1200 to 1500 kilocalories (4800 to 6000 kilojoules) a day to meet the basic metabolic functions necessary for living, and to maintain his activity. When injured, the body has increased requirements for nutrients to meet the needs of the healing process: protein to lay down new tissue and carbohydrate to meet increased metabolic needs. Patients undergoing surgery may be fasted for a few hours or for a number of days and their requirements during this period are met from their body store. Initially the store of glycogen in the liver is used and then, after about 24 hours, adipose tissue (i.e. fat stores) is drawn upon. Patients with minimal fat stores will then metabolise body protein to meet their needs.

The return to normal eating and drinking habits will be directed by the patient's physical condition and his ability to absorb what is taken in. To allow the gastro-intestinal tract time to adjust after surgery, the patient should be given a dietary regime which will gradually lead back to full diet and

Table 24.6. *Summary of Mrs Archer's diet and fluid programme*

Post-operative day and relevant data	Food	Fluid	Evaluation and assessment
3rd Bowel sounds	–	15 ml water hourly for 2 hours	Well tolerated
Flatus from colostomy		30 ml water hourly for 4 hours 60 ml water hourly for 4 hours	3200 ml intake with IVI
		Free clear fluid	Discontinue IVI
4th IVI discontinued	Lunch: Soup and ice cream	3 litres in 24 hours	Intake 2800 ml in 24 hours
Remove catheter	Supper: Soup and semolina		Micturition reinstated SG 1010 Colostomy – faecal fluid
5th Colostomy – very loose stools	Soft light diet and bran in soup	3 litres in 24 hours	Intake 1900 ml Output 900 ml SG 1015
	Weetabix for breakfast		Pain on micturition MSU taken
6th Possible urinary tract infection	Soft diet, brown bread and extra bran	3.5 litres in 24 hours	Intake 3000 ml Output 1200 ml SG 1010 Pain on micturition
Colostomy – liquid faeces	Note any food that makes flatus	Restrict intake of fruit juices No Lucozade	Colostomy – acted x4 soft formed stools
	Restrict milk to 250 ml in 24 hours		
7th Urinary tract infection confirmed Prescribed septrin tabs 2. b.d	Normal diet plus extra fibre and protein e.g. egg milk Try fresh fruit	4 litres in 24 hours	Input 4000 ml Output 2500 ml SG 1005 Colostomy – acted x4 soft formed stool
8th Colostomy acting – soft formed stool	Normal diet Try fresh orange	4 litres in 24 hours	Input 4000 ml Output 2500 ml Colostomy – runny stools x 5
9th Colostomy – loose stools	Normal diet plus extra fibre	4 litres in 24 hours	Urine clear SG 1000 Colostomy – soft formed stools x 3
	Avoid fresh fruit Try again in a few days		Patient changed flange and bag with supervision

10th No further monitoring or intervention required as the patient is meeting these needs herself

normal intake of fluid. For a summary of this progress in one patient see Table 24.6.

It should also be remembered that psychosocial problems, as well as a poor physical state, may prevent the patient from taking in the requirements necessary for recovery. Some 48 hours after Mrs Brown's surgery, an interview with her son enables the nurse to add the following information to her history. Mrs Brown's husband died 18 months ago, since when she has been generally anorexic. She very rarely cooks for herself and, as her son eats a meal at work, she does not have to cook for him. She lives on sandwiches, toasted snacks, biscuits and crackers and drinks vast quantities of sugared tea. Apart from the tea she has no milk intake. She eats little meat and no eggs. She also takes three to five senna tablets every night before going to bed.

Mrs Brown is physiologically stable 48 hours after surgery, but her general physical well-being is in jeopardy. Her needs for nourishment and fluids have not been met over a period of time and this has created many problems, both actual and po-

tential, for her other activities of living (see Fig. 24.14.).

A summary of factors which may affect the activity of eating post-operatively is given in Table 24.7.

Finally it would be rare to find a patient whose normal eating habits coincided exactly with both hospital routine and diet, and furthermore who normally eats all his meals dressed in pyjamas and in the company of other people at various stages of ill health. The individual nurse has little control

Table 24.7. *Factors affecting the patient's ability to eat post-operatively*

(1) Fasting
(2) Paralytic ileus
(3) Specific dietary needs (e.g. high fibre diet following haemorrhoidectomy)
(4) Permanent physical changes to gastro-intestinal tract (e.g. stomas, partial gastrectomy)
(5) Psychosocial problems

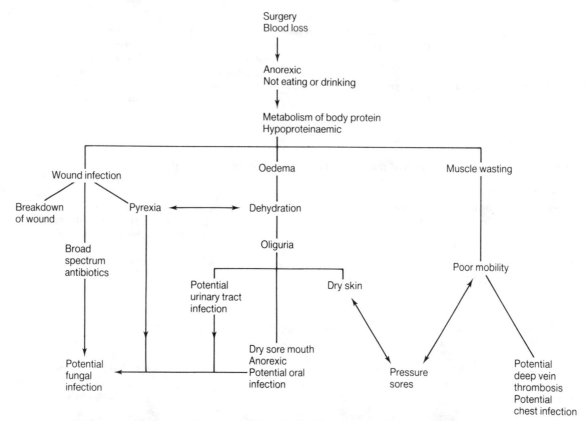

Fig. 24.14 *Actual and potential problems identified 48 hours post-operatively for Mrs Brown*

over these factors but an awareness of them should help in assessing patients who present with problems.

Elimination

Patients normally pass urine within 24 hours after surgery, depending on a variety of factors mentioned above. They may require assistance to meet this need if they are in pain or are in the wrong position – for example, many men find it difficult to micturate lying down. A temporary disruption to normal function may arise from the particular surgery that has been performed – for example, dribbling incontinence may follow prostatectomy.

Resumption of bowel function occurs over a much wider time scale and invariably involves a temporary change of habit due to a reduced amount of privacy, the period of fasting, change of diet and specific disruption caused by surgery – for example, diarrhoea following colonic surgery.

There is also the small group of patients (like Mrs Archer in the profile given in Fig. 24.2) who undergo a permanent change following surgery. The nurses have cared for Mrs Archer's colostomy over the first nine days, gradually letting her do more. The nurse responsible for her care knows that the colostomy is functioning normally and producing formed stools. She re-assesses Mrs Archer's needs on the tenth day and finds that although the patient accepts the physiological function of the colostomy and is pleased that it is not as bad cosmetically as she had expected, she still has worries about how she will cope socially. After discussion with the patient, the nurse decides to change the model of care to the self-care model (Orem, 1990). With guidance and support, Mrs Archer will now be able to start the process that will eliminate her self-care deficit.

Figure 24.15 shows part of the care plan drawn up for Mrs Archer from the tenth day postoperatively. The problem areas are highlighted by the patient. A further section of this care plan can be seen in Fig. 24.20 on page 764, illustrating that despite success within the hospital environment she was still identifying needs that she felt unable to meet only two days before discharge.

Other problems with elimination may arise from anxiety or lack of privacy. The immediate postoperative period can be depersonalising. The patient is usually still in a hospital gown. His immediate surroundings are unfamiliar. He feels pain, and he is bombarded by nurses administering care which may necessitate exposure. He is allowed no physical comfort from food or fluid and contact with those closest to him is restricted. It is therefore little wonder if he feels anxious enough for his ability to eliminate urine and faeces to be affected.

Finally, education forms an increasingly important part of the nurse's role. She may help the patient to meet his own elimination needs in a more healthy way, thus avoiding many of the problems that he may have experienced in the past.

Maintenance of a safe environment

In order to maintain a safe environment, an individual needs a certain amount of knowledge about where and what the hazards may be. Much postoperative nursing intervention, like pre-operative care, is carried out as a direct result of the nurse's knowledge of actual and potential hazards to the patient. With her skills, and with the help of equipment and drugs, she can help maintain his physical safety. This physical safety will in turn give him mental security.

This section looks at some of the hazards that may be encountered, and at how they may affect other activities of living.

Physiological instability

This has been looked at in depth in the content of this chapter.

Pain and vomiting

Uncontrolled pain may lead to the patient harming himself physically through restlessness, shallow breathing and inability to concentrate on and co-operate with nursing instructions.

Pain is also mentally debilitating and in extreme cases may produce abnormal psychological behaviour.

In assessing the needs for pain control, the nurse should consider not only the effectiveness of any analgesia used but all those factors that either exacerbate or temper pain (see Chapter 15).

Persistent, copious vomiting can have a detrimental effect on oral hygiene and cause erosion of tooth enamel.

Increasingly, non-pharmacological methods of

Fig. 24.15 Care plan (2) for Mrs Archer: self-care model

Date	Self-care deficit	Objectives/goals	Nursing intervention	Type of nursing action	Evaluation
25.1	Feels that she will look 'odd' in public	To discover what is comfortable to wear	(1) Move to a side room to promote privacy	Providing suitable environment	
	Feels that appliance will be noticed when she wears clothes	To mix with general public before discharge	(2) Give a copy of colostomy handbook (section on clothing)	Teaching	27/1 Is dressed in the afternoon. Had an accident with the bag whilst at shop. Very distressed
			(3) Plan any formal nursing care in morning – allowing the afternoons free to go to shop, grounds, WRVS canteen	Support	29/1 Much more confident. Feels in retrospect that the accident was not as bad as she thought. Was asked directions by a hospital visitor today – very pleased
	Is worried about smell	Choose an effective deodorising method for colostomy	(4) Provide with all the alternatives and discuss daily how she is getting on	Guidance and support	29/1 Having read colostomy book has kept a diary of what she has eaten.
			(5) Show section in colostomy handbook	Teaching	Notes root vegetables increase flatus. Has chosen a liquid deodorant for her bag

NAME: Dorothy Archer   **Date of Birth:** 7.4.28   **Signed:** *J. Smith*

controlling pain are being introduced. Research has indicated that a combination of both pharmacological and non-pharmacological pain control often gets the best results (McCaffrey, 1990). Non-pharmacological methods, such as distraction with humour, music and relaxation and cutaneous stimulation with hot and cold, can have beneficial effects. Whilst they are not all appropriate to post-operative surgical patients, the nurse with a knowledge of both can bring greater relief to her patient.

Complications

The risks of chest infections and deep vein thrombosis are highlighted on the standard pre-operative procedure (see Table 24.4). The biggest potential hazard is that of breakdown of the wound, usually due to infection. When predisposing factors are considered (see Fig. 24.4), not all patients can avoid a post-operative wound infection. However, 5.7% of all hospital acquired infections are wound infections (Lascelles, 1982). The sources of those infections are the environment, hospital personnel, the patients themselves and other patients. Prevention of wound infection can be discussed under two headings: hygiene and local wound care.

(1) *Hygiene* includes the standards both of the environment and personnel. It includes the responsibility of personnel in identifying themselves as potential sources of infection – if they have a sore throat or diarrhoea for example. For more details, see the references and suggestions for further reading lists at the end of this chapter; also Chapter 16.

(2) *Wound healing* by primary intention involves the skin layer being closed either with sutures or with clips (see Figs. 24.16 and 24.17). It is important to know what sort of sutures have been used in order to effect their safe removal. When removing them, care should be taken to ensure that no part of the suture material above the skin passes through the skin. The choice of sutures or clips is that of the surgeon. Clips are usually used in areas subject to little muscular tension, for example in the neck following thyroidectomy.

Some wounds will also have a drain *in situ* to remove exudate and stale blood from the bed of the wound. The drain may consist of a piece of rubber or plastic material that forms a tract along

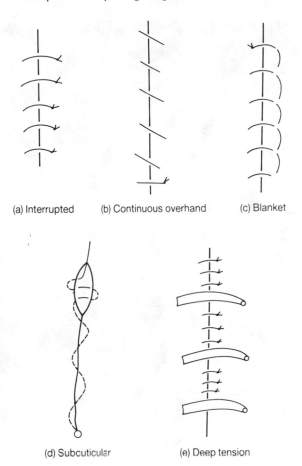

(a) Interrupted (b) Continuous overhand (c) Blanket

(d) Subcuticular (e) Deep tension

Fig. 24.16 *Methods of skin suturing*

which the exudate can run to be soaked up by the dressing. Ragnall or corrugated drains are examples of this type. Alternatively, a closed system which allows gentle suction to be applied may be used – the Redivac drain is an example. There are also specific occasions when a drainage tube will be inserted to assist temporarily in the anatomical function of the area, allowing drainage of normal body fluids from that area. The insertion of a T-tube following exploration of the common bile duct is an example of this.

Wounds are usually covered with a dressing. Those without drainage or with a Redivac drain have a waterproof dressing whilst those with open drainage require a padded sterile dressing which allows the passage of air but not of micro-organisms. Once the outer layer is breached by moisture the effective barrier is lost and the wound will require redressing.

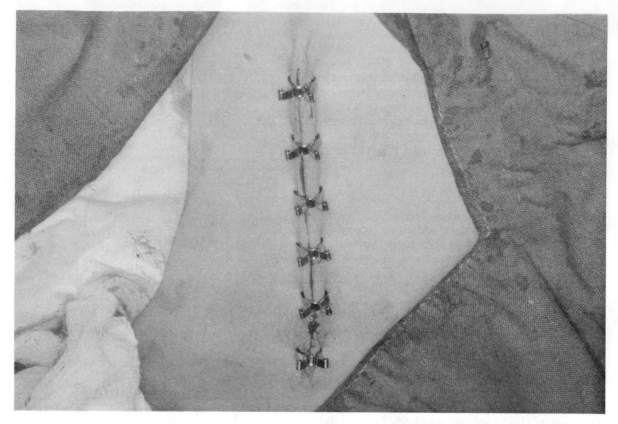

Fig. 24.17 Skin closure with clips

When a wound is covered with a waterproof dressing, the longer the dressing is left intact the faster the wound will heal. Redivac drains should be checked for patency (i.e. the existence of an effective vacuum) and their contents should be examined for signs of underlying infection. All wound drains are usually removed within 48 hours.

The signs and symptoms of a wound infection are: an increase in wound pain after a period of improvement, swelling and redness visible around the dressing, and a swinging pyrexia. Under these circumstances the wound should be examined for purulent discharge and signs of breakdown.

The wounds of patients with rubber or plastic drains may require daily dressing. Such drains are often inserted into a designated 'dirty' area (for example, the perineum following abdominoperineal resection of the rectum). All dressings, including removal of drains, clips and sutures, are conducted using techniques that maintain asepsis. (See also the suggestions for further reading at the end of this chapter.)

Wounds that break down through infection are cleaned and then may be resutured using deep tension sutures (Fig. 24.16). These are also used when dehisence of an abdominal wound (burst abdomen) occurs.

Dehisence of an abdominal wound is a medical emergency. It is often associated with obesity. A total breakdown of all layers of the wound occurs, exposing the bowel. First aid measures by nursing staff should be the aseptic application of gauze soaked in warm, isotonic, sterile saline. Immediate medical aid should be sought.

Wound healing by secondary intention and the appropriate management of these wounds has received much attention in the last ten years. Whilst not able to address this in detail, the following information may give the reader some insight.

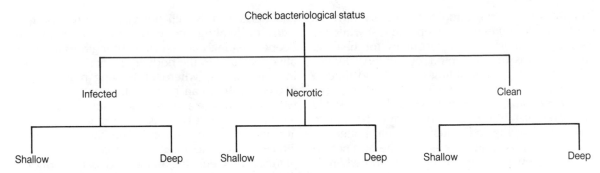

Fig. 24.18 *A method of wound assessment (adapted from Johnson, 1988)*

There are also a number of recommended articles suggested for further reading at the end of this chapter.

Wounds healing by secondary intention are open wounds. Healing occurs by granulation from the bottom upwards. Care of these wounds is aimed at reducing and removing infection and not allowing ridges of granulation tissue to form, creating potential spaces for abscess formation. With the wealth of preparations offered to treat wounds, it is essential that wounds are assessed and appropriate treatment used. One method of assessment is described by Johnson (1988) (see Fig. 24.18). Treatment is then chosen, which can vary from the simple laying on of saline-soaked gauze to the use of a proprietary agent. Bale and Harding (1991) divide these into four main categories:

(1) Foam dressings
(2) Hydrocolloids
(3) Hydrogels
(4) Alginates.

Further information on these can be found at the end of the chapter and full details of use and effect are supplied by the individual manufacturers. Local policy will determine which types of dressings are used, but nurses must avail themselves of the knowledge regarding wound care and play a full part in the management of such wounds.

As with closed wounds, exposure to the air should be kept to the minimum. The use of antiseptic cleaning agents is generally considered inappropriate and wounds should be cleaned with normal saline. 'The ideal wound dressing should "remove excess wound exudate, maintain high humidity on the wound/dressing interface, allow gaseous exchange, provide thermal insulation, be impermeable to micro-organisms, be free from contaminants and allow removal from the wound without causing trauma"' (Spenser and Bale, 1990, quoting Johnson, 1988).

It is essential that the treatment chosen and used is fully documented on the patient's care plan and not changed without full evaluation. Many districts now employ wound management specialists and these can be consulted.

With his needs for physical safety met, the patient may express the need to achieve goals in the higher levels of Maslow's theoretical hierarchy. Some patients will have no problems meeting these needs with a minimal amount of support from their relatives and friends and the nursing staff. Other patients may need to be re-assured that much of what they are experiencing is completely normal following surgery.

To re-establish self-esteem the patient must be able to like himself, to accept himself, and to be confident that others feel the same way.

In the following activities of living, problems can arise which may stop the patient meeting higher level needs. Nursing intervention is aimed at *education*, at giving the patient some idea of when he can expect a return to his normal way of life. It is aimed at *supporting* the patient through a period of temporary inability to meet his own needs and at *assisting* the patient to adapt to any permanent changes created by the surgery.

Sleep, rest and mobility

All these activities, sleep, rest and mobility, are affected to a greater or lesser degree by surgery. It may be a temporary disruption of the activity, a total cessation for a period, or a permanent change.

Patients who have undergone surgery have an increased requirement for sleep and rest while the body is using its energy resources for healing. Sleep patterns are disrupted by surgery. Drugs, anaesthesia, the withholding of food and fluid, a change of environment, and anxiety all disrupt *circadian rhythms*, and rest is virtually impossible during the first 24 hours. Nursing care should aim to re-establish the individual's normal pattern of sleep and rest as soon as possible. The best person to decide how much rest is needed, and when, is the patient. This may necessitate the nurse re-organising her plan of care.

Factors that may inhibit sleep and rest over which the nurse has *some* (discretionary) control include noise, overstimulation, post-operative 'blues' and physical discomfort.

(1) *Noise* is one of the most stressful occurrences for an inpatient. Nurses are often the biggest perpetrators of noise.

(2) *Overstimulation* can cause anxiety. Although initially beneficial, visitors can be too many and stay too long. Likewise, repeated interruptions for nursing procedures followed by doctors, *phlebotomists*, etc. can mean that the patient does not get a continuous period of rest. With the increased tendency for open visiting hours and a family's natural desire to be with someone undergoing surgery, it is the nurse's responsibility to ensure, in the early post-operative period, that all the patient's needs are met. This will require firstly skills in managing work and the environment, and secondly interpersonal and communication skills in conveying the patient's needs to visitors.

(3) *Post-op 'blues'* are commonly experienced around the fourth post-operative day. The patient can be reassured that this is not only normal but will resolve itself within 24 hours.

(4) *Physical discomfort* includes pain, vomiting, position in bed and the other physiological disruptions that have been discussed.

A relaxed mind leads to a relaxed body and the nurse can play a large part in creating a calm and ordered atmosphere within which the patient may sleep and rest.

As the patient starts to mobilise, his thoughts may turn to his outside activities, his job, his home and his social life. It should be stressed to all patients that although the visible and superficial signs of healing are evident at discharge, the deeper healing and return of strength to the operative area and to the body in general takes longer. In many cases, where underlying muscle is involved healing can take six to eight weeks. This will vary with age and the type of surgery and again the patient's own body is the best guide to when activities may be resumed. The care plan in Fig. 24.19 shows the long term goals set and care planned between the nurse and patient prior to discharge. The care plan passed to the district nurse will allow her to cope with any problems that may arise after discharge.

Other problems may present as a result of permanent change, as in Mrs Archer's profile (Fig. 24.2). Mrs Archer's anxiety is focused on her acceptability to her drama group where there is communal changing of costume, etc. This is a situation where the nurse is not in a position to forecast what will happen, and as such problems are outside her experience she may find it best to refer the patient to a self-help group or society that can help the patient. In this case an appropriate society would be the Colostomy Welfare Group, whose address can be found at the end of this chapter. Most of the stoma appliance manufacturers also produce booklets which carry useful advice for patients and can be obtained from the manufacturer.

By the time patients are discharged, most feel fairly well and are looking forward to going home. It is advisable to tell them that they may have days in the coming weeks when they will feel low, both physically and mentally, and that this is common for up to six months, especially following major surgery.

Finally there are those patients in whom permanent change as a result of surgery (for example, the amputation of a limb) requires a permanent change in their activities of living. The nurse can help these patients by meeting their immediate post-operative needs and by playing a role as part of a team in helping them adjust to a new lifestyle.

Expression of sexuality

In any hospital ward a loss of personal identity can occur, particularly during the few hours before and after the operation. It is important that clothes and other personal effects are restored to the patient as soon as possible, although obviously this must be

Fig. 24.19 *Care plan (2) for Mr Singh*

Date	Identified needs/problems	Objectives/ goals	Nursing intervention	Evaluation
18.1.92	**Work and play**			
	For discharge today	Reassure patient that he will be able to resume fully all activities	Explain through interpreter that complete healing will take about six weeks	
	Is worried about being able to play squash and train for next season's athletics programme	Devise with patient a timetable for return to activities	No physical exertion for three weeks	
			Start some gentle stretching exercises in the middle of February	
			Re-start running in March	
			Recommence squash in April	
			Slow down if pain or excessive fatigue experienced	

NAME: Raj Singh   **Date of Birth**: 4.11.72   **Signed**: *J. Smith*

balanced with other needs that may override the need to replace teeth, glasses and personal clothing.

Post-operative problems may arise that relate to the patient's perception of his own body. Scars may worry some patients – especially young patients for whom appearance and presentation is particularly important. Much of this anxiety can be relieved by pointing out that the scar will eventually shrink somewhat and the surrounding skin area will return to its normal colour. The nurse should point out that scar tissue will not tan due to loss of melanocytes in that area.

For other patients the problems may be more serious, being related not only to the physical acceptability of the surgery but also to their perception of how those closest to them will accept the results of surgery.

Mrs Archer's self-care deficit (Fig. 24.20) identified two days prior to discharge after several conversations with the nurse, shows her anxiety to be centred on her ability to fulfil her role as wife and grandmother. She was particularly anxious about the need to maintain hygiene and about cuddling and picking up her baby grandson. The care prescribed indicates how she is helped towards resuming these two roles, discovering that surgery has not changed her role fulfilment or how those closest to her perceive her. It should be noted that most of the problems were self-perceived and had no basis in fact apart from one and that the conversation initiated by the nurse was the only action required before Mrs Archer could start to meet her own needs again.

Problems related to the sexual relationship between the patient and his partner may occasionally arise. These vary from a simple desire to know when sexual activity may resume following surgery to an altered perception of body image and how that will affect the relationship, or a fear of inability to resume sexual function and therefore fulfil his perceived role. In many instances, the nurse will be able to answer these questions and allay anxieties. She should, however, be alert to the fact that she may occasionally encounter a problem that she does not have the expertise to deal with. When

Fig. 24.20 Care plan (3) for Mrs Archer: self-care model (two days prior to discharge)

Date	Self-care deficit	Objectives/goals	Nursing intervention	Type of nursing action	Evaluation
28.1	Mrs Archer is still unsure of how acceptable she will be to her family. She is particularly worried about hygiene aspects when cuddling her grandson. She feels unable to approach this subject with her family	To initiate (with patient's permission) dialogue to identify any problems that may actually exist	(1) Arrange a meeting with staff nurse, Mrs Archer, husband and daughters, stomatherapist – for 29/1	Acting for	29/1 Husband and youngest daughters have no qualms at all but eldest daughter is also worried about baby and very glad that there is a chance to discuss it
			(2) Ensure visitors room is empty	Providing suitable environment	
			(3) After identifying the perceived problem to all present, let stomatherapist help plan future care	Guidance	Stomatherapist to call at patient's home on 31/1 to see patient, daughter and baby

NAME: Dorothy Archer   **Date of Birth:** 7.4.28   **Signed:** J. Smith

this happens, the patient should be referred for specific counselling. The nurse may also refer the patient to specific publications. An example that would suit Mrs Archer can be found at the end of this chapter in the suggestions for further reading.

Communication

Communication cannot be viewed in isolation: it is intrinsic to every aspect of care discussed. It is not only important in reducing post-operative pain, speeding recovery and in observing for post-operative complications; it is also crucial to the creation of an atmosphere and environment which generate confidence in patients. Furthermore, open communication is highlighted by learners as a key component of good ward management where individual patient care is practised effectively, and an environment exists which fosters a caring attitude towards both staff and patients (Fretwell, 1980). Good communication also enables learners to share their experience. It enables them not only to meet the needs of patients, but to learn to recognise and meet their own needs. To give specific examples would be ineffectual. While this text may supply instances of the value of verbal communication, it is impossible to convey the richness and depth of communication that can be achieved through touch, eye contact and listening. Communication could and should try to be in all walks of life:

> 'A sensitive ability to hear, a deep satisfaction in being heard; an ability to be more real, which in turn brings forth more realness from others; and consequently a greater freedom to give and receive love'
>
> (Rogers, 1980; page 26)

Future trends

Surgical intervention continues to be a necessary and useful medical tool but there is an increasing body of knowledge and skill which allows this intervention to be less traumatic and sometimes redundant.

Twenty years ago, surgery for gastric and duodenal bleeding ulcers was common. With the development of H2 (hydrochloric acid) blocking drugs it has become a rarity and when surgical intervention is required, it is often approached via endoscopy (Taylor, 1991). In this manner, the patient requires only a light anaesthesia and is protected from a surgical wound.

Similarly, the development of endoscopic crushing of gallstones and keyhole surgery with a laparoscope for performing cholecystectomy drastically reduces the amount of time normally required for recovery from this procedure (Keanne *et al.*, 1991).

Other recent developments have seen the use of photodynamic therapy (PDT) which has the 'potential for selective destruction of cancer' (Boulos and Barr, 1990). Although only suitable for some cancers, it uses a systemic administration of photosensitising agents which are picked up by malignant cells and then exposed to specific wavelengths of light. This is currently being used to treat malignant skin lesions and recurrent bladder tumours.

Laser treatment is also being developed in other areas of surgery, most notably in cervical cancers where, with early detection, there is a 96% cure rate (Boulos and Barr, 1990).

Conclusions

This chapter has endeavoured to give a brief insight into the care that patients undergoing surgery might require. It is by no means definitive nor are the models of care suggested the only ones suited to the type of patient that will be encountered. For more in-depth study, learners are urged to consult such texts as those given in the references and suggestions for further reading list.

With the development of alternative surgical treatments and an increasingly shorter stay in hospital, nurses with a surgical orientation will need to meet the challenges of the changes with new skills and increased knowledge. They may also find that their skills are required not only in the hospital, but increasingly in the community.

Glossary

Abdominoperineal resection of the rectum: Surgical procedure to remove the rectum performed by two surgeons, one approaching through the abdominal wall, the other through the perineum, resulting in colostomy formation

Anastomosis: Artificial joining of a tubular structure (for example the colon) following surgery

Appendicectomy: Surgical excision of the appendix

Aseptic technique: Method of changing dressings to minimise the risk of infection using sterile equipment and a non-touch technique

Cholecystectomy: Surgical excision of the gall bladder

Circadian rhythms: Repeated cycles (for example, of hormone secretion) that occur approximately every 24 hours

Colostomy: A section of the colon is brought to the surface of the abdominal wall to form an opening for the excretion of faeces

Diathermy: Heat treatment by means of high frequency electric current. Used in surgery to coagulate blood vessels or dissect tissues

Dyspnoea: Difficulty with breathing

Functioning and defunctioning colostomies: Both ends of the colon are brought to the surface of the abdominal wall following *hemicolectomy* to allow the inflammation within the peritoneal sac to subside before *anastomosing* the colon together and returning it to the peritoneal cavity

Hemicolectomy: Surgical removal of half of the colon

Hypoproteinaemic: Low circulating levels of plasma proteins causing a reduced osmotic pressure

Hypoxia: Reduced oxygen supply to the tissues

Ligature: A thread (of silk, catgut, etc.) tied around a blood vessel to stop it bleeding

Oliguria: Insufficient urine output

Paralytic ileus: Absence of *peristalsis* and hence bowel sounds – usually resulting from handling of gut during surgery

Partial thyroidectomy: Surgical excision of part of the thyroid gland

Peristalsis: Muscular contraction and relaxation of the wall of the small bowel propelling the contents along the gut

Peritoneal lavage: Washing out of the peritoneal sac (usually with isotonic normal saline) during surgery to remove faecal contents that have leaked due to perforated bowel

Phlebotomist: Technician who takes blood samples

Scar tissue: Avascular, acellular tissue formed from collagen and granulation tissue

Subphrenic abscess: Encapsulated area of infection in space left by the excised gall bladder below the diaphragm

Tachycardia: Heart beating in sinus rhythm at more than 100 beats per minute

Tachypnoea: Rapid shallow breathing

Tekmar: Electronically controlled machine giving prescribed intravenous fluid in measured doses

Thyrotoxicosis: Medical condition with symptoms brought about by oversecretion of thyroxine causing an increased metabolic rate

References

Bale, S. and Harding, K. (1991). Foam still finds favour. *Professional Nurse*, 6(9), 510–518.

Balfour, S.E. (1989). Will I be in pain? Patients' and nurses' attitudes to pain after abdominal surgery. *Professional Nurse*, 5(1), 28–33.

Baughen, R. (1989). Hospital food – a literature review. *Surgical Nurse*, 2(3), 18–22.

Biley, F.C. (1989). Nurses' perception of stress in pre-operative surgical patients. *Journal of Advanced Nursing*, 14(7), 575–581.

Boore, J. (1976). *A Prescription for Recovery*. RCN, London.

Boulos, P.B. and Barr, H. (1990). Lasers and their application to surgery. In *Current Surgical Practice, Vol. 5*, Hadfield, J., Hobley, M. and Treasure, T. (eds.). Edward Arnold, London.

Carr, E.C.J. (1990). Post-operative pain; patients' expectations and experiences. *Journal of Advanced Nursing*, 15(1), 89–100.

Central Statistical Office. (1988). *Social Trends No. 18.* HMSO, London.

Child, D. (1981). *Psychology and the Teacher* (3rd ed.). Holt, Eastbourne.

Copp. L.A. (1986). The nurse as advocate. *Journal of Advanced Nursing*, 11(3), 255–263.

Dallison, A. (1991a). Improving pain relief. *Nursing*, 4(34), 34–35.

Dallison, A. (1991b). Self-administration of oral pain relief. *Nursing*, 4(35), 30–31.

Department of Health. (1989). *A Guide to Consent for Examination and Treatment.* HMSO, London.

Egan, G. (1990). *The Skilled Helper* (4th ed.). Brooks Cole, Andover.

Fairclough, J., Evans, P.D., Elliot, T.S.J. and Newcombe, R.G. (1986). Skin shaving: a cause for concern. *Journal of the Royal College of Surgeons of Edinburgh*, April, 76–78.

Fretwell, J. (1980). *Ward Teaching and Learning.* RCN, London.

Hamilton-Smith, S. (1972). *Nil by Mouth.* RCN, London.

Hayward, J. (1975). *Information: A Prescription against Pain.* RCN, London.

Henderson, V. (1978). Nurses' unique function. *Journal of Advanced Nursing*, 3(2), 113–130.

Holmes, S. (1991). Nutrition and the surgical patient. *Nursing Standard*, 5(44), 30–32.

Johnson, A. (1988). Standard protocols for treating open wounds. *Professional Nurse*, 3(12), 498–501.

Kalldeen, D. (1990). Preparing skin for surgery. *Nursing*, 4(15), 28–29.

Keanne, F.B.V., Tanner, W.A. and Darzi, A. (1991). Alternatives to cholecystectomy for gallbladder stones. In *Recent Advances in Surgery*, Taylor, I. and Johnston, D. (eds.). Churchill Livingstone, Edinburgh.

Lane-Franklin, B. (1974). *Patient Anxiety on Admission.* RCN, London.

Lascelles, I. (1982). Wound dressing techniques. *Nursing*, 2(8), 217–219.

Llewellyn-Thomas, A. (1990). Pre-operative skin preparation. *Surgical Nurse*, 3(2), 24.

McCaffrey, M. (1972). *Nursing Management of the Patient in Pain.* J.B. Lippincott, Philadelphia.

McCaffrey, M. (1983). *Nursing the Patient in Pain.* Harper and Row, London.

McCaffrey, M. (1990). Nursing approaches to non-pharmacological pain control. *International Journal of Nursing Studies*, 27(1), 1–5.

Maslow, A. (1970). *Motivation and Personality* (3rd ed.). Harper and Row, Philadelphia.

Orem, D. (1990). *Nursing: Concepts of Practice* (4th ed.). McGraw-Hill, New York.

Rogers, C. (1967). *On Becoming a Person.* Constable, London.

Rogers, C. (1980). *A Way of Being.* Houghton Mifflin, Boston.

Roper, N., Logan, W. and Tierney, A. (1990). *The Elements of Nursing* (3rd ed.). Churchill Livingstone, Edinburgh.

Rutter, P., Murphy, P. and Dudley, H.A.F. (1980). Morphine: controlled trial of different methods of administration for post-operative pain relief. *British Medical Journal*, 280, 12–16.

Shireff, A. (1990). Pre-operative nutritional assessment. *Nursing Times*, 86(8), 68–72.

Spenser, K. and Bale, S. (1990). The logical approach; management of surgical wounds. *Professional Nurse*, 5(6), 303–308.

Taylor, I. (1991). A review of recent advances in surgery. In *Recent Advances in Surgery*, Taylor, I. and Johnston, D. (eds.). Churchill Livingstone, Edinburgh.

Tingle, J. (1990). Patient consent: the issues. *Nursing Standard*, 5(9), 52–54.

Torrance, C. (1991). Pre-operative nutrition, fasting and the surgical patient. *Surgical Nurse*, 5(4), 5–8.

Tschudin, V. (1989). Informed consent. *Surgical Nurse*, 2(6), 15–17.

Winfield, U. (1986). Too close a shave. *Nursing Times*, 82, 64–68.

Suggestions for further reading

Altschul, A. (1983). The consumer's voice: nursing implications. *Journal of Advanced Nursing*, 8(2), 175–183.

Ayliffe, G., Collins, B.J. and Taylor, L.J. (1982). *Hospital Acquired Infection.* Wright, Bristol.

Bale, S. (1991). A holistic approach and the ideal dressing. *Professional Nurse*, 6(6), 316–323.

Barkes, P. (1979). Bioethics and informed consent in American health care delivery. *Journal of Advanced Nursing*, 4(1), 23–38.

Collins, B.J. (1981). Infection and the hospital environment. *Nursing*, 1(26), Supplement.

Griffiths-Jones, D. (1991). Wound care: can the nursing process help? *Professional Nurse*, 6(4), 208–212.

Long, B.C. and Phipps, W.J. (1985). *Essentials of Medical and Surgical Nursing.* Mosby, St Louis.

Piper, S. (1989). Effective use of occlusive wound dressings. *Professional Nurse*, 4(8), 402–404.

Salter, M. (1988). *Altered Body Image: The Nurse's Role.* John Wiley and Sons, Chichester.

Schindler, M. (1981). *Living with a Colostomy*. Thetford Press, Norfolk.

Stronge, J.L. (1984). Principles of wound care. *Nursing*, 2(26), Supplement.

Taylor, L.J. (1984). Skin disinfection. *Nursing*, 2(26), Supplement.

Tootla, J. and Easterling, A. (1989). PDT: destroying malignant cells with laser beams. *Nursing*, 89, 48–49.

Torrance, C. (1990). Sleep and wound healing. *Surgical Nurse*, 3(3), 16–20.

Useful addresses

National Association for the Welfare of Children in Hospital (NAWCH)
Argyle House, 29–31 Euston Road, London NW1 2SD

British Colostomy Association (Colostomy Welfare Group)
38 Eccleston Square, London SW1V 1PB

Stoma Advisory Service
Abbott Laboratories Ltd, Queensborough, Kent ME11 5EL

Coloplast
Peterborough Business Park, Peterborough, Cambs PE2 0FX

Convatec
Squibb House, 141–9 Staines Road, Hounslow, Middlesex TW3 3JB

25

CARE OF THE PERSON WITH CHRONIC HEALTH PROBLEMS

Ann Mackenzie

This chapter will consider the diverse nature of chronic health problems and their impact on the life of the individual. It will explore handicap in terms of a socially constructed problem rather than a medically diagnosed problem inherent in the individual. Health needs of people with chronic health problems will be identified in the light of research and with particular reference to community health care. Issues for nurses will be raised and will include:

- Demographic and epidemiological change
- International classification of impairment, disability and handicap
- Characteristics of chronic illness and their impact on the aims of health care
- Inter-relationship between physical, social, psychological and emotional aspects of chronic health problems
- Prevalence of disability and

consequences on lifestyle, e.g. rheumatoid arthritis

- Assessment and planning of care for individuals and their families, emphasising partnership with patients and carers, e.g. alleviation of chronic pain. Utilisation of dependency measures
- Policy towards community care and disabled people with reference to services for black people and the needs and roles of informal carers

Extent of chronic health problems

Chronic health problems are generally associated with degenerative disease and chronic illness and are the primary causes of mortality and morbidity in advanced societies. These problems can impose major changes and difficulties upon the lifestyle

of individuals, their families and their immediate social contacts (Patrick and Peach, 1989).

An increasing ageing population, for whom chronic disorder and deterioration is endemic, together with the increased survival from acute illness and trauma, have resulted in a shift from problems associated with acute illness to those involving long term and chronic illness or disability. Although disability clearly affects all age groups, the majority of chronic health problems related to

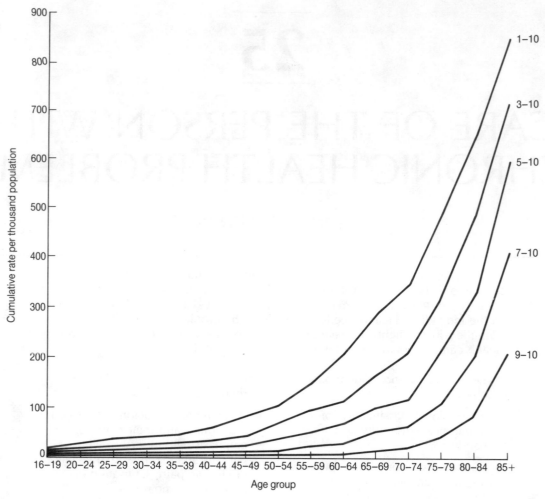

Fig. 25.1 *Estimates of prevalence of disability among adults in Great Britain by age and severity category (OPCS, 1988)*

disability occur in those over 50 years of age and almost one third of the 6 million disabled people in Great Britain are over 75 years old (OPCS, 1988) (Fig. 25.1). The severity of the disability has been categorised on a scale from 1 to 10, from very slight to very severe respectively.

Need is related to the severity of the disability and the majority of the needs are met by informal carers, that is, by family, relatives and friends. In the most dependent groups only 28% received formal help from services such as the district nursing service or home helps (OPCS, 1988). Therefore chronic health problems have consequences for individuals, their carers, their social contacts and society.

However, this does not mean that all individuals with similar conditions have the same health problems, or indeed that individuals see themselves as having any health problems if their needs are being met. Differences between individuals are influenced by such factors as age, economic circumstances, environmental factors and family support. Chronic health problems range across a broad spectrum from mild impairment of sight requiring the use of spectacles for reading, to advanced multiple sclerosis requiring help with many aspects of daily living activities.

Classification of chronic illness

For the purpose of studying chronic illness and associated health problems, varying classifications and categorisations are used. In common use and employed for the most recent national survey by the OPCS (1988) is the International Classification of Impairments, Disabilities and Handicaps by the World Health Organisation (Wood, 1975):

- Impairment is any loss or abnormality of psychological, physiological or anatomical structure or function.
- Disability is any restriction or lack (resulting from an impairment) of ability to perform an activity in the manner or within the range considered normal for a human being.
- Handicap is a disadvantage for a given individual, resulting from an impairment or disability, that limits or prevents the fulfilment of a role that is normal (depending on age, sex, social and cultural factors) for that individual.

This type of classification is useful in separating out these three aspects of chronic health problems. The terms are often used interchangeably but they are clearly not the same, as this definition demonstrates. *Impairment* refers to the loss of function, *disability* refers to the restricted ability to carry out certain activities as a result of impairment, and *handicap* is the consequence of the impairment or disability. Handicap, then, is the social disadvantage, the severity of which will depend upon the extent of the limitations to the social activities of the individual and upon the perception and definition of that handicap by society. Handicap is defined by groups in society and meets varying degrees of acceptability. It carries with it judgements based on values of the group and this in turn is dependent on such things as the individual's age, social activities, work, access to finance, family support and role expectations. For instance, the impairment of muscle weakness resulting in the disability of restricted mobility may be a devastating handicap to the social activities of a young adult of 18 unable to join in a game of football, but may be perceived as less of a handicap by a man of 60, who may not expect to play football or wish, as part of his normal activities, to take part in strenuous physical exercise.

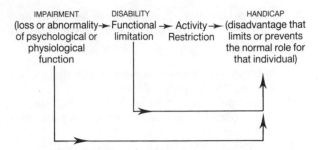

Fig. 25.2 *Links between impairment, disability and handicap (adapted from Wood, 1980)*

Figure 25.2 helps to illustrate the linear relationship between impairment, disability and handicap. It also adds further to our understanding of chronic health problems. On the one hand handicap, the social disadvantage, may result from the linear process of disability, the restrictions of function and activity, and on the other hand handicap may arise from impairment such as facial disfigurement, which does not limit functional activity but still causes social disadvantage through embarrassment or self-consciousness.

Disability is therefore the term most frequently used in relation to the identification of chronic health problems, since restrictions or lack of function to perform a range of normal activities may arise from the impairment of a physical or mental disease, disorder or trauma, and may result in the handicapping physical, psychological and social problems which affect a person's health.

Characteristics of chronic illness and related health problems

The social consequences of these types of problems are frequently linked to illness behaviour and the characteristics of chronic ill health, and pose some difficulties for professionals and lay public in the rehabilitation of people with chronic health problems.

Chronic health problems are related mainly to characteristics of chronic illness and to illness behaviour. Medical sociology (Morgan *et al.*, 1985) and the work of Talcott Parsons (1951) offer a starting point for considering the sick role in society (see also Chapter 10). From the functionalist perspective, Parsons identifies rights and obligations of the role which can be summarised as follows:

(1) Individuals are exempt from their normal obligations and responsibilities;
(2) Individuals are not to be held responsible for their condition and are to be given sympathy and support;
(3) Individuals are expected to desire health;
(4) Individuals are expected to cooperate with prescribed treatment and seek professional advice.

This is not the only perspective, but it has been influential in our thinking about the roles and behaviours of those who are ill.

The sick role depicted by Parsons is familiar and carries the traditional expectations by the patient of treatment and cure and of the professional who will give treatment. It appears to offer a dominant role to the nurse or doctor and a submissive and passive role to the patient. Occupation of the sick role is short-lived with the expectation that treatment will effect cure or return the individual to full health – however health is defined (see Chapters 1, 2 and 3).

Definitions of chronic illness and any corresponding health problems do not therefore fit easily into these expectations which reflect disorders of an acute nature.

In contrast, characteristics of chronic illness drawn from the sociological (Peroni, 1981; Strauss, 1984) and the nursing (Kratz, 1978) literature can be summarised as follows:

- Slow insidious onset; the signs and symptoms are often slow in developing;
- Length of the illness is usually over a period of at least six months;
- Course is episodic, the development of symptoms is variable in severity and duration, resulting in an unpredictable prognosis;
- No obvious cure but rather emphasising control of symptoms and tertiary prevention with long term rather than short term goals for improvement;
- Permanence producing handicap and usually disability of varying severity.

In comparing the two sets of characteristics above it can be seen that the Parsonian model is limited, as it assumes that everyone will behave in the same way from the beginning of their illness. It does not distinguish between impairment and acute illness as starting points. For the person with chronic illness, the impairment and the disability are part of their way of life. Complete cure is not an appropriate goal; it is rather the maintenance of health to an optimum achievable level dependent on the disability of the individual and the social and psychological consequences of the handicap. Independence and resolution of accompanying chronic health problems are dependent on the individual taking control of the situation, rather than relying solely on professional intervention.

There are always exceptions to such categorisation. Some chronic illnesses are sudden in onset, as is frequently the case with cerebrovascular accidents. Others leave very little discernible disability, as in the case of uncomplicated diabetes mellitus.

The important issue for nurses when considering the above points is that the aims of health care for patients with chronic illness and resulting health problems will be different from those for patients with acute illness. Furthermore, disability arising from chronic illness will have different consequences and require different interventions to maintain health compared with disability arising from sudden trauma such as that caused by a car accident (Oliver, 1988).

Inter-relationships between chronic health problems

The multiple chronic health problems which may result from disability and handicap are usually inter-related. There is interplay between the physical, social, psychological and emotional difficulties that makes assessment, and therefore alleviation, of chronic health problems complex and demanding. This can be demonstrated by examining some of these links.

Social isolation and loneliness can result from mobility problems and loss of social contacts. Self-concept, depending on the consequences for the individual, may produce varying degrees of low self-esteem. A person may feel and look different due to the disability.

Stigma, a social reaction which 'spoils' normal identity (Goffman, 1968), can result in long term isolation. Some illnesses are more stigmatising than others; for instance, epilepsy can evoke negative feelings and even fear in the minds of other people. The reactions of those who have been diagnosed as epileptic and of others who know of the diagnosis may lead to restriction in employment and in other social activity (Scambler, 1984), and to a reluctance on the part of the sufferer to disclose any impairment. On the other hand, heart disease may be perceived as non-stigmatising and receive empathetic reactions.

Social relationships may also be at risk. The disability will almost certainly produce some change in the immediate family environment — according to the extent of the dependency and the need to change routines. All chronic illness will require change from other family members or relatives. This may result in variation in role relationships. The man who one day is the main wage earner may be forced to relinquish that role if heart disease inhibits his capacity to remain in paid employment. The young mother with increasing weakness caused by multiple sclerosis may find herself becoming dependent on her children or spouse for help with personal hygiene. Sexual relationships may be disrupted. Outside social relationships with friends who are unsure how to respond to disability can become strained. A previously confident and socially active person may become embarrassed and self-conscious in the company of others. The lack of control over bodily functions, such as continence, speech and movement, may disturb any social relationship.

Feelings of self-worth are complicated by the disruption in reciprocal patterns of support and low self-esteem results when the individual is always dependent on the support of others and feels unable to contribute to the relationship. This type of interdependence is also affected by financial factors. Financial difficulties due to increased expenditure on extra fittings and adaptations in the home or on equipment, together with unemployment, all add to feelings of low self-esteem.

Powerlessness is a further aspect of dependence and occurs when people no longer feel they can influence their life or their future. The lack of involvement in the usual rituals and activities of normal life gives a feeling of lack of control.

Prevalence of disability and effect on normal life

The effect of disability on normal life caused by chronic illness is well described by Locker (1983):

'To the non-disabled person many, if not all, the activities of daily living are non-problematic; they are simply taken for granted, performed with hardly any awareness that they are being performed at all. This contrasts vividly with the experience of people disabled in some way'

(page 70)

Indeed, the most common disabilities identified in the most recent survey of adults (OPCS, 1988) are those which affect activities normally taken for granted — locomotion, followed by hearing and personal care disabilities (Fig. 25.3). Locomotor problems are the most common type of disability, affecting over 4 million adults. Around 2.5 million have hearing and personal care disabilities. Both types of chronic health problems are experienced predominantly by those living in private households.

Locker's (1983) study, in which he interviews 24 people with rheumatoid arthritis, demonstrates the consequences of one disabling condition — the most common cause of disability of adults who live at home (OPCS, 1988). It describes, through finely drawn extracts, the real situations of people struggling and coping with disability.

One important point emphasised by this study is that 'mundane activities' cannot be performed and therefore become all the more frustrating. As Locker (1983) points out, such achievements as climbing Everest or swimming the English Channel are beyond most physical capabilities and we live happily without achieving them. However, for disabled people even moving from chair to toilet may be a major operation for both the disabled person and carer, requiring a great expenditure of energy.

Respondents in Locker's study describe how they undertake intricate routines of movement, involving rolling and transferring body weight in a predetermined sequence to enable changes in position, and slow mobility from one place in the room to another, extending over one or two hours. Such activities as dressing are achieved in stages; first the top half of the body is dressed and then,

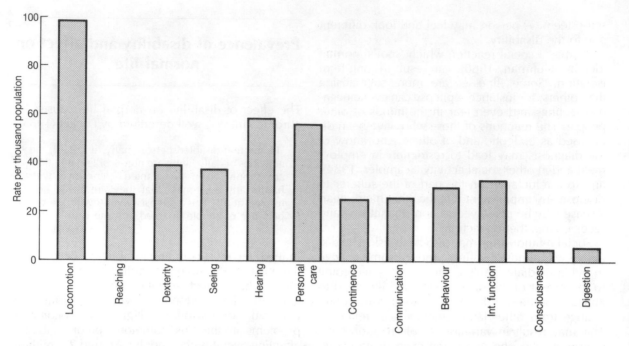

Fig. 25.3 Estimates of prevalence of disability among adults in Great Britain by type of disability (OPCS, 1988)

when help arrives, the awkward garments like underpants or stockings are added. Compromises in everyday activities are usual, such as sleeping in stockings because they are difficult to change, not having a bath, not visiting the hairdressers, or shaving once a week rather than every day.

The outside environment is no less hazardous, but not so easy to influence. Two small steps outside the Post Office may prevent access to a necessary service, or a high kerb may present an unsurmountable obstacle to negotiating the local High Street.

The discriminatory nature that society has towards those with disability leads to the lack of provision for individuals to carry out everyday activities such as shopping. This discrimination extends to all aspects of life such as housing, travel, employment and leisure facilities (Finkelstein, 1980). Chronic health problems may then be seen to involve not only those problems of chronic illness for which medical and nursing intervention are appropriate, but also problems arising from disability and handicap which are more to do with changes in attitudes and in society generally (Oliver and Zarb, 1989).

For the 6.5 million adults in Britain with one or more disabilities and for the 360,000 children

under 16 and their carers (OPCS, 1988), difficulties such as these are everyday occurrences which are not easily solved. For the older age groups the picture is complicated by the morbidity pattern of multiple diseases which affect older people.

Planning to meet individual health needs

The difficulty in definition and the complexity of chronic health problems make it daunting for the nurse who is charged with the responsibility for care. Assessment, planning, implementation and evaluation need to address particularly the maintenance and rehabilitative aspects of care, having in mind the inter-relationship between physical, emotional, psychologial and social problems.

Paralysis, one of the common residual physiological impairments following a stroke, may also be associated with a loss of social contacts normally gained when working, visiting friends, shopping or participating in sporting activities. This effect on normal activities may in turn result in emotional problems associated with changed relationships within the family group, or result in more severe psychological problems, such as anxiety or depression, caused by social isolation and loss of earnings. The disability associated with suffering a stroke is clearly therefore not just of a physiological nature, but is also frequently interlinked with social, emotional and psychological problems. This makes assessment a complex procedure which calls for knowledge and sensitivity on the part of the nurse. Planning, implementing and evaluating the care of people who have suffered a stroke is a case not only of meeting the physiological needs, but also of considering the chronic health problems related to social, emotional and psychological factors, which for some may constitute more of a handicap than the lack of physiological functioning. In this instance the nurse, by enabling social contacts for the patient, may also alleviate other problems relating to isolation and loss of self-esteem.

It is important to note that assessment of need of people who are disabled is not just undertaken on an individual level. However, it is at the interface between the nurse, the client and the informal carers where most nursing assessments are made and where the outcomes of such assessments are evaluated in the first instance.

In undertaking assessments, and in making subsequent decisions about care, the nurse must recognise the characteristics of chronic illness and assess the implications for the individual and their carers. Connelly (1987) states:

'Essentially the role of the nurse in working with chronically ill patients is less as a provider of direct treatment and more as a facilitator and supporter of effective self-care behaviours performed by patients'

(page 623)

It requires close working with patients and the encouragement of participation in care. The difficulty for the patient in self-care is that self-care behaviours have to be maintained over lengths of time and motivation may be difficult to sustain.

Planning is concerned with the maintenance of care acceptable to the patient – not just with short term goals to be achieved in a week or a month, but with a mix of both short and long term goals of relevance to the patient and supported by knowledge of the condition from the nurse. Mainten-

ance of care is also a difficulty for nurses, as demonstrated by Kratz (1978) in her study of district nurses caring for the long term sick in the community. It is one of the many issues raised by this study of people who have suffered a stroke and is relevant for all nurses caring for people with long term illness as it concerns the relationships between the aims of care and the needs of the patients. When the aims of care were clear and focused, the observed needs of the patient were met, but when the aims were not identified the care was diffuse and did not correspond to the needs of the patient. Setting aims or goals for care became increasingly difficult when the district nurses could not see the patient 'getting better' and the expectations of the traditional sick role of cure and improvement were not therefore being met.

A further pertinent issue raised was the predicament of the carers who were frequently expected to cope. Despite their own needs, they were often expected to make a major contribution to any rehabilitation – the whole process of restoring a person with chronic health problems to a condition in which he is able, as early as possible, to resume a normal life.

Participating with patients and carers in planning care

To enable any sort of rehabilitation the patient has to agree with the plan which is being drawn up. Decisions about priorities have to be discussed and agreed with the patient. There is no room here for the standardised plan of acute care which is predetermined and based on the predictable. The starting point for identifying chronic health problems is the subjective view of the patient, after which the knowledge of prevention and promotion of health from the nurse is added.

Patients may be very knowledgeable about their condition, more knowledgeable in fact than the nurse. For example, many societies and associations provide in-depth literature for those suffering from such conditions as diabetes mellitus or multiple sclerosis. Individuals and their families who have coped with the problems associated with such conditions for years should therefore be respected as an important and unique resource and nurses should be prepared to work in equal partnership with patients when planning care and setting goals. In this respect, it is important to remember that not all goals are long term. Some activities may return quickly, such as the ability to stand following a stroke. Plans for rehabilitation should therefore ensure that progress is documented, and that goals attainable in the short term are set in order to maintain motivation.

Re-assessment needs to be frequent, framed by the unique situation of the patient, responsive to the uncertain and often unpredictable course of the condition and cognisant of the importance of keeping disruptions to established and daily routines to a minimum. Chronic illness results in a change to previous routines and lifestyles. Therefore an important function of assessment is to establish what the patient regards as desirable daily activities. This should be followed by planning and implementing care that can be evaluated through outcomes which are realistic and appropriate to patient and carers. The imposition of a professional framework is not effective, although some sort of framework or model, for instance those of Orem (1991) or Roper *et al.* (1990), may be a useful reference point once the patient's view has been identified.

There are many instruments for assessing loss of independence. The inclusion of any measuring instrument in the assessment process should be dependent upon the purposes of the assessment. Scales and scoring systems have been devised to measure activities of daily living and are frequently referred to as dependency scales. Some have been devised or adapted for specific purposes, such as research studies or the planning of services, and need to be carefully appraised for suitability if used in individual assessment of disabled people. It is important to have in mind the distinctions between impairment, disability and handicap, none of which may result in dependency. Also consideration should be given to the inter-relationship between the unmet needs that result in chronic health problems requiring a multidimensional measurement scale.

For instance, the Index of Activities of Daily Living (ADL) (Katz and Akpom, 1976) was developed to measure and evaluate the degree of functional incapacity or independence of people, especially the elderly, suffering from chronic conditions. This measure includes six main activities – bathing, dressing, toileting, transfer, continence and feeding. Individuals are observed, perhaps by a nurse or a physiotherapist, and the observer records the degree of dependence in each area. For example, in bathing the degree of dependence

or independence is assessed according to the extent to which the individual needs assistance while bathing. The results of the observations are then converted into a scale.

As one can see, the basic physiological functions of ADL scales are fairly easy to assess, but few problems associated with chronic diseases are solely concerned with the lack of ability to perform physical functions. However, other activities which are also part of daily life, such as shopping, working or taking part in leisure activities, are more difficult to assess in absolute terms and depend more on what is accepted as normal in a particular culture or social group. As Wilkin *et al.* (1992) state, 'The further one moves from basic physiological function the more difficult it becomes to define such norms in any absolute sense'.

Therefore multidimensional measures need to be used in order to incorporate physical, psychological and social aspects of daily activities.

The Sickness Impact Profile (SIP) (Bergner *et al.*, 1981) was developed to assess the impact of disease across a range of severities and across various cultural groups, and has been used particularly with people with chronic illness. This measure has in turn been adapted by Patrick and Peach (1989) in a study which took a very broad definition of disability, to include economic and psychosocial activities, such as recreation, social interaction, communication and work. Of necessity, the evaluation of the use of these types of multidimensional measures is a complex activity. A possible starting point for appraisal could be the work of Wilkin and Thompson (1989) and Charlton (1989).

In order for patients to be able to make decisions they need to be informed not only about their condition, but also about the resources and services available. For instance, the lack of information about important aids and equipment is an unnecessary obstacle to people who are disabled and to their carers. In a recent study on this subject, Campbell and Ross (1990) found that information about aids and equipment available to patients and carers was incomplete and fragmented. In some cases the equipment did not meet patients' needs because their condition had changed and provision of equipment was delayed. In other cases equipment was not acceptable because it was too large, or ugly, or because no instructions were given as to its use. Clearly there are implications here for continuous assessment and involvement of patients and carers in the planning of care.

A recognition of patients' perspectives and priorities and of the way in which these relate to patients' social life will influence the extent to which any goals for maintenance of health and prevention of further deterioration are achieved.

The roles of passive patient and dominant professional must not be sustained if the patient is to be actively involved in the rehabilitation that leads towards gaining and maintaining independence. Care and alleviation of chronic health problems is only a possibility with full cooperation of the client (Cameron, 1987).

The importance of planning care to meet the needs of patients is nowhere more obvious than in the case of rheumatoid arthritis. As described above, one of the symptoms in a common disabling condition such as this is chronic pain resulting in a number of further health problems that affect daily activities and relationships.

Meeting health needs of people with chronic pain

The cause of chronic pain is not easy to identify and therefore, like chronic illness itself, the goals or outcomes of intervention are likely to be indeterminate and uncertain. In pain associated with acute illness, the cause is usually identifiable and alleviation occurs when the physiological condition is resolved and healing has taken place. In contrast, chronic pain is often not affected by the treatment of the condition or disease. The long-standing nature of chronic pain, which may last for months or years and have episodes of extreme severity, may give rise to further related conditions, such as immobility, anxiety, depression, sleeplessness, loss of appetite and irritability. For instance, in rheumatoid arthritis, the pain may be more disabling than the damage to joints caused by the disease (Locker, 1989).

Each individual will experience and cope with pain in a different way. Their previous experiences of pain (Walker *et al.*, 1989), their cultural background, and their family (Snelling, 1990) are all factors known to influence chronic pain. One guiding principle in pain assessment and management is the subjective view of the person who is feeling the pain (Beyerman, 1982). Pain is 'what-

ever the person says it is and exists whenever he says it does' (McCaffrey, 1979). Clearly the accuracy of pain assessment is crucial to its management, but as research studies indicate (Anderson, 1982; Seers, 1987), nurses are not good at assessing patients' pain.

However, as Walker *et al.* (1990) point out, the procedures in hospital for assessing pain and acute conditions may not be suitable for assessing pain at home, where most people who suffer chronic conditions are living. This study of the nursing management of elderly patients with persistent pain in the community shows that a multidimensional assessment of pain is the most likely approach to take account of all the factors associated with pain. Within this approach a measurement scale such as the McGill Pain Questionnaire (Melzack and Wall, 1988) may be useful in the estimation of changes in pain over time. Use of assessment tools may help the nurse, patient and carer to gain a shared understanding of the location, frequency, severity and nature of the pain. In this respect it may be helpful for the patient and carers to map out or catalogue the pain by using a diary, a body chart or a simple analogue scale such as the one shown in Fig. 25.4.

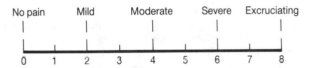

Fig. 25.4 *Visual analogue scale (VAS)*

Changes in severity may be recorded and seen in graphic form. Together with a pain diary to record timing, nature and interference in social activities, and with a body chart to note location, this leads to a more comprehensive assessment of pain (Raiman, 1988).

However, the crucial factor here is 'What matters to the patient is not the actual level of pain, but whether or not he feels that it is under control' (Walker *et al.*, 1990). In controlling pain the patient's own coping strategies are important.

The chronic health problems and subsequent coping strategies caused by pain and stiffness of joints – common symptoms of rheumatoid arthritis – are clearly described by the patients in Locker's study (Locker, 1983). Restlessness due to pain and stiffness meant disturbed sleep patterns for partners as well as patients. Different strategies were adopted to overcome this, e.g. relieving the weight of heavy blankets, patient getting up into the wheelchair for a change of position or sleeping in a chair, partner having a single bed. Clearly the nurse must be able to recognise and encourage such coping strategies, which will at the very least complement drug regimes and in some instances be more appropriate. Giving information is a further aid in helping patients to gain control of chronic pain (Marcer *et al.*, 1990) and in improving their ability to cope and consequently their quality of life (Walker *et al.*, 1990).

Needs of carers

As previously mentioned, the needs of disabled people are complex and relate not only to individuals, but also to immediate family and carers who support the person with chronic health problems living at home. The term 'carer' can be defined as:

> '. . . someone who regularly helps a relative or friend who is disabled or ill with tasks like dressing, shopping or household tasks, or who offers other sorts of practical or emotional support'
> (Robinson and Yee, 1991; page 116)

There is mounting evidence to show that the needs of carers are not acknowledged (National Carers Organisation, 1990). It is estimated that there are 6 million carers in Great Britain (Green, 1988), many of them women, some of whom have given up a career or personal ambitions to care for their relatives. Men may also be carers, in the older age groups particularly, and in this group the carer may be the same age or older than the dependent.

Professionals are criticised for their lack of understanding of the needs of disabled people (Oliver, 1988). Frequently this criticism refers to the lack of flexibility of the service. For instance, district nurses who are only able to visit at times determined by their workload and who are not available to undertake tasks such as washing and dressing. In situations such as this the disabled person has to rely on carer, family and friends to contribute to the establishment and maintenance of independence – the main goal of the disabled person or those with chronic health problems.

According to Borsay (1990), the family are still the mainstay for the disabled person living at home, despite the general view from professionals and lay public that family support is in decline.

In an effort to provide individualised care assessment, there is a danger that nurses may concentrate on the needs of the disabled person at the expense of the carer. Therefore the nurse should not only assess the needs of the disabled person or, as now often known, 'the service user', but also consider the needs of the carer.

Privacy is important here and nurses may well agree to meet carers outside the home to discuss their own problems. 'Listening, clarifying and offering advice and information' (Robinson and Yee, 1991) are major aspects of the role of all service providers, including nurses. Again, the giving of information about services and referral to other agencies may be frequently overlooked as appropriate interventions (Badger *et al.*, 1988). In this respect nurses working in primary health care should be disseminating information not only to individuals and families, but also to the community at large (Cameron *et al.*, 1988). Nurses should also be aware that carers may feel guilty about their own needs and be reluctant to ask for help. Indeed, some families and relatives may not wish to be categorised as carers, having developed their helping and supporting role as a natural part of their relationship. Others may not wish to be part of the personal care of their relatives and may be embarrassed to find themselves in situations where they are expected to undertake tasks for which they are ill equipped (Wade, 1983).

A growing concern is developing for carers in the black population. These people are often overlooked due to myths about the black and ethnic minority communities – that they look after their own relatives or that they are young and geographically mobile (Baxter, 1988). It is clear from those who work with such communities that there are now well-established families living in this country and among these families are old and disabled members. Indeed the OPCS survey (1988) found that there was no significant difference in the prevalence of disability between adults in West Indian and Asian households and those of the white population. Assessment and planning must be sensitive to the cultural differences among black carers, without using these differences as an excuse for not recognising that the disabled black population have similar needs to other communities.

Ethnocentrism – aimed mainly at the white majority population – is one of the reasons why the services are under-used by black elderly

(Donaldson, 1986) and disabled people (Cameron *et al.*, 1988). Access can be improved by multilingual information and more involvement of black people in the delivery of the service to those who are disabled and those with chronic health problems. An example of trying to improve accessibility to information is the publication of a booklet by the British Diabetic Association aimed at both Asian and English-speaking people and written in six languages. The King's Fund is also involved in improving services for black populations through its work in the Primary Health Care Group. This group aims to help health authorities to develop a sensitivity to race issues in their contracts and service agreements, by involving black users in assessing need and by targetting resources to black communities.

Policy and community care

Clearly the contribution of carers and families underpins the policy on community care and is the 'central principle' in health and social services for people with chronic illness (Anderson and Bury, 1988). Indeed the most recent White Paper on community care (DoH, 1989), now embodied in legislation, acknowledges that:

'The great bulk of community care is provided by friends, family and neighbours. The decision to take on a caring role is never an easy one. However, many people make that choice and it is right that they should be able to play their part in looking after those close to them. But it must be recognised that carers need help and support if they are to continue to carry out that role; and many people will not have carers readily available who can meet all their needs'

(para 1.9)

The White Paper on community care identifies priorities in government policy promoting 'community based services which encourage and prolong independent living for disabled people' (DoH, 1989). The priorities may be summarised as follows:

(1) Promoting positive and healthy lifestyles through health surveillance and screening programmes;

(2) Promoting networks of local services to encourage and assist people to live dignified and independent lives in their own homes;
(3) Providing a full range of health care and social service facilities for those who require it;
(4) Avoiding unnecessary institutional care by providing services based on careful assessment of need;
(5) Ensuring improved access to information about local and national facilities with greater involvement of patients, clients and carers in the development of services.

(taken from para 2.12)

The context of this provision, within the NHS and Community Care Act 1990, is underpinned by a mixed economy of care, in which varying agencies in the community have a contribution to make.

In 1992 local authorities, health authorities and other agencies drew up community care plans and developed their joint assessment and care management programmes for those in need, including those with disabilities (see Chapter 4). This involves a multidisciplinary approach in which nurses play a major role. Needs assessment is not new, being a requirement of the local authority under the Chronically Sick and Disabled Persons Act 1970 and the Disabled Persons (Services, Consultation and Representation) Act 1986. However, the responsibilities for Social Services within the new Act have much greater implications for the close collaboration of services and for those working in them. Indeed, it is hoped that identification of people in need, assessment of care needs, planning and securing delivery of care, monitoring quality of care, and review of needs (DoH, 1989) through care management will offer a better mechanism for meeting the needs of disabled people than was previously the case.

Care management is concerned with putting together packages of care, planned to take account of individual social and health needs, that are frequently provided by a number of different agencies, such as Social Service authorities, health authorities and voluntary agencies. One person, employed by any of the agencies involved, would be responsible for managing and coordinating the care package. How the provision of services within this new framework is implemented still remains to be evaluated. A number of different models will be used dependent on local arrangements (Beardshaw and Towell, 1990), although strong guidelines are now available for implementation within the purchaser, commissioner and provider roles (DoH, 1991) (see Chapter 4).

Conclusion

It is at the interface between professionals, including nurses, and lay carers that the implications of primary health care in the community come into sharp relief. The identification of individual needs cannot be undertaken in isolation from the health needs of the family and of a wider defined population, e.g. the caseloads of community nurses or a general practitioner's list.

The current emphasis on a market economy in health care, the demands of value for money and the certainty that resources are finite require nurses to enter into a political climate in which they must consider the best use of the limited resources available. Cooperation not only with patients and carers but also with other agencies, both voluntary and statutory, is mandatory if unmet health needs demonstrated as chronic health problems are to be met or, at the very least, identified. The involvement of the community itself in meeting health needs of different groups who live within the locality is part of the nurse's role in primary health care (see Chapter 4).

There has been an obvious fundamental shift of health care philosophy, escalated by the global concerns about health and the declarations of the World Health Organisation (1974). This shift has been made obvious by the explicit declaration of partnership between the professional and the lay populations as an approach to the promotion of good health. Knowledge of the health and resources of the locally defined population will be a prerequisite to planning health care in order that family and community resources can be appraised and utilised.

The diversity of health needs will therefore require innovative and flexible approaches to service provision. Cooperation across agencies such as health units, voluntary groups and Social Service departments is an important aspect of primary health care and of the nurse's role in caring for the person with chronic health problems.

References

Anderson, J.L. (1982). Nursing management of the cancer patient in pain.: a review of the literature. *Cancer Nursing*, 5(1), 33–39.

Anderson, R. and Bury, M. (eds.). (1988). *Living with Chronic Illness. The Experience of Patients and Their Families*. Unwin Hyman, London.

Badger, F., Cameron, E. and Evers, H. (1988). Care at the crossroads. *Health Service Journal*, 98(5130), 1454–1455.

Baxter, C. (1988). Black carers in focus. *Carelink*, 4, 4.

Beardshaw, V. and Towell, D. (1990). *Assessment and Case Management Implications for the Implementation of 'Caring for People'*. Briefing Paper 10, King's Fund Institute, London.

Bergner, M., Bobbitt, R.A., Carter, W.B. and Gibson, B.S. (1981). The Sickness Impact Profile: development and final revision of a health status measure. *Medical Care*, 19, 789–805.

Beyerman, K. (1982). Flawed perceptions about pain. *American Journal of Nursing*, 82, 302–303.

Borsay, A. (1990). Disability and attitudes to family care in Britain: towards a sociological perspective. *Disability, Handicap and Society*, 5(2), 107–122.

Cameron, K. (1987). Chronic illness and compliance. *Journal of Advanced Nursing*, 12, 671–676.

Cameron, E., Evers, H., Badger, F. and Atkin, K. (1988). *District Nursing, the Disabled and the Elderly: Where are the Black Patients?* Community Care Project. Working Paper No. 6, University of Birmingham.

Campbell, F. and Ross, F. (1990). Aids and equipment. *Journal of District Nursing*, 9(5), 4–10.

Charlton, J.H.R. (1989). Approaches to assessing disability. In *Disablement in the Community*, Patrick, D.L. and Peach, H. (eds.). Oxford Medical Publications, Oxford.

Connelly, C.E. (1987). Self-care and the chronically ill patient. *Nursing Clinics of North America*, 22(3), 621–629.

Department of Health. (1989). *Caring For People. Community Care in the Next Decade And Beyond*. HMSO, London.

DoH. (1991). *Implementing Community Care. Pur-*

chaser, *Commissioner and Provider Roles.* HMSO, London.

Donaldson, L. (1986). Health and social status of elderly Asians: a community survey. *British Medical Journal,* 293, 1079–1082.

Finkelstein, V. (1980). *Attitudes and Disabled People: Issues for Discussion.* World Rehabilitation Fund, New York.

Goffman, E. (1968). *Stigma: Notes on the Management of Spoiled Identity.* Penguin Books, Harmondsworth.

Green, H. (1988). *Informal Carers.* General Household Survey, Supplement 16, OPCS. HMSO, London.

Katz, S. and Akpom, C.A. (1976). A measure of primary sociobiological functions. *International Journal of Health Services,* 6, 493–507.

Kratz, C.R. (1978). *Care of the Long-term Sick in the Community.* Churchill Livingstone, Edinburgh.

Locker, D. (1983). *Disability and Disadvantage: The Consequences of Chronic Illness.* Tavistock Publications, London.

Locker, D. (1989). Coping with disability and handicap. In *Disablement in the Community,* Patrick, D.L. and Peach, H. (eds.). Oxford Medical Publications, Oxford.

Marcer, D., Murphy, E.J.J., Pounder, D. and Rogers, P. (1990). The pain relief clinic: how should we define success? *Journal of Intractable Pain Society of Great Britain and Northern Ireland,* 7(2), 9–13.

McCaffrey, M. (1979). *Nursing The Patient in Pain.* Harper and Row, London.

Melzack, R. and Wall, P. (1988). *The Challenge of Pain* (2nd ed.). Penguin Books, Harmondsworth

Morgan, M , Calnan, M, and Manning, N. (1985). *Sociological Approaches to Health and Medicine.* Croom Helm, London.

National Carers Organisation. (1990). *Opportunities for Women. Carers at Work.* NCO, London.

Office of Population Censuses and Surveys.(1988). *Surveys of Disability in Great Britain. Report 1 The Prevalence of Disability Among Adults.* HMSO, London.

Oliver, M. (1988). Flexible services. *Nursing Times,* 84(14), 25–29.

Oliver, M. and Zarb, G. (1989). The politics of disability: a new approach. *Disability, Handicap and Society,* 4(3), 221–239.

Orem, D.E. (1991). *Nursing Concepts of Practice* (4th ed.). McGraw-Hill, New York.

Parsons, T. (1951). *The Social System.* Free Press, Glencoe, Illinois.

Patrick, D.L. and Peach, H. (eds.). (1989). *Disablement in the Community.* Oxford Medical Publications, Oxford.

Peroni, F. (1981). The status of chronic illness. *Social Policy and Administration,* 15(1), 43–53.

Raiman, J. (1988). Pain and its management. In *Nursing Issues and Research in Terminal Care,* Wilson-Barnett, J. and Raiman, J. (eds.). John Wiley and Sons, Chichester.

Robinson, J. and Yee, L. (1991). *Focus on Carers. A Practical Guide to Planning and Delivery of Community Care Services.* King's Fund, London.

Roper, N., Logan, W.W. and Tierney, A.J. (1990). *The Elements of Nursing* (3rd ed.). Churchill Livingstone, Edinburgh.

Scambler, S. (1984). Perceiving and coping with stigmatising illness. In *The Experience of Illness,* Fitzpatrick, R., Hinton, J., Newman, S., Scambler, G. and Thompson, J. (eds.). Tavistock Publications, London.

Seers, C. (1987). Perceptions of pain. *Nursing Times,* 83(48), 37–39.

Snelling, J. (1990). The role of the family in relation to chronic pain: review of the literature. *Journal of Advanced Nursing,* 15, 771–776.

Strauss, A.L. (ed.). (1984). *Chronic Illness and the Quality of Life.* Mosby, Toronto.

Wade, B., Sawyer, L. and Bell, J. (1983). *Dependency with Dignity.* Bedford Square Press, London.

Walker, J.M., Akinsanya, J.A., Davis, B.D. and Marcer, D. (1989). The nursing management of pain in the community: a theoretical framework. *Journal of Advanced Nursing,* 14, 240–247.

Walker, J.M., Akinsanya, J.A., Davis, B.D. and Marcer, D. (1990). The nursing management of elderly patients with pain in the community: study and recommendations. *Journal of Advanced Nursing,* 15, 1154–1161.

Wilkin, D., Hallam, L. and Doggett, M.A. (1992). *Measures of Needs and Outcome for Primary Health Care.* Oxford Medical Publications, Oxford.

Wilkin, D. and Thompson, C. (1989). *User's Guide to Dependency Measures for Elderly People.* Joint Unit for Social Services Research, University of Sheffield.

Wood, P.H.N. (1975). *Classification of Impairments and Handicaps.* World Health Organisation, Geneva.

Wood, P.H.N. (1980). The language of disablement: a glossary relating to disease and its consequences. *International Journal of Rehabilitative Medicine,* 2, 86–92.

World Health Organisation. (1974). *Community Health Nursing.* Technical Report No. 558. WHO, Geneva.

Useful addresses

Association of Carers
First Floor, 21–23 New Road, Chatham, Kent ME4 4QJ

Association of Crossroads Care Attendant Schemes
10 Regent Place, Rugby, Warwickshire CV21 2PN

Carers Unit
Kings Fund Centre, 126 Albert Street, London, NW1 7NF
Provides information and publications for and about carers.

Disability Alliance
25 Denmark Street, London, WC2 8NJ
Publish the *Disability Rights Handbook* annually

Disabled Living Centres (DLC)
Within health authorities where displays of equipment, modifications and adaptations may be seen, and where information, education and training may be provided.

Disabled Living Foundation (DLF)
380–384 Harrow Road, London W9 2HU
Advise and offer useful information about aids and equipment.

DHSS Leaflet Store
Honeypot Lane, Stanmore, Middlesex
For leaflets about allowances (leaflet HB1).

Primary Health Care Group
King's Fund Centre, 126 Albert Street, London NW1 7NF
Information about improving services for black populations.

RADAR
25 Mortimer Street, London W1N 8AB

SPOD (Sexual and Personal Relationships of the Disabled)
286 Camden Road, London N7 OBJ
Publishes useful leaflets on sexual and personal relationships.

26

CARE OF THE ELDERLY PERSON

Margaret Ostro

The aim of this chapter is to introduce the nurse learner to an understanding of the various concepts of ageing so that she can deliver sensitive and appropriate care to elderly patients. It is assumed that nurses working permanently with old people would consult further sources which are pertinent also to community care.

The chapter will include the following topics:

- An ageing population
- Nursing elderly people
- Demographic trends
- Ageism
- Concepts, theories and processes of ageing
- Changes in body systems with ageing
- Ageing and psychological functioning

- Sociology and ageing
- Dependency
- Retirement
- Medical services and elderly people
- Illness in elderly people
  - presentation of disease
  - aims of care
  - special considerations in nursing elderly people
- The rights of elderly people

'When you were young you fastened your belt about you and walked where you chose; but when you are old you will stretch out your arms, and a stranger will bind you fast, and will carry you where you have no wish to go' (St John, Chapter 18, verse 21).

An ageing population

The populations of all the developed nations of the world are ageing because:

- The fertility rate (the average number of children born to women in their childbearing years) is falling;
- The infant mortality rate (the number of deaths of infants under one year of age per 1000 live births per year) is falling;
- The life expectancy rate is rising; and,
- Many people are alive today who were born before the fertility rate began to fall. The inevitable consequence is that developed nations face today a greater increase in the numbers of

older people within the populations than there has ever been before.

This situation will continue well into the second half of the twenty-first century. At that point the effects of a lower fertility rate will produce a more balanced age grouping of the populations. The increase in the number of elderly people alive within the populations already has, and will continue to have, profound social and economic effects on all countries.

In 1972, the United Nations Economic and Social Council (UNESCO) organised the first World Assembly on Ageing to consider the effects that the rising numbers of elderly people within populations were creating. As the then Secretary General said, 'For the first time in human history this generation has seen the creation of a new human age group – the ageing'. Such a significant social event obviously produces new health needs, which in turn challenge attitudes, change working practices, and alter existing arrangements for the care of elderly people.

Nursing elderly people

One such change occurred in nursing in Great Britain in July 1979. In order to comply with European Community (EC) nursing directives, all student nurses entering general training after that date were required to have planned experience during the three years training period in 'the welfare of elderly people and the care of the elderly sick' (General Nursing Council, 1977).

This chapter is intended to inform and therefore help the student who is required to nurse elderly people.

Growing old is not easy: changes occur which demand both physical and psychological adjustments and much stamina and flexibility are needed by an individual if inevitable losses are to be balanced by gains. Yet stamina and flexibility are too often lacking as the capacity to maintain homeostasis is reduced, old ways become set as though in concrete, and finance is frequently severely reduced.

Nursing those growing old is not easy either, and requires sophisticated communication skills, a substantial amount of specialised knowledge, and great maturity on the part of the nurses. 'To encourage and nurse an elderly person so that they may return to their normal habits demands not only

patience, but teaching and counselling skills far in excess of the ability to control a patient on a life support machine' (Castledine, 1982). But the rewards of such work are great, both for the elderly person and the nurse.

The elderly person

In the developed countries of the world, the age at which a person becomes elderly is usually linked to that of the official retirement age from work. This is an arbitrary age set by the government, and may vary from country to country. In Britain a person is considered elderly when he has reached the age of 65 – the official retirement age for men – and he may draw his old age pension. Because more people are surviving past their 65th year, old age pensioners now form a large group of the population with unique problems, interests and rights. There are enough of them today to create a considerable socio-economic and political impact on their own.

Demographic trends

Why are more people living longer?

There are three concepts to be understood before considering this question. These are the differences inherent in the words lifespan, longevity and life expectancy.

Lifespan means the number of years it is possible for a human being to survive. Only in rare instances is this more than 100 years.

Longevity is species specific: a human being lives and dies within a 100 year span, a mouse within three years, a fruit fly within 75 days. No fruit fly lives for 100 years!

Life expectancy is calculated by studying present death rates with regard to future progress in medicine and science. Life expectancy rates have increased because child mortality rates have decreased. The care of pregnant women, and the care of the young child, have ensured that those born can look forward to a longer lifespan and have an increased life expectancy rate.

This care of the young has been aided by the much improved standards of housing, heating, sanitation and, especially, nutrition that have been achieved for all during the last century. Medical care for all sections of the population has improved since the introduction of the NHS in July 1948. The discovery of antibiotics, and the increase in vaccination and immunisation with improvements in anaesthesia and surgical techniques have either prevented illness or been able to cure it. Therefore, more people are living longer.

Statistics relating to elderly people in the UK

From 1900 to 1951 the growth of the pensionable age population of the United Kingdom rose from 6% of the total population to 14% (Table 26.1). Unfortunately, the figures from the 1991 census will not be available until 1993; however, projected figures in Table 26.1 for 1991 and 2001 are borne out by Warnes (1989): 'Since 1951, the growth (of the elderly numbers) in the relative share of the population has slowed, though until the 1970s the absolute annual increase remained substantial. Not until the first decade of the next century, when the high post-1945 birth cohorts reach retirement, will there again be a further substantial increase in the elderly population of Britain'. Today, the ratio of elderly people to the total population is reducing.

However, for those who plan or care for elderly people, it is the changes occurring within the over-65 age population that are important. Firstly, elderly people are dividing into two distinct groups – the young-elderly (those aged from 60–75 years) and the old-elderly (those over 75 years of age).

Within the total population of elderly people an increasing number are surviving into very old age.

Whereas in 1901, half a million elderly people were over 75 years of age (21%), in 1951 this figure had risen to 1.8 million (26%). By 1981 there were 3.2 million people over 75 years of age (32% of the elderly population). For 1991 the projected figure for very old people is 3.6 million or 36%; and by 2001 it is expected that 38% of the elderly population as a whole will be over 75 years of age (Tinker, 1984).

The very old are more frail, less likely to have living, active relatives, more likely to live alone, and more subject to ill health than the younger elderly. It is this division of elderly people into two distinct groups which is, for carers, the most significant development of the latter half of this century; the grouping of young-elderly (a great number of whom are active and self-sufficient, needing minimum help, or who only intermittently require formal care) and the separate group of old-elderly (an increasing group where large numbers are frail, dependent and who require continuous care).

Secondly, because of the earlier lifestyle of many elderly people, when women remained in the home and men went out to work, the life expectancy rates of the two sexes are different. The life expectancy rate for women is 76 years, and for men 71 years (Warnes, 1989). These figures represent the average – many people of course live longer than this. As women change their lifestyle, though, their life expectancy rate may also change. At present, however, the numbers of elderly women and men in hospital care are usually in a ratio of four women to every one man.

For this reason, the female pronoun is used for the patient throughout the chapter, unless this is clearly inappropriate.

Table 26.1. *The elderly as a proportion of the total population (figures taken from Tinker, 1984)*

	Year	Total population in millions	Elderly* in millions	Elderly as % of total
	1901	38.2	2.4	6
	1951	50.5	6.9	14
	1981	56.3	10.0	18
Projected figures on current trends	1991	57.2	10.0	17
	2001	58.3	9.5	16

* males over 65, females over 60

Ageism

'Ageism is the notion that people cease to be people, cease to be the same people, or become people of a distinct and inferior kind, by virtue of having lived a specific number of years'
(Comfort, 1977)

Ageism is a prejudice similar to sexism or racism.

'No society can call itself civilised if it treats its older generation with a lack of consideration. But consideration requires understanding and everyone needs to know more about the process of ageing and the difficulties it may bring. Ultimately, the quality of life of elderly people, especially the very old and frail, rests on the attitudes and perceptions of those younger than themselves'

(DHSS, 1981)

Attitudes play an all-important role in determining behaviour. They affect judgement and perception of other people; they influence the speed and efficiency of learning; and they help decide which groups one becomes friendly or identifies with. The feelings and thoughts which activate behaviour are themselves moulded by the culture and traditions of the society in which we all live, and are fashioned by our experience, education and training.

A common attitude of society towards elderly people is that something must be done, but that someone else should do it. Student nurses need to increase their knowledge of the world elderly people live in, and the concepts and processes of ageing, in order that they, at least, can care more effectively for elderly patients. Problems that occur are frequently caused by understimulation and overprotection so that elderly patients become dependent; by becoming authoritarian – not listening, giving orders ('you *have* to have a bath', 'you *must* take these pills'); by treating adults as children; or by the generation and educational gap between elderly patients and young students which hinders communication.

Gerontology – the study of ageing

Ageing is normal and inevitable for any living organism. Ageing starts at conception and continues until death. In this chapter ageing is considered to be the process which occurs as the adult passes from maturity to older ages.

Chronological age

Chronological age is often the only concept people have about ageing: 'How old are you?'. In human terms chronological age is represented by birthdays. However, these birthdays represent only the number of times the earth has revolved around the sun during the person's lifetime. Time is, of itself, neutral; it is what happens to the person during that time that is significant. Knowing a person's age gives minimal information about that person.

Ageing in everyday speech

Here the common concept is that ageing equals decline. It is this connotation that introduces the surprise into a commentator's speech as an older person completes a marathon or launches himself into a second career after retirement. Yet decline in function and ability can often be observed in individuals well before their sixty-fifth birthday. Professional sportsmen may have to enter veterans' competitions after the age of 30; some gymnasts are 'old' at the age of 20; a young person crippled with rheumatoid arthritis may have joint damage more usually associated with an 80 year old.

Biological age

Biological age depends on biological efficiency. The passage of time brings irreversible changes which make the individual increasingly unable to cope with the stresses of his environment. *It is biological efficiency which is altered if a person becomes ill.* Also parts of the body can become less efficient biologically, while other parts remain efficient.

It is unfortunate that many decisions about patient care are made on a chronological age basis alone – for example, in some centres no person over 65 will be admitted to the intensive care unit, or no patient over 65 will be allowed to get out of bed at night. An understanding of the difference between a patient's chronological age and his biological age is essential in planning care for elderly patients. Knowledge and experience is also vital before making judgements as to the extent of irreversible damage (Birren, 1964).

Psychological age

The way a person ages psychologically refers to the adaptive capacity of the individual towards his environment. The psychological age of a person is closely linked to the state of such key organs as heart and lungs, but also involves memory, learning, intelligence, skills, feelings, emotions, and motivation. It therefore depends heavily on the state of his brain – which may have nothing to do with his chronological age. Indeed, the phrase 'an old head on young shoulders' suggests disadvantages to psychological youthfulness (Birren, 1964).

Functional age

Functional age represents an individual's capacity to function in society relative to others of his (chronological) age. Perhaps this concept can best be understood by comparing the skills of car driving/road sense of men aged 75 or 80 years today, with women of the same age. The same could be done by contrasting women's skills in meal preparation with those of men. It is the unwise medical team that discharges an elderly, recently widowed, gentleman home to shop for and prepare his meals, without considering his functional age in this capacity. It may be that of a small child (Birren, 1964).

Social age

Social age refers to the social behaviour of an individual relative to his chronological age. Recently, an elderly man was refused entry into several discotheques 'because discos are for young people'. The phrase 'mutton dressed as lamb' refers, cruelly, to a person who is considered to be at variance in her dress with her perceived chronological age (Birren, 1964).

An alert, well-adjusted and healthy individual would produce the pattern indicated by Fig. 26.1. This pattern can be constructed for many senior citizens over 60, who continue to work efficiently and to function effectively. It is alterations in this pattern that show why two patients of the same chronological age are so different. Understanding of the various concepts of ageing enables nurses to deliver sensitive and appropriate care for elderly patients.

Theories of ageing

No two individuals age at the same rate. The cells within each individual age at different rates. No one has yet discovered an Elixir of Youth (though many have tried). No theory has been proved absolute to the exclusion of all others. These four facts should be remembered when one considers theories of ageing.

Biological ageing

What causes biological ageing? Schneider et al., in 1987, wrote 'While gerontology, the study of ageing, is an old discipline, it has had significant funding only in the past ten years. As a result, we are just at the earliest stages of our understanding

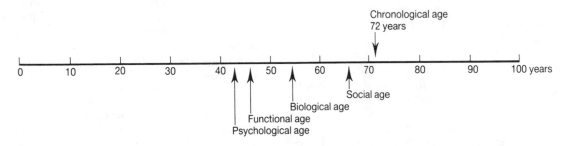

Fig. 26.1 *A positive pattern of ageing*

Table 26.2. *Theories of ageing (adapted from Schneider et al. 1987)*

Theory	Proponent
Collagen theory	Verzar (1957)
Cross-linking theory	Bjorksten (1968)
Endocrine theory	Korenchevsky and Jones (1947)
Error catastrophe theory	Orgel (1963)
Free radical theory	Harman (1955)
Immunological theory	Walford (1969)
Metabolic theory	Carlson *et al.* (1957) Johnson *et al.* (1961)
Programmed senescence theory	Hayflick (1968)
Rate of living theory	Pearl (1928)
Somatic mutation theory	Sziland (1959)
Waste product theory	Carrell and Ebeling (1923)
Wear and tear theory	Pearl (1928)

of the basic nature of ageing processes'. They have produced a useful table of the most prominent theories, reproduced in Table 26.2.

There is today, especially in the United States, much research that is ongoing both to prove and/or disprove further refinements of the above theories, and to create new theories. It is doubtful, however, that any single theory will be found to explain all the mechanisms of ageing.

Ageing processes appear to involve many different genes and to occur separately at molecular, cell and organ levels. 'Ageing is more complex than cancer and will probably require more theories to explain its multi-causal nature' (Schneider *et al.*, 1987).

A brief explanation of the theories

(1) *Theories based on genetics*
Examples include:
– an inherited genetic programme. When this programme is complete, the cells die (*Programmed Senescence*);
– a 'growth' substance (other than, or similar to, growth hormone) fails to be produced;
– a gradual malfunction of the ability of DNA or RNA to synthesise and translate messages (*Error Catastrophe*);
– a steady accumulation of *lipofuscin* (a nonfunctional, non-soluble lipoprotein) which builds up in the liver, heart, ovaries and neurones.

(2) *Theories based on the auto-immune system*
As the body ages, there is a gradual breakdown in the body's immunochemical memory – as for example, in rheumatoid arthritis or maturity onset diabetes.

(3) *Collagen-linked theories*
Collagen is a protein. Collagen in connective tissue, one of the most prevalent tissues in the body, becomes distorted and cross-linked as the person ages. This distortion reduces the rate at which nutrients are absorbed and waste disposed of, and reduces the efficiency of nerve pathways.

(4) *Wear and tear theory*
This is a mechanistic theory: stresses and/or continual work lead to less efficient functioning. Machines wear out eventually, however carefully they are serviced.

(5) *Free radical theory*
Oxygen is essential to life but the byproduct of oxygen metabolism, free radicals, are toxic. Free radicals left in the body will damage cell membranes, DNA and proteins. Normally the antioxidant system (a homeostatic mechanism) mops up free radicals. Vitamins C and D and a number of enzymes are anti-oxidants, but if these substances are deficient or unable to be synthesised, free radicals and damage increase.

(6) *Disease-producing organisms* – such as bacteria, viruses and fungi – which shorten life.

(7) *Radiation*
Low level radiation appears to have no immediate effect, but has been shown to shorten life span in animals. Excess ultraviolet light exposure eventually causes 'old age' type skin wrinkling.

(8) *Nutrition*
Excess nutrition, beyond that which the body needs to grow and replace cells, causes obesity. Rats have been shown to increase their lifespan if their nutrition is reduced from free feeding levels (McCay *et al.*, 1956, cited by Hall, 1984). It is quality of nutrition that counts, not quantity.

(9) *Environmental influences*
Ingesting non-lethal doses of substances (such as mercury, lead, arsenic or pesticides) produces pathological changes similar to ageing. Tobacco smoking and excessive alcohol drinking 'age' the lungs and the liver. Crowded living conditions,

excessive stress, and overload of coping mechanisms also shorten life.

Psychosocial theories of ageing

Cumming and Henry (1961) hold that people gradually disengage themselves from life as they get older. Disengagement is sometimes encouraged by society which says, 'You're too old. It's time you retired', or sometimes by the person who says, 'I'm too old. You do it.' Disengagement can be seen as producing an orderly transfer of power from the old to the young.

Maddox and Eisdorfer (1962) hold that it is the maintenance of *activity* that keeps older people young in heart. Interest in what is going on in the world helps to keep people up to date. Contact with children, grandchildren or other young people is helpful. However, activities and interests outside the home are difficult to maintain if income is limited.

Some theorists (e.g. Neugarten, 1973) believe that personality and basic patterns of behaviour are unchanged as people age. Others believe that women become more assertive and aggressive as they get older, and that men become more nurturing and expressive. It is obvious that all not old ladies are sweet and gentle, nor all old men kindly and loving, just as not all young people are thoughtful or passive. It is what has happened to people as they age which may change their personalities, or reflect what opportunities were available to them during their lives.

For a comprehensive explanation of the above theorists — and many others — read Chapter 10 of *Adult Development and Aging* by Hayslip and Panek, 1989.

Processes of ageing

These processes are *normal* developments in human beings as they age. Some start before maturity is reached, depending upon the genetic inheritance, the lifestyle and environment that individuals have.

Homeostasis

Homeostasis, or the ability of the body to maintain a constant internal environment despite a constantly changing external environment, is necessary for life. A constant internal environment is achieved by 'a complex series of physiological and biochemical changes and responses and almost all the organs of the body participate in this process . . .' (Herbert, 1986).

When illness occurs, the ability to maintain homeostasis is disturbed. Fortunately, with treatment and support, the ability can be restored and the body has been provided with an extensive reserve capacity to maintain homeostasis (for example, reserves of lung and kidney tissue which, normally, are not called into use).

Though an elderly person is usually able, unless ill, to maintain homeostasis, the reserve capacity may be much less than it was. Repeated insults coupled with ageing processes can produce the situation where homeostasis can be maintained in normal 'resting' states but not under conditions of sudden stress.

It should always be remembered that ageing processes take place at different rates; that not all people 'age' at the same time or in the same way; and that previous lifestyle or illnesses may 'age' some parts of the body yet leave other parts unaffected. There is no typical 70 or 80 year old. Older people are much more unlike each other than, say, two year olds are.

Changes in body systems that occur with ageing

In the following section, nursing considerations are included in the discussion of each system.

Surface areas of the body

In the *skin* the elasticity of the collagen layer of the dermis is reduced and altered by cross-linkage, and changes occur in the amino acid structure of collagen. The water content of cells is reduced. The effect of this is to produce thinner, more fragile, dry and wrinkled skin.

Nursing considerations
The use of hard water and poor quality soap with inadequate, rough drying causes further damage. Moisturising creams, emulsifying ointments and bath oils should be used. Gentle, thorough drying is essential. An electric hair dryer on a warm setting can be employed to help dry awkward areas.

Do this at the bedside, not in the bathroom, for safety.

Hair loses its original colour and becomes grey or white. It becomes thinner and more brittle. Baldness may occur. Due to decreased oestrogen production after the menopause, however, women may show an increase in facial hair.

Nursing considerations
Heat is lost very quickly from the head. When outside in cold weather, elderly people should wear hats or caps, or at least have their heads covered. Heads should also be covered in strong sunlight to avoid burning, especially if the head is bald.

Hair should be washed as necessary, and attractively cut and arranged. Hairdressers should be encouraged to visit elderly patients. Facial hair on women should be removed, provided the patient agrees.

Mouth and teeth: accumulated tooth decay and the build up of **plaque** may cause teeth to fall out and gums to recede. Dentures made many years ago may no longer fit.

Nursing considerations
Elderly people should be encouraged to visit their dentist regularly. Transport may have to be arranged and appointments made. New dentures may be necessary. Denture fixative may be a novelty to them. Dentures need cleaning just as frequently as natural teeth. If there are dentures, the mouth also needs cleaning and rinsing.

Nails become harder and more brittle. Many elderly people cannot reach down to cut their own toe nails.

Nursing considerations
It is better to file nails short than cut them. Visits to or from the chiropodist should be encouraged.

Special senses

Vision: changes in the crystalline lens of the eye make it unable to change shape to focus on near objects (Kritzinger, 1989). This is called *presbyopia*. Eventually a pathological condition may develop, as more and more layers of tissue are laid down on the lens surface, causing **cataract**. Intra-

ocular pressure rises with age, and this may develop into the pathological condition of **glaucoma**.

With age comes an increasing inability to accommodate the amount of light let into the eye, because of increasing rigidity of the iris. Peripheral vision ceases to be so wide.

Nursing considerations
Objects (including speaking faces) must be held at the correct distance from the elderly person for them to be seen. Eye contact – at the right distance – should be ensured before speech is begun. Glasses should be clean, available, and worn.

When possible, approach patients from in front. Try not to use high winged chairs which cut down side vision. Do not sit patients in straight rows side by side and expect them to talk to each other.

Lighting should be arranged so that it shines over patients' shoulders, and should be strong. A dimly lit ward at night means most patients will have difficulty in seeing, and will need more time to adjust their eyes if lights or torches are switched on. Not seeing properly is a sure recipe for inducing confusion and is unsafe.

Notices should be clear, and at an appropriate height.

Hearing: the tympanic membrane gradually becomes less effective in transmission of sound. The ability to hear high frequency sounds is usually the first to diminish. Wax builds up and becomes harder (Eliopoulous, 1987).

Nursing considerations
It is counterproductive to become excited and raise the tone of one's voice in order to make a patient understand. Lower the tone, speak more slowly, stand in front and obtain eye contact. Do not bellow into the ear from the side. Make sure background noise (for example, from radios, television, cleaning equipment, multiple conversations) is reduced. It is because the ward is quiet and the patient is concentrating that she suddenly understands what the helpfully tenor or baritone voice of the male doctor says.

Hearing aids should be in good working order, and worn in the correct ear. Wax should be softened and then removed by a nurse who is experienced in this technique.

Taste and smell are two senses which are closely connected. There is an 80% reduction in the functioning of taste buds from that of the youthful level. Sweet and salt tastes are the first to diminish, which may be why many elderly people add large quantities of sugar and salt to their food.

Loss of acute smelling ability affects taste and appetite. It also may be dangerous. If an elderly person turns on the gas but forgets to light it, the smell of escaping gas does not warn her of what is happening. Subsequent attempts to light the gas result in lethal explosions (Rai *et al.*, 1989).

Nursing considerations
Tempting appetites requires skill. What people like and dislike in food has roots well into their past and in their culture. Many elderly people do not think of rice as a vegetable substitute, or find pizza too foreign. Sloppy mashed potato, mushy peas and soft white fish may be easily swallowed, but usually taste like cotton wool. More savoury foods, such as sardines, bananas – rather than a hard, unpeeled apple – or tender roast meat, rather than the eternal mince, should be offered.

Sense of touch: because of alteration to the dermal layer of the skin, the tactile sense may lose some of its acuteness. This alters awareness of pain, temperature discrimination and the sense of pressure. Scorch marks may be seen on legs from sitting too close to the fire, or elderly people may remain in one position too long – and are therefore at risk of pressure sore development.

Nursing considerations
It is essential to help elderly people to change their position frequently. It is often easier to do this if the person is in bed. The trend is to get patients up early and 'mobilise' them, but this should not mean getting them out of bed in the morning, and then leaving them for hours on end sitting in a chair. Mobilising implies *movement*.

Respiratory system

Lungs gradually lose elasticity and the smooth muscle strength in the airways diminishes. Lungs therefore become less effective. Gradually, alveoli are reduced, along with cilia and goblet cells (Villar *et al.*, 1991).

Nursing considerations
There is increased shortness of breath on exertion. Rehabilitation has to be taken slowly. There will be a slower recovery from bouts of chest infection, and increased difficulty in expectoration (i.e. the coughing up of mucus). Exercise has to be carefully planned and unhurried.

Cardiovascular system

The valves of the heart become gradually thicker (i.e. more fibrous) and more rigid. Blood vessels lose their elasticity. Deposits of *atheromatous plaque* on the inner lining of blood vessels increase in number (Green, 1985). Muscle action is weaker. The effects of this are a rise in blood pressure resulting from the increased **peripheral resistance** necessary to maintain **cardiac output**. Sudden stress – such as rising from a lying position to walk, when blood pressure has to be adjusted quickly – is not well managed and under such circumstances the person may faint. The extremities may become colder.

Nursing considerations
Blood pressure should be carefully monitored – especially the difference between that recorded in a standing position and that recorded in a lying position. If the need to sit up, stand up, and walk slowly is not recognised, enforced incontinence may occur when the person wishes to get to the toilet in a hurry. Hands, legs and feet should be kept covered and warm.

Gastro-intestinal system

The production of saliva may gradually be reduced – often because smell is reduced (saliva is produced as a conditioned reflex). Stomach motility and **peristalsis** slow. The production of gastric acid and intestinal secretions diminishes (Steen, 1985). This impedes digestion, especially if chewing is difficult; fewer vital nutrients are absorbed and slower peristalsis leads to a longer resting time for food waste in the large intestine. As a result more water is absorbed in the colon which can lead to constipation (Eliopoulous, 1987).

Nursing considerations
An adequate fluid intake is essential. Many elderly people do not like to drink too much because they are afraid of accidental incontinence. Sensitive, thoughtful nursing avoids this situation. Enough time has to be allowed for meals; small, frequent meals are better than large, infrequent ones. Simple

foods – such as sandwiches, fruit and ice cream – should be available at night.

Genito-urinary system

In the kidneys there is a gradual reduction of nephrons. There is also a reduction in renal blood flow. **Glomerular filtration** may become less effective, and there may be some albumin loss through the kidneys. Tubular function may be damaged resulting in less concentrated urine production. The kidneys lose some of their ability to balance electrolytes (Eliopoulous, 1987).

In the bladder, muscle strength weakens and capacity diminishes. The effects are that less concentrated urine has to be passed more often in smaller quantities. The prostate gland enlarges in men. Sexual organs gradually atrophy.

Nursing considerations

Elderly people need to go to the toilet more often than when they were young. The provision and accessibility of toilets in wards and residential homes is usually inadequate. This should be the *first priority* in planning new units. Much so-called incontinence occurs because the person cannot get to the toilet in time. Commodes should be used. The elderly person can be wheeled to the toilet and walking can be practised on the return journey.

Musculoskeletal system

Muscles atrophy and become replaced with fibrous tissue especially if they are not used. Intervertebral discs thin, and are therefore less effective as shock absorbers to the spinal column (Green, 1985). Height is lost. The bone marrow gradually becomes less effective, and there is reduction in calcium absorption by the bones. Joints may enlarge and fibrose. There is a decrease in physical strength, a reduction in new blood cell production, and bones are more brittle. Movement is affected and the body, without sufficient exercise, becomes stiffer. The head bends forward and **kyphosis** develops (Eliopoulous, 1987).

Nursing considerations

Elderly people need exercise within their limitations. A walk up a boring ward is unmotivating. A walk to a pub or shop may be much more interesting. Falling has to be foreseen and planned for

– by installation of suitable floor surfaces to reduce damage. A highly polished ward floor looks slippery and frightening. Suitable shoes which grip the floor are essential. Chairs, beds and toilets should be of a height to allow easy entrance and exit – or be easily adjustable to suit individual height and/or disability. If walking aids are used, they should be examined regularly to check for worn ferrules, etc.

Nervous system

There is no further neurone production after childhood. It is thought, moreover, that brain cells are lost gradually (Green, 1985). As neurones disappear, response time diminishes and reaction time to sudden stimuli lengthens. All the control centres become less effective. Sleep patterns change: many elderly people seem to sleep for shorter periods at night, but nap during the day. The person may have to get up several times during the night to pass urine (Green, 1985).

To balance without support in an upright position depends on the coordination of postural reflexes through efficient proprioception by sensory nerves, basal ganglia and cerebellar functions, and muscular strength. Any person who has watched a child learn to crawl, sit, stand and walk can see how complex this coordination is, and how much practice it takes to get it right. It is also greatly assisted by normal vision. If neurones diminish, if changes occur in the dermal layer of the skin, due to cross-linkage of collagen, which therefore interferes with the smooth passage of sensory and motor nerve impulses, if muscular strength weakens and if vision is impaired, is it surprising that elderly people may have increased problems with walking and standing, and an increased number of falls? Sway also increases (Brocklehurst and Hanley, 1981).

Ageing and psychological functioning

Psychological development depends on a number of factors: sensory ability, general health, genetic factors, education and activity.

Personality changes may occur through losses such as that of a spouse, a job, independence in the activities of living, a home, money or abilities.

The gradual loss of ability may not be such a great shock as the sudden loss of a dearly loved husband, wife or friend. Gradual decline in function may be seen as inevitable but is still not welcomed – especially if the elderly person does not feel any different inside.

Memory

We are dependent upon what we have learned for survival. One hallmark of learning is memory, which is why memory is so often tested in examinations. Remembering is a function of the brain by a series of interlocking systems. Even if one has 'lost' one's memory, the abilities of talking, thinking and doing are often retained. Any one or more of the links may be faulty, but not all at the same time. Retrieval from memory becomes more difficult as one grows older – there is more on file to retrieve from. It is becoming clearer that the difficulty many older people have with short-term memory is due to a diminishing ability to *encode* new material, which then makes the retrieval less easy, if not impossible (Hayslip and Panek, 1989).

Learning abilities are affected by motivation, the length of the attention span, the difficulties inherent in extinguishing old learning and the ease with which motor performance may be achieved. All these factors may make it less easy to 'teach an old dog new tricks', but it can be done.

The following poem was written by an elderly lady in her 80s who attended a writing course and subsequently published a book entitled '*Old Age Ain't No Place for Sissies!*'

No Freedom

The world will never be free for me
Because I'm on Social Security—
Social life is out, you see
And secure I know I'll never be.

(McGee, 1986)

Table 26.3 lists some practical considerations in teaching an elderly person new material. Next time a patient is discharged, try to remember these points when explaining the drugs she should take. It is useless to give her a paper bag with several bottles in it, and say cheerily, 'Don't forget to take your tablets' (Shulman, 1989).

Table 26.3. *Practical considerations in teaching an elderly person new material*

(1) Do not think in an age-specific way (e.g. a 60 year old can learn this, but an 80 year old cannot)
(2) Avoid tasks that have to be performed under time pressure. Let the elderly person work at her pace, not yours
(3) Avoid creating anxiety. Allow plenty of time for the person to become familiar with the equipment
(4) Do things her way. Keep changes small. Explain slowly
(5) Teach in small steps. Instructions should be written to help memory retrieval
(6) Allow for difficulties in hearing, sight or physical discomfort
(7) Expect slower reaction time
(8) Praise and reward success

Sociology and ageing

Some understanding of the sociological aspects of ageing is important if elderly people are to benefit from holistic nursing care.

Old age in history

In the pre-industrial era, early death was commonplace. Survival over the age of 40 was uncommon; those who did survive, therefore, became venerated. In a society that changed slowly, the wisdom of those that had lived the longest was apparent. Under the Elizabethan Poor Laws, parishes were obliged to support those who were too old or too young or otherwise incompetent to support themselves. As today, the majority of old and young were supported by their families, but literature is full of stories of workhouses, orphanages and madhouses for those without family support. Gradually, because there was little that could be done to prevent the spread of infection when these, the frailest members of society, were placed together in this way, these institutions became more like hospitals.

It was the efficient, orderly Victorians who separated the groups, and who, in the main, built large satellite mental hospitals and workhouses ringing the major cities. They also separated out the infectious cases, and built fever hospitals. Many of these buildings still exist today, and many are now geriatric units. Even though upgraded, the physical plant is often so old and inefficient that many of the difficulties nurses face in caring for elderly patients stem from this Victorian legacy.

It was not until 1908 that old age pensions were first introduced. People had to be 70 years old, with 20 years of residential qualifications in one area, because the scheme was administered by a local pension committee. Those receiving poor relief were disqualified from receiving a pension. Ten years had to pass after a prison sentence (this was later reduced to two years in 1911), there was a moral code to be passed, and the pension was five shillings a week. One had to be very old, very poor, and very respectable to receive the pension.

Gradually, this system has been amended by successive governments to today's rate (1992) of £54.15 for single people and £86.70 for couples per week. National Insurance contributions are levied on all those who work during their lifetime to help pay for their (eventual) pension.

Also today there exists a complex range of supplementary benefits available to those in need. However, you have to know about them to apply for them. It takes knowledge, time, patience, the ability to travel to offices or to have someone to travel for you, and much form-filling to succeed.

All are means-tested and unfortunately many elderly people are unwilling to accept what they consider to be charity or are frightened that their small savings will be taken away (see section entitled Governmental Help for more details).

Currently, health screening targets are set for general practitioners and health authorities, e.g. with regard to cervical smears and mammography. It would probably be more beneficial in the elderly age groups to offer 'social screening' in order to achieve a greater pick-up rate in extra benefits. This would create improvements in general health.

Changes in family structure

Family size has gradually been shrinking. Changing from an agricultural society, where many children were needed to work the land, to an industrial society where many hands were needed to work machines, to today's technological society, has reduced the need for manpower. Today, the nuclear family, of two parents and two children, is the norm. However, because of increased lifespan, more people live longer. Therefore it is possible to have four generations of a family alive together for a longer time. Great-grandparents, grandparents, parents and children may all live together.

Families have always been the main carers for their elderly relatives. This is as true today as it ever was. Only 6% of elderly people today live in hospitals, residential homes or nursing homes. The remaining 94% either live alone, or with relatives and friends (Tinker, 1984). Again, the 1991 census figures are not yet available, but the percentages are not thought to have changed significantly.

As the numbers of domestic servants and children decrease and more people live further away from their workplace, as travel has become easier, faster and more available, houses have become smaller and many younger families have moved into suburban areas leaving their elderly relatives behind in inner city areas. When an elderly person needs care, the family may be too far away, or their house too small, to accept another family member.

Wealth versus poverty

It is not the wealthy elderly that present the NHS and its staff with problems. If the wealthy are sick, need a housekeeper, cannot walk, cook, shop, and take care of themselves, or are alone, they can buy the services that they require. They become employers and are therefore valued. Why are the elderly poor or those not so well-to-do considered burdens, or 'bed-blockers', by many doctors and nurses? It is usually because their poverty makes attempts to alter their living conditions so difficult, and therefore the elderly person outstays his welcome in the acute NHS sector. As acute hospital care becomes ever more costly, government is shifting responsibility for care for those unable to make a quick, efficient recovery onto the community. This means an increased workload and costs to both local authorities and the community-based NHS service, such as health centres, district nurses and health visitors (see Community Care Act (1990) later in the chapter).

Students who follow a Project 2000 training will be qualified to work in either the acute hospital service or the community service. It is inevitable that many of their patients or clients will be elderly, whichever branch of the service is chosen.

Local authorities

The major providers of services to elderly people have been the Social Services and Housing departments of local authorities. These provide residential services, day care services, domiciliary services, and a variety of other services.

Residential services

There are two main types of residential services: *old people's homes* – run by the Social Services department – and *sheltered housing* (sometimes called *warden-controlled units*) – run by the Housing department.

The best old people's homes offer residents a single room into which they may introduce some smaller items of their own furniture. Many, however, have been converted from larger houses – often old and inconvenient – and require residents to share a room with others. Consider for a moment how distasteful it may be to an elderly person to share a room, when the desire of most children is to achieve a room of their own! There should be a lift and plenty of bathrooms and toilets. Old people's homes are run by officers, with care assistants to help the residents. There is usually a communal dining room and sitting room(s). Residents may remain under the care of their GP.

Old people's homes are sometimes called Part III homes, because they exist under Part III of the National Assistance Act 1948 – which requires local authorities to maintain homes for those in need.

Sheltered housing units have increased in number over the last ten years. Here, each resident has her own self-contained flat or bed-sitter, with her own cooking and bathroom facilities. She has the key to her own front door, and furnishes and maintains her home herself. Originally there was a resident warden, who was responsible for making daily contact with each resident, and whose assistance could be summoned by an alarm system in each flat. There may be some communal facilities, such as washing machines or meeting rooms. Residents in this type of accommodation must be reasonably self-sufficient, able to cook, clean and care for themselves. However, they may receive help from *home helps, meals on wheels, or district nurses*.

In the last few years, to reduce costs, many wardens have been replaced by radio/telephone systems. This transition has not been without problems – many residents miss the daily contact with a friendly person; some inappropriately test that the system is working every hour; some find it difficult to remember how the system operates at all. The housing complex may also suffer from increased vandalism or even assaults on residents because of the absence of a warden.

There has been a substantial increase in the number of private residential and sheltered housing schemes that have opened in the 1980s.

Domiciliary care services

The *home help* service is of great value in providing a lifeline to many elderly people. Home helps are usually younger women living locally. The tasks they undertake include cleaning, tidying, lighting fires, washing up, shopping and bedmaking, but some will help with cooking and washing. Often a warm, personal relationship is established between the elderly person and the home help. Home helps are often the best source of information about the normal capabilities of an elderly person if she becomes ill and is admitted to hospital. Many local authorities are piloting new schemes which offer intensive domiciliary help for short periods. Elderly people, therefore, can be discharged earlier from hospital or avoid hospital admission.

Most local authorities make an hourly charge for the home help service.

The *meals on wheels* service usually consists of a cooked meal delivery to the old person's house. Outside large metropolitan areas this service is often run by the Women's Royal Voluntary Service (WRVS), Age Concern or the British Red Cross Society, with the support of the local authority. It is important for nurses to understand that meals on wheels is a *back-up service*; an elderly person cannot live on this service. It is almost impossible to get meals on wheels seven days a week; two or three days is the norm and seldom at weekends. An elderly person cannot be discharged from hospital to live alone if he cannot – as an absolute minimum – boil and pour a kettle of water safely, or has no help to do this. There is usually a charge for this service.

Laundry service is obtainable from some local authorities to help with the washing of increased quantities of sheets and other bedlinen. Some other authorities have special rubbish collections to cope with incontinence pads or colostomy bags.

Day care

Local authorities also run *day centres*. These are more like clubs, and provide meals (lunch), some kind of recreational activity, and give opportunities for elderly people to meet. Many authorities now run *pop-in centres* in towns where elderly people may rest, have a cup of tea, and meet others while out shopping.

Other services

Table 26.4 gives a list of other services which may be run by local authorities, often in conjunction with voluntary agencies. A major problem is that all or none of these services may be in operation in any given local authority. Development depends on the money available and often the creativity of local authority staff.

The social worker

The social worker can provide the vital link between the elderly person and the availability of any of the local authority services. The social worker should be included in the multidisciplinary team involved in the discharge of an elderly person who needs Social Services from hospital. Nurses cannot order meals on wheels five days a week for a patient, nor decide that Mrs Jones must be admitted to the Rosy Old People's Home. The social worker is the link between the hospital sector and the Social Services or Housing department of the local authority.

Voluntary groups which help the elderly

Many groups work in conjunction with local authorities; some work on their own.

Special interest groups

There are numerous special interest groups. Examples are: the Royal Association in Aid of the Deaf and Dumb; the Royal National Institute for the Blind (RNIB); the Royal Society for Mentally Handicapped Children and Adults (MENCAP); all denominations of religious organisations; the Women's Royal Voluntary Service (WRVS); the British Red Cross Society, and the Salvation Army. Some groups, such as Age Concern or Help the Aged, are age-specific and work only with elderly

Table 26.4. *Services for elderly people*

- Installation of telephones
- Installation of alarm systems
- Provision of aids and adaptations to housing – such as banister rails, widening doors, etc.
- Good neighbour schemes
- Holiday schemes
- Short-stay residential accommodation so that relatives of an elderly person may go away on holiday
- Day-sitting, evening-sitting or night-sitting schemes
- Roof insulation

people. Without the work and time given by voluntary agencies, many elderly people would be totally alone and bereft.

The major carer

Despite all the available assistance, the greatest amount of care is delivered by the families of elderly people. This care is informal, mostly given with love and is, usually, the best form of care.

Friends and neighbours also give much of this type of care. The social network that any old person has created around herself is very important when her discharge from hospital is being planned. A patient's *social network* must be explored when she is admitted. The elderly person often arrives in the hospital only because the social network around her has – for some reason – broken down or become unable to cope.

Government help

The social worker is usually the key to obtaining extra financial help for an elderly person, or such help may come following visits to the local Social Security office. The basic old-age pension may be drawn after the age of 60 years for women and 65 years for men. An extra amount is available for those over 80. There is a host of further additional benefits for those who have only the basic pension to live on. The major one is income support which is means-tested (i.e. the level is set according to the recipient's existing financial resources). Free prescriptions and remission of charges for spectacles, dentures and dental treatment are currently available only to pensioners on low incomes.

Local authorities are permitted to allow Council

Tax reductions and rent allowances to some pensioners, although this may depend on the amount that the elderly person has in savings. The Community Charge is shortly to disappear and will be replaced by a modified rating system dependant upon property.

Special heating allowances and attendance allowances may also be available. Travel at a reduced rate is often possible and British Rail allows pensioners to travel at half-price with a special card which they have to purchase.

The take-up of special allowances is variable, and many elderly people do not know what may be available. Many Post Offices and public libraries provide leaflets, but these may not always be easy for elderly people to understand – or to find. All hospitals with elderly patients should have a supply of leaflets freely available for patients and their relatives. Nurses should make certain they are aware of what is on offer and be able to direct patients or relatives to the information. They should also be sure that their information is up-to-date as financial allowances not infrequently undergo changes. The social worker should also be consulted.

The NHS and Community Care Act 1990

This Act was preceded by two governmental White Papers, *Working for Patients* (DoH, 1989) which set out changes in the National Health Service, and *Caring for People* (DHSS, 1989) which sought to change the way care in the community operated.

Caring for People was developed from a report by Sir Roy Griffiths (1988) which suggested that individual 'packages of care' should be organised/devised for all those in need of community care. These would range, for example, from providing a home help for a couple of hours a week to finding a permanent placement in a nursing home.

Griffiths hoped that this would mean that (i) people with disabilities or in long term care could go home, and (ii) families keeping relatives at home would be helped. He further suggested that the finance would come from central government.

The White Paper *Caring for People* (1989) said that (i) local authorities would become the lead agency for community care, (ii) the priority would be to keep people in their own homes, (iii) there was to be maximum use of the private and voluntary sectors, but (iv) the finance would come from the standard revenue support grant to local authorities (i.e. that there would be no extra money for implementation).

Shortly after the passage of the NHS and Community Care Act 1990, the Secretary of State for Health announced that the community care part of the Act would have to be implemented over a three year period beginning April 1st 1991:

1st Phase: (April 1991) New specific grants were to be made for services to people with mental illnesses and to drug and alcohol abusers. Local authorities should concentrate on these areas first.

2nd Phase: (April 1992) Local authorities should publish their first community care plans, having discussed them with health authorities, professional workers and consumers, etc., to determine need.

3rd Phase: (April 1993) Local authorities were to take on full responsibility for care in the community (Turner, 1989).

Care for elderly people will obviously be greatly affected but, at the time of writing, Phase 2 has just begun. How local authorities will manage their new responsibilities remains to be seen.

Dependency

One of the major problems for an elderly person as she ages is that of increasing dependency. The dependency of elderly people on the State, the Social Services, the family, or the goodwill of others, frequently has its roots in poverty. Many elderly poor prefer to live in poverty rather than accept what they see as 'charity'.

Other types of dependency that bedevil elderly people are listed in Table 26.5.

Table 26.5. *Types of dependency*

Life-cycle dependency	Their previous life experience has made them dependent *now* (for example the widower who cannot cook)
Inherited defect dependency	Traits or familial tendencies which they inherited from their parents either in the physical sense (e.g. poor eyesight) or the psychological sense
Acquired defect dependency	Usually resulting from illness or trauma (a stroke, for example)
Incomplete family dependency	They have no nearby or helpful relatives, or no children of their own, or no living family or friends

Retirement

'One of the commonest mistakes people make about retirement is to assume that it requires no effort, no preparation . . .'

(Pilch, 1974)

How people feel about their retirement depends on whether they are forced to retire because a certain chronological age has been reached, whether they are happy to retire whatever age has been reached, or whether, because of the nature of their work, they do not have to retire. Work gives shape, meaning and interest to life. Going to work is a habit formed over 40–50 years. For some, retirement may bring a sharp drop in income. To argue that retirement automatically brings the freedom to do whatever one wants to do is nonsensical if there is no money with which to do it. Retirement represents loss for many, and it may accompany the individual's first realistic look at his own ageing. Many go through bereavement and grieving processes following retirement. **Sudden death syndrome** has been classified as 'death within one year of retirement'.

It is necessary to prepare for retirement by widening interests and friendships outside the workplace, and by trying to save some money throughout life to supplement the basic State pension.

Medical, nursing and paramedical services and the elderly

Nursing homes

Since the proposed shift from hospital to community care was recommended, there has been an increase in nursing home provision. These are developed, run and staffed by three different groups – the NHS directly, housing associations or groups backed by church organisations, and the private sector for profit.

All nursing homes, whoever owns and runs them, have to be licensed and inspected by the health authority in which they are situated. There has to be a Registered General Nurse on the premises at all times. Each home must be inspected – a 'notified' inspection – annually, with a minimum of two unannounced inspection visits. In practice, most nursing homes are visited more frequently, especially if the inspectors are concerned about the standards of care provided. Only establishments with three or fewer residents should escape inspection.

The majority of staff in the homes are care assistants – some with minimal or no training. The standard of care within the homes can vary widely and there are usually long waiting lists for the best homes.

Most health authorities run separate homes for the elderly mentally ill (EMI) client. Here the provision of suitable homes lags seriously behind the numbers needing care and the special needs of this type of client.

There are a number of different health professionals with whom elderly people are likely to come into contact.

General practitioners

GPs provide the bulk of medical care for elderly

people. In November 1989, effective from April 1990, the government introduced a new General Practitioner Contract as part of the reforms of the health service. For patients over 75, the Contract stipulates that each patient on the GP's list is to be invited to participate in a consultation, or offered a domiciliary visit, annually in order to assess any matter which appears to be affecting the patient's general health. An assessment of sensory functions, mobility, mental condition, physical condition, continence, social environment and use of medicines as appropriate should be completed (Pereira-Gray, 1990). Obviously, if pathological conditions or other problems are discovered these should then be treated or brought to the attention of the appropriate agency or health professional.

Many GPs are consequently employing more practice nurses and some health visitors and district nurses directly to assist with compliance with the Contract. Planning for the additional educational input for nurses and the development of a systematic assessment scheme is of current concern to doctors, nurses and managers (Sparkes and Kelsey, 1991).

Too often the insidious onset of disease is explained away by the elderly person as 'to be expected at my age'. The consequence is that disease is not diagnosed early – until the sufferer has become unstable, immobile or incontinent, or until the social network cannot cope any longer. By this time rehabilitation has become even more difficult.

District nurses

District nurses provide a nursing service for sick elderly people at home. For many, their visits and the care they provide become a key support. Their work may be preventive – giving the regular maintenance doses of drugs such as digoxin or thyroxine – or curative (for example, dressing venous ulcers). In areas where many elderly people live, this service can easily be overwhelmed by the demand.

Health visitors

Historically, health visitors have concentrated most of their work on children but since 1984 there have been some welcome additions to the community nursing service, in the form of health visitors specialising in care of elderly people.

Allied health professionals

Chiropodists provide an invaluable service to the elderly. The inability simply to cut one's toenails can be the first slip towards total immobility and social isolation. Physiotherapists, occupational therapists, and speech therapists are vital members of any multidisciplinary team providing care for elderly people.

Geriatricians

Geriatricians are consultant doctors who specialise in the diseases and problems of ageing, and who are responsible for geriatric departments. Unlike most other hospital-based consultants, geriatricians make domiciliary (home) visits, at the request of GPs, to advise on treatment for elderly patients. They are also responsible for *day hospitals* – usually attached to district general hospitals – where elderly patients can attend daily for physiotherapy, occupational therapy, nursing or medical care, returning home in the late afternoon. The existence of a day hospital means that patients can be discharged earlier from hospital yet continue a course of treatment.

In hospital, some geriatric departments divide patients into *assessment/**rehabilitation** wards* or ***continuing care** wards*; others mix shorter and longer stay patients in the same ward. Some hospitals organise geriatric beds within medical wards. In all hospitals, many elderly patients are to be found on all types of wards (other than paediatric).

Since 1982, the NHS has been experimenting with the development of *nursing homes* for patients who cannot return to their own homes. This is a welcome development as sensitive, home-like care for longer stay patients may be difficult to achieve within a hospital devoted to rapid turnover.

Multidisciplinary teams

Effective teamwork is essential for effective care. The range of physical, psychological and social problems, let alone the disease processes, become so complex with elderly people that no discipline can work effectively in isolation. The social worker provides a vital link with the Social Service department of the local authority, and the Geriatric Liaison Nurse works both in hospital and out in the community. The team has to set up good communication links and the members must respect each other's expertise. It is essential that the patient and/or his relatives are aware of, and agree to, the plans of the team, a simple point which is sometimes, unfortunately, forgotten.

Nurses, who care for patients 24 hours a day, have to understand the work of other professional colleagues, and to coordinate the work of the team.

Illness in elderly people

Whenever an elderly person becomes ill, the normal ageing processes should always be considered when planning nursing care and giving treatment since they increase the complexity of the patient's needs. The disease may have an acute or insidious onset, or may be chronic – progressing slowly but inexorably, and forcing the sufferer from activity to inactivity.

Presentation of disease

The presentation of illness in an elderly person may differ in a number of ways from the presentation of illness in someone younger.

Awareness of pain

Pain in the elderly person may seem less severe to the observer than that seen in a younger person. The severity of a myocardial infarction may not be immediately apparent, or the effects of prolonged pressure on tissues may go unnoticed until it is too late to prevent the development of a pressure sore because of age-related changes in the skin, control centres and nervous system. The localisation of pain may be capricious and therefore misreported. Pain may be forgotten, or accepted stoically as inevitable, and therefore ignored.

Alteration in body temperature

The rise in body temperature in response to infection is frequently less effective in an elderly person, due to a slowed homeostatic response. Significant pyrexia may not be an early response to pneumonia or urinary tract infection. The shivering re-flex may no longer be fully effective, letting the elderly person become very cold without the usual warning. It is even possible for an elderly patient who is severely immobile to suffer from hypothermia in a heated hospital ward, especially if the hands, feet and head are uncovered.

The *first* warning sign of impending disease is sudden mental confusion.

Sudden mental confusion

The appearance of mental confusion in an otherwise alert person is *always* a warning sign that must be taken seriously. This is the time to call or consult the doctor. It should never be ignored or thought of as 'just old age catching up with the person at last'.

The presence of chronic disease

The existence of a known chronic disease can mask the onset of another illness or injury; for instance, a person with hemiplegia following a cerebrovascular accident can be discovered with a dislocated, paralysed shoulder. This unfortunate occurrence can happen if the patient has been lifted incorrectly. Because sensation and the normal protective muscular response are absent, dislocation may occur *without* pain if the shoulder is inexpertly raised. Suddenly, one observant onlooker notices the unusual way the arm is hanging, and dislocation is diagnosed. **Pathological fractures** can occur in limbs already distorted by joint or bone disease, but because the person limps anyway, this further damage may remain unreported until the sufferer becomes totally immobilised.

Increased incidence of falls

An increase in falls is often considered by the elderly to be due to paying insufficient attention, to failing eyesight, or to 'just tripping'. If increased falls occur without proper investigation, the elderly person only comes to medical attention when bones are broken or severe lacerations are caused (see also Nervous System earlier).

'I can't cope: we can't cope'

Only too often elderly people are presented to the doctor in these terms – either by themselves or more often by relatives, friends, neighbours, home helps or other carers. People say (for example):

'We could manage her increasing frailty, but now she's incontinent, it's too much'

'We could cope until she began falling without warning; but now we're afraid to let her out of our sight'

'I know the old are forgetful, but now she forgets to light the gas or lock the door; it's too risky to let her live alone any longer'

'He doesn't recognise me any more'

'She doesn't know day from night'

'It takes me over two hours just to get dressed'

'I'm afraid'

'We can't go on like this'.

Regardless of the underlying disease process, it is, above all, the introduction of any one of the 'four great I's of geriatric medicine', in the phrase coined by Professor Bernard Isaacs, that forces the inability to cope out into the open (Coni *et al.*, 1988). Families, friends, informal carers, or all forms of carers in the community find it increasingly difficult to manage if the elderly person has begun to suffer from: *Incontinence, Instability, Immobility,* or *Intellectual impairment.*

Aims of care

There are three main aims of care which are common for all patients who are elderly, on which their individual care plan should be based. These are the promotion of independence, the establishing of a key supporter, and the identification and achievement of a realistic outcome.

Independence

The first aim of care is to achieve the optimum level of independence possible. Skilled planning, with frequent evaluation and re-assessment, are required to achieve this aim. It is easy to write on a care plan 'encourage independence', but it is much less easy, and very time-consuming, to put this maxim into practice. Motivation may have been lost. Other losses may appear insuperable. The new learning necessary has to proceed at a slow, steady pace, and the gains may appear very small at first. Nurses faced with too much to do and too little time in which to do it find it quicker and easier to do things *for* patients. It is here that hope of achieving independent functioning begins to be lost, and ultimately the situation is created where the elderly person is subjected to long term hospitalisation and thought of as 'blocking' a bed needed for patients requiring acute care. Much patience and skill are required to teach, encourage, wait, and give only the help necessary to avoid frustration. The goals negotiated with the patient should be realistic and achievable – for example, 'By the end of the week Mrs Smith should put on her cardigan unaided' rather than a global goal such as 'restore full mobility in dressing' (see Fig. 26.2). The latter goal is unclear and set too far into the future; it may remain on the plan unchanged for weeks, if not months, and may never be achieved. Yet nothing succeeds like success. Praise for achievement realised is a far more effective motivator than recrimination, impatience and failure, so set small achievable goals.

Key supporter

The second aim of care is to identify and note the key supporter(s) for each patient.

The key supporter is the entity or person which enables the patient to remain independent, and without which she will inevitably return to care. It is often failure of the key supporter which has brought the patient into the hospital.

Once the key supporter has been identified, it may be necessary to support the supporter, as well as the patient, in order for a successful return home to be achieved. For example, a frail elderly lady can remain at home as long as her daughter is with her, but the daughter cannot be there 24 hours a day, year in year out, without some respite. It may be necessary to arrange respite care for the mother so that the daughter can go on holiday, or attendance at a day centre, giving the daughter free time for herself, or a night-sitter so that the daughter can rest properly. With this type of help, the daughter may continue to cope and the elderly lady remain at home.

Very careful assessment of the patient and her social networks, and understanding of the methods of usual functioning and of what has gone wrong, are necessary.

Many different people and things serve as key supporters. Relatives, friends and neighbours, and often home helps, are examples. Many pets serve

Fig. 26.2 *Care plan: concerned with the activity of personal cleansing and dressing*

Mrs Smith: Third week following admission for left cerebrovascular accident.
Right hemiplegia

Activity of Living: PERSONAL CLEANSING AND DRESSING (Roper, Logan and Tierney, 1990)

Goal (long term): To restore maximum ability and/or compensate for loss

Liaise with: Physiotherapist, occupational therapist, family

Problem	Goal (short term)	Nursing intervention	Evaluation
Movement of right arm restricted making self-dressing difficult	(1) By end of the week Mrs Smith will be able to put on and take off her cardigan herself	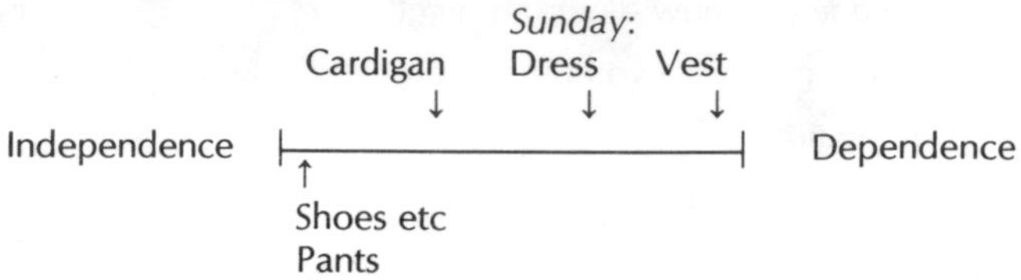	

Independence

Cardigan   *Sunday:* Dress   Vest
   ↓   ↓   ↓
├─────────────────────────────────────┤   Dependence
   ↑
Shoes etc
Pants

	Goal (short term)	Nursing intervention	Evaluation
	(2) Maintain progress with dress and vest	(Occupational therapist to teach method Monday and Tuesday) (a) Mrs Smith to be washed etc. and sitting out of bed by 10 am (b) 10 am visit by OT (c) Arrange further practice after lunch and in evening (d) Supervise (c) and follow method taught by OT (e) Do not let Mrs Smith become frustrated. Be patient (f) Encourage with praise when successful	(from previous week) *Wednesday:* Very slow but finally managed (half an hour) *Friday:* Much quicker. Physiotherapist helping with exercises *Saturday:* Success (5 mins) *Sunday:* Achieved except for buttons. Ask daughter to sew on new larger ones

Signed: *D. Potter* 26/2/92

---

the same function, giving interest, companionship, a reason for activity, and motivation to keep going. The welfare of these pets needs to be considered if the owner is admitted to hospital. If Blackie, the cat, is out wandering the streets, no wonder his elderly owner refuses to settle in hospital and keeps trying to climb out of bed or leave the unit.

Spectacles, hearing aids, dentures, walking sticks, Zimmer frames, etc. are other examples of key supports. The moment the patient says 'I can manage as long as I have . . .', the nurse should be alert. A key supporter is being identified. Another useful clue is a sentence beginning 'It doesn't seem to work properly any more . . .' A key supporter is failing. It is the wise nurse who checks to see

that the prescription for the spectacles is current, that the lenses are not hopelessly scratched, nor the frames broken; that the batteries for the hearing aid are strong, the connecting wires in place, and the ears not full of hard wax. The dentures may have been made many years ago and no longer fit, or they may be broken, and some patients have never heard of dental fixatives which help dental plates to stay in place; walking sticks may have been mislaid, they may not be strong enough or ferrules may get lost; Zimmer frames get bent out of shape or are the wrong height. Patients who live both upstairs and downstairs need two Zimmer frames – otherwise one has to be dragged upstairs, sometimes fastened by a piece of string to the patient's waist, then hurled downstairs in front of the patient so that it can be used on the lower floor!

Wishes can be powerful key supporters. The desire for a message from the Queen; the wish to finish a piece of work or embroidery; the determination to outlive a relative or friend; the longing to see a grandchild born, or for a relative to arrive after a long absence abroad, are some examples of powerful motivators, which keep the elderly person going. Again, it is the thoughtful nurse who considers, and anticipates, what is likely to occur if the desire is achieved. Another key supporter could be encouraged.

Realistic outcome

It may seem obvious but the aim of planning for a realistic outcome is sometimes forgotten. Recognition of the fact that for some elderly patients, planning care for *dying* (rather than care for living) should be identified (see also Chapter 27).

For the nurse this situation should not be a period of inaction or maintenance of the same old routines. Every effort should be made to sustain, comfort and remain with patients and their relatives during this period. Routine should be forgotten. Individual wishes, whenever possible, should be considered, catered for, listened to, and supported.

Realistic planning should be a multidisciplinary team effort with each professional group contributing its knowledge and experience to help solve the patient's problems.

Problem areas which require special planning

Whenever an elderly person becomes ill there are three potentially difficult or highly stressful areas that have to be considered in order for suitable plans to be made.

(1) *Admission to hospital*, where familiar surroundings vanish and the patient may not understand why she is where she is, increases the risk of mental confusion, falling, incontinence or immobility. Elderly patients may take several days to settle. It is very helpful if someone they know can stay with them.

(2) *A change of home* becomes necessary. This is a stressful event for many. Some may pass through classic stages of bereavement and grieving if a change of home becomes inevitable. One lady, struggling to explain what the home she had lived in with her husband and children for 60 years meant to her, said, 'It is not just bricks. It is walls of laughter and tears – my life'. Any change of home that is not willingly entered into must be prepared for long before the event takes place, if it is to be successful. Much multidisciplinary teamwork revolves around this very difficult problem.

(3) *Discharge from hospital*. If discharge is not properly planned the return of the patient to hospital is almost inevitable. Geriatric departments pay great attention to discharge planning. Nurses are responsible for coordinating the greater part of the plans, and the work can be very time-consuming. Discharge from hospital may mean many elderly people return to isolation and loneliness. It is important to ensure that heat, food and help are available, and that drugs, exercises and medical regimes are thoroughly understood and practised *before* discharge.

Care planning

Successful care planning depends on accurate assessment. Assessment of elderly patients is complex. Processes of ageing, which are normal, have to be recognised and allowed for. Disease processes have to be understood. Because sight and hearing may be failing, communication can be difficult – even if the person is only temporarily confused in time or space, this adds to the difficulty. The social situation has to be properly investigated, otherwise unrealistic plans are made. Other disciplines have to be consulted and all have to work together.

The model of nursing used should be chosen to suit individual patient needs. Whichever model is used, nurses must make allowance for the following:

(1) A different timescale of expectation
(2) The presence of normal processes of ageing
(3) The altered response to disease that may occur.

The six year old who has his appendix removed may be trampolining on his bed the following day. The younger adult can usually walk upright without clutching his abdomen within two days, but the older adult may take much longer to walk freely, and may become incontinent or immobile if the nursing care has not been planned sensibly.

The elderly person with some short term memory impairment may forget to take her drugs, she may take them twice, or she may take some of them sometimes and others not at all. She may take them at the wrong time, or in the wrong sequence. She may not be able to open the containers, or she may be unable to obtain refills when necessary.

If an elderly person becomes ill but also is unable to raise his temperature in response to cold or infection, or has reduced ability to feel undue pressure on his skin, these altered responses need to be recognised and planned for. Nursing skills need to be adapted with experience and sensitivity in order to give the best possible care to the elderly person. For this reason, it is better that student nurses do not practise nursing on geriatric wards too early in a three year training programme.

Care for the elderly person should be planned jointly, not only with the patient and the nurse, but also with each member of the team that contributes to the total pattern of care.

Two sample care plans, each relating to one activity of living, are given in Figs. 26.2 and 26.3.

Special considerations in nursing elderly people

It is important to be aware of some specific points when caring for elderly people as there are certain conditions or situations which are more likely to occur among this age group.

Hypothermia

Hypothermia occurs when the core body temperature falls below 35° Celsius.

Care must be taken to warm patients *slowly*. This should be done at a rate of 0.5°C an hour, therebye avoiding too rapid peripheral vasodilation and shock. Use of a **rectal probe** to monitor temperature is best, or a low reading rectal thermometer can be used. A **space blanket** is useful, warm drinks may be given, and the use of a ripple mattress and bed cradle will help to alleviate pressure. Fluid intake and output need accurate calculation. In the initial stages life-saving measures may be necessary. Nurses should remember that elderly patients can become hypothermic in warm hospital wards.

Bone disorders (osteoporosis, Paget's disease, osteomalacia)

The alteration in bone structure that occurs with ageing can often not be reversed when bones fracture in old age. It is for this reason that more health knowledge and health screening, especially bone scanning of adults before they become old, would be helpful (Purdie, 1990).

Changes to bone structure in *osteoporosis* usually begin in woman after the menopause, probably due to alterations in hormone levels at this time. The disease can affect both men and women although it is more common in women. The balance between osteoblast cell activity (bone building) and osteoclast cell activity (bone resorption) is not maintained, resulting in a reduction in bone mass. The bone structure on X-ray resembles a honeycomb. The bones become fragile and break easily (Medcalf, 1989).

The most common sites for disabling fractures are the neck of femur and vertebrae. The former produces instant immobility and requires surgery. The latter produces intense, often overwhelming, pain in the lower back or neck regions. Adequate levels of pain control are essential, as usually lumbar vertebrae have collapsed and many nerve pathways have been affected.

Hormone replacement therapy (HRT) for women at the menopause is recommended by some doctors to halt the process of osteoporosis. The therapy does not suit all women (Fairlie, 1989). What *is* recommended is the maintenance of load-bearing exercise throughout life. The simplest form of this is walking, and all elderly people should be encouraged to walk to boost bone-building activity. They should walk at a pace and distance to suit their general health.

Paget's disease occurs when bone breakdown is excessive yet bone replacement is too rapid, with consequent replacement of bone by immature cells. Bone deformity is common, and fragility increases. Pain occurs at or over the site of the deformed bone. The hormone calcitonin can be given with some success. Again, control of pain to encourage movement is essential.

In *osteomalacia* the bones become soft due to inadequate calcification. The disease (in children, it is called rickets) has been almost eradicated in the United Kingdom due to an improved diet. It occurs when there is a lack of vitamin D or its metabolites, either in the diet or in the pathways which synthesise the vitamin. In elderly people, osteomalacia can develop from a straight dietary deficiency; from malabsorption problems, e.g. post-gastrectomy; from impaired metabolism of vitamin D because of changes in liver or renal function; from the effects of some drugs, especially anticonvulsants; or from a simple lack of sunlight because the person is housebound. Once the cause is identified the treatment is relatively simple, though existing deformity cannot be reversed. Again, more extensive health and dietary education is needed to prevent the disease ever occurring (Brocklehurst and Hanley, 1981).

Nursing considerations
It requires considerable skill by nurses to persuade elderly people to walk and to help them to do so safely. Liaison with the physiotherapist is essential. Pain control has to be achieved at the right time. The risks of falls must be minimised. This involves obtaining suitable footwear, proper consideration of suitable floor surfaces, the removal of articles that might cause tripping, the provision of stable things to hold on to such as rails in corridors, furniture on wheels that can be braked, easy, quick access to toilet facilities and *some activity should be out of doors*.

None of these are simple in large Nightingale type wards or in old adapted nursing homes, however. Consequently, the need for exercise is too often ignored or left to the physiotherapist's visit.

Continence

A major problem in nursing elderly people is that either they are admitted to hospital with continence difficulties alongside all their other problems, or that they become incontinent as a result of their admission.

In either case the lack of continence has to be addressed. The pattern to follow is that of assessment, planning, implementation and evaluation. There exist many charts and schemes for the assessment of incontinence patterns. It is essential that all staff are aware that an assessment scheme is in use and follow the instructions. Too often only parts of the scheme are followed and the chart ends up being used as a check list for a 2-hourly toileting regime. Along with the nurse's assessment should go a medical assessment and urodynamic tests. The end result should be the establishment of the cause, type, pattern and degree to which

the incontinence damages or restricts the patient's lifestyle. Once the cause, type and pattern are established a plan can be made, implemented and evaluated to promote continence (Fig. 26.3) (Norton, 1986). The assistance of a Continence Adviser – often a specialist nurse – is invaluable.

Nursing considerations
Why do so many elderly patients become incontinent on admission to hospital? The first response to disease, especially infections, is so frequently the sudden onset of mental confusion or a change in the level and type of existing confusion. The change in surroundings may in itself be confusing, and some elderly people may have difficulty in remembering where they are, where to go, or what has happened. Although they may have been continent in their own homes, the admission to large ward areas coupled with long walks to toilets or having to wait tips the fragile hold they may have on maintaining continence into incontinence.

Diuretic medicines are frequently prescribed to treat heart failure or oedema but incontinence may result. Also a significant number of people have developed coping strategies for maintaining continence by restricting their mobility (fear of distance from toilet) or their fluid intake, especially after 6pm. If infection is present nursing instructions frequently are 'to encourage fluids'. Days of struggle may ensue and the patient can become incontinent.

Additionally many elderly women already have pelvic floor damage following childbirth and many elderly men develop enlarged prostate glands. Both these conditions create difficulties with the maintenance of continence. If an increased fluid intake is necessary, for whatever reason, the bulk of the increase should be given before 2pm to reduce the frequency of urination during the night. Access to toilets should be close to the bed or sitting area and well marked. Clothing should be easily manageable.

An interesting study by Jirovec (1991) considered the impact of a daily exercise regimen on the mobility, balance and urine control of a group of elderly mentally frail patients. Subjects were able to walk significantly greater distances without tiring and the incidence of urinary incontinence was significantly decreased, following a month of daily assisted walking (balance was not altered). The need to walk all elderly patients whenever possible cannot be overemphasised. All nurses,

Fig. 26.3 *Care plan: concerned with the activity of elimination*

Mrs Jones: Admitted with urinary tract infection, incontinence   2nd week
Walks with stick – very slow

Home situation: small flat (approx. 25 square feet)
toilet

Activity of Living: ELIMINATING (Roper, Logan and Tierney, 1990)

Goal (long term) (1) Mrs Jones will be continent within her flat.
(2) Mrs Jones will be able to walk to the corner shop and back

Liaise with: Physiotherapist, continence adviser, home help, doctor

---

Problem	Goal (short term)	Nursing intervention	Evaluation
(1) Only one minute warning of need – or less	(1) That Mrs Jones is not incontinent using commode in toilet area	(a) Keep commode at bedside (b) Ensure stick always available (c) 1000 ml oral fluid by midday (d) Take Mrs Jones to the toilet on a commode. Walk back	*Tuesday*: One episode of incontinence at 6.30 am
(2) Walks very slowly (3) Toilet is at end of ward	(2) Walks from toilet area after eliminating	*Evening* (a) Restrict fluid to 200 ml after 6 pm. Mrs Jones agrees (b) Ensure that Mrs Jones eliminates before bedtime (c) Ensure Mrs Jones gets up within one minute of waking (d) No night sedation (see also MOBILISING, NUTRITION)	*Friday*: Can now walk length of ward Getting out of bed is easier and quicker *Sunday*: No incontinence. Needs reminding to drink plenty before midday

Signed: *J. Pritchard* 6/2/92

---

whether in the hospital or community setting, should know how to promote continence with sensitive and successful assessment and carefully planned programmes.

Energy expenditure

World marathon records show that at the ages of 70+, some people can still run the distance in under three hours. The energy needed for marathon running is that of steady, not explosive expenditure. This suits an elderly person because the reaction time of the body to any stimulus is slower, making it difficult for them to react quickly. This is true whether one considers the energy rise necessary to complete a 100 metre sprint successfully, or that needed to raise the body from a hori-

zontal position to the upright and walk (e.g. to get out of bed and go the toilet). All activities for elderly people have to be carefully planned and carried out steadily without hurry.

Hypothyroidism and pernicious anaemia

Although these two conditions have quite different causes, clinical features and pathology, there are certain similarities in their nursing care. Both conditions are due to the slow decline in the production of essential substances by the body (endocrine theory). In hypothyroidism, the thyroid gland fails to produce enough thyroxine. In pernicious anaemia there is a failure to secrete enough gastric intrinsic factor with a resulting deficiency in vitamin B_{12}. In both conditions the effects of the deficiencies in the early stages are often associated with what are thought of, by the elderly person herself and/or her carers, as inevitable age-related changes, e.g. slowing down, gradual failure to thrive, lost interest in food, difficulty in walking, or a lack of motivation generally (Coni *et al.*, 1988).

Often it is only when an inevitable crisis occurs that the underlying pathology becomes apparent. Once the crisis is over (and this may require much skilled medical and nursing care to correct) both conditions can usually be managed by medicines (thyroxine tablets for hypothyroidism and hydroxocobalamin injections for pernicious anaemia).

Nursing considerations

The problem is that the medicines must be taken regularly for life. Difficulties may occur in getting the patient to understand and remember to comply with the regime. The ability of the patient to do this must be tested and monitored before the patient leaves the hospital or care. If compliance is impossible, other solutions to medicine-taking must be explored. It becomes essential, then, that relatives or carers understand the importance of maintaining the regime and are able to take on the responsibility of maintaining it for the elderly person.

Maturity onset diabetes

Sufferers from **maturity onset diabetes** are rarely acutely ill. Nursing intervention, with the assistance of dieticians, pharmacists and social workers, should be directed towards helping clients understand the nature of the illness. The client also has to be educated how to manage her diet, drugs, urine testing, and the avoidance of, and recognition of, complications – for example, in the skin, the eyes, or the feet. Relatives may also have to be taught.

Medication

The accumulation of often large numbers or varieties of drugs is sometimes discovered. This may be the result of overprescription which is known as *polypharmacy*. The elderly may have difficulty in elimination of drugs if any degree of kidney or liver failure is present. Drugs tend to remain in the body for longer periods and their **half-life** is extended.

Compliance in drug-taking regimes may be seri-ously diminished for a variety of reasons – physical, mental or social. Containers may be difficult to open; drugs may be difficult to swallow; timing cannot be remembered; apathy may be felt; or the client cannot get out of her high-rise flat to renew the prescription because the lifts are broken.

Nutrition

Elderly people can become malnourished because of poverty, or because they cannot prepare meals. They may forget to eat, they may gradually reduce food intake to cups of tea with sliced white bread and margarine, or they may do nothing but eat sweets and biscuits all day.

The DHSS (1969) published recommended daily intakes of energy and nutrients for people over 65 years (assuming they led a sedentary life). With the exception of energy there was little difference in the amount of protein, thiamine, riboflavine, nicotine acid, vitamin C, vitamin A, vitamin D, calcium and iron that were recommended compared with other age groups, with the obvious exception of children and pregnant women. Further research, notably by Steen (1985) and Debry *et al.* (1977), agrees. Energy requirements obviously depend on energy expenditure.

What often seems forgotten by many when considering the actual nutrition of elderly people is that firstly, there is often, for numerous reasons, decreased intake of the recommended levels and secondly, if illness occurs, increased levels of all nutrients *and* energy (K calories) may be necessary.

Reasons for deficiencies include lack of money; isolation and loneliness; lack of shopping, preparation and cooking skills; lack of knowledge; apathy and depression; becoming housebound; reduced taste and smell; lack of mobility; ill-fitting dentures or lack of teeth; some medicine regimes, e.g. steroids, anticonvulsants; influences of culture and/or religious beliefs; old habits; dislike of new things; and the onset of pathological conditions such as hypothyroidism, maturity onset diabetes, cerebrovascular accidents, rheumatism, arthritis, venous ulcers, etc.

In itself the above list demonstrates the size of the problem of ensuring that elderly people at home obtain adequate nutrition for health. However, in hospitals and institutions the situation can be equally complex. Kirk (1990) showed that the food *served* to patients was deficient in fibre, energy, iron, vitamin D, vitamin C and folate, and that is before one begins to consider the problems of eating the food and/or wastage.

Nursing considerations

Barnes (1990) examined nurses' feelings about patients with specific feeding needs and concluded: 'The fussy patient and the patient who is difficult to feed provide little reward for carers. . . . one problem which staff consistently spoke of as insoluble was "patients who just won't eat anything" either because they did not like the food or because they were difficult to feed. Organisational constraints which limit nurses' freedom to provide greater choice. . . . or to spend more time with difficult patients could further compound the problem'.

Yet wounds will not heal – whether caused by pressure or venous ulcers – unless the patient takes in sufficient energy and vitamin C. Patients will not walk if they have an insufficient energy intake. It takes energy to get better! Shift patterns should ensure that the nurses' 'changeovers' or own meal times do not coincide with patients' meal times. Weighing should be regular. Elderly people with mechanical difficulties with eating and/or feeding themselves must be identified, and a plan made to solve the problem and to help them. It may be necessary to run *food* intake measurements. Liaison with dieticians and catering staff is essential.

- Some food must always be available for those who eat little but often. This is especially important at night.
- Likes and dislikes should be catered for, help given with menus, and there should be opportunity for choice.
- Sufficient *time* should be allowed for meals, and thought given to keeping food hot.

Multiple pathology

It is not uncommon to find elderly people with multiple diagnoses such as hypothyroidism, chronic renal failure, osteo-arthritis, Paget's disease, duodenal ulcers, *and* a urinary tract infection. Planning care can be very complex and present a real challenge to all concerned. If motivation is lost and cannot be restored, or the drive to achieve homeostasis is overwhelmed, care for dying has to be substituted for care for living (see also Chapter 27).

Elderly people have rights

Nurses should never forget that elderly people – whatever their medical condition – are adults with *all the rights and freedoms* of any adult. Too often, elderly patients become dependent because nurses (and others) are too protective and do not look at or plan for the safe management of risk. Elderly patients should *never* be imprisoned in their beds by cot-sides. They should *never* be penned or tied into chairs, forced into baths against their will, or toileted in public. They should *not* be incorrectly addressed by name or title, nor forced to eat or drink, nor treated as children.

What is needed is 'an underlying shift in attitudes towards the old – away from a patronising and paternalistic over-protection from risk and towards acknowledgement of their right to as much self-determination as possible . . .' (Norman, 1987)

Curtin (cited by Blythe, 1981) remarked that the ideal way to age and suit society 'would be to grow slowly invisible, gradually disappearing from sight without causing worry or discomfort to the young'.

Nursing elderly people requires skill, knowledge, and much patience and understanding. If all else fails, the nurse should adopt the philosophy 'Do as you would be done by' expressed by Charles Kingsley in his classic book *The Water Babies*. Read again the quotation at the beginning of this chapter. Remember that life expectancy is increasing. If the stranger that helps you in old age is a nurse, let us hope that he or she will not carry you where you have no wish to go.

Glossary

Cardiac output: The amount of blood ejected from the left ventricle of the heart per minute, which depends upon the heart rate and the stroke volume

Cataract: Opacity in the lens of the eye resulting in blurred vision

Continuing care: Units or wards in hospitals which become the patient's home – sometimes called *long stay units*

Glaucoma: A condition in which loss of vision occurs because of an abnormally high pressure in the eye. Can be of insidious or sudden onset

Glomerular filtration: The primary filtration of products and water from the blood by the glomerulus of the kidney into the kidney tubule

Half-life (of drugs): All drugs taken into the body have an active life before being broken down and eliminated. If elimination processes are inefficient, the drugs remaining are semi-active for a longer period than normal

Kyphosis: An excessive outward curvature of the spine causing hunching of the back

Maturity onset diabetes: Diabetes mellitus that commences in mature or elderly adults

Pathological fractures: Breakage of an already diseased bone which may occur as a result of only a minor injury.

Peripheral resistance: Resistance occurring at the periphery of a system causing the central

pump to work harder to achieve the same effect

Peristalsis: A wave-like movement that progresses along some of the hollow tubes of the body. It occurs involuntarily and is characteristic of tubes that possess circular and longitudinal muscles (such as the intestines)

Plaque (dental): A layer that forms on the surface of a tooth, composed of bacteria in an organic matrix. The purpose of oral hygiene is to remove plaque

Rectal probe: A probe inserted into the rectum which gives a continuous temperature reading without the need to remove it from the rectum to ascertain the reading

Rehabilitation: Any means employed for restoring independence after disease or injury. A vague term which has to be given a precise meaning via medical, nursing, paramedical or social services personnel care plans for each individual patient

Space blanket: A large, light-weight blanket made of synthetic fibres. One side has a reflecting, shiny surface. The blanket is placed with the shiny side next to the patient. Any body heat lost by the patient is reflected back to the patient and not dissipated

Sudden death syndrome: Death within a year of retirement from work

References

Barnes, K.E. (1990). An examination of nurses' feelings about patients with specific feeding needs. *Journal of Advanced Nursing*, 15(6), 703–711.

Birren, J.E. (1964). *The Psychology of Aging*. Prentice Hall, New Jersey.

Blythe, R. (1981). *The View in Winter*. Penguin Books, Harmondsworth.

Brocklehurst, J.C. and Hanley, T. (1981). *Geriatric Medicine for Students*. Churchill Livingstone, Edinburgh.

Castledine, G. (1982). Sorry, I haven't got time. *Nursing Mirror*, 155(13), 17–20.

Comfort, A. (1977). *A Good Age*. Mitchell Beazley, London.

Coni, N., Davison, W. and Webster, S. (1988). *Lecture Notes on Geriatrics* (3rd ed.). Blackwell Scientific Publications, Oxford.

Cumming, E. and Henry, W.E. (1961). *Growing Old: The Process of Disengagement*. Basic Books, New York.

Debry, G., Bleyer, R. and Martin, J.M. (1977). Nutrition of the elderly. *Journal of Human Nutrition*, 31, 63–83.

Department of Health. (1989). *Working for Patients* (Cmnd 555). HMSO, London.

Department of Health and Social Security. (1969). *Recommended Daily Intakes of Energy and Nutrients for the Elderly in the UK*. HMSO, London.

DHSS. (1981). *Growing Older*. HMSO, London.

DHSS. (1989). *Caring for People* (Cmnd 849). HMSO, London.

Eliopoulous, C. (1987). *Gerontological Nursing* (2nd ed.). Lippincott, London.

Fairlie, J. (1989). HRT and the menopause. *Health Visitor*, 62(10), 321.

General Nursing Council. (1977). *A Statement of Educational Policy*. GNC, London.

Green, R. (1985). Old age. In *Variations in Human Physiology*, Case, R.M. (ed.). Manchester University Press, Manchester.

Griffiths, R. (1988). *Community Care: Agenda for Action*. HMSO, London.

Hall, D.A. (1984). *The Biomedical Basis of Gerontology*. Wright, Bristol.

Hayslip, B. and Panek, P.E. (1989). *Adult Development and Aging*. Harper and Row, New York.

Herbert, R. (1986). The biology of ageing: maintenance of homeostasis. *Geriatric Nursing*, 6(6), 14–16.

Her Majesty's Stationery Office. (1990). *NHS and Community Care Act*. HMSO, London.

Jirovec, M.M. (1991). The impact of daily exercise on the mobility, balance and urine control of cognitively impaired nursing home residents. *International Journal of Nursing Studies*, 28(2), 145–150.

Kirk, S.F.L. (1990). Adequacy of meals served and consumed at a long stay hospital for the elderly. *Care of the Elderly*, 2(2), 77–80.

Kritzinger, E.E. (1989). The elderly eye I. Series of 14 parts beginning in *Care of the Elderly*, 1(6).

Maddox, G.L. and Eisdorfer, C. (1962). Some correlates of activity and morale among the elderly. *Social Forces*, 40, 254–260.

McCay, C.M., Pope, F. and Lunsford, W. (1956). Experimental prolongation of the lifespan. *Bulletin of the New York Academy of Medicine*, 32, 91.

McGee, G. (1986). *Old Age Ain't No Place for Sissies*. THAP Books, Whitechapel.

Medcalf, P. (1989). Osteoporosis. *Care of the Elderly*, 1(5), 210–215.

Neugarten, B.L. (1973). Personality changes in late life: a developmental perspective. In *The Psychology of Adult Development and Aging*, Eisdorfer, C. and Lawton, M.P. (eds.). American Psychological Association, Washington DC.

Norman, A. (1987). *Rights and Risk* (2nd ed.). National Corporation for the Care of Old People, London.

Norton, C. (1986). *Nursing for Continence*. Beaconsfield Publishers, Beaconsfield.

Pereira-Gray, D. (1990). The care of the elderly in general practice. *Care of the Elderly*, 2(9), 342.

Pilch, M. (1974). *The Retirement Handbook*. Hamish Hamilton, London.

Purdie, D. (1990). Osteoporosis screening: only the beginning. *Care of the Elderly*, 2(12), 13–14.

Rai, G.S., Stewart, K., van der Cammen, T. and Veenendall, D. (1989). Impairment of smell and taste in normal elderly and inpatients with Alzheimers dementia. *Care of the Elderly*, 1(6), 280–281.

Roper, N., Logan, W.W. and Tierney, A.J. (1990). *The Elements of Nursing* (3rd ed.). Churchill Livingstone, Edinburgh.

Schneider, E.L., Butter, R.N., Sprott, R.L. and Warner, H.R. (1987). *Modern Biological Theories of Ageing*, Vol. 31. Raven Press, New York.

Shulman, J. (1989). Informing the patient. *Nursing the Elderly*, 1(1), 142.

Sparkes, T. and Kelsey, A. (1991). A flexible contract to care. *Nursing the Elderly*, 3(6), 14–16.

Steen, B. (1985). Nutrition. In *Principles and Practice of Geriatric Medicine*, Pathy, M. (ed.). John Wiley and Sons, Chichester.

Tinker, A. (1984). *The Elderly in Modern Society*. Longman, London.

Turner, T. (1989). Opening the package. *Nursing Times*, 85(49), 15–16.

Villar, M. *et al.* (1991). The structure and function of the ageing lung. *Care of the Elderly*, 3(3), 129–130, 132.

Warnes, A.M. (ed.). (1989). *Human Ageing and Later Life*. Edward Arnold, London.

Suggestions for further reading

Davies, I. (1983). *Ageing*. Edward Arnold, London.

Davies, L. (1981). *Three Score Years . . . and Then? A Study of the Nutrition and Well-being of Elderly People at Home*. Heinemann, London.

Easterbrook, J. (1987). *Elderly Care: Towards Holistic Nursing*. Using Nursing Models Series. Edward Arnold, London.

Fielding, P. (1986). *Attitudes Revisited: An Examination of Student Nurses' Attitudes towards Old People in Hospital*. Royal College of Nursing, London.

Greengloss, S. (1986). *The Law and Vulnerable Elderly People*. Age Concern, London.

Holden, U.P. and Woods, R.T. (1988). *Reality Orientation* (2nd ed.). Churchill Livingstone, Edinburgh.

Philipson, C., Bernard, M. and Strang, P. (1986). *Dependency and Interdependency in Old Age: Theoretical Perspectives and Policy Alternatives*. Croom Helm & British Society of Gerontology, London.

Pitt, B. (1982). *Psychogeriatrics* (2nd ed.). Churchill Livingstone, Edinburgh

Wells, N. and Freer, C. (eds.). (1988). *The Ageing Population: Burden or Challenge?* Macmillan Press, London.

Wells, T. (1980). *Problems in Geriatric Nursing Care.* Churchill Livingstone, Edinburgh

Wright, S.G. (ed.). (1988). *Nursing the Older Patient.* Harper and Row, London.

Useful addresses

Voluntary organisations which help the elderly are listed below. The addresses and telephone numbers of local branches of these organisations can be found in your main telephone directory or in Yellow Pages under 'Charitable and Benevolent Associations'.

It may be helpful to give such information to the elderly patient, where appropriate, or to his carer.

In addition voluntary organisations often provide information and learning materials which might be useful in your studies.

Age Concern England

Astral House, 1268 London Road, London SW16 4ER. Tel. 081-679 8000

Alzheimers Disease Society

Bank Lodges, 158–160 Balham High Road, London SW12. Tel. 081-675 6557

British Red Cross

9 Grosvenor Crescent, London SW1. Tel. 071-235 5454

Disabled Living Foundation

380 Harrow Road, London W9. Tel. 071-289 6111

Help the Aged

St James Walk, London EC1. Tel. 071-253 0253

Womens' Royal Voluntary Service

234–244 Stockwell Road, London SW9. Tel. 071-733 3388

27

CARING FOR THE DYING PATIENT

Judith E. Hill

The aim of this chapter is to introduce the reader to a range of issues concerning the care of the dying patient and his partner, carers and friends. The purpose is to help prepare nurses to meet the needs of a particularly vulnerable group of people.

The chapter includes the following topics:

- Concepts of death
- Quality framework for care of the dying patient
- Team concept
- The nurse's role in caring for the dying patient

- What happens after a death
- Support needs of nurses
- Services for the care of the dying
- Bereavement

In her definition of nursing, Virginia Henderson (1966) states that it is part of the nurse's role to assist the patient to a peaceful death. Up to 60% of deaths take place in hospital, 30% at home and 10% elsewhere, including nursing homes and hospices. This chapter seeks to prepare the nurse to care for dying patients and to support their partners, carers and friends in hospital or at home. A considerable amount of knowledge has been gathered in the last 25 years about the needs of the dying and the bereaved. Increasingly this area of care is being researched and more knowledge added to the store. The aim of the chapter is to draw on this knowledge in discussing the care of the dying and those being bereaved, thus giving the nurse a range of strategies to meet the needs of the patient and his carers.

Different concepts of death are presented. The importance of teamwork and the nurse's role in meeting the patient's physical, emotional, social and spiritual needs is explored, with guidance on the care of the patient in the final days.

The nurse is often relied upon to guide partners/ carers on what to do after a death, therefore information on how death is diagnosed, how to register a death, and how to arrange a funeral have been included. The needs of nurses, as they care for dying patients, are explored and suggestions made for ways of handling the stresses experienced. The range of services for care of the dying, including the contribution of voluntary organisations, is presented and a list of useful addresses included at the end of the chapter.

The process of grief and ways of helping the

bereaved are discussed at some length, bearing in mind that it is not only grieving partners, carers and friends for whom the nurse will have to care; some of her other patients may have experienced a recent bereavement themselves and the way they respond in their illness may be influenced by their grief reaction.

Caring for dying patients and bereaved people can be very rewarding once the nurse knows some of the things to expect and has learned some interventions which enable her to plan effective care.

Concepts of death

The Western view of death in the latter part of the 20th century has been shaped in large measure by what is seen on television, heard on radio or read in newspapers. It is frequently presented as the sudden removal of people in the midst of life or as something against which people have fought bravely, enduring pain, discomfort and weakness. Only occasionally is it presented as appropriate, usually when the person who has died is in their eighties, having pursued a successful career well into old age. Death is seen as an unnatural intrusion into life. In the past many nurses, doctors and other professional helpers in the health field viewed death as a failure of their skills and rejected the dying person as a reminder of the limitations of their abilities to cure ailments and sustain life. Yet death is as much a part of the world as birth. Just as there is a health/illness continuum along which people move, so there is a life/death continuum. The length of that continuum varies. For some it is short; for others it covers many years over the full range of developmental stages. Life is full of letting go and moving on; death is the final stage of the journey. The baby leaves the womb, the infant leaves the breast, the toddler leaves its mother for school, the teenager leaves childhood, the adult leaves parents, the older person leaves work. Different cultures recognise these milestones and often have ceremonies and rituals which denote the changes in status and role which occur as the individual matures. Thus, death is seen as appropriate for those who have completed the different developmental stages. Should it occur earlier it is seen as cruel and out of place, sometimes more by the people who are left behind than the ones who are actually dying, many of whom, even young children, feel they have fulfilled their purpose and potential in life.

The taboos and prohibitions surrounding the topic of death have much to do with the way people see and value life. The major religions of the world have certain rites and practices concerning death and the nurse needs to be aware of how to deal with death in such a way that she supports the person who is dying and does not offend any particular group. The nurse will come across death in a variety of forms (see Table 27.1). Some will be sudden, others will follow a long period of illness with recurrent hospitalisation and different treatment regimes and the death may occur anywhere within the developmental process.

Table 27.1. *Common causes of death*

Sudden

Cerebral haemorrhage

Myocardial infarction

Trauma—haemorrhage
 —respiratory arrest

Anaphylactic shock

Pulmonary embolism

Predictable
Infection—pneumonia
 —*septicaemia*
 —meningitis
 —auto-immune deficiency disease (AIDS)

Cancer

Cerebral haemorrhage

Drug overdose

Cardiac failure

Respiratory failure

Renal failure

Liver failure

Congenital conditions

Multiple sclerosis

Motor neurone disease

Huntington's chorea

Quality framework for care of the dying patient

Quality can be defined as a degree or standard of excellence. The difficulty is that we may all perceive excellence in different ways. In health care, at least four groups of people will have different perspectives of quality: the recipients of care, the providers of care, the commissioners of care and the general public or society. In care of the dying, the types of issues that will be important to patients and their carers are likely to be in the following areas:

- Was the patient's pain controlled and other symptoms managed?
- Did the care received lead to a peaceful and dignified death?
- Was there honest and open communication about the patient's condition and the benefits of likely treatment?
- Did the carers feel that their needs had been addressed?
- Was there continuing support for the partner or carers after the death?
- Was the patient able to choose the place of their death?
- Were the necessary services available for care at home?

For the providers of care of the dying, the quality issues are likely to be:

- Are there adequate referral systems to specialist care?
- Is there a range of skills available to provide care?
- Are there adequate processes for respite care, domiciliary care, inpatient care?
- Are sufficient facilities available to offer choice to patients and their partners and carers?
- Are the staff adequately trained and skilled to provide care for the dying?

- Are there good communication processes between the different providers, i.e. inpatient, hospice, domiciliary services?
- Is the environment suitable for care of the dying?
- Are services available locally to individuals and in sufficient number to meet the needs of the population?
- Do clinical and other staff have the appropriate attitudes and skill to care for the dying and are resources allocated to this important area of care?
- Are plans in place to meet identified need?

Developing quality measures in the care of the dying requires a multidisciplinary approach involving the consumers, both patients and their partners and carers, and also other professionals who refer patients to services. The work needs to progress through all the components of the quality cycle which will now be explored in relation to care of the dying. The quality cycle can be applied at different levels in the health service (Fig. 27.1).

The commissioner of services may set out their values for a quality service to care of the dying and develop a range of standards which can then be audited and the results fed back to the providing organisations who can develop their services further to meet the requirements of the commissioning authority. An example of this approach has been developed by several regional health authorities (NAHAT, 1992). Such a quality initiative is about ensuring access to services, equity of distribution, and effectiveness of the service to meet identified local and individual need.

Working within such a quality framework, the provider of services for care of the dying can develop their own quality cycle. Firstly, a multidisciplinary group of professionals involved in providing care can be drawn together to set out a statement of values and beliefs that underpin their work. The membership of the group that produces these value statements would be usefully enhanced by the inclusion of partners or carers or other representatives of the recipients of care. Once the group have identified their values and beliefs, which are likely to include statements in relation to the patient, the carers and the staff involved in care, areas in which standards should be set can be clearly identified. The value statements are likely to cover issues relating to the rights of

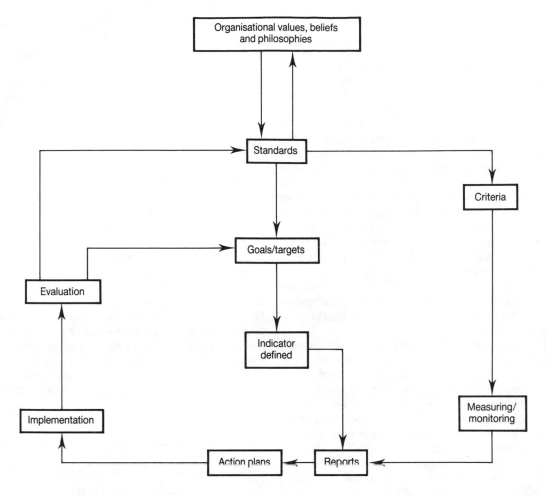

Fig. 27.1 *Quality cycle or review process*

the individual, the relief of suffering, the opportunity for choice, the recognition of the role and needs of staff for support, education and training, the importance of information and the principles of equity. Thus, the areas to be addressed through standards are likely to be those which are seen as important in order to provide care which would meet the requirements of such beliefs and values or areas where there are likely to be difficulties in meeting the values and beliefs.

In most services for care of the dying you are likely to find standards that relate to pain control, choice of place of care, needs of the carers, communication with the patient and their partners/carers, bereavement care, multidisciplinary working, discharge procedures, the environment of care, the education of staff and the support of staff. The standards may be set for the multidisciplinary team and from these nurses may develop standards that relate to their particular role. Within the standards, criteria should be established in relation to the resources that need to be available to achieve the standard, the processes that will need to be carried out to meet it and finally some statement on the outcome for the patient, relative or staff member.

Once the standards have been written and agreed for the work of individuals or teams in care of the dying, then some measures of the quality of care will have to be developed. Outcome measures can be very difficult in this area of care as the issues that are being addressed are mainly to do with the quality of life rather than a demonstrated health gain or improvement of the status of the patient.

Attempts can be made to identify patient satisfaction and carer satisfaction with the care given and also the staff views. Finding out the response of other professionals such as general practitioners to the service provided to the patients are other ways of measuring the care given. To help the work of the development of quality within care of the dying, a range of guidelines for professionals and managers has been produced in recent years. *Care of People with Terminal Illness*, a report by a joint advisory group to the National Association of Health Authorities and Trusts (1992), sets out some guidelines in relation to palliative care and services which can be helpful for both commissioners and providers of services. The document also looks at nursing home provision for people with a terminal illness. The King's Fund Centre has produced a study of bereavement support in NHS hospitals in England (Wright *et al.*, 1988). The paper includes information from relatives and health authorities and produces a check-list to enable hospitals to review their services.

The Office of Health Economics has produced a report (Griffin, 1991) which reviews the issues in relation to place of care and the provision of appropriate care for the terminally ill. It recognises that, although hospices have provided an example of good quality care, there needs to be more work done to see how the standards from hospices can be transferred into ordinary hospital wards. The Royal College of Nursing has produced some standards in cancer nursing which includes a section on palliative care (RCN, 1991). Several regional health authorities have produced frameworks for the care of the terminally ill, for example Trent, South West Thames and Yorkshire. By using all of these sources, nurses can begin to identify for themselves what constitutes good quality care for the dying in particular areas in which they work.

Promoting quality is an ongoing process. Once values have been agreed, standards set, measuring tools developed and audit carried out, the results need to be analysed and reviewed and the continual striving for excellence, based on these results, will go a long way to improve the care for the dying.

Team concept

As indicated in the quality framework, one of the principles to emerge from the pioneers in developing specialist skills for the care of the dying person and their partners and carers is that an interdisciplinary approach involving a wide range of professionals and voluntary helpers is required. In the team involved in the patient's care, each person fulfils their own professional role, with the roles of different team members dovetailing and overlapping in the provision of care and support. It is important that the team member to whom the patient relates most easily coordinates the care, rather than this being a prescribed function of one particular discipline. The professional team includes nurses, doctors, physiotherapists, occupational therapists, social workers, pharmacists, administrators, clergy, domestic and portering staff. The nurses and doctors may be generalists or specialists in the care of the dying. The team may be involved with dying people simply as part of their work, such as the team on general medical and surgical wards or the primary health care team in the community, or it may be their sole activity. Good communication between the team members and a supportive attitude to one another are essential features of the way the team functions. It is important that the multidisciplinary group of professionals and volunteers involved in providing care work to agreed values and beliefs as the basis for their work.

The nurse's role in caring for the dying patient

The quality framework for care of the dying indicates the various components of care which make up the service to the patient and their carers. This section will explore the specific role of the nurse.

Where death is the result of a sudden, catastrophic event, the nurse will have certain practical things to do relating to the care of the body, but her main role will be in supporting the partners/carers of the person who has died. These issues will be discussed later. When death is the end of an illness, whether long or short in duration, her role is much more complex and she will be required to identify and plan care for the physical, emotional, social and spiritual needs of the patient, as well as provide support and advice to the carers and social group surrounding the patient. The nurse will need to develop certain skills, knowledge and attitudes to enable her to give a high quality of care to the dying patient and his family. She will need to be a competent clinical nurse, with good communication skills, motivated by a genuine compassion for a very vulnerable group of people.

An approach to the nurse's role which is particularly helpful in caring for the dying is the one described by Benner and Wrubel (1989) which identifies 'the nature of the caring relationship as central to most nursing interventions'. They describe caring activities within a trusting relationship which will enable 'the one cared for to appropriate the help offered and feel cared for'. The nurse shows she cares by firstly recognising the uniqueness of the patient's experience of illness and secondly, by being 'present' with the patient in their situation in a way which shows she is engaged with his individual situation 'Non-caring amounts to not being present with the patient but rather being there only to get the job done.' Thirdly, caring activities include 'doing for' the patient by providing comfort and supportive measures; fourthly, 'enabling' the expression of feeling, and finally 'maintaining belief' in the ability of the sick individual to cope and be themselves, i.e. to maintain hope.

Benner and Wrubel (1989, page 9) describe nursing as concerned with the relationships between disease and the lived experience of health and illness. 'Even when no treatment is available and no cure is possible, understanding the meaning of the illness for the person and for that person's life is a form of healing, in that such understanding can overcome the sense of alienation, loss of self-understanding and loss of social integration that accompany illness.'

In describing the nurse's role in caring for the dying patient, consideration will be given to ways in which the nurse individualises care to recognise the uniqueness of what is happening for the individual and behaviours that demonstrate that she is engaged with the individual in their dying. 'Doing for' activities in the provision of comfort and support are carried out through symptom management, positioning and establishment of a therapeutic environment. 'Enabling the expression of feeling and maintaining belief' will be addressed in the discussions in relation to meeting emotional and spiritual needs of the dying person. One of the principles that underlies nursing care for the dying is creating an environment in which patients can

live as fully as possible rather than concentrating on the confines of the disease process.

Table 27.2. *Physical needs of the dying patient*

Need	Actual/potential problems
Breathing	**Dyspnoea**, pleuritic or rib pain, infection, cough, retention of sputum, 'death rattle'
Nutrition	Anorexia, **dysphagia**, nausea, vomiting, hiccough, dry/sore mouth
Mobility	Weakness, lethargy, muscle and joint stiffness, pressure sores, paralysis, fractures, pain, **ascites**, **lymphoedema**
Elimination	(Bladder) Urinary retention/ incontinence. **Dysuria**, infection **haematuria**. (Bowel) Constipation, faecal incontinence, colic
Hygiene	Sweating, inability to self-care, incontinence
Skin integrity	Pressure sores, incontinence, **fungating lesions**, fistulae
Rest	Anxiety, nightmares, hallucinations, confusion, depression

Physical needs

The dying person has many physical needs (Table 27.2). Symptoms may arise as a result of specific disease processes, for example, pain, nausea, vomiting, paralysis, breathlessness. Symptoms may also arise as the result of increasing weakness, loss of function and deteriorating ability to maintain daily living activities. Thus the patient's experience of the symptoms and the consequent distress is aggravated if all aspects of the patient's care are not attended to (Baines, 1981). Many patients will not admit to distressing symptoms, feeling they cannot complain about too many. Actively questioning about different symptoms is important to obtain a full picture of the various sources of distress to the patient. The nurse must pay meticulous attention to detail. No problem is too small for her to try to alleviate in the dying person. In Hockley's study (1983), and more recently in Finlay's (1991), symptoms such as anorexia, sore mouth, and sleepless nights came top of the patients' list of concerns, most of which could be alleviated by properly focused nursing care. Involving the patient and carers in working out ways of dealing with such problems means that care can be planned to tackle the problems that are of most concern to the patient.

In meeting the physical needs of the dying patient, the nurse will draw on the knowledge and skills required to care for the dependent patient and exercise her ability to observe and monitor changes in the patient's condition. She will require specialised knowledge in the area of symptom control to understand the use of drugs to relieve symptoms and to know the side effects of treatment. Such knowledge will enable her to identify the need for certain medication and to report the need to the doctor. She will also be able to observe the effect of treatment on the patient, monitor the relief experienced and report any adverse side effects. It is this specialised knowledge which is presented here with some comments on the general care required by the patient.

Breathing

Dyspnoea can be relieved by positioning the patient to allow freedom of movement for the respiratory muscles. This includes supporting the patient sitting up in bed with adequate pillows, or the patient may be more comfortable in a chair, with his arms and feet supported. His clothing should be loose and not restricting in any way. A fan or open window (where appropriate) will increase air circulation and may ease the sensation of breathlessness. The physiotherapist can teach the patient relaxation techniques which can help him control his breathing, exercises that will make breathing more effective by increasing air intake, and may teach the patient how to expectorate and clear the lungs of excessive secretions. If the patient is breathing through his mouth, frequent mouth washes or drinks will keep the mouth moist, and a little white paraffin will prevent the lips drying and cracking.

Some doctors will prescribe a small dose of morphine or diamorphine which has been found to ease the sensation of dyspnoea without causing problems of respiratory depression (Regnard et al., 1983). Depending on the cause of the dyspnoea, other drugs may be prescribed. In cardiac failure or bronchospasm the usual measures of **diuretics** or **corticosteroids** respectively may be effective. When infection is present, the decision to treat with antibiotics will be judged on the degree of distress experienced by the patient from such symptoms as pyrexia, cough, pleuritic pain or foul-smelling sputum. The nurse may assist the doctors in reaching a decision by careful assessment and observation of the patient for signs of distress. If there is **superior vena cava obstruction** present the doctor may prescribe corticosteroids which reduce inflammation and local oedema. Anxiety and dyspnoea are often related and one will affect the other. An **anxiolytic**, such as diazepam, has been found helpful in treating the dyspnoeic patient, along with a calm, unhurried approach to care by nursing staff. When the patient is dying, secretions from the lungs collect and produce noisy breathing (sometimes known as the 'death rattle') which can be distressing for relatives and carers, though the patient seems to be unaware at this stage. Hyoscine given subcutaneously will help to dry up these secretions and reduce the noise.

Nutrition

Food has a number of meanings and values to different people. It carries 'biological, emotional and sociological meanings' (Gallagher-Allred, 1991). The values, which give meaning to the way that food is served and eaten, may be religious, cultural or ethnic.

From the physical point of view, terminal illness can alter a patient's nutritional needs in several ways. Firstly, the disease process can decrease absorption and nutrient requirements. Secondly, as the body functions are slowed by the dying process, so the person will not feel as hungry and may develop intolerance to certain foods. Thirdly, medical intervention, especially the use of drugs, can alter a person's response to food. Anorexia is a very common problem in the terminally ill. The patient will benefit from a large measure of choice in what he eats and when he eats it. Small, easily eaten meals taken frequently are often appreciated. An alcoholic drink before a meal can make a social occasion of the event and tempt the appetite. The doctor may prescribe a low dose of corticosteroid which will lift the patient's mood and increase his appetite (Baines, 1986). The overall approach to nutritional care should thus include the relief of troublesome symptoms, the enhancement of the pleasurable experiences of living and the prevention or treatment of malnutrition (Gallagher-Allred, 1991).

Nausea and vomiting in terminal illness have a large number of causes, including the drugs used to control pain. An ***anti-emetic***, such as prochlorperazine, may be prescribed to be given with the analgesic drugs. Different anti-emetic drugs act at different sites, such as the vomiting centre or the chemoreceptor trigger zone in the brain, or the upper bowel. For example, prochlorperazine acts on the chemoreceptor trigger zone, metoclopramide also acts on the chemoreceptor site and in addition the upper bowel, and cyclizine acts directly on the vomiting centre. If the patient has persistent vomiting which is difficult to control, the doctor may prescribe two drugs with different sites of action (Regnard *et al.*, 1983). The drugs may have to be given parenterally, at least initially, until the vomiting is controlled. The subcutaneous route using a ***syringe driver*** (Fig. 27.2) can be used for anti-emetic drugs apart from the ***phenothiazine*** group which are irritant to the skin and require intramuscular injection. The rectal route can be used for prochlorperazine in suppository form.

Many dying patients suffer from a sore mouth (Hockley 1983), often as a result of monilial fungal infection. The nurse needs to examine the patient's mouth every day for redness or coating of the tongue or mucous membranes. Fungal infection responds well to betadine mouthwashes and nystatin suspensions, administered two-hourly. If the patient has dentures these should be removed before the nystatin is given.

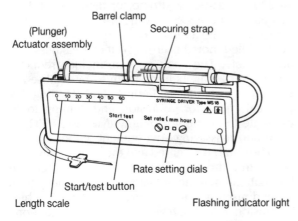

Fig. 27.2 *Syringe driver*

Elimination

Constipation can occur when the patient is less active, taking a limited diet and receiving narcotic drugs. Encouraging the inclusion of more fibre and fluid in the diet, when possible, can help, or the doctor can prescribe a faecal softening preparation, e.g. lactulose, or stimulant laxatives, e.g. senna. To clear the bowel the nurse may be asked to administer glycerine and/or biscodyl suppositories. If these measures prove unsuccessful an enema will usually be required.

Rest

Anxiety and depression are part of the normal reaction to loss, as discussed in the next section. However, counselling and empathetic care may need to be supplemented by the administration of anxiolytic and antidepressant therapy. Drugs from the ***benzodiazepine*** and phenothiazine groups may be prescribed to control anxiety. Slow-release amitriptyline and mianserin are examples of drugs given to clinically depressed patients.

The management of pain, both in hospital and at home, is one of the greatest challenges of terminal care. However, considerable advances have been made in our understanding of the principles by which to manage pain relief, particularly that associated with dying from cancer. The nurse has a major role to play. An accepting and understanding attitude on the part of the nurse will help support the patient in pain.

The principles which underlie the management of terminal pain include assessment, which should involve taking a full detailed history and an accurate measurement of the different kinds of pain and the consideration of the patient's total situation, not only their physical pains but their emotional and social distresses. There needs to be constant review of the management of the patient's pain relief measures. In developing a plan of care to control the patient's pain, realistic goals need to be set. Firstly, achieving a good night's sleep should have priority. Then, reducing pain on movement and finally putting pain to the periphery of the patient's consciousness. Patients will need a range of therapies to be available to them. ***Analgesic*** drugs, co-analgesics, psychological approaches such as sensitive listening and relaxation therapy, distraction and imagery, physical therapies such as heat and cold, the use of massage and acupuncture. Medical treatment such as radiotherapy and interventions such as nerve blocks (Corcoran, 1991) may be appropriate.

Evidence suggests that most pain is treatable and

controllable. The reasons for failure to relieve pain include lack of factual knowledge of the use of analgesics with an unfounded fear about addiction, tolerance, and respiratory depression in the use of the **narcotics**. There may be inaccurate assessment and perhaps a lack of re-assessment or review of the patient's situation. Co-analgesics may not be used appropriately and there may be a lack of emotional support or adequate communication to deal with the patient's fears and anxieties. There may be also a lack of understanding of the use of non-drug measures.

The different kinds of pain require different drugs to be prescribed by the doctor. Nerve compression pain may respond to corticosteroids, such as dexamethasone. Gastro-intestinal colic requires **antispasmodic** drugs, such as loperamide or hyoscine. Nerve pain responds well to the non-steroidal anti-inflammatory drugs, such as indomethacin or flurbiprofen. In other situations the doctor may start pain control by prescribing a mild analgesic, such as paracetamol or aspirin. If these are not effective, compound drugs such as co-codaprin or co-proxamol may be tried before prescribing narcotic drugs, such as morphine and diamorphine. This approach to pain control is called the use of the pain ladder (WHO, 1986). Morphine and diamorphine are controlled drugs and their administration requires special recording procedures.

Mobility

Lethargy and weakness are commonly felt by the dying patient. Nursing tasks need to be performed at a pace which does not exhaust the patient and rest periods planned to enable him to do the things which are of importance to him. The physiotherapist plays a large part in keeping the patient active but the nurse needs to know the exercise programme which has been devised for the patient so that she can encourage him to persist when the physiotherapist is not available. Likewise, when the patient is being treated for lymphoedema the nurse should familiarise herself with the equipment and elasticated garments so that she can support the patient during treatment.

Skin integrity

Prevention of pressure sores in the dying patient can tax the nurse's ingenuity, as many patients are only comfortable in a limited number of positions. She needs to apply the general principles of prevention whilst allowing the patient some freedom of choice in position.

The stoma care nurse will advise on appliances which may help control leakage from fistulae and the continence adviser may have some helpful ideas to enhance the quality of life for the patient with problems with continence.

Fungating lesions present a considerable challenge to the nurse, especially in the control of odour. A different set of care goals than those required for surgical wounds will need to be set in relation to fungating lesions that will not heal and will look worse as the tumour grows. The containment of odour and exudate must become the markers of successful therapy (Finlay, 1991). The general principles include keeping the lesion clean and free from secondary infection. Sometimes, following microscopy and culture of a swab from the lesion, the doctor will prescribe a course of systemic antibiotics. Charcoal pads and yoghurt have been used to absorb odour and superficial radiotherapy can help reduce the size of the lesion and seal bleeding points. It is essential that pain relief measures are used prior to redressing of lesions.

Confusional states

Confusion in the dying patient may result from several situations. There may be delirium as part of an acute organic syndrome, or there may be dementia as in AIDS. Brain disease, such as a tumour, may be a further cause. Finally, there may be muddled thoughts arising out of weakness, fear and anxiety. The goals for care include reducing the patient's fear, helping them to rationalise any underlying anxieties, finding and treating the physical cause for confusion and helping to re-orientate the patient to reality (Mannix, 1991). A calm and reassuring environment, either at home or in hospital, is required and the patient may need some drug therapy. The aim is to try to reassure the patient that he is safe and that the people around are trying to understand and to help him. Confusion can be reversed in many situations. However, if it cannot be completely resolved there can be understanding and the situation can be managed.

Emotional needs

The emotional needs of the patient focus around their ability to adapt to loss and cope with their fears and anxieties. 'Illness as the human experience of loss or dysfunction has a reality all its own' (Benner and Wrubel, 1989). Illness brings with it a variety of losses (Table 27.3). The ill person becomes dependent upon others for certain things, for example food and shopping, and is unable to fulfil his normal social roles at work, home or in the community. He has to accept the dependent, inferior role of the sick person and accept help from others, and is expected to obey doctor's orders and get better quickly and take up his normal activities as soon as possible (Parsons and Fox, 1961).

Table 27.3. *Losses experienced in illness*

Independence
Status
Self-image
Family roles
Social contacts and activities
Work responsibilities and rewards
Money
Mobility
Plans for the future

Hospitalisation brings further losses such as privacy, self-determination, routines of life, family, home, status, lifestyle, body image, and body function. On admission, the person's privacy is invaded in a variety of ways; he has to divulge information about himself, including intimate details; there is the exposure of the body during medical examination; possibly collective sleeping arrangements; enforced relationships with staff and fellow patients and exposure of the patient's own personal relationships (Goffman, 1961). Thus, illness and hospitalisation lead to loss of independence, the right to control the situation and to the stripping of family, occupational and recreational roles.

How much these losses produce emotional reactions depends on their significance to the individual. They constitute the psychosocial losses of illness and contribute to the loss of a person's self-image. Pain, incontinence, loss of mobility, and alteration of body image by disease, drugs and other therapies represent losses in the physical sphere and compound the total feelings of loss. In providing emotional support to the dying person, the nurse has to try and assess the predominant feelings that the person is experiencing in relation to his condition, and determine those losses which are currently affecting him to the greatest degree.

Studies with dying people have identified a range of feelings which have much in common with a grief reaction (Kubler-Ross, 1970). There is denial – 'This cannot be happening to me'; anger – 'Why me?'; bargaining – 'Surely I can prevent this happening to me; someone, somewhere must be able to help'; depression – 'It is happening to me and I'm sad about it'; acceptance – 'It is happening and I'm ready'. Similar reactions have been demonstrated by people who lose a limb or a home, and by young children deprived of their mothers. Thus a loss which represents the removal of a valued object or attribute of an individual will be followed by a process of mourning. So the dying person will experience loss reactions related to the illness, the loss of those close to him (family) or work role and, if transferred from home to die, the loss of a familiar environment. The dying person will also experience grief at the ending of his relationships with loved ones.

Meeting the emotional needs of the dying patient presents a considerable challenge to the nurse. Firstly, there is the need to form a trusting relationship. The nurse often does this by listening to the story of the patient's experience. Hunt (1989) described nurses visiting the dying as asking questions which enabled the patient to tell the story of their illness as they understood it. As the story unfolds the nurse is able to identify plans in a person's life that have been thwarted, relationships that have been disturbed, and the meaning that the patient is attaching to symptoms depending on what else is happening in their life (Benner and Wrubel, 1989). By showing acceptance of the patient and a non-judgemental attitude, valuing the person as an individual, the nurse can allow expressions of feelings. She can help the person to explore what is happening and allow him to voice fears and anxieties.

The nurse needs to be careful to avoid responding to unanswerable questions with platitudes and trying to reassure the dying patient prematurely. By recognising and acknowledging the unfairness of much suffering, she can help the person to move from asking, 'Why is this happening to me?' to 'How can I cope with what's happening to me?'. She can work with the person on his fears and anxieties, keep him company and offer hope by agreeing with him realistic, achievable goals. Thus, enabling hope is about helping the individual to find meaning and purpose in their existence and the nurse must consider attitudes, values and support systems and coping mechanisms of the patients and their families that will help the patient to retain a reason for living (Hesswell and Bramwell, 1989).

It can be helpful to use the technique of life review to create situations which enable the patient to see the significance of past life events in terms of accomplishments, milestones and unresolved issues. The significance of these things in the context of the current situation, in particular the review of past positive endeavours, can heighten awareness and confirm a sense of personal worth (Hesswell and Bramwell, 1989). In using this approach the nurse needs to ask questions that encourage the patient to share his thoughts and feelings about being seriously ill (Ufema, 1991).

Social needs

The social needs of the dying patient concern practical issues: finance, housing, Social Security benefits, work-related issues, and social support and relationship networks. Voluntary organisations, charities, professional and trade union benevolent funds will often provide gifts of money or items to relieve financial stresses and provide extra comforts. Such benefits include grants for heating to keep an invalid warm; payments for the redecoration of a room to give a better environment; nursing home fees, even a holiday. When the terminal illness is prolonged and the ill person is dependent on care, he can apply for State benefits. A number of benefits may also be available for the person providing care, who should enquire at their local DSS office.

Family relationships today can become complex with the rise in divorce rates, the large numbers of one-parent families and the large population of elderly people who live alone at a distance from relatives. There are a number of partnerships, e.g. homosexual or common law relationships, which exist with varying degrees of commitment between the partners. This has implications for the amount of social support families are willing or able to give.

Where children under 16 years of age have only one parent, providing for the future care of these children after the death of that parent may present difficulties and heighten emotional tension. Such children may have to face not only the loss of a parent but also home, school and friends.

The social worker will be the key person in helping with some of these situations, but the nurse needs to be aware of available support and advise the patient and family appropriately. One area the nurse can advise the family about is how to visit the dying person in institutional care and spend time with him without overtiring him or putting extra stress on themselves. It is not necessary for visitors to sit and talk all the time with the dying and plague them with lots of questions. Sitting with the patient, knitting or doing a crossword, sharing a favourite television programme or simply being quiet, holding hands, are all supportive activities. When involving the family in the patient's care, care must be taken not to ask too much of tired relatives, and similarly, the patient's wishes must be taken into account. A young person, newly independent of parents, may prefer the nurses to give intimate personal care, however much the parent may wish to be involved. Ensuring relatives get adequate rest and refreshment is also a nursing responsibility, as is arranging overnight accommodation for those wishing to remain near the patient. Some services provide a double bed for couples to remain close. Where this is not possible, an extra bed in a side ward can usually be arranged.

Spiritual needs

Spiritual needs of the dying patient and their carers have historically been the domain of the clergy and, in hospital, the chaplain. In an increasingly secular and multifaith society it can be difficult to define the chaplain's role. The chaplain is involved in helping those patients who wish to maintain religious rites and practices and to administer the sacraments of the Church. Other patients with no definite Church allegiance may still need to be reassured of forgiveness and life after death and would look to the chaplain for help. For some, the chaplain will be seen as the representative of the God who has permitted the suffering that accompanies death and he may have to deal with anger and resentment from the patient and family. For others the chaplain may be a useful person with whom to explore the meaning of what is happening and to share thoughts and feelings.

Spiritual needs include the beliefs and practices associated with a religion and the need of individuals to find some meaning and purpose in their lives. Where a person belongs to a particular religious or cultural group, the nurse will need to identify how firmly he holds to the beliefs and tenets of the religion, and how much he wants to follow the normal pattern of behaviour associated with that group. Listening to the patient's and family's wishes will guide the nurse to what is required (Walker, 1982).

Within the *Christian Church* there are many divisions and therefore differing practices to support the dying patient, the bereaved, and in making arrangements for a funeral. Eastern Orthodox Christians may arrange for a priest to visit their dying relative to hear a last confession and give communion. The priest may anoint the patient with a special oil, known as the oil of the sick. Once the person has died there are no restrictions on the nurses handling the body. The family may arrange for the body to lie in state in the church with the coffin open for people to pay their respects. The body is usually buried.

Roman Catholic Christians who practise their religion are often regular churchgoers and appreciate bedside communion services. The patient may have religious symbols attached to the bed or placed nearby. The dying person receives the sacrament of the sick from the priest, which includes the priest anointing the patient with oil, praying for them and administering absolution (a statement of God's forgiveness for the patient's sins). Once dead, the patient's hands may be placed in an attitude of prayer, holding a crucifix or rosary.

There are many Protestant churches with varied practices. The hospital chaplain or the patient's own minister or church leader can be asked to visit the patient and family. The traditional sacraments of baptism, confession, communion, laying on of hands and anointing may be administered on request. The nurse needs to ask the family about any particular practices they would like carried out when the patient dies.

Muslims have a number of traditions related to the care of the sick and the dying. Personal hygiene is regarded as being equivalent to spiritual purity. Washing is carried out before prayer which is performed facing Mecca. Muslims have strict dietary laws which ban pork and alcohol. A relative will recite verses from the Koran to the dying, so that these are the last words heard in life. After death the family will wash and prepare the body. The nurse should only straighten the body and remove any drainage tubes. The head is turned towards the left shoulder and the person is buried facing Mecca. The body is buried without a coffin within 24 hours. Organ donation, cremation or post mortems are forbidden. Every Friday for 40 days the grave will be visited and alms given to the poor. Grief is a family affair which is openly displayed.

When a person of the *Hindu* faith is dying a priest will tie a thread around the neck of the person and readings will be given from the Bhagavad Gita. Hindus prefer to die at home, often lying on the floor in order to feel close to the earth. The eldest son will arrange the funeral. Cremation is usual for the Hindu, the ashes being scattered over water. There is a set pattern to mourning with a final service being held on the eleventh day. Relatives and friends will visit the bereaved with gifts of money, food and clothing.

The *Sikh* religion combines elements of Hindu and Muslim beliefs. The body is cremated and a series of services held for ten days. The final service marks the end of the official mourning period.

Buddhists require quiet and privacy for meditation during the period preceding death. They aim for a calm, hopeful and alert frame of mind, and are therefore often reluctant to take drugs which they feel will cloud the mind. There are no special rituals concerning the body and cremation is common.

The *Jewish* patient may belong to the liberal or orthodox category of Judaism. The orthodox Jew will keep certain dietary laws while the liberal Jew may not follow the customs so rigidly. Again, asking the patient and family will help the nurse ensure that he receives the appropriate food. There are no last rites in Judaism (Neuberger, 1987); however, the patient may request the presence of a rabbi and prayers may be said. The family too may be comforted by the presence of a rabbi as he can guide them on the practices to be followed once death has occurred. After death, the nurse may remove any drainage tubes if present, straighten the limbs and bind up the jaw, if there is no near relative to perform these tasks. The family will arrange for the care of the body which should not be left alone. Burial takes place within 24 hours, unless a Sabbath intervenes. There is a seven day intensive mourning period, when the bereaved stay at home and are visited frequently.

The visitors bring food with them and encourage the bereaved to talk about the dead person.

Mutual integrity and respect should characterise communications about religion and cultural matters between the nurse, the patient and his family. For those with no formal beliefs there may still be spiritual matters to be discussed as they struggle to find some purpose in their lives and deaths, and the nurse is often chosen to be the confidante to share in that struggle.

Care in the final days

During the last days and hours of a person's life, the nurse is in a privileged position, sharing a very sensitive time with the patient and those close to him. How she acts and what she says will be observed by those left behind after death, and will be remembered as good or bad depending on the quality of the care she offers to the patient and the support she gives to the bereaved.

As the patient becomes weaker the process of letting go accelerates. He becomes more and more dependent on those around him to meet physical, emotional and other needs. Dying patients are easily exhausted, so care needs to be spaced to allow time for rest. The minimum hygiene and pressure area care necessary for patient comfort is offered, and timed so that the patient has the opportunity of resting before social activities. Visitors are encouraged to come at a time when the patient is less tired and more able to talk or do things with them. The patient will sleep more, eat less and often be satisfied with small amounts of fluids. It is unnecessary to force those who are dying to eat and drink; rather, let them dictate what they would like, and when they are unable to swallow, moistening the tongue and lips is generally all that is required for comfort. Preventing constipation and faecal impaction in someone who is inactive, eating and drinking little, and possibly receiving drugs which are constipating requires constant vigilance and appropriate intervention such as the use of suppositories and enemas without unduly disturbing the patient. Catheterisation may be necessary to relieve urinary retention. If the patient has been taking narcotic drugs to relieve pain these are continued subcutaneously, perhaps via a syringe driver, or rectally in the form of suppositories to ensure maintenance of adequate serum levels.

The dying person often appreciates the company of those he knows and trusts. These may be relatives, friends, priests, or nurses who can sit and keep him company, not necessarily talking, but holding his hand and listening to whatever he wants to say. Carers may find this time difficult and the nurse needs to guide them on how to act, when to touch the patient, and when to be silent. She may act as an intermediary between family members, helping them to support one another.

The emotional strain of caring at home can be considerable. Many people will not have had experience of nursing a very sick person at home and may be concerned with a number of worries and anxieties.

When the nurse in the community first meets the relative or carer it may be difficult to make an accurate assessment of their ability to cope with the care of the dying person. The relative may be exhausted from managing on their own, or frightened by suddenly having back home a sick person the doctors in the hospital are unable to cure. They may still be adjusting to the news that their relative is not going to recover and feel very vulnerable and helpless. As the nurse begins to work with the carers and gain their confidence she will try to reduce their anxiety level and enhance their ability to cope. Carers are often likely to become housebound. They may also be anxious about the medication that is prescribed. Herd (1990) emphasises the importance of clear instructions on the purpose of different drugs and written instructions on a simple drug sheet to aid the relatives. The family or carers will require an increased amount of support from the professional team, especially the district nurse. They may need careful explanation and continuing support to make the experience of caring for their relative at home a rewarding one.

The nurse will advise the patient and carers on how to set up the patient's room for easy living and will teach the carers how to meet the patient's needs. For example, she may suggest adapting a downstairs room so the patient will feel part of the family and the carer will not get overtired going up and downstairs, and will be able to keep a close watch on the patient. Preferably the room should be well lit and ventilated with a pleasant outlook. A hospital type of bed can be ordered through a community occupational therapist and the local medical team service will loan a commode, backrest, bathing aids or a wheelchair. Some areas have an incontinence laundry service and the community nursing service will loan pressure-relieving equipment such as ripple beds or sheepskins. A small table, within the patient's reach, can hold a bedside lamp, a small bell, tissues, a glass and drinks. A flask will keep a drink hot or cold according to preference, and is particularly useful overnight. The nurse can advise the carers about ways of diverting the patient and filling time, such as reading, jigsaw puzzles, crosswords, radio, television and tapes. She can teach the carers how to observe and report any pain or other symptom the patient may experience, and how to give the medicines prescribed. The nurse can also advise on diet, the amount of exercise the patient may take, and how to cope with sleepless nights (Doyle, 1983).

A major concern of carers is, 'What will happen when the person dies? Will it be obvious that death has occurred?'. The nurse can explain that the person's breathing will slow and become irregular before it finally stops, then it will be obvious that the skin is paler and the eyes lose their lustre. At home, the family will need to be told who to inform and what will happen next after death.

In hospital or hospice, once the patient has died the carers or relatives may like to spend some time at the bedside to say goodbye and to begin to take in the fact of the death. They may then be offered refreshment and some time in a private room with a nurse to help them plan what to do next.

If the carers or relatives have not been present at the death, a message must be sent as quickly as possible to inform them of the event. Opinions differ as to whether to inform the next-of-kin over the telephone. Sometimes if the nurse knows the carer well and the death is expected she may give the news over the telephone. However, if the death has been sudden and unexpected it is kinder to ask them to come as quickly as possible to the hospital and to ask for the nurse in charge by name. Alternatively, the police will carry a message to those at home. This latter means of conveying news ensures that someone is on hand to make a cup of tea, send for neighbours or contact other members of the family.

Breaking bad news requires some thought and awareness of the likely reaction of the recipient. We all feel uncomfortable about telling people something they would rather not hear and in the desire to unburden herself the nurse should not be too hasty, but give information gently and slowly, allowing time for the individual to grasp what is being said and offering sympathy and acknowledgement of the loss.

The relatives may want to see the body and most hospitals have a viewing chapel where this can be done. The head porter will arrange for the body to be available and the relatives are accompanied by a trained nurse – preferably one familiar to them – and/or the hospital chaplain. The nurse should check the body is well positioned and that chairs are available for the relatives to sit for a while by the body.

Each hospital has guidelines on how to prepare the body for removal from the ward. Care must be taken to remove infusions and drains and to seal any wounds. The body should be clearly labelled and the property of the dead person should be listed and stored in a secure place. There may be local policy restrictions concerning handing over valuables to relatives and these should be observed. Usually, wedding rings are given directly to the spouse, if it is the wish that they be removed.

Patients in nearby beds need to be informed of the death and given the opportunity to talk and express their own fears and anxieties. This should be done not only at the time of death, but again the following day.

When the death has occurred at home, the nurse usually calls the following day after a death, to offer sympathy and to collect any equipment. She may continue to visit the carers over the next year, timing her visits according to the needs of those bereaved.

What happens after a death

There are certain events which take place after a death which the nurse needs to be aware of in order to guide and support relatives. As described later, the bereaved are often stunned and bewildered, especially if the death was unexpected, and they look to nursing staff to tell them what to do. In the community in particular, the family may ask the nurse about arrangements to register the death and plan the funeral. In the hospital the question of organ donation may arise in certain circumstances and, again, it is helpful if the nurse has some understanding of the procedures involved so she can support relatives and junior colleagues.

Confirmation of death

There is no legal definition of death. Normally, death is diagnosed as a result of irreversible cessation of respiration and heartbeat. The patient is seen by a doctor to confirm death. He will listen for a heartbeat with a stethoscope, observe for breathing movements and examine the pupils — which will be fixed and dilated. In hospital, if the doctor on call looked after the patient prior to death and knows the cause of death, he will issue the Death Certificate to the next of kin. If the patient is not known to the doctor, the Death Certificate is not issued until the doctor who normally looks after the patient is on duty. Thus the relatives will have to come back the following day to collect the Certificate.

In the community, if the doctor who is in attendance also looked after the person in his last illness, he can issue the relatives with the Death Certificate, providing he knows the cause of death. The Death Certificate may be withheld pending a Coroner's inquest, for the reasons given below.

Table 27.4. *Reasons for which death is reported to the Coroner*

(1) If the cause of death is uncertain
(2) If death was sudden, violent or caused by an accident
(3) If death was caused by an industrial disease
(4) If death occurred while the patient was undergoing an operation or was under the effect of an anaesthetic
(5) Where the deceased was not attended by a doctor in his last illness — generally a single attendance is insufficient
(6) Where the patient has not been seen by a doctor for 14 days before death
(7) If death occurs within 24 hours of admission to hospital.

If the death at home was violent, accidental or there are suspicious circumstances, the police will have to be informed.

The Coroner may arrange for a post mortem examination of the body to establish accurately the cause of death. Relatives do not need to give consent for this but a doctor of their choice may be present. The Coroner's inquest is an enquiry into the medical cause of death. It is held in public, sometimes with a jury present.

Registration of death

Once the Death Certificate has been issued, the death must be registered within five days at the Registrar's office in the district where the death took place. The death may be registered by the next of kin, any relative or friend, or the executor of the dead person's estate. The death may also be registered by the occupier of the house in which the death took place, or a member of hospital staff when the hospital is responsible for the funeral. The person registering the death should take the Death Certificate together with the dead person's National Health Service card and any war pension order book. It is sometimes necessary to make an appointment to register the death and the Registrar will require certain information listed below.

Table 27.5. *Information for the Registrar*

(1) The date and place of death and the deceased's usual address
(2) The full names and surname (and maiden name where appropriate)
(3) The date and place of birth (town and county or country if born abroad)
(4) Occupation (and the name and occupation of her husband if the deceased was a married woman or widow)
(5) Whether the deceased was in receipt of a pension or allowance from public funds
(6) If the deceased was married, the age of the surviving widow or widower.

The person registering the death will be issued a Certificate for Disposal to be given to the funeral director and a Certificate of Registration of Death for Social Security purposes only, which is sent to the local office to make application for Widow's Benefit, where appropriate. Copies of the Certificate of Registration for insurance purposes can be obtained from the Registrar at a small cost.

Funeral arrangements

There is a National Association of Funeral Directors who work to an agreed code of practice and it is advisable that people choose a funeral director registered with the Association. Funeral costs can vary considerably depending on whether someone is buried or cremated and the sort of service required. Burial and funeral services carry set fees, with an organist, choir and erection of a headstone being purchased as extras. No one can be cremated until the cause of death is established. The funeral director will supply the forms and a small fee is charged (DSS, leaflet D49). The relatives will find it is usually best to get details from several funeral directors with the likely charges set out in writing. The cost of the funeral is the first charge on the estate of the dead person and it is often possible to pay by instalments. The Will, where there is one, may contain some instructions about the funeral, although these are not binding. If the person died in hospital and his relatives cannot be traced or cannot afford to pay for the funeral, the health authority will take responsibility for the arrangements.

Brain death and organ transplantation

Transplantation techniques have been developed which mean that an individual who has incipient failure of a major organ can have his life prolonged by the donation of an organ from a person who is diagnosed as brain dead, i.e. there is irreversible cessation of brain stem functions. Brain death may be diagnosed in the following situations:

(1) The patient is deeply comatose and the coma is not due to depressant drugs (e.g. narcotics, hypnotics or tranquillisers), primary hypothermia, metabolic or endocrine disorders;

(2) The patient is being ventilated because respiration has become inadequate or has stopped completely;

(3) There is no doubt that the patient's condition is due to irremediable structural brain damage, as in severe head injury, cerebral haemorrhage, or cerebral anoxia following cardiac arrest, air or fat embolism.

A series of tests are performed by two senior doctors on two occasions to confirm brain death. These include tests which examine the function of a series of reflex arcs which pass through the brain stem and tests to exclude drug, metabolic or endocrine causes of coma or respiratory difficulties (Simpson, 1987). The time of death is recorded as the time brain death is diagnosed, not when artificial respiration is discontinued or the heartbeat ceases. Diagnosis of brain death is not usually contemplated until at least six hours after the onset of coma or 24 hours after cardiac arrest.

The kidneys, liver or heart and/or lungs may be transplanted under the following conditions:

(1) The diagnosis of brain death is confirmed in the donor;

(2) There is no objection from the relatives or next of kin;

(3) The Coroner or, in Scotland, the Procurator Fiscal, has no objection in cases which would be referred to him.

A Code of Practice has been drawn up and revised by a Working Party on behalf of the Health Departments in Great Britain and Northern Ireland (DHSS, 1983) which gives guidance on the choice of donors, the approach to relatives, the premortem tests and tissue-typing, the diagnosis of death and the removal of organs, including corneas.

Confidentiality concerning the donor and the recipient is to be maintained at all times.

Support needs of nurses

Caring for the dying person is physically demanding and emotionally draining. The nurses's own views of life, death and the meaning of suffering will be challenged. There will be a need to live with uncertainty at times. It is not always possible to do what one would like in a situation; the resources may not be available, time may run out or help may be rejected. When it is not possible to meet all the goals of care, stress occurs for the nurse. Because patients are very vulnerable, it is easy for them and their families to become dependent on the nurse who is sharing in such a sensitive part of their lives. The nurse has to be able to judge the amount of involvement, the degree of dependence, and the level of demand that is appropriate in each situation. The nurse will need to be open enough to empathise with the patient and family, but she takes the risk of being hurt by her involvement. The team concept of care can help keep the involvement within limits, allowing the nurse to feel she has made a contribution without burning herself out, trying to be all things to all people. The way the team functions should provide for individual members to be able to voice their fears and anxieties concerning a particular patient and family, and there should be a forum set up to look at care and the demands that it is making upon team members.

Signs of stress in a person include: tiredness out of proportion to the work, low morale, irritability, anxiety about small things and overconscientiousness (Stedeford, 1984). Apart from the possibility of being hurt by her involvement with the patient and family, the nurse may be stressed as a result of a number of other factors. She may identify the patient or family with herself or one of her own family, so she begins to think of them as if they really were herself or her mother, sister or husband.

She may experience an irrational fear about illness or death, becoming over-anxious when she experiences symptoms similar to those of the patient. The nurse may be struggling to meet high ideals she has set for herself, personally or professionally. As a person is coming to the end of his life, the nurse may feel she has only one opportunity to get the care right. Stedeford (1984) gives some valuable help by suggesting that how a person dies depends on three factors: the life they have lived, the nature of their illness, and the quality of care being given. The staff may be concerned about the first two but can only be responsible for the last. Stresses may also come from personal conflicts and difficulties outside of work (Tschudin, 1987).

Each team member will have to develop her own ways of handling stress and looking for support. Maintaining good general health is important. The nurse will be able to cope better with stressful conditions if she takes holidays at reasonable intervals and arranges her off-duty times to avoid long stretches of unbroken work. Charles-Edwards (1983) suggests that learning relaxation techniques or meditation may help some nurses handle stress, whilst others prefer physical exercise or creative activities such as singing in a choir or participating in amateur dramatics. Others find support through spiritual activities such as prayer and sharing in small Bible study or fellowship groups.

Further support measures may be provided by the employing authority (Tschudin, 1987), including a counsellor for personal consultations or work with groups. Peer groups may be organised where individuals are able to raise anxieties with their colleagues. Occupational Health departments may offer opportunities for nurses to go and discuss, in confidence, personal or work-related stresses. Finally educational programmes may be offered which are designed to equip staff with the skills they require to fulfil the changing expectations and demands of their work.

Services for the dying

Care may be provided in a variety of settings – the patient's home, the hospital ward or in a hospice. Hospice is the term given to a service which provides inpatient care and home support for terminally ill patients. Day care services, pain and symptom relief clinics as well as respite and home sitting services, counselling and educational services may also be included. The majority of patients in hospice care are dying from cancer, but some may have other long term illnesses, such as multiple sclerosis or motor neurone disease. In more recent years hospice provision has been made for people with AIDS. The modern hospice movement stemmed from the pioneer work of Dame Cicely Saunders, who founded St Christopher's Hospice in London in 1967. Hospice care has been instrumental in increasing the understanding of the needs of the dying person and their family and has pioneered research into pain and symptom control and the support of the bereaved. Many hospices are charitable foundations raising money from local committees, others are funded through the National Health Service and still others are joint funded. It has been the policy of the Department of Health for each health authority to increase its links with the charitable organisations and formulate policies on the provision of care to dying patients (DoH, 1987).

As our understanding of the needs of the dying has grown, questions are being asked concerning the access to hospice type care for groups of patients other than those with cancer (Seale, 1989). It would seem that the medical diagnosis is being used as the main criterion for admission to hospice services, the reason being given that there are different patterns of symptoms associated with dying from other diseases. However, there does seem to be a stigma attached to age and those with AIDS. Goddard (1991) states that hospice services will accept patients only if they already have cancer and others specify that only home care is available for AIDS patients. It is important to view hospice care as a philosophy rather than to associate it with a particular place or type of service. As Seale (1989) indicates:

'Where nurses have the time to get to know dying patients and where nurses are assigned responsibility for the care of individual patients rather than just tasks, where a supportive and non-hierarchical relationship exists between staff, and when a policy of open disclosure of diagnosis and prognosis prevails, nursing care for the dying approaches the ideals of hospice care.'

Sometimes the access to services is limited because people do not realise that they or their relatives are beginning to die. From a study in Eastbourne, Cowley (1990) identified a number of individuals attributing symptoms to age rather than to underlying disease and so did not contact the doctor until an illness was far advanced. Cowley states:

'It seems possible that some of those who are most in need of help with facing their diagnosis and expected death are barred from the very services which have developed the skills for helping such people to cope . . .'

because either the relatives or the doctor do not wish to share the true nature of the diagnosis with the patient. Where there is chronic disease it is often difficult to predict the projection of the dying process. If the medical diagnosis is used as the means to predict the need for care, it can mean that individuals with symptoms that could be addressed through the skills of those experienced in care of the dying do not receive effective treatment and support, especially in the elderly.

There has been much criticism of the way death is dealt with in hospitals and a number of complaints are being brought to the fore by the **National Health Service Ombudsman**. As a result of this, a circular (DoH, 1992) has been issued by the Department of Health asking health authorities to review their policies in connection with the death of patients, the handing over of property and the information given to relatives.

Research (Parkes, 1978; Hinton, 1979) has been carried out comparing the care of dying patients in hospital, at home, and in a hospice. The early studies showed a marked difference between care in home and hospital in comparison with the hospice. The patient received better treatment, symptom control and emotional care, and the relatives' needs were met much more successfully in the hospice. In the home the patient was more likely to have uncontrolled pain and the anxiety levels of both patient and family were high. The hospital gave slightly better symptom control than in the home but was still behind the hospice, and the emotional needs of the patient and family were largely unmet. Studies undertaken by Lunt (1985), Hockley (1983) and Parkes and Parkes (1984) have shown that symptom control in hospital and home is improving, but there is still a great need to improve emotional care for patients and relatives.

The majority of patients still die in hospital but as specialist knowledge increases and is more widely available across the country, home care is becoming a real alternative for those with terminal illness. Recent trends show that the time spent at home before death has increased (Dicks, 1989). Deaths at home overall do not appear to have increased. Admissions to hospice or hospital care are often due to non-medical problems, either the patient having no family or the family or carers being unable to cope (Walsh and Kingston, 1988). Sometimes a planned admission for respite care allows the family to rest and the patient to remain at home longer or even to die there. Another reason for admission is often connected to poor communication between hospital and domiciliary services, with either the patient's family, GP, district nurse or support services unaware of the patient's medical and nursing requirements. In a comparison of hospice and conventional care (Seale, 1991), hospice patients were reported:

'more likely to know that they were dying and individuals' level of satisfaction with hospice home nursing and inpatient hospice care was significantly higher than other forms of care. When final admissions were considered, inpatient hospice care involved fewer medical interventions and, in the last year of life, those receiving hospice services were less likely to have an operation'

In a study to assess the preference of terminally ill patients with cancer for their final place of care (Townsend et al., 1990), half of the patients dying in hospital would have preferred to have been at home and 28% of their carers also wished for them to be at home.

'It was assessed that nearly two thirds of the patients in hospital for their last admission did not need 24-hour care but would have been looked after adequately with the supportive visits from the Continuing Care and District Nursing Service, short-term use of equipment such as pressure-relieving mattresses when needed, and some home care support. For the future, with appropriate provision of domiciliary service and the opportunity for respite care, more people should be able to choose to die at home'

(Townsend *et al.*, 1990)

There may be a difference between the ability to provide home care within a rural area as compared with the city. Herd (1990) found that marriages were stable and neighbours and relatives were able to offer good support in a rural area. Also, the primary care teams are used to dealing with serious illness at home and, as there are fewer deputising services, the patients and their carers are likely to be cared for by a familiar doctor when emergencies arise. This may not be the case in the cities although with the changes to the contracts for general practitioners they are more likely to be available out of hours to their patients. Herd (1990) states:

'The availability of a person who is willing and able to undertake the work of caring is fundamental to the provision of home care'

Both patient and family may feel it is not possible to give a good standard of care at home. They may feel the hospital has the best equipment and staff to care for the dying. However, with support and the services which are now available in many areas, more people are finding it possible to have the dying person at home for much of their illness and even to die there. The role of specialist nurses in the community is discussed later in this section. The district nurse, with the backup of specialist advisory and medical services, continues to be the mainstay of the provision of home care. She is recognised as the key planner of care. She is involved in providing practical nursing care and, although there is an indication that more time is needed to spend with the terminally ill, especially in providing counselling and support (Bergen, 1991).

The role of the specialist nurse

In recent years the specialist nurse role in the care of the dying has been developed in the hospital and community. In the hospital a variety of approaches have been adopted, such as a *hospital support team* in terminal care, consisting of specialist nurses with doctor, chaplain and social worker support. The team is called for consultation by ward staff. The nurses will advise their colleagues and teach, often by example, the best way to approach the patient, their carers and their problems. A second approach consists of a *clinical nurse specialist* who carries a caseload of patients and works as a primary nurse, formulating plans of care with ward staff. She participates in the patient's care and offers counselling and support to partners/carers. She liaises with community nursing staff and/or specialist nurses in the community, aiming to provide continuity of care between hospital and home. A further example is the clinical nurse specialist who fulfils a specialist role in the hospital and the community in some of the smaller health districts.

Finally, some hospitals, such as the Royal Marsden Hospital and the Brompton Hospital in London, have set up small *hospice type units* within the hospital, with senior nurses from the unit acting as advisers to their colleagues on other wards where there may be dying patients.

Much of the development of the specialist nurse role has been funded by the Cancer Relief Macmillan Fund. Some *Macmillan nurses* work as clinical nurse specialists in hospital, but the majority are in the community working alongside the primary health care team. *Macmillan nursing teams* operate to meet local needs, therefore there is some variation in the way they work. Some are attached to inpatient hospice services, others work as part of local community nursing services and can arrange with the patient's general practitioner to admit the patient to small community hospitals should it become necessary. The Macmillan nurse has developed skills in helping people to understand their illness and how their lives will need to be adapted as a result of it. They also have a responsibility to keep up to date with methods of controlling pain and other symptoms, so they can suggest alternatives to their medical and nursing colleagues.

Some local charitable foundations have developed home care nursing teams along the lines of Macmillan nursing services, but they operate outside the health service management structure. They may have access to day care facilities and small inpatient units, and often have medical, social work and volunteer members. Examples of such services are the Dorothy House Foundation at Bath (Clench, 1984), Hospice at Home in Tunbridge Wells, and the Prospect Foundation at Swindon. The Hospice Information Service at St Christopher's Hospice, London, keeps an up-to-date list of all the services available to the terminally ill and will supply details on request (see useful addresses).

In a review of the literature, Bergen (1991) found that district nurses and other health professionals value the specialist services, despite the potential conflicts over responsibility for care.

> 'The majority of the specialist nurses have a primary advisory/liaison counselling resource role'

Carers and patients found this role particularly helpful. It is thought that many patients have been able to stay at home longer or to die there because of the availability of a specialist service. Early referral is thought to be critical to ensure a high standard of care.

In her review of hospice nursing, Dobratz (1990) found that the hospice specialist nurse spent most of her time in:

> 'case management and counselling activities, that include care co-ordination, record keeping, telephoning, bereavement counselling, pain and symptom management, advocacy, and instruction. In addition to these management and collaborative aspects large amounts of time were spent in patient/family instruction which was needed to facilitate the care of the patient's death at home'

Dobratz discussed the nursing functions within hospice nursing as being of four kinds. Firstly, intensive caring, 'managing the physical, psychological, social and spiritual problems of dying persons and their families'. Secondly, collaborative sharing, 'co-ordinating the extended and expanded components that constitute hospice care services'. Thirdly, continuous knowing, 'acquiring the counselling, managing, instructing, caring and communicating skills and knowledge that compose the role of hospice nursing'. And finally, continuous giving, 'balancing the hospice nurse's

own self-care needs to the complexities and intensities of repeated death encounters'.

The Marie Curie domiciliary nursing service will supply nursing care for cancer patients in their own home, day or night, the greater demand being for help at night to allow relatives to rest. Application for a Marie Curie nurse is made to the senior nurse managing the community nursing services, as the local health districts share the costs with the Marie Curie Memorial Foundation and administer the service on its behalf. There is no charge for this service which is jointly funded by the Foundation and the health authorities. Donations are welcomed from patients, relatives and other interested people. The local health authority recruits nurses who are willing to care for cancer patients at home and they receive some training. These nurses are placed on a register and are called in response to requests from families or nursing colleagues.

The role of voluntary organisations

The care of the dying person and his family relies on competent and compassionate professional skill supported and complemented by all kinds of voluntary help. Different groups of patients and relatives are the focus of interest for particular organisations. Some organisations will fund research and professional education, others will make grants to patients and their families. Some are national enterprises, others operate locally.

The Cancer Relief Macmillan Fund provides money for a wide variety of activities in connection with cancer. The Macmillan nursing service has already been discussed. The fund also provides inpatient continuing care units which are managed by the health service and supports many local voluntary hospice projects. Patient grants are given for any reasonable request, e.g. clothing, bedding, telephone connection, holiday and travel expenses. The Macmillan Fund also aims to make a swift response to requests. Applications are received via Social Services departments, community nurses, health visitors or social workers in the hospital, or by contacting the Patient Grants department direct. More recently, the Fund has made grants for posts to be set up to provide medical, nurse and professional education programmes.

Marie Curie Cancer Care is another organisation active on behalf of cancer patients. Apart from the domiciliary nursing service, it runs residential nursing homes and has a welfare department which gives funds for such items as extra heating, dietary requirements and a wide range of comforts. An information and advisory service is run in conjunction with BACUP – the British Association of Cancer United Patients.

Other terminal illnesses such as multiple sclerosis, motor neurone disease and Huntington's chorea have similar societies.

Many local communities have developed voluntary groups to support people with special needs or to supply a particular service. Examples might be night-sitting services, transport facilities, care attendant schemes and day centres. Most local services are listed in the telephone directory or the local Citizens Advice Bureau may be able to give guidance on how to contact a particular service.

There are now a number of voluntary groups set up to help the bereaved, as mentioned earlier, often started by people who have been bereaved and become aware of the associated problems. Parents who have suffered the loss of a baby may find help from the Stillbirth Society; others who have lost a child of any age may be referred to the Compassionate Friends. The Gay Bereavement Switchboard is open 24 hours a day to receive calls from homosexual men and women who have lost their partners by death.

The Lisa Sainsbury Foundation provides support to health professionals caring for patients for whom there is no cure in two ways; firstly, the Foundation runs workshops and seminars; secondly, it supplies bibliographic information on books, journal articles, tapes and videos, with details of pain relief clinics and other available resources.

Bereavement

The death of a loved person gives rise to emotional reactions which will vary in intensity, depending on the significance of the loss to the individual. The loss may be of parent, spouse, child, sibling, partner or friend. The level of reaction appears to have more to do with how much a part of someone's life the dead person represented than with the emotional involvement (Marris, 1986), Thus the widow of a man who worked, say, on a oil rig, however much she may have loved her husband, is likely to adapt to his death more

quickly and with less disturbance to her life than the woman who was wife and business partner of a newsagent and worked and lived 24 hours a day with her husband. In the latter case the death means that everything in her life will be different. They may have had a difficult relationship but her adjustment to his death will cause considerable stress.

Grief is a recognised pattern of emotional reactions following bereavement that reflects the individual's attempt to take in the loss, cope with it and make the necessary psychological adjustments (Engel, 1962). Various stages have been identified but the common aspects include shock, disbelief, numbness, denial of the loss, physical symptoms, anger, guilt, sadness, identification and preoccupation with the image of the lost person (Parkes, 1972).

The initial period of disbelief and denial of the loss is usually brought to an end by the necessity of making practical decisions and plans for the registration of the death, settling of financial affairs and planning the funeral. The ritual of the funeral gives shape to the family and friends' acknowledgement of the life of the person who has died and gives the opportunity of saying goodbye. As the reality of the loss is taken in by the bereaved, there will come pangs of grief, feelings of fear, anxiety, butterflies in the stomach, tears, palpitations and sweating (Stroebe and Stroebe, 1987).

The bereaved may feel that these physical symptoms mean that they are ill and visit their general practitioner for reassurance. Often they are afraid they have the same illness as the person who has died, as they may have similar symptoms. For example, palpitations with sweating may equate in their minds with having a heart attack. Abdominal discomfort may equal cancer to them; headaches equate with having a stroke.

The bereaved are full of regrets. They may have a great need to review the circumstances of the death, especially if it was sudden and unexpected. By rehearsing the events, the bereaved begin to take in the reality of the death. Some want to talk a lot about the dead person and feel hurt if others will not use the person's name. Others will not have them mentioned and avoid people and situations where it is likely memories of the dead person will be revived. Often the dead person is idealised with no mention being made of their faults. Their room may be made into a shrine with nothing being altered. Sometimes, the bereaved will see, hear or smell the dead person. They are often frightened by these sensory perceptions and feel they are going mad. Others find it hard to remember the dead person's face or how they looked before they were ill (Lewis, 1961).

A sudden death can be very difficult to take in, particularly if there is no body to identify, such as in sea, air and some fire disasters. If the person dies and is buried abroad, the bereaved may find they cannot believe the person will not return, or they are concerned that a mistake might have been made. The bereaved may search for the dead person in a physical way, literally looking at faces in a crowd to try and spot them, or they may search mentally, going over their last meeting with the person who died, or they may simply be very restless, unable to concentrate in their thinking or settle down to anything. These feelings persist for many months, gradually fading into the background, but they can be triggered off again by the discovery of a forgotten photograph, visiting a place which was connected with the dead person, or finding an old letter.

Dealing with the strong emotions and practical outworkings following a death can be very tiring and stressful. Bereavement carries a high risk of becoming physically or mentally ill, or of actually dying from a stress-related illness (Stroebe and Stroebe, 1987).

The bereaved person has to adapt in a number of areas of life. Emotionally, there is the working through of feelings, adjusting to a new identity. Spiritually, there may be a struggle of faith, adjusting their philosophy of life to take into account the meaning and purpose of the situation in which they find themselves. Physically, they are coping with symptoms related to anxiety, the flight and fight response. Socially, there may be changes in status and role. There may be financial loss or gain, the need to go out to work for the first time, becoming both mother and father in a one-parent family, being treated by friends and social contacts as a single person instead of one of a couple. Practically, they may need to develop new routines and learn new skills related to home work or social activities.

The first year of bereavement brings constant reminders of the dead person – events such as birthdays, anniversaries, festive occasions, holidays and dates of significance to the individual family. Full resolution of grief is achieved when the dead person can be remembered with emotional stability and the positive and negative aspects of the relationship can be discussed.

Children's reactions to bereavement depend on their age. To the toddler or pre-school child, time is a difficult concept. Separation from a loved person will bring a small scale grief reaction. When the mother leaves the toddler, he may cry violently and search for her before settling into a withdrawn, depressed state. Finally the toddler will be distracted by things around and appear to forget the mother (Bowlby, 1979). On her return, the toddler will ignore her for a while until the relationship is re-established.

If the mother dies, the toddler will become bonded to a significant other person who is a continuous feature of his environment. The early school child is very concrete in his thinking and will take the practical approach and worry about what happens to the body and what the dead person will be doing. The middle school child may feel guilty and responsible. They may feel the person died because of something they did or did not do, or because they thought something bad or expressed a feeling of hatred. The teenager will react similarly to adults but may have ambivalent feelings, especially if it is a brother or sister who has died, as they may feel guilt about the jealousies and rivalry which are a natural part of family life.

Children need to be told the facts openly and honestly. They require a lot of reassurance about their own survival and the fact that they are loved and accepted in the family. It often helps for them to attend the funeral and to be part of their parent's grief. Sharing feeling and grieving together can be very supportive. Trying to protect the child by not including him or talking to him about the dead person may give rise to all sorts of fantasies and fears. It is often hard for parents who are grieving themselves to support their children. Perhaps a family friend or relative, not closely affected by the death, can help in offering support to them all and in identifying the children's feelings. Teachers need to be aware of a death in the family, especially if it is a parent, brother or sister who may have died, as deterioration in the child's school work and lapses of concentration may be the only outward signs of the child's grief, which is perhaps not being openly expressed elsewhere.

Abnormal grief

For a few, the grief process does not run an average

course. It may be unduly prolonged and the bereaved person may become stuck in a particular phase.

Anger and bitterness over the circumstances of the death may leave a bereaved person resentful, helpless and hopeless, unwilling to make new relationships or to let other family members help to resolve their grief. Grief may be suppressed and unacknowledged with feelings not worked through, so that when another crisis or loss comes, the bereaved person may be overwhelmed and express feelings out of proportion to the new situation (Parkes, 1986; Worden, 1983).

Feelings of guilt, depression, loneliness and hopelessness may lead to the contemplation of and/or attempt at suicide. Those close to the bereaved person or visiting to support them in their grief should be alert to signs of depression, such as early waking and poor sleep patterns, lack of eating, neglect of house and personal appearance, expressions of hopelessness. Those exhibiting such signs require skilled counselling and psychiatric help. There is a fine balance between normal and abnormal behaviour in grief. The dead person may be idealised to the point of idolisation. Their memory becomes sacred and the place where they lived enshrined. Queen Victoria's reactions following the death of Prince Albert are an example of this type of behaviour (Gorer, 1965). Whilst it is inadvisable for the bereaved to move residence and clear out belongings very early after the death, it is equally inadvisable for someone to remain in a situation which is not practical or suitable and to do so borders on the abnormal.

Working with the bereaved

The bereaved need an empathetic listener who can tolerate expression of feelings and does not mind stories being repeated again and again, who is familiar with the grief process and can advise on practical arrangements. Most people will cope with their grief through the help of supportive families, friends and social groups such as churches.

There are a number of agencies which have been set up to offer help and advice and to act on behalf of the bereaved. The help may range from personal befrienders and counsellors to group meetings, newsletters, access to professional legal and financial advice. Some are national organisations with local branches, others have arisen out of the interest of local people. Some hospices have bereavement services run by volunteers and professional staff to support the families of patients who have died. Examples of national organisations are CRUSE, the National Association of Widows, Compassionate Friends, the Gay Bereavement Project and the Stillbirth Association. Addresses of these organisations can be found at the end of this chapter.

Conclusion

The dying patient, his family, partner and friends have many varied needs. They are all facing a crisis in their lives which represents a considerable challenge to their mental and physical health. Care of the dying patient and his family requires a high level of commitment by the nurse to tailor her care to the individual's goals and needs. As has been shown, the dying patient can have a large number of problems, some related to the primary diagnosis and others to increasing weakness. Every part of his life is affected and so the nurse needs to listen carefully to how the patient feels about things. His family, too, are facing a major crisis and the nurse can be involved in preventive care by reducing the stress on the family as they adjust to the inevitable changes coming into their lives. She needs to develop good communication skills and the ability to work closely with other disciplines, sharing the decision-making and caring process with the patient, his family, other professionals and volunteers.

Caring for the dying patient and his family is challenging and rewarding as the nurse sees the effectiveness of her care in assisting the patient to live until he dies and the family begin to adjust to their loss.

Glossary

Analgesic: A drug which relieves pain

Anaphylactic shock: Collapse of the patient with low blood pressure, raised pulse rate, respiratory disturbance and, possibly, a rash, as the result of an allergic reaction

Anti-emetic: A drug which controls nausea and vomiting

Antispasmodic: A drug which relieves spasm

Anxiolytic: A drug which controls anxiety

Ascites: Abnormal collection of fluid in the peritoneal cavity

Benzodiazepines: A group of drugs, including diazepam, nitrazepam and temazepam, which have a sedative effect

Corticosteroid: A substance derived from the cortex of the adrenal gland

Diuretic: A drug which increases the production of urine

Dysphagia: Difficulty in swallowing

Dyspnoea: Difficulty in breathing

Dysuria: Difficulty in passing urine

Fungating lesion: An open sore with a fungus-like appearance resulting from the growth of a cancer tumour

Haematuria: Blood in the urine

Health Service Commissioner: NHS Ombudsman – a person appointed by Parliament to receive and investigate complaints from patients or their families which have not been dealt with adequately by a local health authority

Huntington's chorea: An inherited disease of the central nervous system which occurs in late middle age, giving rise to involuntary movements and dementia

Lymphoedema: Oedema (excess fluid in the tissues) which is the result of blockage or destruction of the lymph vessels

Motor neurone disease: A condition of the motor nerve fibres which leads to progressive paralysis

Narcotic: A drug which induces drowsiness, usually with pain relief

National Health Service Ombudsman: See *Health Service Commissioner*

Phenothiazines: A group of drugs including chlorpromazine and prochlorperazine which have sedative and anti-emetic effects

Pulmonary embolism: Blockage of a pulmonary blood vessel, usually by a blood clot

Septicaemia: Severe infection of the blood with large numbers of bacteria present in the blood

Superior vena cava obstruction: External pressure on the superior vena cava, usually from a tumour mass in the chest, resulting in congestion of the facial and upper trunk veins

Syringe driver: A battery-operated machine which delivers drugs to the patient over a controlled time period

References

Baines, M. (1981). The principles of symptom control. In *Hospice: The Living Idea*, Saunders, C.M., Summers, D.H. and Teller, N. (eds.). Edward Arnold, London.

Baines, M. (1986). *Drug Control of Common Symptoms*. St Christopher's Hospice, London.

Benner, P. and Wrubel, J. (1989). *The Primacy of Caring*. Addison Wesley, New York.

Bergen, A. (1991). Nurses caring for the terminally ill in the community: a review of the literature. *International Journal of Nursing Studies*, 28, 89–101.

Bowlby, J. (1979). *The Making and Breaking of Affectional Bonds*. Tavistock Publications, London.

Charles-Edwards, A. (1983). *Nursing Care of the Dying Patient*. Beaconsfield, Bucks.

Clench, P. (1984) *Managing to Care – Community Services for the Terminally Ill*. Patten, Richmond.

Corcoran, R. (1991). The management of pain. In *Palliative Care For People with Cancer*, Penson, J. and Fisher, R. (eds.). Edward Arnold, London.

Cowley, S. (1990). Who qualifies for terminal care? *Nursing Times*, 86(22), 29–31.

Department of Health. (1987). *Circular HC(87)4*. DoH, London.

DoH. (1992). *Patients Who Die in Hospital*. HSG(92)8. DoH, London.

Department of Health and Social Security. (1983). *Working Party on Cadaveric Organs for Transplantation*. DHSS, London.

Department of Social Security. Leaflet D49. *What to Do After a Death*. DSS, London.

Dicks, B. (1989). Palliative care – a vital cornerstone. *Nursing Times*, 85(44), 45–47.

Dobratz, M.C. (1990). Hospice nursing. *Cancer Nursing*, 13(2), 116–122.

Doyle, D. (1983). *Coping with a Dying Relative*. Macdonald Publishers, Edinburgh.

Engel, G. (1962). *Psychological Development in Health and Disease*. W.B. Saunders, Philadelphia.

Finlay, I. (1991) The management of frequently encountered symptoms. In *Palliative Care for People With Cancer*, Penson, J. and Fisher, R. (eds.). Edward Arnold, London.

Gallagher-Allred, C. (1991). Nutritional care of the terminally ill patient and family. In *Palliative Care for People with Cancer*, Penson, J. and Fisher, R. (eds.). Edward Arnold, London.

Goddard, M. (1991). Hospice services. In *Health Care UK '90*, Harrison, A. (ed.). Policy Journals, Newbury.

Goffman, E. (1961). *Asylums*. Anchor Books, New York.

Gorer, G. (1965). *Death, Grief and Mourning in Contemporary Britain*. Cresset, London.

Griffin, J. (1991). *Dying with Dignity*. Office of Health Economics, London.

Henderson, V. (1966). *The Nature of Nursing*. Macmillan, London.

Herd, E.S. (1990). Terminal care in a semi-rural area. *British Journal of General Practice*, 40, 248–251.

Hesswell, K. and Bramwell, L. (1989). The supportive role of the staff nurse in the hospital palliative care situation. *Journal of Palliative Care*, 5(3), 20–26.

Hinton, J. (1979). Comparison of places and policies for terminal care. *Lancet*, 1, 29–32.

Hockley, J. (1983). *An Investigation to Identify Symptoms of Distress in the Terminally Ill Patient and His/Her Family in the General Medical Ward*. Nursing Research Papers 2, City and Hackney Health District, London.

Hunt, M. (1989) Caring for the terminally ill at home. *Nursing Standard*, 4(39), 23–26.

Kubler-Ross, E. (1970). *On Death and Dying*. Tavistock Publications, London.

Lewis, C.S. (1961). *A Grief Observed*. Faber and Faber, London.

Lunt, B. (1985). *A Comparison of Hospice and Hospital Care for Terminally Ill Cancer Patients and Their Families*. Unpublished research report.

Mannix, K.A. (1991). Confusional states. In *Palliative Care for People with Cancer*, Penson, J. and Fisher, R. (eds.). Edward Arnold, London.

Marris, P. (1986). *Loss and Change*. Routledge and Kegan Paul, London.

National Association of Health Authorities and Trusts. (1992). *Care of People with Terminal Illness*. NAHAT, Birmingham.

Neuberger, J. (1987). *Caring for Dying People of Different Faiths*. Austen-Cornish/Lisa Sainsbury Foundation, London.

Parkes, C.M. (1972). *Bereavement: Studies of Grief in Adult Life*. Penguin Books, Harmondsworth.

Parkes, C.M. (1978). Terminal care as seen by surviving spouses. *Journal of Royal College of Practitioners*, 28, 19–30.

Parkes, C.M. (1986). *Bereavement: Studies of Grief in Adult Life* (2nd ed.). Penguin Books, Harmondsworth.

Parkes, C.M. and Parkes, J. (1984). 'Hospice' versus 'hospital' care – re-evaluation after ten years as seen by surviving spouses. *Postgraduate Medical Journal*, 60, 120–124.

Parsons, T. and Fox, R.C. (1961). Illness therapy and the modern urban family. In *A Modern Introduction to the Family*, Bell and Vogel (eds). Routledge and Kegan Paul, London.

Regnard, R. (1983). *A Guide to Symptom Relief in Advanced Cancer*. Haigh and Hochland, Manchester.

Royal College of Nursing. (1991). *Standards of Care: Cancer Nursing*. Scutari Press, London.

Seale, C.F. (1989). What happens in hospices: a review of research evidence. *Social Science and Medicine*, 28(6), 551–559.

Seale, C.F. (1991). A comparison of hospice and conventional care. *Social Science and Medicine*, 32(2), 147–152.

Simpson, A. (1987). Brain stem death. *Nursing Times*, 83(8), 41–42.

Stedeford, A. (1984). *Facing Death*. Heinemann, London.

Stroebe, W. and Stroebe, M.S. (1987). *Bereavement and Health*. Cambridge University Press, Cambridge.

Townsend, J., Frank, A., Fermont, D., et al. (1990). Terminal cancer care and patient's preference for place of death: a prospective study. *British Medical Journal*, 30, 415–417.

Tschudin, V. (1987). *Counselling Skills for Nurses* (2nd ed.). Baillière Tindall, London.

Ufema, J. (1991). Meeting the challenge of a dying patient. *Nursing*, February, 42–46.

Walker, C. (1982). Attitudes to death and bereavement among cultural minority groups. *Nursing Times*, 78(50), 2106–2109.

Walsh, S. and Kingston, R. (1988). The use of hospital beds for terminally ill cancer patients. *European Journal of Surgical Oncology*, 14, 367–370.

Worden, J.W. (1983). *Grief Counselling and Grief Therapy*. Tavistock Publications, London.

World Health Organisation. (1986). *Cancer Pain Relief*. WHO, Geneva.

Wright, A., Cousins, J. and Upwood, J. (1988). *Matters of Death and Life*. King's Fund, London.

Suggestions for further reading

Ainsworth-Smith, I. and Speck, P. (1982). *Letting Go.* SPCK, London.

Buckman, R. (1988). *I Don't Know What to Say.* Papermac, London.

Corr, C.A. and Corr, D.M. (1983). *Hospice Care.* Faber and Faber. London.

De Boulay, S. (1984). *Cicely Saunders.* Hodder and Stoughton, London.

Hill, S. (1974). *In the Springtime of the Year.* Penguin Books, Harmondsworth.

McCaffery, M. (adapted by Sofaer, B.) (1983). *Nursing the Patient in Pain.* Harper and Row, London.

Penson, J. and Fisher, R. (1991). *Palliative Care for People with Cancer.* Edward Arnold, London.

Robbins, J. (1983). *Caring for the Dying Patient and the Family.* Harper and Row, London.

Saunders, C. (1983). *Beyond All Pain.* SPCK, London.

Saunders, C. (ed.). (1984). *The Management of Terminal Disease* (2nd ed.). Edward Arnold, London.

Torrie, M. (1975). *Begin Again.* J M Dent and Sons Ltd, London.

Twycross, R.G. and Slack, S.A. (1984). *Therapeutics in Terminal Cancer.* Pitman, London.

Useful addresses

Cancer Relief
Anchor House, 15–17 Britten Street, London SW3 3TY. Tel. 071-351 7811

Marie Curie Cancer Care
28 Belgrave Square, London SW1X 8QG. Tel. 071-235 3325

Lisa Sainsbury Foundation
8–10 Crown Hill, Croydon, Surrey CRO 1RY. Tel. 081-686 8808

Hospice Information Service
St Christopher's Hospice, 51–59 Lawrie Park Road, Sydenham, London SE26 6DZ. Tel. 081-778 9252

Help The Hospices
The Secretary, General Office, Help the Hospices, BMA House, Tavistock Square, London WC1H 9JP. Tel. 071-388 7807

Age Concern
Astral House, 1268 London Road, London SW16 4ER. Tel. 081-679 8000

National Association of Widows
Stafford District Voluntary Service Centre, Chell Road, Stafford ST16 2QA. Tel. 0785 45465

Gay Bereavement Project
Tel. 071-837 7324

Foundation for the Study of Infant Deaths
5th Floor, 4 Grosvenor Place, London SW1. Tel. 071-235 1721

Stillbirth and Neonatal Death Association
Argyle House, 29–31 Euston Road, London NW1 2SD. Tel. 071-833 2852

Compassionate Friends
6 Denmark Street, Bristol BS1 5DQ. Tel. 0270 292778

INDEX